Large Animal Medicine for Veterinary Technicians

Second Edition

Edited by

Sue Loly, LVT, VTS (EVN)
University of Minnesota, St Paul, MN, USA

Heather Hopkinson, RVT, VTS (EVN), CCRP
North Carolina State University, Raleigh, NC, USA

WILEY Blackwell

This second edition first published 2022

Edition History
John Wiley & Sons Inc., (1e, 2014)

Registered Office
John Wiley & Sons, Inc., 111 River Street, Hoboken, NJ 07030, USA

Editorial Office
111 River Street, Hoboken, NJ 07030, USA

For details of our global editorial offices, customer services, and more information about Wiley products visit us at www.wiley.com.

Wiley also publishes its books in a variety of electronic formats and by print-on-demand. Some content that appears in standard print versions of this book may not be available in other formats.

Library of Congress Cataloging-in-Publication Data Applied for

Cover Design: Wiley
Cover Images: © Charles Novotny, Sue Loly, Heather Hopkinson

Set in 9.5/12.5pt STIXTwoText by Straive, Pondicherry, India

Printed in Singapore
M106734_161221

Contents

Contributors

Erin Matheson Barr, RVT
Ophthalmology Clinical Technician, North Carolina State University
College of Veterinary Medicine
Raleigh, NC
USA

Myra F. Barrett, DVM, MS, DACVR
Assistant Professor of Radiology
Colorado State University
Fort Collins, CO
USA

Kara M. Burns, MS, MEd, LVT, VTS (Nutrition)
Academy of Veterinary Nutrition Technicians
Lafayette, IN
USA

Celina M. Checura, DVM, MS, PhD, Dipl ACT
Clinical Assistant Professor of Theriogenology
University of Wisconsin-Madison
Madison, WI
USA

Jamie DeFazio, AS, CVT, VTS (EVN)
Nursing Supervisor, New Bolton Center
University of Pennsylvania School of Veterinary Medicine
Kennett Square, PA
USA

Sian Durward-Akhurst, BVMS
Large Animal Internal Medicine Resident
University of Minnesota
St. Paul, MN
USA

Sheryl Ferguson, CVT, VTS (LAIM)
Large Animal Hospital Manager
University of Minnesota
St. Paul, MN
USA

Derek Foster, DVM, PhD, DACVIM (LAIM)
Associate Professor of Ruminant Medicine, North Carolina State University
College of Veterinary Medicine
Raleigh, NC
USA

Carrie J. Finno, DVM, PhD, DACVIM
Postdoctoral Fellow and Associate Veterinarian
University of Minnesota
St. Paul, MN
USA

William Gilsenan, VMD, DACVIM (LAIM)
Clinical Assistant Professor, Production Management Medicine
Virginia-Maryland Regional College of Veterinary Medicine
Blacksburg, VA
USA

Sergio Gonzales, BS
Large Animal Hospital Crew Supervisor
University of Minnesota
St. Paul, MN
USA

Ann Elizabeth Goplen, DVM
Assistant Clinical Professor, Small Ruminant Specialist
University of Minnesota
St. Paul, MN
USA

Jennifer Halleran, DVM, DACVIM (LAIM)
Food Animal Medicine and Surgery Clinician, North Carolina State University
College of Veterinary Medicine
Raleigh, NC
USA

Scott R. R. Haskell, DVM, MPVM, PhD
Director Veterinary Technology Program
Yuba College
Marysville, CA
USA

Leslie Hiber, CVT, BS
Veterinary Technician Practitioner (Infection Control)
University of Minnesota
St. Paul, MN
USA

Heather Hopkinson, RVT, VTS (EVN), CCRP
North Carolina State University
College of Veterinary Medicine
Raleigh, NC
USA

Lauren Hughes, DVM
VMED PhD Student, Equine Genetics and Genomics Laboratory
University of Minnesota
St. Paul, MN
USA

Amy L. Johnson, DVM, DACVIM (LAIM & Neurology)
Assistant Professor of Large Animal Medicine and Neurology
University of Pennsylvania School of Veterinary Medicine
Kennett Square, PA
USA

Shana Lemmenes, CVT, VTS (EVN)
University of Minnesota
St. Paul, MN
USA

Laura Lien, MS, CVT, VTS (LAIM)
Instructional Laboratory Planner
Madison Area Technical College
Madison, WI
USA

Bonnie L. Loghry, BAS, MPH, RVT
Professor Veterinary Technology Program
Yuba College
Marysville, CA
USA

Sue Loly, LVT, VTS (EVN)
Large Animal Hospital Technical Supervisor
University of Minnesota
St. Paul, MN
USA

Zach Loppnow, DVM
Anoka Equine Veterinary Services
Associate Veterinarian
Elk River, MN

Fernando J. Marqués, DVM, DACVIM (LAIM)
Associate Professor
University of Saskatchewan
Saskatoon, Saskatchewan
Canada

Annette M. McCoy, DVM, MS, DACVS
Postdoctoral Fellow
University of Minnesota
St. Paul, MN
USA

Erica McKenzie, BSc, BVMS, PhD, DACVIM, DACVSMR
Associate Professor
Oregon State University
Corvallis, OR
USA

Rolf B. Modesto, VMD
Large Animal Surgery Resident
University of Minnesota
St. Paul, MN
USA

Harry Momont, DVM, PhD, Dipl ACT
Clinical Associate Professor of Theriogenology
University of Wisconsin-Madison
Madison, WI
USA

Danielle Mzyk, DVM, PhD
Associate Veterinarian
Janesville Animal Medical Center
Milton, WI
USA

Stephanie Rutten-Ramos, DVM, PhD
Senior Biostatistician
Minneapolis Heart Institute Foundation
Minneapolis, MN
USA

Shirley Sandoval, BAS, LVT, VTS (LAIM)
Head Instructional Technologist
Comparative Large Animal Theriogenology
Washington State University
Pullman, WA
USA

Kurt Selberg, MS, DVM, DACVR
Veterinary Biosciences and Diagnostic Imaging
University of Georgia
Athens, GA
USA

Stacie K. Seymour, DVM
Animal Connections Integrative Care
Minneapolis, MN
USA

JoAnn Slack, DVM, MS, DACVIM (LAIM)
Clinical Studies, New Bolton Center
University of Pennsylvania
Kennett Square, PA
USA

Meagan Smith, RVT, VTS (Anesthesia and Analgesia)
Veterinary Specialty Hospital of the Carolinas
Raleigh, NC
USA

Kirsten Wegner-Fowley, DVM, DACVAA
GCAS Veterinary Anesthesia and Pain Management
Wilmington, DE
USA

Kimberly Schreiber Young, BS, DVM
Resident Candidate – DACVIM (LAIM)
North Carolina State University, College of Veterinary Medicine
Raleigh, NC
USA

Preface

The journey to complete a Veterinary Technician Specialty (VTS) is long and laborious, no matter what the specialty area. Completing this process includes many long hours poring over references and textbooks to soak up the knowledge contained within them. The editors of this book have completed their VTS in large animal species; that process is further complicated by the limited availability of large animal textbooks written at the appropriate level for VTS technicians and veterinary technician students. It is due to these frustrations that this text came into being.

Books are such a valuable resource. Our first edition needed enhancements in some areas, and, from the moment it was published, we set our sights on improvements, collecting pictures and experiences from our clinical work. The binding of a single book limits what we can include, and this is why we have greatly expanded the companion online resource in the second edition, to include more references to abnormals, forms, and references. Whether you are moving through your education process on the associate or bachelor level, a fresh graduate studying for the VTNE, or out in the field for a few years, we hope you will find this book to be a valuable reference that you will pull from the shelf frequently during your time as a credentialed veterinary technician.

It takes a totally driven person to commit to writing on specialized subjects, and, for that, we would like to thank all of our contributors from both the first and second editions, who persevered in authoring their chapters despite insanely busy schedules. A great thank you to the editors of the first edition, Laura Lien and Sheryl Fergson, who were instrumental in establishing a solid foundation to build the second edition on. Thank you from the bottom of our hearts.

The text is only a part of the book; we needed many photos to illustrate difficult concepts. Special thanks go to Dr. Kimberly Young for her photo contributions, Dr. Lauren Hughes, as well as Erin Matheson Barr for her picture and contribution for ophthalmology. For the illustrations, we wish to thank Michele Pico and Lisa Haviland for their contributions from the first edition in the radiology chapter. To all the technicians and veterinarians at both NCSU and UMN CVMs, thank you for supporting our efforts – it truly takes a team. We also thank our family and friends for their patience and support throughout the writing, editing, and production processes.

Finally, we would like to thank everyone at Wiley-Blackwell – and Erica Judisch and Merryl Le Roux specifically – for guiding us through the process with encouragement and support.

Sue Loly
Heather Hopkinson

Abbreviations

Ab	Antibody
ACT	Activated clotting time
AD	Right ear (auris destra)
Ad lib	As much as desired
AGID	Agar gel immunodiffusion
ALT	Alanine aminotransferase
AS	Left ear (auris sinistra)
AST	Aspartate aminotransferase
AU	Both ears (auris uterque)
BID	Twice a day
BP	Blood pressure
Bpm	Beats per minute
BUN	Blood urea nitrogen
BW	Body weight
BV	Biological value
°C	Celsius
C1, C2. . .	Cervical vertebrae
C/M	Castrated male
CAD	Cricoarytenoideus dorsalis
CBC	Complete blood count
cc	Cubic centimeter
CK	Creatine kinase
cm	Centimeter
CNS	Central nervous system
CO_2	Carbon dioxide
CPD	Citrate-phosphate-dextrose
CPDA	Citrate-phosphate-dextrose-adenine
CPK	Creatinine phosphokinase
CPR	Cardiopulmonary resuscitation
CRI	Constant rate infusion
CRT	Capillary refill time
CSF	Cerebrospinal fluid
d	Day
dl	Deciliter
DA	Displaced abomasum
DNA	Deoxyribonucleic acid
DSO	Daily sperm output
ECG	Electrocardiogram or electrocardiographic
EDTA	Ethylenediaminetetraacetic acid
ELISA	Enzyme-linked immunosorbent assay
EMG	Electromyography
ET	Embryo transfer
°F	Fahrenheit
FFD	Focal film distance
FNA	Fine needle aspirate
g	Gram(s)
GI	Gastrointestinal
grain	Grain(s)
h	Hour
Hct	Hematocrit
Hgb	Hemoglobin
Hpf	High-power field
hr	Hour(s)
ID	Intradermal
IFA	Indirect immunofluorescence antibody testing
IM	Intramuscular
in	Inch
IN	Intranasal
IP	Intraperitoneal
IV	Intravenous
IVF	in vitro fertilization
kg	Kilogram
L1, L2. . .	Lumbar vertebrae
lb	Pound
LDA	Left displaced abomasum
liter	Liter
Lpf	Low-power field
m	Meter
m^2	Square meter
MAC	Minimal alveolar concentration
MCH	Mean corpuscular hemoglobin
MCHC	Mean corpuscular hemoglobin concentration
MCV	Mean corpuscular volume
mg	Milligram
min	Minute
ml	Milliliter
MRI	Magnetic resonance imaging
NPO	Nothing by mouth (nil per os)
NSAID	Nonsteroidal anti-inflammatory drug
O_2	Oxygen
OD	Right eye (oculus dexter)
OS	Left eye (oculus sinister)
OU	Both eyes (oculus uterque)
oz	Ounce
PCV	Packed cell volume
PE	Physical exam
pH	Measure of the acidity of a solution
PMI	Point of maximum intensity
PO	By mouth (per os)
PRN	As required
PSI	Pounds per square inch
q	Every
QD	Once a day
QID	Four times a day
QOD	Every other day
RAV	Right abomasal volvulus
RBC	Red blood cell
RDA	Right displaced abomasum

RDVM Referring Doctor of Veterinary Medicine
RER Resting energy requirement
RLN Recurrent laryngeal neuropathy
RNA Ribonucleic acid
Rx Take, receive – used to indicate a prescription or treatment
S Second
SC Subcutaneous
SGOT Serum glutamic-oxaloacetic transaminase
SGPT Serum glutamate-pyruvate transaminase
SID Once a day
T3 Triiodothyronine
T4 Thyroxine
TID Three times a day
TIVA Total intravenous anesthesia
TP Total Protein
TPR Temperature, pulse, respiration
TSH Thyroid stimulating hormone
WBC White blood cell
wk Week
wt Weight
yr Year

About the Companion Website

This book is accompanied by a companion website:

www.wiley.com/go/loly/veterinary

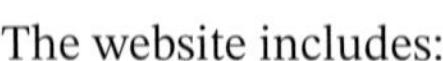

The website includes:

- PowerPoints of all figures from the book for downloading.
- A large animal breed ID image bank.
- Printable forms.
- Review questions and answers.
- Case studies.

Chapter 1

Hospital Biosecurity

Leslie Hiber, CVT, BS

Learning Objectives

- Describe the life cycle patterns of pathogens.
- List and describe the three main routes of transmission.
- List and describe ways to prevent disease in a patient.
- Describe the biosecurity steps that should be taken prior to patient arrival and on arrival.
- List and describe types of barrier precautions.
- Outline the steps of putting on and taking off the personal protective equipment when entering/exiting mini-isolation and isolation areas.
- List categories of products used for good hand hygiene, and describe how to perform hand washing.
- Compare and contrast disinfection and sterilization in preventing nosocomial infection.
- Describe the role of the infection control team and the function of the veterinary technician on this team.

Clinical Case Problem 1.1

An eight-year-old quarter horse mare is presented to the clinic with colic-type clinical signs. The owner reports no history of infectious diseases and has no history of traveling. The patient is treated medically and is hospitalized overnight in the main clinical area. The following day, she begins having diarrhea and a fever. What steps would you take in order to protect the other patients and staff? What type of communication needs to be dispersed and to whom? How would you follow up with cleaning?

See Clinical Case Resolution 1.1 at the end of this chapter.

Key Terms

Active surveillance
Aerosol transmission
Antibiotic stewardship
Antiseptics
Asymptomatic carrier
Biosecurity
Direct contact transmission
Disinfection
Hazard identification
Incubation period
Indirect contact transmission
Multidrug-resistant organism (MDRO)
Nosocomial
Passive surveillance
Personal protective equipment (PPE)
Risk communication
Risk management
Risk perception
Sterilization
Vector-borne transmission
Zoonotic diseases

Large Animal Medicine for Veterinary Technicians, Second Edition. Edited by Sue Loly and Heather Hopkinson.

Companion website: www.wiley.com/go/loly/veterinary

Introduction

Biosecurity is security from exposure to harmful biological agents. It is emerging as a hot topic in veterinary hospitals and clinics throughout the world. As more diseases and superbugs are being discovered due to new technology, clients and communities are becoming more aware of what protocols are in place to ensure that their animals are safe while under the care of a veterinary care team. As a valuable member of this team, veterinary technicians need to understand the basics of disease transmission and how to protect the patients while in the clinic. Veterinary technicians are also evolving to become the leaders of the biosecurity team, and are referred to as the *infection control* (IC) team. They are often in communication with all members of the veterinary care team and fully understand the day-to-day operation of the hospital/clinic. It is the mission of this team to protect all staff, clients, and patients that enter the hospital/clinic.

TECHNICIAN TIP 1.1: In order to protect the patients when visiting the clinic, the veterinary technician should understand the basics of disease transmission.

Cycle of Infection

A pathogen has a very specific purpose in its life cycle, that is, to infect as many hosts as possible in order to maintain the disease in a population. In order to complete this task, the pathogen must:

- find a portal of exit from the current host;
- find a method of transmission;
- find a portal of entry into a host;
- seek a susceptible host; and
- multiply within the host (the reservoir).

The likelihood of a pathogen's success depends on a variety of factors: the pathogen, the environment, and the host (Figure 1.1).

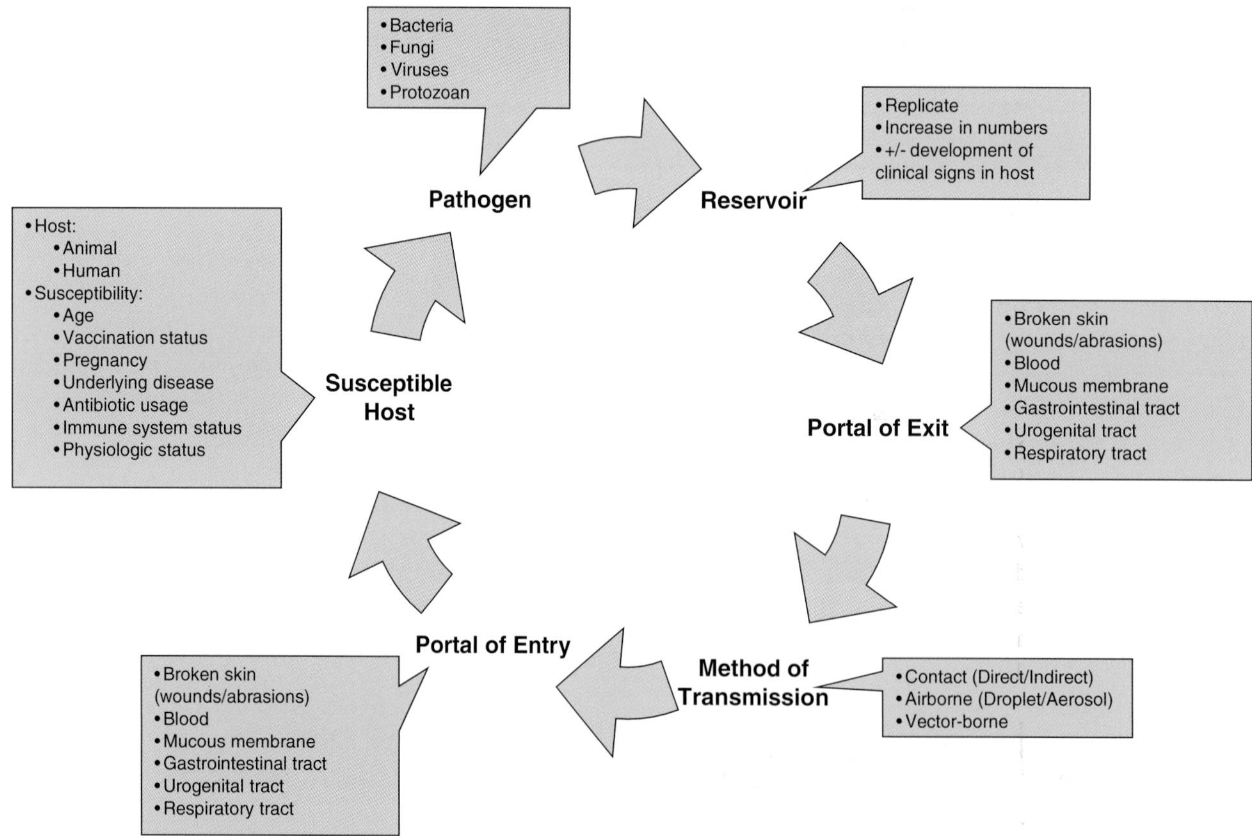

Figure 1.1 Cycle of Infection: Each component of the cycle must be present in sequential order for an infection to occur. At any point, the cycle can be broken, decreasing the risk of disease transmission and infection.

For the pathogen to infect other susceptible hosts, it must first leave the host that has been serving as the reservoir. The portals of exit from the host can include: gastrointestinal tract, urogenital tract, respiratory tract, blood, broken skin (wounds/abrasions), and mucous membranes. Some hosts may be an accidental host in that the pathogen does not have a strong specificity to that species. This may cause clinical disease in the patient, but it will not be able to exit the host. Accidental hosts are often referred to as a "dead-end" host for the pathogen because it is unable to replicate enough to exit the host. The more routes that a pathogen is able to utilize to exit the animal, the more successful it will be in finding a new host to start the infection process.

If a pathogen is able to successfully leave the host, it must move to another host. Contact, airborne, and vector-borne are the three main routes of transmission. These routes are discussed in further detail later on in the chapter. Environmental conditions and hardiness of the pathogen must be ideal for the pathogen to survive long enough to find the next host. Those pathogens that cannot withstand adverse environmental conditions must find a susceptible host in a short period of time or else it will die. Pathogens will succeed if there are a number of vulnerable hosts living closely together. Transmission may also occur if cleaning and hand hygiene is not adequate. Pathogens that are resistant to adverse environmental conditions can survive for years and cannot be eradicated unless appropriate disinfectants are used.

Once the pathogen is successful in finding a method of transmission, it must find a portal of entry into a host. Entry points are the same as exit portals out of a host (mucous membranes, abrasions/wounds [broken skin], blood, respiratory tract, urogenital tract, and/or gastrointestinal tract). More sites available to a pathogen increases the chances that it will progress to the next stage in the infection process.

The infection process into a new host is only successful if the host is susceptible to infection. Susceptibility of the animal can include, but is not limited to, age, vaccination status, pregnancy, underlying disease, immune system status, antibiotic usage, and/or physiological status. Those patients that are being exposed to any immune-suppressant medications (i.e. radiation therapy, chemotherapy, steroids) are at a higher risk of infection.

> **TECHNICIAN TIP 1.2:** Age, vaccination status, pregnancy, underlying disease, immune system status, antibiotic usage, and/or physiologic status are all factors that come into play regarding the susceptibility of an animal to a pathogen.

Some pathogens can only infect one species of animal, while others can infect many. This is known as species specificity. The more diverse numbers of species that the pathogen is able to infect, the greater the chance that the pathogen has to survive. This is especially true when dealing with smaller populations of animals in a given area. It is important to know if the pathogen is zoonotic so that people working with infected animals can take proper precautions to protect themselves from disease.

> **TECHNICIAN TIP 1.3:** It is important that the veterinary technician use proper precautions to protect themselves when working with animals that have a zoonotic disease to keep from becoming infected.

During the final phase, the pathogen will stay in the reservoir host to try to replicate and increase in numbers to eventually exit the host to start the chain of infection all over again. As the organism replicates and increases in the population, it will often cause a disease response in the host, which will begin to exhibit clinical signs of infection.

The time period between exposure to an infectious agent and the appearance of the first clinical signs is called the incubation period. This time period can vary significantly from one pathogen to another. If the host has a good immune response to the pathogen (either due to health status and/or vaccination against the pathogen), then the pathogen can be destroyed before causing any harm. A pathogen contains virulence factors or properties that enable it to establish itself on or within a host and enhance its potential to cause disease. The virulence factor plus immune status of the host will determine how clinically ill the patient will become.

Not all hosts present clinical signs of disease once infected. Some may be asymptomatic carriers or subclinical and may shed the pathogen without any apparent knowledge that they are infected. If you picture an iceberg, the part one can see from the surface depicts the clinical or obvious infections. Underneath the surface, the iceberg is an even larger mass and depicts the subclinical or colonized patients. This is why it is extremely important to take standard precautions to prevent exposure or movement of the potential pathogen.

Transmission

Routes of transmission can occur via three main pathways: contact (direct/indirect), airborne (droplet/aerosol), and vector-borne transmission. Interrupting the transmission of a pathogen from the reservoir to the susceptible host is an important component of eliminating nosocomial infections.

Contact Transmission

Contact transmission is the most common route and is divided into either direct or indirect contact. Direct animal-to-animal transmission can occur through a variety of different behaviors including, but not limited to, biting, touching, and grooming. The best way to break this cycle of transmission is by preventing patient-to-patient interaction.

Indirect Transmission

Indirect transmission occurs by contact with a contaminated piece of equipment, surface, or objects called fomites. High touch/patient contact areas, surgical instruments, fluid pumps, grooming aids, and endoscopes are just a few examples of contaminated areas/equipment that are commonly found to be responsible for indirect transmission of pathogens. Performing good hand hygiene and environmental decontamination are extremely important ways to prevent transmission via indirect contact.

TECHNICIAN TIP 1.4: To prevent transmission via indirect contact, good hand hygiene and environmental decontamination are extremely important.

Good hand hygiene should be performed before touching other objects such as clipboards, pens, and other pieces of equipment. Washing with soap and water and utilizing hand sanitizer are two methods of hand hygiene. Washing with soap and water is the preferred method as it eliminates all types of pathogens including non-enveloped viruses and parasites, in which hand sanitizer has no effectiveness. More information on hand hygiene is discussed later in the chapter. There are often times when hand hygiene cannot be performed directly after working with a patient. This is very common in barns and on farms where no sink is readily available. Antibacterial hand wipes followed by the use of hand sanitizer is a great alternative in these types of environments. If good hand hygiene is not completed, then these surfaces can cause indirect transmission (Figures 1.2 and 1.3).

TECHNICIAN TIP 1.5: The preferred method of hand hygiene is to wash with soap and water. A great alternative for environments where sinks are not readily available is the use of antibacterial hand wipes along with hand sanitizer.

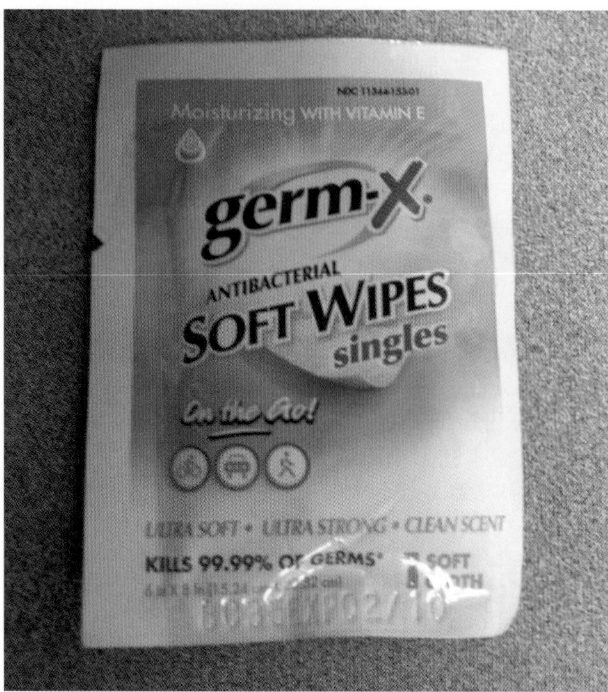

Figure 1.2 Antibacterial hand wipes are a great alternative when sinks are not available.

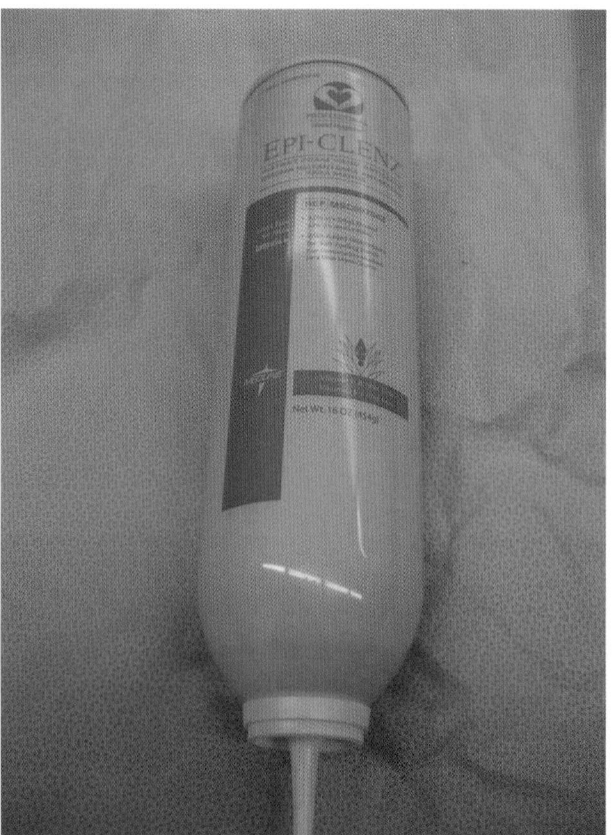

Figure 1.3 Foam hand sanitizer.

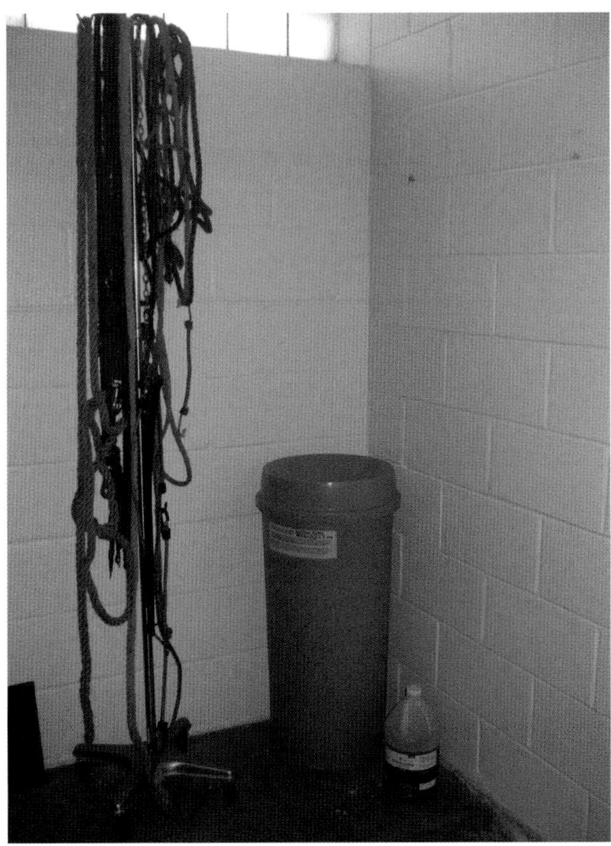

Figure 1.4 A dunk tank setup used for soaking porous equipment after the patient leaves. Items are hung to dry.

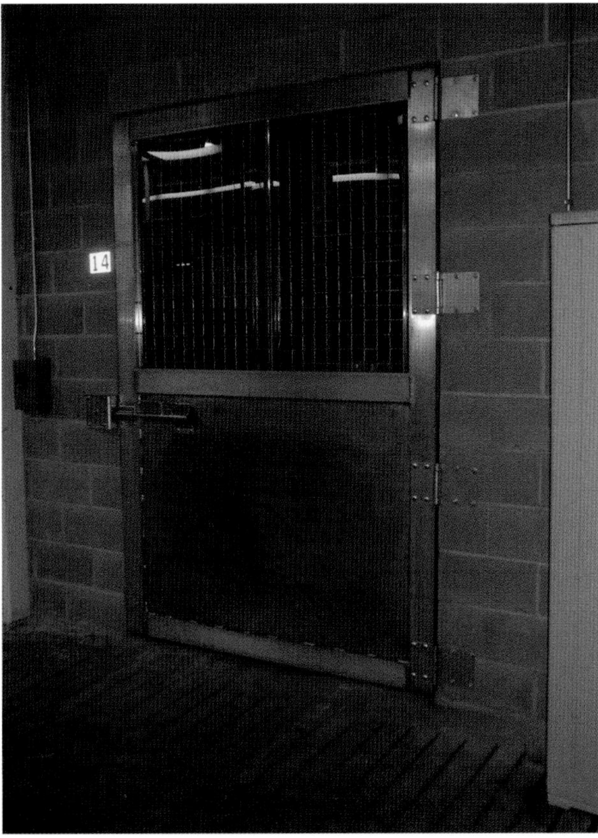

Figure 1.5 An isolation stall with its own ventilation system.

Disinfectant wipes are great for quick decontamination of high touch surfaces. Fluid pumps, stethoscopes, pens, thermometers, sink handles, and keyboards are a short list of the items that should be decontaminated after every patient/room use. It is important to have a protocol that identifies how to thoroughly clean items that are not easily cleaned. Items such as halters and ropes (porous items) should be soaked in disinfectant solution and left to dry after patient discharge (Figure 1.4).

Airborne transmission occurs when a pathogen in droplet or aerosol form travels through the air to find a host. Droplets are usually projected less than 3 ft (due to size and weight), and can be deposited on mucous membranes (i.e. conjunctiva, nasal, mucosa, oral cavity) and open wounds of the susceptible host. When droplets are 5 μm or less in size, they can be classified as aerosols. The smaller the droplet size the farther it may be able to travel via air currents, therefore, increasing the area of contamination. The risk of transmitting a pathogen by air also increases with proximity to the initial source and the duration of exposure. The length of time pathogens remain infectious in the droplet or aerosol form depends on the following factors:

- physiochemical properties of each individual pathogen (particularly environmental stability);
- concentration of infectious particles;
- air currents; and
- temperature and humidity.

The best way to decrease the likelihood of droplet transmission is to make sure that high-risk patients are kept at least 3–6 ft away from other patients, and that stall cleaning also includes the area outside of the stall. For pathogens that produce smaller droplet sizes, patients should have an isolated stall with its own ventilation system. See Strict Isolation Precautions for further details (Figure 1.5).

> **TECHNICIAN TIP 1.6:** The best way to decrease the risk of droplet transmission includes keeping high-risk patients at least 3–6 ft away.

Vector-Borne Transmission

Vector-borne transmission utilizes a vector such as mosquitos, fleas, ticks, and rodents in order to transmit the pathogen. These carriers transmit the pathogen either via biting the host (mosquitos) or by transporting the pathogen to an area that a susceptible host will be present (cockroaches). If the facility is able to provide good pest control, then the risk of vector-borne transmission decreases. The type of vector will vary geographically. Regardless of the vector, it is important that these offenders be identified and eliminated.

Preventing Disease Occurrence in the Host

There are a number of options available to prevent disease occurrence in the host. Vaccinations, prevention of malnutrition in the host, prevention of poor environmental conditions, and good antibiotic stewardship are all ways to stop a host from being susceptible to infection. Vaccinations provide protection by stimulating the immune system in the host. Vaccines are made from dead or inactive organisms that are unable to cause disease. This specific organism, when introduced into an animal, causes the immune system to produce antibodies against the specific antigen in the vaccine. When that specific live pathogen finds a portal of entry into a previously vaccinated host, the host is then able to fight off the pathogen before the pathogen is able to reproduce and cause a disease response.

Each clinic/hospital should establish an immunization protocol, based on species seen and types of problematic diseases. A patient's vaccination status is a vital component of the history that should be taken at admission to the clinic/hospital. This information will help in deciding patient placement in the hospital and will also help the clinician when ruling out diseases.

> **TECHNICIAN TIP 1.7:** Upon admission to the hospital/clinic, it is vital to get the patient's vaccination status when taking the history.

Malnutrition and vitamin deficiencies in a host can lead to an increased susceptibility to infection. Ensuring that animals are receiving the right nutrients and in correct amounts are easy ways to increase host resistance.

> **TECHNICIAN TIP 1.8:** Ensuring that animals are getting appropriate nutrition and adequate food supply are easy ways to increase host resistance.

Poor environmental conditions for the host are often an ideal environment for pathogens to thrive. Stalls should be kept clean and disinfected periodically. Food and hay should be inspected for mold, and obvious reservoirs for pathogens (i.e. standing water, rodents, and insect pests) should be eliminated. Removing pathogen reservoirs will decrease the likelihood that pathogens are either shed in the environment or directly transmitted to the host.

Good antibiotic stewardship is another way to prevent disease occurrence in the patient. Antibiotic stewardship follows four basic factors:

- give the right antibiotic;
- at the right dose;
- at the right time; and
- for the right duration.

The prevalence of antibiotic resistance commonly increases in proportion to the frequency of use. The goal of antibiotic administration is to achieve optimal clinical outcomes while minimizing adverse effects in the patient and limiting the selection for antimicrobial-resistant strains. Ideally, a culture of the infected area or suspected area should be taken prior to administration of any antibiotics. If a culture cannot be obtained, then antibiotics should be chosen dependent on the type of organism suspected of causing the infection. Gram stains can provide some help in narrowing down the type of bacteria present (Figure 1.6). Based on the Gram stain, a narrow spectrum low-level antibiotic should be given until culture results are available. Antibiotics should never be prescribed randomly. Antibiotics may also be given as a prophylactic prior to surgery. Surgical procedures disrupt the skin's normal defensive barrier and can become an easy entry point for pathogens if the sterile surgical field is broken. An antibiotic for this purpose should be safe and provide adequate coverage for broad-spectrum contaminants that might be found in the environment. For an antibiotic to be effective, it needs to be administered to the patient within 60 min of cut time to provide therapeutic levels at the time of the first

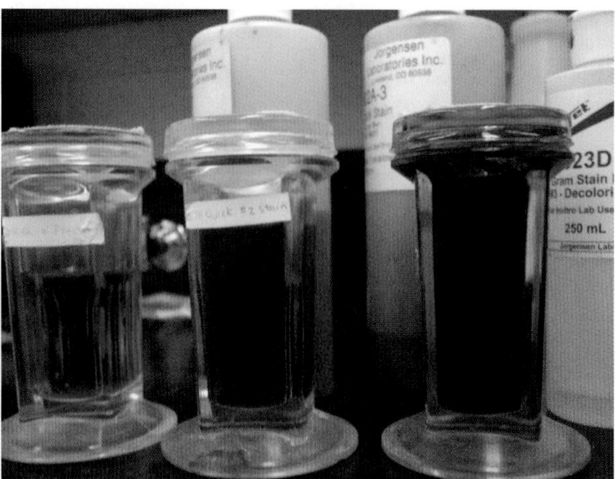

Figure 1.6 Gram stains are used to narrow down types of bacteria.

surgical incision. If surgery time is longer than one to two times the half-life of the drug, then additional doses should be given during the surgery. If IC protocols are followed throughout the prep and surgical procedure, then post-op antibiotics may not be needed.

> **TECHNICIAN TIP 1.9:** Antibiotic stewardship includes: giving the right antibiotics, at the right dose, at the right time, and for the right duration.

Patient Placement in the Hospital

Prescreening Patients

Patient screening should begin before the patient reaches the hospital. Knowing the patient's clinical signs before he or she comes into the hospital will give the clinic/hospital staff a general idea of what to expect before arrival. A stall can be prepared in the correct location and appropriate personal protective equipment (PPE) can be arranged. Patient placement ultimately depends upon the type of infection, the ability to provide appropriate care, and appropriate staffing.

Prescreening questions should include, but are not limited to:

- travel history including any fairs or shows recently attended;
- any clinical signs including fever, nasal discharge, open sores, coughing, and diarrhea;
- other members of the herd having similar clinical signs; and
- history of infectious disease in the patient or on the farm/homestead.

At arrival, a brief physical exam should be completed before entry into the hospital. This can occur in the trailer or outside. The physical exam should include noting any open sores, nasal discharge, diarrhea, coughing, and other infectious clinical signs.

Species Separation

When placing patients in the hospital, they should be separated according to species, reason for admission, and desired contact precautions. Correct patient placement is necessary to control disease transmission.

> **TECHNICIAN TIP 1.10:** Correct placement of the patient within the hospital or clinic is necessary to control disease transmission.

All species should be separated within the clinical setting (Figures 1.7 and 1.8). In an ideal situation, each species would have separate buildings/barns. Most clinics/hospitals do not have that luxury so species need to be separated by hallways or other physical barriers. Separation needs to occur because each species may shed infectious organisms in varying amounts, length of time, and based on different stressors. For example, bovine patients shed *Salmonella* (in feces) and often without clinical signs. Environmental contamination can occur easily with salmonellosis, creating a higher potential of transmission to other species and patients. Housing of species together can also cause stress to some animals, such as llamas with horses. Stress can cause a prolonged healing time and can often increase shedding of infectious pathogens.

Within the different areas of the hospital/clinic setting, each species should be separated based on their risk level

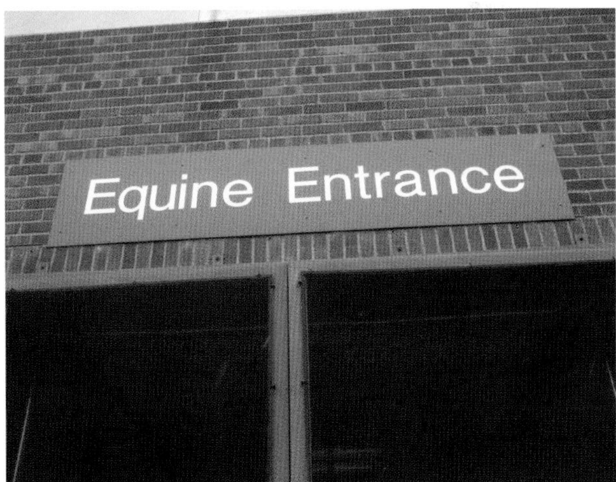

Figure 1.7 Equine entrance separate from other species is ideal.

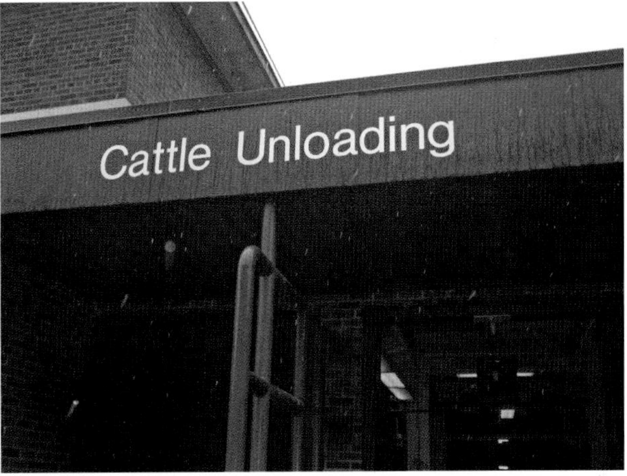

Figure 1.8 Bovine entrance is separate from other species.

of spreading or acquiring infectious diseases. Patients undergoing orthopedic surgery generally have a lower potential of shedding infectious organisms but have a higher risk of acquiring them. In an equine facility, it has been shown that colic patients tend to have a higher risk of shedding *Salmonella*. Orthopedic and colic patients should ideally be placed in different areas of the hospital/clinic or separated by physical or virtual barriers.

> **TECHNICIAN TIP 1.11:** It has been shown that colic patients tend to have a higher risk of shedding *Salmonella* within an equine hospital.

Barrier Precautions

Once the risk level of spreading or acquiring infectious diseases is determined, then barrier precautions can be assigned depending on the patient's risk level. In the large animal setting, four different levels of precautions are:

- standard
- contact
- mini-isolation
- strict isolation

Reevaluate the risk level of the patient on a daily basis, as it can change dependent on the patient's clinical status. If the risk level increases, then the barrier precautions should reflect that change (Figures 1.9 and 1.10). It is important to note that with all levels of precautions, hospital personnel should be wearing clean outerwear and, if working with horses, all hooves need to be picked prior to transporting them outside of the stall environment.

> **TECHNICIAN TIP 1.12:** Daily evaluation of the patient is important as the risk level of the patient can change on a daily basis.

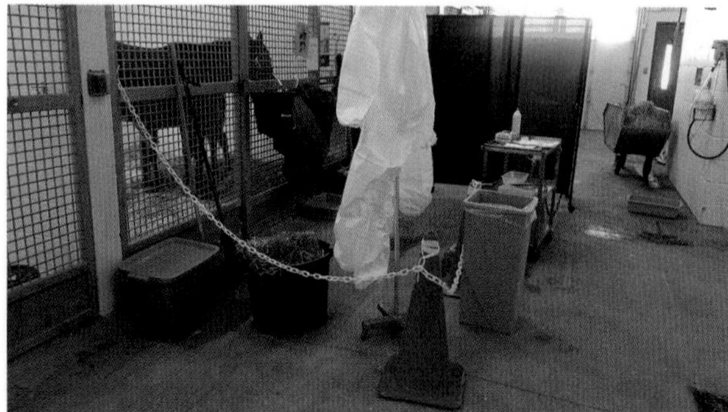

Figure 1.9 Mini-isolation stall.

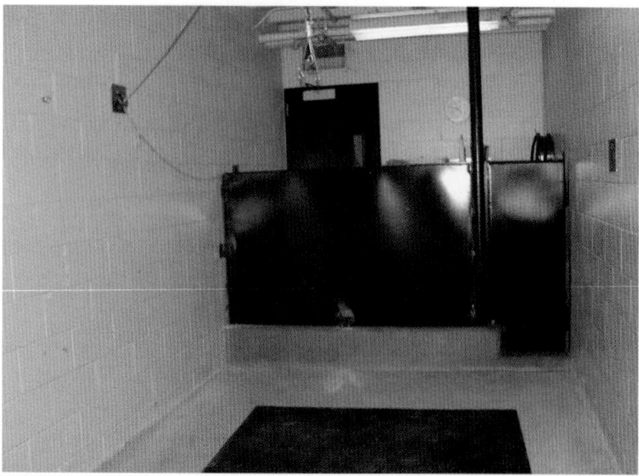

Figure 1.10 Strict isolation stall.

Standard Precautions

The basic precautions are called standard precautions. Standard precautions include good hand hygiene before and after handling the patient. Standard precautions should be used with all patients, even if they appear to be healthy, as they can be asymptomatic carriers.

Contact Precautions

Contact precautions are the next level in the precaution recommendations. Contact precautions include good hand hygiene before and after patient contact, wearing of gloves while handling the patient, and the addition of a footbath at the front of the stall. Gloves add an additional barrier between the personnel and the patient, which can decrease the risk of disease transmission. It is important to remember that gloves are not an adjunct for good hand hygiene and that hand hygiene still needs to be performed after gloves are removed. The same pair of gloves should not be used on more than one patient, and gloves should be switched if moving from a dirty to a clean area of the patient. For example, personnel should not handle a catheter after touching an open wound. Whenever possible, clean procedures should be performed before procedures in dirty areas of the patient. In addition, best practices would include a "clean" technician and a "dirty" technician. The "dirty" technician should deal with all the isolation/restriction cases and not go in with any patients that are immunocompromised including foals and young animals.

Mini-Isolation Precautions

Mini-isolations should be used only in cases where transferring a patient to a strict isolation facility/stall cannot be done safely or patient care would be compromised. Mini-isolations are not to be used for the sole purpose of staff convenience.

Mini-isolation includes the previous steps plus a perimeter barrier, gowns/coveralls, boot covers, multiple footbaths, and with or without face shield. A barrier should extend far enough out from the front of the stall so that there is adequate room for personnel as well as necessary equipment and supplies. A stall should also be left vacant on either side of the infectious patient. A footbath should be placed at the entrance to the barrier and also at the front of the stall door. The area on the outside of the barrier chains is considered the clean area. The space between the chains and the stall front is considered the semi-clean area. All items used with the patient should be kept neatly in this area and should not be removed unless they are completely disinfected or sent for sterilization. This includes, but is not limited to, stethoscopes, thermometers, hoof picks, manure shovels, bins, and so forth. All personal items should be left in a neutral non-clinical area. The inside stall area is considered the dirty area, and all PPE needs to be used anytime personnel enter this space. Proper gowning will be discussed later on in the chapter. It is also important to remember good hand hygiene before and after patient contact even though additional PPE is being utilized. Movement of patients out of the mini-isolation area should be restricted to necessary procedures only. Limiting traffic of infectious patients in a hospital/clinic reduces the possibility of environmental contamination.

Strict Isolation Precautions

The fourth and final type of precaution is known as strict isolation precautions. This includes all of the previous items discussed in the mini-isolation step, but adds an additional space factor. All strict isolation patients should be placed in an area that has a separate ventilation system and has no communication to other stalls or patients. Isolation facilities are often located in a completely separate barn or clinic (Figure 1.11). Isolation patients are those that are considered extremely infectious and require the highest barrier precautions and PPE available (i.e. equine herpesvirus myeloencephalopathy, strangles, *Salmonella*, etc.). The isolation area is set up similar to that of the mini-isolation area, except facility walls, and doors will be in place rather than chains as a barrier to ensure that there is no risk of aerosol transmission to the outside area. As mentioned in the previous section, no items should be removed from the isolation area unless they are thoroughly disinfected or placed in a clean bag to be transported for sterilization.

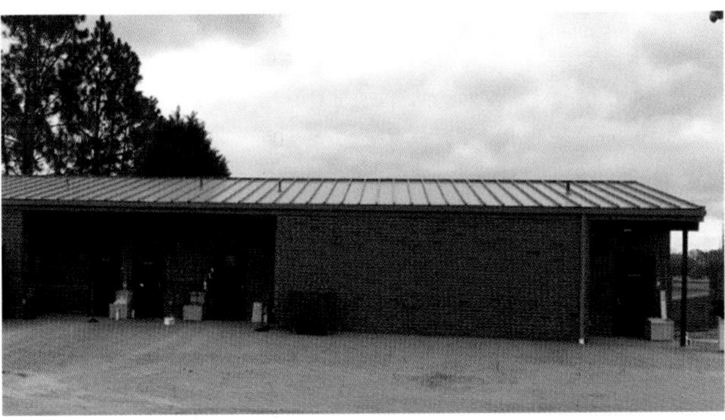

Figure 1.11 A strict isolation building.

Patient placement will ultimately depend on the type of infection, the ability to provide appropriate care, and appropriate staffing.

Proper Gowning Techniques

Proper dressing and undressing of personnel entering/exiting the isolation (and mini-isolation) areas need to occur in a specific order to prevent contamination to clothing and equipment/items in the area. Note that institutions may have slightly different orders dependent on protocols, preferences, or facilities. Any refrigerated medications or disposable items should be brought to the changing area before putting on PPE. While in the clean area, gloves, boots, and coveralls are donned. The staff member may now enter the semi-clean area after stepping into and through the first footbath. A second pair of gloves and a facemask (if needed) can be put on at this time. Gather the items needed for the patient and cross through the second footbath to enter the dirty area. It is helpful to have another staff member on the clean side to be the runner if additional items are needed or to record findings in the patient's record.

To exit the dirty area, the first stage is to step into and through the footbath at the stall front and enter the semi-clean area. The first item to be removed is the facemask (if used) and then the first layer of gloves that had direct patient contact. If the inner gloves are also soiled, discard them and replace them with a clean pair before going onto the next step. The next item to be removed is the coveralls and the boots. First take both arms out of the coveralls, being careful to only touch the clean side (inside). Again, only touching the clean side of the coveralls, carefully balance on one foot and remove the first leg from the coveralls along with the boot from that leg as well. Step that foot into the footbath and then balance on this foot in order to remove the leg and boot from the other foot. Step into the footbath, now with both feet in the footbath, and discard the coveralls and boots. Step into the clean area and finally remove the last pair of gloves. It is important to remember to perform good hand hygiene before going to the next patient or documenting anything on the treatment sheet. The process of gowning and de-gowning can be a little tricky and will take some practice to become efficient at the process (Figures 1.12–1.23).

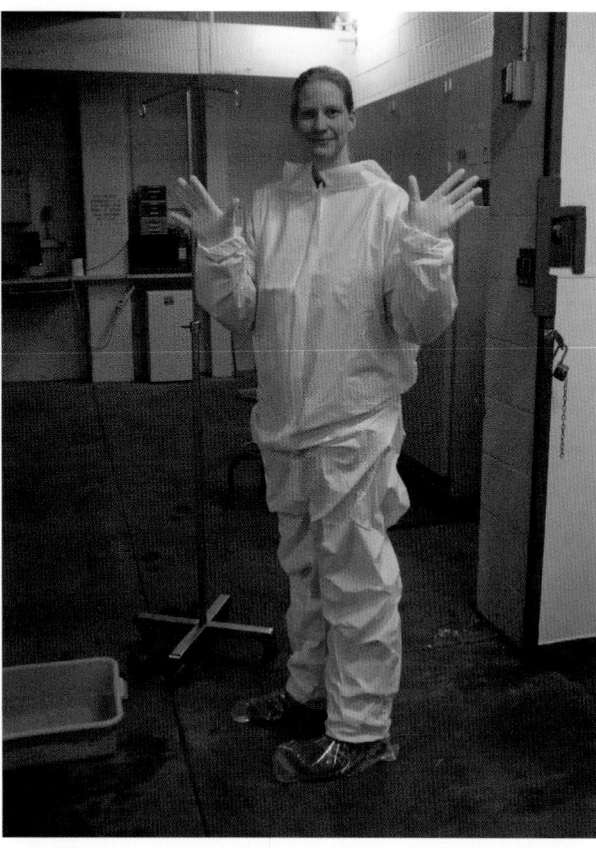

Figure 1.12 Full PPE on a technician who is ready to enter isolation.

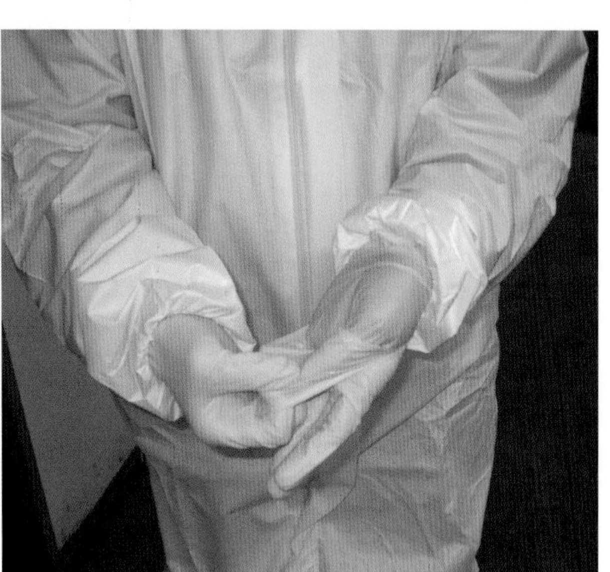

Figure 1.13 Exiting isolation step one: Remove soiled gloves and replace.

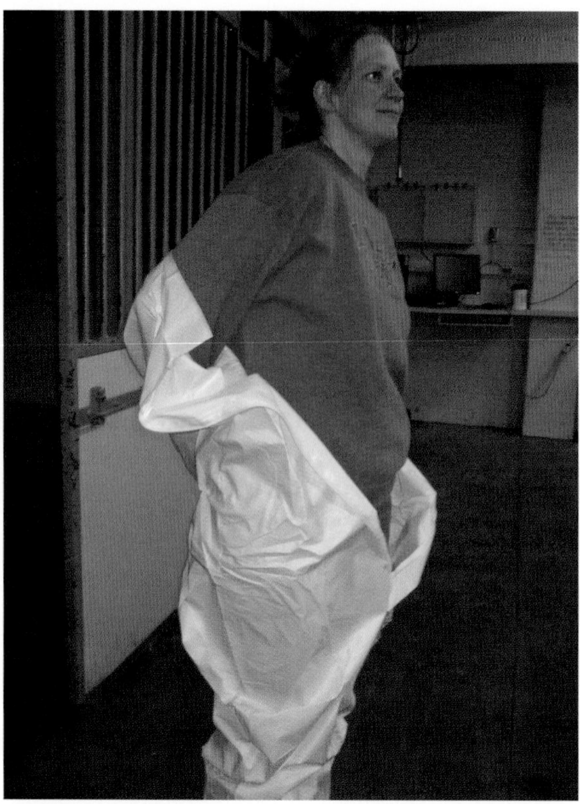

Figure 1.14 Exiting isolation step two: Remove gown with clean gloves by pulling your hands through, touching only the clean inside of the gown.

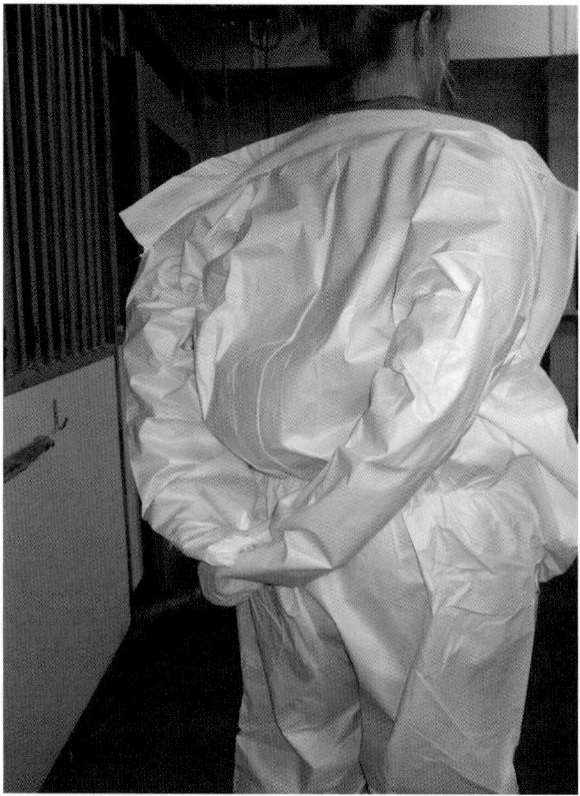

Figure 1.15 Continue taking off the isolation suit being sure to touch only the inside of the gown.

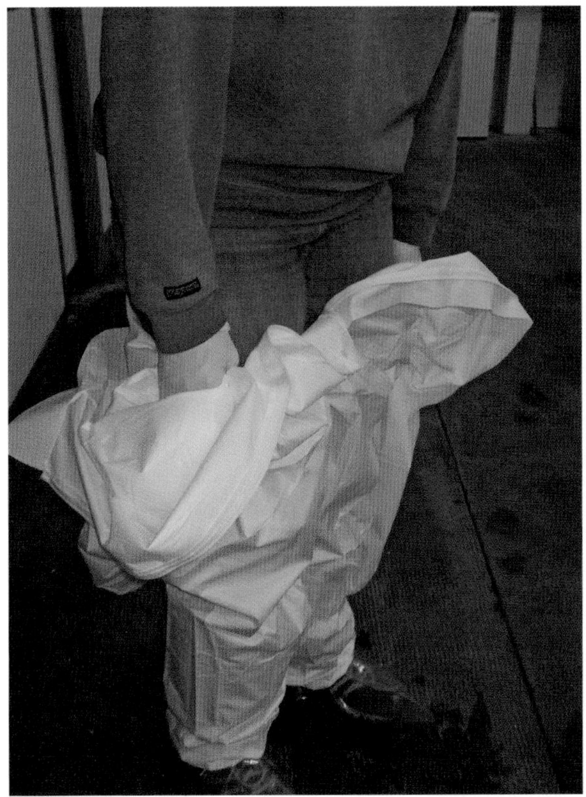

Figure 1.16 Move the isolation suit down to the boots.

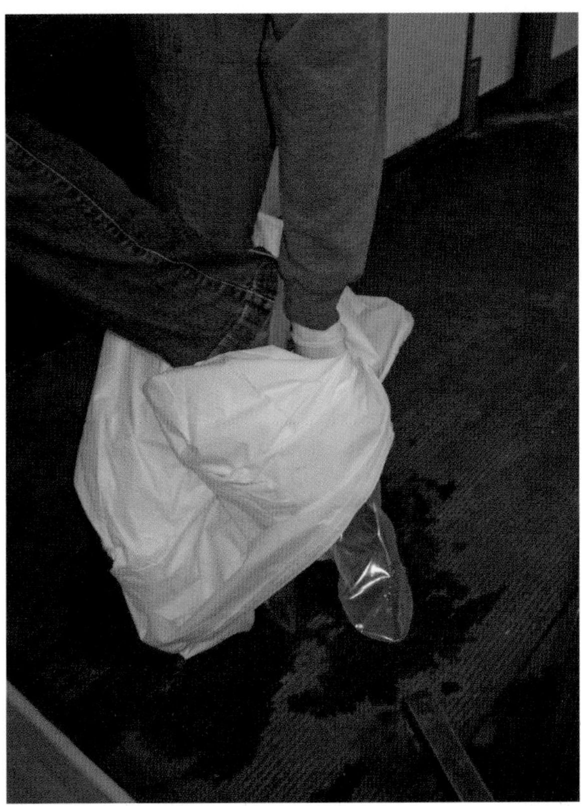

Figure 1.17 Remove the suit and one boot.

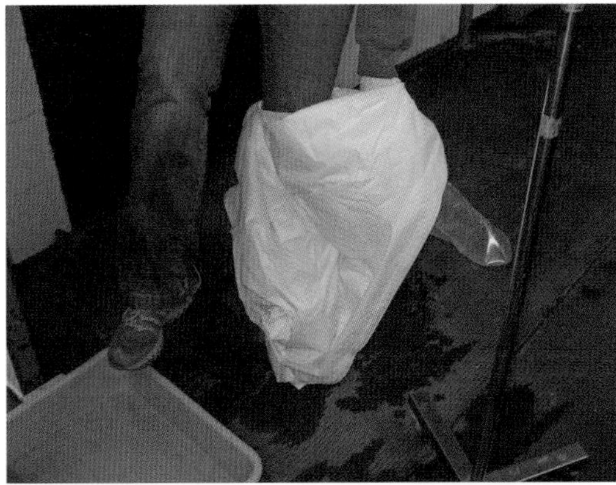

Figure 1.18 With one boot loose, step into the footbath.

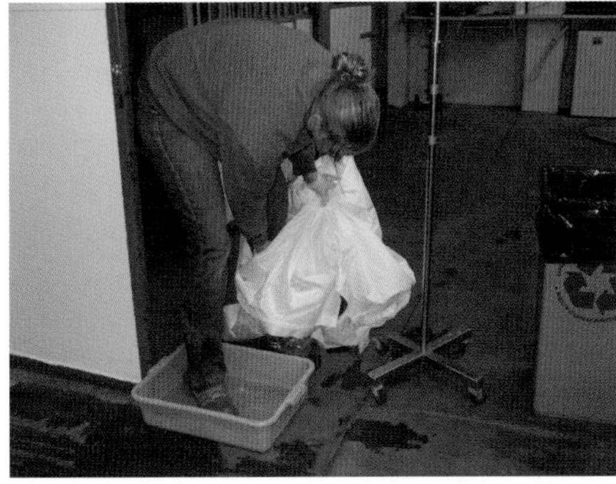

Figure 1.19 Continue ungowning by removing the second boot.

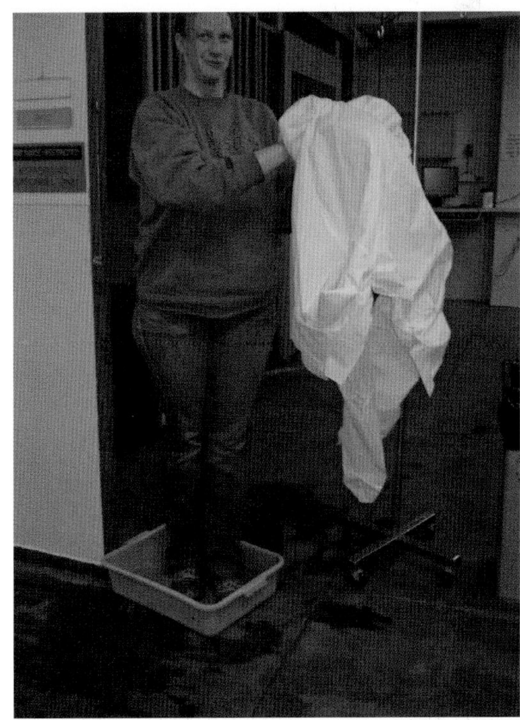

Figure 1.20 Place second loose foot into the footbath.

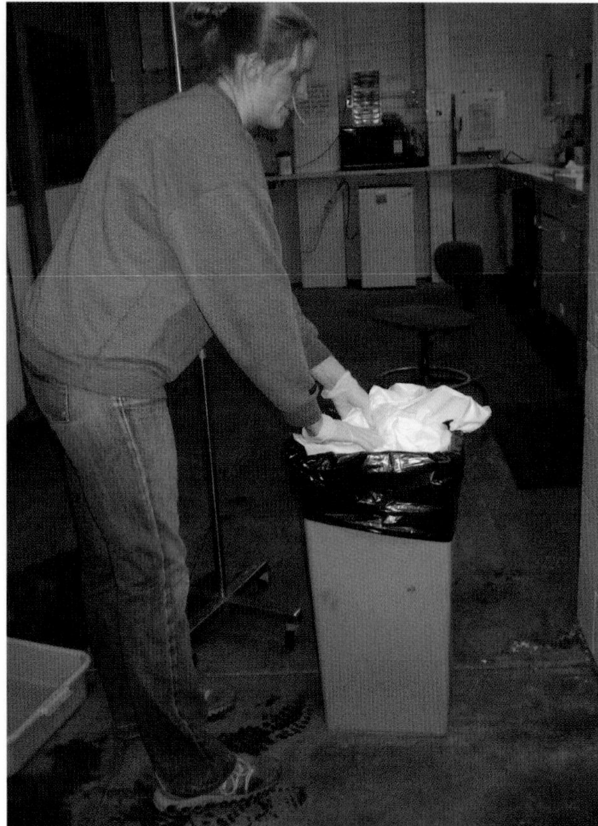

Figure 1.21 Dispose of contaminated suit.

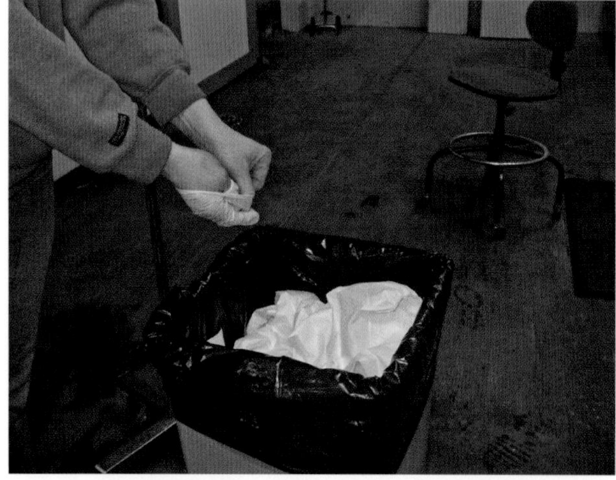

Figure 1.22 Dispose of gloves.

Hand Hygiene

As mentioned earlier, hand hygiene is the number one way to prevent transmission of disease with environmental decontamination coming in as a close second. Performing both of these tasks correctly and timely will dramatically decrease the risk of contamination to patients and personnel.

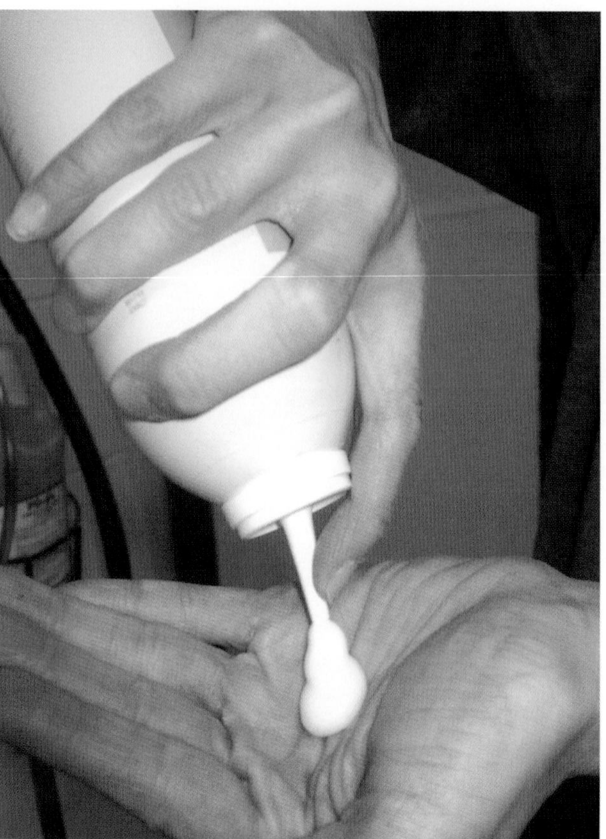

Figure 1.23 Use hand sanitizer after taking off PPE.

Hand hygiene can be completed with the use of soap and water and/or alcohol-based hand sanitizer. It should be done before and after patient contact, after using the restrooms, before and after eating, when entering and leaving the hospital/clinic, and many other times during the day. See Figures 1.24–1.29 for a proper hand washing technique.

Soap and water is always the best option for hand decontamination and should always be done in place of sanitizer if the hands are visibly soiled. Some hand soaps may contain an antiseptic. Antiseptics are antimicrobial substances that are applied to the skin or mucous membranes to reduce the number of microbial flora. In addition to hand soaps, antiseptics can also be found in surgical scrubs that are used to prepare a surgeon's hands and to prepare the skin of patients for sterile procedures.

Hand Sanitizer

Hand sanitizer is an alternative to soap and water only if hands are not visibly dirty, as it is deactivated by organic material. It is common in barns and large animal hospitals/clinics to have a large amount of organic material in the environment and on the patient; therefore, in this

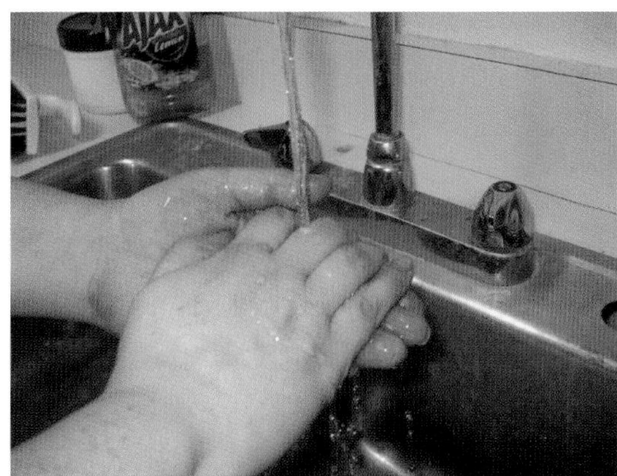

Figure 1.24 Wet hands.

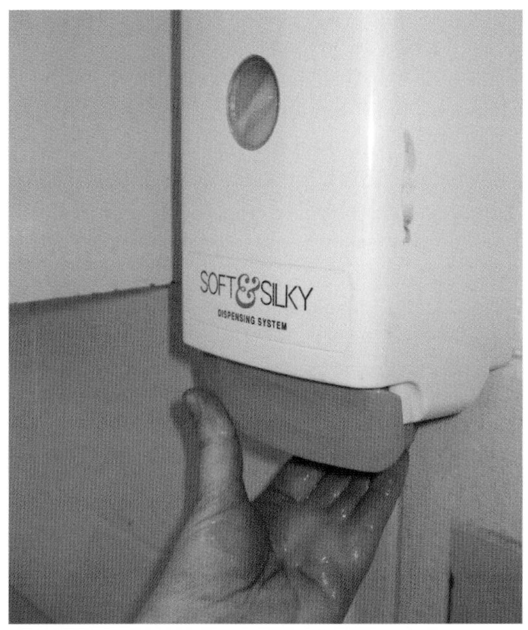

Figure 1.25 Add soap.

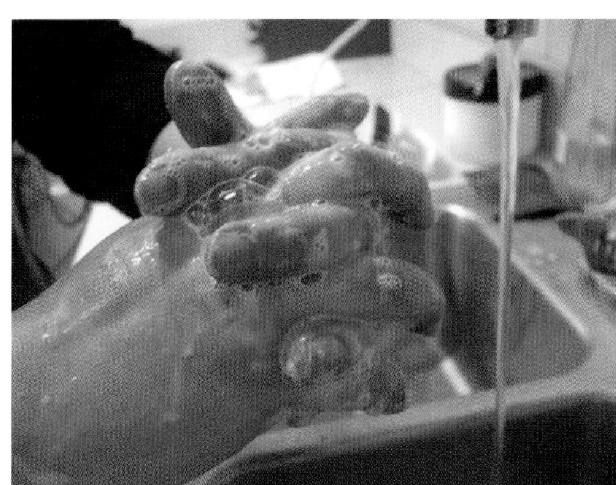

Figure 1.26 Wash for 20 S.

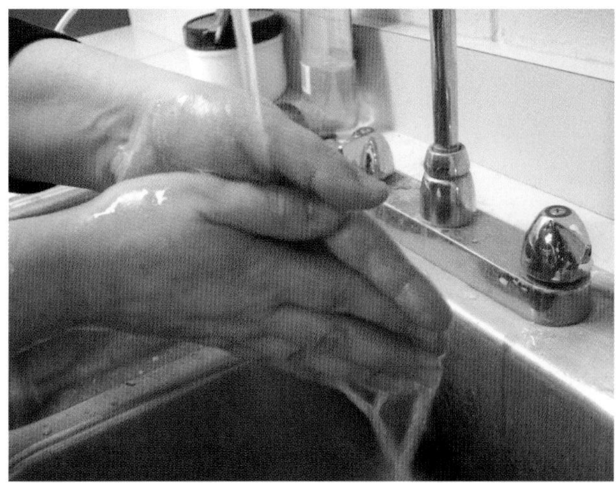

Figure 1.27 Rinse.

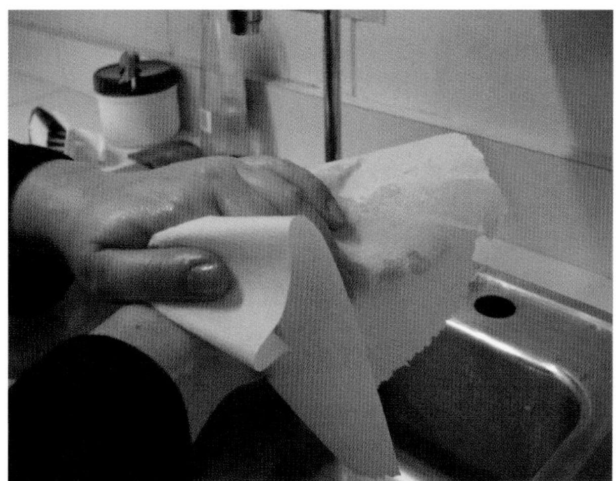

Figure 1.28 Dry.

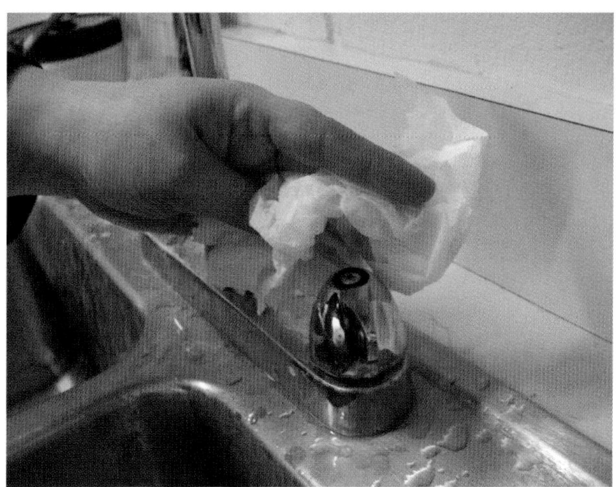

Figure 1.29 Turn off water with paper towel.

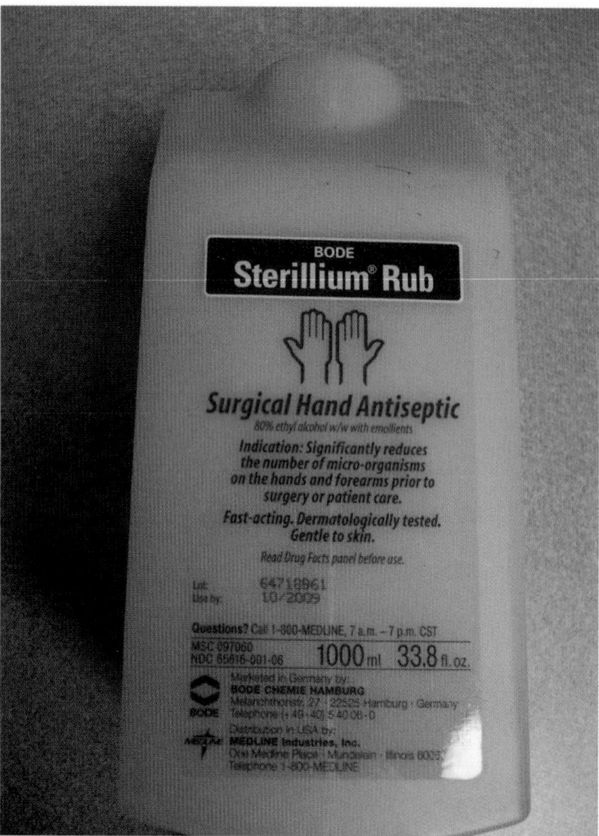

Figure 1.30 Surgical hand scrub.

situation, it is better to have access to hand washing stations rather than simply using hand sanitizer. Hand sanitizer should contain at least 70–90% alcohol content to be considered appropriate for a hospital environment and should contain some type of emollients and moisturizers to keep hands from drying out. Before purchasing a sanitizer, it is important to ensure that staff will utilize the product. If personnel do not like the product due to fragrance, too much alcohol smell, foam versus gel, and so forth, they will not use it. Lack of personnel compliance will render this ineffective. Note that hand sanitizers kill most pathogens but not all of them. It will not kill parasites or non-enveloped viruses, including *Norovirus*, which is a common human virus causing gastroenteritis.

The last component to good hand hygiene is maintaining hand health and skin integrity. Dry and cracked skin provides pathogens an entryway to infect personnel. Hand lotion should be used frequently to maintain skin health.

Disinfection and Sterilization

Disinfection and sterilization are two extremely important concepts that aid in interrupting the cycle of infection. When performed properly, environmental surfaces and equipment can be safe and free of pathogens.

Disinfection

Disinfection is a process that eliminates many or all pathogenic microorganisms on inanimate objects. All cleaners/disinfectants are composed of chemicals that fall into different categories of effectiveness. For each category, there are different kill times, levels of effectiveness, and types of pathogens they affect. Table 1.1 illustrates chemical types and their properties. Each clinic/hospital should have a low-level or intermediate-level disinfectant (kills most types of bacteria and viruses but it will not kill bacterial spores) and a high-level disinfectant (kills all microorganisms except for some bacterial spores). All personnel need to be trained when to use each chemical and the safety precautions needed when using them.

It is critical that chemicals are diluted correctly. Over-diluting chemicals will render them ineffective, while under-diluting them will not make the cleaners/disinfectants more powerful. Using higher concentrations of chemicals is hazardous to personnel, causes more wear and tear on surfaces or equipment, and is not cost-efficient. Resistance can develop in some pathogens when certain disinfectants are misused over long periods of time.

> **TECHNICIAN TIP 1.13:** The misuse of disinfectants may develop resistance in some pathogens.

For the chemical/disinfectant to be completely effective, the organic material must first be removed. All surfaces should be cleaned of shavings, manure, and visible dirt. Once the object/surface is visibly clean, the disinfectant of

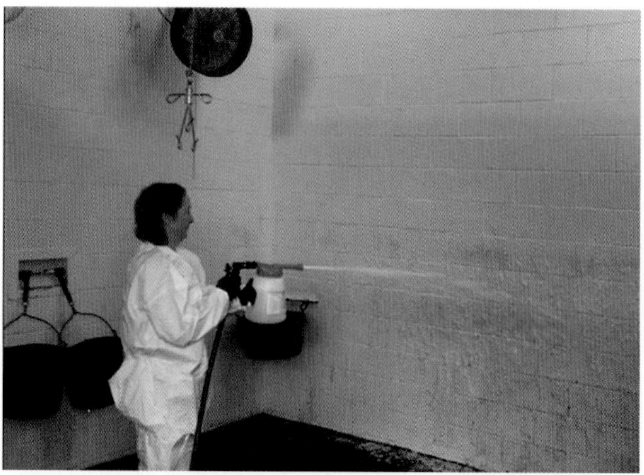

Figure 1.31 A stall being disinfected that was first stripped of all organic material.

Table 1.1 Characteristics of selected disinfectants.

Disinfectant category	Alcohols	Aldehydes	Biguanides	Halogen:hypochlorites	Halogen: iodine compounds	Oxidizing agents	Phenols	Quaternary ammonium compounds (QAC)
Sample trade names	Ethyl alcohol Isopropyl alcohol	Formaldehyde Glutaraldehyde	Chlorhexidine Nolvasan® Virosan®	Bleach	Betadyne® Providone®	Hydrogen peroxide Peracetic acid Virkon S® Oxy-Sept 333®	One-Stroke Environ® Pheno-Tek II® Tek-Trol®	Roccal® DiQuat® D-256®
Mechanism of action	Precipitates proteins Denatures lipids	Denatures proteins Alkylates nucleic acids	Alters membrane permeability	Denatures proteins	Denatures proteins	Denature proteins and lipids	Denatures proteins Alters cell wall permeability	Denatures proteins Binds phospholipids of cell membrane
Advantages	Fast acting Leaves no residue	Broad spectrum	Broad spectrum	Broad spectrum Short contact time Inexpensive	Stable in storage Relatively safe	Broad spectrum	Good efficacy with organic material Non-corrosive Stable in storage	Stable in storage Non-irritating to skin Effective at high temperatures and high pH (9–10)
Disadvantages	Rapid evaporation Flammable	Carcinogenic Mucous membranes and tissue irritation Only use in well-ventilated areas	Only functions in limited pH range (5–7) Toxic to fish (environmental concern)	Inactivated by sunlight Requires frequent application Corrodes metals Mucous membrane and tissue irritation	Inactivated by QACs Requires frequent application Corrosive Stains clothes and treated surfaces	Damaging to some metals	Can cause skin and eye irritation	
Precautions	Flammable	Carcinogenic		Never mix with acids; toxic chlorine gas will be released			May be toxic to animals, especially cats and pigs	
Vegetative bacteria	Effective	Effective	Effective	Effective	Effective	Effective	Effective	YES—Gram Positive Limited – Gram Negative

(Continued)

Table 1.1 (Continued)

Disinfectant category	Alcohols	Aldehydes	Biguanides	Halogen:hypochlorites	Halogen: iodine compounds	Oxidizing agents	Phenols	Quaternary ammonium compounds (QAC)
Mycobacteria	Effective	Effective	Variable	Effective	Limited	Effective	Variable	Variable
Enveloped viruses	Effective	Effective	Limited	Effective	Effective	Effective	Effective	Variable
Non-enveloped viruses	Variable	Effective	Limited	Effective	Limited	Effective	Variable	Not Effective
Spores	Not Effective	Effective	Not Effective	Variable	Limited	Variable	Not Effective	Not Effective
Fungi	Effective	Effective	Limited	Effective	Effective	Variable	Variable	Variable
Efficacy with organic matter	Reduced	Reduced	?	Rapidly reduced	Rapidly reduced	Variable	Effective	Inactivated
Efficacy with hard water	?	Reduced	?	Effective	?	?	Effective	Inactivated
Efficacy with soap/detergents	?	Reduced	Inactivated	Inactivated	Effective	?	Effective	Inactivated

For more information, see the "disinfection 101" document at http://www.cfsph.iastate.edu.
? Information not found.
DISCLAIMER: The use of trade names does not in any way signify endorsement of a particular product.
For additional product names, please consult the most recent Compendium of Veterinary Products.
Source: Adapted from Linton et al. (1987), Quinn and Markey (2001). ©2008 CFSPH.

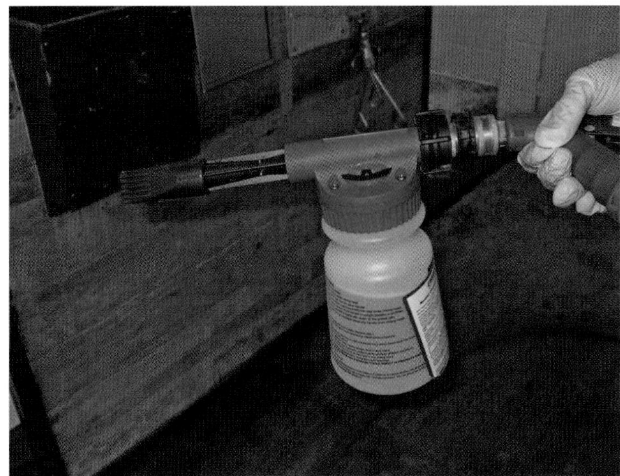

Figure 1.32 Foam gun used to apply disinfectant solution to a stall.

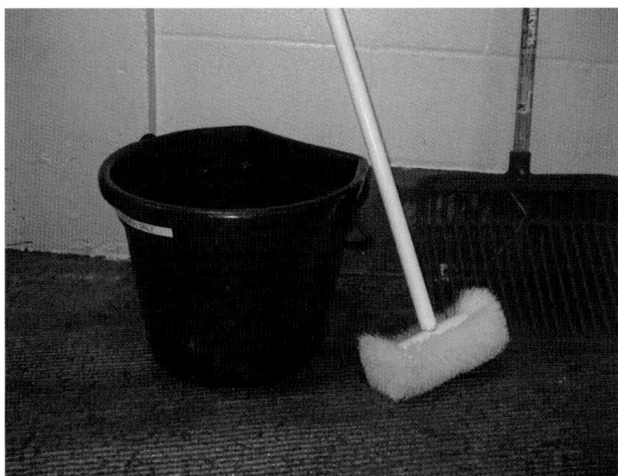

Figure 1.33 Scrub brushes can help remove soiled areas on stall surfaces.

choice should be applied and left to sit on these surfaces for a minimum of 10 min (or as recommended by the manufacturer). Spray/rinse with water and let dry. If the area was heavily soiled, repeat the process to ensure that all pathogens are eliminated.

Sterilization

For items that need a higher level of disinfection for sterile procedures, sterilization is utilized post-cleaning. Sterilization is a process that destroys or eliminates all forms of microbial life via physical or chemical methods. Steam under pressure, ethylene oxide gas, hydrogen peroxide gas plasma, and liquid chemicals are the main types of sterilization utilized in hospitals/clinics.

Deciding which option to use is primarily dependent on the type and composition of the equipment itself and the manufacturer's specifications. Regardless of the method utilized, all items must be thoroughly cleaned, and all gross material must be removed from the surface in order for the process to be effective.

TECHNICIAN TIP 1.14: Thorough cleaning and removing of all organic material from surfaces before disinfecting or sterilizing must be performed in order for the process to be effective.

Steam Sterilization

Steam sterilization requires four conditions to be met in order to be effective:

- type of steam
- pressure
- temperature
- time

To kill all pathogens, spores, and heat-resistant organisms, the steam inside of the autoclave must contain a relative humidity of 97–99%. The pressure of the steam must be forceful enough to penetrate wrapped items to quickly kill microorganisms. The two common steam-sterilizing temperatures are 121 °C (250 °F) and 132 °C (270 °F). Temperature correlates with time in that the length of time at the predetermined temperature must be maintained for a minimal time to kill microorganisms. Recognized minimum exposure periods for sterilization of wrapped supplies are 30 min at 121 °C (250 °F) or 4 min at 132 °C (270 °C). It is important to remember steam sterilization is only safe for items that are heat and moisture resistant. A low temperature sterilization alternative may be used for heat or moisture sensitive equipment.

Gas Sterilization

Gas sterilization utilizes ethylene oxide (EtO) to provide low temperature sterilization. The four essential parameters are:

- gas concentration (450–1200 mg/l)
- temperature (37–63 °C)
- relative humidity (40 to 80%) (water molecules carry EtO to reactive sites)
- exposure time (1–6 hr)

After the cycle is complete, the items must undergo an aeration period to remove any residual ethylene oxide that was absorbed by the items.

Gas Plasma Sterilization

Hydrogen peroxide gas plasma is a fairly new sterilization practice that has only been marketed in the United States since 1993. It is safer than ethylene oxide while sterilizing items that are heat or moisture sensitive. A hydrogen peroxide vapor solution is released into the sterilization chamber at a concentration of 6 mg/l. Microorganisms are initially inactivated by the hydrogen peroxide before a microbicidal substance is applied to the items in the chamber. An electrical field is created by a radio frequency that is applied to the chamber creating gas plasma. Free radicals are generated in the gas plasma that are capable of interacting with essential cell components disrupting the metabolism of the microorganism. The hydrogen peroxide plus the gas plasma create a deadly combination for microorganisms. This method is safer for handling items immediately post cycle. The process operates in the range of 37–44 °C and has a cycle time of 75 min.

Hospital Management

Every veterinary clinic or hospital should have an IC program in place to ensure that nosocomial infections are caught quickly and that IC guidelines are in place and followed. Infection control programs will differ between facilities dependent on the size of the clinic/hospital, number of personnel, risk of nosocomial infections in the practice, amount of funding available, personnel available to dedicate themselves to the program, and overall willingness of administration and personnel to put forth effort to build and maintain a program.

Key components of an infectious disease program include:

- Determining which diseases are to be controlled and understanding the ecology of these diseases.
- Grouping animals based on their infection status.
- Maintaining hygiene of the facility, personnel, and patients.
- Monitoring the occurrence of infectious disease.
- Instituting an immunization program for patients and staff.
- Optimizing the overall health of the animals by minimizing stressors, optimizing nutritional status, optimizing specific immunity through vaccination, and minimizing treatments that may make the animal more susceptible to disease.

Infection Control Programs

Leadership is a key component of a successful IC program. Historically, most programs have been chaired by a clinician. However, times are changing in that veterinary technicians are becoming vital parts and leaders of the IC programs of their clinics/hospitals. It is not only more cost-effective for the clinic to give this responsibility to a technician, but it also gives the program a different insight as technicians generally have a better idea of what is actually occurring in the clinic in regard to IC. Technicians are key personnel for direct patient care, cleaning (including sterilization and laundry), and oversight of patient placement.

A good IC program begins with an IC committee that consists of essential personnel in the hospital. Which personnel are deemed essential will differ from clinic to clinic. However, it should include a range of people including technicians, clinicians, clinical pathology personnel, hospital epidemiologist, administrators, and cleaning personnel.

The committee should have clearly defined goals and objectives that are based on ways to protect patients, hospital personnel, owners, and the community. Goals and objectives should be in writing and reviewed annually. The committee needs to be involved in policy development and in the review of standard operating procedures. This can range from having simple policies and procedures to organizing routine surveillance programs. Regardless of the complexity of the program, protocols and procedures should be adjusted and tweaked to ensure that it is a good fit for the clinic and the personnel that need to follow these policies. If people do not support or understand the reasoning behind the protocols, they will not follow them, and the goals of the committee will therefore not be met.

The committee should complete a risk analysis of key areas of concern. The steps in the analysis include determining risk perception, hazard identification, risk management, and risk communication.

Risk perception would be the real or perceived risks for infectious or zoonotic disease. This may be based on what has historically caused problems in the hospital/clinic and community, on what has affected other hospitals, and on what the media and medical journals are portraying as potential risks. It is important to remember that all the potential risks that might occur cannot be predicted. However, by having a strong foundation in place, the magnitude of the outcomes of an outbreak can be significantly reduced.

Hazard identification involves identifying what infectious and zoonotic diseases are most likely to affect the hospital. There are some diseases that all hospitals/clinics should be concerned about such as salmonellosis, strangles, and equine herpes virus; however, large animal risks will vary by geographic location. Pathogens endemic to the area should be identified, measures to control and prevent them should be taken, and personnel should be educated about them. All exposures or outbreaks carry varying degrees of risk in regard to disease in animals and/or humans. This does not take into account lost revenue, decrease in client confidence, public image, and staff morale. The committee

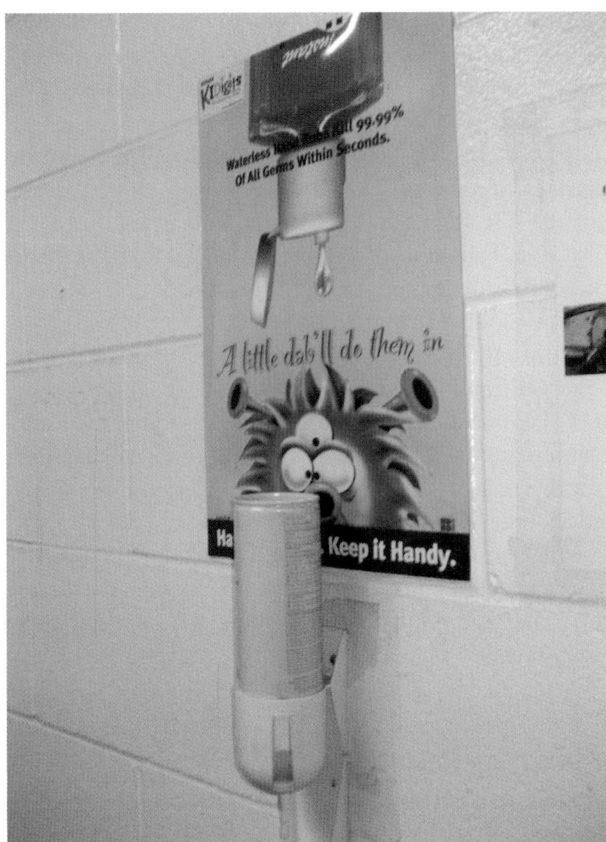

Figure 1.34 Signage should be strategically placed so that personnel are likely to read them.

must decide which diseases are the most detrimental to its patients, to its staff, and to the hospital.

> **TECHNICIAN TIP 1.15:** *Salmonella*, strangles, and equine herpes virus are diseases that all hospitals and clinics should be concerned about.

Risk management is the process of identifying, selecting, and implementing measures that can be applied to reduce the level of risk. Managing risks centers on enforcing or changing protocols or procedures to improve hospital IC. This includes looking at ways to improve hygiene (both hand and environmental), promote better barrier precautions, and implement better training and education for all staff and clients. Surveillance is an important piece of risk management and will be discussed later on in the chapter.

Risk communication is the final piece in risk analysis and involves ensuring that all personnel understand, support, and adopt the protocols and procedures developed to improve hospital IC. A training program that includes the reasons behind the protocols will help to persuade the staff that these measures are important and are a vital component of patient care.

Technicians are essential in the creation of the training program and in how it is presented to all staff. A training program will not be effective if staff cannot apply it directly to the work that they will be performing. Generally, veterinary technicians know the ins and outs of the clinic/hospital and are able to adapt the training and deliver it in a manner that staff can relate to (i.e. visual or hands-on-based training). Training should include basics, such as how to perform proper hand hygiene and environmental decontamination, but should be specific enough so that all staff executes all tasks in the same manner leaving no room for self-interpretation. Never assume that personnel know how to wash their hands or clean out a stall properly. Training needs to be documented and repeated annually.

> **TECHNICIAN TIP 1.16:** Veterinary technicians are essential in the creation of a training program and in how it is presented to all staff.

Once training is complete, posters and signs are easy ways to provide staff a constant reminder on how to complete tasks or to alert them to precautions that need to be taken. Signs should be simple and concise. They should

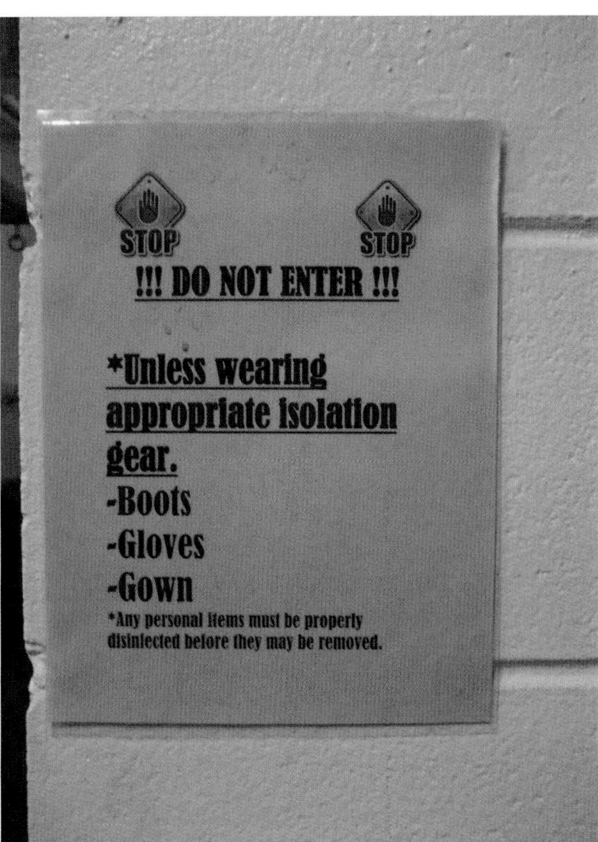

Figure 1.35 Signs should be simple and concise.

also be big enough and strategically placed so that personnel are likely to notice and read them.

Communication is essential. Keeping open lines of communication between all clinicians, technicians, and cleaning staff is one of the most important jobs of the IC technician. Being the central "go to" person is important so that ideas, comments, and complaints are not lost and can be pieced together and brought forward to the IC committee. If something is not working, then it needs to be changed. As long as the basics remain consistent, the program can be molded to meet the needs of the hospital.

Surveillance

Surveillance is an important part of any clinic's IC program and is a key responsibility of an IC technician. This may include monitoring of organisms, environmental hygiene, surgery site infection rates, and other factors deemed important by the IC team as necessary. Surveillance is either passive or active. Either type can be used alone or in combination dependent on the pathogen, program, and available money.

Passive Surveillance

Passive surveillance is the easier of the two types and is often adequate for most clinics/hospitals. Passive surveillance involves gathering, organizing, and analyzing data that is already present. To ensure that nosocomial events are not occurring within the patient population, the IC technician would gather culture reports on a routine basis and watch for common organisms or patterns. The frequency of reports should be determined, whether daily, weekly, or monthly, and followed consistently. If this is performed often and by one individual, then nosocomial events can be identified before an outbreak occurs. The gathering of all the culture data can also be analyzed to look for changes in disease patterns and to calculate infection rates of specific procedures, such as post-operative surgical site infections.

Active Surveillance

Active surveillance is more time-consuming and expensive than passive surveillance; however, it produces high-quality data that is extremely useful for larger clinics/hospitals. It also may be more beneficial in detecting potential events earlier. Active surveillance can involve collecting environmental samples or contacting owners to identify potential surgery site infections.

Obtaining environmental or patient samples can be very beneficial only if there are protocols in place that lay out exactly what is to be done if there is a positive sample result. If a positive environmental sample is found, the written protocols should determine what areas need to be deep cleaned, what further cultures need to be taken, if patients located in the area need to be sampled, and what needs to be communicated to hospital staff, clinicians, and possibly clients. If a positive patient sample is cultured, the next steps should be determined in regard to: the patients (move to isolation, put in mini-isolation, or enforce PPE); the environment (what type of cleaning needs to be completed); and other patients around the positive patient. Communication is again critical in this scenario to ensure that all personnel are aware of what was found, why contact precautions may or may not have changed, and what exactly needs to be communicated to clients or others outside of the clinic/hospital environment.

Whichever type of surveillance or combination the IC team decides to utilize, the IC technician is vital to identifying trends and notifying IC personnel (the hospital director, clinicians, staff, and cleaning crew) to unusual events.

Multidrug-Resistant Organisms, Methicillin-Resistant *Staphylococcus* sp., and Zoonotic Diseases

Multidrug-Resistant Organisms (MDRO)

Multidrug-resistant organisms (MDRO), methicillin-resistant *Staphylococcus aureus* (MRSA), zoonotic, and other infectious diseases that affect different regions are often motive for veterinary personnel to create IC programs. It is extremely important to become familiar with the organisms that are found in the local area.

One area of particular concern is MDROs. These are organisms resistant to three or more antibiotics. These organisms are important as they limit the antibiotics that can be given and often require more expensive ones or some other course of treatment.

Methicillin-Resistant *Staphylococcus aureus* (MRSA)

Staphylococcus sp. are gram-positive organisms that are considered normal flora and generally do not cause disease. Staph organisms can cause disease when the bacteria are found in abnormal locations and can precipitate tissue inflammation and pathogenic changes. These organisms can be multidrug resistant and/or methicillin resistant. MRS organisms are mediated by the production of an altered penicillin-binding protein (PBP), which confers resistance to all beta-lactam antimicrobials. Methicillin is an antibiotic drug of the penicillin family that was used as a marker for resistance to all beta-lactam antimicrobials and also Carbapenems. The drug companies have since phased out this drug, and oxacillin has taken the place as the new marker for this type of resistance. Methicillin-resistant staph species are usually not considered a zoonotic agent unless dealing with MRSA.

MRSA is a concern in human hospitals and recently has become important in veterinary medicine. As in humans, equine infections with MRSA can be subclinical (colonized), which can put other patients and hospital staff at risk. The most common site for colonization in equines is in the nasal passage. Colonization is transient in most adult horses, and MRSA colonization is eliminated in most horses within weeks (some longer than others and a small percentage have lifetime colonization), provided that measures are taken to prevent reinfection from other horses or people.

To treat or not to treat for colonization is dependent on a variety of factors, including traveling and housing situations. It is important to note that MRSA develops resistance rapidly, which may leave few treatment options for persistent or reinfected patients; therefore, antimicrobial treatment needs to be limited to those patients that are a key component in the method of transmission.

MRSA surveillance and protocols should be tailored to the degree of risk that is seen in that area. Regions that have a higher prevalence of MRSA tend to take a more active surveillance protocol. This may include a protocol in which all horses admitted are screened and swabbed for MRSA (via the nasal passage), then swabbed routinely during their hospitalization. If a positive MRSA isolate is cultured at arrival, then the MRSA infection is more likely to be community acquired (picked up outside of the hospital environment). If after being hospitalized for more than 72 hr, one can speculate this to be a hospital-acquired infection. A more passive approach to surveillance is often instituted in regions with a low occurrence of MRSA. At a minimum, all hospitals and clinics should ensure that all *S. aureus* pathogens are tested for oxacillin resistance.

Strict isolation precautions need to be enforced for all MRSA positive cases. Cleaning should occur as soon as the positive result is revealed, paying close attention to buckets, hay nets, and other objects/surfaces with which the nose of the horse or affected area had the most contact. It is possible that clinic personnel can become colonized or, if immunocompromised, can become ill. The decision to test human personnel for MRSA colonization is a decision to be made by the IC team. It is a key component in events where there is evidence that links human transmission with nosocomial events. Personnel that are colonized or have been diagnosed with an active MRSA infection should be seen by a physician to prevent transmission to other staff and patients.

Zoonotic Diseases

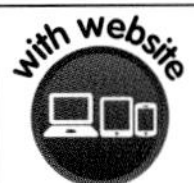

Check out a list of common zoonotic diseases.

Zoonotic diseases are diseases that are communicable from animals to humans. Acquiring an infectious pathogen is a risk that all personnel face daily as a result of working with sick animals. Immunocompromised personnel should not work with known zoonotic patients and should take extra precautions to ensure that they are keeping themselves safe and healthy. These individuals require additional PPE while working with patients and should consult with a human physician in regard to what these extra precautions may be. Hospital administration and the IC team have a responsibility to protect their employees. Vaccinations are also available to protect staff from specific diseases. Records of immunizations should be recorded and monitored to ensure that all personnel are current. Rabies and tetanus are two significant diseases that staff members should be protected against with vaccination regardless of the species that they are working with. Initial prophylactic rabies immunization should be administered before working with patients. A titer every two years thereafter is drawn to ensure that antibody levels in the blood are still adequate for protection. If levels fall below the required titer (less than 1 : 5 as determined via the rapid fluorescent foci inhibition test method), then a booster shot is recommended. A tetanus immunization should be administered and updated every 10 years. Influenza vaccinations are also important for those staff working with poultry and swine to protect their patients.

TECHNICIAN TIP 1.17: Staff members should be protected against rabies and tetanus regardless of the species that they are working with.

Transmissions of zoonotic diseases are preventable. Education and knowledge of zoonotic diseases that affect your local area is essential to the protection of staff and patients. Please see the "Diseases" chapter for specific disease information.

Many zoonotic diseases are reportable (i.e. rabies). Reportable diseases also include diseases that can have an effect on a large population of animals in the affected area (i.e. equine infectious anemia). A list of reportable diseases should be available and easily accessible to all hospital staff, and required reporting procedures should be included in the IC protocols. Contact your state department of health for more information on what diseases are reportable in your state.

Summary

The mission of the biosecurity (IC) team is to protect all staff, clients, and patients that enter the hospital/clinic. The chain of infection and ways to break this chain are important concepts that all hospital staff should be educated about and trained in. Leadership is a key component of a successful IC program. Veterinary technicians are evolving into this leadership role and are key to keeping the lines of communication open, to ensuring that protocols and procedures are being followed, and to looking for continual ways to improve and enhance biosecurity.

References

Bender, J. (2004). Horses and the risk of zoonotic infections. In: *Veterinary Clinics of North America: Equine Practice*, vol. 20 (Number 3) (eds. A. Turner, F. Bain and J. Weese). Philadelphia, PA: Elsevier Inc.

Caveney, L. and Jones, B. (eds.) (2012). *Veterinary Infection Prevention and Control*. Oxford, UK: John Wiley & Sons, Inc.

Greene, C. (ed.) (2006). *Infectious Diseases of the Dog and Cat*. St. Louis, MO: Elsevier Inc.

Ikram, M. and Hill, E. (1991). *Microbiology for Veterinary Technicians*. St. Louis, MO: American Veterinary Publications, Inc.

Linton, A.H., Hugo, W.B., and Russel, A.D. (1987). *Disinfection in Veterinary and Farm Practice*. Oxford, England: Blackwell Scientific Publications.

National Association of State Public Health Veterinarians (NASPHV) (2010). Compendium of veterinary standard precautions for zoonotic disease prevention in veterinary personnel. *JAVMA* 237 (12): 1403–1422.

Quinn, P.J. and Markey, B.K. (2001). Disinfection and Disease Prevention in Veterinary Medicine. In: *Disinfection, Sterilization and Preservation*Lippincott, 5e (ed. S.S. Block). Philadelphia: Williams and Wilkins.

Rutala, W. and Weber, D. (2007). An overview of disinfection and sterilization in health care facilities. In: *Disinfection, Sterilization and Antisepsis* (ed. W.A. Rutala). Washington, DC: Association for Professionals in Infection Control and Epidemiology.

Rutala, W., Weber, D., & Healthcare Infection Control Practices Advisory Committee (HICPAC). (2008). Guidelines for Disinfection and Sterilization in Healthcare Facilities, 2008. Atlanta, GA: Centers for Disease Control and Prevention. Retrieved from www.cdc.gov.

Santschi, E. (2006). Prevention of postoperative infections in horses. In: *Veterinary Clinics of North America: Equine Practice*, vol. 22 (Number 3) (ed. L. Southwood). Philadelphia, PA: Elsevier Inc.

Spickler, A. (2011) *Methicillin Resistant Staphylococcus aureus*. Retrieved from Iowa State University, Center for Food Security & Public Health Web site: http:// http:// www.cfsph.iastate.edu/DiseaseInfo/factsheets.php

Steneroden, K. (2005). *Stationary Veterinary Clinic Biological Risk Management*. Ames, IA: Center for Food Security and Public Health.

Traub-Dargatz, J., Dargatz, D., Morley, P., and Dunowska, M. (2004). An overview of infection control strategies for equine facilities, with an emphasis on veterinary hospitals. In: *Veterinary Clinics of North America: Equine Practice*, vol. 20 (Number 3) (eds. A. Turner, F. Bain and J. Weese), 507–520. Philadelphia, PA: Elsevier Inc.

Weber, D. and Rutala, W. (2007). Use of germicides in the home and healthcare setting: is there a relationship between germicide use and antibiotic resistance? In: *Disinfection, Sterilization and Antisepsis* (ed. W. Rutala), 248–271. Washington, DC: Association for Professionals in Infection Control and Epidemiology.

Weese, J. (2004). Barrier precautions, isolation protocols, and personal hygiene in veterinary hospitals. In: *Veterinary Clinics of North America: Equine Practice*, vol. 20 (Number 3) (eds. A.S. Turner, F.T. Bain and J.S. Weese), 543–559. Philadelphia, PA: Elsevier Inc.

Weese, J. (2004). Methicillin-resistant *Staphylococcus aureus* in horses and horse personnel. In: *Veterinary Clinics of North America: Equine Practice*, vol. 20 (Number 3) (eds. A.S. Turner, F.T. Bain and J.S. Weese), 601–613. Philadelphia, PA: Elsevier Inc.

Yang, J. (2013). *Virulence Factors of Pathogenic Bacteria*. Retrieved from www.mgc.ac.cn/VFs/main.htm

Clinical Case Resolution 1.1

Salmonella would be a suspect pathogen in this case; therefore, it would require isolation to prevent spreading to other patients and to the staff. The patient needs to be transported to a separate isolation stall. If one is not available, move the patient to a stall that is away from all other patients and follow the steps for mini-isolation; however, moving the patient into full isolation is the best option. During transport, be sure to disinfect the path the horse has taken to the new stall, as well as those of all members of the veterinary care team, including cleaning crew, staff working in the area, and clinicians of the other patients housed in the same area. The hospital IC team needs to be notified and needs to decide on what to tell the owners of the patients housed in the same area, if they are notified at all. The IC team should also determine if those patients need to have further monitoring (i.e. twice daily temperatures) to watch for any signs of possible *Salmonella* infection.

All areas that the infectious patient visited need to be thoroughly cleaned and disinfected. This includes any treatment areas as well as the hallways and the stall area. It is not a bad idea to block off the stall and/or the treatment area (if it was heavily used or soiled) until the fecal cultures have returned to normal. If there is a positive *Salmonella* result, environmental cultures should be taken (focusing on high touch surfaces, walls, and the floor) to ensure that the areas were cleaned properly and there is no apparent risk of contamination left when a new patient is admitted.

Activities

Multiple Choice Questions

(Answers can be found in the back of the book.)

1. Factors that account for how clinically ill a patient may become include:
- **A** immune status of the pathogen
- **B** route of transmission
- **C** virulence of the pathogen
- **D** portal of entry for transmission

2. What host factor will not affect disease prevention?
- **A** vaccinations
- **B** mode of transmission
- **C** malnutrition in the host
- **D** good antibiotic stewardship

3. Good antibiotic stewardship refers to which of the following:
- **A** Give antibiotics to mitigate infections before potential exposure.
- **B** Give the right antibiotics, at the right dose, at the right time, and for the right duration.
- **C** Antibiotics prescribed randomly during periods of potential exposure.
- **D** Give heavy dose antibiotics for extended periods of time.

4. Which of the following is not considered a portal of exit for pathogens?
- **A** gastrointestinal tract
- **B** urogenital tract
- **C** mucous membranes
- **D** central nervous system

5. Patients in the hospital should be separated according to which factor?
- **A** their risk level of spreading or acquiring infectious diseases
- **B** clinical symptoms that are present at the time of admission
- **C** species and breed specifications
- **D** color and size

6. Which of the following precautions should be used for hospitalizing a patient with equine herpesvirus type 1 (EHV-1)?
- **A** standard precautions
- **B** contact precautions
- **C** mini-isolation precautions
- **D** strict isolation precautions

7. What is the number one way to prevent transmission of disease?
   A antibiotic therapy
   B environmental decontamination
   C hand hygiene
   D elimination of fomites

8. In order for steam sterilization to be effective, the following conditions must be met:
   A type of chemical used and time
   B type of steam, pressure, temperature, and time
   C type of packaging items are wrapped in
   D gas concentration, relative humidity, and exposure time

9. In order to kill all pathogens, spores, and heat-resistant organisms, the steam inside of the autoclave must contain a relative humidity of:
   A 50–60%
   B 60–80%
   C 80–90%
   D 97–99%

10. Which of the following is not true of MRSA?
   A gram positive
   B normal flora
   C multidrug resistant
   D species specific

Test Your Learning

1. Describe three things that factor into a pathogen's success.
2. Describe what a dead-end host is and its effect.
3. Describe the three common routes of disease transmission.
4. Describe the difference between disinfection and sterilization.
5. List the key components of an infectious disease program.

Answers can be found in the back of the book.

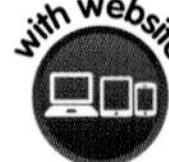

Extra review questions, case studies, and a breed ID image bank can be found online at www.wiley.com/go/loly/veterinary.

Chapter 2

Restraint

Ann Elizabeth Goplen, DVM, Sergio Gonzales, BS,
Sheryl Ferguson, CVT, VTS (LAIM),
Darcy DeCrescenza, CVT, Laura Lien, MS, CVT, VTS (LAIM), and
Sue Loly, LVT, VTS (EVN)

Learning Objectives

- Describe how to apply the concepts of flight zone, point of balance, and flocking instinct to animal-handling situations to reduce animal stress.
- Outline the basic methods of catching and restraining large animal species safely and effectively.
- Compare the major behavioral and physical differences in how large animals respond to handling and restraint.
- Create plans for working groups of animals or individuals that take into account the handler, the animal's condition and temperament, procedure being undertaken, and the working environment.

Clinical Case Problem 2.1 Hobby Farm Call

You are making a farm call to a small hobby farm that has 12 female sheep for ultrasound pregnancy checks and blood collection. They have no chute or race for handling the animals. What will you tell the owner to have set up and prepared for your visit and what is your plan for restraining the ewes?

See Clinical Case Resolution 2.1 at the end of this chapter.

Key Terms

Casting
Catch pen
Chemical restraint
Chute
Cow kick
Ear-ing
Flight zone
Flocking instinct
Front leg hopple (hobble)
Halter
Kush
Neck Twitch
Nose tongs
Point of balance
Setting up
Sheet bend
Shepherd's crook
Stanchion (See Chute)
Twitch

Large Animal Medicine for Veterinary Technicians, Second Edition. Edited by Sue Loly and Heather Hopkinson.

Companion website: www.wiley.com/go/loly/veterinary

Introduction

Large animal restraint requires considerable forethought; for some species, heavy-duty restraint devices are necessary as these animals are able to inflict serious trauma to humans, herd mates, and themselves. The veterinary team must be careful and routinely evaluate the facilities they are using either in hospital or during ambulatory calls. Use of restraint devices depends on species, breed, sex, age, and training of individuals or groups. Proper maintenance of facilities and equipment is essential to the welfare of all involved in procedures.

The goal in working with all large animal species is to gather, restrain, and handle animals safely and efficiently with minimal stress to animals and humans. The method chosen depends on several factors: animals, humans, facilities, and task at hand. It is always preferable to use the least possible amount of restraint to perform a procedure. If the safety of the animals or humans is in jeopardy, the procedure should be reevaluated and a different technique, additional assistance, or chemical restraint should be employed.

TECHNICIAN TIP 2.1: The least amount of restraint to perform a procedure is best.

Knots

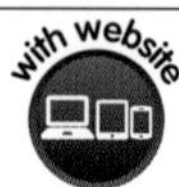

Check out how to tie knots step by step.

Knots are important to know when needing to restraint a patient. Basic knots and rope procedures that are included in the online resource that accompanies this book are:

- Bowline
- Square Knot
- Sheet Bend
- Clove Hitch
- Half Hitch
- Quick Release
- Temporary Horse Halter
- Tail Tie
- Cleat Hitch

Rope Care

Rope care in the veterinary field is important to ensure safety of all veterinary personnel and the patient. It is important to inspect ropes before use, looking for any deterioration due to age, chemicals, and misuse, which can lead to decreased rope strength. Measures should be taken to protect the rope and should include practices such as protecting the ends from unraveling and storing the rope in a coiled position. There are different techniques to coiling a rope, but the end result is the same, namely a rope that is kink-free, knot-free, and twist-free. Ideally, ropes should be stored off the ground to keep them clean and avoid twists and kinks if grabbed in a hurry. Ropes should be washed by hand in cold water with a mild soap. After soap is rinsed off, the rope should be hung to air-dry; a dryer should not be used. Direct sunlight and excessive heat can deteriorate fibers and should be avoided. Using chemicals to clean is not advised. How long a rope lasts can vary depending on its care.

Basic Behavior of Large Animals

Prey animals will naturally move away from perceived threats. The amount of space the animal allows between the threat and itself before the animal moves is called the flight zone. If the threat is outside the flight zone, the animal will turn and look. Once the flight zone is penetrated, the animal will move away. The flight zone will vary in size depending on species, presence of offspring, space confinement size, individual temperament, and threat level.

TECHNICIAN TIP 2.2: To keep the animals calmest, stay just on the edge of the flight zone without entering too deeply or quickly.

The point of balance is situated at the level of the animal's shoulder. If the handler is in front of the point of balance, the animal moves backward. If the handler is behind that point, the animal moves forward. The concepts of flight zone and point of balance are used to move and handle these species. Ruminants, in particular, will readily follow one another but will refuse to move forward if they see people, shadows, sharp corners, darkness, or a dead end in front of them.

Sheep, goats, and camelids all have strong flocking instincts (Figure 2.1). When possible, they should be moved as an entire group. Watch for the animal that lags behind or cannot keep up; these often warrant further evaluation for ailments (lameness, respiratory disease) that become apparent upon examination. Sheep tend to have the strongest flocking instinct, naturally clumping together when threatened. This can cause problems with pileups in corners and against walls, leading to crushed individuals or breakouts. Separated sheep will make heroic attempts to rejoin the main group. Goats tend to spread out more when grazing and when threatened may scatter and run every which way. Most goat herds are not accustomed to being worked by a stock dog, whereas sheep rapidly become

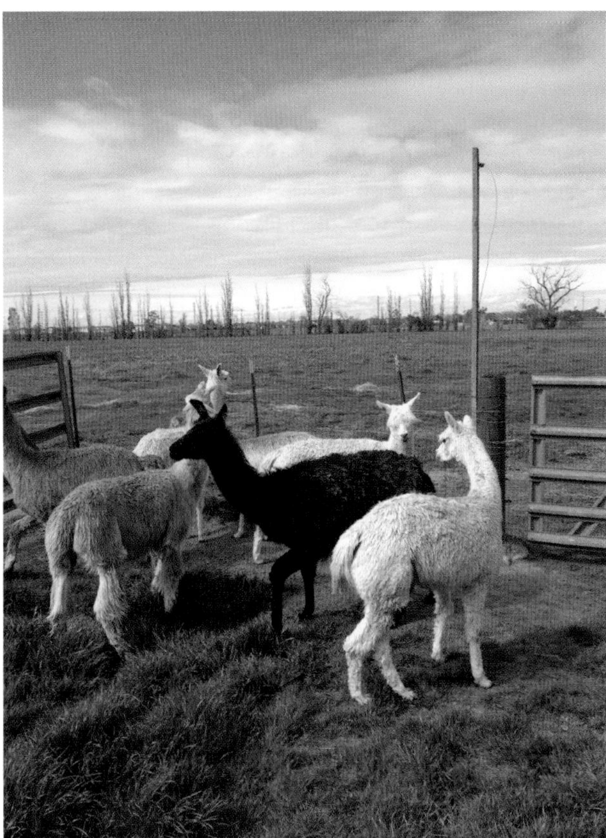

Figure 2.1 Sheep, goats, and camelids have strong flocking instincts. *Source:* Courtesy of Scott R.R. Haskell, DVM, MPVM, PhD.

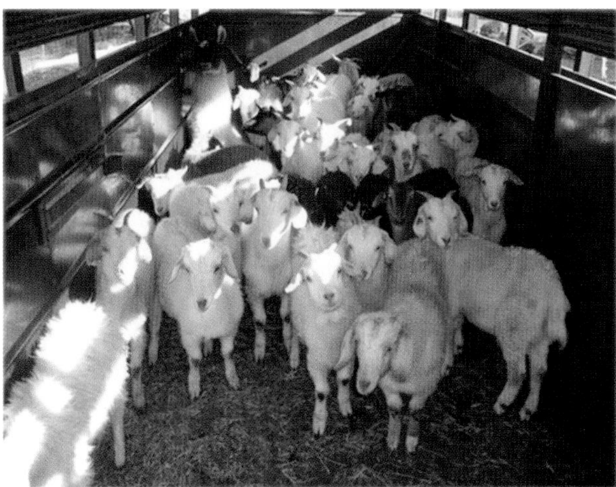

Figure 2.2 A guard llama is transported along with its flock. *Source:* Courtesy of Scott R.R. Haskell, DVM, MPVM, PhD.

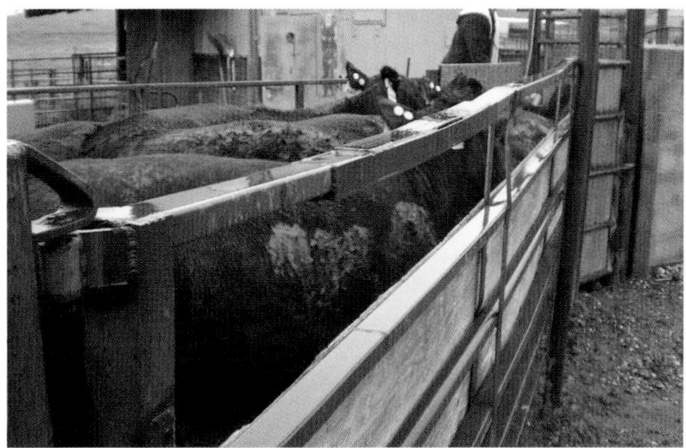

Figure 2.3 A funnel system that narrows cattle down into a single lane. *Source:* Courtesy of Scott R.R. Haskell, DVM, MPVM, PhD.

acclimated to their use. Herding dogs are generally not used with alpacas and llamas as it is too stressful for the latter. Livestock guard dogs that live with the flock or herd may not be socialized to humans and should not be approached or handled without first consulting with the herder or flock owner.

Bovids, sheep, and alpacas tend to retreat and watch when strangers enter their spaces, whereas goats and llamas exhibit more curiosity, approaching and investigating the newcomer. This behavior makes llamas effective guard animals for herds and flocks of sheep, goats, or alpacas. Rams and bucks can be extremely aggressive during breeding season. It is wisest not to turn your back on any intact males and know where they are while you are in their space (Figure 2.2).

All small ruminants and camelids stay calmer with a companion. If an animal is to be transported or moved to a sick pen, a calm companion should be brought along. If it cannot be housed with the animal, such a companion should in an adjacent pen. Goats form very strong friendship bonds and may need their special buddy with them.

Low-stress handling and restraint start with planning and good facilities. Facilities should be well lit, clean, dry, and in good repair. Animals should be trained to the handling process. Ruminants and camelids do well in a system that funnels them down into a narrow single-file lane (race or chute) or small catch pens (Figures 2.3 and 2.4). A small catch pen makes it easier to catch an individual animal. Handling equipment can be placed at the end of the race or lane (tilt table, tipping cradle, ultrasound crate, etc.). Some treatments like vaccination or deworming can be done while the animals stand single file in the race, with no additional handling. Dairy animals familiar with a stanchion or the milking parlor will often come voluntarily into these areas.

Ruminants and camelids are intelligent animals with good memories. They have a good memory for both humans and their own herd mates. They are good at remembering and associating negative experiences with places and peoples. Individual llamas can develop a dislike for an individual person offering a less-than-welcoming spit on subsequent visits. Their strong flocking and flight

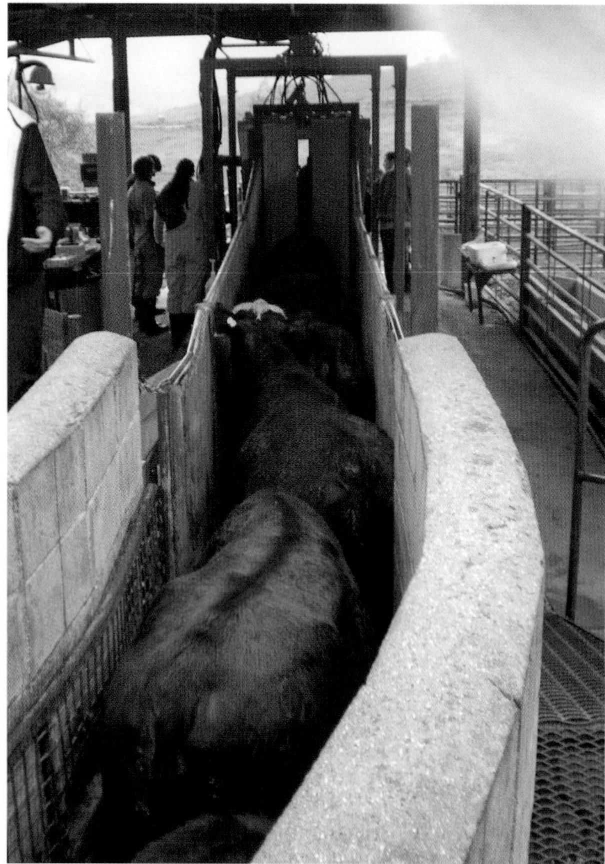

Figure 2.4 A single-file lane is known as a race or chute. *Source:* Courtesy of Scott R.R. Haskell, DVM, MPVM, PhD.

instincts often make their behaviors seem irrational. Negative experiences should not occur in places where routine herd work or milking is done. Goats often respond to the call of their caregiver; some will respond to their own name. They all can learn the sound of food in the bucket or feeder. All of these species can be taught to lead on a halter.

Understanding equine, ruminant, and camelid psychology and using their behavioral instincts rather than overpowering them with brute strength will lead to lower stress and easier handling. Good handling is more a matter of knowing "how to do it" and finesse rather than overpowering the animal. Human handlers need to be calm, confident, and patient. You cannot hurry or force these animals, as it leads to frustration and increased stress for both animals and handlers.

Equine Restraint

Equine behavior is similar to that of other livestock, yet it is important to consider equine-specific behaviors and handling techniques. It is imperative to know the general characteristics of horses and equine behavior. The greatest tool we have in keeping ourselves safe while working on horses is our brains. It is important to assess every situation logically, even in high-speed, high-stress situations, to make sure we are providing the utmost safety to coworkers, owners, patients, and ourselves. Watching a horse's expression can be a great tool in assessing the safest place to stand, how to get them to travel, and how to encourage the desired response. Like other livestock, horses are flight animals and have evolved into ideal creatures for escaping scary and uncomfortable situations. The veterinary visit is often just that. As in other species, it is important to achieve the desired effect from the patient using the least amount of restraint and creating as little patient stress as possible. Horses are strong, large animals with the capability of becoming very dangerous in situations they deem frightening. Utmost care and consideration must be given to understanding the horse's natural responses to these types of situations.

Halter

Halters and lead ropes are perhaps the best-known and effective way to handle a horse effectively in the veterinary setting. Halters and lead ropes generally provide you with the ability to control the direction of a horse's head and momentum. Horses are strong and most certainly can overpower even the strongest, most experienced handlers.

Adding a chain (often referred to as a lead shank) to the halter provides even greater control of a horse's head. Chains can be placed through the ring of one side of the halter and clipped to either the opposite most rostral cheek ring or run through the opposite rostral cheek ring and diagonally to the caudal cheek ring, creating a larger, more sensitive area of pressure. Chains placed over a horse's nose create pressure when a horse tries to move forward, as well as help keep their heads down when necessary. Chains should be used with quick "pull and release" pressure, and all pressure on the horse should be removed as a reward when they do what is asked. Chains have also been used under a horse's chin, which causes them to lift their head and must be used carefully as they can cause a horse to rear up. Chains can also be placed through a horse's mouth or on their top lip, but great caution must be used as there is a high potential to cause injury to the horse's lips, gums, or tongue. It is also important to always allow enough room between yourself and the horse's head to ensure enough time to escape if the horse becomes fractious. The lead should be held approximately 10–12 in from the halter to allow ample space. Always make sure the rope is not wrapped around your fingers or hand, or any other part of the body (Figures 2.5–2.8).

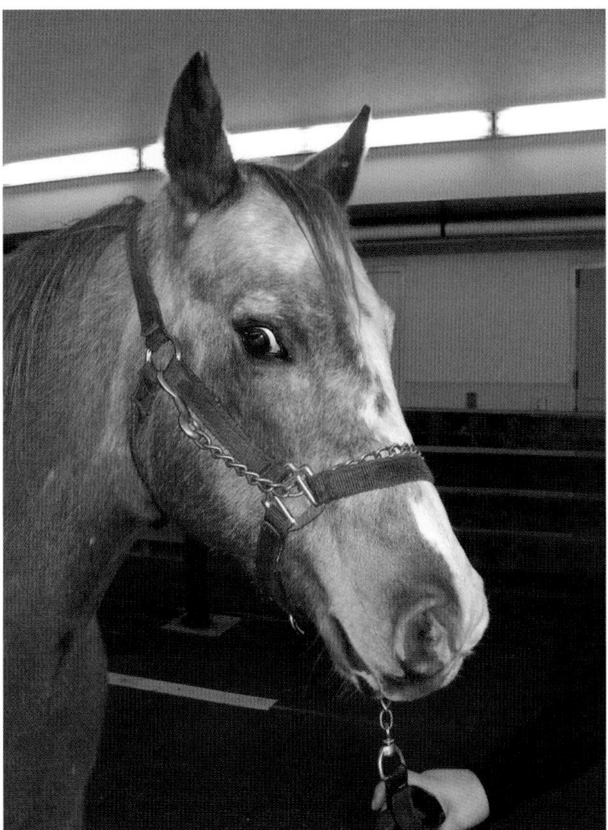

Figure 2.5 Chain placement over a horse's nose using the rostral cheek ring.

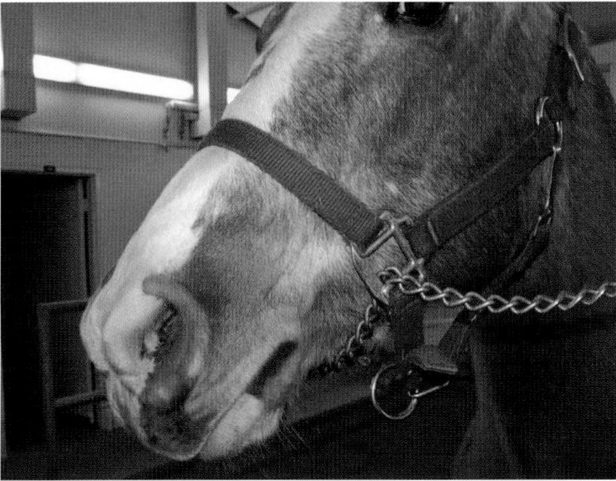

Figure 2.6 Chain placement under the horse's chin.

TECHNICIAN TIP 2.3: A chain placed under the horse's chin may cause it to rear up.

TECHNICIAN TIP 2.4: It is dangerous to allow a lead rope to wrap around your fingers, hands, or other parts of the body.

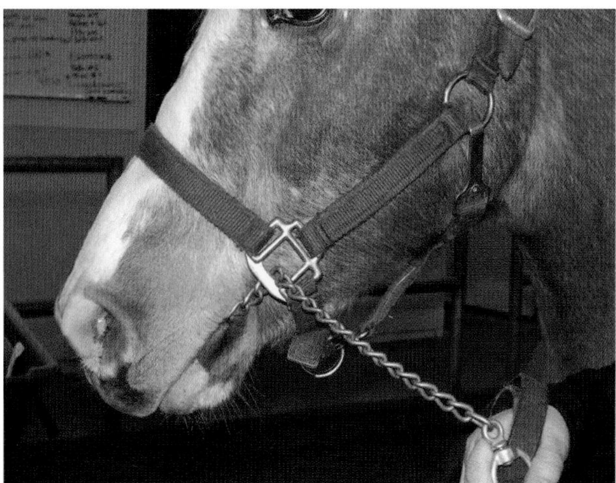

Figure 2.7 Chain placement through a horse's mouth.

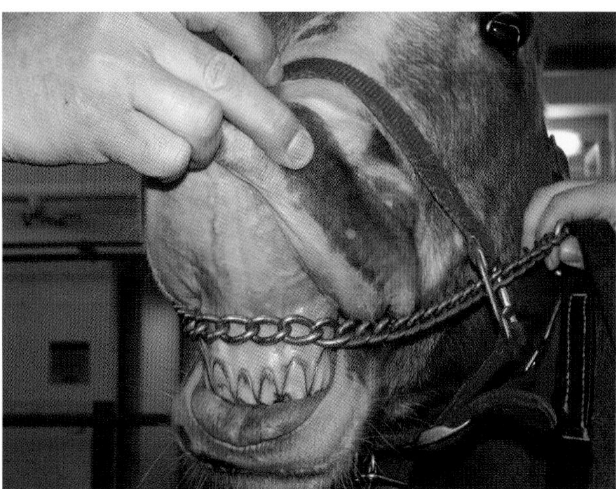

Figure 2.8 Lip chain placement.

When handling a horse, you should not stand directly in front of or behind it. Unlike cows, horses kick directly back rather than to the side. When working around the hind end of a horse, the safest place to be is close to them. When leading or holding a horse, it is generally accepted that horses should be handled primarily from the left side, although veterinary medicine can create challenges with this theory, as doctors often have to address issues on the right side of the horse as well. Handling horses from the same side as the veterinarian or staff member who is working is necessary to create the ability to move the horse's hindquarters away from the human if it kicks or becomes fractious. A great deal of care should be taken to switch sides as the veterinarian or staff member does (Figures 2.9 and 2.10).

TECHNICIAN TIP 2.5: Horses kick directly back, and one should never stand directly behind them when working on them.

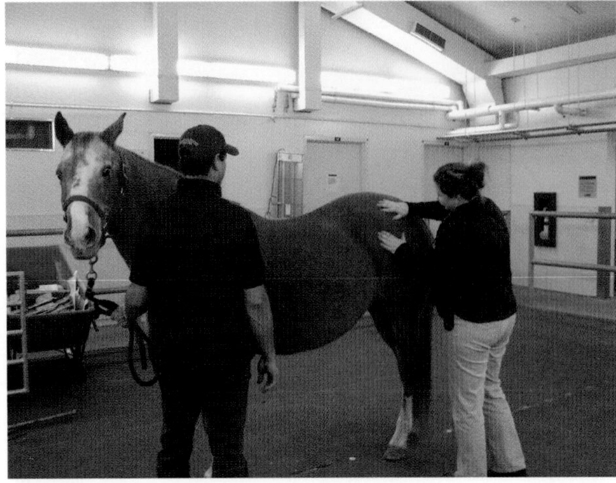

Figure 2.9 The restrainer should always stand on the same side as the person performing a procedure.

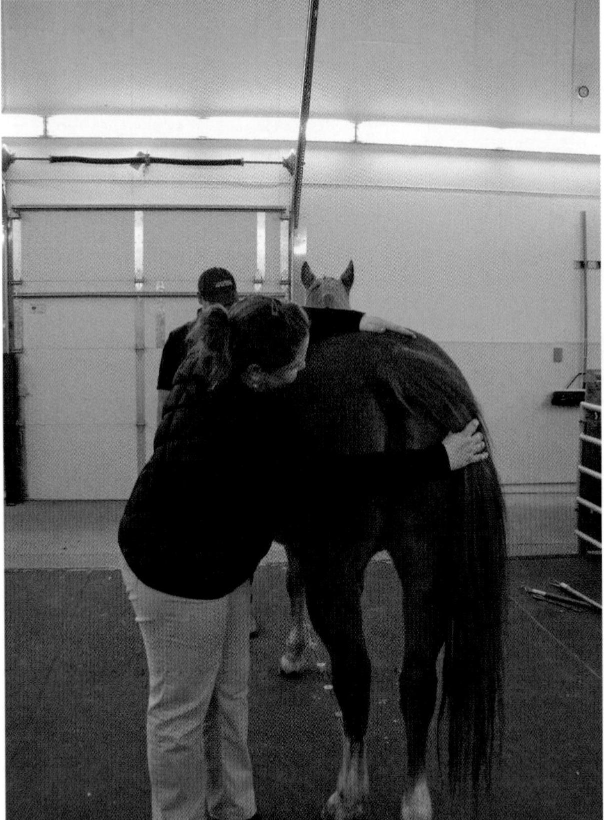

Figure 2.10 When inspecting a horse, care should be taken to never stand directly behind them to avoid being kicked.

Twitch

Twitches are a device that can be applied to the horse's nose to provide restraint. Several models are available. One type of a twitch is called a humane twitch and is made of bent metal, similar in action to a nutcracker. Opening the hinge and placing the horse's upper lip within the pliers-like grip applies the necessary pressure to keep the twitch in place. Two other types of twitches consist of a stick with rope or a chain at the end, which are twisted around the nose, providing an endorphin release for the horse. Twitches place the patient into a relaxed state, allowing for ample time to complete short tasks such as nasogastric tubing or injections. Twitches are only effective for 10–15 min; if they are removed before the effects wear off, horses are often left with a "high" feeling and so they rarely build an aversion to the twitch when used properly (Figures 2.11–2.14).

Neck Twitch

Neck twitches are an effective manner to distract the horse from an event for a short time. Grabbing a handful of skin at the junction of the neck and shoulder of a horse and pulling firmly applies the neck twitch. A neck twitch generally causes the horse to bend away from the twitch and causes a paralytic effect on the horse for a short time (Figure 2.15). As with any type of touch, horses can respond either in a positive, calm way or they can "blow up," resulting in handling becoming even more difficult. It is

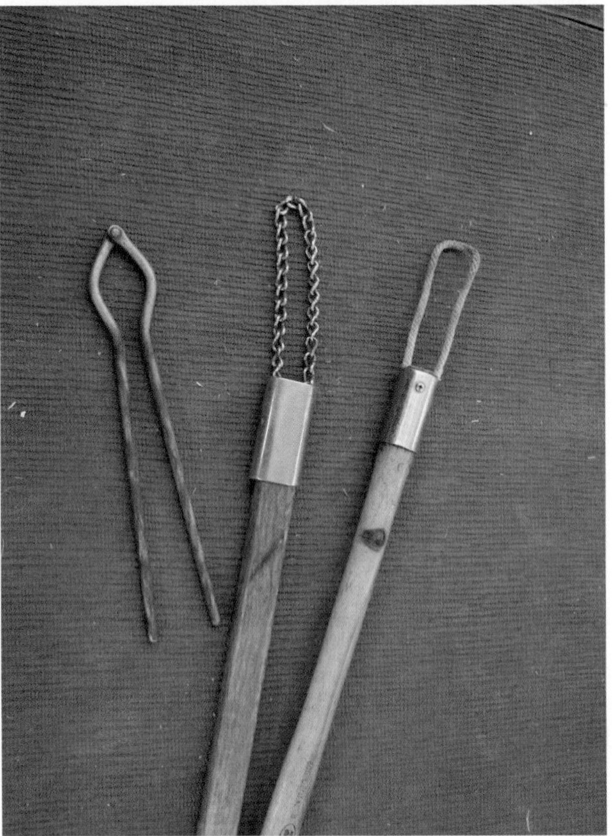

Figure 2.11 Three different types of twitches from left to right; humane, chain, and rope.

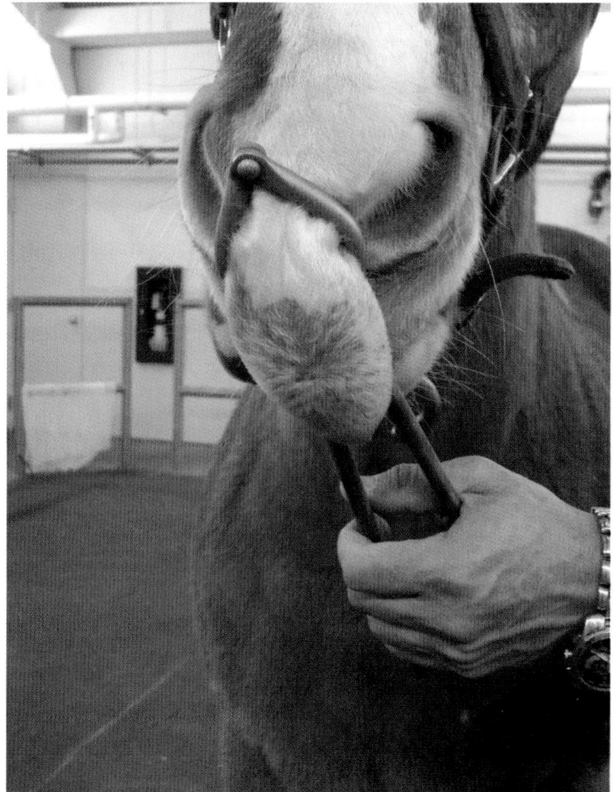

Figure 2.12 A properly applied humane twitch.

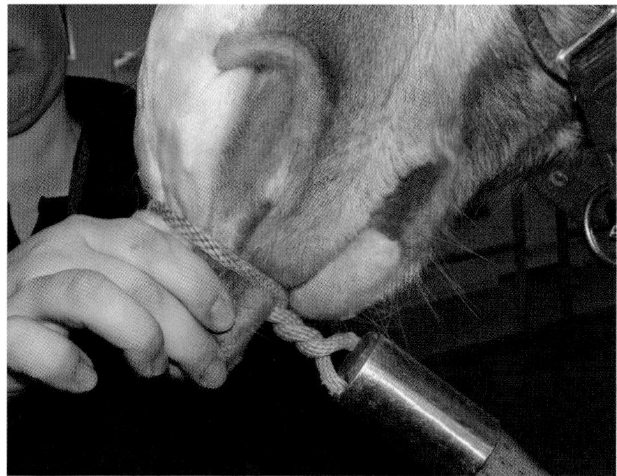

Figure 2.13 A properly applied rope twitch.

important to read a horse's body language and make note in the patient's file if they are known to react negatively to specific restraint methods.

> **TECHNICIAN TIP 2.6:** If a horse reacts negatively to restraint, make sure to note in medical records for future reference.

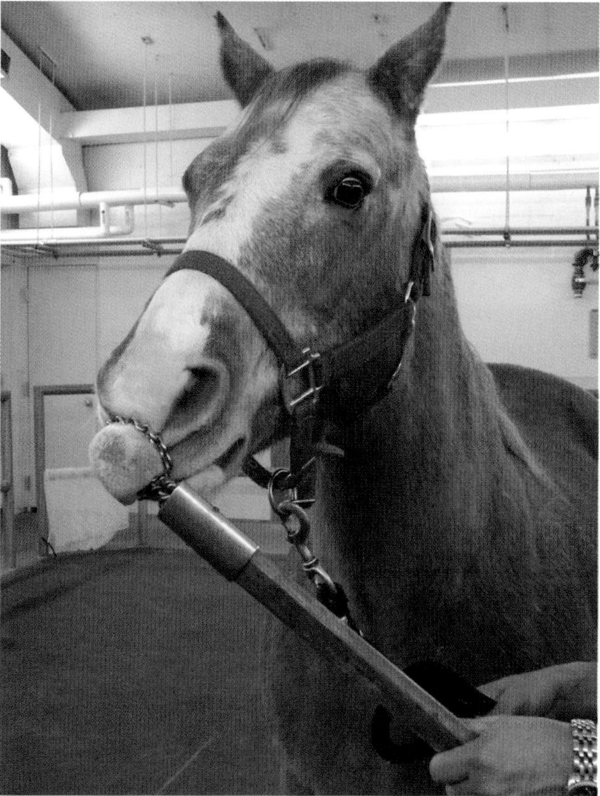

Figure 2.14 A properly applied chain twitch.

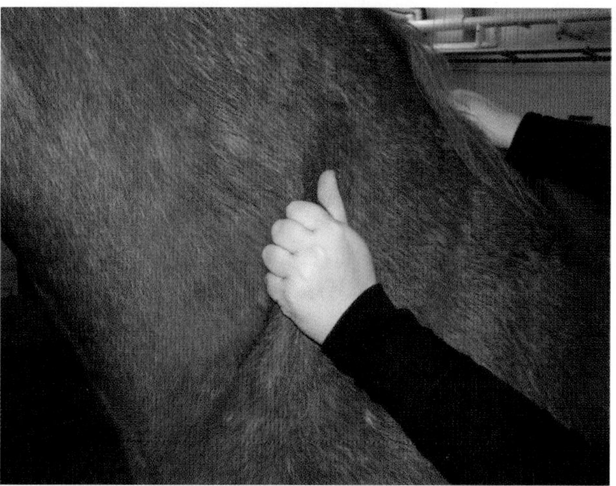

Figure 2.15 A neck twitch.

Stocks/Chutes

Stocks and chutes are also a useful tool in veterinary practice. For especially fractious or dangerous horses, stocks are a great restraint tool. Many styles of stocks have adjustable side bar height and, in some, length. Bars should be adjusted to a height that approximately matches the horse's point of shoulder height. Safety precautions should be taken to ensure safety to both veterinary staff and the horse. It is recommended that two people be used whenever loading a horse into the stocks. Only halter-broken horses should be led into stocks. If horses are not halter-broken, a chute may be more appropriate.

Before entering the stocks with the horse, ensure they are wide open on both the entrance and exit. This will keep the veterinary staff from becoming crushed against the front bar or door in the event the horse panics and rushes forward. It is highly recommended to remove blankets as they may be caught or "hung up" as the horse enters the stocks.

Horses often move backward in the stocks when the front gate is closed in front of them. This can endanger any person who is standing at the rear of the stocks. The correct steps for loading a horse are as follows (Figures 2.16–2.20):

1) The horse handler walks through the stocks with the front and rear gates wide open.
2) The horse handler stops just before the front gate.
3) The person standing at the rear of the stocks closes and secures the rear gate, never standing directly behind but off to either side. This will keep them safe in case the horse decides to bolt backward or kick.
4) Once the rear gate is secured, the person handling the horse should secure the front gate so it is closed between themselves and the horse.

A horse should never be left unattended when in the stocks or have its halter tied to the stocks. The horse handler should always be alert as a horse can still try to rear over the top and, in some instances, may even try to get under the bars. Horses can also collapse while in stocks, so

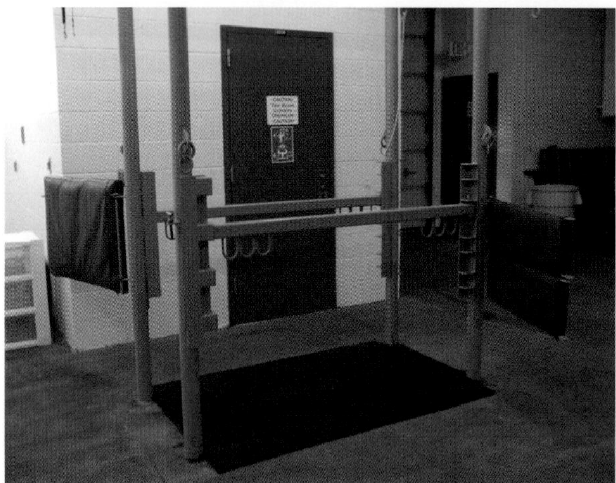

Figure 2.16 Horse stocks with both front and rear gates wide open and ready for a horse to enter.

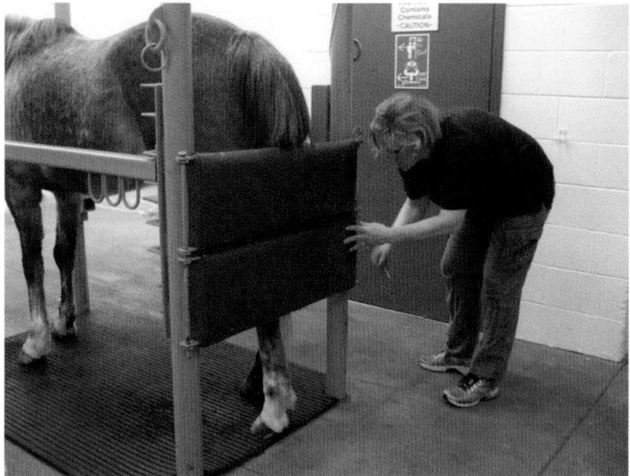

Figure 2.18 The person at the rear gate closes the rear gate while not standing directly behind.

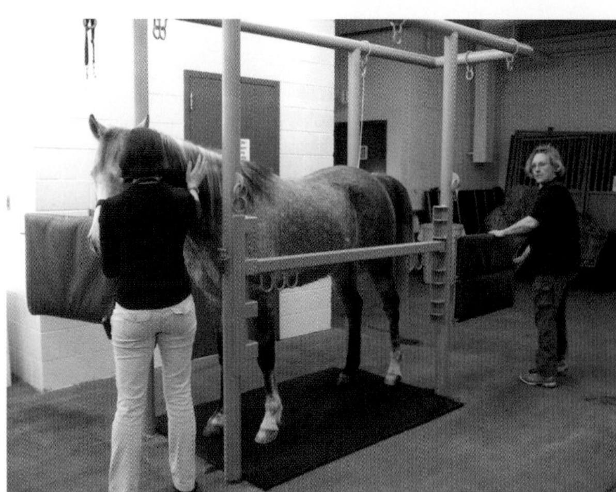

Figure 2.17 The horse handler enters the stocks with the horse and stops just short of the front gate.

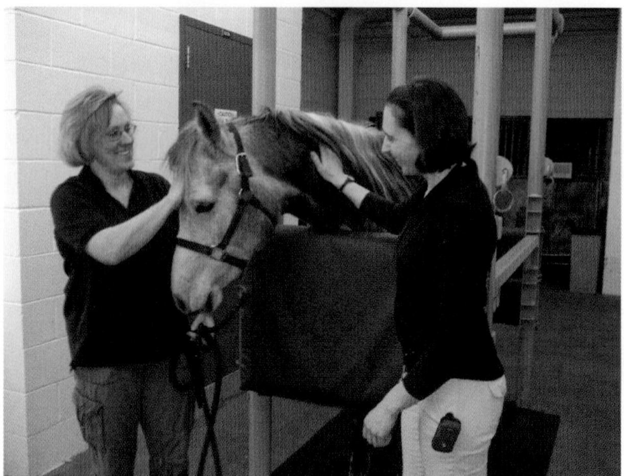

Figure 2.19 The person in the front closes the front gate after the rear gate is closed and secure.

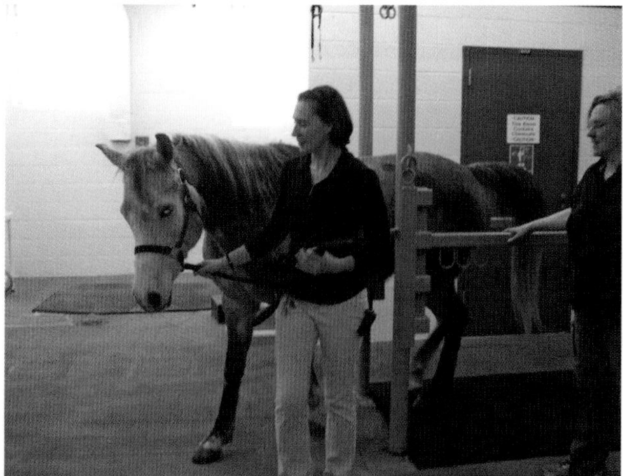

Figure 2.20 The front gate is open, and horse is led out of the stocks.

additional help should be within hearing distance in case assistance is needed in an emergency.

A chute is much different from stocks in that horses are usually not halter-broken and are generally driven forward into a chute through a serious of gates, creating both distance and safety for the handler. It is important to note that horses are still often able to kick or bite through the bars of a chute. Veterinarians and staff need to be aware of chute openings and slats at all times. Chutes provide the ability to keep the horse in a small area and keep it from moving forward, backward, or laterally. While the horse can still move to some extent, it is generally contained enough to administer some type of chemical restraint.

TECHNICIAN TIP 2.7: Horses are still often able to kick or bite through the bars of a chute.

Foals

Restraining foals requires care and consideration for the foal's size and age. Foals often are not halter-broken and generally do not lead. Foals less than two weeks of age can be "folded" into a lying-down position by placing one hand on their muzzle, another hand on their tail, and bending them by moving their muzzle and tail together. This creates a response in the foal that causes them to relax and go limp so they can be gently placed or slid into lateral recumbency. By placing a towel over the foal's eyes and keeping environmental stimulation to a minimum is often effective for keeping them calm while in this position. For foals that are older than two weeks of age, and for procedures that require the patient to be standing, placing an arm under the foal's chin and tail and jacking them often works to restrain them. Extra-large horse halters can be placed upside down over their heads, with the nose band at the thoracic inlet. This can give the handler an additional "handle" to move a foal a short distance. Miniature or small foals can be picked up and carried but always hold in front of the chest and behind the rear. DO NOT pick up foals under the abdomen as this can lead to a ruptured bladder (Figures 2.21–2.25).

Keeping the mare's disposition in mind is necessary when working on foals. Reading a mare's body language is important; some mares could not care less when you are handling their baby, whereas others become nervous and agitated. Some mares prefer to stand over their baby while personnel work on them; other mares are so aggressive they must be sedated, segregated, or tied while working with their foal. Never put yourself between the mare and the foal. Learning to interpret subtle gestures from the

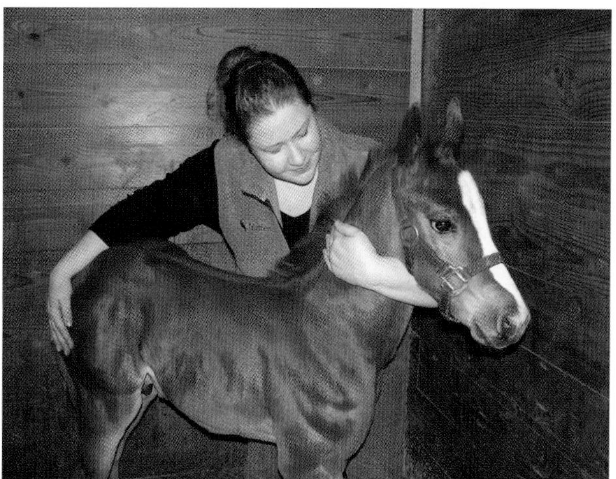

Figure 2.21 A foal with minimal restraint performed with the front arm wrapped under the foal's chin and the rear arm wrapped around the back.

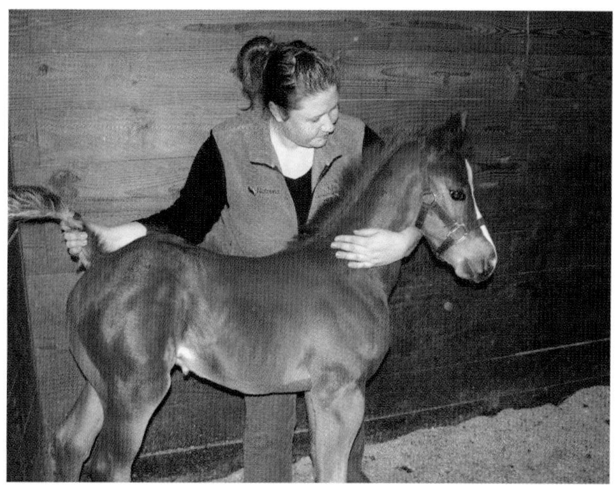

Figure 2.22 A tail jack placed on a foal.

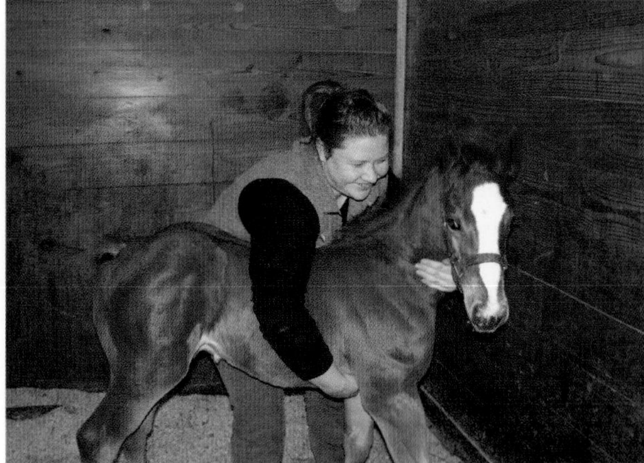

Figure 2.23 Foals often resist arms placed around their girth area.

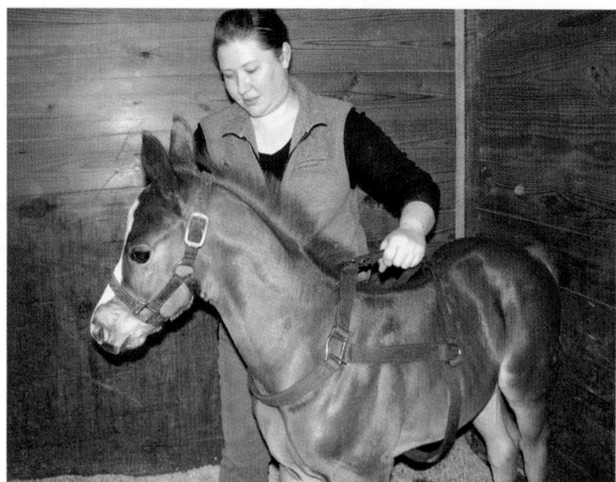

Figure 2.24 An upside-down horse halter used on a foal for a harness type of restraint.

mare is essential to providing a safe environment for those working on the foal.

Stallions

Stallions require increased caution during handling. Stallion behavior can often be unpredictable and erratic, especially during breeding season. Keeping stallions separate from mares and other stallions can reduce their stress and anxiety levels compared to when they are housed in general population. Stallions should be handled with a lead shank, and the handler should always be prepared for unpredictable actions from the stallion. Vocalizing, prancing, biting, and striking are commonplace with stallions. Handlers should be alert to these behaviors and expect them at all times, even with a seemingly harmless stallion.

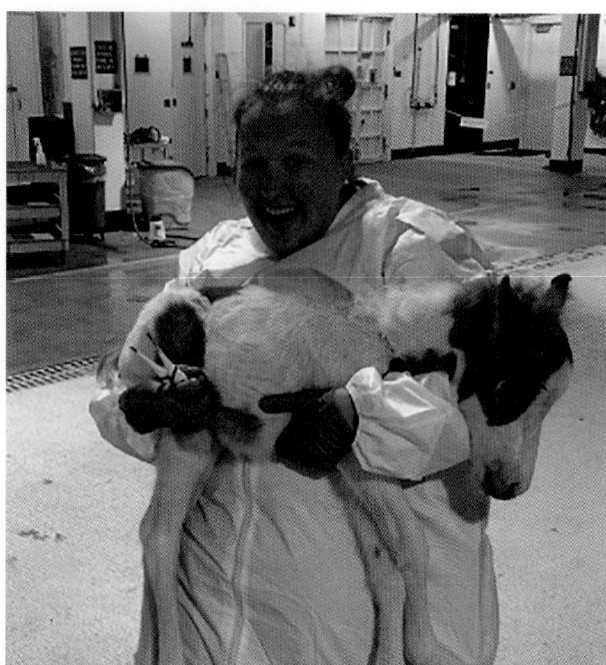

Figure 2.25 The proper restraint for miniature or small foals.

> **TECHNICIAN TIP 2.8:** During breeding season, a stallion's behavior is often unpredictable.

Chemical Restraint

Chemical restraint can be achieved with various drugs, with many different outcomes. Chemical restraint can provide a range of reactions from slowing a horse down (acepromazine maleate) to head-hanging sedation (xylazine, detomidine) or full injectable anesthesia (xylazine and ketamine). Depending on the procedure and duration of procedure, the veterinarian can decide which drugs or combination of drugs can produce the desired effect. For example, castrations are often performed with a combination of xylazine and ketamine to produce lateral recumbency and complete disassociation (Figure 2.26).

> **TECHNICIAN TIP 2.9:** The veterinarian will decide on the type of chemical restraint depending on the procedure, the duration of the procedure, and the desired effect.

Xylazine

Xylazine is an Alpha 2 – adrenergic agonist used for its sedative and analgesic effects in horses. Xylazine can cause central nervous system depression in horses and produces adequate visceral analgesia. Sedation signs in horses include lowering of the head, relaxed facial muscles,

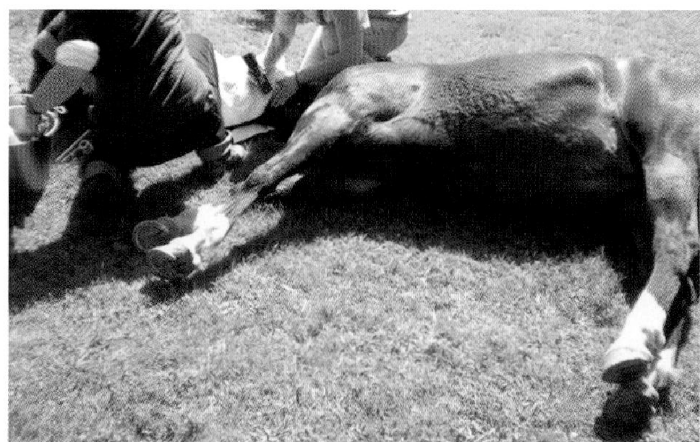

Figure 2.26 A horse that is anesthetized with a combination of drugs that place it in lateral recumbency. *Source:* Courtesy of Scott R.R. Haskell, DVM, MPVM, PhD.

drooping of the lower lip, and a relaxed retractor muscle in male horses. Horses have been known to kick (xylazine aggression) or become aggressive, so caution should be used. Xylazine has a wide variety of dosages for intramuscular and intravenous routes, as well as for desired effect (sedation vs. field anesthesia). Doses vary from 0.2 to 2.2 mg/kg. The reversal for xylazine is yohimbine.

TECHNICIAN TIP 2.10: Horses have been known to kick while on xylazine.

Detomidine

Detomidine HCl is another analgesic that is primarily used on horses. Similar to xylazine, detomidine is an Alpha 2 adrenergic antagonist that produces dose-dependent sedation, but it also has respiratory and cardiac effects. Appropriate caution should be used with detomidine, because, as with xylazine, horses have been known to kick out spontaneously. Doses of 0.2–0.4 mg/kg are generally used. Higher doses of sedation have been noted to last for 120 min, with analgesia working for up to 75 min. The reversal for detomidine is atipamezole.

Acepromazine

Other drugs such as acepromazine maleate are known to "aid in controlling fractious animals" and have a wide dose range varying from 0.01 to 0.05 mg/kg. Onset of action is between 15 and 30 min depending on IV or IM route, respectively. Combinations of drugs can also be used to achieve different levels of sedation and analgesia.

Chemical restraint is the most efficient, practical, and affordable means of completing procedures in modern veterinary medicine (Figure 2.27). Veterinarians have a variety of options to create the desired effect. As with all restraint, the key factor is to use the minimum chemical

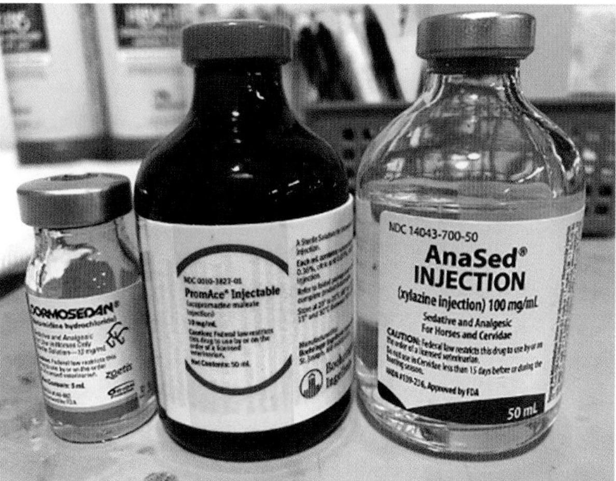

Figure 2.27 Sedation drugs (detomidine, acepromazine, xylazine).

restraint necessary to achieve a low-stress, appropriate environment for the horse.

Bovine Restraint

Although beef and dairy cattle are both bovine species, their temperament and personality are quite different. Dairy cattle tend to be more docile as they are used to being handled, whereas beef cattle are raised on pasture and have minimal handling. Different breeds can also vary in regard to the amount of restraint needed. The size of cattle brings a higher level of safety concerns. Their heavy weight and size can easily crush a body of the handler, and they can butt with their large heads. Veterinary technicians should always take great care to not place themselves between the animal and an object to prevent crushing. The presence of horns should bring extra precaution. It is important to note that although cattle do not usually kick with their front legs, they can step on toes, bruising or breaking the handler's foot. Cattle can and will kick with their hind feet. They more commonly kick sideways, or "cow kick," but have also been known to kick straight back. As with small ruminant and camelids, the presence of herd buddies and keeping noise levels down can be helpful in keeping them calm.

TECHNICIAN TIP 2.11: Use extra caution when working on bovines with horns.

Halter

The halter is the basic tool for restraining cattle. Cattle can be halter trained but it is often difficult to teach them to lead. Proper placement of the halter is important. Correct

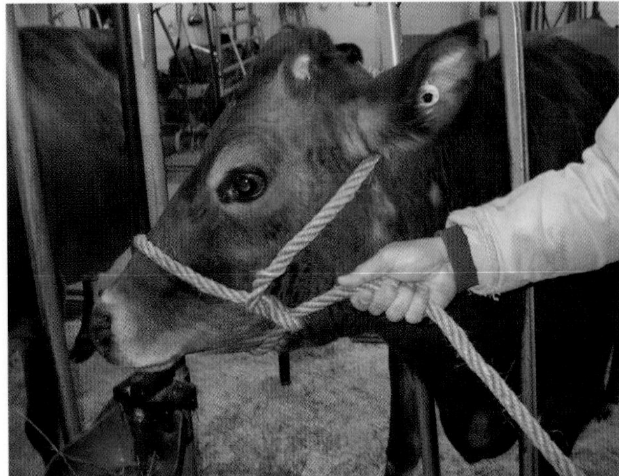

Figure 2.28 A properly placed cow halter with the rope tightening under the chin.

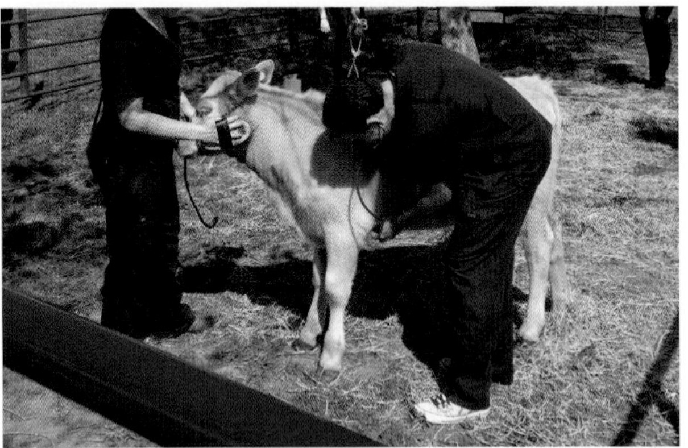

Figure 2.29 Using minimal restraint on a calf that is having a PE performed. *Source:* Courtesy of Scott R.R. Haskell, DVM, MPVM, PhD.

placement has the halter tightening under the chin rather than having it tighten over the nose or behind the ear. In the chute or stanchion, the halter should be tied to something secure like a post or the side of the stanchion. A quick release knot should always be used. If trying to lead, steady pressure works better than jerky movements do (Figures 2.28 and 2.29).

> **TECHNICIAN TIP 2.12:** Correct placement of the halter on bovids has the halter tightening under the chin rather than having it tighten over the nose or behind the ear.

Nose Tongs

Cattle have a sensitive nasal septum. Pinching this nasal septum can be an effective way to help them remain still.

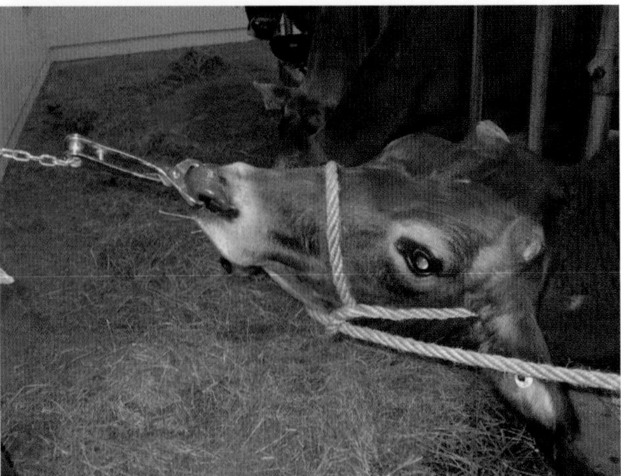

Figure 2.30 Nose tongs placed on a cow.

Your thumb and pointer finger may be used to do this, but it can still be difficult to hold the cattle still, and is usually effective for short periods only. A more effective way is to use a commercially made nose tong. The tongs clamp the nasal septum and are held in place by keeping the rope taught by use of an assistant or by tying to a secure object using a quick release knot. Use of a nose tong alone may tear the nasal septum if the cow thrashes violently. Use of a halter by tying the cattle's head in place is helpful to avoid excessive movement, thus helping avoid any tears. Placement of the nose tongs often takes quick movement. With the patient in the head catch, approach the patient from the side. The tongs should be in the open position. Sufficiently restrain the head, then place first one side then the other into the nares and squeeze the tongs together. Tongs should never be left in place on an animal that is unattended and should never be used in procedures that are significantly painful; those procedures should be performed under anesthesia (Figure 2.30).

> **TECHNICIAN TIP 2.13:** Because bovids have a sensitive nasal septum, it can be an effective way to help them remain still.

Tail Restraint/Tail Jack

Like the nose tongs, tail restraint should only be used in procedures that are not significantly painful. First, restrain the cattle's head either with a halter or by placing it in a chute or stanchion. The tail jack is applied by the handler grabbing the tail close to the base and lifting up, toward the back, while applying steady pressure (Figure 2.31). Lifting the tail too high and other than by the base may result in breaking the tail. The handler should be standing behind,

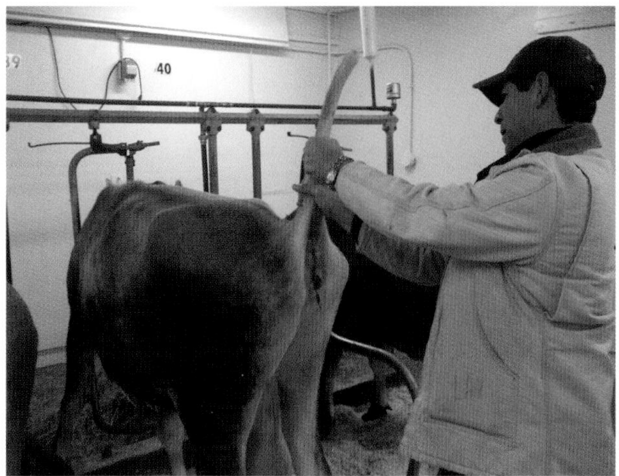

Figure 2.31 Tail jack restraint.

just off to the side, to avoid being kicked. If the cattle are not placed in the chute, the handler should be prepared to step to either side, as the cow may fidget and move sideways.

> **TECHNICIAN TIP 2.14:** Lifting a bovid's tail by the base avoids breaking of the tail.

Flank Rope

Applying pressure to the flank of cattle can help discourage them from kicking. A rope with an eyelet in the end or an eyelet created using a bowline knot is used to create a large loop that encompasses the flank area. Pressure is applied as necessary. Care should be taken to not have the rope directly placed on the udder or prepuce (Figure 2.32).

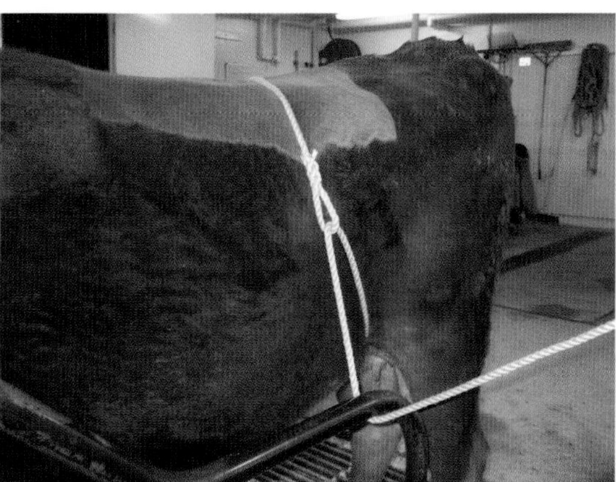

Figure 2.32 Proper flank rope placement with rope in front of the udder.

Front Leg Hobble

The hobble is used for inspecting the front feet for injury and can also be helpful to keep the back legs from kicking. Use a rope with an eyelet at the end or create an eyelet by using the bowline knot. Create a loop around the pastern. The end of the rope is placed over the withers and should be held by another person. An assistant is used rather than tying, as this way the rope can be quickly released in the event that the cow may start to go down (Figure 2.33).

> **TECHNICIAN TIP 2.15:** When placing a front leg hopple, use of an assistant instead of tying is important, as the cow may start to lie down and the rope can be released quickly.

Hind Leg Restraint

Hind leg restraint is used for inspecting the hind legs for foot injury. An overhead beam or hook that is slightly behind the bovid is needed to lift the leg. A rope is placed around the hock using a half hitch. The person placing the rope should kneel, with one leg down and the other knee up, when placing the rope as it allows a quick escape route in the event the bovid decides to kick. The long end of the rope is then placed over the beam or hook and the leg can be lifted (Figures 2.34 and 2.35).

Tilt Table

The tilt table is a valuable tool for examining feet or working on bovids because it allows the animal to be turned on its side. The table is like a chute and can turn in either direction. The bovid is walked on and its head, body, and legs are secured with straps and ropes (Figures 2.36 and 2.37). To avoid the risk of bloat and regurgitation, food and water should be held for

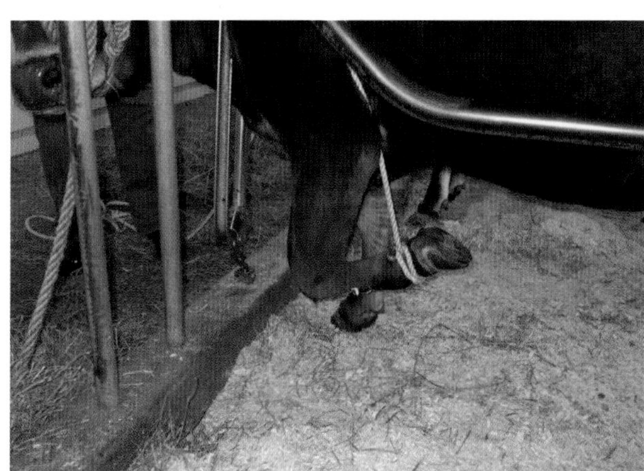

Figure 2.33 Front leg hopple restraint.

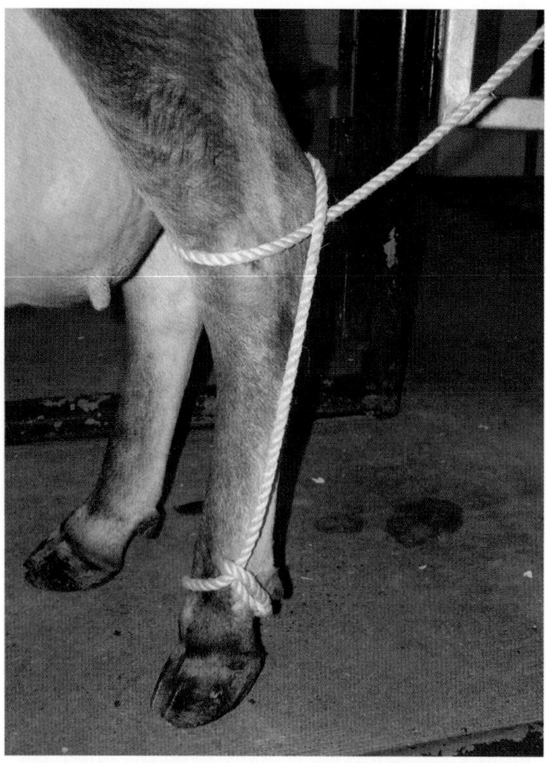

Figure 2.34 Step one of hind leg restraint.

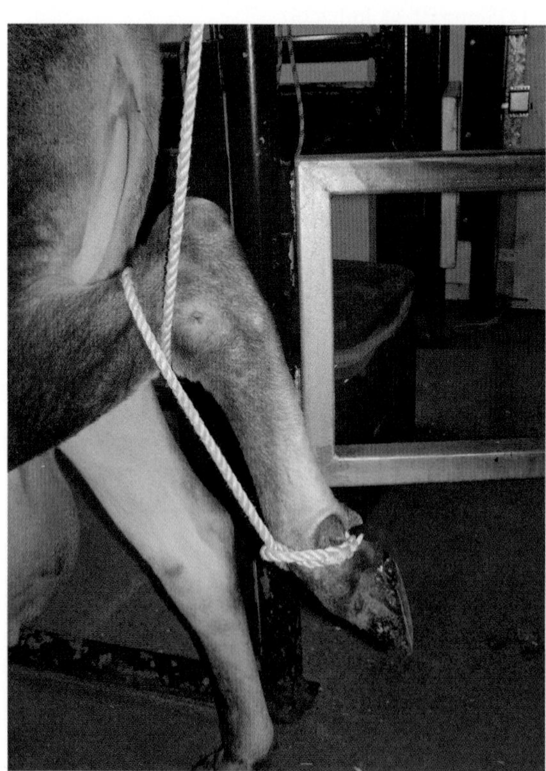

Figure 2.35 Hind leg restraint allows for examination of the rear leg.

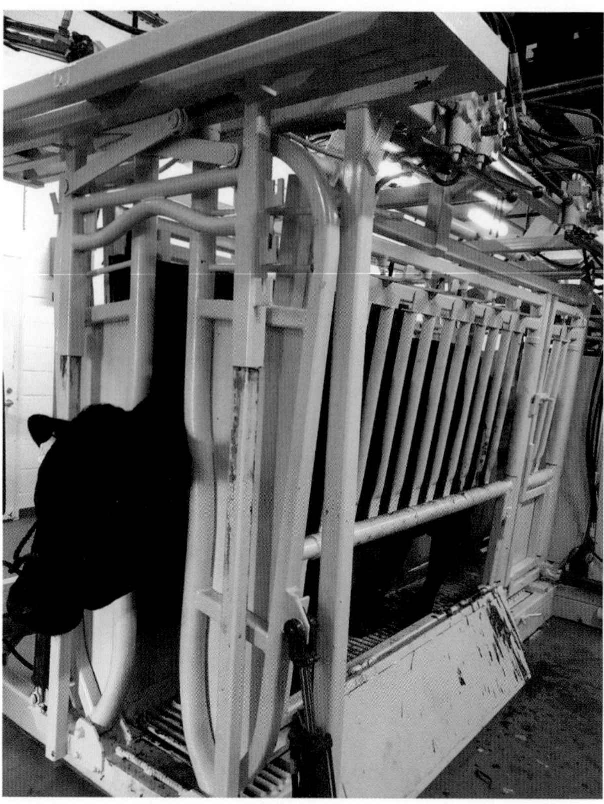

Figure 2.36 Bovine tilt table. *Source:* Courtesy of Kim Bicking.

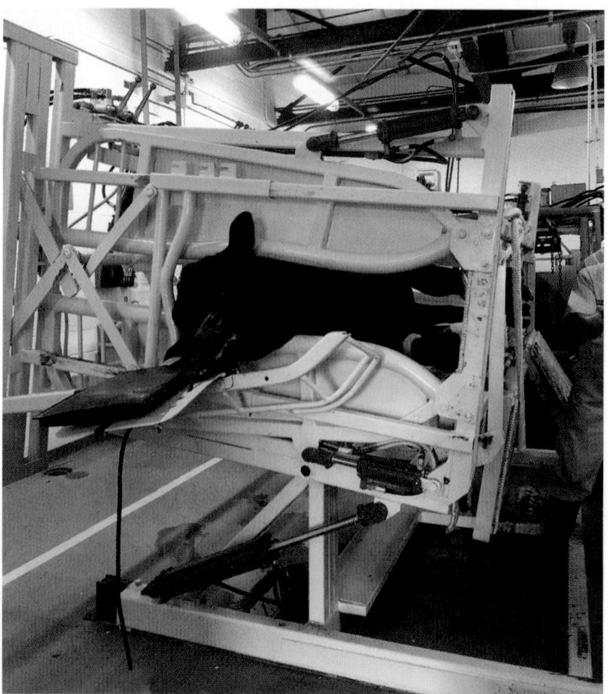

Figure 2.37 A bovine tilt table in use. This cow is placed in right lateral recumbency. *Source:* Courtesy of Kim Bicking.

several hours if the procedure is performed in lateral recumbency and is estimated to take more than 30 min to complete.

Casting

Casting is used on cattle when it is necessary to force them to lie down on the ground. There are two different methods that can be used. Regardless of the method, a halter is first placed, and the head secured to a sturdy post for placing the ropes. The first casting technique described here uses a long rope with eyelet in the end – or you can make an eyelet using a bowline knot – creating a noose around the neck. The rope is brought caudally, and a half hitch is placed around the girth area and then another half hitch around the flank area. As in the flank restraint, care should be taken that the rope is not placed directly on the udder or the prepuce. The end of the rope is then pulled caudally off the back of the bovid. A strong pull forces the cow to lie down (Figures 2.38 and 2.39).

TECHNICIAN TIP 2.16: Casting ropes should not be paced directly on the udder or prepuce during placement.

The second method of casting is referred to the as the Burley casting harness. This is also known as the criss-cross method and avoids pressure on the trachea, prepuce, and milk veins. The ropes are crossed under the brisket and passed between the front legs before coming up over the back and being crossed again. Then both end of the ropes are passed in between the back legs (Figures 2.40 and 2.41). After casting, the bovid should be rolled onto their back as they are less likely to bloat in sternal or dorsal recumbency as compared to lateral recumbency. Items such as bales or wedges can be used to keep them dorsal. For safety to both the bovid and personnel involved, the

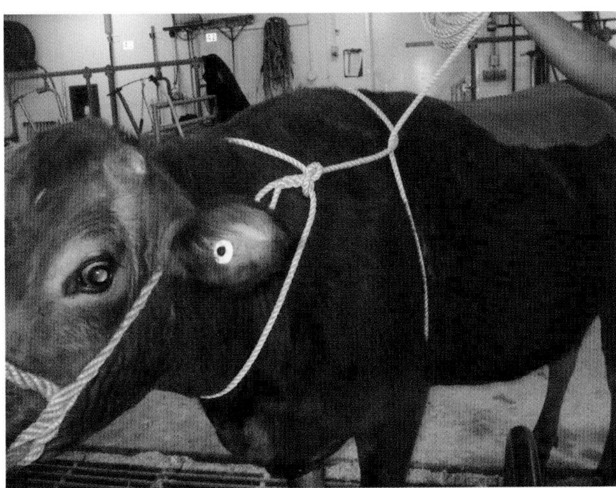

Figure 2.38 Casting rope placement step one.

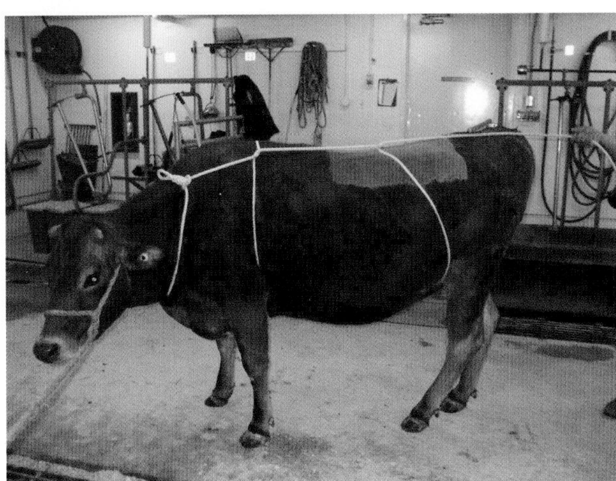

Figure 2.39 Casting rope step two.

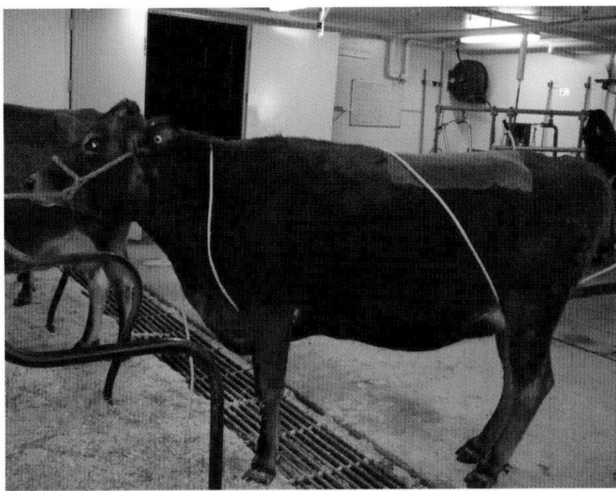

Figure 2.40 The Burley casting harness step one.

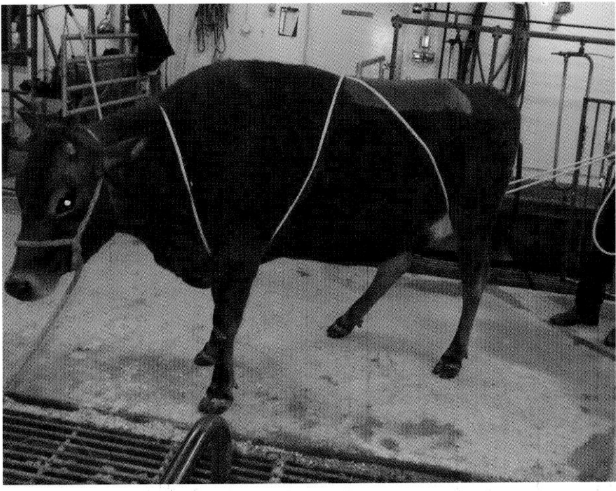

Figure 2.41 The Burley casting harness step two.

front legs should be pulled forward and secured using soft cotton ropes. The rear legs should be extended backward and also tied with soft cotton ropes. If the bovid must be placed on its side, then the right side is more desirable. By being in this position, the rumen can be more readily observed, and signs of bloat may be more apparent. Only short procedures should be done in ruminants placed in lateral recumbency.

TECHNICIAN TIP 2.17: Bovids should be placed in sternal to avoid bloating.

Squeeze Chute

Squeeze chutes are also a useful tool in veterinary practice. Cattle are driven forward into a squeeze chute through a serious of gates, creating both distance and safety for the handler. Veterinarians and staff need to be aware of chute openings and slats at all times. Chutes provide the ability to keep the bovid in a small area and prevent them from moving forward, backward, or laterally (Figures 2.42–2.45).

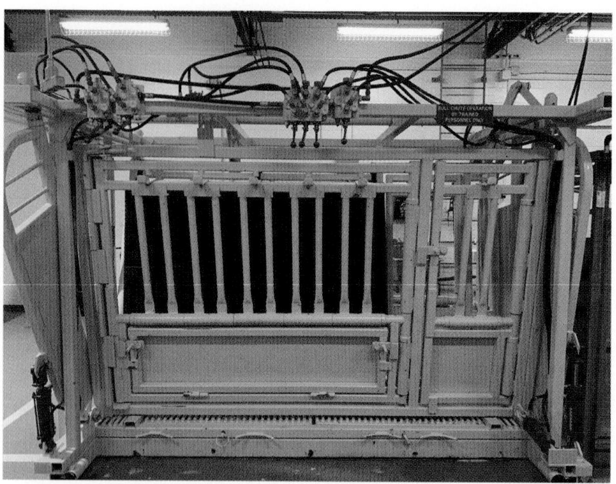

Figure 2.43 A side view of a squeeze chute.

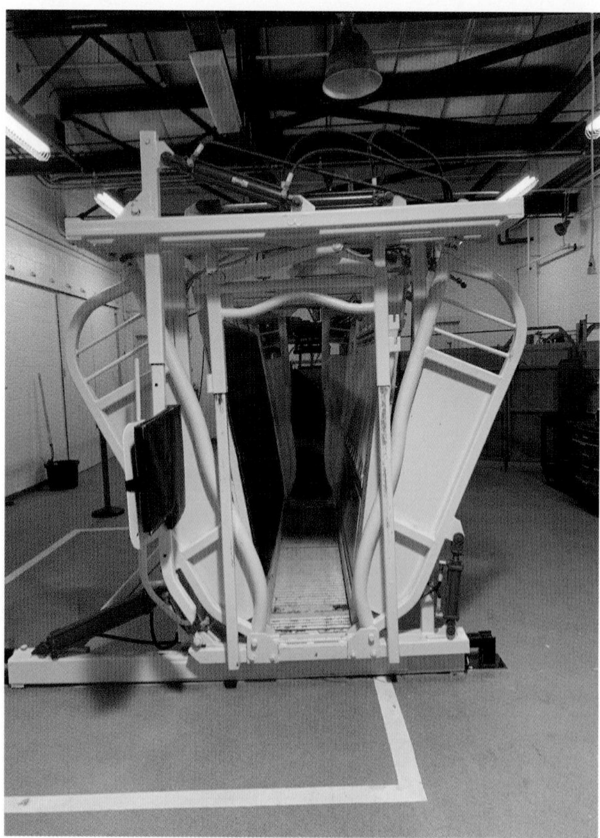

Figure 2.42 A front view of a bovine squeeze chute.

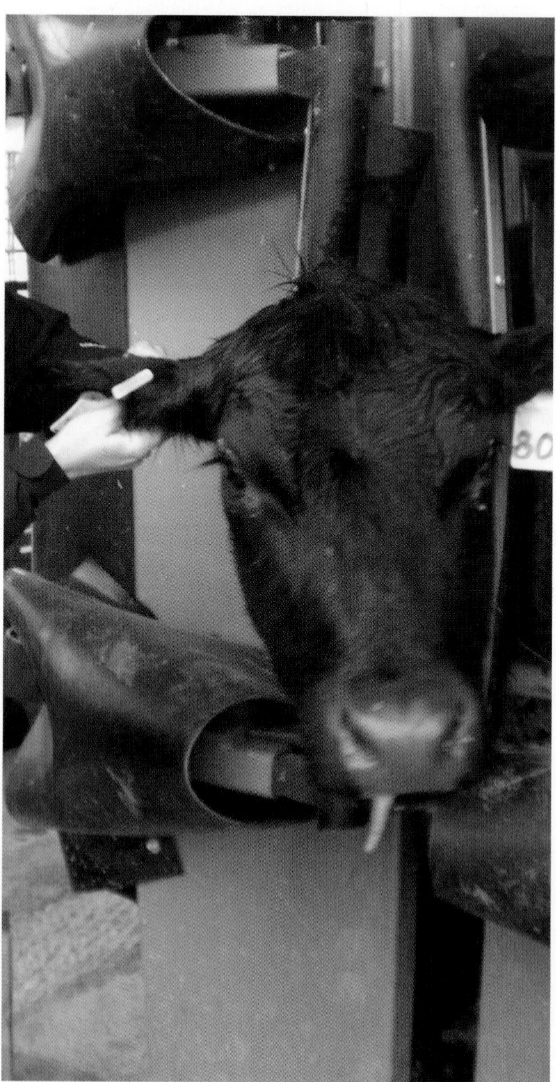

Figure 2.44 A squeeze chute used for ear tag placement on a cow. *Source:* Courtesy of Scott R.R. Haskell, DVM, MPVM, PhD.

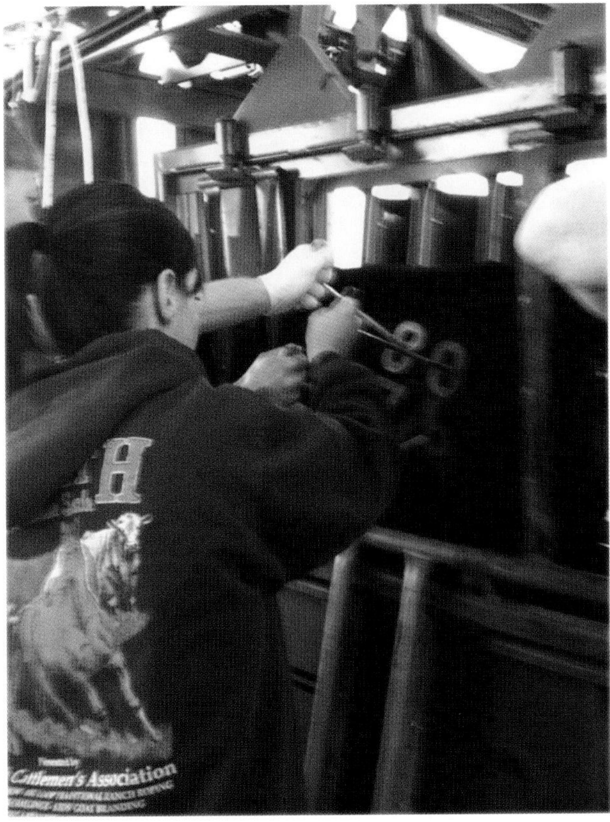

Figure 2.45 Branding cattle in a squeeze chute. *Source:* Courtesy of Scott R.R. Haskell, DVM, MPVM, PhD.

Calves

Cows have strong protective instincts, which should be taken into account when working on calves. Whether dairy or beef, it may be best if the calf can be separated from the cow before working on them, to ensure safety. If the calf cannot be removed, a panel should be used to shield it from the cow. Calves are generally easy to catch once separated, having a natural curiosity. A cow on pasture should be funneled into a smaller containment area. The calf will easily follow the dam. To restrain the standing calf, wrap one arm around the neck or chest with the other arm wrapped around the hindquarters.

> **TECHNICIAN TIP 2.18:** When working on calves, take precautions around the cows as they have strong protective instincts.

If the calf must be restrained in lateral recumbency, the flanking process can be used.

1) Stand on the left side of the calf.
2) Lean over the calf.
3) Grasp the calf's left pelvic limb with the right hand.
4) Grasp the calf's left forelimb with the left hand.
5) Lift the calf and let it lean into the handler's legs.

Slide the calf down the handler's legs to the ground and place one knee on the neck and the other knee on the back or restrain the legs with the hands. Never throw the calf on the ground.

Small Ruminant Restraint

Goats

Goats are very playful and curious and seem to enjoy human attention. Paper is a highly favored consumable, and pocket contents, equipment, tools, and clothing will be thoroughly investigated. They can be very vocal when separated from herd mates and will often become more agitated and struggle against prolonged restraint. Goats are especially food motivated and trainable. Dairy or pet goats can be quite tame, making moving as a group more difficult. They often will wear collars, which makes catching and handling easier. Chasing goats rarely works; they may scatter haphazardly or pile up in corners and crush each other. Horned goats may be wary of narrow races and gates.

> **TECHNICIAN TIP 2.19:** Do not bring clipboards, paper, or equipment into a goat pen. These items will not stay where you leave them. Dangling earrings, strings, clothing, and hair may tempt the goats to pull and tug.

Catching and Holding

Goats are best caught by crowding a small group into a small pen. Quietly and with patience, the individual is caught and moved out of the pen into the work area. The collar can be grasped or an arm can be reached around its neck or torso while the other hand is placed on its tail to direct the animal. Horse halters can be placed upside down over their heads, with the noseband at the thoracic inlet. This can give the handler an additional "handle" to walk or move the goat. Goats should not be held or caught by the hind limb as they may struggle and dislocate a hip (Figures 2.46–2.48).

The basic strategies for holding are the same for goats as they are for sheep. Tame goats will normally stand with minimal effort. Goats may be held against a wall or can be straddled like a sheep. The head is restrained by the use of a collar, halter, jaw hold, or horns.

If horns are present, they should be controlled during restraint to avoid handler injury. Horns are strongest at the base and may break off if handled near the tips. Points are sharp, and horned animals may use their horns offensively. Rough handling of the horns is resented by goats. Scurs

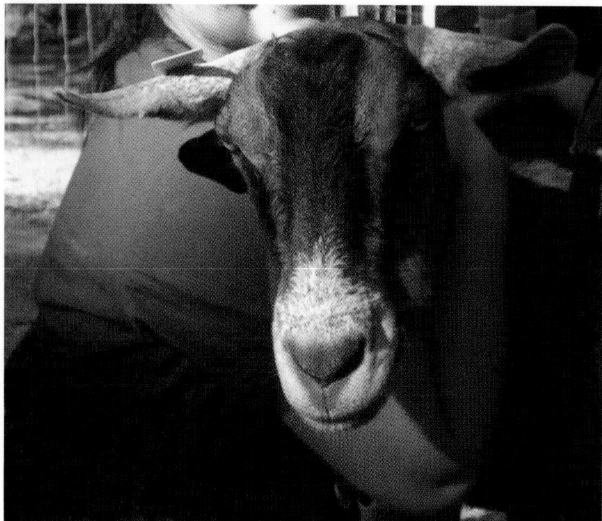

Figure 2.46 A goat is quietly restrained by wrapping an arm around the neck. *Source:* Courtesy of Scott R.R. Haskell, DVM, MPVM, PhD.

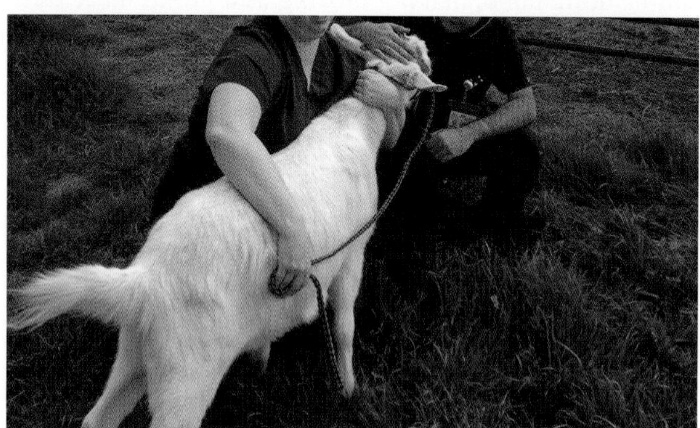

Figure 2.47 Tame goats normally stand with minimal effort. *Source:* Courtesy of Scott R.R. Haskell, DVM, MPVM, PhD.

(abnormal horn growth due to incomplete disbudding) should not be used for restraint as they may snap off and bleed. The beard may be held if the hand is placed close to the jaw (Figure 2.49). Some owners may object to this hold, and during breeding season, bucks urinate on their own beards, making this option unpleasant. Goats find it painful to be held by their ears, so they should not be used as a form of restraint. Goats can be tethered for short period of time by their collar or a halter.

TECHNICIAN TIP 2.20: Horns should be handled near the base of the horn where they are the strongest.

If more restraint is necessary, the goat may be placed in lateral recumbency. They do not tolerate being set up on their rump like sheep. Two methods of achieving lateral recumbency exist. The first is similar to flanking a calf:

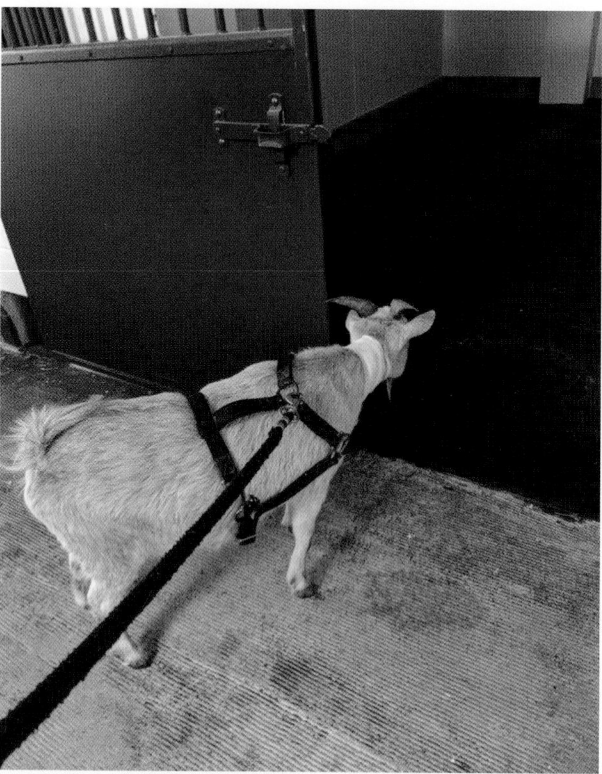

Figure 2.48 Horse halter being used to walk a goat without putting pressure on their trachea.

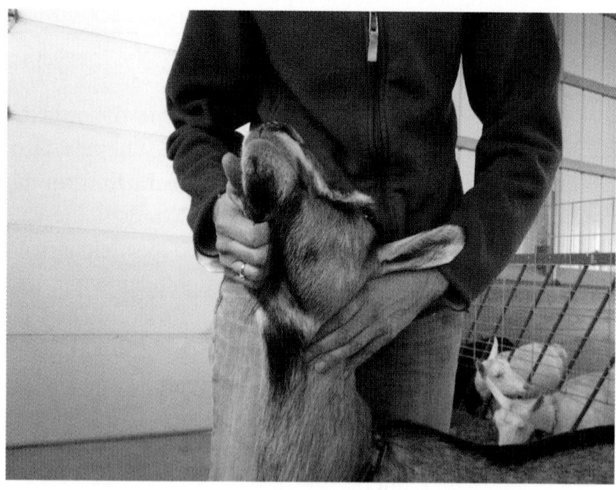

Figure 2.49 Jaw hold on a goat. *Source:* Courtesy of Ann Goplen, DVM.

1) Stand on the left side of goat.
2) Lean over the goat.
3) Grasp the goat's left pelvic limb with the right hand.
4) Grasp the goat's left forelimb with the left hand.
5) Lift the goat and let it lean into the handler legs.
6) Slide the goat down the handler's legs to the ground and place a knee on the neck and restrain the legs with the hands.

Table 2.1 Setting up a Sheep.

1) Stand on the left side of sheep.	
2) Hold the sheep's head in your left hand by placing your hand under its jaw.	
3) Your left knee should be near or just behind the sheep's left shoulder.	
4) Your right leg should be touching the sheep's side near its left hip.	
5) Place your right hand on the sheep's back over the hips.	
6) Turn the sheep's nose away from you toward its right shoulder/flank.	
7) You should feel the weight of the sheep leaning against your legs.	
Rump Pressure Method	**Lift Method**
8) Put pressure on the sheep's hips with your right hand so the animal cannot pick its back feet off the floor.	8) Reach across the back to grasp either the right flank skinfold, the upper portion of the right hind leg, or reaching back under the abdomen, grasp the left hind leg.
9) Take a step back with your right leg and pivot slightly with the other leg to throw the sheep off center.	9) Slightly lift the leg off the ground, outward and slightly forward.
10) The hind leg of the sheep should start to go down, and the sheep will lean on your legs.	10) Set the sheep down (not throw) onto its rump on the ground in front of the handler.
11) Continue to bring the animal's head around and slide the sheep's weight off your legs and onto the ground, keeping the sheep sitting slightly on the side of pelvis vs. directly on tail.	
12) Release the jaw and pull upward on the forelimbs and straighten the sheep until it is reclining with its back leaning against your legs.	
13) Keep sheep slightly off center to reduce struggling.	
14) Sheep can also be lowered from this position into lateral or dorsal recumbency if necessary.	

The second method is more of a gentle "flip" very similar to the lift method of setting up a sheep, but the animal is taken all the way to the ground rather than set up on the rump. Refer to steps 1–11 of the Lift Method of the setting-up procedure in Table 2.1. Then, take a half-step back and allow the goat to slide off the handler's legs onto the ground and restrain as described above.

Feet

Both front and rear legs are lifted by grasping the leg at the level of the fetlock and bending the knee or elbow. The leg can then be held in one hand or rested on the handler's knee. The rear legs are also brought out slightly behind the goat. Avoid over-abduction, especially of the rear limbs. Lift the legs only to a position that is comfortable to the goat, otherwise the animal will resist (Figure 2.50).

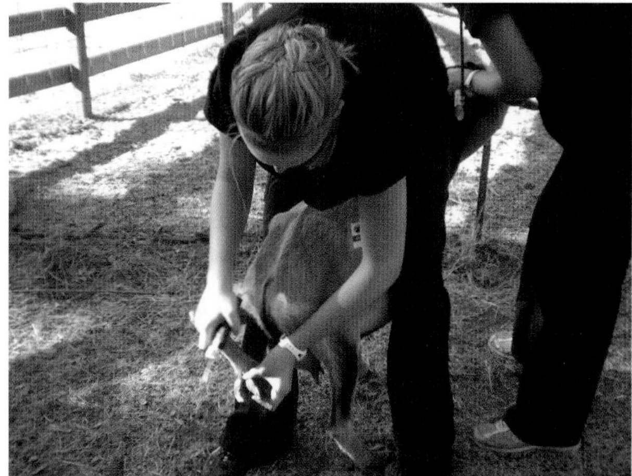

Figure 2.50 Inspect the back legs of a goat, lifting them in a position that is comfortable to the goat. *Source:* Courtesy of Scott R.R. Haskell, DVM, MPVM, PhD.

Kids

Most dairy kids are disbudded early in life and are restrained like lambs. Place them in sternal recumbency or in a "disbudding box" built to contain the kid, and hold the head still. The kid can be held in the lap of an assistant, with the front legs folded beneath the kid, with the handler's forearms placed along the side and back pressing down to keep the kid from rising. The hands control the head with thumbs behind ears, fingers wrapping around the muzzle (Figures 2.51 and 2.52).

Sheep

Catching and Holding

The key to catching sheep is keeping excitement and stress to a minimum. Once panicked, sheep can lead the entire

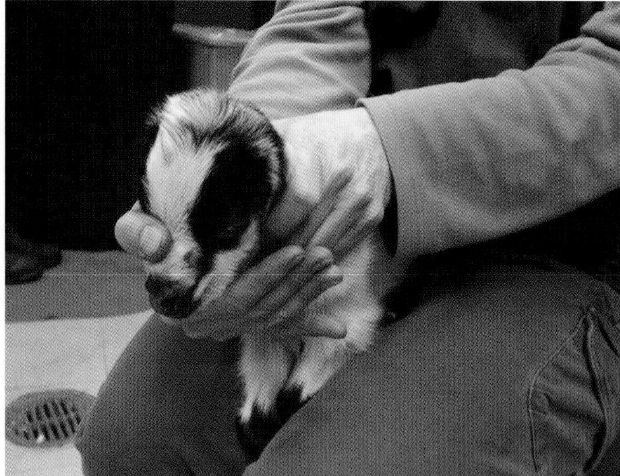

Figure 2.51 A kid restrained for disbudding.

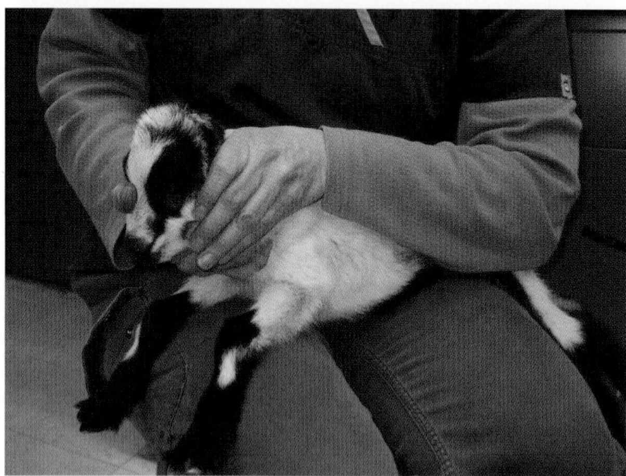

Figure 2.52 An alternative hold for restraining a kid for disbudding.

flock into chaos. A scared sheep may try to jump or climb over or through any human or fence. If a handling facility is not available, drive the flock into a small catch pen. Crowd a group into the corner and then catch the desired animal. To catch a sheep, grab the head under the jaw, grasping the bony part of the mandible (Figure 2.53). Either wrap your fingers around the lower muzzle or place your fingers between the two jawbones. Immediately tilt the nose upward to control the sheep's motion. Place a knee into the flank or behind the elbow and push the animal against the wall. This jaw hold can be maintained with one hand and the other hand can be placed under the jaw from the other side, behind the ears, on the rump, or can grasp around the tail base or the skinfold of the opposite lower flank. Forward or backward pressure with the hands will direct the sheep. The tail or "go button" can be lifted to initiate forward motion. The rump of the sheep can be put into a corner or against the wall to prevent backing.

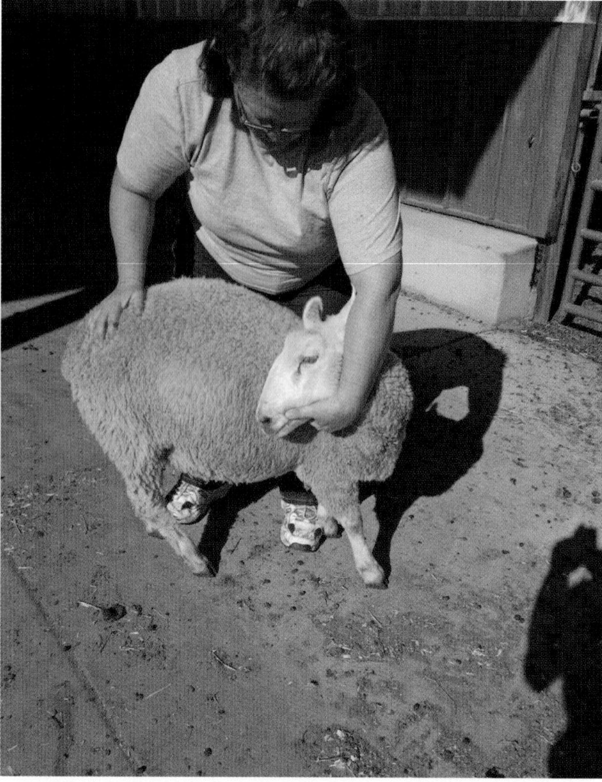

Figure 2.53 Jaw hold on a sheep. *Source:* Courtesy of Ann Goplen, DVM.

> **TECHNICIAN TIP 2.21:** Keeping the sheep's head tilted, "nose up" will allow the handler to maintain control of the animal. The sheep is much more powerful when its head is down.

Avoid grabbing the sheep low on the leg or throwing it to the ground, to avoid fractured legs or vertebrae. Avoid grabbing the horns or wool as clumps of wool can be pulled out or broken, damaging and reducing the value of the fleece and pelt. In addition, skin can be bruised or ripped.

A shepherd's crook can be a useful tool to catch a sheep. The proper use is catching the hind leg at or above the level of the hock. A lower catch runs the risk of fracturing the leg. The crook should never be used to catch a sheep by the neck. Once the leg is caught, quickly wrap an arm around the sheep's neck and move into a jaw hold. A flank catch is another option. The aim is to grab high on the flank with your hand. Quietly approach the sheep directly from the rear. With your strongest hand, grasp the sheep's leg on same side as the hand you are using, anywhere from just above the hock to well up into the flank. Lift upward enough to elevate the leg off the ground. Quickly grasp the jaw with your other hand. The flank can be released, and other handling points (head, rump, tail) can be used to control the sheep.

> **TECHNICIAN TIP 2.22:** When utilizing a shepherd's crook, it is important to catch the hindleg at or above the level of the hock. Catching lower than the hock runs the risk of fracturing the leg.

A straddle hold can be used if the handler's feet can remain firmly on the ground. With the sheep restrained and backed into a corner, swing one leg over its back. The sheep's shoulders should be squeezed firmly between the handler's knees. Place two hands loosely around the muzzle or the jaw control the head.

A halter is a valuable tool after the animal is caught, although they will not lead unless trained. Other equipment that are useful restraint aids are tipping crates, tilt tables, shepherds chairs, and gambrel restrainers. The gambrel restrainers is a simple, W-shaped plastic device that keeps adult sheep immobilized in sternal recumbency by holding the neck and outstretched front legs alongside each other. The shepherd's chair is a device that sits the sheep on their rump, reclining in a mesh sling chair. Tipping cradles and tilt tables squeeze the animal and turn the animal on its side or upside down for easy access to feet.

Setting Up

"Setting up" a sheep sits the sheep down on its rump, facing away from and leaning back into the legs of the restrainer (Figure 2.54). Sheep struggle very little in this position, tend to relax, and are quite easy to handle. It is possible for one person to restrain the sheep and draw blood, examine and trim feet, and perform other tasks without additional assistance. There are several different methods used to set up a sheep. The preferred method will depend on the size and strength of the handler and the sheep. The rump pressure method requires the most finesse and the least amount of lifting. For the sheep that needs a little more encouragement to sit, the lift method is required. The head can be allowed to rest to the side, freeing both hands for use. If more restraint is needed, both forelegs can be held in one hand and the head supported with the other, or the right hand can hold the right foreleg while left hand holds left foreleg.

> **TECHNICIAN TIP 2.23:** Work smarter, not harder. Use the sheep's weight to throw it off balance. Do not try to muscle a sheep to set it up.

Lamb Restraint

To carry a lamb, place one hand under the body with fingers extending between the forelimbs to support the sternum. The forearm can either be under the abdomen supporting the lamb's weight or along the contralateral side of the body cradling the lamb into handler's chest. The other hand supports the head and neck.

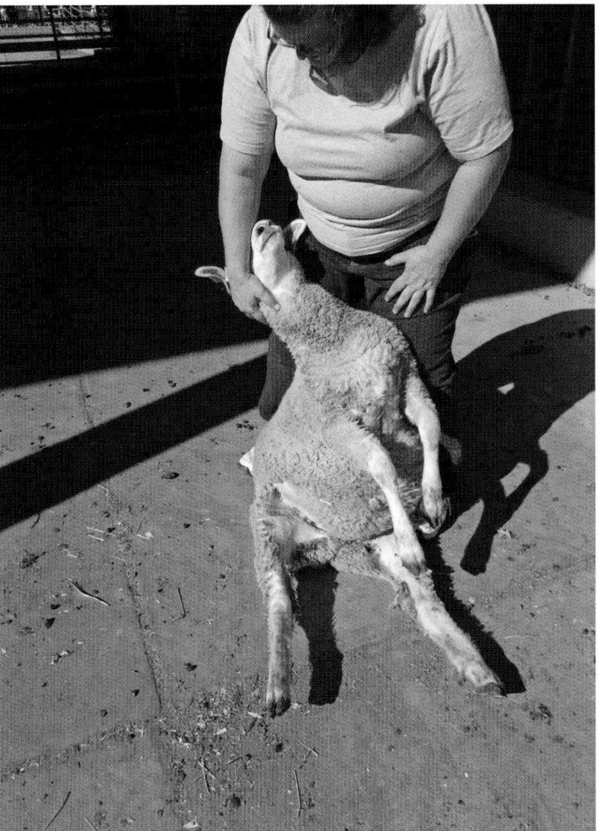

Figure 2.54 "Setting up" of a sheep allows for a relaxed position. *Source:* Courtesy of Ann Goplen, DVM.

Lambs are generally placed in dorsal recumbency for docking and castrating. They may be held in the holder's lap or against the chest or laid on a flat surface. Both right front and rear legs are held in the holder's right hand, while both left legs are held in the left hand. For naval dipping or intraperitoneal injections, the lamb's forelegs are held in one hand at about the level of the handler's waist, with the lamb sitting on its rump or hanging with its back against the holder's legs. If necessary, the lamb's hips can be gently squeezed between the handler's legs. Standing lambs may be restrained by gripping their rib cage or neck between the holder's lower legs. The head is facing forward or backward depending on what access is needed.

Camelid Restraint

The two domesticated species of South American camelids are the llama and the alpaca. Llamas and alpacas are herd animals and do best with other herd mates around. Llamas are generally calmer than alpacas are. Camelid ear and tail

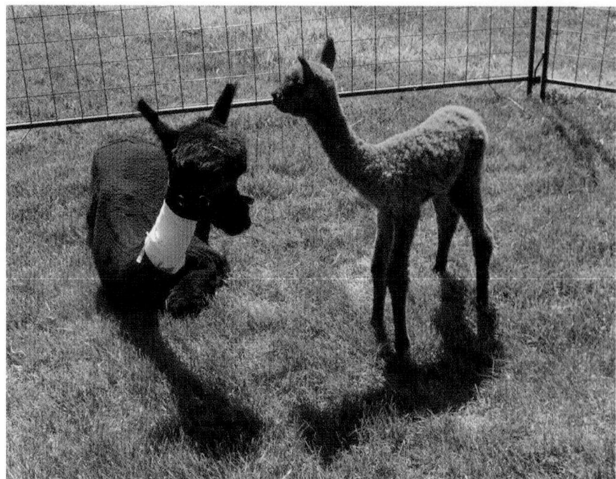

Figure 2.55 The adult llama on the left is in a kush position.

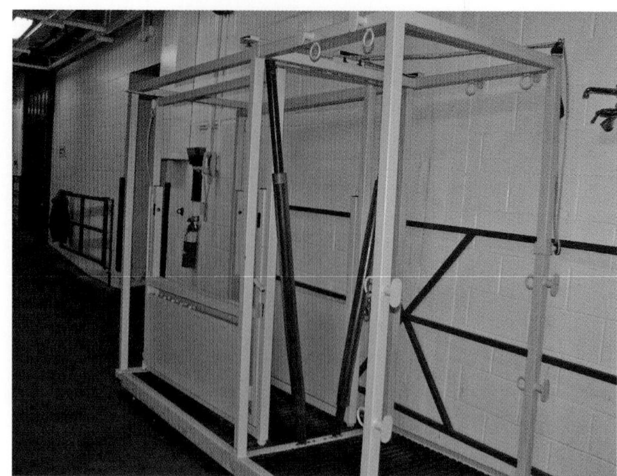

Figure 2.56 A camelid stanchion.

position can express important information about the animal's emotional state. Alpacas may protest loudly during restraint with screams and screeches. They tend to jump more than llamas do when physically restrained, or conversely, spontaneously kush. Kushing is often their default position of submission, indignation, or displeasure (Figure 2.55). They tuck all their legs tightly under their body and can pop up into a standing position very quickly. Some camelids are trained to halters, leading, chutes, or stanchions (Figure 2.56).

Camelid defensive behaviors include spitting, kicking, stomping, and rearing. They can bite but usually reserve this for fighting between intact males. Spitting is the ultimate response if mild threat displays have been ignored. The spitting sequence begins with the ears laid back against the neck and a gurgling or gulping sound coming from the throat, followed by high-force expulsion of stomach contents and saliva. The ingesta can fly as far as 1–2 m in a diffuse pattern, often directly into the face or hair of the handler or unsuspecting bystander. The spitter's head can be directed away from humans once the animal is restrained. A towel can be placed over the nose and mouth to discourage spitting, but it will make some animals more fidgety and upset. Alpacas tend to be more prone to spitting than llamas are (Table 2.2).

Camelids generally "cow kick," reaching forward and outward with their hind legs, but they can kick directly backward as well. The safest place to stand is at the shoulder. Rearing and stomping are rare, but if seen, such behavior indicates a highly aggravated individual. It may be best to stop and reevaluate the procedure for the safety of both the animal and humans.

TECHNICIAN TIP 2.24: The safest place to stand is close to the body at the shoulder of an alpaca or llama.

Table 2.2 Camelid body language.

Attitude	Ears	Tail	Vocalization
Calm	Relaxed, vertical, slightly forward, or lying horizontal and spread laterally from top of head	Lay flat against rump	None, hum
Alert	Cocked forward	Horizontal to 45° above horizontal	Snort (short burst of air through mouth with loose lips) Tongue click
Alarm	Pointed forward	45° above horizontal	High pitch series of whistles or neighing noises
Aggression/threat	Flat against neck, nose pointed skyward	Completely vertical	Grumble, scream (extreme fright), screech (fighting)
Submission (head and neck held low, front limbs slightly bent)	Normal to above horizontal	Curved forward over back	

Catching

It is preferable to have the animals contained in a small catch pen and have the owners catch and halter the animals and lead them to you; however, many owners are unable to do this. A small group or whole herd can be moved easily with two or more people. Ropes, poles, or outstretched hands may be used to direct a small group into a corner or move them along a fence line. If one breaks free, the others will follow. It is best to regroup and start over. Do not chase camelids – this only entertains them. If what you are doing is not working, get reinforcements or change the set.

Once the group is huddled up, the desired animal may be calmly and slowly approached. The simplest catch is to slide the hand nearest the animal up the back of the neck into position behind the ears while the other hand comes around to cup the lower jaw. Another method involves one arm placed around the chest and neck while the opposite hand grasps the tail or applies slight downward pressure to the withers. The animal can be pushed up against a wall or fence for additional restraint. A light rope is sometimes draped behind the neck and brought round in front to assist in catching more wily animals.

> **TECHNICIAN TIP 2.25:** Don't chase camelids. If what you are doing is not working, get reinforcements or change the set.

Holding

If the animal is halter trained, a halter and lead rope can be used to control the head. Grasp the lead rope near the halter to prevent excessive head movement. Short bursts of pressure work better than a constant tug does for leading the untrained animal. A halter must be adjusted properly in order to be safe and effective. The noseband must be placed high on the nose, close to the eye, resting on bone. If the halter is placed too low or slides down, the cartilage and soft tissue of the nose is compressed, shutting off the nasal passages and causing the animal to panic and struggle. Some camelids are in the "less is more" category; they struggle harder when more restraint is applied (Figure 2.57).

> **TECHNICIAN TIP 2.26:** Short bursts of pressure work better than a constant tug for leading the untrained animal.

> **TECHNICIAN TIP 2.27:** The noseband of the halter must remain high up, near the eyes, to prevent pinching off the nasal passage.

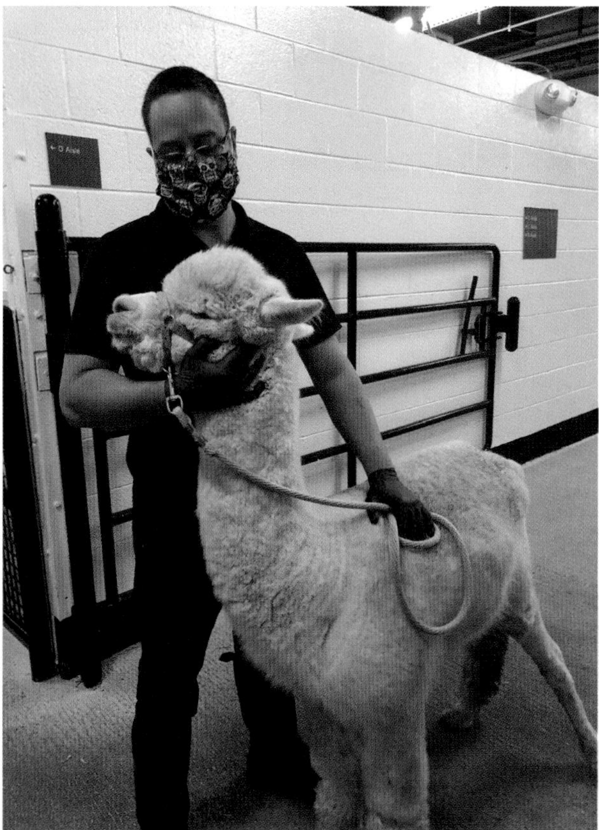

Figure 2.57 A camelid being minimally restrained. *Source:* Courtesy of Kim Bicking.

The "Bracelet hold" is an elegant and effective method developed by Marty McGee Bennett of Camelidynamics. It is accomplished by cupping the lower jaw with the thumb and forefinger of one hand just behind the bottom lip. The other hand rests just below the ears, thumb lateral to one ear and index finger lateral to the other ear. The hands do not squeeze, they just rest. Elbows are out, arms parallel to ground, with the animal and human balanced on their respective feet (Figure 2.58).

An alpaca or smaller llama can be held with its head against the handler's body with one hand, while using the other to apply slight pressure to the withers or hold the base of the tail. Ear-ing immobilizes the head for procedures where stillness is required, such as microchipping or eye exams. Grasp the base of the ear and squeeze up firmly. Do not twist. The nose should be pointed forward, with the head and neck in line with the rest of the body. This should not be painful to the animal, but rather a suggestion that it will be if they move. It is a very subtle action that can be applied as needed by the person holding the head.

Camelids can be cross-tied or placed in a narrow alley, chutes, or stanchions for short-term confinement for veterinary care or examination. They can be cross-tied

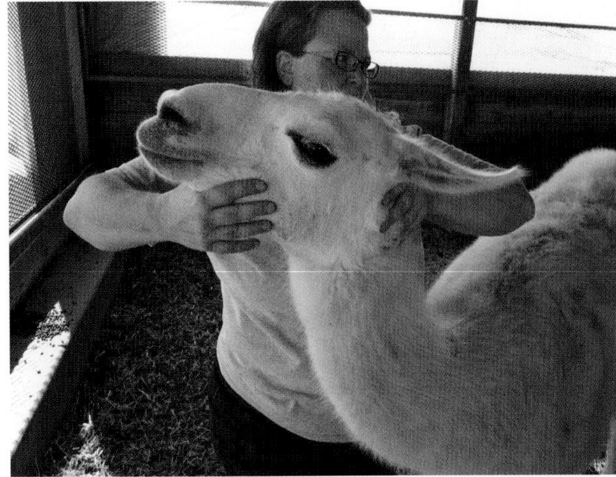

Figure 2.58 The bracelet hold performed correctly on a llama. *Source:* Courtesy of Ann Goplen, DVM.

between two trees, fence posts, or the uprights on chute fronts that will restrict forward and backward movement. The head will be fairly stable, but the hindquarters will be free to swing. A chute is a narrow passage or enclosure in which an animal can be safely held for a brief period. They must be stable and safe for the animal and the handler. Animals need to be trained to enter and stand in the chute or stanchion and should never be left unattended while restrained. Cinches below (for kushers) or over withers (for jumpers) may be added and a back bar can be used to prevent backward motion. A stanchion is a chute with two adjustable poles at the head end. These poles do not pinch the head or neck; they prevent forward movement by pressing against the shoulder. They are close enough to prevent the animal from squeezing between them but remain far enough apart to prevent pinching the neck if the animal kushes. It is preferable to cross-tie the animals in chutes or stanchions with quick release knots or snaps.

Some alpacas are sheared standing, but it is very common for them to be placed in lateral recumbency with their fore and hind legs stretched and tied out away from their body. Some producers have tilt shearing tables that the animal stands next to while a bellyband and leg wraps are placed, and after the table is tilted, the legs are stretched out and tied.

Crias

Crias may be lifted with one arm around the chest and the other arm supporting the abdomen in front of the rear legs or around the rump for crias under 45 lb (20 kg). Crias in a kushed position can be straddled and the head held in the handler's hands. A larger juvenile can be held similar to an adult with one arm around the chest and the other holding the base of the tail or rump. Alternately, two or three people can gently push the cria up against a wall, with each person's knees under the belly, slightly lifting the animal off the ground. A cria may be placed in lateral recumbency similar to goats. To hold a cria in lateral recumbency, lay an arm over the neck and grasp the animal's foreleg, either the downside leg or both. The other arm should pass over the body in front of the hips to grasp the thigh of the down rear limb.

Swine Restraint

Basic principles of swine restraint are similar to other large animal species in that stress levels are lower when less restraint is used. This requires forethought for several concerns when performing procedures on swine, including procedures to be performed, restraint items available at a facility, and handler expertise. Swine are generally friendly when handled regularly and housed in low-stress environments. Speaking with a calm voice to and/or touching a pig before restraint will reduce startling (Figure 2.59).

Moving pigs is similar to other large animal species in regard to flight zone and point of balance. Relying on these concepts will assist in moving pigs or pulling out

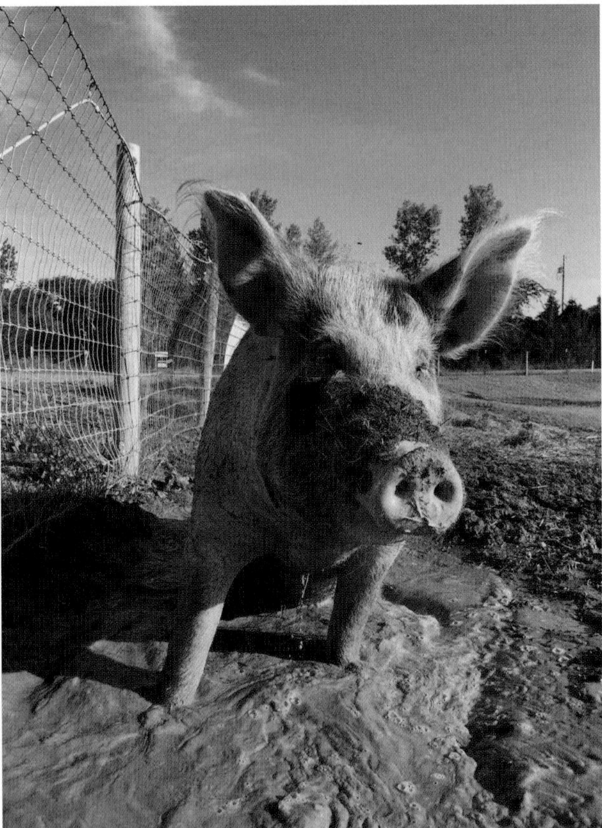

Figure 2.59 Swine are generally friendly when in a low-stress environment. *Source:* Courtesy of Farmaste Animal Sanctuary.

individual pigs from a group. Individual pigs may be moved backward into a corner or another area by placing a blindfold or bucket over their eyes. This principle may assist in handling situations and environments when corners must be utilized for restraint.

TECHNICIAN TIP 2.28: Placing a blindfold or bucket over a pig's eyes can help move an individual pig backward into a corner or another area.

Dr. Temple Grandin's outline for facilities to move cattle can also be used for swine, and includes elimination of shadows, use of light or darkness, and single-file races. These methods can improve safety and reduce animal stress.

Restraint methods and devices used with pigs include pig boards, snares, slings, weighing crates, or food. Each item may be used in various situations depending on procedure performed, animal size, and type of facility. Pig boards are used effectively for restraint during procedures of short duration or that require minimal restraint, such as physical exams or marginal ear blood collection (Figure 2.60). For longer or more invasive procedures such as jugular venipuncture on adults, a hog snare may be necessary. Adult pigs have been successfully trained to the use of a sling, but this is typically used only in research facilities.

Forking a pig is a great way to help them relax. It works on pigs or hogs of any size and any age. It seems to work similar to acupressure. Many use this technique to relax their pigs during stressful situations, hoof trimming, ear cleaning, pregnancy checks, vet visits, belly rubs, or at hospitals when the pig gets overwhelmed. A touch of the fork can relax them just enough. To fork a pig, use a fork or similar object that is blunt and lightly touch the ribs, back,

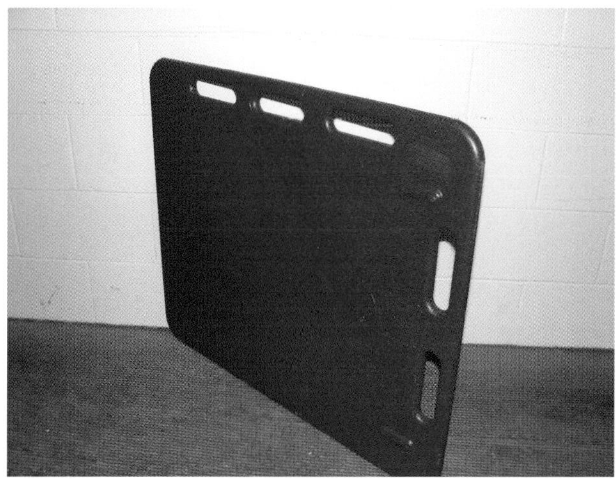

Figure 2.60 A pig board.

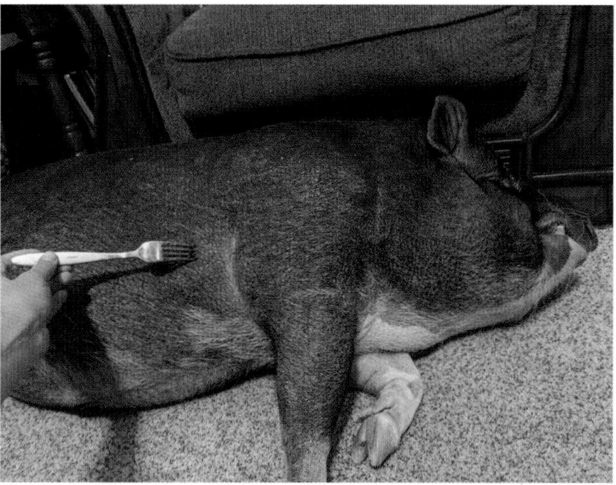

Figure 2.61 Using the forking method to calm a pig. *Source:* Courtesy of Siri Rea and Badger Pig Pig.

thigh, belly, forehead, chin, shoulder, wherever the pig seems to enjoy. You can use the fork to gently poke the pig repetitively or gently scratch it. Many pigs first react by raising their mohawk and then laying down, sometimes rolling to expose their belly (Figure 2.61).

Piglets

When performing neonatal procedures on piglets, all procedural items must be assembled. The sow should be separated from the group of piglets during the procedures. To catch piglets, one may grab the rear leg and, while lifting, place a second hand under the body for support. For minimally invasive procedures, restraint is usually limited to holding the piglet under one arm. Great care must be taken to finish procedures in a timely fashion with minimal stress so that the sow is not overly concerned with stressed piglets, which can lead to maternal attack on her offspring.

Older piglets can be restrained in V troughs, by laying them in dorsal recumbency in a person's lap, or by picking up by their front or hind legs.

Chicken Restraint

To hold and carry, put one hand under the bird so the breast is in the palm of the hand, with the index finger around the hocks and the thumb around one leg and the remaining fingers around the other leg. The other hand is placed on the bird's back to help stead the bird, hold the bird between the arm and body (Figures 2.62–2.64).

Remove from coop – put one hand over the back of the bird and turn it toward you, use the other hand underneath the bird so the bird is resting in the palm of your hand, supporting the breast. Then lift and move the bird.

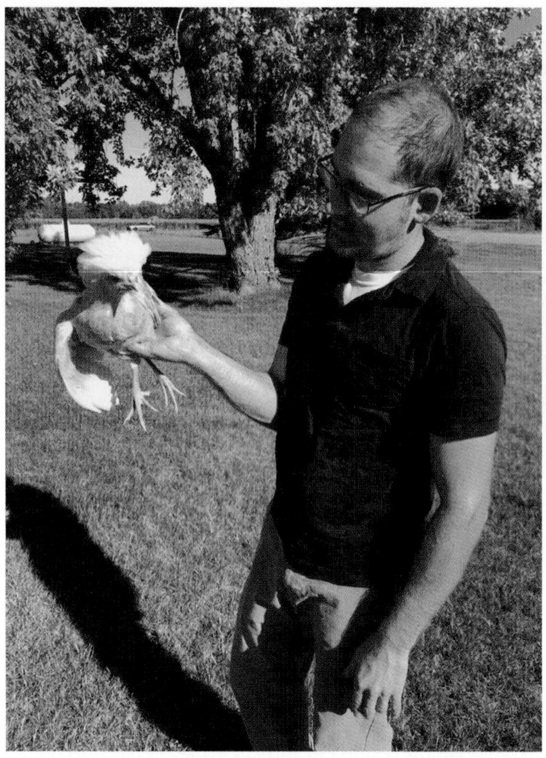

Figure 2.62 The breast is in the palm of the hand with the index finger around the hocks. *Source:* Courtesy of Paul Weinand.

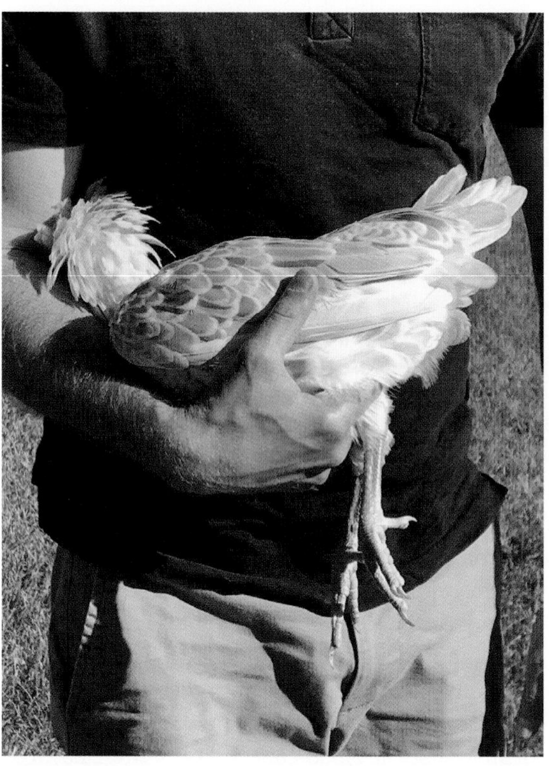

Figure 2.64 Hold the bird between the arm and the body. *Source:* Courtesy of Paul Weinand.

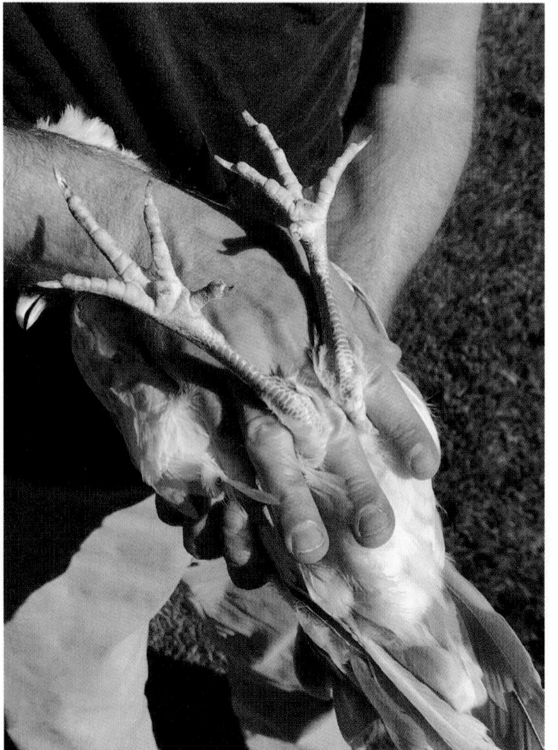

Figure 2.63 The remaining fingers are around the other leg. *Source:* Courtesy of Paul Weinand.

References

Battaglia, R. (2007). *Handbook of Livestock Management*. Upper Saddle River, NJ: Prentice Hall.

Fowler, M. (2008). *Restraint and Handling of Wild and Domestic Animals*. Ames, IA: Wiley Blackwell.

Fowler, M. (2010). *Medicine and Surgery of Camelids*. Ames, IA: Wiley Blackwell.

Grandin, T. (ed.) (1993). *Livestock Handling and Transport*. New York: CAB International.

Grandin, T. (2011). Understanding flight zone and point of balance for low stress handling of cattle, sheep and pigs. Retrieved from https://www.grandin.com/behaviour/principles/flight.zone.html

Grogg, LLC. (2012). Animated knots by Grogg. Retrieved from https://www.animatedknots.com

Holtgrew-Bohling, K. (2012). *Large Animal Clinical Procedures for Veterinary Technicians*. St. Louis, MO: Elsevier Saunders.

Kane, E. (2011). Safety 101: 7 commonly asked questions on how to use a twitch. *DVM 360.com*. Retrieved from https://www.dvm360.com/view/7-commonly-asked-questions-how-use-twitch

McCurnin, D. and Bassert, J. (2006). *Clinical Textbook for Veterinary Technicians*. St Louis, MO: Elsevier Saunders.

McGee Bennett, M. (2006). *The Camelid Companion*. Bend, OR: Raccoon Press.

Plumb, D. (2005). *Plumb's Veterinary Drug Handbook*, 5e. Ames, IA: Wiley Blackwell.

Pugh, D. and Baird, A. (2011). *Sheep and Goat Medicine*. Maryland Heights, MO: Elsevier Saunders.

Smith, M. and Sherman, D. (2009). *Goat Medicine*. Ames, IA: Wiley Blackwell.

Clinical Case Resolution 2.1 Hobby Farm Call

SETUP: The owner needs to have an approximately 10′ × 10′ catch pen adjacent to a work area that is clear of debris, well lit, level, and dry. It should have electrical power or extension cords in place. One solid wall or sturdy fence should be available. Rope halters must be available for the sheep if needed. The animals should be in the catch pen when you arrive.

RESTRAINT: Sheep will be individually caught in the small pen by quietly approaching from behind and grabbing the lower jaw and quickly pointing the nose up. The other hand will grab the tail and use this to direct and encourage movement. A flank catch could be used if all the sheep are standing in the corner with their heads down. The sheep will be moved out of the catch pen to prevent damage to the ultrasound machine and operator. The sheep can be straddled with two hands on the jaw, or one hand on the jaw and another on the rump, with knee on the shoulder pushing the sheep against the wall to accomplish the procedures. The sheep could also be set up on their rumps for bleeding. The sheep should be marked and returned to the catch pen rather than released since there are so few animals to be worked.

Activities

Multiple Choice Questions

(Answers can be found in the back of the book.)

1. While at the edge of the flight zone of a small ruminant, moving from the front to the rear of the animal will make the animal:
   A move backward
   B move forward
   C turn to face you
   D stop

2. While at the edge of the flight zone of a small ruminant, moving from the rear to the front of the animal will make it:
   A move backward
   B move forward
   C turn to face you
   D stop

3. Which of the following will not prevent a sheep from moving forward?
   A person standing in front of its shoulder
   B a dark dead end or right-hand corner
   C flapping coats or cloth on the gates
   D a well-lit opening where it can see herd mates

4. A llama or alpaca:
   A is difficult to halter train
   B should have a well fitted halter with the nose band high on the nose resting on bone
   C will never spit at a human
   D is often worked by stock dogs

5. Acceptable methods of catching a goat include all of the following except:
   A grabbing its collar
   B having it come to the milking parlor or stand
   C looping an arm around the goat's neck
   D using a shepherd's crook on a hind leg

6. Restraining an adult sheep is easily done by all but:
   A setting up on its rump
   B holding its jaw in one hand and using a knee in its flank to hold it against a wall
   C hanging on to handfuls of wool
   D straddling its back and pressing knees into its shoulders and holding its head

7. Where is the best place to stand while restraining an alpaca?
   A directly in front of the head
   B at the shoulder near the body
   C even with the hips and one foot away
   D behind the animal holding onto the tail

8. Why do you need to point the nose of the sheep upward while restraining?
   A because it cannot walk if it cannot see its feet
   B to check for nasal bots
   C because it is much more powerful when its head is down
   D so it does not spit on you

9. When setting up a sheep, you should:
   A lift the sheep 3–6 in off the ground
   B have it sitting straight up directly on its tail
   C use its weight to shift it off balance and slide it down your legs to the floor
   D throw it down onto its rump

10. Signs of increased agitation and displeasure include all except:
   A spitting
   B ears flat against the neck
   C screams and screeches
   D tail curved all the way forward over the back

11. What is not true regarding use of nose tongs in cattle?
   A used alone, may cause tearing of the nasal septum
   B may be used in place of anesthesia for significantly painful procedures
   C if the nose tongs are tied, a quick release knot should be used
   D usually only effective for short periods

12. What is true regarding use of a halter and chain for restraint on horses?
   A pressure should always be removed as a reward when they do what they are asked
   B should never be used as a restraint device on horses
   C can be used over the nose but never under the chin
   D is only effective when used in collaboration with injectable anesthesia

Test Your Learning

1. When working with animals in a race/chute system, what are the best ways to get and keep the animals moving forward?
2. What does it mean to use minimal restraint?
3. Why must an alpaca or llama halter be well fitted?
4. List the different handling points where your hands and legs should go when holding sheep and goats.
5. Describe two ways cria's could be restrained.
6. Describe two restraint methods that can be used to inspect a cow's foot.

Answers can be found in the back of the book.

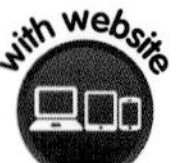

Extra review questions, case studies, and a breed ID image bank can be found online at www.wiley.com/go/loly/veterinary.

Chapter 3

History

Stacie K. Seymour, DVM and Sue Loly, LVT, VTS (EVN)

Learning Objectives

- Describe the role of the veterinary technician in taking a patient history.
- List questions that are commonly asked when obtaining a ruminant history.
- List questions that are commonly asked when obtaining an equine history.
- List questions that are commonly asked when obtaining a camelid history.
- List questions that are commonly asked when obtaining a porcine history.
- Differentiate a herd history and an individual patient history.

Clinical Case Problem 3.1

A large dairy producer has several cows that are off-feed and have decreased milk production. Before the veterinarian goes out to this farm call, a thorough history can be obtained. What questions would you ask this producer in order to obtain a history for the veterinarian?

See Clinical Case Resolution 3.1 at the end of this chapter.

Key Terms

Caseous
Colic
Days in milk
Freshening
Herd health
Lactation
Lameness
Off-feed
Open-ended question
Ruminant

Introduction

Obtaining a thorough history and physical exam is the first step that should be taken when any animal is seen by a veterinary professional. The veterinary technician must be able to ask open-ended questions and based on the client's answers, generate additional questions. The answers to these questions will guide the client to provide further details to create a full picture of what has transpired and therefore a thorough history. A large animal history will include the signalment of the animal or animals. Breed knowledge is important as some breeds are predisposed to certain diseases. The presenting complaint, the onset, the duration, and any clinical signs the animal(s) may be exhibiting are also included in the history.

It is important to note that large animals are usually kept together in a herd. These animals share food, water, and shelter. Living in a herd situation can cause competition for these resources and allow for disease transmission. Because of this, large animal medicine looks at herd health and prevention as well as individual animal health. If many animals are showing clinical signs, the veterinarian will look for a common cause to which all the animals are exposed. This may mean euthanizing one of the sick animals to perform a necropsy to obtain diagnostic answers. This can be done through gross observation and/or sampling and submission for additional testing.

Large Animal Medicine for Veterinary Technicians, Second Edition. Edited by Sue Loly and Heather Hopkinson.

Companion website: www.wiley.com/go/loly/veterinary

Biosecurity is important in large herd situations as many animals can be exposed to an infectious disease if proper precautions are not instituted and followed. Diseases such as brucellosis, contagious ecthyma, and tuberculosis are all zoonotic diseases, therefore veterinary professionals need to adhere to biosecurity precautions to safeguard clients and the veterinary team.

The patient or herd history will usually focus on the current chief complaint, and much of this information can be taken before the veterinarian even sees the animals. Several of the questions being asked will pertain to all large animal species, such as vaccination status, history, and diet. A technician must be knowledgeable about the management practices utilized for each species. Familiarity with terminology that is used for each species and their life stage will allow for better communication with the producer.

TECHNICIAN TIP 3.1: Have a check-off list of questions as a guide while taking a history.

History information that will be consistent among large animal species include:

- Housing: barn, confinement, stall, pasture, comingling species
- Feed and Water: type, source, changes
- Herd health status: disease free, currently being tested, culling program
- Animal contact: new additions, fence line, transportation, shows/competition
- Animal use: dairy, meat, fiber, pet, competition

TECHNICIAN TIP 3.2: Areas of interest in a large animal history include: housing, feed and water, herd health status, animal contact, and animal use.

Table 3.1 Medical species terminology versus common name species.

Species	Term
Equine	Horse
Bovine	Cattle
Caprine	Goats
Ovine	Sheep
Porcine	Pigs
Camelid	Llamas and Alpacas
Poultry	Chickens

Table 3.2 Parturition terms for large animal species.

Species	Term
Equine	Foaling
Bovine	Calving
Caprine	Kidding
Ovine	Lambing
Camelid	Parturition
Porcine	Farrowing
Poultry	Hatching

Production animals are commonly grouped by age and/or reproductive status. This allows the owner/producer to appropriately manage resources and give animals suitable nutrition for their current life stage. It is important to note that feed and bedding may not always be located on the same farm with the animals. Larger operations may have to ship in all feed and bedding resources, sourcing them from multiple vendors. This can present challenges in obtaining consistent feed and bedding quality.

Reproduction constitutes a significant portion of large animal practice. Keeping breeding stock healthy helps to ensure the health of the neonate. A reproductive history can be extensive or very straightforward (Table 3.2). Reproduction of large animal species is covered in Chapter 9.

Equine

Today's horse is primarily utilized for recreational purposes in the United States. Equine events are held across the country and horses travel long distances, crossing state lines, and transporting possibly infectious disease hundreds to thousands of miles. Details that must be included in a history are travel history, dates, and exposure to new horses. As with other species, vaccination and deworming histories are also important. Ask if the horse is insured, as additional paperwork will need to be accessed (Figure 3.1). If the horse needs medical treatment or surgery, the insurance company contacts will need to be available. Horses can be insured for loss of use, mortality, or surgery, and the type of coverage could be a determining factor in patient outcome (Table 3.3).

TECHNICIAN TIP 3.3: Horses can be transported hundreds or thousands of miles to attend equestrian events, possibly carrying infectious disease with them.

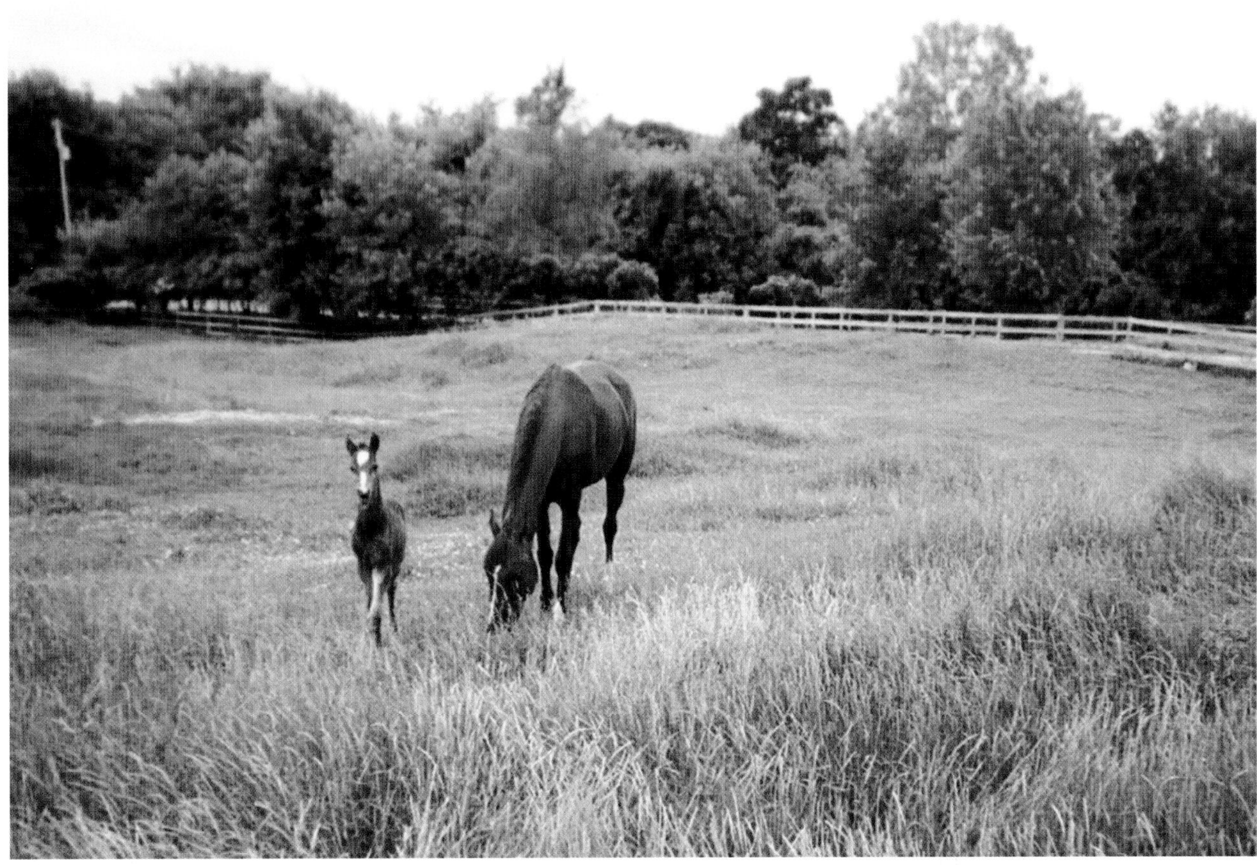

Figure 3.1 Mare and foal grazing on lush pasture grasses.

Table 3.3 Equine age terms.

Life stage	Term
Neonate	Foal
Weanling	Young horse ~5 months to 1 year old
Yearling	Young horse 1–1½ years old
Young female <3 years	Filly
Young male <3 years	Colt
Mature female	Mare
Older mare that has not given birth	Maiden
Mature male	Stallion
Castrated male	Gelding

TECHNICIAN TIP 3.4: Horses may be insured for loss of use, mortality, or surgery.

Horses are used in many disciplines, such as racing, dressage, eventing, polo, endurance, and trail riding. All of these activities require the horse to be sound and physically fit. Lameness is one of the most common reasons horses need veterinary services. Many times, a horse will have chronic lameness issues, and the history for the horse can be very lengthy. Questions should include prior known injury, shoeing changes, joint injections, surgeries, other treatments, and the outcomes of these activities. Ask if previous radiographs have been taken and are available. Lameness exams can be very time-consuming and frustrating, so organizing an extensive history will be beneficial (Figures 3.2 and 3.3).

TECHNICIAN TIP 3.5: For lameness exams, ask whether previous radiographs are available.

Colic is a common ailment among horses and many times, it warrants an emergency call. When dealing with a horse that is experiencing colic, it is very important to note the last time the horse defecated, ate, or drank. In the case of a mare, it is also important to note if she is pregnant. Ask about any client interventions or treatments and about the patient's response as well. Emergencies become hectic, so

Equine Lameness History Form Date________________

Owner______________________________ AnimalName:____________________

DOB______________ Breed:______________ ______Sex__________ Insured? Yes No

Company and Phone #:______________________________________Type: _____________

Intended Use:____

Current level of competition: ____

Duration of lameness? ____

Shod: Front Hind Both Date last shoeing:__________________________________

Wounds or swellings on limbs?____

When is lameness noticed?____

Does the lameness get better or worse with exercise?__________________________

Housing: ____

Previous lameness or trauma: ____

Current medications or supplements:____

____

Previous evaluation of lameness?____

____

Past Surgeries or Injections or other Treatments:_______________________________

____

____

Response to treatment:____

Additional History:____

____

____

____

Figure 3.2 Equine Lameness History Form.

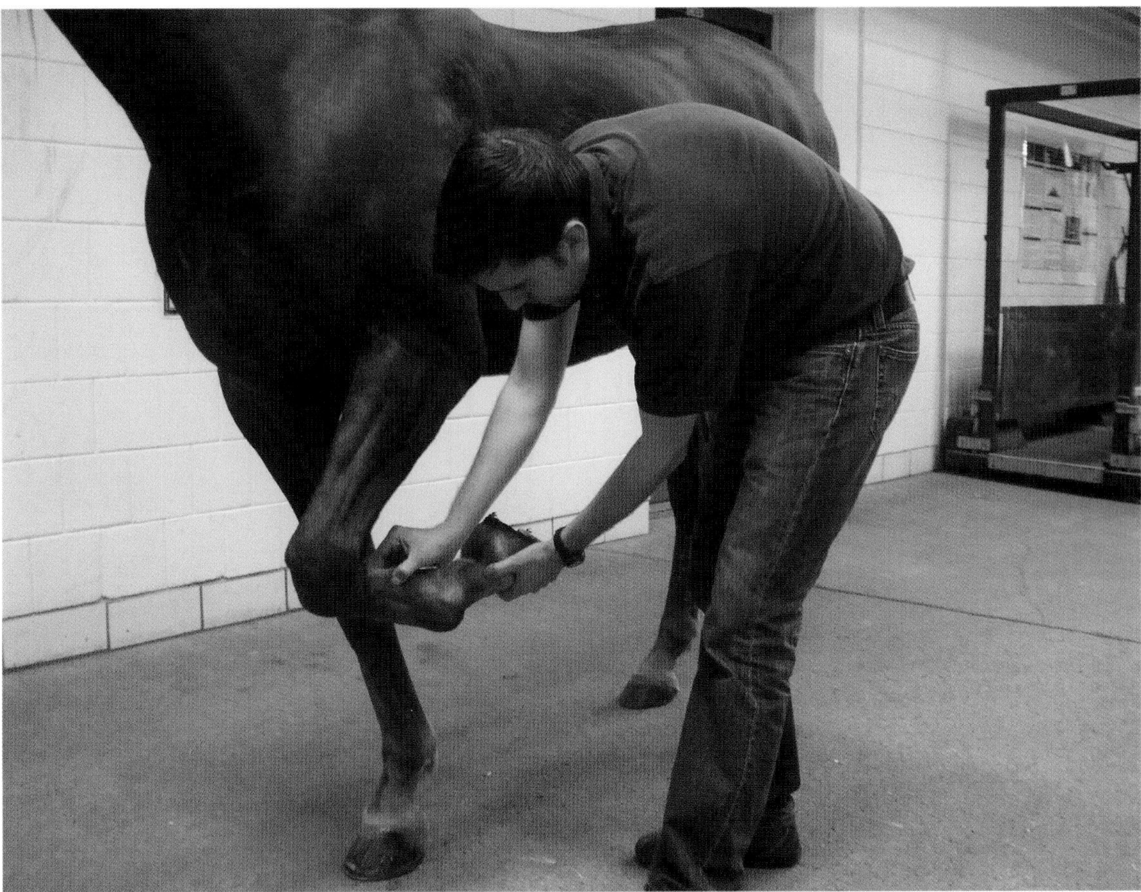

Figure 3.3 Palpation of an equine distal limb during a lameness exam.

using a history form will allow for a thorough history. Check out Chapter 4 for more on colic in the horse (Figure 3.4).

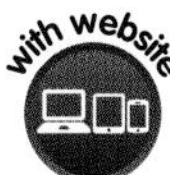

Don't forget to check the website for additional reference including a Breed ID image bank of different species.

Ruminants

Table 3.4 Ruminant age terms.

Life stage	Bovine	Caprine	Ovine
Neonate	Calf	Kid	Lamb
Young female	Heifer	Doe kid	Ewe lamb
Young male	Bull	Buck kid	Ram lamb
Mature female	Cow	Doe	Ewe
Mature male	Bull	Buck	Ram
Castrated male	Steer	Wether	Wether

Cattle

The management practices and the environment of bovine production animals differ greatly from that of small animal species. The difference is herd health and prevention versus individual health. Production animals in the United States are kept in close proximity to each other, and disease can spread quickly in a short amount of time. It is important to note if clinical signs are seen in more than one animal. Environmental factors can affect herd health, and abrupt feed changes may affect several animals at one time. Cattle tend to be housed by age groups and reproductive status, so it is important to tailor history questions to fit the age group. Animals that are presenting with reproductive problems will have very specific history questions regarding their reproductive status. Cattle fall into two production categories: beef or dairy. Beef production medicine deals primarily with young cattle that are destined for slaughter, whereas dairy production medicine focuses on replacement heifers and the adult lactating cow.

All ruminants are foregut fermenters, a unique digestive system where the stomach is divided into four chambers.

Date____________________

Owner__________________________ Animal Name:____________________

DOB____________ Breed:__________________ Sex_______ Insured? Yes No

Company and Phone#:_______________________________ Type:__________

Use of Horse:___________________ Pregnant? Yes No Due date:____________

Prior episodes of colic: how many and type?________________________________

When were the signs of colic first observed?________________________________

When was the horse last seen to be normal?________________________________

What signs is the horse currently exhibiting?________________________________

____

Have any medications been given and what has been the response?__________________

____

When was feces last passed?____________ When did the horse last urinate?________

Current Feed: Type/Amount/Schedule____________________________________

____

Recent changes in feed?:____

Housing:____________________ Bedding used:___________________________

Access to sandy soil?______________ Indiscriminant appetite?_____________________

Access to water, any changes?____

Last deworming and product used:______________________________________

Date of last dental examination:______________________________________

Recent stressors?(transport, foaling, weaning)_____________________________

Current medications or supplements:____________________________________

____

Contact with other horses?____

Any other horses showing signs of colic?_________________________________

Past colic surgery?____

Additional History:____

Figure 3.4 Equine Colic History Form.

The main fermentation chamber is the rumen, and it contains bacteria and protozoa that break down the large amount of cellulose in their diets. There is a delicate balance between the food that is digested and the bacteria and protozoa that will survive and reproduce to maintain the balanced rumen. During a dietary imbalance, bacteria can produce more gas than the animal can expel and cause bloat. Due to this concern, it is important to always inquire about the animal's diet and if the animal has ever suffered bloat.

Dairy Cattle

Generally, cows give birth and start their first lactation by the age of two. The calf is taken from the cow shortly after birth and is bottle-fed colostrum. Bull calves are usually sold, and heifer calves are kept as replacement heifers. Heifers may be reared at the milking facility or shipped to another farm to be raised to breeding age, bred, then returned to the milking facility before freshening.

History questions for dairy cows should include the date of freshening, days in milk, what lactation she is in, and if she is off-feed. Dairy producers keep records of pounds of milk the cow has produced and what lactation she is in based on her age. These records may show trends in milk production and also give an indication of where in her lactation the cow became sick. This is very useful information to provide in the history (Figures 3.5 and 3.6).

TECHNICIAN TIP 3.6: Dairy calves are taken away from their dam shortly after birth.

Beef Cattle

Beef cattle are usually kept on pastures and producers choose to have the cow calves in the spring. Beef calves are kept with the cows as cow/calf pairs until weaning. After weaning, bull calves are castrated and raised for slaughter. Heifers can also be raised for slaughter but may be used as replacement stock.

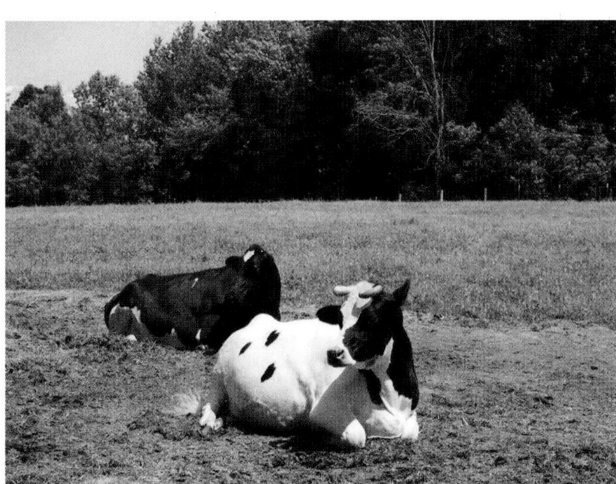

Figure 3.5 Two dry cows on pasture. *Source:* Courtesy of Farmaste Animal Sanctuary.

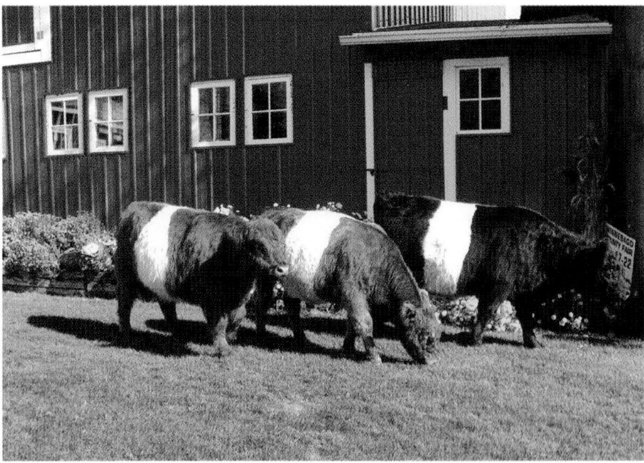

Figure 3.6 Tricolor Belted Galloway cattle on pasture. *Source:* Courtesy of Klover Korner farms.

TECHNICIAN TIP 3.7: Beef calves stay with their dam until weaning.

History questions of importance in beef cattle include a thorough vaccination and deworming history. Feedlot cattle have many stressors: new animals, weather, feed changes, and transportation. All of these can take its toll on the immune system and affect disease state and clinical signs (Figure 3.7).

Goats

Caprine species, like cattle, fall into dairy or meat production categories. They are also popular for 4-H programs where children learn to raise and care for animals. Some goat breeds, such as Angora and Cashmere, are also used for their fiber. History questions that pertain to dairy production will be the same as those listed for dairy cattle. Herd status for caseous lymphadenitis (CL) and caprine arthritis encephalitis (CAE) should also be noted. Hobby farm or homestead owners with only a few pet goats may be less informed about those types of diseases and may also be unaware of the herd of origin's health history.

Goat producers should be asked about vaccination and deworming programs. Internal parasites that plague small ruminants have become more and more resistant to deworming medications; therefore, it is very important to know the dewormers being used, frequency of use, and whether their use is rotated.

Food/ Fiber Animal History Form Date___________________

Owner____________________________ Animal Name/Tag #______________________

Weight:_________ Species________ DOB________ Breed______________ Sex________

Presenting problem:___________________ Duration:__________________________

Feed:____

Change in feed or water intake?__________________________Weight Loss?____________

Changes in urination/defecation?_____________________Activity Level?_______________

Housing:____

Vaccinations Dates and Vaccine:____

____

Herd Disease Status:____

Deworming Dates and Products:____

____

Most Recent Parurition:____

Previous Illness or Trauma:____

Milk Production in #'s_______ Days in Milk:___________ Lactation #:______ Pregnant: No Yes

Date Bred:______________Animals in herd with similar signs:___________________________

New animal contact or recent transport:_______________________________________

Past Treatments:____

____

____

Additional History:____

____

____

____

Figure 3.7 Food/Fiber Animal History Form.

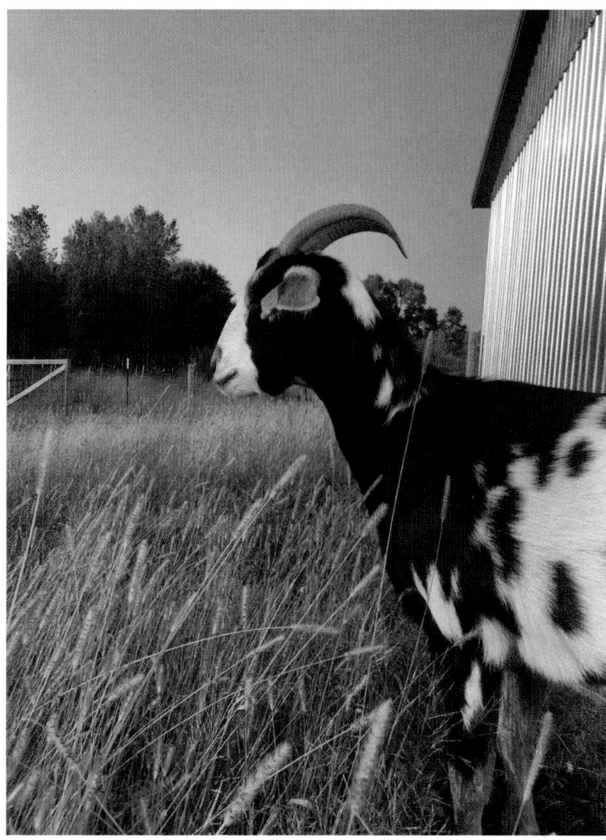

Figure 3.8 Alpine and pigmy goats are common as hobby farm pets. *Source:* Courtesy of Farmaste Animal Sanctuary.

Diet is also important to discuss in the history taking. Diet tends to be regulated with larger herd, but pet goats, especially those housed with other species, may have access to other feeds, such as rich alfalfa hay. Male goats are often culled as pets from dairy farms; they can commonly present for diet-related urinary stones and blockages (Figure 3.8).

> **TECHNICIAN TIP 3.8:** Angora and Cashmere goats are generally raised for their fiber.

Sheep

Ovine species are utilized for meat and/or wool. Goats are more popular for milk production due to their adaptable personalities, although several breeds of sheep can be used for milk production as well. Sheep are also popular for 4-H activities though they are less commonly found as single pets. Questions that pertain to sheep will be the same as those for goats. Two additional questions specific to sheep would be herd scrapie status and availability of copper in the diet (Figure 3.9).

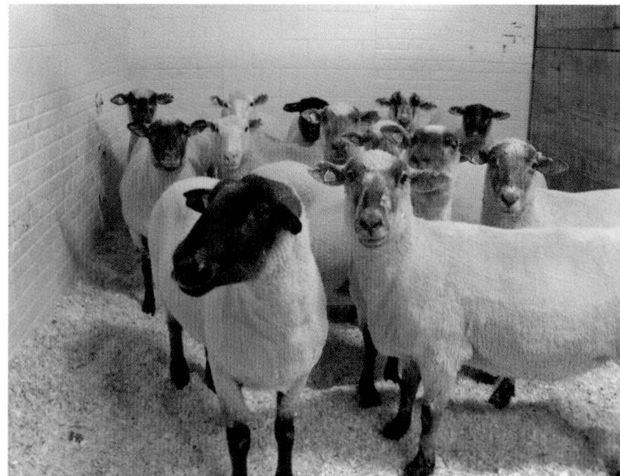

Figure 3.9 Herd of Hampshire sheep.

> **TECHNICIAN TIP 3.9:** Some breeds of sheep are raised for milk production.

Camelids

Alpacas, llamas, and camels comprise most of the common camelids that are seen in veterinary medicine. Llamas and alpacas are shown in competition and utilized for their fiber. These animals are very hardy and do not succumb to many diseases (Table 3.5). History questions that should be asked are similar to that of sheep and goats. Camelids can have dental issues that differ from other ruminant species. Questions about weight loss or problems eating should be included in a camelid history. Some owners may be unaware of weight loss due to the coverage of the animal's fiber; it is often necessary to palpate the back and neck to feel the body condition (Figure 3.10).

Alpacas and llamas are also susceptible to internal parasites; therefore, deworming schedules and deworming medication resistance should be noted on the history form. For the most part, llamas and alpacas use a communal or shared dung (manure) pile. There may be one or two areas in their pen or pasture that they all utilize, much different

Table 3.5 Camelid age terms.

Life stage	Term
Neonate	Cria
Female	Female
Male	Male
Castrated male	Gelding

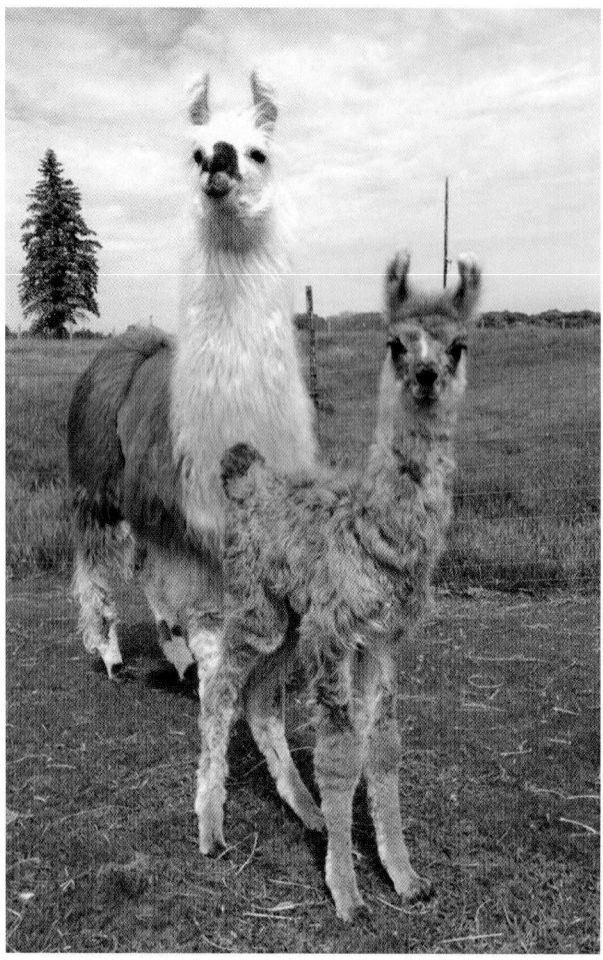

Figure 3.10 A Llama female with her cria. *Source:* Courtesy of Paul Weinand.

than goats and sheep that tend to go everywhere and anywhere. Additionally, male alpacas and llamas urinate backward between the hind legs because the tip of the sheath points caudally and the penis is not extended during urination, unlike the other mammals discussed in this book.

> **TECHNICIAN TIP 3.10:** Llamas and Alpacas commonly share a communal dung pile.

> **TECHNICIAN TIP 3.11:** Male alpacas and llamas urinate backward between the hind legs because the tip of the sheath points caudally and the penis is not extended during urination.

Porcine

Porcine industry medicine focuses on prevention and biosecurity in the herd. Most hogs are raised in a confinement setting, and while this type of management has benefits and challenges, the confinement setting has made successful herd management and biosecurity a top priority. The confinement environment should be evaluated when getting a history. Temperature, air quality, flooring, hygiene, and disinfectants used in the building may give clues as to what is causing herd problems. If automated systems are malfunctioning due to electrical outage or breakage, many animals can be affected. Vaccination and herd disease status should be noted along with antiparasitic protocols.

Table 3.6 Porcine age terms.

Life stage	Term
Neonate	Piglet
Young female	Gilt
Weaner	Piglet that has been weaned from sow 3–5 weeks of age
Starter	Pig that is approximately 5–10 weeks of age
Grower	Pig that is approximately 10–16 weeks of age
Finisher	Pig that is approximately 16–24 weeks of age
Young male	Boar
Mature female	Sow
Mature male	Boar
Castrated male	Barrow

Pet pig are becoming ever popular and are allowed in more urban setting than in years past. Pet pig management can be different from production pig in that, there may be only one rather than a herd. Some owners will keep pet pigs in a barn and in the yard, while others will have them in the home and intermingled with other pets like dogs and cats. They can be house trained like domestic dog, but it is important for owners to realize they are very different from dogs. They naturally enjoy rooting, whether it be under a blanket or some straw. They require special care of their skin/hair coat as well as tusk and toenail maintenance to avoid overgrowth. Pet pigs are more likely to have a varied diet; therefore, it is important to get a detailed nutritional history (Figures 3.11 and 3.12).

> **TECHNICIAN TIP 3.12:** Temperature, air quality, flooring, hygiene, and disinfectants used in swine housing may give clues to herd problems.

Poultry

Poultry production on a large scale can be complex and is not covered in this book; however, backyard/urban fowl and homestead popularity has been on the rise; therefore,

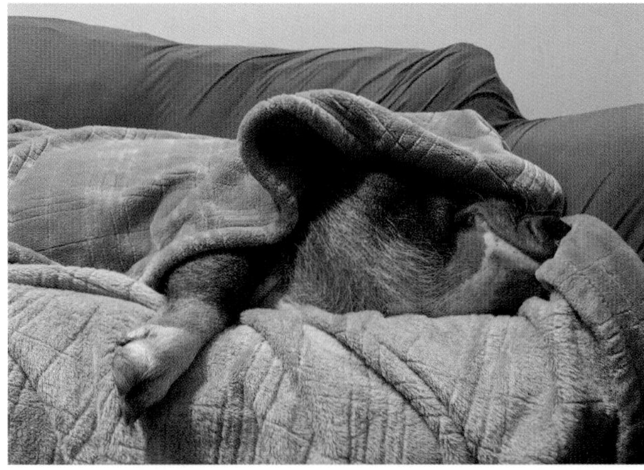

Figure 3.11 Potbelly pig relaxing on a couch and rooted under a blanket. *Source:* Courtesy of Siri Rea.

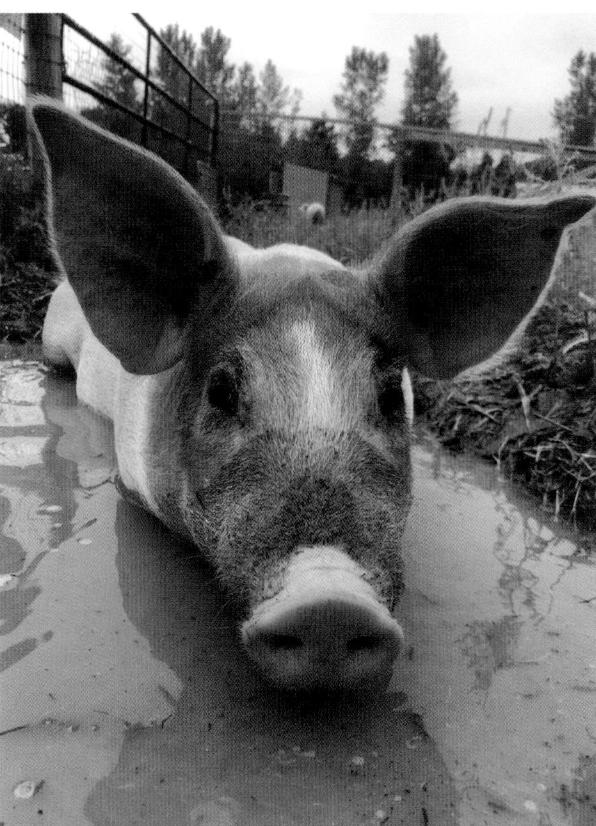

Figure 3.12 Pig enjoying a mud soak. *Source:* Courtesy of Farmaste Animal Sanctuary.

general terms and knowledge are included in reference to small homestead and urban production only.

Backyard poultry medicine focuses on prevention and biosecurity in the flock. Most commercial birds are raised in a confinement setting, while homestead production birds are more often raised in a private coop, usually with a caged run and free-range opportunities. The term "free range" in the production world is quite different than in a private ownership.

Table 3.7 Poultry terms.

Hen	Female bird from the poultry family.
Rooster	A male bird from the poultry family, also known as a cockerel or cock.
Capon	Cockerel (rooster) that has been castrated.
Chick	A young bird, newly hatched with only down feathers.
Starter Pullet	A young hen, 0–6 weeks of age.
Grower Pullet	A young hen, 6–14 weeks, has regular feathers.
Developer Pullet	A young hen, 14–20 weeks, and has not started laying eggs yet.
Layer	Egg laying hens, primarily used for production of food grade, unfertilized eggs.
Breeder	Egg laying hens used primarily for production of fertilized eggs in order to produce offspring for meat production or replacement layers.
Fryers	The smallest sized chicken bred and raised specifically for meat production and are dressed around 4 lb in about 7 weeks of age.
Broiler	Any chicken that is bred and raised specifically for meat production and are dressed around 6 lb at approximately 6 weeks of age.
Roaster	Any chicken that is bred and raised specifically for meat production and are dressed around 8–15 lb in 3–5 months. (12–20 weeks).
Dressed	Poultry slaughtered for human food, with head, feet, and viscera intact, and from which the blood and feathers have been removed.

The coop setting and security of the fenced area environment should be evaluated when getting a history. The coop design can widely vary, and some owners go to great lengths to create a home for their birds. Temperature, air quality, flooring, hygiene, and disinfectants used in the building may give clues as to what is causing flock problems. Vaccination and flock disease status should be noted along with antiparasitic protocols (Figures 3.13–3.14).

A popular way for owners to purchase chickens is to buy unhatched eggs and hatch them out themselves. Batches of chicks are also an option and a good way to diversify the variety. Batches can be ordered as all female, but inadvertently, there can be a male of two that get

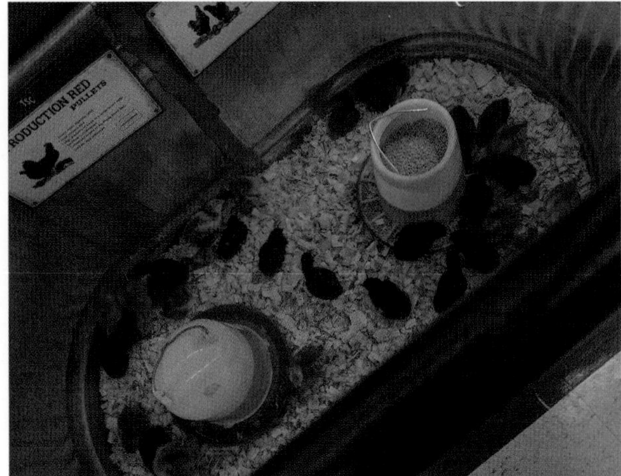

Figure 3.13 Urban Chicken Coop.

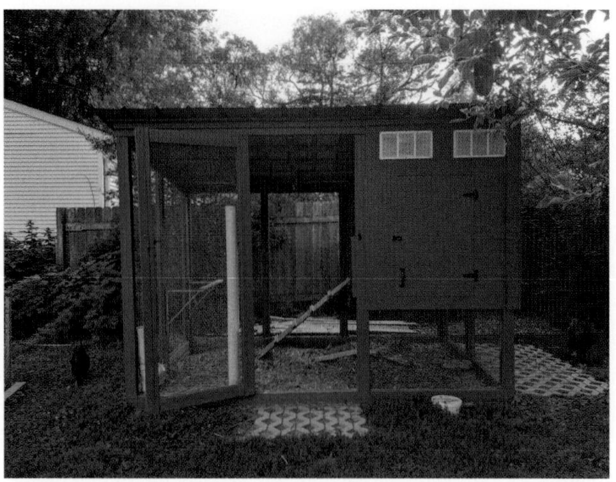

Figure 3.14 Mobile Chicken Coop.

mixed in the bunch. Gender of newborn chicks can be tricky to determine for even an experienced, and owners could easily find themselves with fertilized eggs in the coop (Figure 3.15).

TECHNICIAN TIP 3.13: Hens will naturally slow down egg production around six to seven years of age.

TECHNICIAN TIP 3.14: The decreased daylight in the fall tend to lead hens to stop laying eggs unless supplemented with light and warmth.

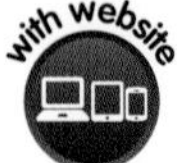

A coop reference guide is available in the online resources.

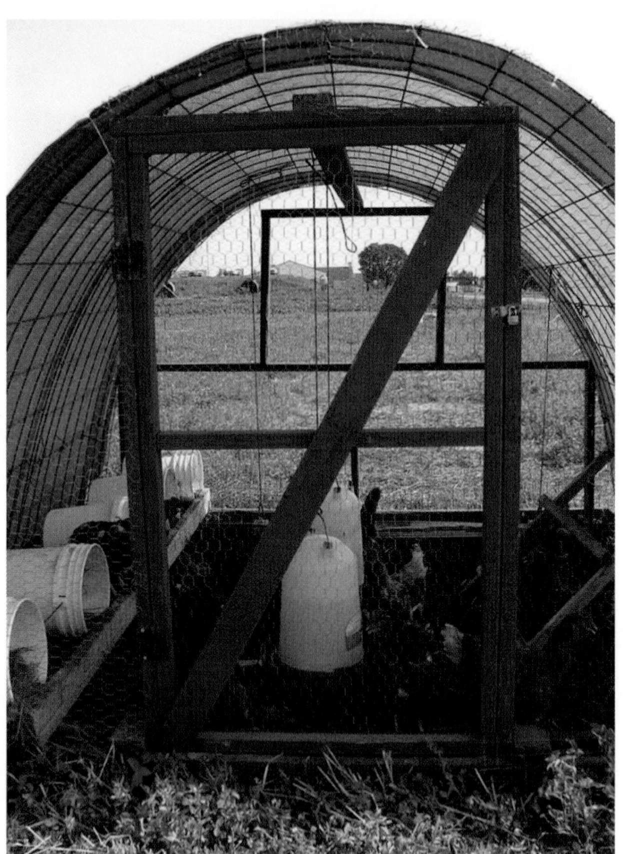

Figure 3.15 Hatchling Chicks in a brooder pen.

Multiple Species Management

Comingling of species in a pasture setting presents a unique challenge to the veterinary team when considering parasite load of a pasture. Animal housing and deworming schedules used by the owner is a required notation in the history, including parasitology testing and deworming medications. Sheep and goats generally comingle well together, as do llamas and alpacas.

References

Fowler, M. (2010). *Medicine and Surgery of Camelids*, 3e. Ames: Wiley Blackwell.

Jackson, P. and Cockcroft, P. (2007). *Handbook of Pig Medicine*, 1e. St. Louis: Saunders Elsevier.

McCurnin, D. and Bassert, J. (2010). *McCurnin's Clinical Textbook for Veterinary Technicians*, 7e. St. Louis: Elsevier Saunders.

Pugh, D.G. and Baird, A.N. (2012). *Sheep and Goat Medicine*, 2e. Maryland Heights: Saunders Elsevier.

"Raising Chickens for Eggs." Accessed January 19, 2021. https://extension.umn.edu/small-scale-poultry/raising-chickens-eggs.

Shapiro, L. (2001). *Introduction to Animal Science*, 1e. Upper Saddle River: Prentice-Hall.

Smith, B. (2009). *Large Animal Internal Medicine*, 4e. St. Louis: Mosby Elsevier.

Smith, M. and Sherman, D. (2009). *Goat Medicine*, 2e. Ames: Wiley Blackwell.

Clinical Case Resolution 3.1

Use Figure 3.7 as a guide to obtain the history. As you ask questions, the farmer may give you information that will help you gain more patient history and formulate additional questions. For this case, the presenting complaint is that several cows have decreased milk production and are off-feed. Based on this information, the following additional questions may prove beneficial as you are gathering a complete and thorough history.

- How many animals are affected?
- Are affected animals housed in the same location?
- What stage of lactation?
- Are there changes in feed sources/manufacturers?
- Are the animals exhibiting other signs?
- What are the ages of the animals affected?

Activities

Multiple Choice Questions

(Answers can be found in the back of the book.)

1. Which of the following is part of the signalment?
A age, breed, farm location
B age, breed, sex
C herd health status, farm location
D vaccination protocol, deworming protocol

2. Biosecurity refers to:
A isolation of bacteria
B measures taken to prevent transmission of disease to other animals
C security measures taken to ensure sterility of an area
D safe usage of biological agents

3. When taking a thorough history for an equine emergency exam, one must include the following:
A herd health status
B what lactation the mare is in
C if the horse is insured
D housing type

4. Bloat refers to:
A gas distension of the rumen, stomach, or cecum
B abnormal eating habits
C lack of feces
D abdominal pain

5. Animals in a herd environment:
A have more injuries than individually kept animals
B have decreased immunity
C share common resources that can increase disease transmission
D are more difficult to obtain a thorough history

6. Caprine refers to which species?
A cattle
B goats
C sheep
D alpacas

7. Ovine refers to which species?
A cattle
B goats
C sheep
D alpacas

8. Which of the following species is not a ruminant?
A horse
B sheep
C cow
D goat

9. Which species are more likely to be kept individually and have an extensive travel history?
A ovine
B camelid
C equine
D porcine

10. History questions that are common among all species include all of the following except?
A feed type and source
B access to water
C animal contact
D herd health status

Test Your Learning

1. Why is it important to note food and water sources in the history?
2. Why is it important to understand management practices when taking a history?
3. Why is biosecurity so important in our large animal species?
4. Large animal medicine leans more toward herd health, how is this different than small animal medicine?
5. Why is the intended use of the animal important to note in the history?

Answers can be found in the back of the book.

Extra review questions, case studies, and a Breed ID image bank can be found online at www.wiley.com/go/loly/veterinary.

Chapter 4

Physical Exam

Scott R.R. Haskell, DVM, MPVM, PhD, Bonnie L. Loghry, BAS, MPH, RVT, Carrie J. Finno, DVM, PhD, DACVIM, Kristen Wegner-Fowley, DVM, DACVAA, Erin Matheson Barr, RVT, Jamie DeFazio, AS, CVT, VTS (EVN), William Gilsenan, VMD, DACVIM (LAIM), and Amy L. Johnson, DVM, DACVIM (LAIM & Neurology)

Learning Objectives

- Describe components of the physical examination.
- Correlate clinical examination findings with pathophysiology and anatomical structure(s) affected.
- List the normal temperatures, pulse, and respiration rates for large animal species.
- Integrate species-specific behavior with abnormal physiologic states.
- Describe behavioral signs that indicate pain in equine patients.
- List the characteristics and clinical signs of disease within specific organ systems.
- Describe diagnostic procedures commonly utilized in the examination process.
- List the components of a SOAP (subjective objective assessment plan) medical record.

Clinical Case Problem 4.1

A five-year-old female alpaca, nine months pregnant, presents to your clinic with a history of acute onset of anorexia, lethargy, and weight loss. She is unable to rise in the stock trailer, has a dark fecal soiled perineal region, and is obviously dehydrated. The animal, though lethargic and nervous, has remained completely still during the transport. What pertinent immediate information do you need from the client? What are the first concerns for the alpaca's survival? How would you proceed with your initial comprehensive veterinary technician examination in light of these clinical signs?

See Clinical Case Resolution 4.1 at the end of this chapter.

Key Terms

Aortic stenosis (AS)
Assessment
Atrial fibrillation
Auscultation
Bacterial endocarditis
Ballottement
Blepharospasm
Body condition score (BCS)
Borborygmi
Bright alert responsive (BAR)
Bruxism
Buphthalmos
Capillary refill time (CRT)
Cornea
Descemet's membrane
Evaluation
Gastrointestinal (GI)
Hydrophilic
Hydrophobic
Interpretation
Left displaced abomasum (LDA)
Mentation
Mitral valve insufficiency (MVI)
Patent ductus arteriosus (PDA)
Pathophysiology
Percussion
Problem list
Pulmonic stenosis (PS)
Pupillary light response (PLR)
Quiet alert responsive (QAR)
Reticulopericarditis
Right displaced abomasal torsion (RTA)

(*continued*)

Large Animal Medicine for Veterinary Technicians, Second Edition. Edited by Sue Loly and Heather Hopkinson.

Companion website: www.wiley.com/go/loly/veterinary

Key Terms (*continued*)

Right displaced abomasum (RDA)
Somnolent
Subjective objective assessment plan (SOAP)
Temperature, pulse, respiration (TPR)
Tenesmus
Tricuspid valve insufficiency (TVI)
Ventricular septal defect (VSD)
Within normal limits (WNL)

Introduction

The veterinary technician performs many duties during the course of a day's work, few so important as the physical exam (PE) that provides a "snapshot in time" health status of the animal. The PE helps determine the exact nature of any underlying illness and monitors disease progression. By determining the animal's condition, the veterinary team can provide diagnostic, treatment, and nursing procedures to improve the patient's ability to heal and return to full health and performance. This chapter will outline many key observational and interpretive methods that veterinary technicians use to determine current health status as well as interpreting and reporting behavioral and physiologic responses of equine patients experiencing pain.

Communicating patient status, especially abnormal findings, is typically done through medical records called SOAPs. SOAP is an acronym that stands for Subjective, Objective, Assessment, and Plan, and is a standardized method to write progress notes in the medical record. Veterinary Technicians typically complete the "S" and "O" of the SOAP, as these portions are based on observations or specific patient data gathered during the PE and fall within the legal abilities of the credentialed veterinary technician. The "A" and "P," or assessment and plan portion of the record, requires a conclusion, whether a presumptive or final diagnosis, prognosis, or further diagnostic testing and treatment, and would require a licensed veterinarian to make these determinations. In some hospitals the medical records may require that each patient problem be SOAP-ed individually, but most hospitals use a system where one SOAP is written for the patient.

Signalment

The physically distinguishing features of the large animal patient or herd should be specifically recorded at the outset of the examination to establish legal and logistical identity. Establishing each animal or herd's identity is important regardless of outcome, but in cases where evidence may need to be collected for toxic death, feed-related issues, mismanagement, or cruelty/neglected cases, precise identification is vital (Figure 4.1). When including data from a herd check, adequate animal identification may be difficult, such as with range cattle or poultry. Repeat visits warrant some form of individual animal identification for follow-up purposes. Patient observation and treatment require that the correct patient or pen/lot number be recorded and easily traced. Tracing animals is important when drug residue violations may be detected or in the event that an exotic or reportable disease outbreak has occurred. Additionally, repeat visits from the veterinary team require adequate patient identification (Table 4.1).

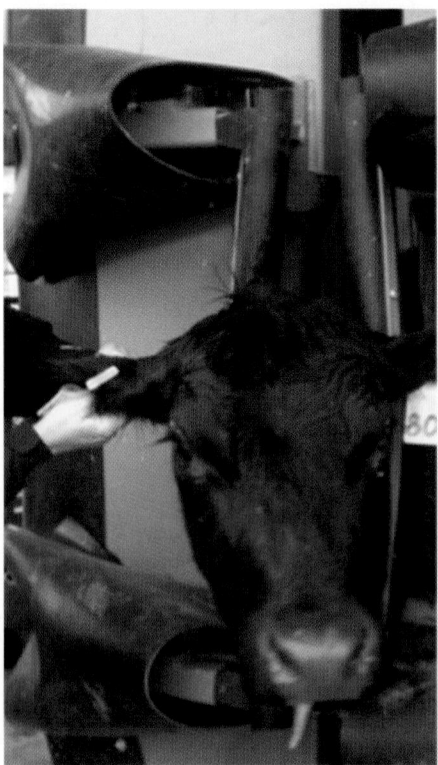

Figure 4.1 Establish individual or herd identification through distinguishing marks, color, or tags for legal and logistical identity.

Table 4.1 An animal's signalment contains information about the animal, such as species, breed, age, and sexual status and should be included in the patient's medical record.

Components of signalment
Species
Breed
Name/number
Sex
Color/markings
Weight
BCS
Identification: tattoos, ear tags, microchip, brands

Dependent on species and farm or ranch management, the PE may be performed for an individual and/or herd. PEs should be performed in a systematic manner using a body system approach, unless an emergency necessitates a limited examination.

When performing a PE on the farm, a quick evaluation on where the animal is kept, past or current treatments, how the animal is used, and other results from a comprehensive history (described in Chapter 3) can provide clues as to how to proceed with the PE. Thoroughly understanding the normal physical examination parameters for each species is necessary to identify any abnormalities (Table 4.2).

Interpersonal communication skills are extremely important to clarify essential issues and to determine the desires and concerns of the client. Results of the PE as well as the wishes of the client can lead the veterinary technician to discuss with the veterinarian possible laboratory or diagnostic testing or nursing procedures that would need to be performed to improve or optimize animal and herd health.

Equine Physical Exam

A complete physical examination of the horse is necessary to determine the exact nature of underlying illness and to monitor disease progression. The veterinary technician must understand normal findings in adult horses and foals to accurately identify and prioritize abnormal findings. A systemic approach is necessary to perform a thorough physical examination. By organizing the examination into body systems, the examiner can classify abnormalities according to the body system they are associated with and thereby provide important insight into the underlying disease process. The examination can be broken into sections: signalment; observational examination; examination of the head, neck, thorax, forelimbs, abdomen, hindlimbs, and perineum; and an ambulatory examination. These sections allow the examiner to move around the horse in a systematic manner while completely evaluating all the body systems. Remember to always include the weight in the PE (Figure 4.2).

Signalment

As previously mentioned, signalment is absolutely essential in the identification of patients, whether as individuals or as herd members.

Table 4.2 Normal TPR parameters.

	Temperature range		Pulse	Respiration
	°F	°C	(beats/minute)	(breaths/minute)
Camelid (Alpaca)	99.5–102.0	37.5–38.9	70–120	10–30
Camelid (Llama)	99.5–102.0	37.5–38.9	60–90	10–30
Bovine (Mature)	100.0–102.5	37.8–39.2	40–80	10–30
Bovine (Yearling)	101.5–103.5	38.6–39.8	100–120	15–30
Ovine/Caprine	102.0–104.0	38.9–40.0	70–90	20–30
Swine (Mature)	100.0–102.5	37.8–38.9	70–90	10–24
Swine (Juvenile)	102.0–104.0	38.9–40.0	100–130	<50
Equine (Adult)	98.5–101.5	36.9–38.6	28–40	8–20
Equine (Neonate)	99.0–101.5	37.0–38.6	75–100	30–40

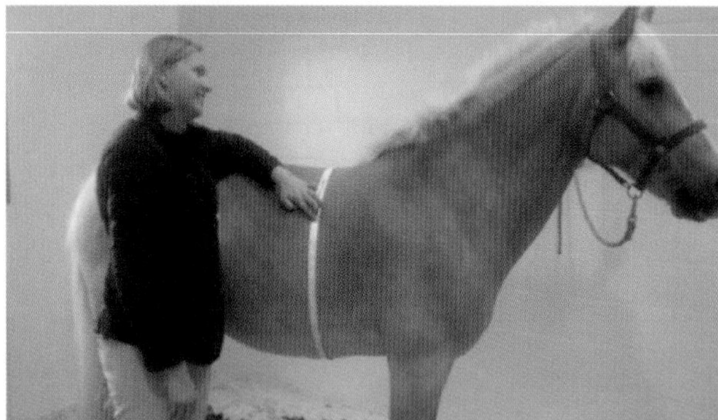

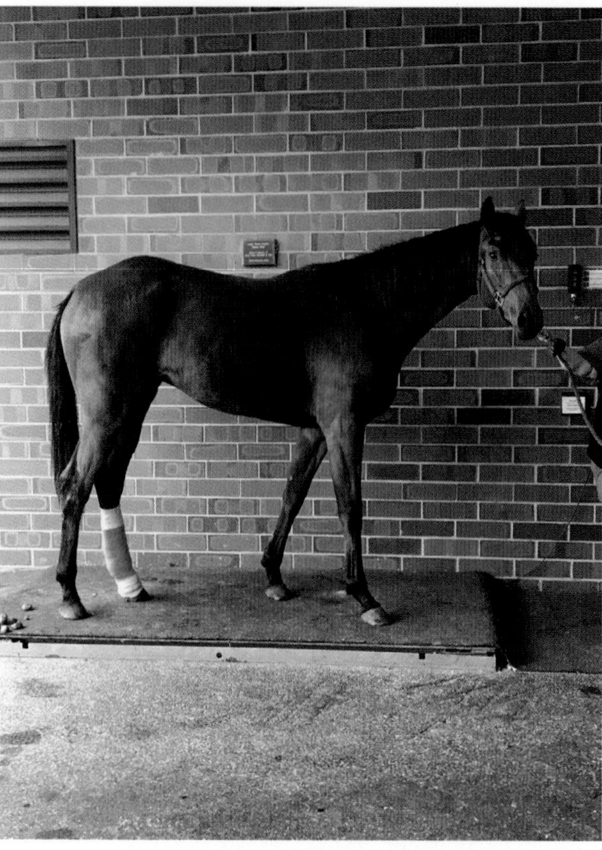

Figure 4.2 (**Left**) The use of a weight tape to measure the weight. (**Right**) Horse on a scale to get a more accurate weight.

Observational Examination

A complete physical examination of the horse begins with observing the patient either in the stall or paddock by using a hands-off approach. The horse's mentation and behavior should be noted before stimulation and can be classified into the following categories.

Mentation/Behavior

- Bright, alert, and responsive (BAR)
- Quiet, alert, and responsive (QAR)
- Agitated or painful
- Excessively quiet but able to be roused back to a normal state (somnolent; refrain from using the term depressed to describe a horse's behavior, lethargy can be substituted)
- Excessively quiet and unable to be roused back to a normal state (obtunded)
- Comatose

Additional Observations and Respiratory Rate

During this observation period, also note the presence of any manure in the stall and its consistency. Additionally, is there feed in the stall and does it appear that the horse has been eating?

> **TECHNICIAN TIP 4.1:** It is recommended to take a resting respiratory rate while observing the horse from a distance to obtain an accurate baseline reading.

Next, examine the horse's overall hair coat quality and length. Is it appropriate for the time of year and climate? Horses with excessively long hair coats that do not shed out could have a metabolic problem known as Cushing's disease. Finally, assign the horse a body condition score (BCS) on a scale of 1–9 with 5 being the perfect weight, 1 is excessively thin, and 9 is obese (Figure 4.3 and Table 4.3).

Adequate Restraint

After the observation period, place a halter and lead rope on the horse and have a handler provide adequate restraint for you to complete the rest of your examination. A handler must stand on the same side of the horse as the examiner. If the horse spooks suddenly, it will most likely move its haunches away from the side on which the handler stands and therefore away from the examiner. For the remaining portion of the physical examination, it is helpful to categorize PE findings into body systems.

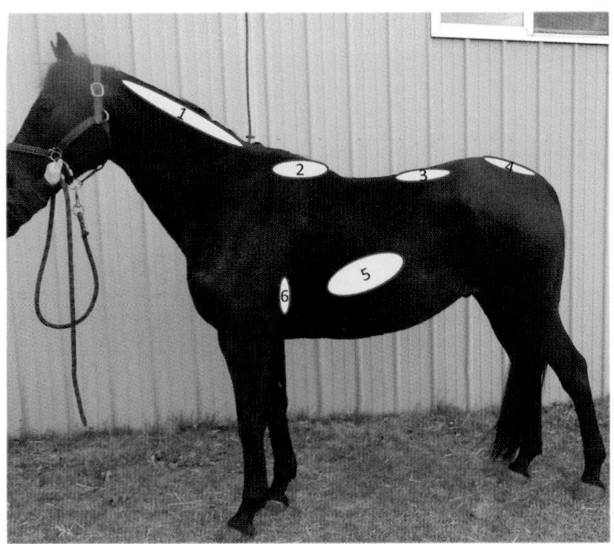

Figure 4.3 Locations used to determine a horse's BCS. Numbers correspond to anatomical locations in Table 4.3 as follows: 1 = neck; 2 = withers; 3 = loin; 4 = tailhead; 5 = ribs; 6 = shoulder.

Examination of the Head

Unless the horse is extremely head shy, the examination generally starts at the head. Stand directly in front of the horse and examine the face for symmetry. Are the eyelids symmetrically open and the ears symmetrically erect? Does the muzzle droop or pull to one side?

Is there any nasal or ocular discharge? If so, the discharge needs to be characterized and described by:

- Location (which side of the horse)
- Appearance (serous, mucoid, mucopurulent, or hemorrhagic)
- Presence or absence of any odor

While examining the nostrils, place your hand over each nostril to determine if there is adequate and symmetrical airflow. Percuss the maxillary and frontal sinuses. Sinus percussion is performed by tapping the end of the index finger over the sinus location. Normal sinuses produce a hollow sound whereas dull sounds may indicate fluid or soft tissue

Table 4.3 Body condition score.

Determine score in all 6 areas; divide total by 6						
Condition	**Neck**	**Withers**	**Loin**	**Tailhead**	**Ribs**	**Shoulder**
1 POOR	Bone structure easily noticeable	Bone structure easily noticeable	Spinous processes project prominently	Tailhead (pinbones) and hook bones project prominently	Ribs projecting prominently	Bone structures easily noticeable
	Animal extremely emaciated: no fatty tissue can be felt					
2 VERY THIN	Bone structure fairly discernible	Fairly discernible	Slight fat covering over base of spinous processes	Tailhead prominent	Ribs prominent	Bone structures fairly discernible
	Animal emaciated		Transverse processes of lumbar vertebrae feel rounded. Spinous processes are prominent			
3 THIN	Neck accentuated	Withers accentuated	Fat buildup halfway on spinous processes but easily discernable. Transverse processes cannot be felt	Tailhead prominent but individual vertebrae cannot be visually identified. Hook bones appear rounded but are still easily discernible. Pinbones not distinguishable	Slight fat cover over ribs. Ribs easily discernible	Shoulder accentuated
4 Moderately THIN	Neck not obviously thin	Withers not obviously thin	Negative crease along back	Prominence depends on conformation; fat can be felt. Hook bones not discernible	Faint outline discernible	Shoulder not obviously thin

(Continued)

Table 4.3 (Continued)

Determine score in all 6 areas; divide total by 6						
Condition	**Neck**	**Withers**	**Loin**	**Tailhead**	**Ribs**	**Shoulder**
5 MODERATE	Neck blends smoothly into body	Withers rounded over spinous processes	Back level	Fat around tailhead beginning to feel spongy	Ribs cannot be visually distinguished but can be easily felt	Shoulder blends smoothly into body
6 Moderately FLESHY	Fat beginning to be deposited	Fat beginning to be deposited	May have slight positive crease down back	Fat around tailhead feels soft	Fat over ribs feels spongy	Fat beginning to be deposited
7 FLESHY	Fat deposited along neck	Fat deposited along withers	May have positive crease down back	Fat around tailhead is soft	Individual ribs can be felt, but noticeable filling between ribs with fat	Fat deposited behind shoulder
8 FAT	Noticeable thickening of neck	Area along withers filled with fat	Positive crease down back	Tailhead fat very soft	Difficult to feel ribs	Area behind shoulder filled in flush with body
	Fat deposited along inner buttocks					
9 Extremely FAT	Bulging fat Fat along buttocks may rub together. Flank filled in flush.	Bulging fat	Obvious positive crease down back	Building fat around tailhead	Patchy fat appearing over ribs	Bulging fat

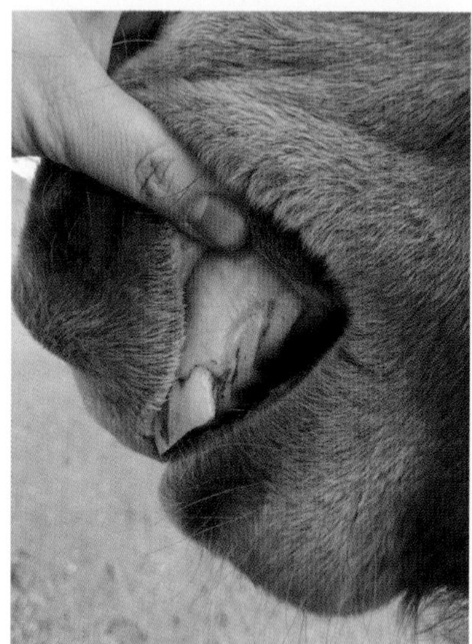
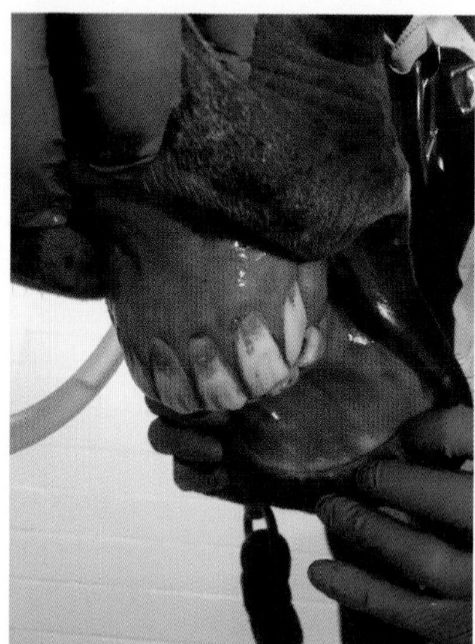
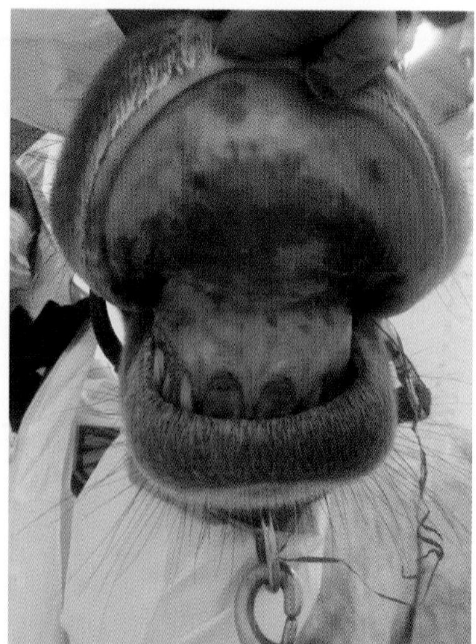

Figure 4.4 **Left**: normal gums **Middle:** toxic gums **Right:** purpura. *Source:* Courtesy of Kate L. Hepworth, DVM, DACVIM (LAIM).

formation in the sinuses. From the side of the horse, gently lift the upper lip or pull down the lower lip to examine the horse's gingiva. This is the best location to adequately assess mucous membranes in the horse, although other areas can be utilized such as vulva and conjunctiva. Examine the gingiva for color, consistency, and capillary refill time (CRT) (Figure 4.4).

These observations assess the horse's hydration status and blood volume. Examine the gingiva for any evidence of ulcerations, petechiations, or a toxic line. Note the presence of malodorous breath, halitosis, which could indicate a tooth root or sinus infection. Palpate the quality of the pulse, either under the jaw or adjacent to the eye below the zygomatic arch. The pulse should have a consistently strong quality. As previously mentioned, the pulse should be taken simultaneously with the heart rate to determine that there are no pulse deficits (Figures 4.5 and 4.6).

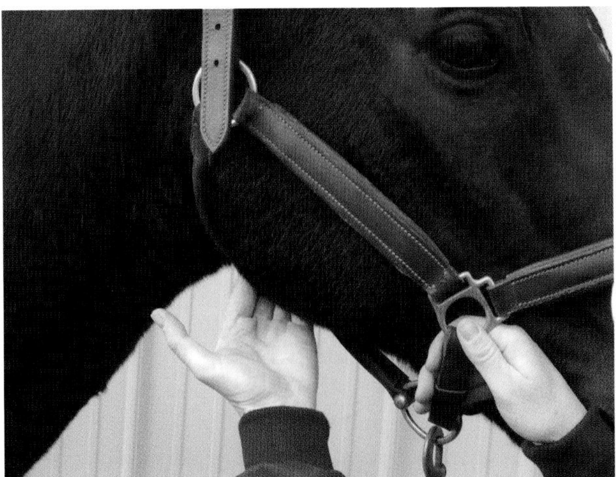

Figure 4.5 The facial artery can be used to determine a horse's pulse quality and rate.

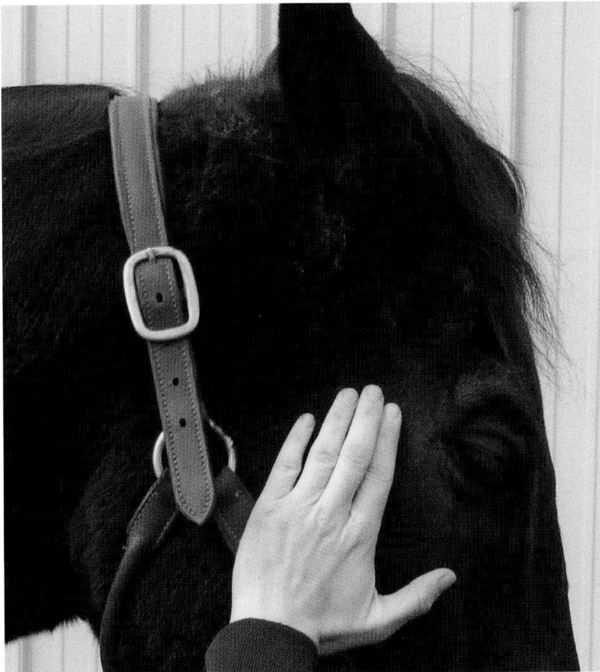

Figure 4.6 The transverse facial artery can also be used to determine a horse's pulse quality and rate. The examiner's index and middle fingers lie over this artery.

TECHNICIAN TIP 4.2: Petechiations are small red dots most commonly seen along the gum line that may indicate a clotting abnormality; a toxic line is a bright pink line outlining the upper incisors.

Assess the ears with a gentle touch knowing that many horses do not like their ears examined. Are there any white plaques inside the ears? These may be aural plaques and are usually benign but can be esthetically unpleasing to owners. Look for any small skin growths that could be benign tumors called sarcoids, which are frequently seen in the ears. Examine the region under the horse's jaw. Submandibular lymph nodes reside between the rami of the mandible and can be found by gliding your hands along the inside of the mandible on each side. In this region and along the parotid region, where the neck begins adjacent to the mandible, it is important to examine for any subcutaneous growths, especially in gray horses. Melanomas are frequent tumors in gray horses, and this tumor will often develop in the parotid region and also around the anus and under the tail.

TECHNICIAN TIP 4.3: Melanoma tumors are frequently found in gray horses.

The Ophthalmic Examination

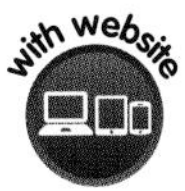

Check out how to perform a full ophthalmology exam including a list of examination supplies.

Typical ophthalmic exam order following general physical exam (Figure 4.7):

1) Assess head set, comfort level, palpebral, retropulsion of globe if appropriate, menace, dazzle prior to sedation if possible.
2) Assess visual acuity if indicated with ground poles, entering/exiting stalls, doorways, navigation of terrain/obstacles.
3) Administer IV sedation if indicated.
4) Apply Auriculopalpebral +/− Supraorbital eyelid nerve blocks with Lidocaine – both eyes almost always should be examined whether new patient or recheck.
5) Assess pupillary light response (PLRs), examine each eye thoroughly with light sources (if painful, apply Proparacaine to cornea to facilitate exam).
6) Photograph lesions.
7) Apply Fluoroscein stain, rinse excess dye with Proparacaine if needed, Blue light exam.
8) Check Intraocular pressure (IOP) with tonometer.
9) Tropicamide if indicated to dilate pupil.

TECHNICIAN TIP 4.4: It takes 15 min typically for full dilation effect. This is a great time for the practitioner to chat with owners and show them photos of the eye to point out important exam details and for the technician to set up for additional procedures or enter charges on the bill.

10) Examine retina.

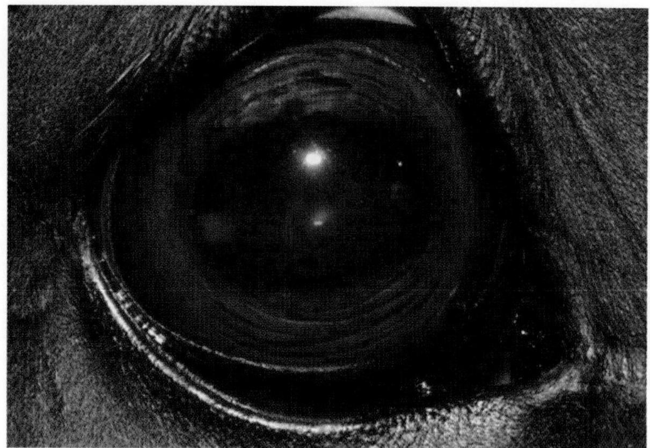

Figure 4.7 Normal equine eye. *Source:* Courtesy of Erin Matheson Barr, RVT.

The first step is to observe the animal, which can be done while obtaining the history. Often it is telling to see how the animal reacts to being caught and led around. It is less concerning if they are spooking and uncomfortable in a new environment, but you would not necessarily expect that in the home environment. Horses that have had visual loss over a long period of time in a stable and unchanging environment may not obviously demonstrate their deficits.

At this point, the technician should take over. Before starting the examination, the animal should have a safe and well-fitting halter on with a lead line in good repair. The horse should not be tied to a fence or in crossties for the exam. It is best if the ambient lights can be adjusted for different sections of the exam but obviously is not always feasible, depending on the client's barn or lack thereof. Being in a stall can also help manage the horse during the exam and keeps other curious animals away. Supplies for the exam should be available and already prepared.

The examiner should begin by standing directly in front of the horse and compare symmetry from one side of the skull to the other. Keep in mind a crooked halter, an offset forelock, or a difference in eye color between left and right may create visual illusions in comparing symmetry. Look at the orbit and surrounding adnexal tissues. Note eyelash position, as downward facing eyelashes often indicate squinting or blepharospasm, as an indication of pain. A mild amount of squinting generally indicates a mild amount of pain, whereas an eye held completely shut can be interpreted as being very painful. If the horse is fairly comfortable and holding the eye open, compare globe size and shape as well as where the globe is sitting within the orbit (Figure 4.8).

TECHNICIAN TIP 4.5: If a horse has been having some ocular pain or frequent past treatments, they will quickly learn to protect the eye(s) when a human comes near, by keeping it closed.

The next part of the exam is to interpret specific reactions known as the menace, dazzle, pupillary light, and palpebral reflexes. It is best to have not sedated the animal at this point unless necessary for safety. Menacing is done by waving one hand at one eye about 6 in away from the eye at the medial, axial, and lateral approaches *without* causing wind movement or touching any of the longer eyelashes, known as vibrissae, that surround the eye. The cornea is highly innervated and therefore very sensitive. It is important that the reaction is due to seeing the motion of the hand, not by a sensation of air movement caused by the hand. The horse should blink and possibly move their head slightly away from the motion. This should be repeatable to be considered consistent and performed on one eye at a time.

TECHNICIAN TIP 4.6: The menace is a learned response and may not be appreciable in young foals.

To test for a dazzle reflex, it is safest to keep one hand on the halter or head as the other shines the Finoff transilluminator or bright penlight at the eye from about 3–6 in away. The dazzle is a subcortical brain reflex that occurs when one shines a light into the eye. The horse should blink that eye almost immediately depending on how bright the light source (very dim lights may not create a strong reaction, but should get some reaction nonetheless). This is a test of the retina's ability to sense the light. This can be noted on the exam as a+ or − for presence or absence.

If possible, the pupillary light reflexes are assessed next. If an eye is painful, it may be necessary to wait to assess these reflexes until after the horse has received eyelid nerve blocks, sedation, and/or topical analgesia. Standing somewhat to the front of the horse, shine the Finoff transilluminator or bright light source a few inches directly to the eye from several inches away. It is good practice to have the non-dominant hand on the horse's head or halter in case of sudden movement or spooking. When the light source is directed into the eye, the pupil should constrict. This is known as a positive direct pupillary light reflex or direct PLR. This positive reaction indicates proper motor function of the iris due to sensory function of the retina. In horses, the normal pupil will somewhat close down in an initial fast phase, followed by a more complete constriction at a slower rate (Figure 4.9).

TECHNICIAN TIP 4.7: It is good practice to have the non-dominant hand on the horse's head or halter in case of sudden movement or spooking.

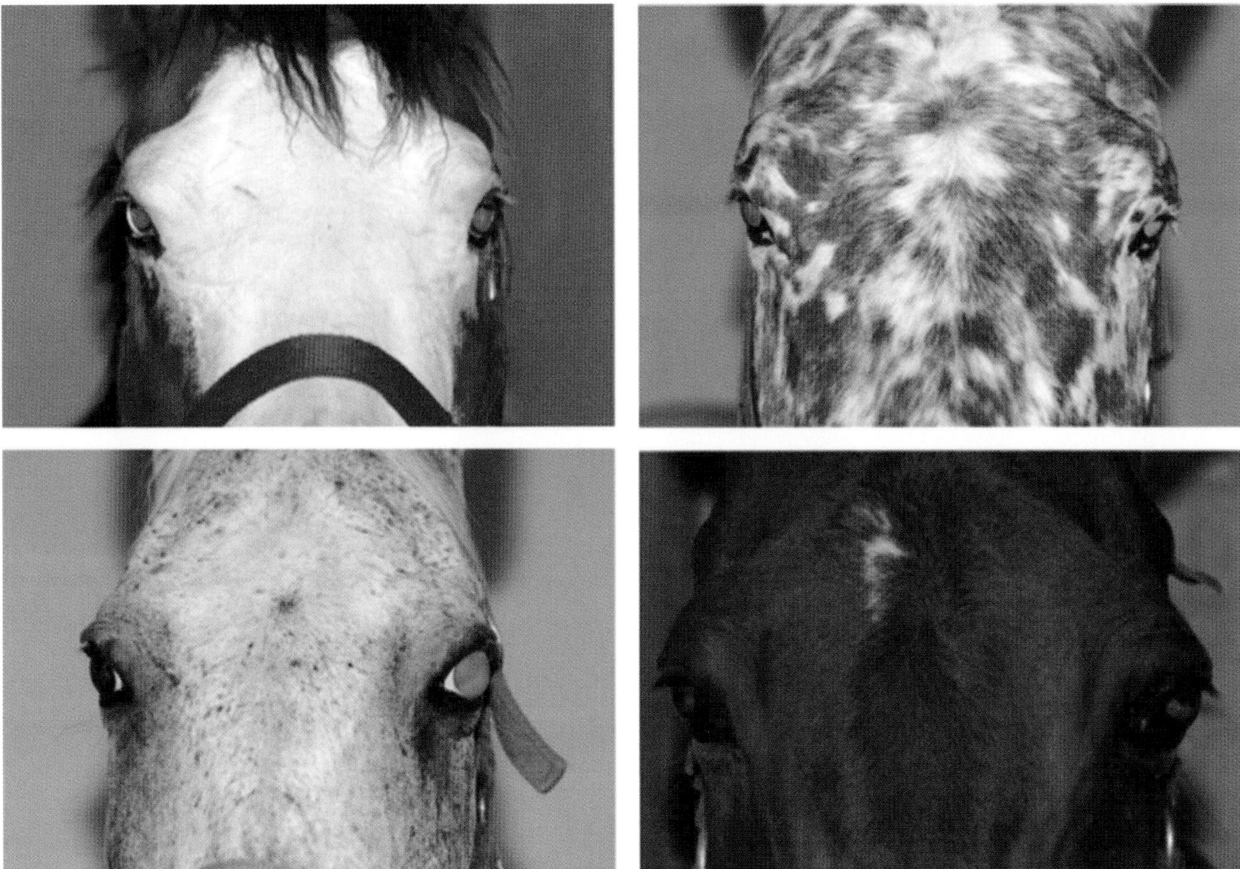

Figure 4.8 **Top Left:** At first glance, this horse may not seem anatomically symmetrical due to the blaze, different colored irises, and tapetal (retinal) reflections, but is normal. Note the normal position of the eyelashes. **Top Right:** Blepharospasm of the left eye is apparent with the downward position of the superior eyelashes as compared to the right eye. **Bottom Left:** Buphthalmos, the left globe is enlarged due to chronic glaucoma (increased IOP), and the cornea has become edematous causing a blue color. **Bottom Right:** Compare symmetry from the front of the face. The left eye is exophthalmic as it is pushed forward due to a sinus mass. *Source:* Courtesy of Erin Matheson Barr, RVT.

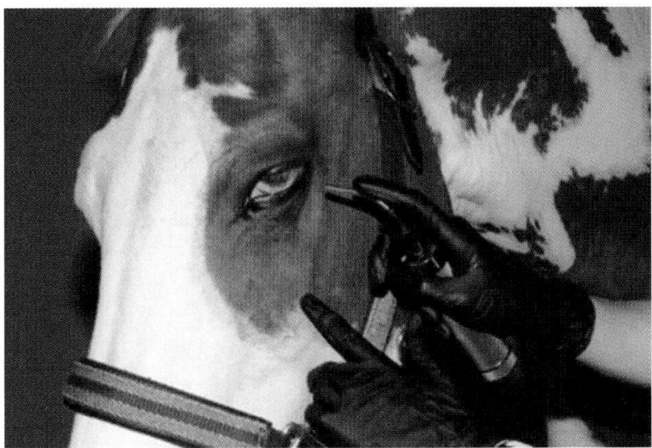

Figure 4.9 Using the Finoff transilluminator, the light is held close to the eye to test a dazzle and direct pupillary light response. Note the guarding hand on the halter and pointer finger directing the tip of the light. It would be even better to cover the entire tip with the finger in case of sudden patient movement. *Source:* Courtesy of Erin Matheson Barr, RVT.

The consensual PLR is assessed next by completing the direct PLR and then quickly swinging the light source over to the opposite eye. Shine the light further back on the contralateral eye, at least a foot away from the globe, so as to not cause a direct PLR and confuse the test outcome. This opposite pupil should also have constricted due to reaction from the light in the original eye. In other words, when light shines directly into the right eye, the iris of the left eye should also constrict down almost at the same time (Figure 4.10).

The palpebral reflex is a test of the ability of the eyelids to sense contact and then fully shut. Lightly tap a finger about an inch or two away from the eyelid margin at dorsal, lateral, ventral, and medial points of the superior and inferior eyelids of each eye. Note if any particular spot yields an incomplete blink. Some animals with repeat testing will cease to blink completely, as they become used to the tapping.

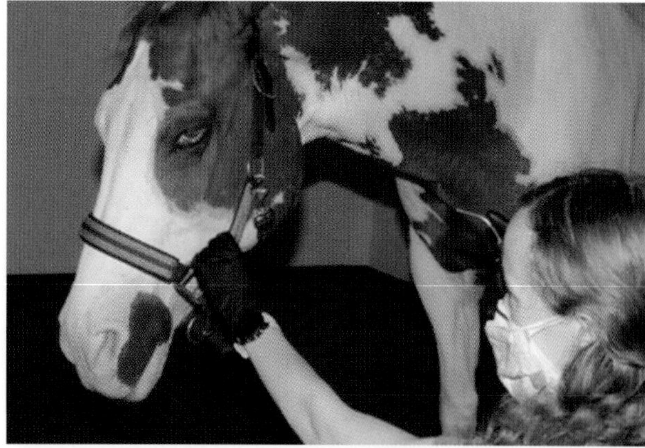

Figure 4.10 When assessing the consensual PLR, the light source should be farther away so as not to inadvertently cause a direct PLR. (In reality, another person would be shining a light into the eye as in the previous photo to cue the consensual.) *Source:* Courtesy of Erin Matheson Barr, RVT.

Sedation may be necessary to complete the rest of the exam. As sedation takes effect, the horse will slowly lower its head to the ground, depending on the dosage given. An accurate ophthalmic exam is *not* possible unless either someone holds the head up or other physical support is used. The outstanding technician will hold the head at the level of height so the practitioner can examine the eye without great effort (Figure 4.11). A respectful veterinarian will also give the technician rest breaks as needed. Head pads or even bales of hay covered in clean towels can be used to provide head support, especially with large patients with heavy heads, or for prolonged procedures. Sedation causes slight relaxation of the extraocular muscles, and it may be useful to tilt the poll or chin toward or away from the examiner to expose each part of the eye for thorough evaluation (Figures 4.12 and 4.13).

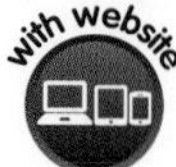

Check out all of the nerve blocks used to perform a more in-depth ocular exam.

You can evaluate the cornea for ulcers by performing the fluorescein dye test (FDT) by gently squirting up to 0.2–0.5 ml of diluted fluorescein dye in eye wash onto the cornea. The presence of a corneal ulcer indicates disruption of the epithelium and will result in a positive bright green uptake of stain at the affected area. This is due to the hydrophilic dye binding to the hydrophilic stroma. Both the epithelium, being the outermost cell layer, and Descemet's membrane, the innermost cell layer, are hydrophobic so will not take up stain (Figure 4.14).

TECHNICIAN TIP 4.8: Be mindful of using gauze near the cornea as it can scratch it, unlike cotton balls.

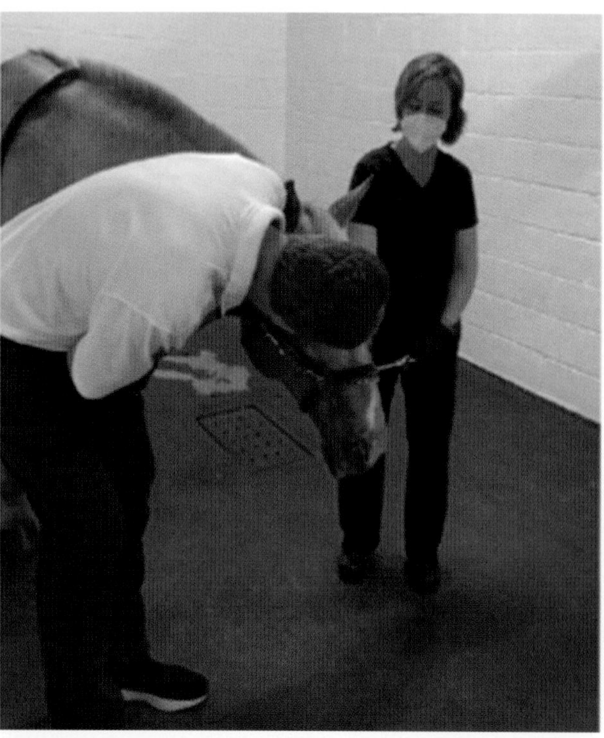

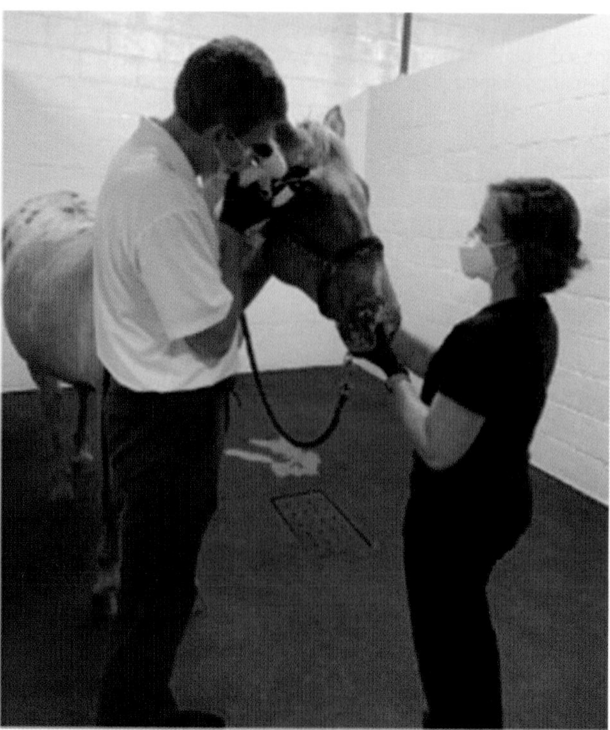

Figure 4.11 **Left:** Once a patient is sedated for the exam, the head drops, and it is unreasonable for a practitioner to perform a quality assessment if the head is not held in an appropriate manner. **Right:** Here, the veterinarian is in a much better position to thoroughly examine the eye. *Source:* Courtesy of Erin Matheson Barr, RVT.

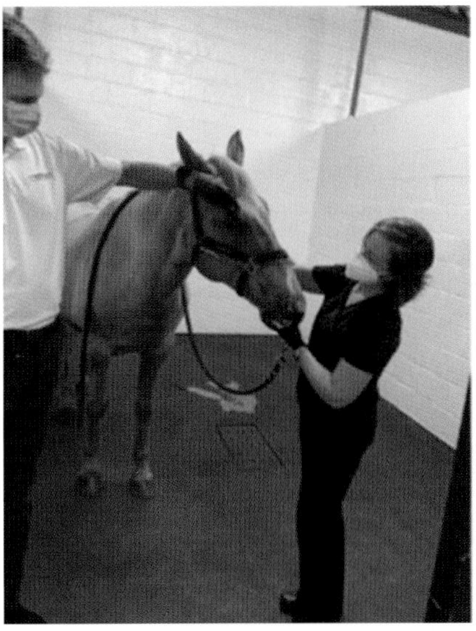
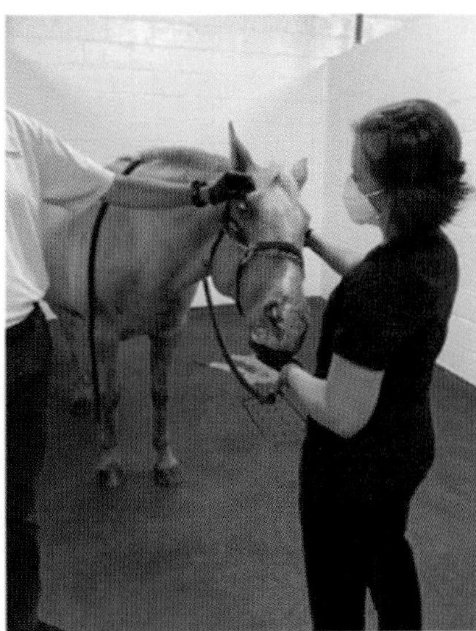
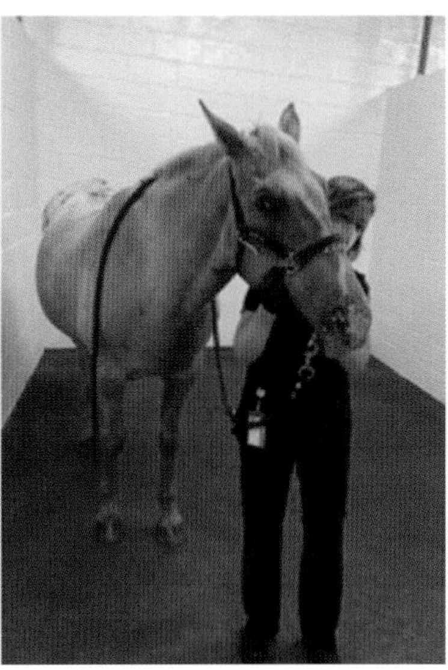

Figure 4.12 **Left:** The sedated patient's poll is pushed toward the practitioner while the nose is pulled toward the technician, allowing the globe to rotate dorsally so that more of the ventral cornea is in view. **Middle:** The opposite effect is achieved when the directions are reversed. The poll comes away and the muzzle toward the practitioner clearly showing the dorsal limbus and hemisphere of the cornea. **Right:** Another method of supporting the head for examination. *Source:* Courtesy of Erin Matheson Barr, RVT.

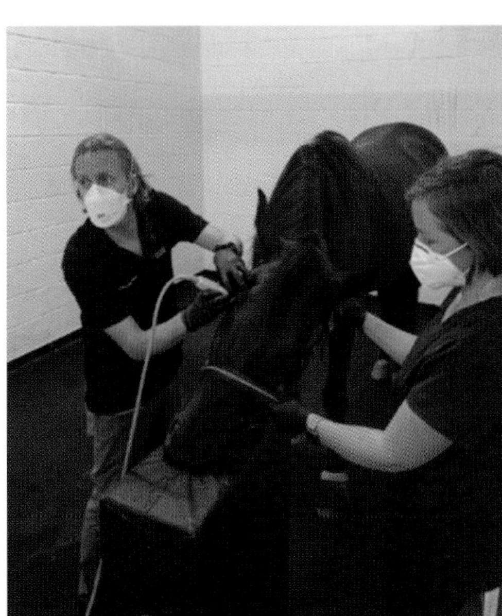
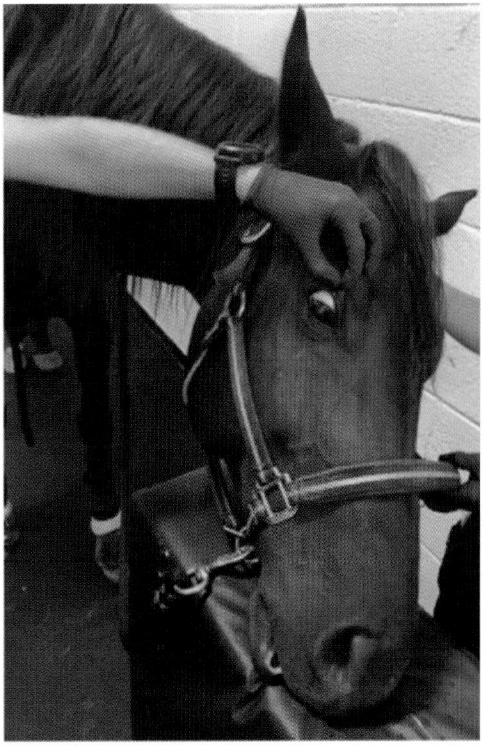

Figure 4.13 **Left:** A large covered foam pad supports this heavily sedated 600 kg horse for a lengthier ultrasound procedure. **Right:** With the head tilted, it is easy to appreciate the globe rotation that may be helpful in accessing a different part of the eye. *Source:* Courtesy of Erin Matheson Barr, RVT.

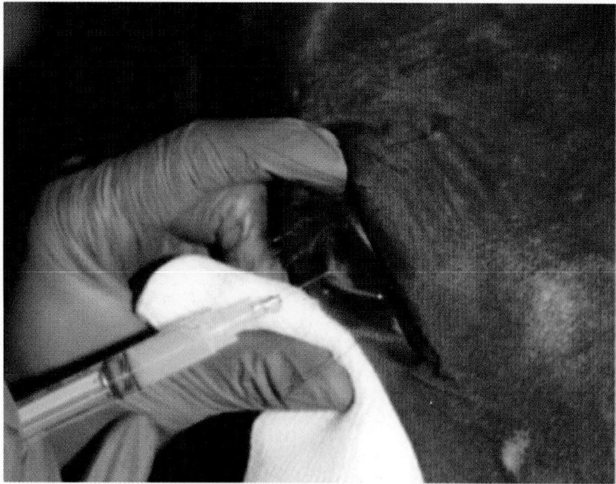

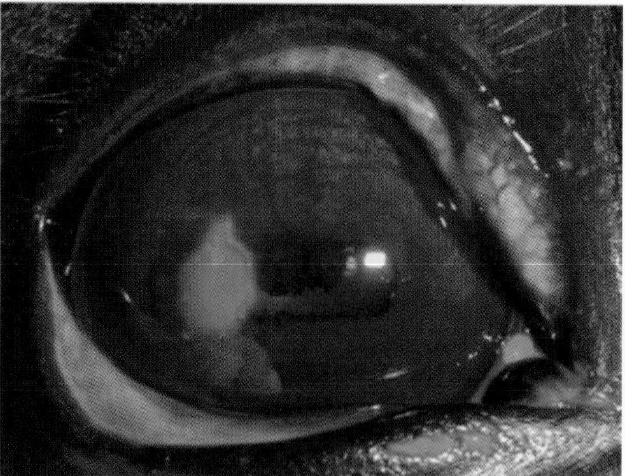

Figure 4.14 **Left:** Fluorescein dye is sprayed onto the cornea to check for ulcers. Note again the guarding hand. Excess liquid is captured with gauze so as not to drip down the face. **Right:** Positive fluorescein dye uptake at the site of a corneal ulcer. The green dye sticks to the underlying corneal stroma and the irregular lip denotes the edge of the epithelium. *Source:* Courtesy of Erin Matheson Barr, RVT.

The colors associated with corneal lesions are also important observations to make. Cellular infiltrate and infection can cause a yellow or white color. A yellow cast of color in particular can be associated with fungal infection of the cornea. Fungal infections in horses are a leading cause of enucleation and are very common in the Southeastern United States and other areas of warm, humid climates. Melting corneal ulcers from a bacterial infection are often circular, malacic in appearance and white, and have purulent ocular discharge associated with them. Blue color in the cornea can be indicative of corneal edema. Healed, fibrotic cornea can be white. Melanin pigment can migrate in, is brown in color, and can indicate disease chronicity. Iris protruding through the cornea can also be brown. Blood vessels growing into the cornea are red, fingerlike projections and grow in from the limbus at 1 mm/day. Location of all these colors should be noted (Figures 4.15 and 4.16).

Next check the IOP of each eye. If a deep ulcer or perforation is apparent, abstain from this test unless a specialist is involved. Previous applications of Proparacaine should still have numbing activity in the cornea. Two different tonometers are commercially available. The Tonopen®, an applanation tonometer, requires an anesthetized cornea. The normal IOP range for the horse is 15–28 mmHg with normal eyes relating to each other +/− 5–8 mmHg.

If the horse is sedated heavily enough to cause the head to hang below the heart, the handler should lift the head to

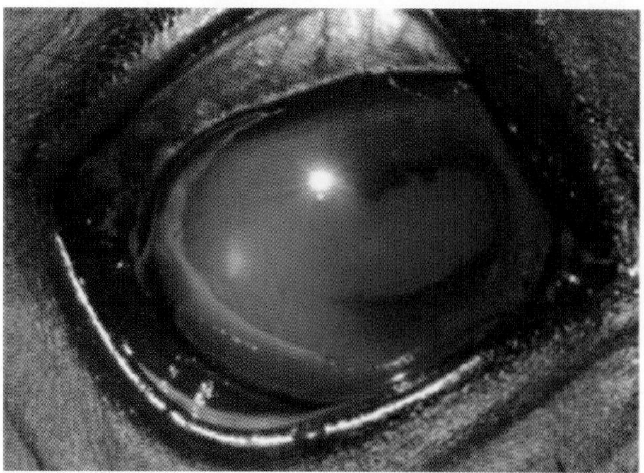

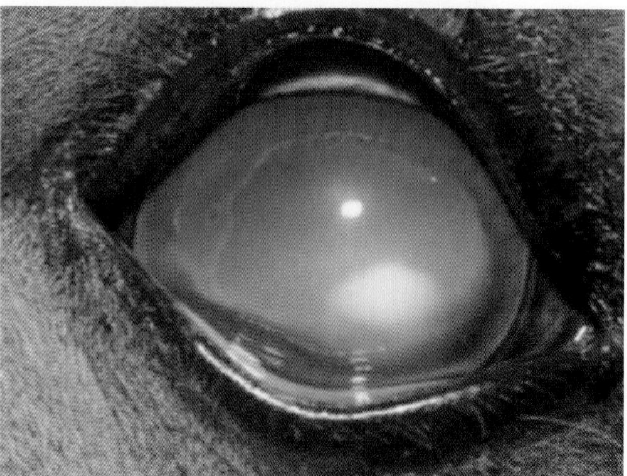

Figure 4.15 Yellow and white can be indicative of infection as inflammatory cells move in to fight the infectious agents. The patient on the left has a focal whiter abscess with surrounding corneal edema. The patient on the right has a large yellow corneal abscess, and many blood vessels have grown into the cornea. *Source:* Courtesy of Erin Matheson Barr, RVT.

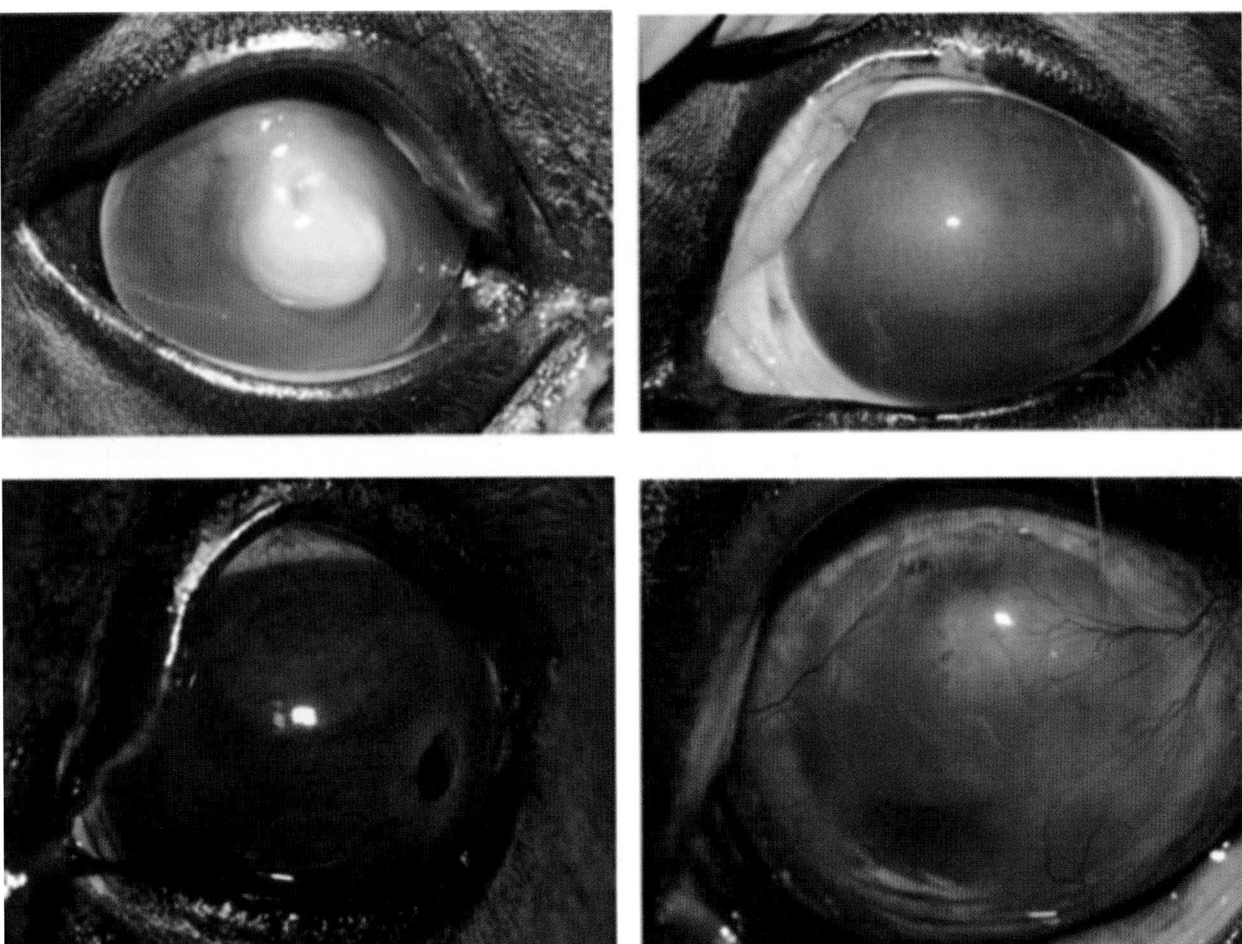

Figure 4.16 **Top Left:** A large melting corneal ulcer. **Top Right:** Corneal edema is a diffuse blue color with "cobblestone" appearance. **Bottom Left:** An ulcer has progressed to corneal perforation with iris prolapse. The iris is the dark tissue in the center of the lesion. **Bottom Right:** Blood vessels have grown into the cornea as a result of chronic immune-mediated corneal inflammation or keratitis. *Source:* Courtesy of Erin Matheson Barr, RVT.

at least chest level to avoid causing an inaccurately elevated IOP. Ensure the disposable cover is resting flat against the tip of the pen with no air bubbles, but also not stretched tightly. Use a new cover for each patient and test the more normal eye first, especially when an infectious corneal ulcer is present. Gently open the superior eyelid and press it against the orbital bone to avoid pressure on the globe which will also falsely elevate the IOP. Press the only button on the Tonopen to activate, and two dotted lines will appear in the window indicating readiness to read measurements. The Tonopen will work best if it is held parallel to the ground and the entire tip contacts the axial cornea at the same time. Brace the heel of the hand holding the tonometer on the horse for better fine motor control of the device and look to the side so as to view the tip contacting the surface of the cornea. If the cornea indents upon application of the Tonopen, too much force is being applied and will cause a false elevation of measurement (Figure 4.17).

Lightly tap the cornea multiple times in the axial cornea if possible while avoiding areas of corneal disease. Each time a reading is taken, a short beep will be heard. A long beep will emit from the tonometer once five readings have been taken. The final reading will appear in the window along with a percentage of error. Any readings with 10% error or greater should be repeated until a reading of 5% or less is obtained. The lowest of two or three final readings is the reported measurement. It is not possible to falsely lower the reading. It is possible to falsely increase the result due to head position, pressure on the globe from elevating the eyelids, or incomplete eyelid nerve blocks that cause resistance to opening the eye and thus pressure on the globe.

The Tonovet® is a rebound tonometer and is not as frequently used in practices, due to being newer on the market. A much smaller surface area is touched with the Tonovet, therefore a numb cornea is not always necessary to achieve a correct result. A small pin ejects repeatedly, as

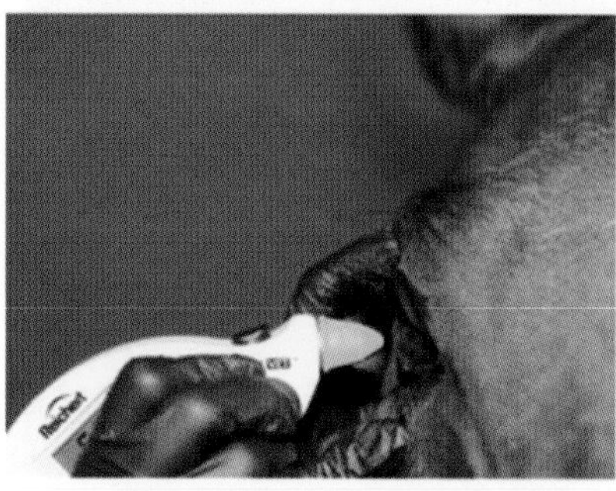

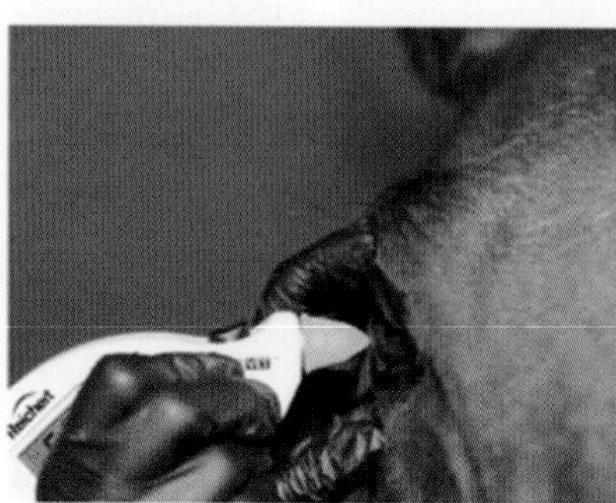

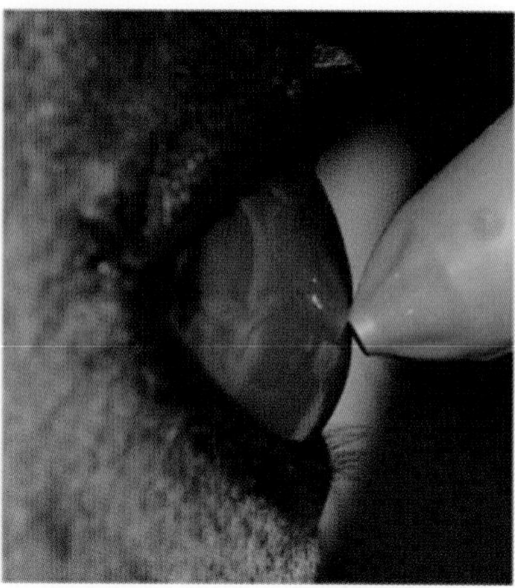

Figure 4.17 **Left:** Advancing the tip of the Tonopen correctly toward the cornea for a reading. The hand holding the Tonopen is braced on the hand holding open the eyelids for better fine motor control. **Middle:** Contact the Tonopen tip to the cornea without indenting the globe for an accurate reading. It is helpful for the practitioner to look from the side, as the camera shot has, to gauge proximity to the cornea as readings are made. **Right:** Incorrect approach of the Tonopen tip to the cornea will not result in any readings. *Source:* Courtesy of Erin Matheson Barr, RVT.

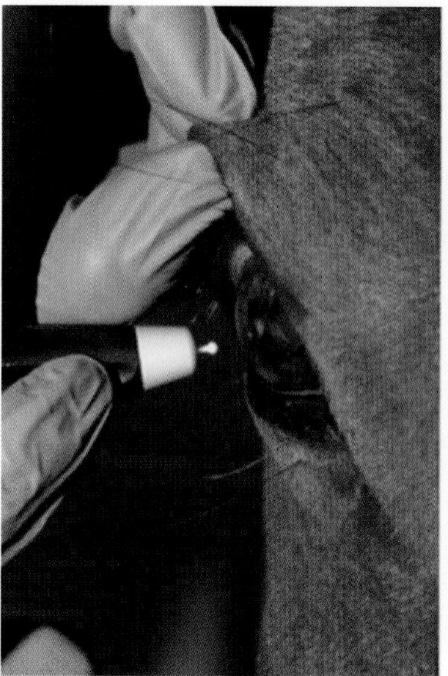

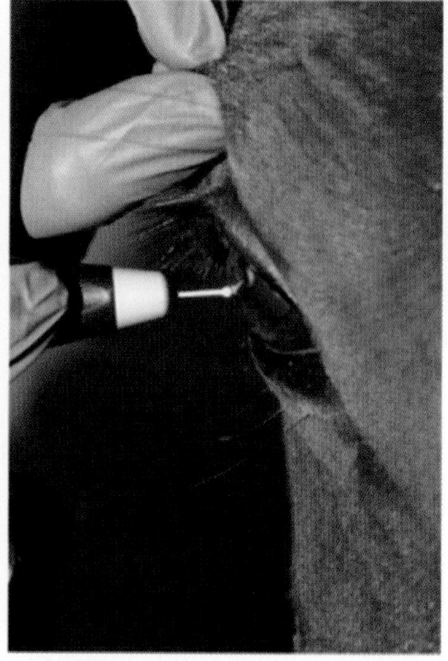

Figure 4.18 The Tonovet uses a tiny white pin that comes forward to touch the cornea and rebounds back to the machine to take a reading with the press of a button. *Source:* Courtesy of Erin Matheson Barr, RVT.

the contact button is pushed, to capture readings with this device. This machine can also be calibrated specifically for the horse, unlike the Tonopen (Figure 4.18).

TECHNICIAN TIP 4.9: Modern day technology has allowed a small hand-held camera to be in many people's back pockets. These devices can help document the patient's lesions and progress and be sent to a veterinary ophthalmologist to help with a telemedicine consultation. Share these tips with clients as well so they can be empowered to share photos of updates with the practitioner (Figure 4.19).

- Take photos inside a barn if possible.
- Do not position the horse in front of or near a window or doorway.
- Have another person hold the patient.
- Hold the phone horizontally 6–10 in from the eye.
  - Hold phone parallel to the eye.
  - Turn off sound notifications.
  - Turn the flash ON.

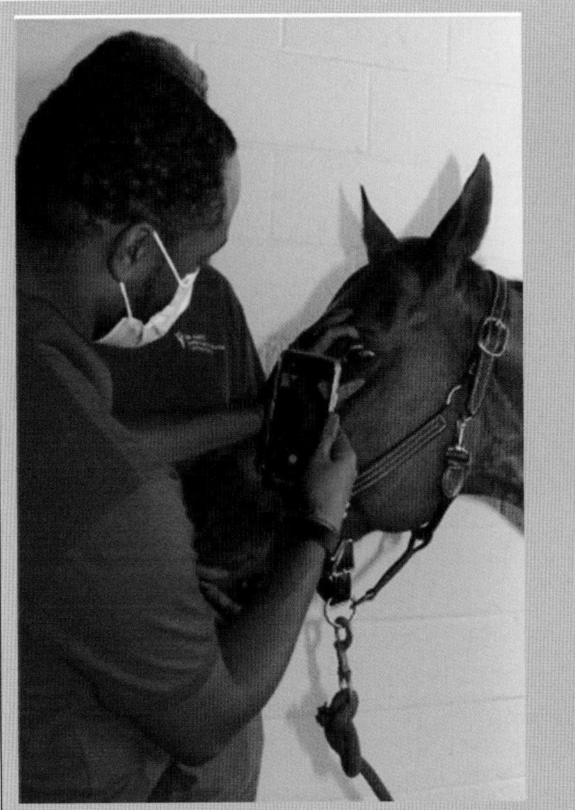

Figure 4.19 With modern day cell phone cameras, decent photos can be taken and used to track progress of consult with veterinary ophthalmologist. *Source:* Courtesy of Erin Matheson Barr, RVT.

- Tap the eye on the phone to make sure the eye is in focus instead of the background.
- Take multiple photos: front, middle, and side.

- If photos are too hard to acquire, then video may be better.
- Send the largest files possible when emailing to a veterinary ophthalmologist for consultation.

Examination of the Neck

The nuchal ligament or crest is a site for excessive fat deposition in obese horses. Palpate the nuchal ligament and along the cervical vertebrae. Note any swelling or asymmetry. Identify the jugular groove and hold off the jugular vein on both sides to assess that the vessel can fill normally. This is a good measure of the horse's overall blood volume. A skin tent is another test that can also be performed along the neck to test for hydration status.

Assess the muscle along the neck between the cervical vertebrae and the nuchal ligament for any atrophy (muscle loss) or patchy sweating, which could indicate a neurologic problem.

Examination of the Thorax

The heart should be ausculted on both the left and right sides. It may be useful to move the horse's forelimb forward to allow better access for auscultation, as it is located under the triceps muscle (Figure 4.20). While ausculting the heart, note whether the rhythm is regular or irregular. Horses were bred to be incredible athletes and their heart rate can be so low that they may drop beats at times. If the dropped beat occurs in a regular rhythm, meaning the drop happens when a normal beat should occur and the returning rhythm remains the same, this is termed second-degree atrioventricular (AV) block and is a normal finding in the horse. If, however, the drops occur at irregular intervals, the horse may have an arrhythmia and further investigation is warranted. The presence of any abnormal sounds, such as turbulence, may indicate a possible heart murmur. It is important to auscult the heart from both the left and right sides as some cardiac murmurs may only be audible from one side.

TECHNICIAN TIP 4.10: It may be useful to move the horse's forelimb forward to allow better access for listening to the heart.

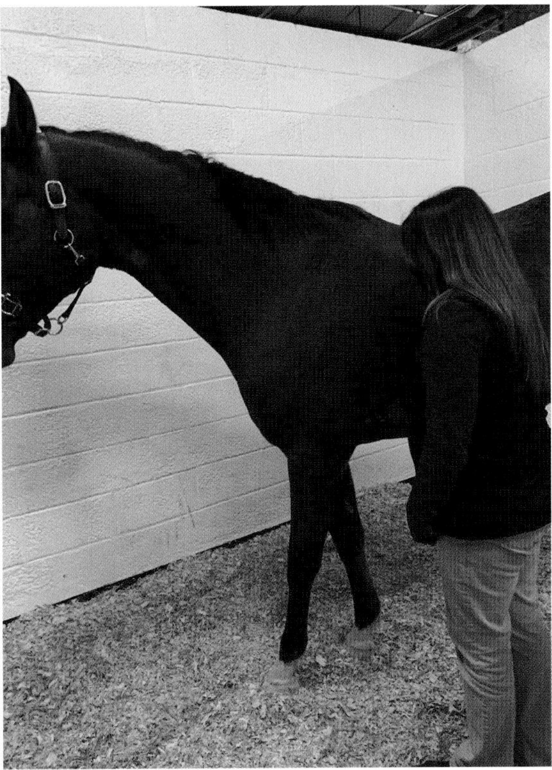

Figure 4.20 Move the left leg forward to allow for better access to listen to the heart.

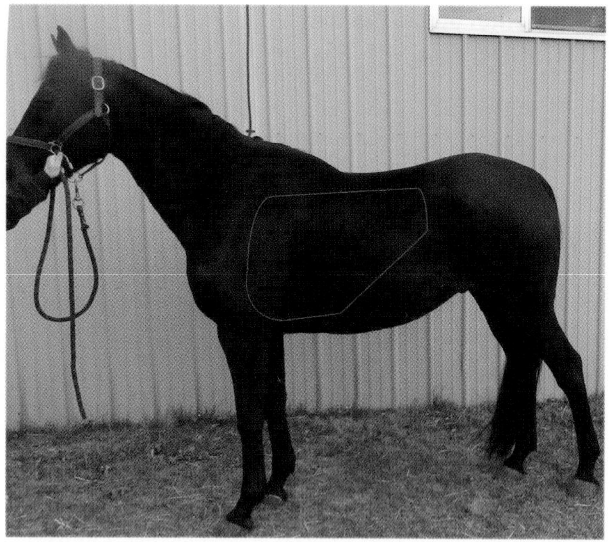

Figure 4.21 Lung fields in an adult horse.

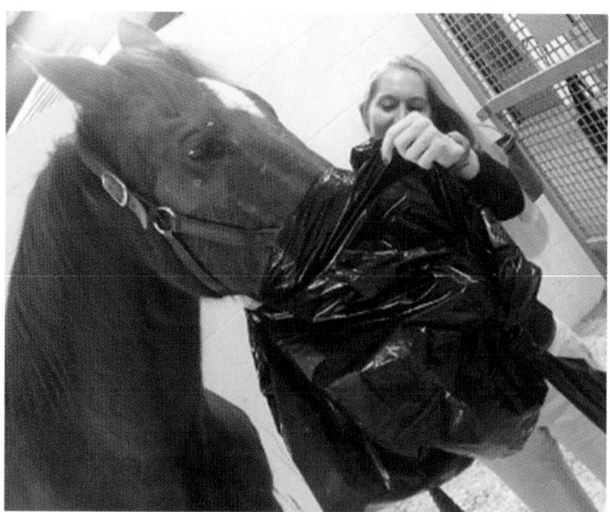

Figure 4.22 For a rebreathing exam, use a trash bag to encourage the horse to take deeper breaths to mimic exercise.

Lung Auscultation

Horses have quite an extensive lung field, extending from the point of the elbow back and upward toward the flank (Figure 4.21). A quiet environment is necessary to hear lung sounds in a normal horse, and even under perfect conditions lung sounds may be impossible to hear in an overweight horse. Abnormal sounds (also known as adventitial sounds) include crackles, wheezes, and friction rubs, which is a sound similar to rubbing your finger on a balloon. A complete absence of lung sounds may indicate fluid in the chest cavity or severe pneumonia in the lower lung fields. If further investigation of the respiratory tract is required, a rebreathing examination should be performed. This procedure uses a plastic bag placed over the horse's nose for three to five min to mimic a horse under exercise and to encourage deeper breaths. The examiner should auscult all lung fields and the trachea at this time. During the procedure, note any coughing that occurs or increased effort for inspiration or expiration, as these findings could indicate respiratory disease. Be sure to listen carefully when the rebreathing bag is removed, as the horse will take several large, deep breaths before returning to a normal rate and depth in their respirations (Figure 4.22).

Examination of the Forelimbs

Palpate the withers for any asymmetry or pain. Continue down the shoulder and antebrachium to the carpus. Palpate the carpus for any joint effusion or heat. Continue to palpate the metacarpus, flexor tendons, the fetlock and pastern joints, and the coronary band for any abnormalities. Digital pulses should be palpated, either on the palmar aspect of the fetlock or the pastern. This pulse is created from the digital artery and should be barely palpable in a normal horse. Increased digital pulses indicate inflammation in the hoof. In addition, the hoof wall should be palpated because increased temperature could indicate inflammation. In laminitis cases, digital pulses are often increased and should be closely monitored. The horse should be moved around the stall to assess for any severe lameness or discomfort. If the horse does not have pain on its forelimbs, pick up each foot and examine the bottom of the hoof (sole) for any abnormalities.

Examination of the Abdomen

Examine the horse's abdominal profile. Does the horse appear distended on one side or both sides? Does the paralumbar fossa appear normal? Using your stethoscope, auscult the abdomen. Listen to all four quadrants carefully and note the absence of sounds or markedly increased sounds, which could indicate impending diarrhea (Figures 4.23 and 4.24).

> **TECHNICIAN TIP 4.11:** Normal gastrointestinal motility in the horse is characterized by two to three borborygmi/min in each of the four quadrants: the upper and lower quadrants on the left and right sides just cranial to the paralumbar fossa.

In geographic regions where horses eat on sandy soil, it is useful to also auscult along the ventral abdomen at the lowest region. Listen for two to three min in this region for any sounds compatible with sand in the ventral colon. While in this region, visually assess the sheath in geldings/stallions and testicles in stallions for any masses or swellings.

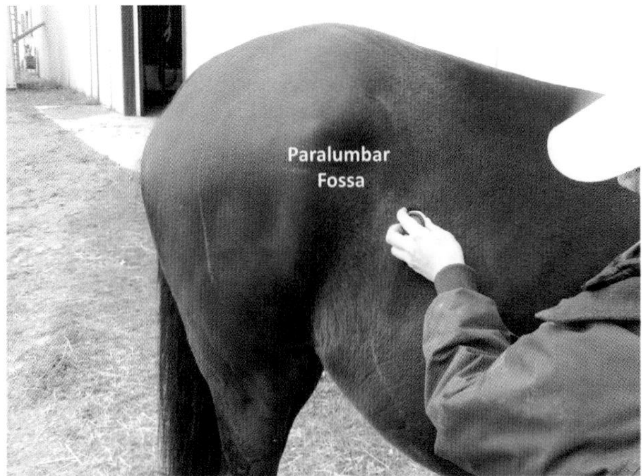

Figure 4.23 Location of the paralumbar fossa in the horse. The examiner is ausculting gastrointestinal sounds in the right dorsal quadrant.

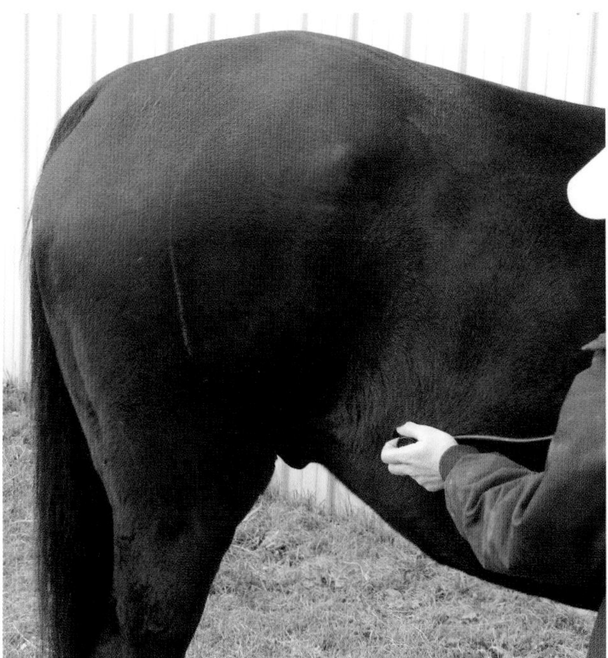

Figure 4.24 The examiner is ausculting gastrointestinal sounds in the right ventral quadrant.

Examination of the Pelvic Limbs

The hind limbs should each be examined in a similar manner to the forelimbs, by careful palpation of joints (stifle, hock, fetlock, pastern) and along the entire limb for any abnormalities. Digital pulses should be assessed on the hind limbs and the hooves examined as previously mentioned.

Examination of the Perineal Region

The perineal region encompasses the tail, anus, and vulva in mares. While standing on the side of the horse, lift the tail to assess tail tone. A normal tail should maintain some strength and resistance upon lifting. Take the horse's rectal temperature at this time. Assess rectal tone while taking the temperature. The anus should constrict around the thermometer. In gray horses, evaluate this region carefully for any masses that could be melanomas. In mares, examine the vulva for any masses, swelling, or discharge.

> **TECHNICIAN TIP 4.12:** Use caution when taking a rectal temperature and evaluating the perineal region. Stand to the side of the horse when lifting the tail.

Ambulatory Examination

Even within the confines of a stall or small paddock, the horse should be moved around to assess comfort level and to determine if there are any neurologic deficits, such as incoordination or weakness, which warrant a full neurologic examination.

Neurologic Examination

Neurologic disease can present with a wide array of clinical signs. The goal of every neurologic examination is to assess the patient's clinical signs to arrive at two primary conclusions. The first of these goals is to decide if the patient's neurologic system is normal or abnormal. Secondly, if the patient is considered neurologically abnormal, neurolocalization of the lesion must be determined. Neurolocalization is the process of assessing a patient's clinical signs and neurologic deficits to determine what region of the nervous system is most likely abnormal. This is further completed by assessing mentation, reflexes, including cranial nerve reflexes, and the animal's gait. Asking the horse to perform simple maneuvers such as backing, circling, or walking up and down inclines can assess balance, proprioception, and strength. It is extremely important to assess all reflexes on both sides of the body because some neurologic deficits may be unilateral (Figure 4.25).

Possible sites of neurolocalization include the forebrain (cerebrum), cerebellum, brainstem, or spinal cord, and, lastly, the neuromuscular system (including the nerves that innervate muscle, the neuromuscular junction, and the muscle itself). The spinal cord is further subdivided into the cervical spinal cord (C1–C5), cervical intumescence (C6–T2), thoracolumbar spinal cord (T3–L3), and lumbar intumescence (L4–S1). Determining the location of a neurologic lesion can sometimes be difficult and might not always be possible. In some situations, it is apparent that multiple regions of the animal's neurologic system are affected. In these cases, neurologic disease is considered multifocal in nature.

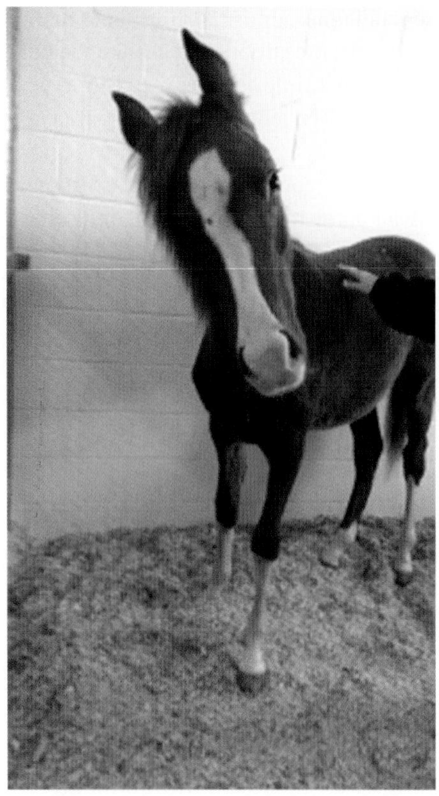

Figure 4.25 A head tilt can be indicative of a neurologic lesion or trauma.

Lesions in the forebrain might lead to numerous neurologic deficits. Most prominently, a change in mentation and attitude usually occurs. Additionally, there might be decreased responsiveness to painful stimuli and the patient might be unilaterally or bilaterally blind. The patient's gait is normal on a flat and straight surface but deficits indicative of loss of proprioception become apparent when more complicated maneuvers are demanded. Seizures are a sign of forebrain disease.

Cerebellar lesions result in a different clinical presentation than forebrain lesions. Animals affected by cerebellar disease do not have any changes in mentation. They are ataxic but not weak. Ataxia is characterized by tremors that worsen with intention and a dysmetric/hypermetric (spastic, uncontrolled, exaggerated) gait. Because cerebellar disease affects motor control, these animals may have difficulty coordinating the menace response despite having no visual deficits. Likewise, horses with cerebellar disease have a tendency to rear in response to minimal stimuli due to poor motor control. Anatomically, the brainstem is the site in the central nervous system (CNS) from which the cranial nerves arise and extend peripherally. As a result, one of the hallmarks of brainstem disease is cranial nerve deficits. The deficits observed in a particular case are dependent on the brainstem region that is affected. It is highly unusual to have all 12 cranial nerves affected. Because areas of the brainstem are responsible for wakefulness, patients with brainstem disease often have a dull or obtunded mentation, such as what could be seen with forebrain disease. Lastly, patients with brainstem disease might be ataxic due to the importance of cranial nerve VIII in the vestibular system as well as the presence of proprioceptive tracts. Unlike cerebellar ataxia, patients with central vestibular ataxia are also weak.

Refer to Table 4.4 for a summary of clinical signs and neurologic deficits observed when different segments of the spinal cord or the neuromuscular system are abnormal.

In addition to neurolocalization, neurologic deficits can be further characterized. Specifically, reflex responses can be exaggerated (hyperreflexive), normal, decreased (hyporeflexive), or absent. Spinal cord lesions identified on gait analysis are also categorized by grading the severity of neurologic deficits. The standard grading system operates on a scale of 0–5. This system allows a concise means by which veterinarians and veterinary technicians can communicate to one another the severity of an animal's status; likewise, it serves as a means of comparison over points in time with animals that have resolving or progressing

Table 4.4 Gait deficits observed on neurologic examination.

Location of lesion	Cervical spine (C1–C5)	Cervical intumescence (C6–T2)	Thoracolumbar spine (T3–L3)	Lumbar intumescence (L4–S2)	Neuromuscular system
Mentation	Normal	Normal	Normal	Normal	Normal
Cranial nerve reflexes	Normal	Normal	Normal	Normal	Normal
Forelimb gait	Stiff, long-strided	Weak, short-strided	Normal	Normal	Normal/weak
Hind limb gait	Stiff, long-strided	Stiff, long-strided	Stiff, long-strided	Weak, short-strided	Normal/weak
Proprioceptive reflexes	All limbs abnormal	All limbs abnormal	Hindlimbs abnormal	Hindlimbs abnormal	Normal

Table 4.5 Clinical grading system for neurologic examinations.

Neurologic Grades	
Grade 0/5	Normal animal; no neurologic deficits.
Grade 1/5	Neurologic deficits are subtle and are only noted when the animal is asked to perform complicated maneuvers.
Grade 2/5	Neurologic deficits are observed during complicated and uncomplicated maneuvers, including when walking a straight line.
Grade 3/5	Neurologic deficits are obvious during uncomplicated maneuvers. During complicated maneuvers, the animal is at risk of falling down.
Grade 4/5	Neurologic deficits are severe enough that the animal may fall over when walking in a straight line.
Grade 5/5	Neurologic deficits are severe enough that the animal is unable to rise or stand.

neurologic disease. Following gait analysis, neurologic grades can be defined as shown in Table 4.95.

After the neurologic examination and neurolocalization have been performed, additional diagnostic procedures are often recommended. With many neurologic diseases, the process of neurolocalization will likely narrow the list of differential diagnoses. As such, additional diagnostic procedures can further differentiate those possible diagnoses. The most commonly performed diagnostic procedures for neurologic disease in large animals include cervical radiography, myelography, cerebrospinal fluid (CSF) collection and analysis, and electromyography (EMG). Advanced imaging such as computed tomography (CT) and magnetic resonance imaging (MRI) allow detailed evaluation of the brain and parts of the spinal cord and might be available at specialty centers (Table 4.5).

CSF bathes the brain and spinal cord; its composition can be altered in states of disease. Sampling CSF may aid in diagnosis of neurologic disease. Aspiration of CSF can be performed at either the lumbosacral space or at the atlantooccipital space. Of these two sites, CSF can only be collected safely from the lumbosacral space in the standing horse. The CSF collection procedure is outlined in the Diagnostic Procedures (Chapter 7) (Figure 4.26).

It is important to stress that in many cases neurologic diseases cannot be diagnosed definitively antemortem. The CNS is well-protected and consequently somewhat inaccessible. Additionally, while sampling an organ is a common method of diagnosis in diseases involving other organ systems, sampling the brain, spinal cord, or peripheral nerves is not routinely performed in large animal medicine due to technical difficulties and risk of complications. As a result, definitive diagnosis is often only achieved in the event that a postmortem examination is performed. However, a provisional diagnosis can often be made following neurologic examination and interpretation of diagnostic testing. As a result, treatment for neurologic disease is usually pursued empirically.

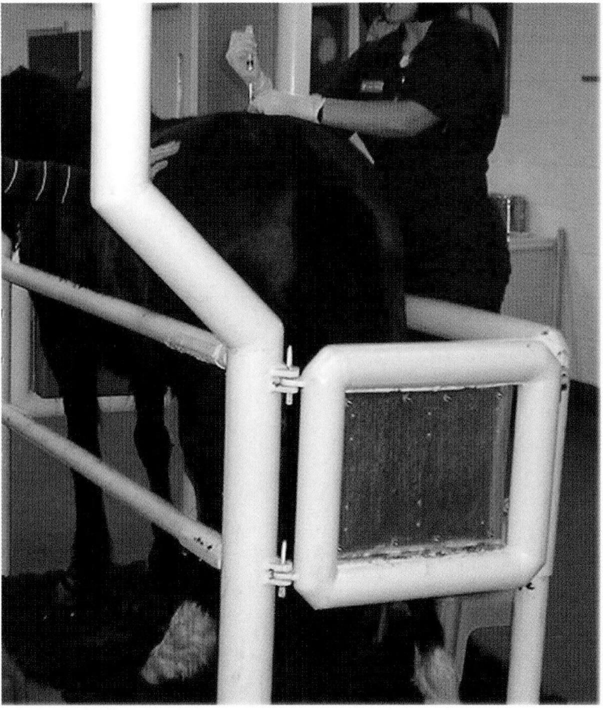

Figure 4.26 Collecting cerebrospinal fluid from the lumbosacral space in a standing horse. This procedure should be performed with the horse standing in sturdy stocks with an experienced handler. *Source:* Reproduced with permission of Dr. Katherine Wilson.

An extremely important consideration in the diagnostics and treatment of neurologic large animals is ensuring protection of the staff members who are working with the animal. Neurologic large animals pose serious dangers to staff members for two primary reasons. First, animals with certain neurologic disorders (primarily, disease of the brain) may behave abnormally and unpredictably, which can lead to serious injury and harm to unprepared or complacent staff members. Ideally, only experienced personnel should work with encephalopathic large animals; regardless of experience level, personnel should never handle these animals alone due to the high risk of injury. Measures to minimize self-inflicted injury by the animal are also important. These include housing the animal in a secure and padded area and using specially designed protective foam helmets for the animal's head (Figure 4.27).

Secondly, rabies is a zoonotic neurologic disease. While transmission of the disease to humans from large animals

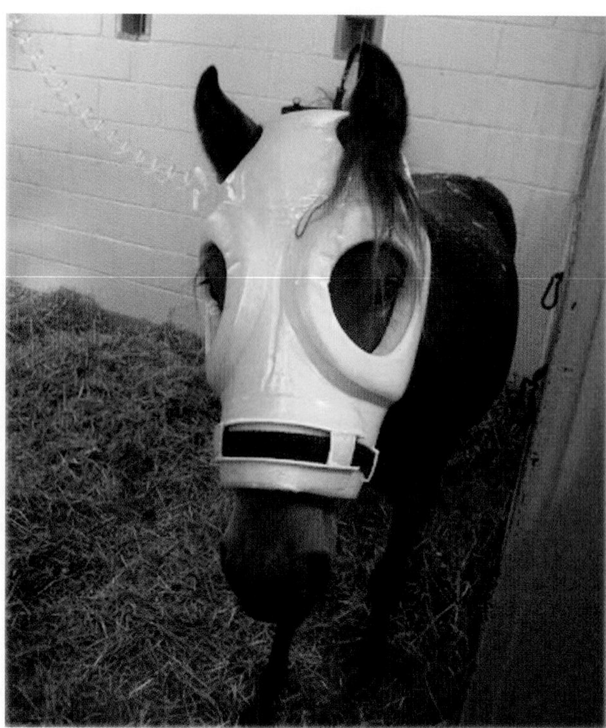

Figure 4.27 Specially designed protective foam helmets can be used on horses or other large animals demonstrating signs of encephalopathy. They are helpful for horses prone to aggressive or unpredictable behaviors that are at risk of injuring themselves. *Source:* Reproduced with permission of Dr. Jennifer Bauquier.

Box 4.1 Documenting Physical Examination Findings

The most useful way to document findings on a PE is to categorize them by body system. Shorthand terms and acronyms are common in veterinary medicine to quickly summarize examination findings. Although many veterinarians and veterinary clinics have various shorthand methods, an example with common acronyms is listed below.

GEN: BAR, T = 100.1 °F, P = 36, R = 12; BCS = 5/9
INTEG: haircoat appropriate for season, no masses/growths apparent, no other lesions observed
EENT: corneas clear OU, menace intact OU, PLRs intact OU, no nasal or ocular d/c, face appears symmetrical, and ears clean AU
C/V: mm = pk, moist, CRT < 2 S, hydration adequate, jugular fill normal, heart rhythm regular and no murmurs ausculted, pulse strong and synchronous
Resp: eupnic, no nasal d/c, bilateral nasal airflow, trachea auscults wnl, normal BV sounds ausculted in all lung fields, no coughing observed
G/I: excellent appetite, G/I motility active × 4, no abdominal distension observed, fecal consistency wnl
M/S: no lameness observed at the walk, DPs wnl × 4, no joint effusion noted; full lameness exam not performed
Lymph: submand LN palpate wnl
U/G: gelding; sheath appears normal, no urination observed
Neuro: mentation appropriate, no neurologic deficits observed; complete neuro exam not performed

Translation

GENERAL FINDINGS: BAR. Rectal temperature 100.1 °F, pulse 36 beats/min, respiratory rate 12 breaths/min; BCS 5/9 (appropriate weight)
INTEGUMENTARY (i.e. skin): as stated EARS, EYES, NOSE, THROAT: both corneas clear, menace, and papillary light responses intact (OU = both eyes, OS = left eye, OD = right eye), no nasal or ocular discharge, both ears clean (AU = both ears, AS = left ear, AD = right ear) CARDIOVASCULAR: mucous membranes = pink, moist; capillary refill time < 2 S
RESPIRATORY: eupnic (normal respiratory rate; tachypneic = increased respiratory rate), no nasal discharge, trachea auscults within normal limits, normal bronchovesicular sounds ausculted in all fields
GASTROINTESTINAL: normal gastrointestinal sounds in all four quadrants, fecal consistency within normal limits
MUSCULOSKELETAL: digital pulses within normal limits on all four limbs
LYMPHATIC: submandibular lymph nodes palpate within normal limits

(horses, cattle, and small ruminants) is considered extremely rare, the potential remains. Rabies is almost uniformly fatal in people. Although the rabies vaccine is extremely effective, rabies should never be completely ruled out in a large animal exhibiting acute onset of neurologic disease. As such, it is often prudent to don personal protective equipment, such as gloves and face masks, when handling neurologic large animals. Personal protective equipment is mandatory when handling neurologic large animals that have not been recently vaccinated for rabies. More details regarding personal safety are discussed in the Disease (Chapter 12) relating to rabies.

The Equine Pain Score

Introduction

To assess is to determine a value for a particular situation or condition. An assessment is an important part of pain management and leads us toward appropriate pain treatment and control. Pain assessment should be included as part of the patient's standard hospital record. To make a proper assessment, there must be a guide that includes what to monitor and how to monitor it. To track pain assessments, metrics are commonly used, in conjunction with pain behaviors. When trained technicians make assessments consistently, the change from one observation point to another can be a very sensitive indicator of increasing, static, or decreasing pain in a horse. When the qualities assessed are quantitated, or assigned some weight or number, actual numeric pain scoring is possible.

Animals, much like people, have different tolerance levels when it comes to pain. We see this variance between breeds, as well as gender. For example, an older Belgian broodmare may have a severe colon torsion yet only show very mild signs of colic, while a young Thoroughbred colt with an impaction could be in violent pain and unresponsive to analgesics.

It is because of the broad range of pain tolerance that it is important to score each patient consistently and based on his or her own parameters. There is no "gold standard" for pain scoring in horses; pain scoring is not cut and dry, and each patient will have its own set of normal and abnormal values.

Evaluation is an overall review of individual values gathered from the patient. When evaluating an animal for pain score assessment, it is important to tailor an evaluation criterion based on an area of injury. An animal undergoing treatment for an orthopedic repair is going to be monitored for specific signs that would not be pertinent to the colic patient, ophthalmic patient, or even the animal suffering from respiratory distress. However, there are certain PE parameters and common behaviors that may be shown by horses experiencing pain or discomfort no matter the cause.

Areas to Assess

Physical Parameters

Metrics are used in a pain assessment as a way to track measurable data, and this includes heart rate and respiratory rate. The normal equine heart rate is 28–40 beats/min and respiratory rate is 8–20 breaths/min. An increase in either value can indicate pain. Pain can cause the heart rate to be consistently elevated in the resting animal. These metrics can be used to track comfort level over time, and also to track the animal's response to analgesia. However, as other conditions can cause elevations in both heart rate and respiratory rate, neither metric should be the sole indicator of pain. Similarly, horses with heart and respiratory rates at the lower end of the normal range may have considerable pain despite values within the normal range. Blood pressure has consistently been linked to comfort level in horses, but may not be the most reliable metric to use due to many variables associated with this measurement.

Appetite

Appetite can be a useful tool in assessing pain, as animals that are in pain are less likely to eat as readily as those who are comfortable. Normal animals tend to eat all of the concentrate feed offered in about 15–30 min, and should eat hay steadily throughout the day. A change in appetite can be seen in concentrate and hay consumption in patients that are in pain.

Demeanor

Observing the animal's overall demeanor can also be a good indicator of an animal's pain level, because animals experiencing pain are likely to become withdrawn and dull, and sometimes appear irritable. Horses, especially in a hospital or clinic setting, should have an alert demeanor, and found to be taking in their surroundings. Horses should have their head up when just standing, should be moving their ears around, and be BAR. Even resting horses should be rousable and responsive when approached or stimulated by sound. Horses experiencing signs of pain are likely to have a lowered head carriage, still ears, as well as a dull or disinterested demeanor. Some appear just the opposite and look obtunded or sleepy. Horses may also become manic with pain, and appear aggressive or mad by pinning back their ears. Animals in pain may bite at themselves, their water and feed buckets, or the wall. Animals in pain may also appear sweaty, especially those suffering abdominal pain, or severe limb pain. When interacting with a horse in pain, it may try to bite or kick at observers, or simply just try and move away from an observer.

Body Language

Demeanor and body language in horses are closely linked. Recumbency and location in the stall are important to monitor because horses tend to be creatures of habit. Any change in their routine could indicate that something is wrong. Horses all have distinct "personalities," and those personalities should be evident, even in the event of hospitalization. The same rule applies to behavior, as horses tend to keep a fairly consistent temperament. A pain-free horse should be standing much more than lying down, and is less likely to spend much of the time down in lateral recumbency. Horses are more likely to lie in sternal recumbency, and be facing the front of the stall when standing, even at rest. Animals experiencing pain, especially those with severe pain, are found lying in lateral recumbency and often facing a back wall or corner whether standing or recumbent. Some horses in pain may appear tense, showing tension in their facial muscles, or tension and trembling of muscle groups in their body. Tail swishing, head shaking, bruxism, and head bobbing or nodding can also be expressions of pain (Figure 4.28).

Orthopedic/Foot Pain

With orthopedic or laminitis cases, it is important to know if the animal is favoring a limb. When a horse is recovering from an orthopedic procedure, it is important to monitor both the operated and the contralateral limb for pain. One way to track if horses are favoring a limb includes measuring the number of hoof lifts or weight shifts per minute. Weight shifts and small hoof lifts can be a very subtle and often an early indicator that there is a change in leg comfort, or an increase in pain. By palpating digital pulses, problems may be detected in a specific limb or limbs; qualitatively "strong" or "bounding" pulses are common with laminitis. Horses with limb pain may also point the affected limb, or alternate pointing if more than one limb is affected. They may also tap, paw, or kick with a painful limb, or appear hyperesthetic when one or more limbs are touched (Figure 4.29).

Abdominal Pain

Some signs to monitor that are common with abdominal discomfort include: pawing, stretching out, flank watching, sweating, rolling (abruptly from lateral to sternal or from sternal to lateral), bruxism, grimacing, and spending excessive time lying down. Animals experiencing abdominal pain are also likely to stand with their abdomen "tucked up," as to protect their abdomen, and may also experience abdominal muscle tremors (Figure 4.30). It is important not only to note these signs but also to track if the signs are progressing in frequency or duration. Marking the frequency and duration of pain behaviors and noting the response to analgesics and sedatives can help give a reliable assessment of the animal's comfort level.

Thoracic Pain

For an animal experiencing thoracic pain, you are likely to see a trend of increased or increasing respiratory rate. In addition, there may be an increase in respiratory effort and perhaps an abdominal component to the breathing. Horses

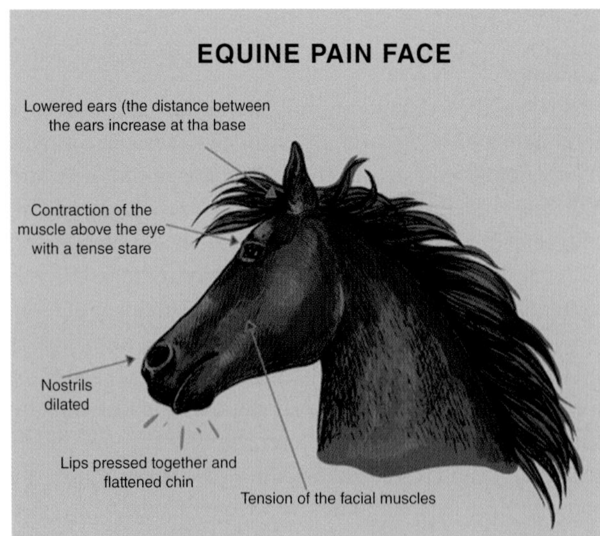

Figure 4.28 These are signs that can be shown in a horse's face when they are painful.

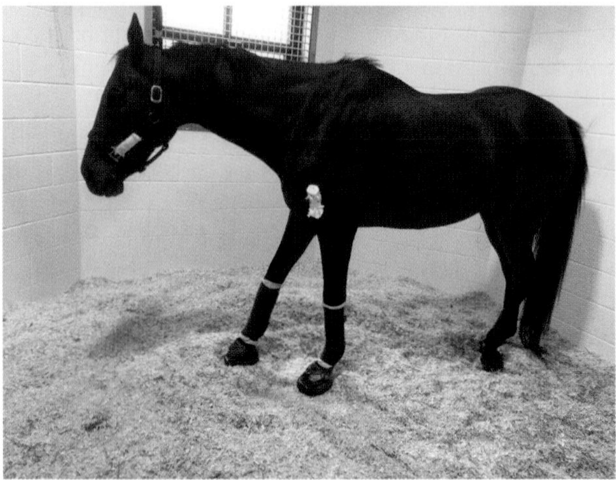

Figure 4.29 Horses with limb pain may point with the affected limb.

Detailed General Comfort Score Sheet q 2h			Observe horse for 1 – 2 min
Medical Record #	Patient:	Clinician:	Record the **NUMBER** for
Date:	Date:	Date:	each behavior and response

	< Recumbency	Location in Stall
4	4	4: back, facing side, back (E = eating)
3	3	3: back, facing front (E = eating)
2	2	2: side, diag, facing front (E = eating)
1	1	1: front, facing front, or moving (E = eating)
	< See Chart	Observed Demeanor
4	4	4: Depressed, unaware
3	3	3: Dull or anxious, min R, not sleepy, ± mad
2	2	2: Q, aware, not anxious, R, ± mad, ± sleepy
1	1	1: B, A, Attentive, R, not mad
	< D = eats down	Appetite
4	4	4: no appetite
3	3	3: eats treats when offered, not hay
2	2	2: eats hay slowly when offered
1	1	1: eats hay readily
		Average Head and Ear Position
4	4	4: H held below withers, E still or back
3	3	3: H held at withers, E still or back
2	2	2: H moving (or eating), E forward, moving
1	1	1: H held above withers, E forward, moving
20	20	Pain behaviors noted per one minute observation (see pg. 2)
15	15	
10	10	
5	5	
0	0	
90	90	Heart Rate and (resp rate)
75	75	
60	60	
45	45	
30	30	
	< Analgesic Tx	A____________________
4	4	4::
3	3	3::
2	2	2::
1	1	1::
		B____________________
4	4	4::
3	3	3::
2	2	2::
1	1	1::
hr	< Time and AM or PM	
	<<< VAS (1 no pain to 10 worst pain)	
	< Initials of observer	

General Comfort Score Sheet q 2h Scoring Notes

Observe the horse for one to two min, then enter the stall and interact with the horse. Record the **NUMBER** for each category in the proper box for that time.

Location in Stall Use 1. if horse is moving voluntarily. Indicate **Recumbency (LLR, L** Sternal, **RLL, R** Sternal in the top shaded square) as well as location in the stall if horse is down.

Observed Demeanor

1: Bright, Alert, Attentive, Responsive, Not angry

2: Quiet, Aware, Somewhat responsive, Not anxious, ± Angry, ± Distracted

3: Dull or Anxious, Angry or minimal response to stimulus, ± Stereotypic behavior that persists around observer

4: Depressed, Unresponsive, Unaware, ± Obtunded

See Chart – Indicate if there is detailed information or change in treatments from previous orders. Use an **X** in the top shaded square.

Appetite

1. = spontaneous eating, 2. = eating when fed but not unless fed. **D = eats down** – write a **D** in the top shaded square if the horse eats while lying down.

Head and Ear Position

1: Head held above withers, moving, looking around. Ears forward or orienting quickly on sounds of interest.

2: Head down (eat, rest), raised occ. to withers level. Ears forward, neutral, or orienting slowly on sounds.

3: Head held at withers, mostly still (not sleeping). Ears neutral or back, orienting intermittently and slowly on sounds.

4: Head held below withers consistently (not sleeping) and still, ±rigid or tense. Ears still, neutral, and droopy or back, not orienting on sounds.

Pain behaviors per 1 min (other than the specific behaviors in A and B)

Note number of pain behaviors (same behavior repeated or multiple behaviors) displayed during a 1-min observation outside the stall. See list of pain behaviors below. Describe behaviors in Chart where applicable.

Heart rate and (respiratory rate) () are to differentiate values.

A: Quality or behavior unique to this patient and grades of "severity" where appropriate

Analgesic Tx – Indicate if an analgesic was given (e.g. Phenylbutazone) or a CRI is continued at the time of scoring. Use an **X** in the top shaded square.

B: Quality or behavior unique to this patient and grades of "severity" where appropriate

Modified VAS score: If 1 = no pain and 10 = the worst pain possible for this horse, pick a number that best describes this horse's pain at the time you FINISH your observations and exam.

Pain Behaviors (PARTIAL list; overlap between categories is common; add additional behaviors as needed)

General discomfort and pain behaviors: Limb pain behaviors: Abdominal pain behaviors:

Weight shifting between limbs, muscle frequent weight shift between front, sweating, abdominal muscle tension, trembling or tension hind, or all limbs trembling

Swishing tail, nodding or shaking head pointing, toe tapping, or pawing with pawing, bruxism, grimacing, vigorously, bruxism one or more limbs flehmen, head shaking

Lip flapping, grimacing, flehmen, touching muzzle to affected front lying down and rising repeatedly, stretching head and neck repeatedly limb(s) often abruptly

Biting at stall walls, bars, buckets, or flinch when one or more limb is rolling from sternal to lateral hay/grain (without chewing) touched (hyperesthesia) recumbency repeatedly

Sweating, pinning ears at observer rolling from lateral to dorsal (sight, or approach and touch) Ocular pain behaviors: recumbency repeatedly

Trying to bite, kick, strike at, or moving squinting, lacrimation OS, OD, OU, buckling one or both front limbs rapidly away from observer photophobia abruptly

Facial muscle tension (periocular, slow reluctant chewing, jaw movement, nostril, chin) or twitch/tremble head held low, still

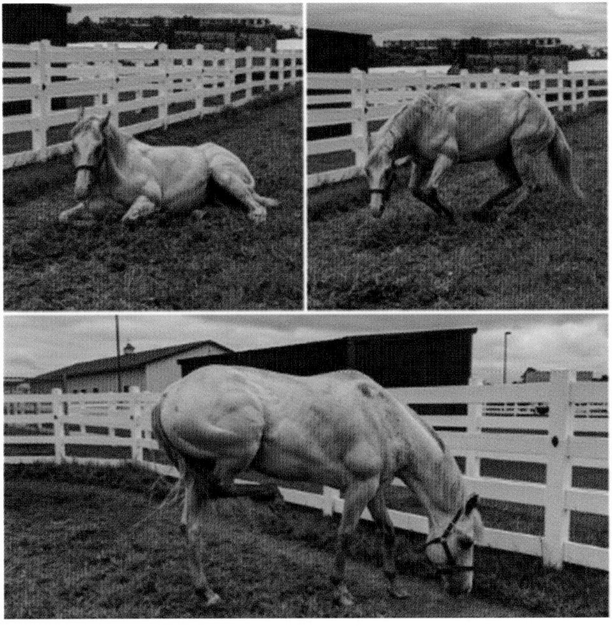

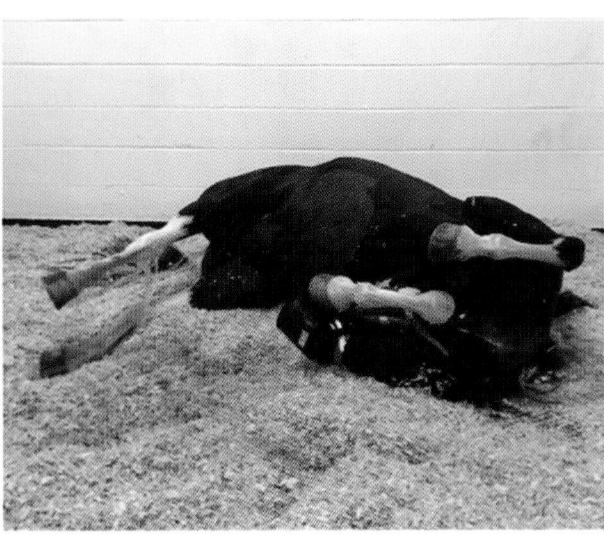

Figure 4.30 Signs of abdominal pain include rolling, kicking, pawing, and spending a lot of time lying down.

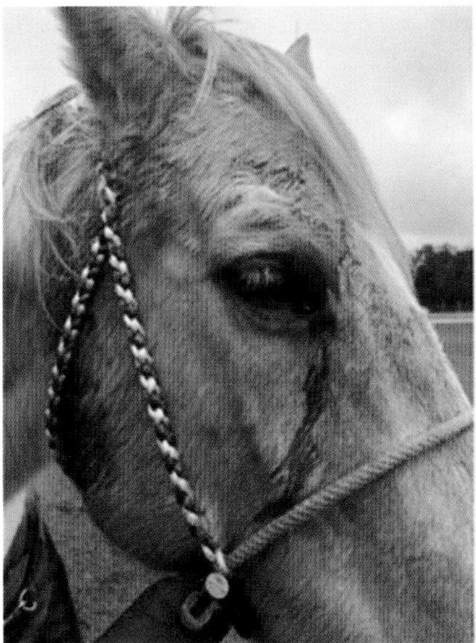

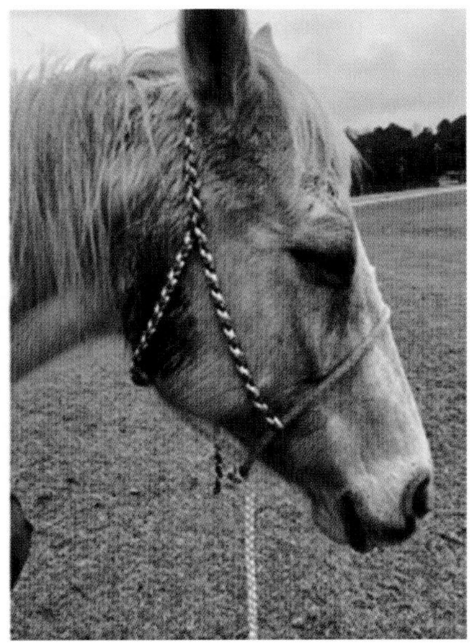

Figure 4.31 Signs of ocular pain can include weeping, squinting, eyelashes pointing downward. *Source:* Courtesy of Sarah Novotny.

with pleural pain may take rapid, shallow breaths and stand with their elbows adducted from their body.

Ocular Pain

There are unique ways to monitor ocular pain in horses. Horses with ocular pain are likely to keep their eye closed or partially closed (Figure 4.31). This is especially true when stimulated with light or medication administration. Horses in pain will tend to rub their eye, and often have increased lacrimation. Sometimes these animals will blink more frequently, and most will be averse to someone looking at the eye. They may sometimes appear to have a head tilt or to chew their feed slowly and reluctantly.

It is important to review pain assessment with respect to any analgesic treatment, because improvements in assessment parameters are an indicator that the analgesic support is appropriate. Whenever a pain assessment is conducted, it is also important to note any procedures that were performed. These procedures vary from farrier treatments, to bandage or cast changes, to repeat surgical procedures under anesthesia. When making use of specific pain assessments, such as those previously mentioned, several methods may be used to quantitate your evaluation. Simple pain scores use a number scale to indicate no pain (as zero, 0) to the worst possible pain (as ten, 10). Other scales use descriptions of behaviors associated with worsening pain states and assign numbers to each category. More involved pain scores make use of both observed and interactive assessments. Observed assessments such as the horse's demeanor and body language are seen from outside the stall. Interactive assessments may be a collection of metrics, such as heart and respiratory rate, or conducting a specific test, such as the horse's willingness to lift a hoof. One example of a specific pain score is the Modified Obel Lameness Score for laminitis patients.

The Modified Obel Lameness Score

The Modified Obel Lameness Score can be used as an evaluation tool for patients showing orthopedic or laminitic pain, and focuses on how the animal moves voluntarily, and when asked to move. The Modified Obel Lameness Score looks at the willingness of the animal to move around the stall, its willingness to stand if recumbent, as well as its willingness to lift feet. A normal horse should rise when asked, pick up all four feet when asked, and be willing to move around the stall, even in a circle. A horse experiencing pain may be reluctant to stand, even with significant coaxing, may not be willing to be led around the stall, and may be reluctant to pick up the hoof opposite the painful limb. Horses with multiple painful limbs will shift their weight repeatedly to avoid bearing weight on more than one compromised limb.

Box 4.2 Modified Obel Score

Grade Definition

0) No gait abnormalities at a walk or trot.

1) At rest, the horse exhibited foot lifting. The horse exhibited a normal gait at a walk. The trot showed a shortened stride and showed even head and neck lifting for each foot.

2) The walk was stilted, but showed no abnormal head or neck lifting. The trot showed obvious lameness with uneven head and neck lifting. A forefoot could be lifted off the ground easily.

3) The lameness was obvious at a walk and trot. The horse resisted attempts to have a forefoot lifted and was reluctant to move.

4) The horse experienced difficulty bearing weight at rest or was very reluctant to move.

Source: Adapted from Owens et al. (1995).

Interpretation

The senior veterinary provider should evaluate data collected from the pain assessment. Every part of the veterinary team can help to score the patient, but the collective data shapes the overall pain picture of the animal. When multiple caregivers are assessing pain, there should be a careful group review of that horse's unique behaviors and qualities so there is as much consistency between observers as possible. If the animal shows an improvement shortly after analgesic medications are administered, this may be determined to be a positive response to treatment. If there does not seem to be a change in the animal's comfort level following analgesic treatment, and it is still showing signs indicating pain, the treatment regime should be evaluated and adjusted.

Pain Management

In some mild cases of pain, horses may be managed with analgesics such as nonsteroidal anti-inflammatory drugs (NSAID)s, but in cases where there is more intense pain, the cause of the pain must be explored, and a comprehensive pain management strategy devised. Medications such as opioids and multimodal medication protocols may be necessary. The pain management regimen should be well-thought-out and tailored to the type of pain the patient suffers. One useful strategy when designing an effective pain management protocol is to use a lower dose of a particular medication, then increase the dose until pain assessment parameters are at an acceptable level or the drug is deemed ineffective. Similarly, if medications are changed, a repeat pain assessment should be performed to confirm the anticipated response. A rescue analgesia plan, which is the addition of a stronger medication to the protocol if the horse becomes more painful, should be available. It is important to create a plan to wean a patient from pain medication when their disease process improves.

Food Animal Physical Exam

During the physical examination process for food animals, the evaluator must note animal activity/behavior, herd/flock characteristics, anatomical structures/abnormalities, and physiologic changes within the patient and/or herd. The evaluator also develops an initial problem list and utilizes the case or herd history results to finalize the subjective and objective components of the medical record.

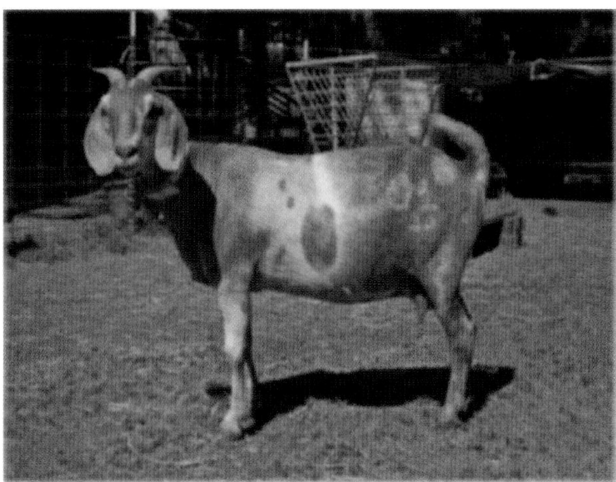
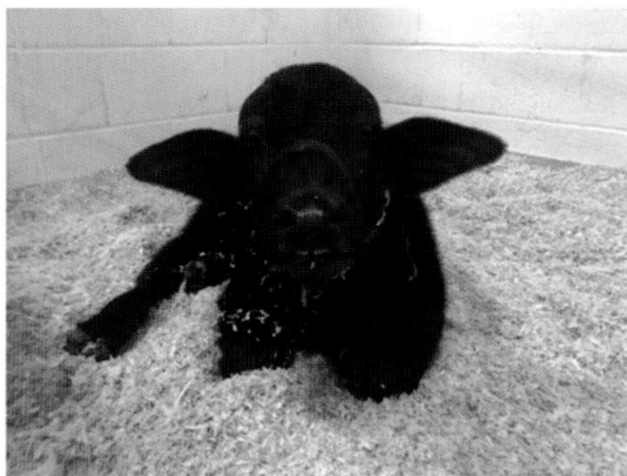

Figure 4.32 A physical examination should begin by using a "hands-off" approach, observing the patient at a distance of a few feet.

Inspection and Herd Examination: General

In the initial step of the examination, the technician should complete a general inspection of the patient or herd utilizing a hands-off approach. This step is best completed with the patient or herd at rest, prior to restraint (Figure 4.32). This allows the examiner to detect subtle details that may not be evident after the animal has been disturbed by capture or removal from a pen or its environment. The general inspection process is usually completed from a distance of a few ft/m (10–15 ft; 3–4.5 m) from the patient or herd. The experienced evaluator observes the patient from the front, rear, right, and left sides. An initial visual examination provides the ability to evaluate many of those characteristics that upon restraint are no longer evident. Sheep, goats, cervids, bison, and camelids are commonly alert and can be flighty, with a strong desire to "bolt" or run away from the observer. Lack of this behavior may signal individual animal health issues. Normal species behavior allows one to compare sick animals with healthy ones during the initial field examination.

In the United States, the majority of swine are raised in closed herds in confinement facilities. As such, one pig is not commonly examined as an individual animal, but as part of a herd. Though patient history is covered extensively in Chapter 3, it is prudent to discuss herd and individual history in this chapter as well.

> **TECHNICIAN TIP 4.13:** History is the most valuable component of the clinical examination, followed by patient observation.

When evaluating swine, the technician should perform much of the initial examination without actually handling the animal. Prior to physically examining the patient, their record, environmental assessment, nutritional evaluation, and a thorough informational history should be completed. Subjective history is the most valuable component of the clinical examination of the swine, followed by patient observation. Once this data is completed, the patient is then restrained and examined. Exotic, research, and pet breeds of swine, such as Vietnamese potbellied pigs and Yucatan, are examined in a similar manner as domestic swine. Management options for these species are far more commonplace. Pet swine prefer to be held firmly and securely with an assistant's hand held under the patient's chin and rump, although other physical restraint techniques may be used. Chemical restraint is often necessary for diagnostic sampling and minor surgical procedures such as foot care. Discuss with the owner and veterinarian any concerns that they may have prior to chemical sedation.

General Appearance Characteristics

The following items should be noted with a hands-off approach. BCS; mental status or mentation; physical or anatomic deformities; posture and gait/lameness; body or physical conformation; animal temperament; animal appetite if eating or animal's distance from feed bunk or water source; respiration (evaluate and record rate, rhythm, type, and intensity/depth); dermatologic issues (skin and coat); abdominal distention/shape; evidence of urination; defecation; tenesmus; regurgitation; or vomiting.

It is imperative to observe the patient's temperament, locomotion capacity, mentation, respiratory rate, urination, and defecation behavior prior to starting the hands-on portion of the examination. For a successful technician's assessment of patient health, the examiner must utilize information from both the history and the actual PE.

Physical Inspection: Regional Inspection for Abnormalities

A thorough PE requires a methodical evaluation of physiologic and anatomic systems function. The physical inspection process generally proceeds methodically either from cranial to caudal or conversely from caudal to cranial. Proceeding from cranial to caudal, the examiner would include:

- Head and neck
- Forelimb and thorax
- Abdomen and hindlimb
- Pelvis, tail, and perineum
- External genitalia and mammary gland(s)

After completing the general inspection process of the patient and/or herd, the technician now captures and restrains the patient. Initial examination data should include temperature, pulse, and respiration rates. These should be performed with as little trauma to the patient as possible to avoid stress-induced physiologic changes. Quietly and gently proceed with the evaluation trying to avoid an increase in animal stress and subsequent changes in heart and respiratory rates.

> **TECHNICIAN TIP 4.14:** Initial PE data should include TPR rates collected with minimal stress to avoid stress-induced physiologic changes.

Specific Physiologic Data: Temperature, Pulse, Respiration (TPR) Rates

Temperature

Vital signs are typically classified as the patient's temperature, pulse, and respiration rate. This data is essential to monitor the animal over time. An elevated or abnormal temperature may reflect disease process, ambient temperature changes, or stress. The veterinary technician should know the normal range of body temperatures for each species prior to determining if the animal's temperature is abnormal (Table 4.6).

Pulse

The normal pulse frequency varies in different food animal species and by individual animals. Factors that may affect the pulse rate include: age variations, BCS, sex, size, breed differences, atmospheric conditions, ambient temperature, time of day, stressful events, disease process, recent exercise, and eating.

The pulse may be defined as the driving rhythmic, periodic thrust felt over an artery over time in conjunction with the heartbeat. The important characteristics to note while taking the pulse are frequency, rhythm, and quality. Frequency is determined by counting the number of beats occurring in 1 min. Rhythm describes a series of rhythmic beats that follow in unison at regular intervals and reflects the interval between contractions; this may be classified as regular or irregular. Pulse quality is the physiologic tension on the arterial wall and it is an indication of the volume of blood flow through the artery. Quality describes the size, amplitude, and hardness of the pulse. Most examiners take a pulse reading for 15 S and multiply it by 4 to determine pulse/min (Table 4.7).

The pulse is a valuable indicator of the health status of the patient's circulatory system. It is palpated with the fingers resting lightly on a superficial artery, preferably with bone directly underlying the palpation site, while simultaneously ausculting heart rate via stethoscope over the left axillary area. Applying too much pressure to the artery at the time of the examination may deeply compress the vessel and eliminate the pulse. This pulse failure is particularly evident in weak, small, and neonatal patients. The technician must be able to evaluate an animal's physiologic state and consider factors such as excitement and stress. The technician should also recognize and correlate pathological irregularities in the pulse and the observed clinical signs (Table 4.8).

Table 4.6 Normal temperature for food animal species.

	Temperature (°F)	Range (°C)
Camelid (Alpaca)	99.5–102.0	37.5–38.9
Camelid (Llama)	99.5–102.0	37.5–38.9
Bovine (Mature)	100.0–102.5	37.8–39.2
Bovine (Yearling)	101.5–103.5	38.6–39.8
Ovine/Caprine	102.0–104.0	38.9–40.0
Swine (Mature)	100.0–102.5	37.8–38.9
Swine (Juvenile)	102.0–104.0	38.9–40.0

Table 4.7 Normal pulse rates for food animal species.

	Pulse beats/minute
Camelid (Alpaca)	70–120
Camelid (Llama)	60–90
Bovine (Mature)	40–80
Bovine (Yearling)	100–120
Ovine/Caprine	70–90
Swine (Mature)	70–90
Swine (Juvenile)	100–130

Table 4.8 Anatomical sites for obtaining pulse rates.

	Camelids	Cattle	Sheep/ Goats/ Calves	Mature Swine
Femoral artery	X		X	X
Brachial artery	X		X	
Facial artery; lateral aspect of mandible	X	X		
Coccygeal artery		X		
Median artery		X		X
Saphenous artery		X		
Aorta/internal iliac artery		X		

TECHNICIAN TIP 4.15: The most common site to take the pulse in cattle is the ventral coccygeal artery.

Respiration

Respiration involves both inspiration and expiration. Respiration rate is usually determined as the number of breaths per minute. In observing the respiratory system of a patient, begin at the nostrils/nares and examine caudally. Observing the movement patterns of the chest/ribs or flanks or dilation/movement of the nostrils/nares can determine the respiratory rate – flow patterns of air on inspiration and expiration. Note any patient abnormalities in respiration, breath, normal/abnormal discharge, nasal cavity evaluation, examination of submaxillary lymph nodes, cough (nature and composition), larynx and trachea auscultation and palpation, surface of thorax, and auscultation of thorax. The respiratory rhythm intervals are normally equal, with expiration being of slightly longer duration than inspiration. Respiratory intensity or depth of breath is barely noticeable in the healthy patient at rest (Figure 4.33).

Generally, an increase of respiratory intensity at rest signifies disease. The type of breathing is also significant to the examiner. When observing an animal breathing, it is normal for movement to be observed in the lower ribs and stomach muscles (costo-abdominal). If breathing has shifted to upper ribs and chest muscles, it is referred to as costal or thoracic. Costo-abdominal breathing is considered normal. When respiratory movements have shifted to primarily costal or thoracic, a disease process should be suspected. Variations in respiration rate can be stimulated by various factors including: body size and BCS, animal age, exertive exercise, induced excitement, ambient temperature, atmospheric conditions, pregnancy, and fullness of ingesta within the digestive tract. If variation in respiration rates are encountered and environmental conditions are suspected as being a possible cause, it is prudent to check the rate of two or three other animals for comparative purposes (Table 4.9).

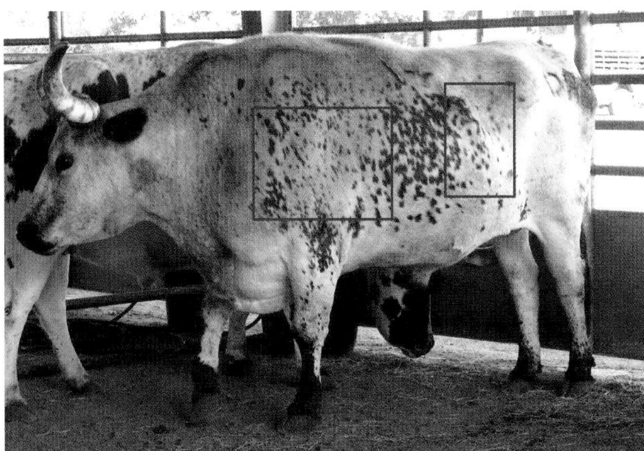

Figure 4.33 Observe the movement patterns of the chest/ribs or flank to determine respiratory rate.

Table 4.9 Normal respiratory rates for food animal species.

	Respiration (breaths/minute)
Camelid (Alpaca)	10–30
Camelid (Llama)	10–30
Bovine (Mature)	10–30
Bovine (Yearling)	15–30
Ovine/Caprine	20–30
Swine (Mature)	10–24
Swine (Juvenile)	<50

Systems Evaluation

The problem list may be reevaluated if interpretive laboratory work is completed. This data is then presented to the veterinarian for the establishment of a differential diagnosis list, a diagnostic plan, and finally a client education plan. The PE contains both subjective and objective components of the SOAP medical record system as well as a technician's assessment. The technician will need to know for each breed and species whether any observation is normal or abnormal. A PE is generally carried out in anatomical order, usually from cranial to caudal. System evaluation includes:

- Cardiovascular
- Respiratory
- Digestive

- Urinary
- Reproductive
- Nervous
- Musculoskeletal
- Integument
- Lymphatic system

Examination of the Head and Neck

Some examiners examine the head last in cattle and swine as these species sometimes resent manipulation of the head and neck, although if dealing with animals that have a contagious diarrheal disease or following a cranial to caudal examination process, the head should come first. The technician should feel the ear pinna for temperature, as milk fever in dairy cattle is commonly reflected in cold ears. Note the head for symmetry as well as nasal, ophthalmic, and otic discharges.

During the physical examination, a dry, dirty nose commonly indicates a sick pig or cow. Evaluate neurologic signs and the cranial nerves through blindness, eye position, constricted pupils, papillary reflexes, head tilt, decreased ear pinna function, facial paralysis and paresis, and eyelid paresis. Monitor the sclera for color and degree of sclera vessel injection. Septic animals generally have large prominent dilated scleral vessels with hypopyon.

Examine the mouth and mucosal papillae for blunting, and the nasal passages for vesicles, ulcerations, and erosions. Palpate the trachea and pharynx as well as retropharyngeal lymph nodes. Mucous membrane assessment should include evaluating the mucous membrane for color and CRT utilizing the conjunctiva, gingiva, or vulva as well as the bulbar or palpebral conjunctiva. Large, congested blood vessels within the bulbar conjunctiva area are a common sequella to bacterial toxemia.

The veterinary technician should assess the eye for papillary light reflex, adequate menace response, and a central position in the orbit with a strong papillary light reflex and menace response. During the examination, the eyelids should be evaluated for size, placement, swelling, symmetry, and position. The presence of a mucopurulent or serous discharge may be indicative of infectious conjunctivitis, trauma, or other infection. Blunt trauma may also stimulate asymmetry (Figure 4.34).

Nostrils or nares should be examined, and the color, quality, and viscous nature of the fluid evaluated. Mucopurulent nasal discharge is not uncommon with respiratory infections. The patient's cheeks should be evaluated for impacted teeth, abscesses, swelling, impacted cuds, and/or salivary gland mucoceles. The dental arcade should be thoroughly inspected, if possible, especially noting broken mouth or tumors. Submandibular fluid accumulation, also known as "bottle jaw," is common with severe parasitism and should be noted. Caseous lymphadenitis abscesses caused by *Corynebacterium pseudotuberculosis* is common at the point of the ramus in sheep and goats. Goiter, trauma, punctures, and abscesses may produce swellings of the lateral neck.

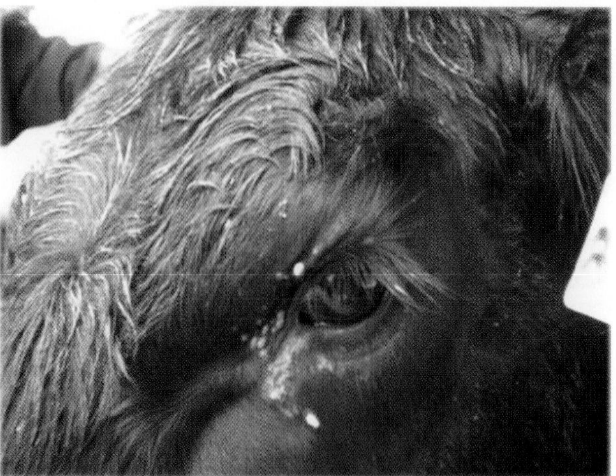

Figure 4.34 Evidence of ophthalmic discharge.

Left Side Examination: The Heart and Lungs

It should be noted that the patient's heart rate is generally elevated during capture and restraint, physiologic stress, pain, excitement, and toxemias. When ausculting the heart in food animal species, apply your stethoscope bell deep into the left axilla between the third and sixth ribs to find the pulmonic (third intercostal space), aortic (forth intercostal space), and mitral (fifth intercostal space) valves. Heart auscultation requires an evaluation of the rhythm, rate, and any irregular heart sounds. While ausculting the heart, the technician should clearly hear the beating on the left side of the animal. If the technician cannot clearly hear the heartbeat, readjust the stethoscope to apply more pressure to the bell or move it into a more axillary position. Heart sounds S1 and S2 are the first and second sound you hear when ausculting the heart. If is often described as a "lub dub." The closing of the AV valves produces these sounds. Heart sounds S3 and S4 are the third and fourth sounds and are less frequently heard. Time and practice improve auscultation skills. While evaluating the heart, muffled or dampened heart sounds can be the result of obesity or pericardial and pleural effusion. Most patients with cardiac disease have tachycardia and many infectious diseases are associated by toxemia, pyrexia, and dehydration resulting in tachycardia. Bradycardia can be associated with vagal indigestion in young stock (Figure 4.35).

Several disease states can change the cardiac pattern during the auscultation process. Bacterial endocarditis may

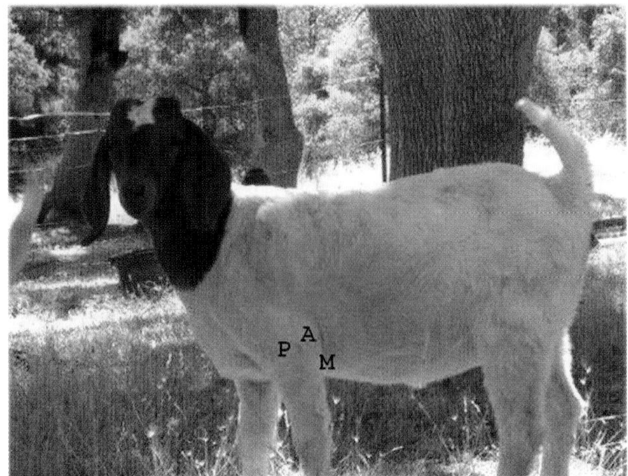

Figure 4.35 Auscultation areas for the pulmonic, aortic, and mitral valves.

occasionally stimulate a regurgitant mitral valve murmur that can be auscultated on the left side. In the bovine patient with cardiac disease as a result of traumatic reticulopericarditis, the technician will note muffled heart sounds and concomitant "washing machine"-like sounds. Gastric disease also affects the cardiac examination. Atrial fibrillation is a common rhythm abnormality causing an irregular heartbeat and is most often associated with gastrointestinal problems such as a left displaced abomasum (LDA). Additionally, auscultation on the left side can detect mitral valve insufficiency (MVI), pulmonic stenosis (PS), patent ductus arteriosus (PDA), and aortic stenosis (AS).

Murmurs are not uncommon in livestock. Endocarditis, congenital heart disease, and intrathoracic masses (e.g. abscesses or thymomas) can cause murmurs. Intrathoracic foreign bodies or masses are often initially detected as a muffled heart sound. Additionally, it should be noted that congestive heart failure is very rare in small ruminant species.

The tricuspid valve on the right side of the heart may be ausculted between the third and fifth intercostal spaces near the costochondral junction. Tricuspid valve insufficiency (TVI) and ventricular septal defects (VSD) can also be noted on the right side of the heart (Figure 4.36).

The veterinary technician should examine the jugular vein for filling by occluding the vein ventral to the palpation/emptying site. The examiner first occludes the jugular vein with a finger; the jugular vein will fail to empty after releasing if cardiovascular disease is present. During the examination process, a distended jugular vein generally indicates a sign of right-sided heart failure and is not usually present in normal animals. Additionally, normal animals do not have significant jugular pulses when the head is elevated above the horizontal plane. Check submandibular

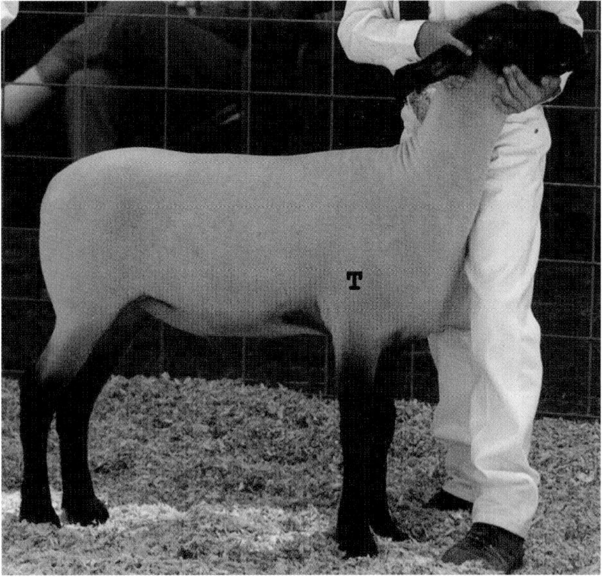

Figure 4.36 Auscultation area for the tricuspid valve.

regions, and in cattle, the brisket area, for edema. Pinch the skin of the neck to assess hydration status.

The patient can be stimulated to take deeper breaths by placing a large plastic bag over the animal's nose and mouth for several minutes or by pinching off the nostril/nares. This technique uses what is commonly called a rebreathing bag and helps to simulate exercise and consequently causes the animal to take deeper breaths at an increased rate. When the bag is removed, most patients will take one to several deep breaths. Auscultation should therefore continue until the animal returns to a more normal respiratory depth and rate after removal of the rebreathing bag. Due to anterior/ventral pulmonary involvement, it is important to auscult well cranial and ventral of the thoracic field on the chest (Figure 4.37).

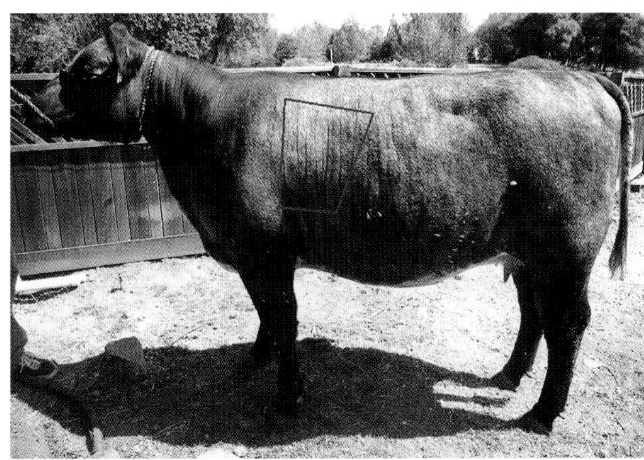

Figure 4.37 Auscult cranial and ventral on the thoracic field on the chest.

Normal respiration rates in livestock generally vary between 12 and 20 breaths/min. This value can be elevated to as high as 60–80 breaths/min during high ambient temperature events. Coughing and open mouth breathing should be examined and noted. Additionally, it may be helpful to take a resting and exercised respiratory rate. Wheezing, rales, crackles, and pleural friction rubs are abnormal sounds and should be noted. Swine commonly have adverse respiratory pathology associated with management and weather changes. Small ruminant pulmonary auscultation can be difficult due to a decreased lung field area. Harsh pulmonary sounds commonly arise from normal bronchovesicular auscultation. The technician must observe not only the rhythm and frequency, but also quality and effort of respiration. Respiratory disease is very common in cattle, sheep, and swine. Obvious signs of respiratory disease include open mouth breathing, coughing, mucopurulent discharge, rales, and apnea.

The technician should auscult the pulmonary field by moving their stethoscope systematically over the entire lung field. It should be noted that normal pulmonary sounds are essentially quiet during the auscultation examination. When evaluating normal pulmonary sounds, inspiration tends to be louder than expiration and ventral lung fields are louder than dorsal fields. When evaluating the trachea, upper airway abnormalities may result in "referred" abnormal inspiratory sounds. Referred means that while a sound may be heard in one area, it could indicate an abnormality within another part of the respiratory system, in this case the lung. In swine and cattle, lung consolidation due to pneumonia may often result in louder than normal large airway sounds, especially in the ventral pulmonary fields. Pleural pain can be observed as shallow and short breaths. The technician should always include tracheal palpation in their respiratory examination. If this pressure elicits a cough, it may indicate bronchitis, tracheitis, or a combination of the two. While in this region, manually examine the superficial cervical lymph nodes (pre-scapular lymph nodes) found just cranial to the patient's point of shoulder.

TECHNICIAN TIP 4.16: Normal pulmonary sounds are quiet during auscultation and inspiration tends to be louder than expiration. Ventral lung fields are louder than dorsal fields.

Left Side Examination: Abdomen

Assessment of the ruminant abdomen usually begins with auscultation of all four quadrants of the flank, each quadrant ausculted for a full minute. The first area to auscult is the left paralumbar fossa, over the rumen, to determine the number of rumen contractions in 60 S. The normal adult rumen contracts one to three times per minute. When ausculting the other quadrants, the character and amount of abdominal sounds or borborygmi should be evaluated and recorded. In camelids, the third chamber sounds should be evaluated for strong contractile efforts.

In addition, the veterinary technician should ping the left side of the patient by simultaneously percussing the examination area and auscultating the left side target region interface. This procedure can be accomplished by firmly flicking the examiner's finger against the body wall. A responding ping may represent a gas-fluid interface. All respiratory and gastrointestinal regions can be evaluated by pinging. This technique can be especially helpful when evaluating the respiratory tract of swine for consolidated regions secondary to pneumonia.

In ruminant species, gas-fluid interfaces may be present in the abomasum as an LDA, rumen tympany, or peritoneal cavity on the left side. When evaluating a potential LDA, the ping can occur in the mid-thorax region on a line between the elbow and the tuber coxae and may extend caudally to the cranial edge of the left paralumbar fossa. LDA pings and rumen pings often occur concomitantly but can be differentiated through location and tonal quality. Patients with vagal indigestion or ruminal bloat will commonly have distention over the rumen and right ventral abdominal quadrant. Percussing, balloting, palpating, and ausculting are all useful tools when evaluating the abdomen.

Right Side Examination: The Heart and Lungs

Initially, the technician should also examine the right jugular vein for filling as was done on the left heart examination. Right-sided heart failure and thrombosis are common causes of distended jugular veins and are never present in the normal patient. When elevating the head in a normal animal examination, jugular pulse is minimal or nonsignificant. The right side of the heart is auscultated in a similar fashion as the left side of the heart. However, the intensity of the heartbeat and subsequent pathology is not as loud on the right side. This can make diagnostic procedures less obvious to the beginning technician. As previously mentioned, the tricuspid valve is located at the third intercostal space and is a very common site for bacterial endocarditis diagnosis through presentation of a persistent murmur. Endocarditis presents to the examiner with a distended jugular vein, submandibular swelling, murmur, and brisket edema in the bovine. In the early course of the disease, tachycardia and fever are evident.

When evaluating the right pulmonary field, the technician must auscult the lungs by moving the stethoscope systematically over the entire lung field from cranial to caudal and dorsal to ventral. Ruminants have a fairly small lung field, whereas swine have a very well-developed pulmonary area. As previously mentioned for the left side thoracic

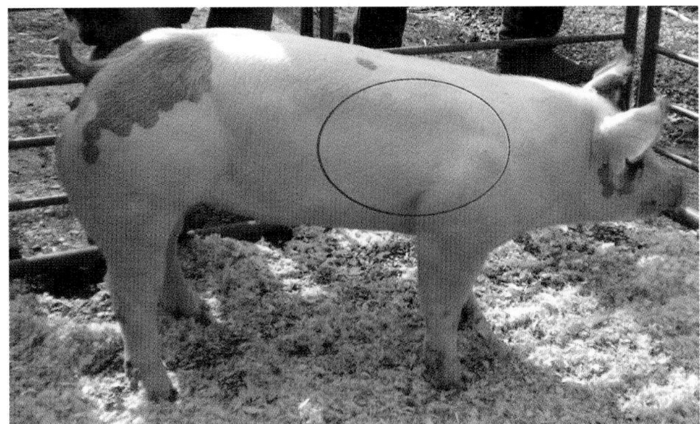

Figure 4.38 The technician should auscult the pulmonary field by moving the stethoscope systematically over the entire lung field, which is well-developed in swine.

examination, the superficial cervical lymph nodes (prescapular lymph nodes) found just cranial to the patient's point of shoulder should be examined (Figure 4.38).

Right Side Examination: Abdomen

The right side of the animal should be auscultated as previously mentioned for the left side, listening to the quadrants for borborygmi. Further evaluation of the right side of the animal is for gas-fluid interfaces, and the technician should ping the right side of the patient and carefully delineate the borders of any abnormal regions. Pings on the right side of the examination can be more confusing as compared to the left side evaluation. Most pings elicited on the right-sided examination are due to organ percussion and not displaced gastric contents. However, right-sided pings may be due to fluid and/or gas accumulation within a number of organs. These organs include the postpartum uterus, cecum, spiral colon, duodenum, small intestine, abomasum, peritoneum, and rectum. In dairy cattle, both right displaced abomasum (RDA) and right displaced abomasal torsion (RTA) can be diagnosed through assessment of the right abdomen. RDA and RTA pings generally are cranial to the eighth rib (much more cranial than the LDA). Right paralumbar fossa pings commonly reflect gastrointestinal disturbances in a number of domestic livestock species. The distended cecum in cattle is palpable on rectal palpation. Both heart rate (elevated) and dehydration (>8%) are additional factors to consider when assessing right-sided gastrointestinal abnormalities. Ballottement is also an important tool for a PE.

The Mammary and Urogenital Tract

Physical examination of the mammary and urogenital tract should first include the collection of diagnostic samples, such as urine and feces. The technician may induce urination in sheep by compressing the nares bilaterally. This technique should not be utilized on critical patients and does not work in goats; however, most small ruminant species will urinate at some point during the physical examination process. The alert technician should always be poised for the impromptu micturition and have sample collection materials close at hand. Male animals with urolithiasis will vocalize loudly while urinating. Additionally, the presence of urine ketone bodies is common in patients with a negative energy balance and may reflect pregnancy toxemia in the female. Free catch urine that is clear and light amber in color suggests normal renal function. A urine sample may be readily obtained from a cow by stroking her perineum or vulva. A field assessment of the urine for ketones, blood, protein, hemoglobin, and bile pigments can be made immediately with a dipstick. Be sure to observe the patient's vulva for any blood, discharge, purulent debris, or fetal membranes. In the male, evaluate the prepuce for fly activity, blood, pus, uroliths, or ventral swelling/edema.

Visual exam of the mammary gland(s) and teats should note color, shape, visual symmetry, texture, and contour. Diseases of the mammary gland and adnexa may cause swelling/edema with concomitant asymmetry and color changes such as reddening or blueness. Each gland should be palpated for heat, loss of function, pain, hardness, fibrosis, tenderness, firmness, edema, or acute swelling. Mastitis in all species will elicit some or all of these findings. Ovine progressive pneumonia (OPP) in sheep and caprine arthritis-encephalitis (CAE) in goats will produce similar mastitic findings but are not associated with a true mastitis. Camelids rarely have udder difficulties. Swine have extensive issues with mastitis following farrowing, including mastitis, metritis, and agalactia (MMA). The technician should always examine the milk whenever possible. Examination and evaluation in cows, sheep, and goats utilizes a strip plate/cup and should be performed routinely. A California Mastitis Test (CMT) in dairy cows, goats, and milking sheep should follow the initial mammary stripping. At this time, the examiner should note the presence of fibrin clots, discoloration, odor, and consistency. Sheep and goats generally have higher milk cellularity than dairy cows, and CMT results should be evaluated accordingly (Figure 4.39). Ulcerated or scabbing lesions may indicate exotic or reportable disease in sheep, goats, and cattle. An enlarged mammary gland in a non-lactating patient is known as a precocious udder and may be common in higher producing small ruminant species. In addition, male goats may develop abnormal mammary tissue, which is referred to as gynecomastia.

TECHNICIAN TIP 4.17: Milk examination and evaluation should be performed using a strip cup and followed by the CMT in dairy animals. Note presence of fibrin clots, discoloration, odor, color, and consistency.

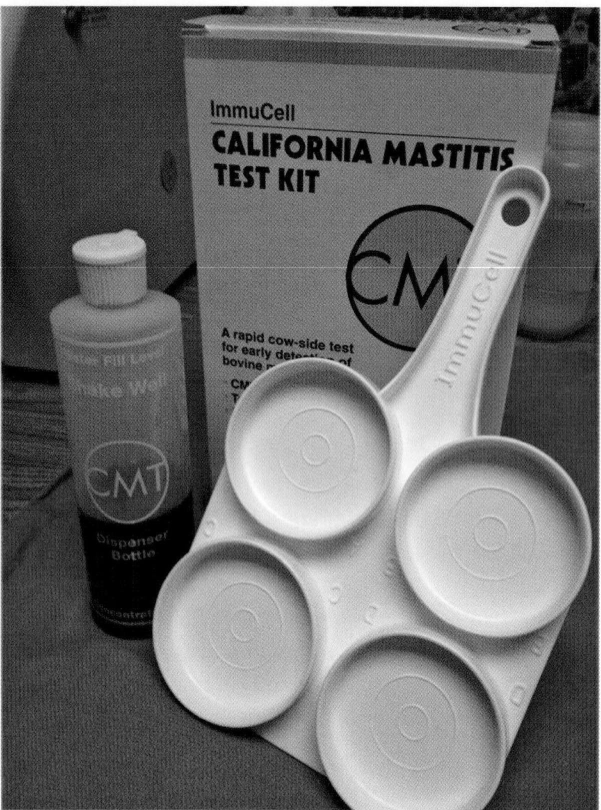

Figure 4.39 California mastitis test.

The technician, whenever possible, should evaluate the penis, testes, and epididymis of male patients via palpation. The size, shape, position, consistency, and texture of the testicles should be noted. Findings such as abnormal texture, shape, or size may indicate a disease process; fibrosis, hypoplasia, orchitis, and epididymitis are common in breeding animals.

Rectal Examination

The technician should examine the perineal region and tail area for evidence of diarrhea, blood, mucus, and feces as this may indicate a digestive disturbance. If the technician is performing the rectal examination, it is important that the exam proceeds in a consistent and repeatable sequence. Within small ruminant species, adding lidocaine to the palpation lubricant gel can facilitate relaxation of the lumen and rectal area. It should be remembered that goats are especially sensitive to the toxic effects of lidocaine; therefore, doses should be calculated carefully and approved by the veterinarian.

In ruminants, palpate the rumen on the left side of midline for shape, size, gas distension, and consistency. Some gas and extensive ingesta levels are palpable. Feed generally palpates as doughy compared to the ventral fluid-filled contents. Next, the technician should palpate the left kidney that is located to the right of the rumen on the midline. Continue the abdominal examination palpating toward the right abdominal wall; this region should feel empty if normal. Finally, if possible, palpate the deep inguinal lymph nodes along each ileum.

When evaluating female patients, locate the cervix on the floor of the pelvis. Examine the uterus and ovaries searching for abnormal pathology. Many times, the bladder may be palpated cranial to the brim of the pelvis if it is fully distended. With intact males, the technician should evaluate the internal and external genital organs. During rectal palpation, the examiner should evaluate the prostate gland, ampullae of the vas deferens, pelvic urethra, bulbourethral glands, and seminal vesicles. Additionally, within the external genital organs, evaluate the penis, scrotum, testes, epididymis, and spermatic cord.

Examination of the Feet and Legs

The examination of the feet and legs is of essential importance. Time must be set aside to differentiate between primary musculoskeletal issues from secondary issues that go beyond musculoskeletal symptoms. These secondary issues include: metabolic, neurologic, organ system failure, and infectious disease. As examples, mastitis may present as hind limb lameness; organ system failure may be a referred lameness condition.

When working in a herd or flock environment, excited animals may appear sound – care must be taken to evaluate the whole animal in a resting or calm state. Physical examination abnormalities may cause changes in body condition, symmetry, patient behavior, posture, and gait, as well as abdominal and thoracic distention. If the patient is initially observed as lame, visibly identify the affected limb or limbs by watching the patient ambulate slowly. The affected limb may be easily identified if the patient is non-weight bearing. Evaluate head carriage as well as hip and leg movement as the animal walks and stands. The patient will lower its head while bearing weight on the non-affected front limb or in layman's terms, "down on the sound." Conversely, the patient will elevate its hip when weight bearing on an affected hind limb.

> **TECHNICIAN TIP 4.18:** Head carriage can assist in lameness evaluations. Patients usually lower their head while bearing weight on the non-affected limb or "down on the sound."

When evaluating lameness in domestic livestock, most cases affect the forelimbs. When evaluating animals for lameness, forelimb lameness is most common in the feet and hind limb lameness is most common in the hocks. When the affected limb is determined, the patient should be restrained, and the affected foot and limb examined ventral to dorsal. The examiner should palpate tendon sheaths, ligaments, and joints. Joint and tendon pain, size, and fluid accumulation are all noted. Septic joints and painful arthritis are common in swine reared on concrete. Stifle joint injuries are commonly seen in breeding bulls and occasionally in older cows.

Overgrown toes and subsequently foot rot, infectious pododermatitis, is common in small ruminants and occasionally feedlot cattle. Inspecting feet for foreign body punctures on initial foot examination is essential to many successful lameness assessments. Interdigital infectious pododermatitis is a painful malady, and the technician may need special restraint equipment to thoroughly examine the feet, especially hind feet in breeding bulls. Interdigital infection with *Dichelobacter nodosus* causes a characteristic swelling, pain, and odor indicative of hoof necrosis. Hoof testers may be useful during this assessment, and many animals are only lame in one foot. In swine and breeding bulls with septic arthritis, palpate joints for heat, swelling, pain, loss of function, redness, and a decrease in range of motion. When evaluating goats for lameness, note painful, enlarged, hot joints, especially carpal joints, and for CAE. Paralysis and paresis are also issues associated with musculoskeletal lameness in domestic livestock.

Examination of the Integument

The veterinary technician should initially observe the patient's skin from a distance to evaluate hair coat, wool, fiber, and skin abnormalities, distribution, consistency, and patterns. Alopecia, hair shaft epilation, erythema, swelling, crusting, scaling, and edema are commonly seen with dermatologic disease. The patient's skin should be evaluated for color, thickness, excoriation, and level of pruritus, elasticity, lesions, and trauma. Testing for ectoparasites should be done at this time via hair shaft epilation and/or deep epidermal scraping. When assessing camelid dermatology, most lesions involve the face and legs. Swine dermatology disease generally involves the face, ears, and neck as well as dorsal and ventral surfaces. Small ruminants commonly are affected with the contagious ecthyma or sore mouth (Figure 4.40).

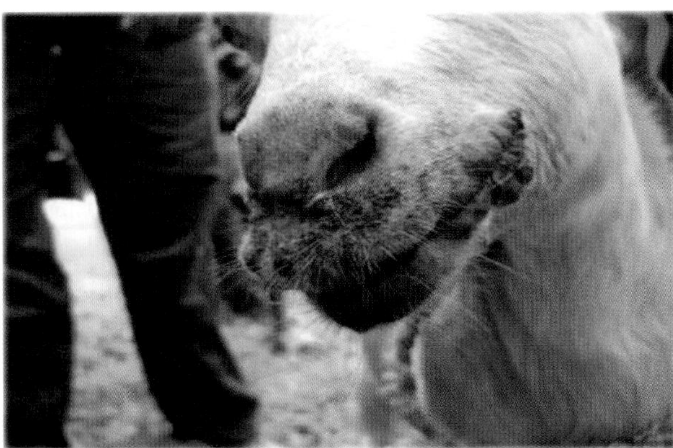

Figure 4.40 Contagious ecthyma or sore mouth.

Summary

The most important aspect of a physical examination is a thorough understanding of what is considered normal. By improving your skills when examining normal large animals, abnormalities noted on future exams will be readily apparent.

References

American Association of Equine Practitioners. (2002). *How Horses Digest Feed*. Retrieved from http://www.aaep.org/health_articles_view.php?id=200.

Andrews, A., Blowey, R., Boyd, H., and Eddy, R. (2004). *Bovine Medicine: Diseases and Husbandry of Cattle*, 2e. Ames, Iowa: Wiley Blackwell.

Bussières, G., Jacques, C., Lainay, O. et al. (2008). Development of a composite orthopaedic pain scale in horses. *Research in Veterinary Science* 85 (2): 294–306.

Dutton, D., Lashnits, K., and Wegner, K. (2009). Managing severe hoof pain in a horse using multimodal analgesia and a modified composite pain score. *Equine Veterinary Education* 21 (1): 37–43.

Fowler, M. (2010). *Medicine and Surgery of Camelids*. Ames, Iowa: Wiley Blackwell.

Graubner, C., Gerber, V., Doherr, M., and Spadavecchia, C. (2011). Clinical application and reliability of a post abdominal surgery pain assessment scale (PASPAS) in horses. *The Veterinary Journal* 188 (2): 178–183.

Haskell, S. (ed.) (2009). *Five Minute Veterinary Consult: Ruminant*. Ames, Iowa: Wiley Blackwell.

Henneke, D., Potter, G., Kreider, J., and Yeates, B. (1983). Relationship between condition score, physical measurements and body fat percentage in mares. *Equine Veterinary Journal* 15 (4): 371–372.

Jackson, P. and Cockcroft, P. (2002). *Clinical Examination of Farm Animals*. Oxford, UK: Blackwell Publishing.

Kentucky Horse Research, Equinews. (2012). *Causes of Poor Appetite in Horses*. Retrieved from http://www.equinews.com/article/causes-poor-appetite-horses

Menzies-Gow, N., Stevens, K., Sepulveda, M. et al. (2010). Repeatability and reproducibility of the Obel grading system for equine laminitis. *Veterinary Record* 167 (2): 52–55.

Orsini, J. and Divers, T. (2003). *Manual of Equine Emergencies, Treatment and Procedures. Management of Special Problems*. Philadelphia, Pennsylvania: Saunders.

Owens, J., Kamerling, S., Stanton, S., and Keowen, M. (1995). Effects of ketoprofen and phenylbutazone on chronic hoof pain and lameness in the horse. *Equine Veterinary Journal* 27 (4): 296–300.

Price, J., Catriona, S., Welsh, E., and Waran, N.K. (2003). Preliminary evaluation of a behaviour-based system for assessment of post-operative pain in horses following arthroscopic surgery. *Veterinary Anaesthesia and Analgesia* 30 (3): 124–137.

Pritchett, L., Ulibarri, C., Roberts, M. et al. (2003). Identification of potential physiological and behavioral indicators of postoperative pain in horses after exploratory celiotomy for colic. *Applied Animal Behaviour Science* 80 (1): 31–43.

Pugh, D. and Baird, A. (2012). *Sheep and Goat Medicine*. Maryland Heights, Missouri: Saunders.

Radostits, O., Gay, C., Hinchcliff, K., and Constable, P. (2007). *Veterinary Medicine: A Textbook of the Disease of Cattle, Horses, Sheep, Pigs and Goats*. Philadelphia, Pennsylvania: Saunders.

Reeder, D., Miller, S., Wilfong, D. et al. (2009). *AAEVT's Equine Manual for Veterinary Technicians*. Ames, Iowa: Wiley Blackwell.

Sellon, D., Roberts, M., Blikslager, A. et al. (2004). Effects of continuous rate intravenous infusion of butorphanol on physiologic and outcome variables in horses after celiotomy. *Journal of Veterinary Internal Medicine* 18 (4): 555–563.

Sherman, D. and Smith, M. (2011). *Goat Medicine*. Ames, Iowa: Wiley Blackwell.

Straw, B., Zimmerman, J., D'Allaire, S., and Taylor, D. (2006). *Diseases of Swine*, 9e. Ames, Iowa: Wiley Blackwell.

Viñuela-Fernández, I., Jones, E., Chase-Topping, M., and Price, J. (2011). Comparison of subjective scoring systems used to evaluate equine laminitis. *The Veterinary Journal* 188 (2): 171–177.

Wagner, A. (2010). Effects of stress on pain in horses and incorporating pain scales for equine practice. *Veterinary Clinics of North America. Equine Practice* 26 (3): 481–492.

Wegner, K. (2012). Detailed General Comfort Score Sheet q2. Modified 8/29/2012 from the orthopedic and laminitis pain score used at The University of Pennsylvania, New Bolton Center.

Clinical Case Resolution 4.1

Final diagnosis: Hepatic lipidosis, a diet and management sequelae in camelids. Initial treatment consisted of supportive care with intravenous fluids, such as dextrose with B vitamins and amino acids added. The patient also received antibiotics, such as ceftiofur hydrochloride, and blood glucose was monitored and managed with insulin. The patient's appetite improved slowly over 10 days. After full recovery, seven weeks later, she gave birth to a live, healthy cria (Figure 4.41).

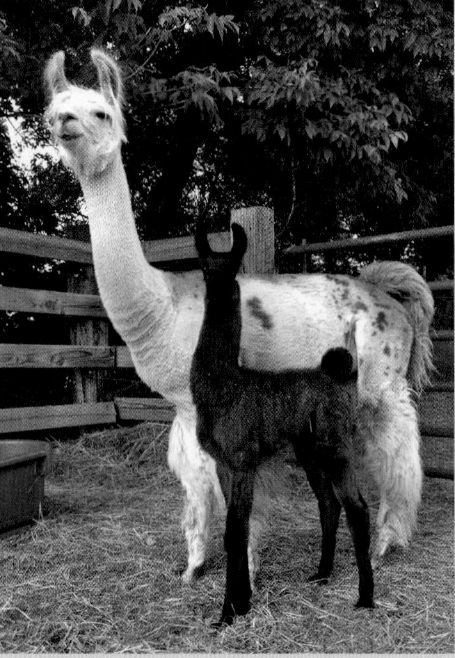

Figure 4.41 A healthy cria.

Activities

Multiple Choice Questions

(Answers can be found in the back of the book.)

1. Where do you properly take a camelid's pulse?
   - **A** ventral coccygeal artery
   - **B** facial artery on the lateral aspect of the mandible
   - **C** median artery
   - **D** saphenous artery

2. What is the normal rectal temperature of feeder pigs in degrees Celsius?
   - **A** 38.9–40.0
   - **B** 37.5–38.9
   - **C** 36.2–37.9
   - **D** 32.4–35.6

3. Which cardiovascular defects can be ausculted on the right side of a patient?
   - **A** bicuspid valve insufficiency (BVI)
   - **B** ventricular septal defects (VSD)
   - **C** mitral valve insufficiency (MVI)
   - **D** patent ductus arteriosus (PDA)

4. In sheep, the presence of ketone bodies in the urine is indicative of what malady?
   - **A** pregnancy toxemia
   - **B** bile pigments
   - **C** gastrointestinal disturbance
   - **D** right displaced abomasal torsion

5. What is the pathophysiology behind polioencephalomalacia in the adult ruminant?
   - **A** thiamin deficiency
   - **B** calcium deficiency
   - **C** copper excess
   - **D** phosphorus excess

6. What are the chambers in the camelid designated as?
   - **A** C1–3
   - **B** C1–4
   - **C** rumen, reticulum, abomasum
   - **D** rumen, omasum, abomasum

7. What pathologic conditions are associated with a severe jugular pulse found during a PE?
   - **A** endocarditis
   - **B** right-sided heart failure
   - **C** caseous lymphadenitis
   - **D** pulmonary parasitic infection

8. Which of the following heart valves can be ausculated on the right side of the patient?
   - **A** aortic
   - **B** pulmonic
   - **C** tricuspid
   - **D** mitral

9. When ausculting heart sounds on a normal patient, which ones are frequently heard?
   - **A** S1 and S2
   - **B** S2 and S3
   - **C** S3 and S4
   - **D** S1 and S4

10. A clinical sign that may indicate septicemia is:
    - **A** cyanotic mucous membranes
    - **B** brick red mucous membranes
    - **C** icteric sclera
    - **D** muddy sclera

Test Your Learning

1. When a pyrexic five-month-old gilt with diarrhea and dehydration is presented for admission to your hospital, what body systems should be evaluated first? How should you approach the rest of the herd?
2. Describe how you would complete a technician's lameness assessment on a three-week-old cria with valgus deformity.
3. Why do small ruminants require a more sedate environment to complete a physical examination?
4. List the areas on a horse where a technician would assess BCS.
5. Outline the use of a rebreathing examination to assess the respiratory system.

Answers can be found in the back of the book.

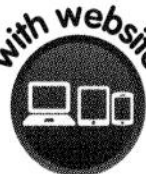

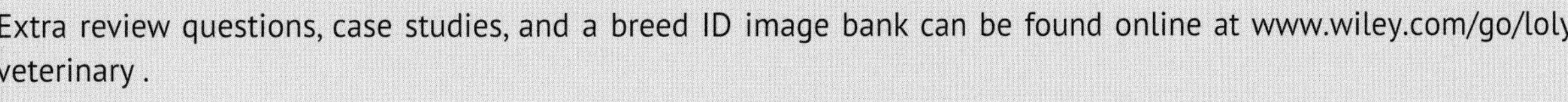
Extra review questions, case studies, and a breed ID image bank can be found online at www.wiley.com/go/loly/veterinary .

Chapter 5

Nutrition

Kara M. Burns, MS, MEd, LVT, VTS (Nutrition) and Sue Loly, LVT, VTS (EVN)

Learning Objectives

- List the six major nutrient groups.
- Describe how each nutrient group affects physiological processes in the body.
- Describe how nutrient excesses produce toxicity.

Clinical Case Problem 5.1 Hobby Farm Call

You will be making a farm call to a medium-sized hobby farm that has 25 sheep. The farm has experienced the sudden death of two of the sheep and the owners are obviously concerned. What questions would you be prepared to ask when taking a history from the owner? What things might you observe in the herd's environment?

See Clinical Case Resolution 5.1 at the end of this chapter.

Key Terms

Amino acid
Average daily gain
Body condition score
Complete feeds
Concentrates
Daily energy requirement
Digestible energy
Dry matter
Enteral nutrition
Insoluble
Kilocalorie
Metabolizable energy (ME)
Nonprotein nitrogen (NPN)
Nutrients
Parenteral nutrition
Roughages
Soluble

Introduction

Nutrition is an area of veterinary medicine that affects every animal. Optimal nutrition is required to attain health and productivity in all livestock, as nutrition has the potential to impact every physiological process in the body. Veterinary technicians should be familiar with the nutritional requirements of various livestock species and how nutritional requirements impact the health and well-being of large animals in their care. Proper nutrition and feeding management are the foundations on which maintenance of health and healing reside.

Nutrients are described as any food constituent that helps support life. There are six major nutrient groups: three that supply energy and three that do not. The energy- producing nutrients include proteins, fats, and carbohydrates; while the nonenergy producing nutrients are vitamins, minerals, and water. Typically, animals, especially non-domesticated animals, eat to satisfy their energy needs.

Large Animal Medicine for Veterinary Technicians, Second Edition. Edited by Sue Loly and Heather Hopkinson.

Companion website: www.wiley.com/go/loly/veterinary

Energy has no measurable size or dimensions, but can be determined by a complete burning of a food sample in a bomb calorimeter and measuring the heat produced, or "gross energy" content of the food. The term "kilocalorie" or kcal is this measurement and is the amount of heat required to raise the temperature of 1 kg of water 1 °C or C. Kilocalories are typically referred to simply as "calories" when discussing food or exercise. The term "digestible energy" refers to the food's gross energy minus the energy that is nonabsorbable and lost in the feces. "Metabolizable energy" is the food's gross energy minus the energy lost in the feces and urine, or the amount of energy that is available to the pet for metabolism after digestion and absorption.

TECHNICIAN TIP 5.1: A kilocalorie (kcal) is the amount of heat required to raise the temperature of 1 kg of water 1 °C or C.

Proteins

Proteins serve as the nitrogen source for animals, which, unlike some plants, cannot utilize atmospheric nitrogen. Besides being primary constituents of many body tissues, enzymes, hormones, and necessary components of hemoglobin and antibodies, plasma proteins are needed to prevent edema and to transport substances in the blood. Proteins supply approximately four (4) kcal of energy per gram, and are composed of combinations of building blocks called *amino acids*. There are 10 essential and 12 nonessential amino acids. Essential amino acids cannot be produced and must be supplied in the diet at proper concentrations. Amino acids consist of nitrogen, carbon, oxygen, and sulfur. The deconstruction or deamination process releases these elements into the body's system and results in either elimination from the body or is used as energy. The amount of required protein is dependent upon species, the animal's age, and the quality of the protein.

Protein quality can be assessed by its digestibility and amino acid profile. Measuring the biologic value (BV) of a protein is one way of determining quality. The more essential amino acids present in a protein, the higher its BV and the higher the protein source quality. The higher the quality of protein, the less protein is required. Protein supplied in excess of body needs is not stored as protein. Converting excess protein into energy and nitrogenous waste product (urea) is the responsibility of the liver. Urea is then excreted by the kidney. Animal source proteins contain more essential amino acids than some plant proteins, although combinations of the two types are often complimentary. When combined in proper proportions, they enhance the overall BV of protein in the diet.

TECHNICIAN TIP 5.2: The amount of protein required is dependent upon species, the animal's age, energy demands, and protein quality.

In ruminants, microbes support digestion and this digestion has the ability to convert most proteins into peptides and amino acids. Subsequently, these are further broken down into ammonia, organic acids, and carbon dioxide. The ammonia released during microbial degradation of protein will be removed from the rumen by absorption through the rumen wall or used by the ruminal microorganisms for synthesis of microbial protein. This protein synthesis results in a consistent protein quality to the lower digestive tract. Protein quality in moderate to poor feed typically improves through rumen metabolism. However, the opposite may be seen in high-quality protein feed as rumen microbes also convert nonprotein nitrogen (NPN) sources into microbial protein. Common NPN sources include: urea, ammonium salts, ammoniated by-products, or free amino acids. These NPN sources should be used cautiously to avoid potential excess or deficiency that may result in toxicity.

Carbohydrates

In livestock feed, carbohydrates are the most commonly used energy source and are typically less expensive ingredients in rations. Dietary carbohydrates provide approximately four (4) kcal of energy per gram, with cereal grains as the most common source in pet and livestock foods. Carbohydrates are classified into two segments based on their digestibility: soluble and insoluble. To increase absorption in the digestive system, carbohydrates must be broken down into simple sugars. For this process to occur, digestive enzymes must be produced by the animal or by microflora populating the digestive system of the host.

Carbohydrate-splitting enzymes are responsible for splitting most complex carbohydrates into simple sugars; the exception is those with beta linkage (i.e. cellulose/fiber). Microflora in the rumen of ruminants and the cecum of some nonruminants, such as the horse or rabbit, produce an enzyme so that cellulose/fiber can be converted into energy. Carbohydrates are commonly categorized as concentrates (grains, high-starch compounds) and forage (grass, hays, legumes). There are no minimum or maximum requirements for carbohydrates; rather, optimal intake is defined in conjunction with an individual's energy needs.

Soluble carbohydrates are also referred to as "nitrogen-free extract" or NFE. Carbohydrates can consist of simple sugars, or monosaccharides, and complex sugars as disaccharides and polysaccharides. Carbohydrates aid in digestion with the help of enzymes such as maltase, sucrase, and lactase, which are found in the intestinal epithelial brush border and break down disaccharides. Soluble carbohydrates in excess of the amount needed to meet an animal's energy requirements are stored in the body as glycogen or fat and may lead to obesity.

Insoluble carbohydrates are sometimes referred to as "dietary fiber," and include cellulose, hemicellulose, and lignin, among others. Monogastric animals lack the intestinal enzymes to completely digest insoluble carbohydrate sources, and rely on key bacterial flora to break down these fibers permitting partial assimilation. Fiber sources have varying degrees of digestibility or solubility. Dietary fiber, especially cellulose, has been shown to normalize intestinal transit time. Components of dietary fiber have also been shown to alter fat and glucose metabolism and to decrease the absorption of other nutrients.

Carbohydrates often used in livestock feeds are as follows:

- Fiber-forage: Structural carbohydrates, cellulose, hemicellulose
- Sugars (molasses, growing plants): Glucose, sucrose, fructose
- Starches: Stored carbohydrates, grains

TECHNICIAN TIP 5.3: Soluble carbohydrates in excess of the amount needed to meet the animal's energy requirements are stored in the body as glycogen or fat and may lead to obesity.

Fats

Fats serve as a more concentrated source of energy in a diet, providing nine (9) kcal of energy per gram. Fats can be a primary energy source of most commercially prepared foods. Fats also:

- enhance palatability;
- serve as a source of heat and insulation;
- are necessary for the absorption, storage, and transport of the fat-soluble vitamins, A, D, E, and K; and
- are a source of essential fatty acids: linoleic, linolenic, and arachidonic acid

Essential fatty acids are necessary constituents of cell membranes. Although linoleic acid is capable of being converted to arachidonic acid, the conversion process is difficult; therefore, arachidonic acid should be considered conditionally essential.

Vitamins

Vitamins are important in metabolic chemical reactions acting as enzyme precursors or coenzymes. Vitamins are divided into two basic categories: fat-soluble vitamins (A, D, E, and K) and water-soluble vitamins (B complex and C). Fat-soluble vitamins can be stored within body fat and in the liver. Dietary excesses of fat-soluble vitamins may result in toxicosis. The water-soluble vitamins are not stored to any great extent in the body. The veterinary healthcare team must be careful of excessive water loss, such as with polyuria and/or diarrhea, as vitamin stores may be depleted and vitamin supplementation may be justified.

TECHNICIAN TIP 5.4: The healthcare team must be careful of excessive water loss, such as with polyuria and/or diarrhea, as vitamin stores may be depleted and vitamin supplementation may be justified.

Minerals

Minerals can be divided into macro or microminerals. Balancing the amount of all minerals in the diet is important. Excess intake of one mineral may be harmful, and any unabsorbed portion may bind with other minerals, adversely affecting their bioavailability and resulting in a deficiency or imbalance (Table 5.1).

Calcium is required in the largest amount in the diet, but must be present in proper proportion and amount in relation to phosphorus. Excess calcium intake in feed will result in decreased absorption of phosphorus, iron, zinc, and copper, and will delay bone growth and maturation.

Phosphorus plays an important role in cell metabolism and composition of bone and teeth. Excess dietary

Table 5.1 Macro and microminerals.

Macrominerals	Microminerals
Calcium	Iron
Phosphorus	Zinc
Potassium	Copper
Sodium	Manganese
Magnesium	Iodine
	Cobalt
	Selenium

phosphorus increases glomerular filtration rate. Excess phosphorus in conjunction with calcium may result in soft tissue calcification, ultimately causing damage to the kidneys. Sodium is the main cation of extracellular body fluids, while potassium is the primary intracellular one.

Water

Water is the most critical nutrient, and all animals should have access to fresh, clean water at all times. A 10% loss in total body water causes serious illness, while a 15% loss may result in death! Owners should not rely on frozen water or snow in cold climates as an adequate source of water. Automatic waterers need to be monitored regularly for function and some animals need to be taught how to use an automatic system if they are not used to it. While convenient, it is not possible to monitor the amount of water consumed when using auto systems but close monitoring of the animals should be sufficient for detecting problems (Figure 5.1).

> **TECHNICIAN TIP 5.5:** A 10% loss in total body water causes serious illness, while a 15% loss may result in death.

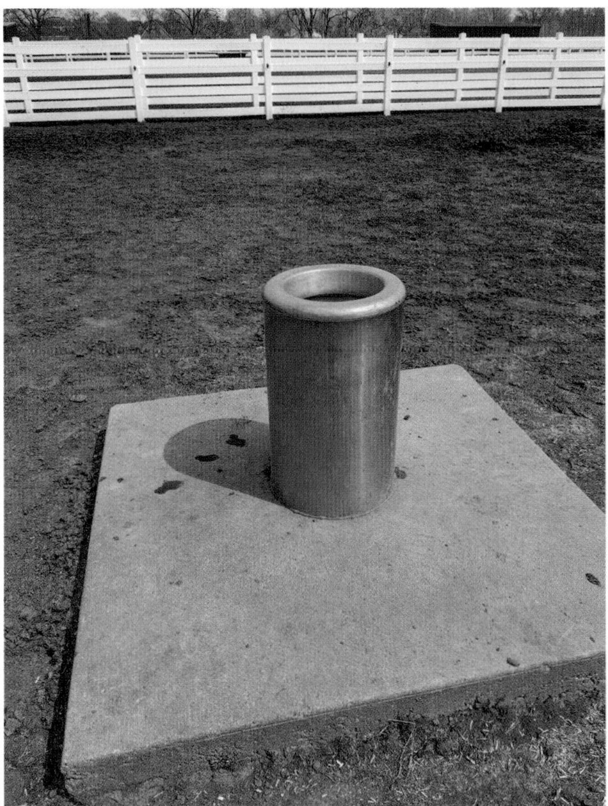

Figure 5.1 Automatic waterer.

Equine Nutrition

Feeding horses is an intricate science that requires providing precise amounts and balanced nutrients. Horses have long been domesticated and are often classified as companion animals. Companion horses today consume a variety of feeds ranging in physical form from forage with a high content of moisture to cereals with a high amount of starch, and from hay in long fibrous stems to salt licks and water. Horses are nonruminant herbivores that when housed on very large pastures or ranges naturally spend 60–75% of their day grazing, and typically ingest approximately 2% of their body weight (BW) (dry matter [DM] basis) per day.

Through domestication of the horse came husbandry changes in feed, feeding times, and feeding methods – more in line with domesticated canines and felines – where the horse is "meal fed" and unfamiliar materials such as starchy cereals, protein concentrates, and dried forages have been introduced. Horses are now confined more often in stalls or smaller pastures; are fed one to two times per day; and as a result, spend less time of the day eating, approximately 40%.

Diets formulated for horses contain on average 5% fat and 7–12% protein, with carbohydrates being the major source of energy (~80%). This is an evolutionary result for horses to eat grass and other forages, thus grass and hays serve as a strong foundation for the feeding of horses. Protein is required to build and replace tissue and although some may consider protein to be an expensive source of energy, dietary protein and fat can contribute to meeting the physiological energy demands of the horse. Protein converts the carbon chain of amino acids to intermediary acids and some carbon chains to glucose. Fat can aid in meeting energy demands following its hydrolysis conversion to glycerol and fatty acids. Subsequently, glycerol can be converted to glucose, and fatty acid chains can be broken down by a stepwise process called ß oxidation in the mitochondria yielding adenosine triphosphate (ATP) and acetate or acetyl coenzyme A utilizing tissue oxygen.

Carbohydrate digestion and fermentation yield primarily glucose and acetic, propionic, and butyric volatile fatty acids. The portal venous system collects these nutrients, and a proportion of them are removed from the blood as they pass through the liver. Both propionate and glucose contribute to glycogen reserves (liver starch) and acetate and butyrate bolster the fat pool and comprise primary energy sources for many tissues.

Nutritional Physiology

The nutritional physiology of the horse differs from that of the cat or dog. There are multiple compartments within the digestive tract of the horse and each compartment has its own function in terms of converting and utilizing ingested feed. The oral cavity is responsible for physically processing foods into smaller particles (~1.6 mm) that allows not only passage through the esophagus but also increases the surface area for small intestine enzymatic action. The oral cavity also breaks down structural carbohydrates for bacterial fermentation in the large intestine. The horse averages 60 000 chews per day and it is only during chewing that the salivation process is activated. Due to the increased amount of chewing in horses, they produce 1–2 gal of saliva per day, which acts as a lubricant for passage into the esophagus.

When an animal appears to be struggling maintaining weight, the healthcare team should recommend checking the dentition of the animal, before making drastic nutritional changes. Because a horse's teeth are always erupting and changing, sharp points and dull grinding surfaces can easily occur. As a horse ages beyond its 20s, a dull grinding surface becomes more common and softer diets that do not require much chewing can be considered. One suggestion of a horse struggling with chewing is to observe dropped feed and "quids" which are parts of hay partially chews and then spat out (Figure 5.2).

TECHNICIAN TIP 5.6: Due to the increased chewing in the equine species, a horse will average 5–10 l per day of saliva, which in turn acts as a lubricant for passage into the esophagus.

The stomach is responsible for ~8% of the total capacity of the equine GI tract, but retention time can range from 2 to 18 hr. The fundus and the pylorus are the two main regions of the stomach, with the pyloric region secreting 2.5–7.5 gal of gastric juice per day. The small intestine of the horse measures 50–70 ft long and has a volume of 10–12 gal. Transit time of the small intestine is on average 2–8 hr. At the proximal portion of the small intestine, pancreatic juice aids in digestion of lipids, protein, and nonstructural carbohydrates. The small intestine is also lined with microvilli, increasing the surface area of the gut. As mentioned earlier, digestion in the small intestine is dependent on oral processing and types of feed (forage is less digested than processed feed).

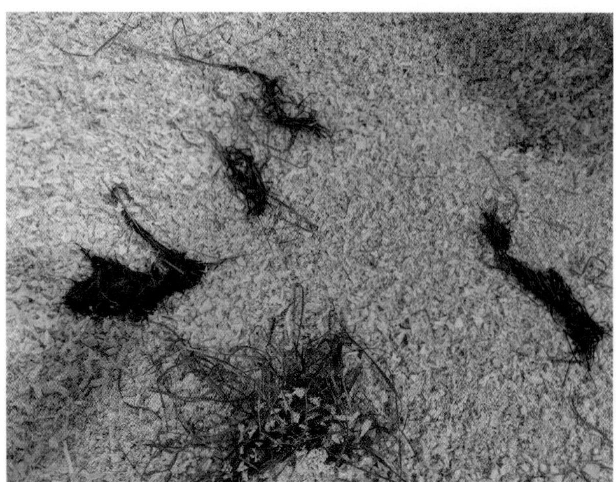

Figure 5.2 Example of hay "quids."

The large intestine has a large volume capacity (25 gal) and a very slow transit time of approximately 50 hr. It is responsible for the fermentation of structural carbohydrates to volatile fatty acids, which is responsible for 50% of the metabolizable energy and absorbs roughly 20 gal of water per day. The bacteria present in the large intestine produce B vitamins. It is also important to note that NPN is not utilized well in the large intestine. The large intestine (cecum and colon) in the equine is an enlarged fermentative chamber that contains an abundant and highly complex microorganism community. Some fermentation of feedstuffs occurs in the stomach and small intestine; however, the majority occurs in the hindgut. The fermentation rate, as well as the microbial and biochemical contents of the large intestine, is influenced by the makeup of the diet and the feeding pattern (i.e. continuous grazing, or small, frequent meals, versus large meals administered twice daily). For example, changing from forage only to a forage and concentrate diet will result in an increased rate of fermentation and marked changes in the microbial population, luminal pH, and the contents of volatile fatty acids (VFA) and lactate.

TECHNICIAN TIP 5.7: In conditions of extreme heat or stress on the horse, the number of liters a horse will drink per day increases to 100.

Key Nutritional Factors for Horses

The main nutrients of concern for the horse are water, energy, protein, minerals, and vitamins. As previously stated, water is the most important nutrient in any mammalian species and should be available at all times. Horses on average will drink 6 gal of water per day. In conditions of extreme heat or stress, this number increases to 25 gal per day. Of note is that technicians should remind owners that the more grain their horses eat, the more water their horses will need.

Energy is measured in terms of digestible energy (DE) and is fed in kilocalories. The amount of DE horses need will be dependent upon various factors: physiologic state, activity level, environment, and the size of the horse. The majority of energy utilized by the horse is provided by

Table 5.2 Kcal of various feeds.

Feed	kcal/kg
Oats	300
Alfalfa (early bloom)	2100
Bermuda grass hay	1800
Corn cob	1250

carbohydrates, which are ingested through the horse's natural feed. Fats provide the horse with high-density energy but should not exceed 20% of the total diet or 30% of concentrates. Exceeding these percentages will likely result in decreased palatability and loose stools.

Protein amounts are typically described as "crude protein" (CP) and are expressed as percent DM. As stated previously, the amount of protein needed by an individual horse is dependent on multiple factors: physiologic state, type of diet, age, quality of diet. The closer the proportions of amino acids in the diet conform to the proportions required by the tissues, the higher the quality of the protein (Table 5.2).

Calcium and phosphorus are evaluated together because of their interdependent role as the main elements of building blocks for the skeletal system. The requirement of calcium and phosphorus is dependent upon the physiologic state of the horse. The average adult horse weighing approximately 500 kg will need ~20 g of calcium and 14 g of phosphorus per day. It is important to balance the calcium-to-phosphorus ratio, as a mature horse needs a ratio of 1.1 : 1 to 6 : 1. The ratio for a growing horse is recommended to be 1.1 : 1 to 3 : 1.

Sodium is the principal determinant of the osmolarity of extracellular fluid, and as a result, the volume of that fluid. Chloride concentration in the extracellular fluid is directly related to that of sodium. Rarely do companion animals have an excess or deficiency of sodium or chloride; however, these are both conditions of which to be watchful. Daily, sodium requirements are recommended to be approximately 0.18–0.36% DM. If the requirements for sodium are met, seldom will a deficiency of chloride occur. Good sources of sodium and chloride can be found in grains with a premixture and in salt blocks.

Potassium is the main intracellular cation. Deficiencies or excesses in equines are rare. However, excess potassium can lead to hyperkalaemic periodic paralysis, a syndrome of episodic weakness accompanied by elevated serum potassium concentrations. This syndrome appears to be confined to descendants of one American quarter horse sire. Forages are approximately 1–4% potassium with cereals being relatively poor sources of potassium.

Selenium is a trace element needed to aid in antioxidant defense. The requirement is 1–2 mg/day for a 500 kg horse or 0.1–2 ppm selenium deficiencies produce pale, weak muscles in foals and a yellowing of the depot fat, known as "white muscle disease." It is imperative that pregnant mares receive adequate amounts of selenium in their diet. Selenium is highly toxic to animals; the minimum toxic dose through continuous intake is 2–5 mg/kg feed. Skin, coat, and hoof abnormalities are the result from excess selenium (Figure 5.3, Tables 5.3 and 5.4).

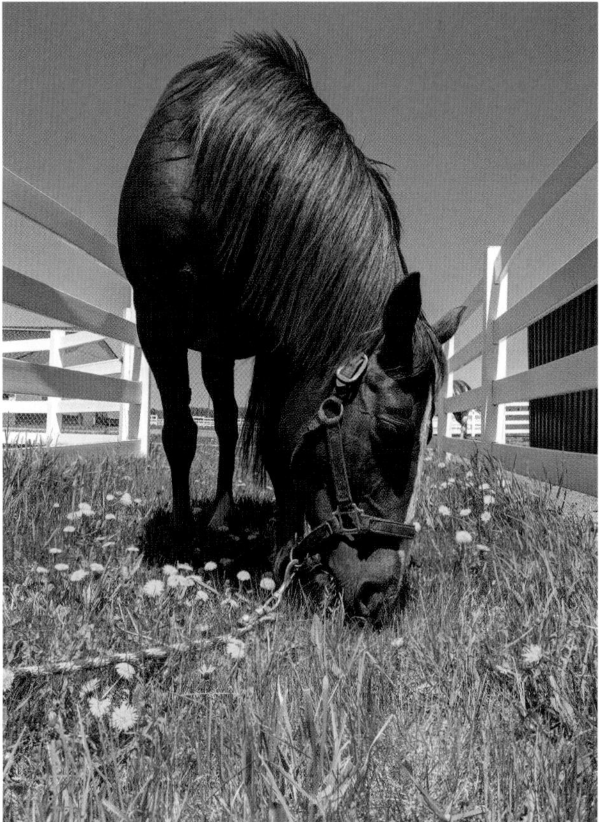

Figure 5.3 Horse grazing.

Table 5.3 Beta-carotene levels (mg/kg DM) amounts.

Pasture grass/alfalfa	300–600
Good hay	20–40
Poor hay	4–5

Table 5.4 Vitamin A requirements for horse life stages.

Mature	30 IU/kg BW
Gestation/lactation	60 IU/kg BW
Growth	50 IU/kg BW

> **TECHNICIAN TIP 5.8:** It is imperative that pregnant mares receive adequate amounts of selenium in their diet to prevent their foals being born with white muscle disease.

Grazing horses derive their vitamin A from the carotenoid pigments present in herbage. The principal one is β-carotene, with 1 mg of β-carotene equating to approximately 400 IU of vitamin A. Horses that graze for four to six weeks build up a three-to-six-month supply of vitamin A in the liver.

Vitamin E functions as a cellular antioxidant in conjunction with vitamin A and is required for normal immune function. Fresh green forage and the germ of cereal grains are rich sources of vitamin E. Adult horses require 80–100 IU/kg DM. Although deficiencies are rare, two neurological disorders of horses have been recognized as influenced by α-tocopherol status, equine degenerative myeloencephalopathy and equine motor neuron disease. These diseases typically are seen in horses that do not have access to pastures, in horses that consume a poor quality of hay, or in horses that have low concentrations of circulating levels of α-tocopherol.

Types of Feed

There are three main categories of horse feeds: roughages, concentrates, and complete feeds. Roughages include grasses and legumes cut for hay. Most common species of grass are suitable, but the preferred and most productive grasses are rye grasses, Kentucky bluegrass, fescues, timothy, and orchard grass. Species found in permanent pastures are satisfactory as well, and these include: meadow grasses, brome, and bent grass. Legumes utilized are red, white, alsike, and crimson clovers, trefoils, and alfalfa. Roughages are relatively low in energy and have >18% crude fiber. Roughages are considered to be the foundation to an equine feeding program and quality hay can provide energy for the maintenance requirements of the horse. Legumes and nonlegume grasses (Figures 5.4 and 5.5) that are well managed and fertilized (proteinaceous roughages) provide >10% CP as opposed to carbonaceous grasses (those that are not well maintained or fertilized) that provide <10% CP. Veterinary technicians can educate clients on the quality of roughage using the following guidelines:

- Free of mold
- Soft and pliable to touch
- Leafy with fine stems
- Pleasant, fragrant aroma
- Bright green, not brown or yellow

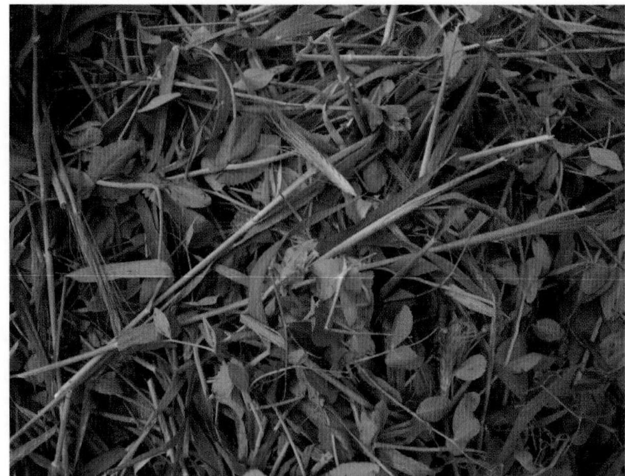

Figure 5.4 Roughage legume alsike.

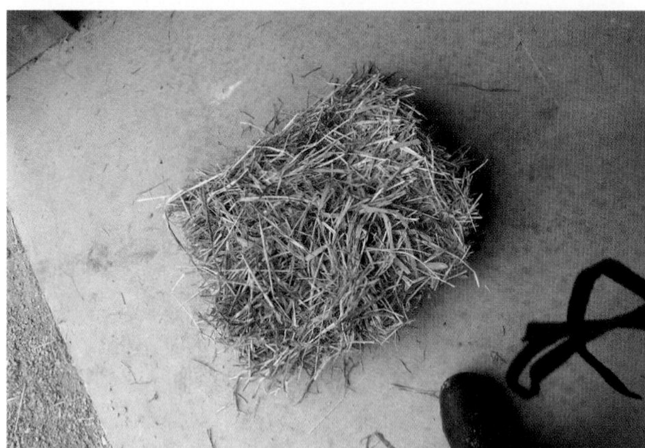

Figure 5.5 Roughage that meets quality criteria.

Another key point to communicate to owners is the fact that excess handling of roughages can result in a loss of 1/4 of the leaves; a loss of 1/4 to 1/3 energy and protein; and a loss of 90% of β-carotene (Figure 5.6).

> **TECHNICIAN TIP 5.9:** Roughages are considered to be the foundation to an equine feeding program.

Concentrates are typically a cereal grain that may or may not have supplemented protein, minerals, and vitamins. Concentrates are high in energy (typically, 50% greater than forage) and are <18% crude fiber. Oftentimes, concentrates are used as a supplement if forage is insufficient in nutrients – especially energy and protein. Concentrates are needed more often in certain life stages, such as gestation (especially, late gestation), lactation, growth, and in workhorses. A rule of thumb would be not to exceed 50 : 50 (wt : wt) concentrate to roughage. Any dietary changes must be introduced and transitioned slowly. It is important for the

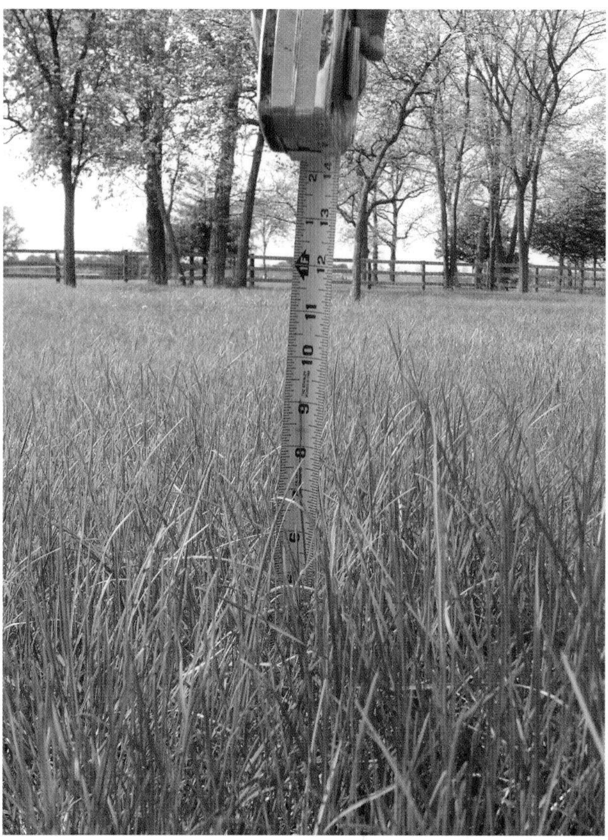

Figure 5.6 Measuring pasture growth. *Source:* Courtesy of Dr. Krishona Martinson.

veterinary team and owners alike to be cognizant of the fact that excess concentrate may lead to laminitis, rhabdomyolysis, developmental orthopedic disease, and obesity.

Complete feeds are typically a mixture of roughage and concentrate – usually an 80% roughage to a 20% concentrate mixture. Complete feeds are manufactured by complete grinding of the ingredients and formulating them into a pellet, thus making them easier to feed. There is often an increased cost for this convenience. Because the complete feed is pelleted or wafered, care must be given to the potential risks associated with inadequate particle size and reduced chewing, including colic and a choking risk (Figure 5.7).

When discussing nutritional management of horses with clients, remember to advocate that fresh water needs to be available at all times. Energy for maintenance can be met entirely with quality hay, but may be supplemented with concentrate if necessary. However, it is important to ensure that the horse is not supplemented in excess of 50% by weight with concentrates. Good-quality green roughage should supply adequate amounts of vitamins A and E. Lastly, nutrition is one area of equine medicine that affects every horse and should be discussed at every visit, every time.

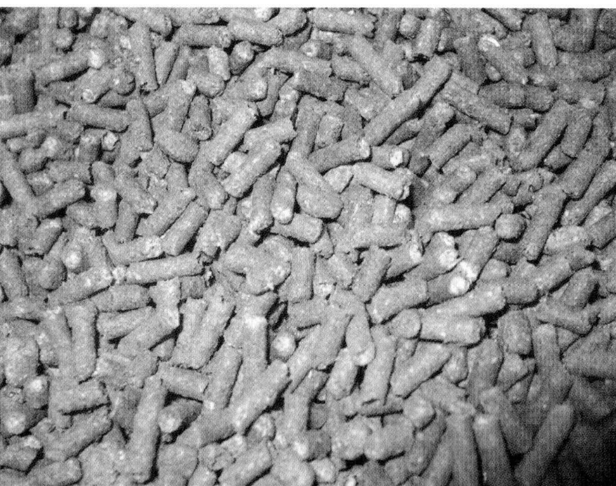

Figure 5.7 A complete feed pellet.

Pediatric Equine Nutrition and Care

The goal of a feeding plan for foals and young horses is to create a healthy animal that will grow into a healthy adult horse. The specific objectives of a feeding plan for a young horse are to achieve healthy growth, to optimize trainability and immune function, and to minimize obesity and developmental orthopedic disease. Growth is a complex process involving interactions between genetics, nutrition, and other environmental influences. Nutrition plays a role in the health and development of growing horses and directly affects the immune system, body composition, growth rate, and skeletal development.

Foals should be assessed for risk factors before weaning to allow implementation of an appropriate diet. A thorough history and physical evaluation are necessary. Additionally, body condition scores (BCS) provide valuable information about nutritional risks. Growth rates of young horses are affected by the energy density of the food and the amount of food fed. It is important that horses be fed to grow at an optimal rate for physiologic development and body condition rather than at a maximal rate.

Nutritional requirements and dietary composition of the foal change markedly from the time they are transitioned from neonate to weanling. The foal is transitioning from a continuous supply of nutrients while in utero to sporadic absorption of ingested nutrients post birth. Concurrently, the neonate's metabolism is no longer dependent upon maternal glucose concentrations to maintain normal glucose levels, and the pancreas must initiate glucose homeostasis. This alteration in energy metabolism is dramatic and does not always occur smoothly, as there are limited energy reserves (glycogen and fat) in the neonatal foal. Even in the "normal" neonatal foal, hypoglycemia occurs frequently, and veterinary healthcare teams must be aware of this fact. In the sick foal, severe hypoglycemia will result if the foal is deprived of energy for even a short period of time.

The neonatal foal has a high metabolic rate, thus frequent ingestion of high volumes of milk are needed to meet its energy requirements for maintenance and growth. During the first week to the first months of a foal's life, calorie needs are as follows:

- First week – ~150 kcal/kg/day
- Three weeks – ~120 kcal/kg/day
- One to two months – ~80–100 kcal/kg/day

Healthy foals younger than seven days old will nurse approximately seven times per hour for 1–2 min a time. After seven days, there is a decrease in frequency, but conversely an increase in the duration of time and amount of milk consumed. The mare's milk averages about 64% sugar (as lactose), 22% protein, and 13% fat.

> **TECHNICIAN TIP 5.10:** Healthy foals less than seven days old will nurse approximately seven times per hour for approximately 1–2 min a time.

After the first 24 hr, foals will start to eat small amounts of hay, grass, and grain along with the mare's feces. It is understood that feces provide the initial microbial flora needed by the foal to aid in the digestion of the hay, grass, and grain. Until several weeks of age, roughages and grains are not well digested by the foal. It is at this time that transitioning from a milk-based to a forage-based diet is gradually occurring. The milk produced by the mare peaks at approximately two months of lactation then begins to decline. Shortly thereafter, the foal will be weaned from the mare and rely on solid feed for an increasing proportion of its nutritional requirements. Complete maturation of hindgut function will occur around three to four months of age.

Energy Requirement

The energy requirement of growing horses is determined by calculating the total energy required for maintenance in addition to the energy required for growth or gain. The daily energy requirement (DER) is dependent upon a number of factors; the environment, the foal's age, the desired average daily gain (ADG), and the individual characteristics of the foal. The veterinary healthcare team members must take into account metabolic and health characteristics. Researchers and scientists have yet to determine the optimal growth rate for horses; therefore, it is difficult to determine the exact energy requirement. If horses grow too quickly and too much weight is added, skeletal integrity and longevity may be adversely affected. Conversely, inadequate energy intake will result in poor or slower growth rates, and young horses will look unhealthy. Most nutritionists and equine specialists will follow the formula recommended by the National Research Council (NRC). This formula calculates the DER of growing horses in the following manner:

$$\mathrm{DE}(\mathrm{Mcal/day}) = \left(56.5x^{-0.145}\right) \times \mathrm{BW} + \left(1.99 + 1.21x - 0.021x^2\right) \times \mathrm{ADG}$$

(x is age in months; ADG is average daily gain; BW is body weight in kilograms.)

The majority of horse owners will feed to achieve an ADG of 1.1–1.4 kg/day with some owners aiming slightly higher. Veterinary healthcare teams and owners must be cognizant of what feed is being fed, how much, other feedstuffs that are being added to the diet, as well as the energy concentration for total diets consumed. The team must perform a nutritional assessment prior to beginning a feeding plan and then on every subsequent patient visit (whether farm or hospital visit). The average energy concentration for the total amount of feed (on an as-fed basis) given to a growing horse can range from 2.5 Mcal/kg with diets consisting of 70% concentrate to 30% hay ratio to 0.72 Mcal/kg for certain pasture-fed growing horses. Young horses have been found to consume sufficient energy from pasture feeding to sustain adequate growth. Many factors must be taken into consideration whether the horse is pasture fed or concentrate and roughage fed. These factors would include the forage type and quality (if pasture fed), training level, environmental conditions, body condition, and overall health. The feed or pasture would also need to be evaluated for protein level, protein quality, vitamin and mineral level, etc. Any and all of these factors will influence the desired rate of growth in young horses. Restrictions in protein have a direct correlation to restrictions in the growth rate of a young horse.

CP requirements for the growing horse can be calculated using the following equation:

$$\mathrm{CP\,requirement} = \left(\mathrm{BW} \times 1.44\,\mathrm{g\,CP/kg\,BW}\right) + \left(\left(\mathrm{ADG} \times 0.20\right)/\mathrm{E}\right)/0.79$$

The "E" in the equation represents the dietary protein efficiency. Estimates from the NRC for the efficient use of dietary protein in the young horse are as follows:

- ~50% for 4–6-month-old horses
- ~45% for 7–8-month-old horses
- ~40% for 9–10-month-old horses
- ~35% for 11-month-old horses
- ~30% for 12-month and older horses

Remember that the quality of protein, as defined by amino acid composition, also plays a huge role in the growing horse, and poor-quality protein sources can have significant effects on growing horses. Inadequate amounts of dietary energy will be consumed if the feed is too low in either DE or protein, even though plenty of feed may be available. Growth rate in the young horse will decrease if inadequate intake of dietary energy or protein occurs. A slower growth rate has the potential to mask other nutritional deficiencies, and if slowed significantly, may reduce the body size of the horse at maturation. At a fast growth rate, a deficiency in minerals may result. If a deficiency of calcium, phosphorus, zinc, or copper occurs, developmental orthopedic disease may result. Conversely, if the young horse has dietary protein and energy intakes that are too high, a rapid growth rate may occur, increasing the risk of developmental orthopedic disease and obesity. When feeding the young horse from nursing to maturity, fresh, clean water should be available at all times.

TECHNICIAN TIP 5.11: Restrictions in protein have a direct correlation to restrictions in the growth rate of a young horse.

Oftentimes as veterinary healthcare team members, we forget to mention the importance of this key nutrient. Owners should weigh growing horses as often as possible (biweekly is recommended), with the use of a weight tape if scales are not available (Figure 5.8). Record BWs, food intake, and BCS at this time. Attention to BCS is important to the development of a healthy growing horse. Regular assessment provides immediate feedback about optimal nutrition. This will prepare the owner to continue to make these observations throughout the life of the horse. Such horses, as adults, should be less likely to experience skeletal diseases, weight problems, obesity, and other related problems. Veterinary healthcare team members should reassess growing horses during farm calls and work in conjunction with the owner's observations to detect potential or actual occurrence of under or overnutrition.

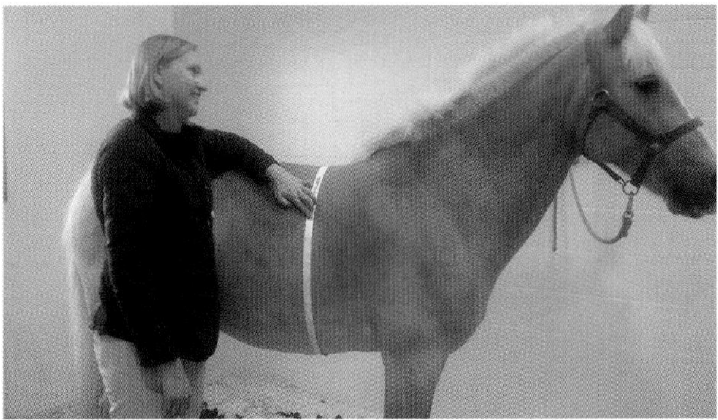

Figure 5.8 Taking a measurement using a weight tape, if a scale is not available.

Critical Care Nutrition in Horses

Nutrition in critically ill horses can be administered enterally or parenterally. It is imperative that nutrition be assessed and administered throughout the entire hospitalization. Enteral nutrition (EN) is considered less expensive and more physiologic, or more natural, for the patient. EN is also believed to provide enhanced immunity to the horse and is somewhat easier and less expensive to administer. The adage, "if the gut works, use it," is a result of research studies that shows EN helps support organ and immune function, improves organ blood flow, and helps the patient gain weight. Current guidelines suggest the use of EN whenever the horse tolerates it over the use of, or in combination with, parenteral nutrition (PN). Veterinary technicians play a large role in the management of nutrition in critically ill horses and should be well aware that early EN with parenteral supplementation (if necessary) is the standard operating procedure for critically ill horses.

TECHNICIAN TIP 5.12: Enteral nutrition helps support organ function, improves organ blood flow, improves immune function, and helps the patient to gain weight.

Nutritional support should be considered in patients that have, or are at risk for, increased metabolic rate. This would include horses that are growing; have experienced a history of malnutrition or hypophagia; have an underlying metabolic abnormality that has the potential to worsen if food is withheld; have experienced trauma or sepsis; or have an increased energy demand. The healthy adult horse can withstand food deprivation (simple starvation) for 24–72 hr with little systemic effects. However, in stressed and injured animals, food deprivation has a greater negative effect.

Stressed or injured horses have increased resting metabolic rates and use their own protein stores as the principal energy source. This is known as catabolism. Increased metabolic rate and catabolism in the equine patient lead to accelerated body wasting. Total body protein synthesis is reduced since the body is using amino acids for energy. Subsequently, the horse has increased metabolic demands, uses protein for energy, develops insulin resistance and glucose intolerance, exhibits poor wound healing and decreased immune function, and becomes extremely weak. Despite protein supplementation, the critically ill horse will continue to experience protein catabolism. Therefore, simply providing protein is not the answer, rather nutritional supplementation as a whole will help to minimize protein loss; provide essential and conditionally essential amino acids, vitamins, and minerals; and subsequently decrease morbidity due to illness.

Enteral Nutrition

EN can be comprised of normal feed, slurry diets made primarily from the patients' normal feed, and liquid diets containing micro- and macrominerals. Typically, the horse does not tolerate normal feed due to decreased appetite, and nutrition must be given through a nasogastric (NG) tube. When implementing the use of an NG tube, making slurry from a complete pelleted feed is advantageous because it is relatively inexpensive and well-balanced for an adult horse. Also, these formulations contain fiber, which aids in gastrointestinal activity, colonic blood flow, and colonic mucosal cell growth and absorption. However, slurry may not easily pass through the NG tube. If slurry is to be made, 1 kg of pelleted complete feed should be soaked with 1.5 gal of water. Administer slurry through a large bore NG tube using a marine supply bilge pump or if pump is not available, pulverize the pellets before the water is added. Take great care and caution and slowly administer the slurry and be cognizant of the horses' reaction as you do so. Each feeding should not exceed 1.5–2 gal, due to the fact that an adult horse's (~450 kg) stomach volume ranges from 2 to 2.4 gal. If prolonged feeding is required (i.e. dysphagia; head, neck, oral trauma; prolonged anorexia with functional gastro-intestinal tract) an indwelling esophagostomy tube is considered a better option for enteral feeding. Longer-term intubation with use of a smaller bore tube will not be conducive to the aforementioned slurry diets. Liquid enteral formulations (human and equine) have been recommended in enteral feedings through an esophagostomy tube. Enteral feeding should be introduced gradually over a period of days, with the goal being to feed the specific calculated DER or Daily Energy Expenditure (DEE) for that patient.

Energy requirements are dependent upon the weight, age, body condition, and metabolic stress of the horse. Maintenance requirements for adult, healthy horses, on average, are 33–40 kcal/kg/24 hr or ~18 000 kcal/day. When attempting to meet the nutritional requirement in a critically ill horse, using the DEE/DER is an acceptable goal. To calculate, use the following equation:

$$\text{Horses} \leq 600\,\text{kg}: \text{DEE}(\text{Mcal/day}) = 1.4 + (\text{BW} \times 0.03)$$

$$\text{Horses} \geq 600\,\text{kg}: \text{DEE}(\text{Mcal/day}) = 1.82 + (\text{BW} \times 0.0383) - [0.000015 \times \text{BW}]$$

(BW = Body weight in kilograms)

The patient should be evaluated daily (and in some instances, multiple times a day) to determine nutritional status and changes. Body condition scoring and weight tapes are recommended. When utilizing the weight tape, technicians should measure the girth just behind the elbow. The circumference determined will correlate with pounds or kilograms. Technicians need to be aware that with critically ill horses, BW can fluctuate dramatically with changes in fluid balance. Diet and hydration status can vary the weight of a horse by 5–10%.

Parenteral Nutrition

When the gastrointestinal tract is obstructed, dysfunctional, damaged, or painful, parenteral nutrition (PN) is indicated. PN is also indicated if there is alteration in plasma electrolytes or acid–base status to the extent that clinical signs are evident. The healthcare team should be aware that if dehydration and/or shock are evident clinically, mesenteric blood flow is commonly inadequate for the intestines to sufficiently absorb fluids for correction of dehydration or shock. Therefore, the veterinary healthcare team must get nutrition into the horse as soon as possible, as delay is not an option. Studies suggest that in patients that cannot tolerate oral nutrition, PN improves wound healing, minimizes muscle loss, decreases the weight loss seen in catabolic patients, and improves immune function. As was stated earlier, using the GI tract is the gold standard, but in times when EN is not tolerated, parenteral feeding must begin as soon as possible.

PN formulations are made up of protein in the form of amino acids, carbohydrates in the form of dextrose, and lipids in the form of long chain fatty acids. Electrolytes, minerals, and vitamins can be added to the formulation. Carbohydrates and lipids meet the energy needs of the horse, breakdown the autologous protein for energy, and work synergistically with the protein for wound healing and increased immune function.

PN is administered for short periods of time, multiple times a day. Total PN is a misnomer in veterinary medicine versus human medicine. Human medicine has a greater ability to prepare nutritional supplementation per individual patient and includes a wider range of microminerals, compared to what is available in veterinary medicine. To begin, the goal is to provide 30–40% of the solution's calories with lipids and 60–70% with protein. Lipid supplementation may be increased to ~60% in those equine cases that are in need of prolonged PN feeding.

When administering PN, the veterinary technician should be aware of the risk of thrombophlebitis, and it should be administered via the horse's jugular vein through a dedicated catheter placed in an aseptic manner. Whether the solution can be administered via a peripheral catheter

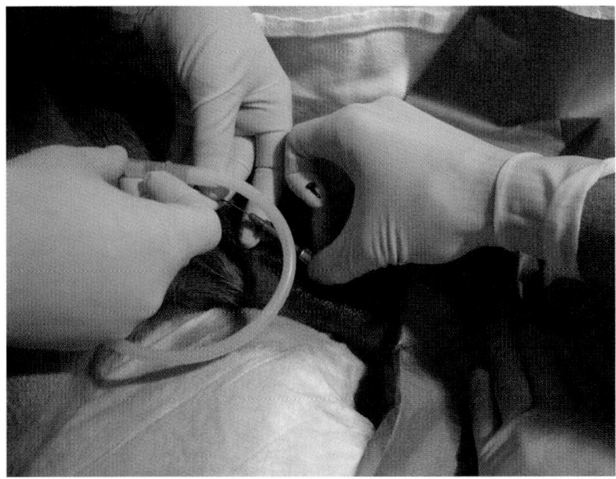

Figure 5.9 Aseptic technique is used for placement of a bilumen catheter, which would be used to administer PN.

or central line is directly related to the osmolarity of the solution (Figure 5.9). Catheters composed of silicone or polyurethane, and are antimicrobial, are also recommended to avoid this complication. Catheters that are multi-lumen are often preferred as they offer dedicated access for PN while still allowing access to the vein for blood draws and allowing access for IV injections. PN solutions are typically administered as a constant rate infusion over a 24-h period. Once the solution is warmed to room temperature, it is recommended to utilize the entire solution in this time frame to prevent contamination and lipid particle destabilization. It is imperative that the veterinary healthcare team reevaluates the nutritional plan every day PN is administered. If the patient is not improving with this modality over several days and remains anorectic, options to institute EN should be considered.

Calculating the patient's caloric requirements is important because feeding more of any food than necessary has the potential for causing metabolic complications. A general rule to remember is that most horses tolerate the food or solution that meets the resting energy requirement. Veterinary patients that are hospitalized have metabolic rates very near their DER. We can estimate the DER of hospitalized patients by using the equations provided previously. Feeding patients at DER is a safe and rational approach as opposed to doubling basal requirements, as this has been shown to result in overfeeding and potential complications, including hyperglycemia, hyperammonemia, and hyperlipidemia. At minimum, veterinary technicians should perform daily nutritional assessments to guide any adjustments to the nutritional plan of the hospitalized patient. At times, a critically ill patient may require more frequent assessments.

Potential complications with PN administration can be classified into three main categories, including mechanical, metabolic, and septic. Mechanical complications usually involve catheter-related problems. Examples include occlusion, premature removal, line disconnection/breakage, and/or thrombophlebitis. These problems can be avoided by the technician's strict adherence to aseptic technique and careful patient monitoring. Metabolic complications are more likely to occur with PN solutions formulated to deliver total caloric requirements. The most common metabolic complication in equines is hyperglycemia and decreases in plasma electrolyte concentrations, especially potassium. Other complications include hypertriglyceridemia, hyperammonemia, or electrolyte changes consistent with refeeding syndrome (e.g. hypokalemia, hypophosphatemia, hypomagnesemia). Reformulation of the PN solution is required if any of these problems occur. The most serious and potential life-threatening complication is sepsis. Technicians need to use strict aseptic technique when placing a catheter. Nursing management of catheters carrying hyperosmolar solutions containing amino acids requires special focus, as the solution is an excellent medium for colonization of bacteria. Aseptic techniques and focused nursing care should be the same for all types of fluid administration, but is especially important in patients receiving PN. If signs of sepsis develop without an identifiable source, contamination of the solution and/or intravenous catheter should be suspected. A culture and sensitivity of both should be considered. It is due to this potential complication that many veterinarians recommend having the PN solution compounded at an outside facility.

TECHNICIAN TIP 5.13: Understanding some of the potential complications that can occur should enhance the effectiveness of EN and PN.

In summary, EN and PN are viable nutritional choices for critically ill equine patients. When applicable, combined enteral and parenteral feeding is recommended to prevent intestinal hypertrophy and to facilitate healing by promoting intestinal growth. Proper nursing care and aseptic technique are also crucial to a positive patient outcome in both EN and PN. The veterinary technician should carefully monitor the nutritional requirements of hospitalized patients. Understanding some of the potential complications that can occur should enhance the effectiveness of EN and PN.

Nutritional History of Large Animals

The veterinary healthcare team should perform a nutritional history on every herd and every animal. The nutritional history provides background for the veterinary healthcare team and is necessary for the veterinary healthcare team to ascertain information on the quantity and quality of the diet that the animals have been receiving. The nutritional history is very beneficial information and assists the team in determining whether the nutrient requirements for that particular species are being met.

Pasture-Fed Livestock

Livestock maintained on pastures differ significantly from stall-fed livestock in that the diet is not easy to control and subsequently may be much more difficult to evaluate. In animals that graze, the potential for parasitic infestation and infectious disease is much greater.

Questions to ask regarding pasture-fed livestock:

- Composition of the pasture
- Nutritive value
- Recent changes brought about by rain or drought
- Whether rotational grazing is practiced
- Fertilizer program
- Potential for minerals and trace elements to be provided by topdressing or mineral mixtures
- Mineral supplementation (i.e. phosphates, which may contain excess fluorine)
- Homemade mixtures (these may have excessive quantities of certain ingredients)
- Authentic examination of the pasture area versus having the owner describe it

Hand-Fed/Stall-Fed Animals

Hand-fed or stall-fed animals are subjected to a relatively controlled feed supply. However, the potential for human error in stall-fed animals does exist; therefore, it is important when taking a nutritional history of stall-fed animals to ask the following questions:

- Types and amounts of feeds.
- Sources of the dietary ingredients.
- Grains from certain areas may be much heavier and may contain a greater proportion of starch to husk versus grains from other areas.
- When feed is measured, as opposed to being weighed, the risk of overfeeding or underfeeding is highly increased.

There are also a number of diseases associated with inadequacies in hand-fed diets and these include:

- osteodystrophia fibrosa – equines on feed comprised of excess grain
- azoturia – equines fed heavy-carbohydrate diets during periods of rest
- lactic acid indigestion – cattle introduced to high-level grain diets too rapidly

Other considerations for the veterinary healthcare team to keep in mind with hand-fed livestock include:

- Using non-milk sources of carbohydrates and proteins (as in milk replacers) may result in indigestion and nutritional diarrhea. Physiologically, the digestive enzyme capacity of newborn farm animals is most efficient in the digestion of whole milk versus milk replacers.
- Exotic diseases (e.g. anthrax, foot-and-mouth disease, hog cholera) have the potential to be imported in feed materials.
- Although not common, food preparation may result in significant variations in feed.
- Foods that are pelleted or cooked have potential for a reduction in the vitamin content.
- Poisoning by chlorinated naphthalene compounds may be the result of the use of lubricating oil in the production line.
- Pressure extraction of linseed has the potential to leave residue of hydrocyanic acid in the residual oil cake.
- Feeding practices may in themselves contribute to the production of disease – for instance, large numbers of pigs being fed in inadequate trough space, or calves being fed in communal troughs.
- Contamination with lubricating oil can result in overeating or inanition.
- High-level feeding and consequent rapid growth may create deficiencies due to increased requirements for other nutrients.

In all animals, changes in diet should be carefully noted. Healthcare team members should document the following in the nutritional history:

- Has there been movement of animals from one field to another?
- Has there been a change from pasture to cereal grazing?
- Has there been a change from unimproved to improved pasture?
- Have there been periods of bad weather or transportation?
- Has there been a change to new/unfamiliar feeds?
- Have there been changes occurring rapidly versus gradually – especially in pregnant and lactating ruminants, as metabolic diseases are more likely to occur in these animals (i.e. hypocalcemia, hypoglycemia, hypomagnesemia)?
- What is the availability of drinking water?

Assessment of Nutritional Status

In addition to a nutritional history taken from the owner, large animal patients should have physical examinations to assist in determining their nutritional needs. It is important for the veterinary healthcare team members to evaluate for potential systemic, mechanical, or neurologic disease that may be associated with or contributing to poor nutrition. Examples would include: foreign bodies, abscess, botulism, and so forth.

All patients should have a BW and BCS taken and recorded. BW measurements should be taken when the large animal patient presents to the hospital or veterinary healthcare team. If hospitalized, BW should be taken frequently throughout the patient's hospitalization.

Oftentimes, the veterinary healthcare team will be faced with obtaining a weight with no access to a scale. In these instances, the team member should utilize a weight tape to take heart girth measurements to estimate the patient's weight.

Another valuable tool to evaluate nutritional status is body condition scoring. BCS allows the healthcare team to subjectively assess the endogenous protein and lipid stores in a large animal patient. BCS tools for various species are found in Figures 5.10, 5.12, 5.14, and 5.15. It is very common for alterations in the animal's weight or BCS to go unnoticed because of the day-to-day interactions with the patient. As mentioned, certain species-specific needs should be noted. Palpation of the animal (ribs, dorsal vertebral processes) is necessary in sheep with a heavy fleece, camelids with long fiber, and horses with a thick winter hair coat. Animals with a low BCS (1–3 of 9; 1–1.5 of 5) have minimal protein and lipid stores and are at greater risk for developing protein calorie malnutrition after a period of anorexia. Large animal patients with a high BCS (7–9 of 9; 3.5–5 of 5) that are anorectic may have an increased risk for developing complications (hyperlipemia, hepatic lipidosis) from abnormal lipid metabolism. It is imperative that dietary therapy be initiated in a large animal patient that has lost 3–5% of its primary BW or whose BCS diminishes by ≥1 grade.

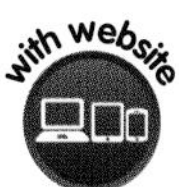

Don't forget to check the website for additional reference pictures, including examples of different body conditioning scores.

Another part of nutritional assessment to be performed by the veterinary healthcare team would be laboratory testing, specifically biochemical analysis. Although few biochemical tests assess protein malnutrition in large animals, physiological response indicative of anorexia manifests as endogenous protein catabolism, thus performing a BCS is critical. Anemia and hypoproteinemia (hypoalbuminemia) may be seen in cases of malnutrition, but typically these are associated with other disease processes (e.g. parasitism or protein-losing enteropathy). Abnormally, low serum urea nitrogen (SUN) concentrations in horses and ruminants may also be linked to severe protein malnutrition. Liver disease may decrease the formation of urea nitrogen and therefore should be ruled out by the veterinary healthcare team when assessing the animal's condition. Protein malnutrition can result in an increase in the urinary excretion of 3-methylhistidine, a myofibril amino acid that is not metabolized. Measurement of this metabolite in the future may be a useful tool to monitor protein catabolism in large animal patients.

Cattle Nutrition

The fact that cattle are ruminants and herbivores has already been established. Herbivores have the ability to convert products such as cellulose in plants into meat products for human consumption. Approximately 42.5 gal can be held in the rumen of a cow. It is also in the rumen that microbial digestion occurs through the utilization of bacteria and protozoans. In the course of the fermentation process, poor-quality forage and NPN (i.e. urea) produce volatile fatty acids, amino acids, and vitamins B and K, which are utilized by the body, as well as methane and carbon dioxide, which are released from the body. Cattle are also able to manufacture their own vitamin C. The pH of the rumen is recommended to stay between 6.2 and 7.2. However, it is important for the veterinary healthcare team to remember that livestock fed a high-grain diet may result in a more acidic rumen. Dietary fiber is key when talking about nutritional factors for cattle, as it is the fiber in the diet that is necessary to keep the microorganisms alive.

The honeycomb reticulum is responsible for regurgitation of food during rumination and can hold up to 2.5 gal. The omasum can contain up to 4 gal and is responsible for squeezing fluid out of the ingesta. The peptic digestion of proteins in cattle begins in the abomasum (true, glandular stomach), which holds up to 5 gal. The small intestine is approximately 150 ft long and can hold about 16 gal, with the cecum measuring approximately 3 ft long with a 2.5-gal capacity. Finally, the GI tract in cattle also includes the large intestine measuring 33 ft long and holding 7.5 gal (Table 5.5).

Key Nutritional Factors in Cattle

Livestock owners must provide water ad libitum, as mature cattle in good physical condition require 10–14 gal of water per day. Dairy cows require 3–5 gal of water to produce 1 gal of milk. Therefore, a cow at peak lactation may need to drink 45 gal of water per day.

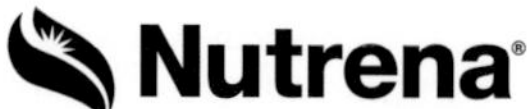

Body Condition Scorecard

This numerical condition scoring system, developed by Henneke et al., provides a consistent measure of the degree of body fat in horses of various breeds and sizes[1].

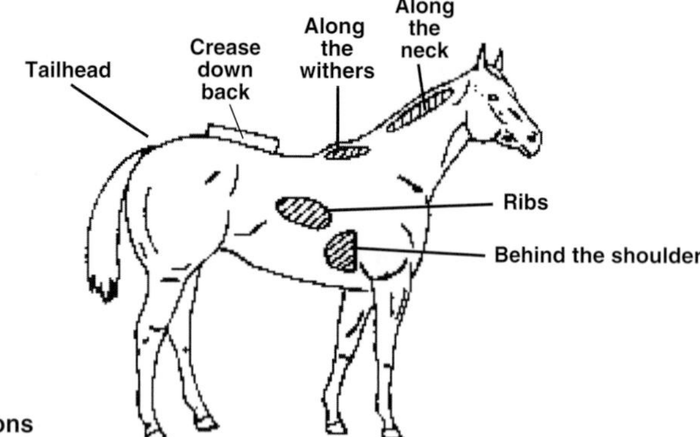

Condition Score	Descriptions
1.	**Poor:** Animal extremely emaciated. Spinous processes, ribs, tailhead and hooks and pins projecting prominently. Bone structure of withers, shoulders and neck easily noticeable. No fatty tissues can be felt.
2.	**Very thin:** Animal emaciated. Slight fat covering over base of spinous processes, transverse processes of lumbar vertebrae feel rounded. Spinous processes, ribs, tailhead, and hooks and pins prominent. Withers, shoulders, and neck structures faintly discernible.
3.	**Thin:** Fat build-up about halfway on spinous processes,transverse processes cannot be felt. Slight fat cover over ribs. Spinous processes and ribs easily discernible. Tailhead prominent, but individual vertebrae cannot be visually identified. Hook bones appear rounded, but easily discernible. Pin bones not distinguishable. Withers, shoulders, and neck accentuated.
4.	**Moderately thin:** Negative crease along back. Faint outline of ribs discernible. Tailhead prominence depends on conformation, fat can be felt around it. Hook bones not discernible. Withers, shoulders and neck not obviously thin.
5.	**Moderate:** Back level. Ribs cannot be visually distinguished but can be easily felt. Fat around tailhead beginning to feel spongy. Withers appear rounded over spinous processes. Shoulders and neck blend smoothly into body.
6.	**Moderate to fleshy:** May have a slight crease down back. Fat over ribs feels spongy. Fat around tailhead feels soft. Fat beginning to be deposited along the sides of the withers, behind the shoulders and along the sides of the neck.
7.	**Fleshy:** May have crease down back. Individual ribs can be felt, but noticeable filling between ribs with fat. Fat around tailhead is soft. Fat deposited along withers, behind shoulders, and along the neck.
8.	**Fat:** Crease down back. Difficult to feel ribs. Fat around tailhead very soft. Area along withers filled with fat. Area behind shoulder filled in flush. Noticeable thickening of neck. Fat deposited along inner buttocks.
9.	**Extremely fat:** Obvious crease down back. Patch fat appearing over ribs. Bulging fat around tailhead, along withers, behind shoulders and along neck. Fat along inner buttocks may rub together. Flank filled in flush.

Recommendations for Assigning Scores
Scoring is based on visual appraisal and handling (particularly in scoring horses with long hair) of horses. Conformation differences between breeds or types do not affect scoring when all criteria are applied. Muscle tone should not be confused with fatness. Scores can be assigned in half-point increments.

[1]Henneke, D.R., G.D. Potter, J.L. Kreider and B.F. Yeates. 1983. Relationship between body condition score, physical measurements and body fat percentage in mares. Equine Vet. J. 15(4): 371-372

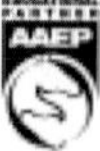

Figure 5.10 BCS equine. *Source:* Nutrition BCS. Courtesy of Nutrena Feeds.

Nutrena®

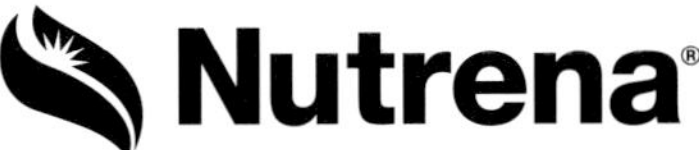

Date	Horse Notes	Condition Score	Weight Trape Measurement

AQHA
AMERICAN QUARTER HORSE ASSOCIATION

AAEP

USEA
Official Equine Feed

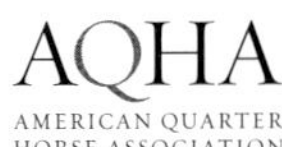

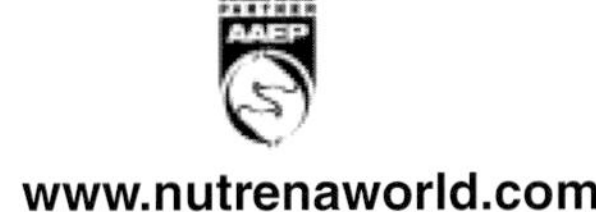

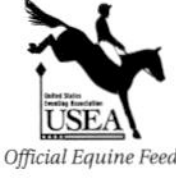

www.nutrenaworld.com

NX-2241 (11/03)

Figure 5.10 (Continued)

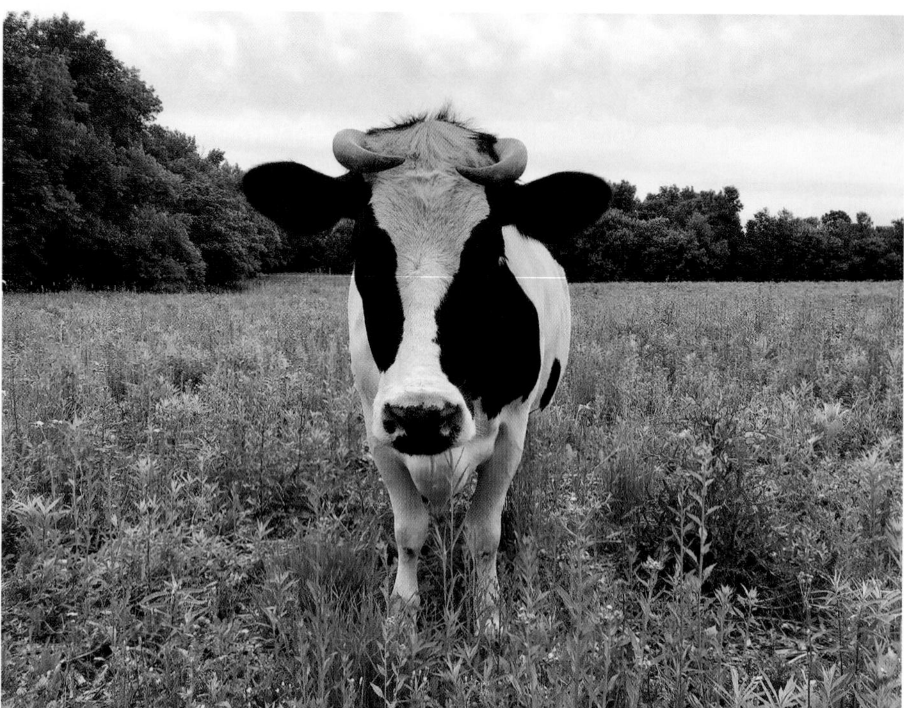

Figure 5.11 Foraging cow. *Source:* Courtesy of Farmaste Animal Sanctuary.

Table 5.5 Cattle gastrointestinal anatomy and fluid volume.

Anatomy	Volume (gallons) held
Rumen	42.5
Honeycomb reticulum	2.5
Omasum	4
Abomasum	5
Small intestine	16
Cecum	2.5
Large intestine	7.5

Cows in good health and condition can be fed good-quality hay or pasture (Figure 5.11). Pregnant cows can remain on this hay feed regimen until approximately two weeks prior to calving. Cows, in their last trimester, characteristically gain the amount of weight that they lose during calving. Obese cows are at risk for complications and health issues as much as underweight cattle, causing reproductive problems and predisposing the cow to ketosis.

As previously mentioned, lactation requires the highest energy needs in cattle. Feed that is fully balanced and has proper dry matter intake (DMI) is essential for optimal milk production. Feed concentrates supply the highest level of energy; however, it is important to balance concentrates with roughages. This balance will help to circumvent problems such as obesity, digestive disorders, and decreased milk production.

Cattle are typically fed what is known as "challenge feeding," which is based on the individual animal's level of milk production. It has been found that the size or weight of the cow does not appear to have much effect on the efficiency of milk production; therefore, most cattle are often challenge fed.

It is recommended that beef calves be creep fed. Creep feeding involves feeding small amounts of grain in a location to which the dam does not have access. The creep feeding method has been associated with less weaning stress and allows calves to start to consume feed, which they will be eating postweaning. At weaning, a 50-lb weight advantage has been shown when utilizing creep feeding.

TECHNICIAN TIP 5.14: Upon weaning, a 50-lb weight advantage has been shown through utilization of the creep feeding method.

Meat, bone meal, and other animal by-products from mammals are not recommended to be fed to cattle and other ruminants. The U.S. Food and Drug Administration established this rule in 1997 to minimize the potential spread of transmissible spongiform encephalopathy. Exclusions to this rule are: tallow, blood by-products,

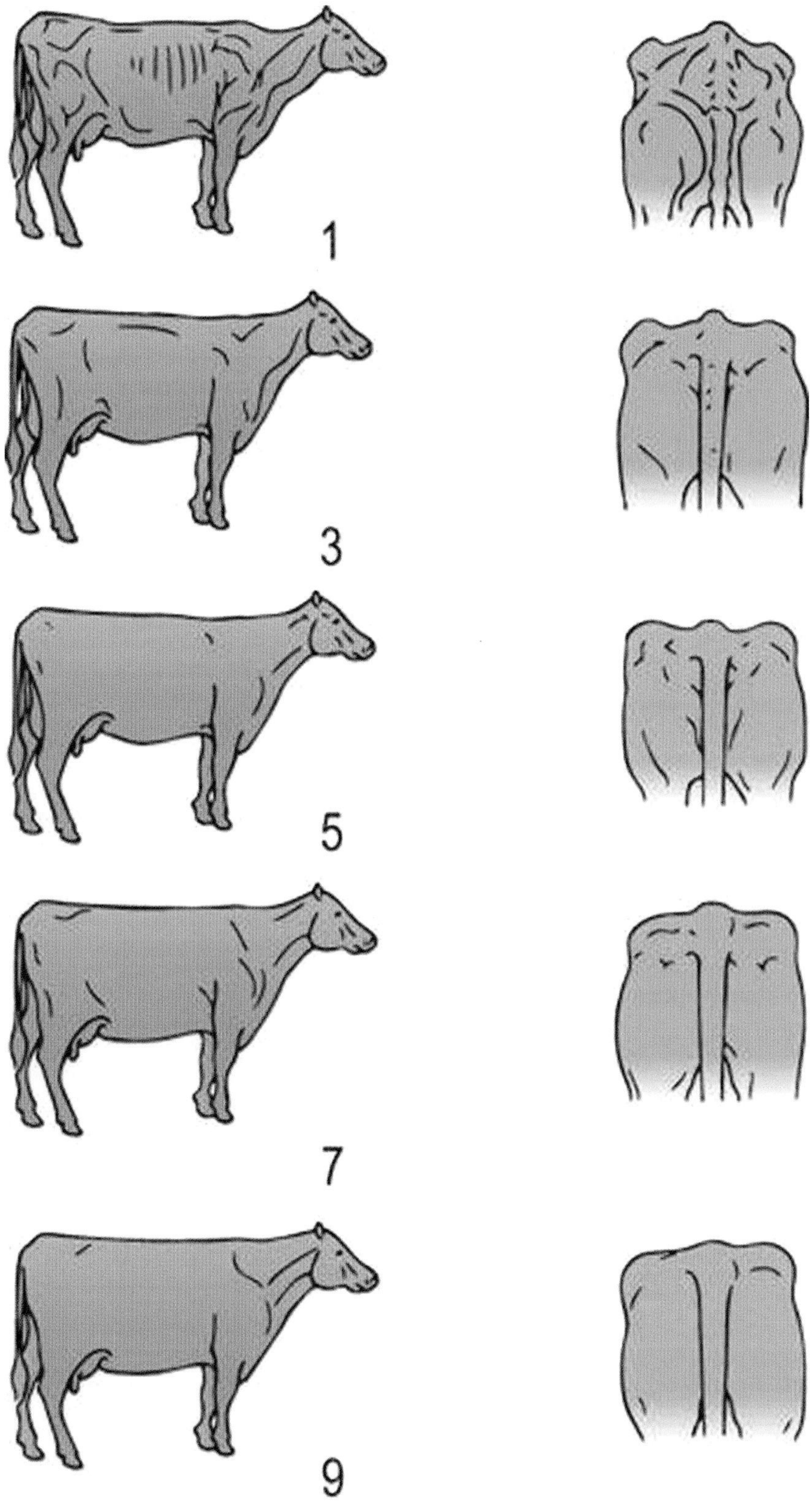

Figure 5.12 BCS bovine. *Source:* Holtgrew-Bohling (2011).

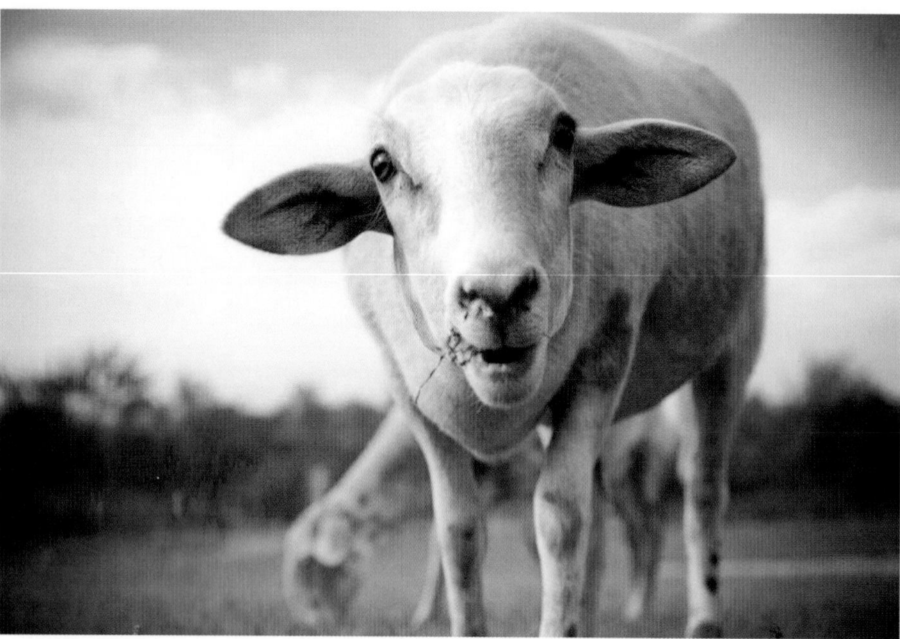

Figure 5.13 Foraging ewe. *Source:* Courtesy of Kara M. Burns.

gelatin, and milk products. These are acceptable for use in ration or ruminant formulation.

Cattle should have free access to sodium and chloride. Also, the use of iodized salt decreases the incidence of iodine deficiency. Iodine deficiencies are most often seen in pregnant animals and have been correlated to increases in stillbirths. In ruminants, deficiencies in calcium occur when fed high-grain diets. When deficiencies are discovered, limestone can typically correct the deficiency. When discussing phosphorus, the amount available to the animal directly relates to the amount in the soil from which their feed is grown. Phosphorus deficiencies in young animals are manifested by poor appetite, slow growth, and an overall unhealthy appearance. Lactating animals may have fragile bones and a poor appetite, as a result of phosphorus deficiency. Only small amounts of cobalt are stored in the body, so owners and veterinary healthcare team members must be observant as cobalt deficiencies could occur rapidly. Typical signs to look for with cobalt deficiencies are: listlessness, ocular discharge, anemia, ketosis, abortions, decreased milk production, and decreased appetite. It is recommended that cobalt be fed with trace mineralized salt. Conversely, feeding too much cobalt can lead to cobalt toxicity. Signs to watch for in cobalt toxicity are: decreased growth rates, incoordination, elevated hemoglobin, and elevated packed cell volume levels. Diets that are deficient in copper may result in neurologic signs, diarrhea, lameness, and anemia. Copper toxicity signs include: liver and kidney disease, increased occurrence of respiratory disease in calves, hemorrhagic diarrhea, and gastroenteritis. Selenium levels vary in the soil. Selenium should also be fed in a trace mineralized salt. Growing cattle fed low-protein diets may require more selenium and vitamin E in the diet to avoid deficiencies. Selenium deficiencies predispose cattle to reproductive problems and immunosuppression. Deficiencies of selenium in pregnant cows may result in the birth of calves that have white muscle disease. Zinc should be added to trace mineralized salt to avoid reduction in growth, reduced conception rates, reduced immune response, bone irregularities, decreased appetite, decreased wound healing, and hoof problems. Young male animals need higher levels of zinc to ensure normal testicular development. An essential component of hemoglobin is iron. Iron deficiencies rarely occur in adults but may be seen in a calf fed an all-milk diet. Treatment of deficiencies includes iron dextran injections in calves.

TECHNICIAN TIP 5.15: Selenium deficiencies predispose cattle to reproductive problems and immunosuppression.

Sheep and Goat Nutrition

Nutrition is believed to have the most profound effect on the general health of both the individual animal and the flock or herd, and this holds true when talking about sheep and goats as well. The veterinary healthcare team must remember the ultimate goal in proper nutrition is healthy animals and herds. In sheep and goats, the results of proper nutrition are seen in productivity and reproductive performance (Figure 5.13).

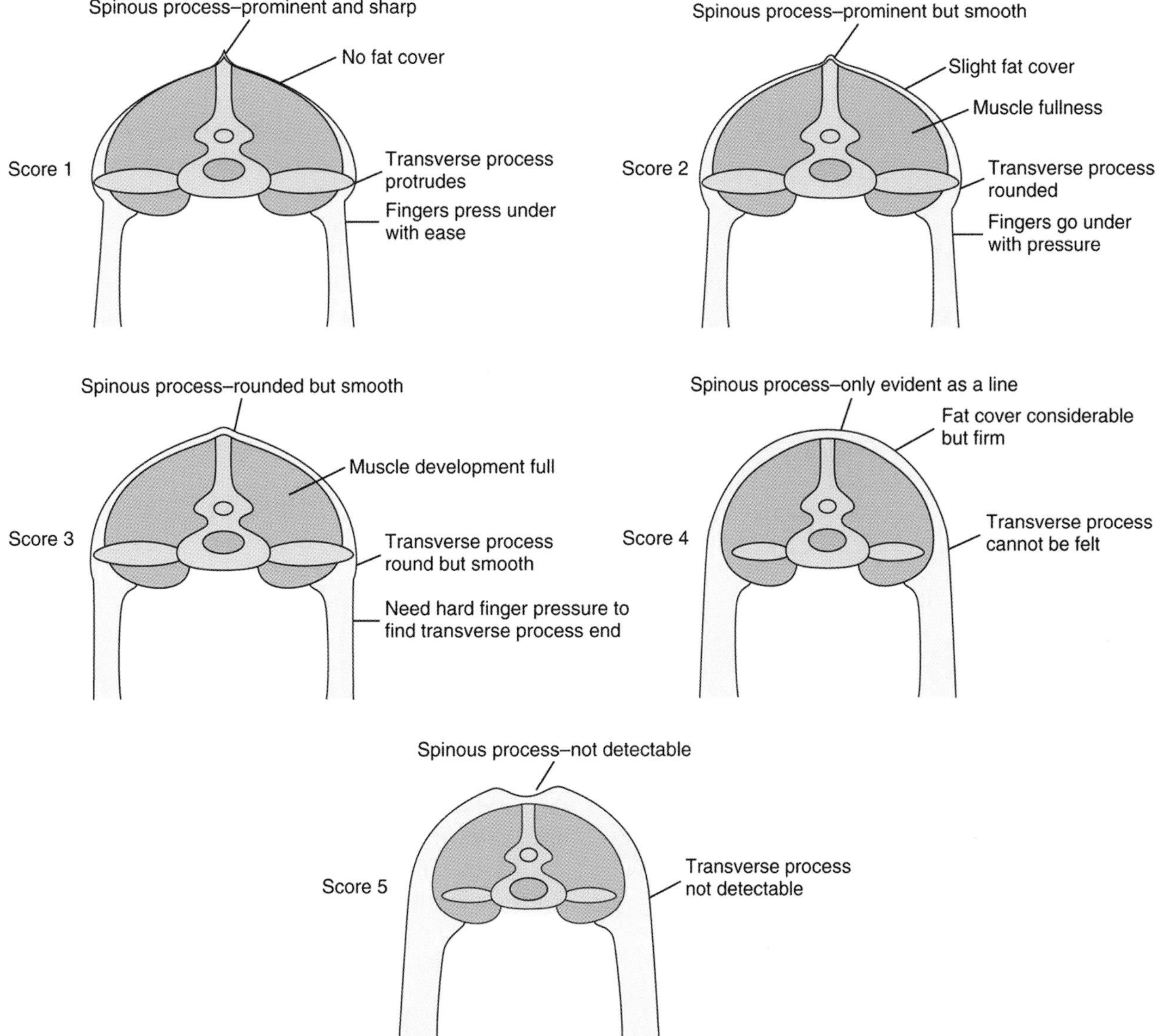

Figure 5.14 BCS Sheep. *Source:* Pugh and Baird (2011).

Sheep and goats have the ability to convert forages and other feedstuffs that may not be usable for more common livestock species into usable animal products (e.g. meat, milk, fiber) or to help the ovine to reach peak performance (e.g. pet, show, breeding).

Sheep and goats have increased mobility of the tongue and the lips, which allows for discrimination during feeding (Figures 5.14 and 5.15, Table 5.6).

Goats do not do as well as sheep or cattle on flat, monoculture pastures, but thrive when grazing in areas featuring browse or numerous plant species. Meat goats (e.g. Kiko, Spanish, Boer, Tennessee Wooden Leg breeds) typically do very well on a diet of 15–20% grasses and 80–85% browse. Goats are very particular creatures, especially where diet is concerned. Goats may refuse to eat feeds that have been soiled. Goats are also commonly used for brush management throughout the world. It is important for veterinary healthcare team members to monitor goats used in brush control for alterations in BW, BCS, and hair coat, and to watch for signs of toxicosis. Browse foraging may lead to greater mineral ingestion compared to grass foraging.

Key Nutritional Factors

Water is the most important nutrient for all animals, and sheep and goats should have easy access to fresh, clean water at all times, especially since sheep and goats are very particular about the quality of their water. Paving the surface 8–10 ft around the water tanks will help to prevent

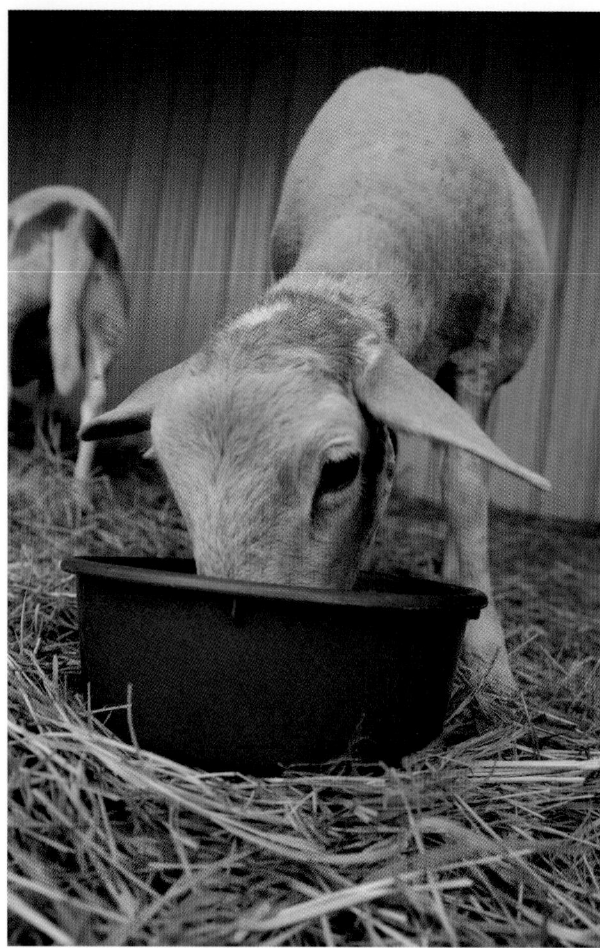

Figure 5.15 BCS goats. *Source:* Modified from Santucci et al. (1991).

Table 5.6 Diets discrimination based on oral cavity.

Sheep	Goats
Roughage grazer	Active forager
Grass	Highly digestible grass parts
High-quality plant parts	Flowers, fruits, leaves

unsanitary conditions, thus reducing the chance of sheep or goats contracting foot rot. Adults generally drink 1–1.5 gal, or 3–5 l, per day with fat lambs and kids drinking approximately 0.5 gal/day.

TECHNICIAN TIP 5.16: Paving the surface 8–10 ft around the water tanks will help to prevent unsanitary conditions, thus reducing the chance of sheep or goats contracting foot rot.

Daily water intake of sheep and goats may be affected by a number of factors. Pregnancy and lactation have a tendency to increase water requirements and consumption. It has been shown that water intake is increased 126% from months 1–5 of gestation. Also, water intake is increased for females carrying twins as opposed to those carrying one. Lactating ewes or does consume twice as much water as opposed to non-lactating females. When grazing lush spring pastures, where the forage water content may exceed 80%, sheep and goats consume much less water as compared to those sheep and goats restricted to dry hay, which may be only 12–15% water. Veterinary technicians also need to remember that lactating dairy animals require even greater quantities of water. When high-protein diets are being fed or when mineral consumption increases, water consumption also increases. Sheep may increase their water intake 12-fold during summer over that during the winter months.

High-protein diets, increased mineral consumption, and summer months all have the tendency to increase water consumption.

Energy

Energy requirements for sheep and goats are dependent upon the production level and stage, the activity level, and the animal's intended use. Energy requirements can most often be met through feeding medium to high-quality forage. The exception to this would be found in those animals where rapid growth rates are desired or in animals where maximum milk production is desired.

Diets that are deficient in energy have the potential for sheep and goats to experience the following:

- reduced growth rates
- lower BCS
- decreased fiber production
- reduced fiber diameter
- diminished immune function
- increased vulnerability to parasitic diseases and other pathologic conditions

The majority of energy that is used by sheep and goats comes from the breakdown of roughage to structural carbohydrates; therefore, roughage should constitute the bulk of their diet. Energy can be expressed in terms of the net energy system (calories) or in terms of total digestible nutrients (TDN) as a percentage of the feed (Table 5.7).

Good to excellent forage should be offered, but in instances where this is not available, energy supplementation may be required, especially in certain life stages or activity level (e.g. lactating ewe). The healthcare team and livestock owner typically have a number of choices. Cereal

Table 5.7 TDN % of various feed.

Feed	% TDN
Grass hay (perennial)	50–54%
Cereal grains	80–90%
Green vegetation forage	62–70%
Lesser quality hay (↑stems)	<50%

grains, with corn being very common, are a consistent choice. Corn is a dense energy source with the majority of the energy coming from starch. Energy from corn will assist in keeping the energy level of the goat or sheep higher, even if a decrease in foraging occurs.

Cereal grains such as corn, oats, grain sorghum, or barley may also be used as an energy supplement for ruminants consuming forage-based diets. Of these, corn remains the highest source of energy density, and most of that energy is in the form of starch.

Soybean hulls and wheat middlings have also been recommended; however, they are not often used. The outermost layer of the soybean is the soybean hull, which is high in digestible fiber. Soybean hulls' advantage over corn is that fiber digestion is not suppressed and an increase in hay digestibility may result. Similar responses are found in wheat middlings, which are a by-product of wheat milling. Beet pulp, citrus pulp, and brewer's grains may also be effective in sheep and goat feeding, and have been found to be more cost-effective than corn. The veterinary healthcare team should analyze the composition of by-product feeds and use accordingly in diet formulation.

Fat

Fat can also be used as an energy source; however, the veterinary healthcare team must remember the risks associated with an overweight animal in any life stage or lifestyle. Consequently, the total fat content must not exceed 8% of the sheep or goat diet, or 4–5% as supplemental fat. Cotton production is widespread in the southern portion of the United States, and whole cottonseed (which contains approximately 24% fat) is used as an energy supplement for both sheep and goats. Not more than 20% of the daily intake should be whole cottonseed in sheep and goats being supplemented. This percentage will need to be lower if there are other sources of fat in the diet.

Protein

In sheep and goats, for normal rumen bacterial growth and proper rumen function, a minimum of 7% dietary CP is necessary. Protein levels below 7% will suppress forage intake and digestibility. Deficiencies in protein intake manifests in the following ways: decreased fiber production, retarded growth, poor immune function, anemia, lethargy, edema, and possibly even death. CP content varies in sheep and goat feed (Table 5.8).

Table 5.8 Protein % in various feed.

Feed	% Protein
Grass hay (perennial)	<6 to >12%
Legumes (vegetative state)	≥28%

As plants age, their protein content declines. CP requirements are also variable depending on the sheep or goat's life stage or production. For maintenance, ewes and does of most weight classes require a diet containing 7–8% protein. Lactating ewes and does require 13–15% CP in the diet. The veterinary healthcare team members should consider the potential for protein deficiency if grass hay is being fed. Signs of protein deficiency to be mindful of in lactating animals are poor weight gain or slow growth in nursing lambs or kids, particularly those with multiple offspring.

TECHNICIAN TIP 5.17: As plants age, their protein content declines.

Protein supplementation in sheep and goats can include:

- oilseed meals as in cottonseed meal or soybean meal
- commercially blended supplements with natural protein and NPN
- range cubes
- pellets
- molasses-based products
- by-products
- whole cottonseed
- corn gluten feed
- dried distiller's grains

In sheep and goats, protein should be fed to meet requirements. Too much protein may lead to excessive cost and higher rates of disease (e.g. heat stress, pizzle rot). NPN is an economical way to increase the protein concentration. As discussed earlier, NPN is nitrogen in the nonprotein form. A commonly used type is urea. Whenever NPN is used, the diet should have appropriate amounts of highly fermentable energy components. Feeding grain with NPN can result in a decrease in rumen pH. This altered environment may depress the ability of the ruminal urease enzyme to ferment urea. This depression then results in a sluggish release of or breakdown to ammonia and carbon dioxide (CO_2). Slowing this metabolic pathway allows more efficient protein synthesis by the rumen microbes. Conversely, poor-quality roughage diets result in a higher rumen pH and enhanced urease activity. If NPN is added to the diet, feeds containing a urease enzyme (e.g. raw soybeans, wild mustard) should be severely limited or avoided.

When urea is fed as a protein source:

1) Urea should not be more than 1/3 of the protein in the diet or >3% of the grain portion of the diet.
2) A highly fermentable source of carbohydrates (e.g. corn, milo) should be fed with NPN.
3) Do not introduce urea into the diet suddenly – allow at least 8–10 days for its introduction.
4) Properly mix feed whenever urea is used.
5) When CP of the diet is >14% of the dietary TDN, NPN is of little value.
6) NPN is best used in sheep or goats with BCSs >2.5 and should be avoided in animals with a BCS <2.
7) If NPN is used in the feeding of animals, make sure it is fed daily; less is used for protein synthesis if the supplement is fed less frequently.

TECHNICIAN TIP 5.18: Do not introduce urea into the diet suddenly. Allow at least 8–10 days for its introduction.

Fiber

Fiber is another key nutritional factor for sheep and goats and is an important dietary consideration for ruminants. Normal rumination cannot occur without adequate amounts of fiber. If sheep are fed a low or limited fiber concentrate-based diet, they will result to "wool pulling" as they search for a roughage source. The dietary fiber content of sheep and goats should be >50%. This level will help promote a healthy rumen. Fiber also is required in the diet to maintain acceptable levels of milk fat. The particle size of the fiber is important. It is generally accepted that a minimum particle size of 1–2.5 cm is appropriate to stimulate normal rumination, although the effect of smaller particles is not well-documented in sheep and goats. Pelleted roughage does not meet this requirement of fiber size. Animals being fed pelleted forage or lush pasture should be offered hay.

TECHNICIAN TIP 5.19: If sheep are fed a low or limited fiber concentrate-based diet they will result to "wool pulling" as they search for a roughage source.

Minerals

Key nutritional factors for sheep and goats should also include minerals – macrominerals and microminerals. Macrominerals are expressed as percentage of the diet. Microminerals are expressed as ppm or mg/kg.

Macrominerals important to the overall health of sheep and goats include calcium, phosphorus, sodium, chlorine, magnesium, potassium, and sulfur. There are eight microminerals important to the overall health of sheep and goats:

1) Copper
2) Molybdenum
3) Cobalt
4) Iron
5) Iodine
6) Zinc
7) Manganese
8) Selenium

Although uncommon, trace mineral deficiencies may occur.

Calcium and Phosphorus

As previously mentioned, calcium and phosphorus are interrelated and work synergistically. The majority of calcium and phosphorus in the body can be found in skeletal tissues. Deficiencies in calcium and phosphorus in young lambs and kids result in slow growth and development and a predisposition to metabolic bone disease (e.g. rickets, osteochondrosis). A severe reduction in milk production is also a result of calcium and phosphorus deficiencies in lactating ewes and does; therefore, supplemental calcium and phosphorus may be needed to meet high milk production demands. Serum phosphorus concentrations are recommended to be between 4 and 7 mg/dl for sheep and between 4 and 9.5 mg/dl for goats. The most common mineral deficiency found in range- or winter-pastured animals is a phosphorus deficiency. Most forage, especially legumes, is high in calcium and low in phosphorus. Beet pulp and legumes (such as clover and alfalfa) are good to excellent sources of calcium. Phosphorus serum concentrations of <4 mg/dl are indicative of a phosphorus deficiency. Phosphorus deficiency manifests in slow growth, lethargy, an "unkempt" appearance, and depraved appetite or pica, which is an abnormal craving or appetite for nonfood substances such as dirt.

TECHNICIAN TIP 5.20: The majority of calcium and phosphorus in the body can be found in skeletal tissues.

TECHNICIAN TIP 5.21: Beet pulp and legumes, such as clover and alfalfa, are good to excellent sources of calcium.

High-grain or high-concentrate diets fed to sheep and goats often require supplemental calcium but not additional phosphorus. This is due to the fact that grains are relatively low in calcium but contain moderate to high concentrations of phosphorus. It has been found that serum calcium concentrations consistently below 9 mg/dl are indicative of chronic calcium deficiency. Chronic parasitism may lead to a decrease in calcium and phosphorus. Calcium supplementation can be achieved through the use of oyster shells and limestone. Defluorinated rock phosphate is an excellent source of phosphorus. Dicalcium phosphate or steamed bone meal provide sources for both calcium and phosphorus. In sheep and goats, the calcium-to-phosphorus ratio should be between 1 : 1 and 2 : 1.

Sodium and Chloride

Sodium and chloride are essential components for many functions in the body. Salt is the primary carrier for most ad libitum mineral supplements and should be offered as such for overall health. If not, it is necessary to add salt into concentrates or grains at a level of 0.5%. Salt blocks are commonly used to promote salt intake, as adults consume roughly 10 g of salt a day, but trace mineral blocks containing copper should not be used due to possible toxicity concerns. Sodium is primarily an extracellular ion and is important for normal water metabolism, intracellular and extracellular function, and acid–base balance. Conversely, chloride is an intracellular ion, functions in normal osmotic balance, and is a component of gastric secretions. Signs for the healthcare team to look for in sheep or goats that are deficient in salt include: wood chewing, soil licking, or consuming other unusual plants or debris. The salt content of feeds may be increased to 5% to aid in increasing water intake and reducing urolithiasis.

> **TECHNICIAN TIP 5.22:** Trace mineral blocks containing copper should not be used in sheep and goats due to possible toxicity concerns.

Magnesium

Magnesium is an important mineral that aids in the normal function of the nervous system and is necessary for many enzymatic reactions in the body. If an animal is deficient in magnesium, the animal can utilize skeletal magnesium; however, the skeletal magnesium reserve is much smaller as compared to calcium reserves. Many fast growing, heavily fertilized cereal grains or grass pastures are deficient in magnesium. High levels of plant potassium or rumen ammonia may suppress magnesium absorption. Livestock owners searching for a good source of magnesium will find it in legume and legume-grass mixed pastures. A deficiency in magnesium may lead to a clinical manifestation known as “grass tetany” in either sheep or goats. Magnesium toxicity is very rare.

Potassium

Potassium is required for normal acid–base balance and is an integral component of many enzymatic pathways; it functions as an intracellular ion. Depending on life stage and level of production, the requirement for potassium is between 0.5 and 0.8% of the diet. Most grains have <0.4% potassium, although fresh green forages generally contain >1%. Deficiencies or toxicities of potassium in sheep and goats are rare; however, the healthcare team should watch for deficiency in stressed animals fed strictly grain diets. It is prudent to recommend supplemental potassium for stressed animals (i.e. weaning) fed mostly grain.

Sulfur

Sulfur makes up many bodily proteins. Higher concentrations are seen in wool and mohair, as there are large amounts of sulfur-containing amino acids (cystine, cysteine, and methionine) in keratin. Deficiency of sulfur in Angora goats specifically can lead to a reduced mohair production. It is recommended that a 10 : 1 nitrogen-to-sulfur ratio be maintained in sheep and goat diets. For both sheep and goats, sulfur deficiency may result in:

- anorexia
- reduced weight gain
- decreased milk production
- decreased wool growth
- excessive tearing
- excessive salivation
- death
- depressed digestion
- decreased microbial protein synthesis
- decreased use of NPN
- lowered rumen microbial population

If signs of marginal trace mineral deficiencies are noticed in sheep or goats, owners and veterinary healthcare team members should measure sulfur concentrations in the forage. High levels of dietary sulfur can lead to a variety of trace mineral deficiencies (e.g. copper, zinc) without causing any overt toxicity problems.

Copper

Copper deficiencies can occur due to low dietary intake or high concentrations of molybdenum, sulfur, and/or iron, or other substances in feedstuffs. In the rumen, copper, molybdenum, and sulfur form thiomolybdates that reduce copper availability. This results in clinical signs of deficiency. High concentrations of dietary cadmium, iron, selenium, zinc, and vitamin C as well as alkaline soils all interfere with copper absorption. Zinc supplementation in the diet (to a concentration higher than 100 ppm) will reduce availability and liver stores of copper. Roughage grown on fertilized and limed pastures is more likely to be deficient. Adding lime decreases the amount of copper uptake by plants, and many fertilizers contain molybdenum. Good-quality lush grass forages have less available copper than that typical for most hays, and legumes have more available copper than most grasses. Copper reserves in the liver last up to six months in sheep.

Signs of copper deficiency seen in sheep and goats include:

- microcytic anemia
- decreased milk production
- faded hair color
- poor-quality fleeces
- heart failure
- infertility
- decreased immune function
- slow growth
- enlarged joints
- lameness
- gastric ulcers
- diarrhea

To aid in prevention of copper deficiency, supplementation may be instituted through the use of oral supplements, trace mineral mixtures, or in some instances injectable copper. Additionally, an appropriate dietary copper-to-molybdenum ratio must be maintained. Dietary copper for sheep and goats should range between 4 and 15 ppm copper toxicity occurs more often in sheep than in goats. Goats are similar to cattle than to sheep when discussing copper toxicity. With sheep, the difference between copper deficiency and copper toxicity is quite small. Toxicity usually occurs from mixing errors during the formulation of mineral premixes or from feeding mineral mixes or trace mineral blocks formulated for species other than sheep. Toxicity may be intensified by the ingestion of toxic plants (e.g. lupines, alkaloid-containing species) and stress (Figure 5.16).

> **TECHNICIAN TIP 5.23:** Copper toxicity occurs more often in sheep than in goats.

Copper toxicity signs to be cognizant of include:

- increased respiration
- depression
- weakness
- hemoglobinuria
- icterus
- sudden death

Cobalt

Cobalt is used by rumen bacteria to assist in the formation of vitamin B12. Organic or poorly drained soils may be low in cobalt. Cobalt deficiency in sheep or goats manifests as

Score	Appearance
0	No subcutaneous tissue seen.
1	Dorsal aspect of vertebral column forms a continuous ridge, hollow flank, ribs easily seen. Sternal fat easily moved laterally. Chondrosternal joints easily palpable. No muscle or fat between ribs or bones. Transverse processes of lumbar vertebrae easily visualized and articular processes easily palpable.
2	Sternal fat moveable but 1 to 2 cm thick. Tissue visible between skin and chondrosternal joints. Some t issue around transverse processes of lumbar spine, but it is more difficult to palpate than in Score 1. Need slight pressure to palpate articular processes.
3	Dorsal aspect of vertebral column is less prominent. Sternal fat is thick and barely moveable. Chondrosternal joints are difficult to palpate. Lumbar vertebrae have thick t issue covering. Articular processes of transverse processes not palpable.
4	Sternal fat, costochondral fat, and rib fat cont inuous. Transverse process difficult to palpate. Spinous processes not palpable.
5	Sternal fat and rib fat bulges between pressed fingers. Spinous and transverse processes not palpable.
From Santucci PM et al: Body condition scoring of goats in extensive conditions. In Morand-Fehr P (ed): *Goot nutrition.* Wageningen, the Netherlands, Pudoc, 1991.	

Figure 5.16 Hand-fed Katahdin lamb. *Source:* Courtesy of Kara M. Burns.

classic B12 deficiency, with signs and symptoms ranging from decreased appetite to emaciation ("wasting disease"), anemia, pale skin, and excessive ophthalmic discharge. Cobalt deficiency is associated with white liver disease, although phosphorus and copper deficiencies and chronic parasitism also play roles in pathogenesis. Typically, a diet with a cobalt concentration of 0.1 ppm is adequate in most instances. Cobalt levels in the diet below 0.06 ppm are deficient. The discovery of a cobalt deficiency should lead the veterinary healthcare team to feed a cobalt-supplemented trace mineral mixture ad libitum. Typically, in North America cobalt toxicity is not of great concern in sheep and goats.

TECHNICIAN TIP 5.24: Organic or poorly drained soils may be low in cobalt.

Iron

Iron deficiency in sheep and goats is rare especially when the herd grazes. The dietary iron requirement generally is 30–40 ppm.

Iodine

Deficiencies in iodine are seen in certain geographic locations – particularly the northern area of North America. The winter months typically are the time when iodine availability in the body is at its peak. Rubidium, arsenic, fluorine, calcium, and potassium are known to interfere with iodine absorption, so veterinary healthcare team members must take these minerals into consideration when discussing nutrition. Signs of iodine deficiency include: goiter, poor growth, depressed milk yield, pregnancy toxemia, and reproductive abnormalities (e.g. abortion, stillbirth, retained placentas, irregular estrus, infertility). Lambs or kids with enlarged thyroid glands are often born to iodine-deficient dams. Recommendations for treatment include three to six drops of iodine (Lugol's solution) every day for seven days.

TECHNICIAN TIP 5.25: Lambs or kids with enlarged thyroid glands are often born to iodine-deficient dams.

Zinc

Zinc deficiency has been seen in sheep and goats. Vitamin C, lactose, and citrate in the diet help to increase zinc availability, while the following suppress zinc availability: oxalates, phytates, large dietary concentrations of calcium, cadmium, iron, molybdenum, and orthophosphate. Zinc concentrations are found to be higher in legumes than in grasses, though legumes invariably contain large concentrations of calcium, which has been determined to depress zinc availability. Zinc does not appear to be readily available in cereal grain feeds. Signs of zinc deficiency include:

- dermatitis and parakeratosis
- decreased milk production
- diminished appetite
- inability to utilize feed
- delayed growth
- susceptibility to footrot
- reduced hair growth on legs and head
- joint swelling
- decreased reproduction
- reduced testicular development
- weakened vitamin A metabolism
- increased vitamin E requirements

An amount of 20–50 ppm of zinc in the diet should be sufficient, except in those animals consuming a high percentage of legumes in their diets. For these animals, a chelated form of zinc is indicated. Providing trace mineral salt mixes with 0.5–2% zinc usually prevents deficiency. Zinc toxicity is very rare.

TECHNICIAN TIP 5.26: Zinc does not appear to be readily available in cereal grain feeds.

Selenium

The absorption of selenium from the small intestine is enhanced by adequate dietary levels of vitamin E, vitamin A, and histidine. Conversely, the absorption of selenium can be inhibited when the diet has large quantities of arsenic, calcium, vitamin C, copper, nitrates, sulfates, and unsaturated fats. Legumes are a better source of selenium than grasses, and grasses are a better source than cereal grains.

The veterinary healthcare team must be cognizant of signs of selenium deficiency including:

- nutritional muscular dystrophy (skeletal and cardiac muscles of fast-growing young lambs or kids)
- retained placentas
- slow growth
- weakness
- premature birth of lambs or kids
- depressed immune function
- mastitis
- metritis

Selenium deficiency is seen most often in lambs between birth and eight weeks of age.

TECHNICIAN TIP 5.27: Selenium deficiency is seen most often in lambs between birth and eight weeks of age.

In the diet, 0.1–0.3 ppm of selenium is recommended. Those regions that are low in selenium should use mineral salt mixes with approximately 24 and 90 ppm selenium. Selenium toxicity is rare, but signs to look for include: wool break, anorexia, depression, incoordination, and death.

Vitamins

Animals with healthy rumen function only need fat-soluble vitamins A, D, E, and K in their diet. There are a number of body functions that require vitamin A, such as growth, reproduction, appropriate skeletal development, vision, and epithelial tissue integrity. The liver can store vitamin A for four to six months. Vitamin A deficiency signs include weight loss, depressed immune function, night blindness, decreased fertility, and hair loss. Sheep and goats need 105 IU/kg of BW/day to meet their vitamin A requirement. This can be attained through the ingestion of green, vegetative forage. Vitamin A requirements increase in late gestation and lactation to 150 and 175 IU/kg/day, respectively.

Vitamin D requirements can be met through sunlight to which pasture animals are exposed. Indoor feeding operations that are located in overcast or cloudy conditions/regions should supplement vitamin D. During the winter months when there are more overcast conditions and shorter daylight hours, blood vitamin D levels may be low. As discussed earlier, calcium, phosphorus, and vitamin D are important for normal bone growth and structure. Rickets is commonly seen in vitamin D deficiencies. Requirements for vitamin D in sheep are 5–6 IU/kg of BW/day. Early weaned lambs have a slightly higher requirement of 6–7 IU/kg/day.

Cell membrane integrity is the major role of vitamin E. Vitamin E is similar in mode of action to selenium. As is true with selenium, deficiencies in vitamin E in sheep and goats can cause white muscle disease, decreased immune function, and depressed fertility. Daily intake of vitamin E is imperative as vitamin E is not stored well in the body. Alfalfa meal, cottonseed meal, and brewer's grains have abundant vitamin E; however, it should be noted that corn, onions, and feeds containing high levels of sulfur will decrease the availability of vitamin E. The recommended amount of vitamin E for small ruminants is 5.3 IU/kg of BW/day.

Vitamin K plays a huge role in proper blood clotting and normal vision. Vitamin K should not need to be supplemented as it is produced in sufficient quantities in the rumen and the lower gut of healthy livestock.

TECHNICIAN TIP 5.28: Browse foraging may lead to greater mineral ingestion compared to grass foraging.

TECHNICIAN TIP 5.29: The veterinary healthcare team must remember the ultimate goal in proper nutrition is healthy animals and herds.

Camelid Nutrition

Camelids are not classified as ruminants, but are considered to be functional ruminants with three compartments instead of the four in cattle, sheep, and goats. Functional ruminants are extremely efficient in their ability to convert roughage to usable nutrients. They do best when allowed to graze on pasture freely. Feed consumption is based on a percentage of BW and is higher in smaller animals and lower in larger animals. Concentrates are rarely needed; if provided, they should be given carefully because obesity is common in overfed camelids (Figure 5.17).

TECHNICIAN TIP 5.30: Camelids are not classified as ruminants, but are considered to be functional ruminants with three compartments instead of the four in cattle, sheep, and goats.

Protein requirements for camelids are very similar to those in sheep and goats. When CP is calculated on a DM basis, camelids require 10% CP for maintenance and 16% for pregnancy, lactation, and growth. Water should be provided *ab libitum* to camelids; they require 9–13% of their BW (kg) in water. When providing water to camelids in cold weather, veterinary technicians should remember that camelids will not break through ice to get to a water source. Trail llamas most often drink water during the evening and will often refuse to drink during the day. Lactating camelids should have ready access to clean water due to the fact that if water is withheld or unavailable, lactating camelids often decrease milk production or stop milking altogether. In extreme cases of water deprivation, camelids may become hyperthermic. Camelids have oval erythrocytes that can swell up to 240% of their normal size without lysing, whereas round erythrocytes in other animals can only swell up to 150% without lysing. This adaptation provides for drinking a large amount of water in a short time period, as their erythrocytes can withstand dramatic changes in osmotic variations.

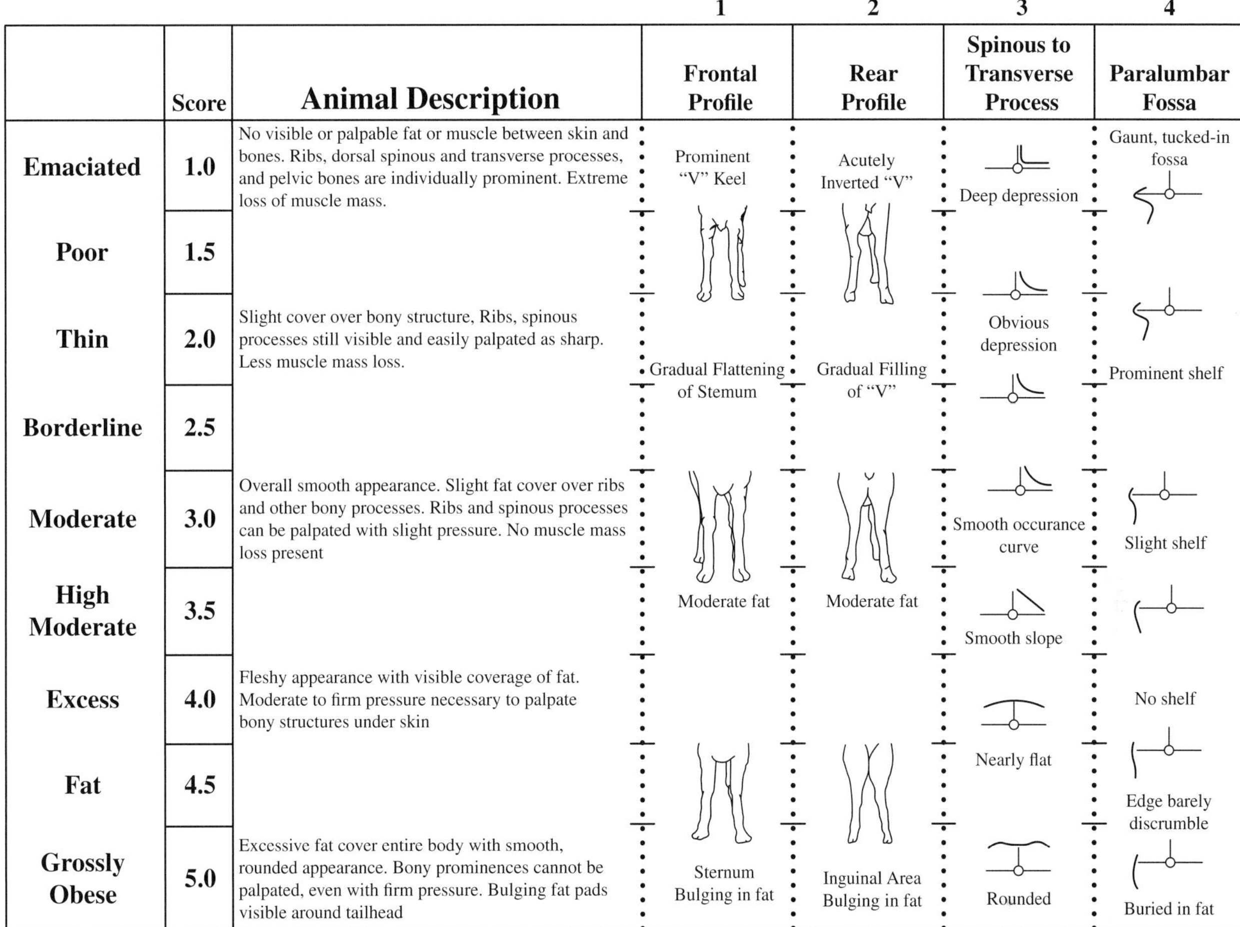

Figure 5.17 BCS camelids. *Source:* Van Saun, Robert J. Veterinary Clinics of North America: Food Animal Practice. Elsevier.

> **TECHNICIAN TIP 5.31:** In extreme cases of water deprivation, camelids may become hyperthermic.

The camelid diet should contain no more than 0.3% calcium on a DM basis and the calcium-to-phosphorus ratio should be no less than 1.2 : 1. Camelids are sensitive to copper, and copper toxicity can be a problem. Iron deficiency is thought to be a factor in the failure to thrive syndrome seen in crias. Zinc deficiency in llamas and alpacas may present as dermatitis. All other mineral requirements are similar to those in other ruminants.

Swine Nutrition

There have been many changes within the swine industry to the point where the industry is vastly different today than it was 30 years ago. Many pigs today are bred and raised in confined areas in an attempt to improve the environment for the pigs and to help offset labor costs for the owner. From a genetics standpoint, the swine industry has become a more prolific breeding herd producing better-muscled and faster-growing progeny. The largest cost associated with breeding and raising swine is feeding, which makes up 60–70% of the cost. The swine industry has become one of the most intensively managed agricultural enterprises.

> **TECHNICIAN TIP 5.32:** The largest cost associated with breeding and raising swine is feeding, which makes up 60–70% of the cost.

Today, swine are typically fed complete high-grain rations with self-feeders rather than grazing on pasture. Those swine in the breeding herd are often limit-fed. Swine production, and thus the nutrition related to swine production, can be better understood by looking at three distinct areas: the breeding herd, starter pigs, and growing-finishing pigs.

The other major factor affecting the swine industry today is feed efficiency. Maintaining high feed efficiency is critical to productivity in the swine industry of today. As with other species, veterinary technicians should be aware of a producer's feed efficiency to help gather a proper history during the physical examination of the pig.

Some pigs may grow fast, and others may grow slowly. The way a pig grows is dependent upon: genetic inheritance, nutrition, and husbandry. Selecting pigs and proper breeding is significant because you cannot grow a good, healthy pig if the breeding and/or genetics are poor. Proper husbandry refers to providing a clean, comfortable place to live. One must also deworm and vaccinate them. It has been shown that healthy pigs grow faster than sick pigs. Weight gain of a growing pig typically averages 1.4–1.8 lb/day. It takes approximately 2–2.5 lb of feed to produce 1 lb of pork.

Remember, technicians are responsible for gathering information on the diet that is being fed as well as its components. The major feed component of today's commercial swine producers is corn, processed in several different ways. Veterinary technicians must perform a BCS on the pigs – at all ages – and assist the owner or swine producer to do the same. This is for the overall health of individual pigs and the herd.

Swine are omnivores and subsequently have capacity for some dietary fiber. Swine diets are mainly comprised of purchased or farm-raised feeds, such as corn, oats, wheat, barley, and sorghum, supplemented with a purchased premix. Swine have been shown to display an increased rate of weight gain when nutritionally balanced feeds are provided.

Grinding feeds increases feed efficiency. However, the veterinary healthcare team must remember that if grain is ground too finely, digestive problems in the pig may result. Therefore, it is best to provide grain that is a medium–fine particle size. To maintain growth gestation or lactation, protein and amino acids are essential to the diet. Growing pigs need the following essential amino acids: arginine, histidine, isoleucine, leucine, lysine, methionine, phenylalanine, threonine, tryptophan, and valine, with the highest importance given to lysine, tryptophan, and threonine. Pelleting of foods helps to increase digestibility and decrease the amount of waste produced.

Clean and fresh water must be provided free choice and available at all times (Figure 5.18).

> **TECHNICIAN TIP 5.33:** Grinding feeds increases feed efficiency in swine, but it is important to know that if ground too finely digestive problems may result.

Breeding Herd

Nutrition plays a key role in breeding sows, especially during lactation. Typically, a swine production sow follows the cycle of:

1) breeding, gestation of 114 days
2) nursing their litter for 21–35 days
3) rebreeding after the litter is weaned

Energy

Breeding sows typically are limit-fed throughout the first two trimesters. During the first two trimesters of gestation, the sow's energy intake should be approximately 6000–7000 kcal ME (metabolizable energy) per day. In the last trimester, the sow's total amount of feed should be increased to approximately 9000–10 000 kcal ME per day. This increase in kcal ME helps to provide extra energy to the developing fetuses. However, a balance must be attained as too much energy during gestation has a direct negative impact on the lactation feed intake. This impact may impair lactation performance.

During lactation, the lactating female may have an increase in the amount of energy intake – pushing upward of 15 000–20 000 kcal ME per day. Typically, it is recommended to feed sows two times a day. This helps to ensure the feed is fresh and helps to improve energy intake. Fat may also be added to the lactating sow's food, as fat enhances palatability and energy density. The milk production peaks between the second and third weeks of lactation; consequently, the sow should be fed to support this peak. For every piglet nursing, it is prudent to offer one additional pound of the base ration to the lactating sow in addition to the 4–5 lb of the base ration she is already receiving.

Protein

Protein requirements for sows during gestation are relatively low (11–12% CP, 0.5 lb of protein per day). Protein is needed for the development of the fetuses and reproductive tissue. However, during lactation, sows require higher levels of protein intake (2–3 lb of protein per day). During lactation, it is recommended to feed a diet with increased protein content. If adequate levels of protein or energy are not supplied to the sow during lactation, then body tissue stores will be utilized to support milk production. Lack of energy or protein may result in the sow losing more than 100 lb in weight during lactation.

Minerals and Vitamins

Throughout the life of the pig, minerals and vitamins will typically need to be supplemented. Breeding herds are typically fed foods supplemented with the minerals calcium, phosphorus, salt, zinc, iron, copper, iodine, selenium, and

Pig condition scoring diagram

Score Number	Condition	Description	Shape of Body
5	Overfat	Hips and backbone heavily covered	Bulbous
4	Fat	Hips and backbone cannot be felt	Tending to bulge
3.5	Good condition	Hips and backbone only felt with difficulty	Tube shaped
3	Normal	Hips and backbone only felt with firm pressure	Tube shaped
2.5	Somewhat thin	Hips and backbone felt without firm pressure	Tube shaped but flat (slab) sides
2	Thin	Hips and backbone noticeable and easily felt	Ribs and spine can be felt
1	Emaciated	Hips and backbone visible	Bone structure apparent (ribs and backbone)

Condition scores from left to right, 1: 2: 3: 4: 5:

Score:
1. Emaciated
2. Thin, backbone prominent
3. Ideal condition during lactation and at weaning, backbone just palpable
4. Slightly overweight, cannot find the backbone
5. Body rotund, over fat

Note: The 'condition score' and 'back fat' correlation does differ between breeds

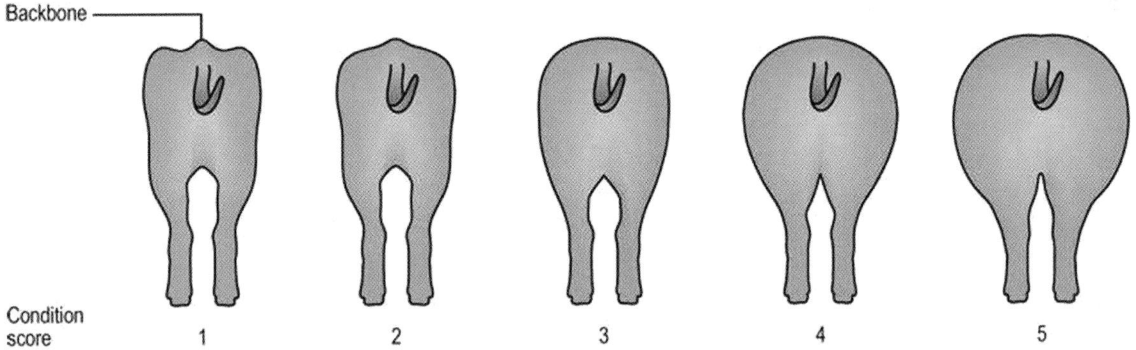

Figure 5.18 BCS swine. *Source:* Holtgrew-Bohling (2011).

manganese. It is important to keep calcium and phosphorus in a balance of 1 : 1 to 2 : 1 during all stages of production. Skeletal fractures and lameness, especially in females, are a result of low levels of calcium and phosphorus in breeding herd diets.

> **TECHNICIAN TIP 5.34:** It is important to keep calcium and phosphorus in a balance of 1 : 1 to 2 : 1 during all stages of swine production.

Supplementing iron is necessary for nursing piglets, as sow's milk is deficient in iron and anemia of nursing pigs will occur unless they are supplemented with another source of iron. The following are common ways to supply additional iron:

1) Three days of age – Injection of iron (150–200 mg) as iron dextran or other iron-carbohydrate complexes.
2) Three days of age – Oral iron solution given or swabbed onto the dam's udder several times during lactation.

3) Allow access to soil that has not been in contact with other pigs.
4) Inject 100–200 mg iron before 72 hr of age.
5) Paint sows' teats lightly with iron solution periodically.
6) Encourage pre-starter ration creep feeding early.
7) Provide iron supplementation in creep feeder.
8) Feeding sows a diet supplemented with 2000 mg iron/kg DM of diet will satisfactorily prevent iron-deficiency anemia in the piglets. The piglets will ingest about 20 g of the sow's feces per day, which will contain sufficient iron and obviate the need for IM injection of iron dextran. The piglets grow and thrive as well as those receiving the iron dextran.

TECHNICIAN TIP 5.35: Supplementing iron is necessary for nursing piglets, as the sow's milk is deficient in iron and anemia of nursing pigs will occur unless they are supplemented with another source of iron.

To ensure proper development of the fetus during gestation and milk production during lactation, the fat-soluble vitamins A, D, E, and K and the water-soluble vitamins thiamin, riboflavin, niacin, pantothenic acid, B6, B12, choline, biotin, and folic acid will most likely need to be supplemented.

Starter Diets

Typically, piglets are weaned between three and five weeks of age. Piglets should remain in the starter phase until their weight reaches 40–50 lb. The earlier the weaning age of the piglet, the more complex the food ration must be to aid in the transition from nursing to solid food. Starter diets are typically 20–24% protein. These diets are a complex and nutrient-dense complete feed. Starter diets use high-quality ingredients, which include milk products, fish meal, spray-dried blood products, oats, corn, and fat. Remember vitamin and mineral supplementation levels will be higher in starter diets. This feed typically is pelleted and the formulation tends to be higher in cost. As the pig ages, the nutrient density of the starter ration decreases and subsequently, the cost of the feed decreases. During the last two to three weeks of the starter phase, the CP requirement decreases to 18–20%. At this point, the diet is often presented as a ground feed.

Growing-Finishing Pigs

Diets for growing-finishing pigs have been revised to complement the changes in the genetic base of current swine. Leaner pigs require higher levels of protein and consume less energy than previous generations.

Energy

Complete grower-finisher rations are based on cereal grains and frequently have fat added to increase caloric intake. Fibrous feed ingredients often are not used or are used sparingly to prevent depressions in caloric intake. Corn, wheat, sorghum, and barley are the more popular cereal grains used to supply energy and comprise 60–85% of the ration.

Protein

Contemporary swine nutrition concentrates not on the protein content of feed, but on the amino acid levels. Lysine typically is the first limiting amino acid in swine formulas. Amino acid levels decrease as a percentage of the diet throughout the growing-finishing phase.

TECHNICIAN TIP 5.36: Contemporary swine nutrition does not concentrate on the protein content of feed.

Amino acid levels are matched to muscle growth throughout the growth period to maximize lean tissue growth. Underfeeding of amino acids depresses muscle deposition, and overfeeding amino acids leads to excess, which is costly.

Typical protein sources in growing-finishing diets are soybean meal, meat and bone meal, and synthetic amino acids. When protein sources are expensive, synthetic amino acids can replace a portion of the protein source with no loss in performance. The most commonly available synthetic amino acids are lysine, methionine, threonine, and tryptophan.

Minerals and Vitamins

Growing-finishing swine are fed diets fortified with the minerals calcium, phosphorus, salt, zinc, iron, copper, iodine, selenium, and manganese. Calcium and phosphorus are kept in a balance of 1 : 1 to 2 : 1 throughout this period. Deficiencies of phosphorus will depress growth performance as the animal grows.

The water-soluble vitamins most likely to be deficient in swine diets formulated with grains and plant protein are riboflavin, niacin, pantothenic acid, and vitamin B12. Additionally, fat-soluble vitamins A, D, E, and K should be added to growing-finishing rations.

Husbandry, housing, and space are important aspects in growing-finishing swine. The veterinary technician's role in a swine facility involves herd health and piglet care. The feed supplier with premixes meets nutritional needs and problems and provides rations tailored to individual operations and life stages of the pigs.

Potbellied Pigs

Potbellied pigs living as pets in a family home are on the rise. Subsequently, diets for potbellied pigs can be purchased commercially. These diets are classified as starter diets, grower diets, breeder diets, or maintenance diets. Maintenance foods for potbellied pigs contain approximately 12% protein, 2% fat, and 12–15% fiber. As with many other mammalian species, the most common disease of potbellied pigs is obesity. Another disease condition that may be seen is cystitis. There are commercially prepared potbellied pig foods with urinary acidifiers to help prevent cystitis available if this problem arises in the potbellied pig for which you are caring. Potbellied pigs should be fed volume according to their body composition. Although potbellied pigs should have a rotund potbelly, as their name implies; potbellied pigs should not have turgid, fat-filled jowls or rolls of fat hanging over the hocks. The healthcare team and owner should be able to feel the ribs, but not see the ribs. Owners will want to treat their potbellied pig, so it is crucial that the veterinary technician educate the owner on amounts of treats to give and types of treats to offer. Suitable treats for potbellied pigs include low-fat, low-salt snack food, such as popcorn (air popped without salt or butter) and small amounts of dried or fresh fruits and vegetables (Figure 5.19). Proper owner education is critical to ensure that a healthy weight is maintained and excessive people food is avoided.

TECHNICIAN TIP 5.37: As with many other mammalian species, the most common disease of potbellied pigs is obesity.

TECHNICIAN TIP 5.38: Suitable treats for potbellied pigs include low-fat, low-salt snack food, such as air popped popcorn and small amounts of dried or fresh fruit.

Clean, fresh water should be provided free choice to prevent cystitis, urolithiasis, and salt poisoning. Pigs spend the majority of their day sleeping unless they are encouraged to forage for their food, which is a natural behavior in swine.

TECHNICIAN TIP 5.39: Foraging for food is a natural behavior in swine.

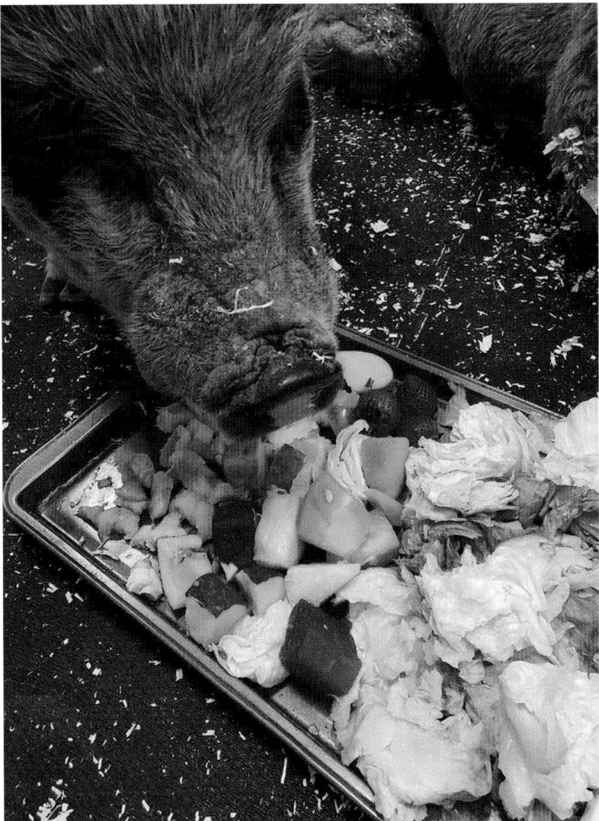

Figure 5.19 Pet pig eating fresh fruits and veggies.

Vitamins

When vitamins are provided in swine diets, stabilized vitamin A is commonly used because natural vitamin A is degraded under normal environmental conditions. Vitamin D is necessary for proper bone growth and ossification. Most vitamin D needs are met by exposing hogs to direct sunlight for a short time each day. Sources of vitamin D include irradiated yeast, sun-cured hays, animal sterols, fish oils, and vitamin A and D concentrates. Vitamin E is required by swine of all ages and is interrelated with selenium found in green forage, legume hays, and cereal grains. Vitamin K is necessary for blood clotting to convert fibrinogen to fibrin. Most producers supplement with vitamin K. Thiamine is not of practical importance in the diet, although riboflavin is a requirement of breeding stock and lightweight pigs. Riboflavin is naturally found in green forage, milk by-products, and brewer's yeast. Pantothenic acid is especially important for females and typically is found in crystalline form within premixes. Natural sources include green forage, legume meals, milk products, and brewer's yeast. Choline is essential for normal functioning of the liver and kidneys. Supplementing choline has been shown to increase litter size. It is naturally found in fish solubles, fish meal, and soybean meal. Young pigs require vitamin

B12 for growth and normal hemopoiesis. Vitamin B12 is present in animal, marine, and milk products.

TECHNICIAN TIP 5.40: Most vitamin D needs are met by exposing hogs to direct sunlight for a short time each day.

TECHNICIAN TIP 5.41: Mulberry heart disease has been seen in both young piglets and in adult sows.

Minerals

Minerals in the swine diet should include calcium and phosphorus primarily for skeletal growth. They also are important for metabolism and are required for gestation and lactation. They are easily supplied by the use of tankage, meat meal, meat, bone and fish meal, limestone, and oyster shells. Sodium chloride is recommended as 0.25% of the total diet. It is supplied by animal and fish by-products in the diet. Iodine is supplied in the diet for use by the thyroid gland to produce thyroxine and typically is supplied with iodized salt. Iron and copper are necessary for hemoglobin formation and to prevent nutritional anemia. Sow's milk is severely deficient in iron. Feeding lactating sows increased levels of iron does not seem to pass sufficiently high levels to the piglets. Cobalt is present in vitamin B12. Manganese is essential for normal reproduction and growth. Potassium requirements are met in the feedstuffs. Magnesium is essential for growing swine. Zinc in swine nutrition is interrelated with calcium. Supplemented zinc is recommended to prevent parakeratosis. The availability of zinc in the diet is adversely affected by the presence of phytic acid, a constituent of plant protein sources such as soybean meal. Most of the zinc in plant protein is in the bound form, thus the zinc is not available to monogastric animals such as the pig. Utilizing meat meal or meat scraps in the pigs' diet will help to prevent parakeratosis because of the high availability of the zinc. Another distinctive feature of the etiology of parakeratosis seen in pigs is an excess of dietary calcium (0.5–1.5%), which can lead to the development of the disease. The addition of zinc to such diets at levels much higher (0.02% zinc carbonate or 100 mg/kg zinc) than those normally required by growing swine prevents the occurrence of the disease. Selenium supplementation is dependent on soil conditions where crops were grown. Many areas of the United States are selenium deficient. Care must be taken when purchasing hay or other feed from a selenium deficient area.

Pig feeding management is similar to beef cattle management in that there are breeding-farrowing (reproductive) and growing enterprises. The farrowing unit produces baby pigs as reproductive replacements or to enter the growing unit for feeding to slaughter weight. The pig industry is one of the most intensively managed agricultural enterprises. Current pig production units are moving to total confinement farrow-to-finish operations containing many animals. Within these operations, feeding groups are segregated according to nutrient requirements, with diets for lactating and gestating sows and gilts, boars, nursery pigs, and growing pigs. For the most part, animals in the farrowing unit are housed and fed as individuals to better control BW and condition. Within the feeding operation, starting with the nursery pigs, all animals are group-housed and fed according to age and moved between groups as an entire unit.

As omnivores, pigs have a digestive tract that can accommodate a certain level of dietary fiber. Given the economics of rate of gain from forages versus grains, pig diets consist primarily of concentrates, along with energy, protein, mineral, and vitamin supplements. All feed ingredients are thoroughly mixed and provided as a single diet, like the TMR for cattle. Dietary ingredients depend on the nutritional requirements of the specific group of animals being fed. The classic pig diet consists of corn grain and soybean meal, with a vitamin-mineral premix. Learning more about the specific nutrient requirements of pigs has resulted in more sophisticated diets for pigs. Crystalline amino acids, high-quality animal by-product protein meals, fiber sources, and vitamin-mineral supplements have been incorporated into specific pig diets to improve growth efficiency.

TECHNICIAN TIP 5.42: Hepatosis dietetica affects young growing pigs up to and including three to four months of age although less commonly seen than mulberry-heart disease (MHD).

Backyard Chicken Nutrition

Chicken feed should supply all the nutrients for growth, development, and productivity for chicken flocks. Most problems encountered with backyard flocks are related to poor nutrition, and the feathers of the birds make it difficult to quickly assess things like weight loss. Nutrient requirements must be catered to bird age, purpose, and environmental conditions such as seasonal changes. A feed that is designed for layer hens is not adequate for optimal growth in broilers. A growing bird will require more protein whereas a layer bird requires increased calcium for shell production. Feeding a grower too much extra calcium can result in kidney failure and potential death for example.

Carbohydrates, proteins, and fats make up the largest nutritional requirement for chickens. Chickens will stop eating when they have met their energy requirement; therefore, it is important that they are eating a balanced diet to meet their other nutritional needs simultaneously.

Egg size is affected by intake of CP, amino acids like methionine and cystine, and total fats and essential fatty acids like linoleic acid. These levels can be adapted to improve early egg size and reduced to control later egg size.

TECHNICIAN TIP 5.43: Egg size is affected by nutrition.

In addition to eating standard chicken feeds like scratch grains and grits, most chickens enjoy the opportunity to forage in the yard, eating things like small insects, garden crops, and even things like watermelon or other fruits and veggies. They can also be given treats like meal worms, but they are a high source of protein, so they should be limited to avoid kidney disease. Provided the birds are consuming the primary nutrition from standard feed sources, extra foraging is a great addition to their diet and for enrichment purposes. Foraging in a yard can also put them at risk to predators including hawks and foxes or even a neighbor's dog.

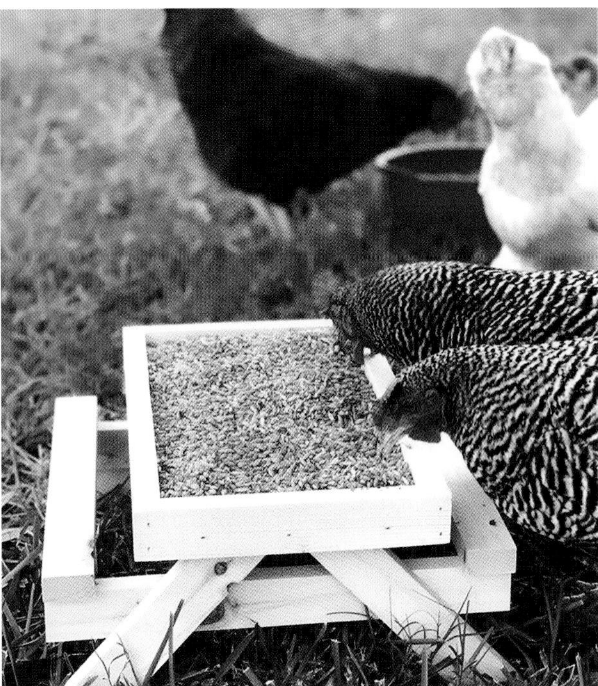

Figure 5.20 Chickens eating scratch grains. *Source:* Courtesy of therapy_chickens.

Types of Feed

Mash – a balanced ration, dusty.

Pelletized – a balanced ration, a mashed feed held together with a binder substance, heat treated, and then cut into pieces.

Crumble – a pelletized feed broken down into much smaller pieces.

Scratch grain – mix of high energy grains, will not meet the DER alone (Figure 5.20).

Fodder – grass can provide xanthophyll, add color to egg yolk and may improve flavor.

TECHNICIAN TIP 5.44: Scratch feed should not be considered a complete feed for any type of bird.

Key Nutritional Factors for Backyard Chickens

See Tables 5.9 and 5.10.

TECHNICIAN TIP 5.45: Seventy percent of the cost of raising chickens is feeding appropriately.

Energy

Carbohydrates represent the largest portion of chicken diet. Their needs vary depending on the life stage, purpose, and even weather. The average standard sized adult bird should require less than 1500 kcal/lb. In hot weather, chickens tend to take less energy but may require additional fat.

Protein

Proteins provide amino acids required for tissue production and egg production. The protein must be a high-quality source in order to produce a high-quality product. The concern with poor source of protein is that the bird may stop eating before it has taken in enough protein, when being fed fillers with low nutritional value.

Corn and soybean are the common protein sources to supply essential amino acids in chicken diets. They complement each other to provide the full spectrum of amino acids needed because corn is high in methionine and low in lysine and soybeans are rich in lysine but low in methionine.

Table 5.9 Average amount of feed required.

Production type	Life stage	Amount of feed
Egg-type	Hatch to 18–22 weeks	13–15 lb
Egg-type	Layers >22 weeks	98–107 g per hen
Meat-type	Hatch to market (7 weeks)	12.5–18 lb[a]

[a] A heavier bird breed will need to eat more.

Table 5.10 Nutrient requirements for production.

Type of feed	ME kcal/lb	CP (%)	Ca (%)	Available protein (%)
Starter	1290–1315	20–22	0.85–1.00	0.40–0.45
Grower	1290–1315	16–18	0.80–0.95	0.35–0.42
Developer	1250–1290	14–16	0.75–0.92	0.30–0.38
Layer	1290–1315	15–19	3.60–4.20	0.32–0.45
Mature	1290–1315	14–18	3.40–4.00	0.32–0.40

Fat

Fats have high energy values and are critical for the absorption of fat-soluble vitamins. They can be supplied through vegetable oils or animal fats. Levels over 5% can quickly lead to rancid development in the feed, particularly when stored improperly. Fats added in the diet can also help reduce the dustiness of a feed and increase palatability.

Vitamins and Minerals

Chickens require all vitamins, except vitamin C unless they are under stress. The vitamins serve as antioxidants and catalysts. Fat-soluble vitamins that include Vit A, D3, E, and K, or water soluble like B complex vitamins are important in growth. The water-soluble vitamin choline is a high requirement in chickens, they manufacture very little; therefore, a content of more than five times should be included in the feed. Failure to meet the vitamin needs of chickens can result in rough feathers, dermatitis, blindness, mouth lesions, foot pad lesions, fatty liver or kidney, and curled toes. They also require specific essential fatty acid linoleic acid.

The macrominerals calcium and phosphorus are the major minerals required for the formation of eggshells in layers. Generally, the grains used in chicken feeds are low in minerals and require supplementation. Limestone or oyster shells are a common source of calcium for backyard chickens and may be available in a mineral premix. It is also possible to break down and offer dehydrated crushed eggs shell to them. Failure to provide adequate mineral supplementation can result in reduced activity, thin shells, reduced egg production, and growth retardation. Feeding an imbalanced calcium-to-phosphorus-to-vitamin D3 ratio can also induce rickets (Figures 5.21).

Grit

In addition to their nutritional needs, chickens should always have access to some grit. Grit may be from granite or flint chipped up into small pieces. If free-ranging, they may find a suitable source in the environment or as mentioned above, ground up dehydrated egg shells can also work. Grit is an important part of digestion. The grit is consumed, and then remains in the gizzard to help grind up their food since chickens do not have teeth for grinding. Oyster shells are a type of soluble grit, where it can function in the gizzard first and later be absorbed to help provide additional calcium to the diet (Figure 5.22).

Water

Critical for body functions like absorption and assimilation of nutrients from the digestive tract. Chickens need approximately 2× the volume of water compared to their feed intake, In other words, two parts water to one part feed. They may need up to 3.5 times in summer months depending on their living conditions and temperatures.

Water sources are a common site for the spread of disease among a flock so it is critical to keep the water source cleaned daily. There are a variety of options for providing chickens with water. Popular option is a stand-alone poultry font, with a center canister that provides continuous

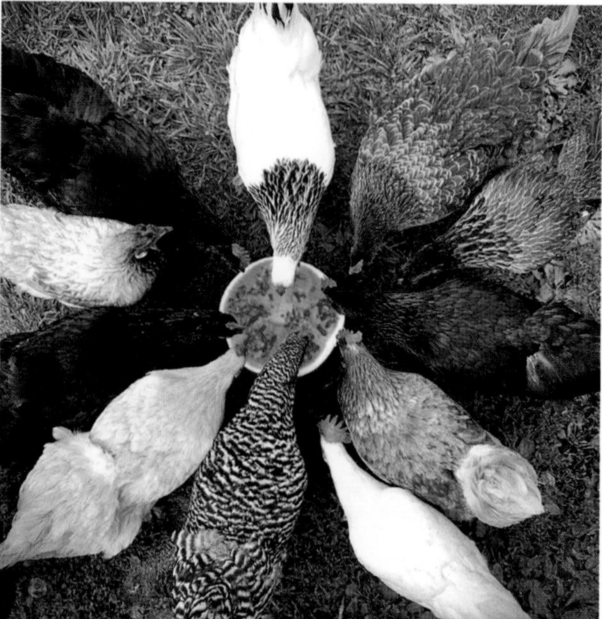

Figure 5.21 Chicken enjoying a watermelon treat.
Source: Courtesy of therapy_chickens.

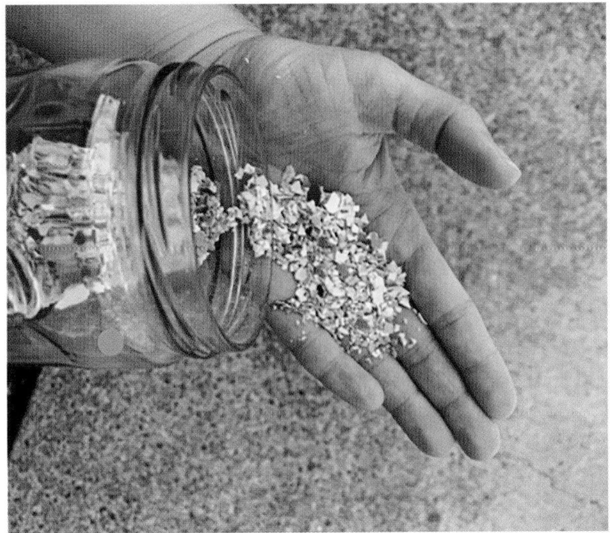

Figure 5.22 Example of ground up shells used for grit.

water and provides fair access from many angles but is subject to getting dirty on the ground. Options to avoid water contamination include small automatic refilling water cups or water nipples that flow down from a continuous source and refill automatically, but these are difficult to share so additional spickets should be provided depending on the number of birds (Figure 5.23).

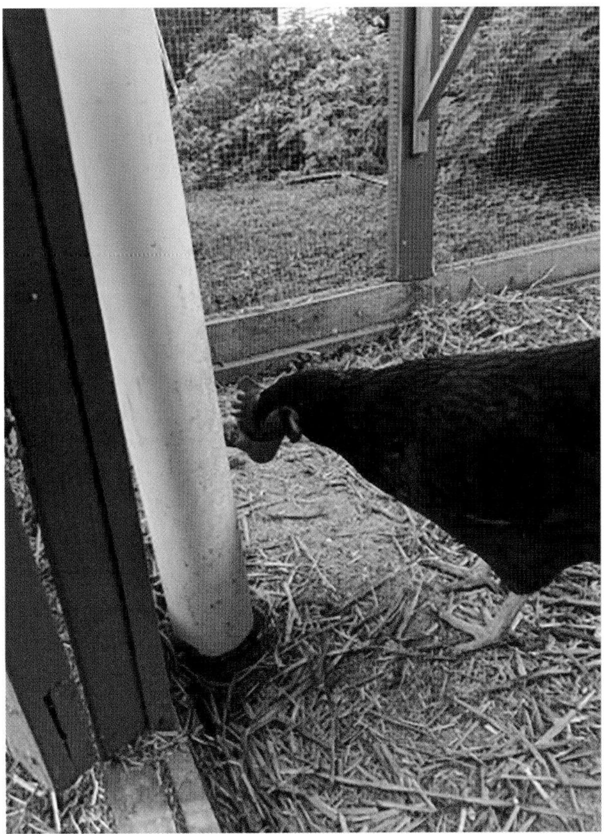

Figure 5.23 Chicken drinking water from a small cup waterer.

TECHNICIAN TIP 5.46: Nutrition is the one area of veterinary medicine that affects every animal.

Summary

Nutrition is vital to the health and well-being of all animals. Proper nutrition and feeding management is the foundation upon which healing and the maintenance of health rests. The veterinary healthcare team, especially the veterinary technician, should be well-versed in key nutritional factors for all large animal species. Appropriate nutrition and proper feeding of livestock will help to increase the quality of life, the longevity, and the productivity of the individual and in the herd.

References

Bassert, J. and McCurnin, D. (2009). *McCurnin's Clinical Textbook for Veterinary Technicians*, 7e. St. Louis, MO: Saunders-Elsevier.

Brotherton, R. (2010). Nutrition. In: *Principles and Practice of Veterinary Technology*, 3e (ed. M. Sirois). St. Louis, MO: Mosby Elsevier.

Burns, K. (2011). Equine nutrition. *Canadian Veterinary Technician*. Fall (3): 4.

Carr, E.A. and Holcombe, S.J. (2009). Nutrition of critically ill horses. *Veterinary Clinics of North America: Equine Practice, Clinical Nutrition.* 25 (1): 93–108.

Davies, Z. (2009). *Introduction to Horse Nutrition*. Ames, IA: Wiley-Blackwell.

Dunkel, B. and Wilkins, P. (2004). Nutrition and the critically ill horse. *Veterinary Clinics of North America. Equine Practice* 20 (1): 107–126.

Frape, D. (2010). *Equine Nutrition and Feeding*, 4e. Ames, IA: Wiley-Blackwell.

Geor, R. (2009). Equine Nutrition. In: *Veterinary Clinics of North America: Equine Practice*. St. Louis, MO: Elsevier/Saunders.

Gross, K., Yamka, R., Khoo, C. et al. (2010). *Macro-Nutrients. Small Animal Clinical Nutrition*, 5e. Topeka, KS: Mark Morris Institute.

Holland, C. and Kezar, W. (1995). *Pioneer Forage Manual. A Nutritional Guide*. Des Moines, IA: Pioneer Hi-Bred International.

Holtgrew-Bohling, K. (2011). *Large Animal Clinical Procedures for Veterinary Technicians*, 2e. St. Louis, MO: Mosby Elsevier.

Lewis, L. (1995). Growing horse feeding and care. In: *Equine Clinical Nutrition: Feeding and Care*. Baltimore, MA: Williams and Wilkins.

Lewis, L. (1995). Sick horse feeding and nutritional support. In: *Equine Clinical Nutrition: Feeding and Care*. Baltimore, MA: Williams and Wilkins.

Lewis, L. (1996). Feeding and care of horses with health problems. In: *Feeding and Care of the Horse*, 2e. Media, PA: Williams and Wilkins.

Lewis, L. (1996). *Growing Horse Feeding and Care. In Feeding and Care of the Horse*, 2e. Media, PA: Williams and Wilkins.

Morand-Fehr, P. (ed.) (1991). *Goat Nutrition*. Wageningen, Netherlands: Pudoc.

Pilliner, S. (2009). *Horse Nutrition and Feeding*, 2e. Ames, IA: Wiley Blackwell.

Pugh, D. and Baird, A. (2011). *Sheep and Goat Medicine*, 2e. St. Louis, MO: Elsevier Saunders.

Qi, K. et al. (1992). Sulfate supplementation of angora goats: metabolic and mohair responses. *Journal of Animal Science* 70: 2828.

Radostits, O., Gay, C., Hinchcliff, K., and Constable, P. (2007). *Veterinary Medicine: A Textbook of the Disease of Cattle, Horses, Sheep, Pigs and Goats*. Philadelphia, PA: Saunders Elsevier.

Reed, S., Bayly, W., and Sellon, D. (2010). *Equine Internal Medicine*, 3e. St. Louis, MO: Saunders Elsevier.

Reeder, D. et al. (2009). *AAEVT's Equine Manual for Veterinary Technicians*. Ames, IA: Wiley Blackwell.

Santucci, P.M. et al. (1991). Body condition scoring of goats in extensive conditions. In: *Goat Nutrition* (ed. P. Morand-Fehr). Wageningen, Netherlands: Pudoc.

Schoenherr, W.D. (2009). Large Animal Nutrition. In: *McCurnin's Clinical Textbook for Veterinary Technicians*, 7e (eds. D. McCurnin and J. Bassert). St. Louis, MO: W. B. Saunders Company.

Smith, B. (2008). *Large Animal Internal Medicine*, 4e. St. Louis, MO: Elsevier Health Services.

Wortinger, A. (2007). *Nutrition for Veterinary Technicians and Nurses*. Ames, IA: Wiley Blackwell.

Clinical Case Resolution 5.1

Upon arrival, the owner meets the veterinary healthcare team at the barn and is quick to point out that another sheep is showing the same symptoms that the other two sheep did before they died. Examination showed increased respiration, weakness, and icteric sclera. A complete history is taken, and the owner is asked to give a detailed description of the feeding practices, including any recent changes in the sheep's diet. The sheep are on pasture but have been supplemented with free choice roughage and a commercially mixed grain diet once daily. Upon questioning the owner further about any changes in diet, it was noted that the sheep had recently been moved into a new pasture that had previously had cattle grazing on it. With this history taken, the veterinary healthcare team inspects all areas of the farm. The food storage areas were found to be unremarkable with quality food storage practices in place. Commercially packaged sheep food was stored properly in rodent proof containers and found to be free of mold. The veterinary healthcare team next inspected the pasture area where they were being housed and discovered a trace mineral block labeled for cattle to be accessible to the sheep. The use of trace mineral blocks labeled for species other than sheep can cause copper toxicity. The signs for copper toxicity include increased respiration, depression, weakness, hemoglobinuria, icterus, and sudden death.

Activities

Multiple Choice Questions

(Answers can be found in the back of the book.)

1. What is one way to determine protein quality?
   - **A** measuring the BV
   - **B** by determining the source as animal proteins are higher quality than plant proteins
   - **C** measuring the calorie content
   - **D** measured by a bomb calorimeter

2. What is the most common source of carbohydrates found in pet and livestock foods?
   - **A** cereal grains
   - **B** any animal by-products
   - **C** dairy products
   - **D** legumes

3. How can good-quality roughage be determined?
   A free of mold
   B soft and pliable to the touch
   C leafy with fine stems
   D all of the above

4. What is considered to be the foundation of an equine feeding program?
   A concentrates
   B minerals
   C roughages
   D vitamins

5. If a decision is made to enterally supplement a 450 kg horse with a slurry via a NG feeding tube, what is the maximum amount the horse should be fed?
   A 0.5 gal
   B 1.5–2 gal
   C 2.5–3 gal
   D 3.5–4 gal

6. What is considered normal rumen pH of cattle?
   A 2.5
   B 3.5
   C 6.5
   D 8.5

7. How many stomach compartments does the camelid have?
   A 1
   B 2
   C 3
   D 4

8. What is important to know when providing water to camelids in cold climates?
   A Camelids will only drink water when the water temperature is greater than 55 °F.
   B Camelids consume double the amount of water that they normally would during warmer temperatures.
   C Camelids will not break through the ice to get to a water source.
   D Camelids do not have any special requirements during cold weather.

9. How many pounds of feed does it take to produce approximately 1 lb of pork?
   A 1–1.5 lb
   B 2–2.5 lb
   C 3–3.5 lb
   D 4–4.5 lb

10. Which of the following chicken feeds can provide xanthophyll, adding color to egg yolk and potentially improving flavor.
    A fodder
    B scratch grain
    C grit
    D crumble

Test Your Learning

1. Define the term kilocalorie.
2. What determines the amount of protein an animal needs?
3. What are the three main categories of horse feeds?
4. What is considered to be the foundation of an equine feeding program?
5. Name two things that may develop if excess concentrates are fed.
6. List the factors that will influence the growth rate of growing horses.
7. List two ways the critically ill can receive nutrition.
8. How many hours can the healthy adult horse withstand food deprivation (simple starvation) with little systemic effects?
9. List two indications for feeding a patient parenterally?
10. What types of questions should healthcare team members ask when documenting the patient's nutritional history?
11. What is the most important nutrient for all animals, especially sheep and goats?
12. Why should trace mineral blocks be avoided in sheep?
13. What is important regarding the practice of grinding feeds to increase feed efficiency in swine?
14. Briefly describe the key differences between a layer's and a broiler's diet.

Answers can be found in the back of the book.

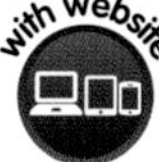

Extra review questions, case studies, and a breed ID image bank can be found online at www.wiley.com/go/loly/veterinary.

Chapter 6

Clinical Procedures

Annette M. McCoy, DVM, MS, DACVS, Erica McKenzie, BSc, BVMS, PhD, DACVIM, DACVSMR, and Sue Loly, LVT, VTS (EVN)

Learning Objectives

- Describe considerations that should be taken into account when choosing a venous catheter.
- List indications for the placement of a urinary catheter.
- Calculate the appropriate volume for a whole blood transfusion.
- List minimum information regarding administration of medication to be included in a patient record.
- Describe methods for determining and monitoring total body hydration status of an individual.
- Calculate the appropriate volume of fluid to be given for replacement or maintenance.
- Describe the potential pitfalls and complications of nasogastric and orogastric intubation, and how to recognize and/or avoid them.
- Describe safety measures that should be taken for all routine dental procedures.

Clinical Case Problem 6.1

A 26-year-old Arabian mare is being brought to the clinic for evaluation of signs of colic that have been rapidly worsening over the past 4 hr. On arrival, the mare has a heart rate of 80 beats/min, bright pink mucous membranes, and a capillary refill time of 4 S. Gastrointestinal sounds are decreased to absent. What diagnostic and/or therapeutic procedures should you be ready to perform or assist with immediately? What concerns might there be for longer-term management of this patient while hospitalized?

See Clinical Case Resolution 6.1 at the end of this chapter.

Key Terms

Alloantibodies
Aseptic technique
Azotemia
Colloids
Coupage
Crystalloids
Dehydration
Dental float
Extracellular fluid
Gastric reflux
Hyperimmune plasma
Hypertonic
Intracellular fluid
Isoerythrolysis
Isotonic
Parenteral
Thrombophlebitis

Large Animal Medicine for Veterinary Technicians, Second Edition. Edited by Sue Loly and Heather Hopkinson.

Companion website: www.wiley.com/go/loly/veterinary

Introduction

A veterinary technician may be called on to perform or assist with a variety of procedures, both in the clinic and in the field. This chapter is intended as an introduction to some of the most common of these clinical procedures used for the treatment of large animal patients, rather than as an exhaustive and detailed listing. Each of these procedures has the common need for adequate restraint of the patient for safe and successful completion.

Understanding appropriate restraint techniques is especially important for individuals dealing with adult large animals, since it is impossible to physically overpower the patient. Even small ruminants, camelids, and neonates of many species can cause significant physical injury to the unwary. The safety of personnel should be always priority – some large animal patients can easily be handled by a single individual, while others require an additional person (or persons) to assist with restraint.

For some patients and procedures, physical restraint may be inadequate and chemical restraint (sedation) must be used. Using chemical restraint does not denote failure or cowardice; instead, recognition of these situations promotes the safety of both the patient and personnel. Our patients do not necessarily understand that we are trying to help them. Thus, for example, administering a sedative to safely place an intravenous catheter so that patient can receive life-saving medication may be warranted. Throughout the course of treatment, patients are often initially listless and weak, accepting treatment quite readily, but as they recover and gain strength, it may become more difficult to manage and to administer the same treatments.

If a patient is proving to be difficult to manage during a procedure, it is important to communicate this to the veterinarian so a new approach may be considered. For example, if a horse does not tolerate oral medications and poses a dangerous threat to the handlers, the veterinarian may change the course of treatment to exclude that form of treatment.

> **TECHNICIAN TIP 6.1:** The safety of personnel should be always priority!

Venous Catheterization

General Considerations

There are a number of indications for placement of intravenous catheters (ICV), including administration of drugs and fluids and collection of blood samples (especially, if repeated). In large animals, the jugular vein is the most common site for catheter placement due to its large size and ease of accessibility. However, other veins, including the cephalic, saphenous, median, lateral thoracic, and auricular veins, can be used if needed. The technician can confirm the course of a vein occluding the vessel at a site appropriate for the planned site of insertion and allowing the vessel to fill proximally ("raising the vein").

> **TECHNICIAN TIP 6.2:** A rubber band placed at the base of the ear can be helpful for raising the auricular vein in a pig's ear.

Catheters are available in a wide variety of sizes and materials. The appropriate choice of catheter depends on the size of the vein; the amount, rate, and viscosity of the fluids/drugs to be administered; and the length of time for which the catheter will remain in place. Short, large diameter catheters will allow for the most rapid fluid administration, while long, narrow-diameter catheters will have a slower flow rate. For adult horses and cattle, 14-gauge, 13-cm (5.25-in) catheters are the most used for jugular catheterization, while in foals, camelids, and small ruminants, shorter 18- or 20-gauge catheters are more appropriate. For extremely rapid fluid administration, as might be needed to treat hypovolemic shock, 10- and 12-gauge catheters are available.

Multi-lumen catheters, with two or three separate injection ports, may be used if several different types of fluids must be administered simultaneously. For example, if a sick foal requires total parenteral nutrition (TPN), crystalloid fluid replacement therapy, and parenterally administered drugs, then a multi-lumen catheter allows a dedicated port for each treatment.

Catheters intended for short-term use (hours to days) are made of polypropylene or Teflon. Polypropylene is highly thrombogenic, while Teflon is less so. In contrast, catheters intended for long-term use (days to weeks) are made of polyurethane or silastic and are significantly less thrombogenic. Teflon and polyurethane catheters are the most commonly available in large animal clinical practice. The former should not be left in place for longer than three days, while the latter can be left in place for up to two weeks. These catheters are available in several different forms, including over-the-needle, through-the-needle, and over-the-wire. Through-the-needle catheters are placed by first putting a short needle into the vessel, then threading the catheter through the needle. This is the least common type of catheter used in large animal practice and has the disadvantage that the venipuncture hole is larger than the catheter, increasing the risk of a hematoma at the insertion site. Over-the-needle catheters have a stylet within the

Box 6.1 Common Supplies Used for IVC Placement

- surgical preparation solutions (iodine or chlorhexidine based and isopropyl alcohol)
- clipper with #40 surgical blades
- sterile gloves
- syringe with 0.9% saline or heparin/saline (20 ml)
- #15 scalpel blade
- local anesthetic (lidocaine or mepivacaine)
- suture material, tissue glue, or tape
- intravenous catheter
- IV extension set and injection port
- bandage material (optional)

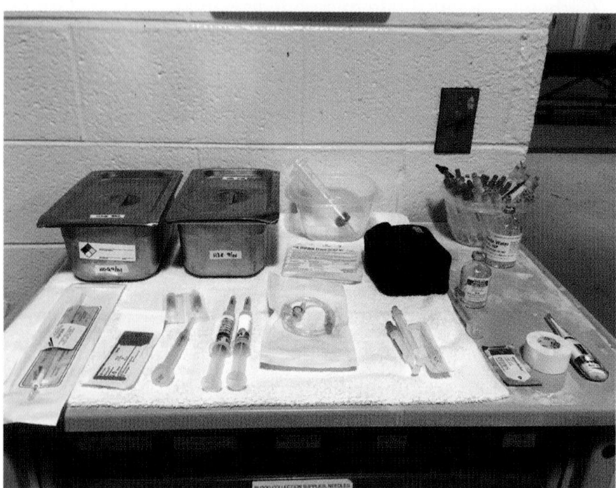

Figure 6.1 Setup for a catheter placement includes various catheters, flush, scrub, sterile gloves, tape, and more.

catheter that is used for venipuncture, which is removed once the catheter is in the vessel. This is the most common style of catheter used in adult large animal patients. Its greatest disadvantages are that the catheter end can become burred during insertion, and the junction between the hub and the shaft is prone to bending and breaking.

Over-the-wire catheters are placed by first inserting a short needle into the vessel, then threading a wire through the needle that is subsequently used to guide the catheter into the vessel. This style of catheter is the most technically challenging to place, but is commonly used in foals, for multi-lumen catheters and for catheters intended to remain in place for a long period of time. Regardless of the type of catheter, sterile technique should be used for placement. See Box 6.1 for general supplies list and Figure 6.1.

Short-Term Catheters

Short-term drug and fluid administration or repeated blood sample collection over a limited time period are the most common indications for short-term catheters in large animal practice. Teflon and polyurethane catheters ranging in length from 5 to 13 cm may be used, depending on the size of the patient and the purpose of the catheter. For a short-term catheter, the choice of catheter material may be largely based on availability or personal preference, but if the catheter will remain in place for longer than three days, then polyurethane is preferred to reduce the risk of thromboembolism.

The jugular vein is most typically used for short-term catheters, and placement in this location using an over-the-needle catheter is described here, although the same general principles apply to catheterization of any vein. Jugular catheters should be placed in the proximal third of the neck. The skin should be clipped with wide margins (i.e. a 10 cm × 10 cm site for a jugular catheter) and aseptically prepared. A small amount (1–2 ml) of local anesthetic is placed subcutaneously at the site of insertion and at any site at which a suture will be placed to secure the catheter, after which a final scrub and alcohol wipe is applied. For animals with very thick skin (i.e. camelids), a stab incision may need to be made through the skin at the anesthetized insertion site to prevent burring of the tip of the catheter. Sterile gloves should be worn for placement of all catheters. The catheter should be filled with 0.9% sterile saline after removal of the cap and sleeve, and a similarly filled extension set with injection cap should be prepared. Holding a fingertip over the hub of the catheter will prevent leakage of the saline. Care should be taken to only touch the hub of the catheter so that the shaft remains sterile. Using one hand to raise the vein, insert the stylet through the anesthetized skin and into the vein at a 45° angle, removing the fingertip from the catheter hub to look for blood. Once this is seen, the angle of insertion should be reduced so that the catheter is nearly parallel to the vein and the stylet and catheter inserted an additional 5–10 mm to ensure that the catheter is within the vein. The vessel can then be released, and the catheter slid off the stylet, being careful not to advance the stylet in any further. The stylet is then removed, and the extension set attached. Use a syringe of 0.9% sterile saline attached to the extension set to confirm placement of the catheter within the vessel – pull back on the plunger until blood enters the extension set ("flash"), then flush with 10–20 ml of saline unless it is a particularly small patient, such as a cria in which smaller volumes (3 ml) should be utilized to flush the catheter. The catheter can be secured in place using suture, cyanoacrylate tissue glue, or tape. In young animals, or those prone to rub at the catheter site, an elastic bandage should be placed to keep the catheter site clean and to prevent accidental removal of the catheter. The extension set should exit the bandage along the side of the neck for ease of access (Figures 6.2–6.4).

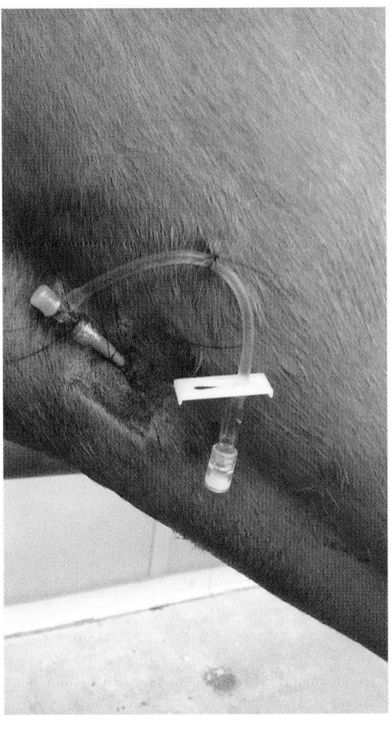

Figure 6.2 Correctly placed and secured jugular catheter in an equine patient.

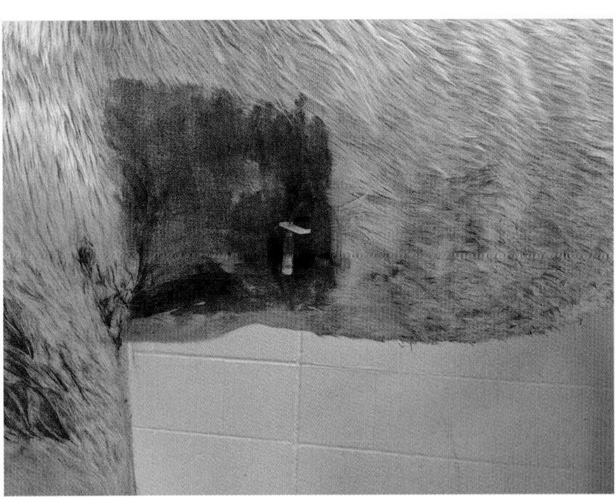

Figure 6.3 Lateral thoracic catheter placement in a horse.

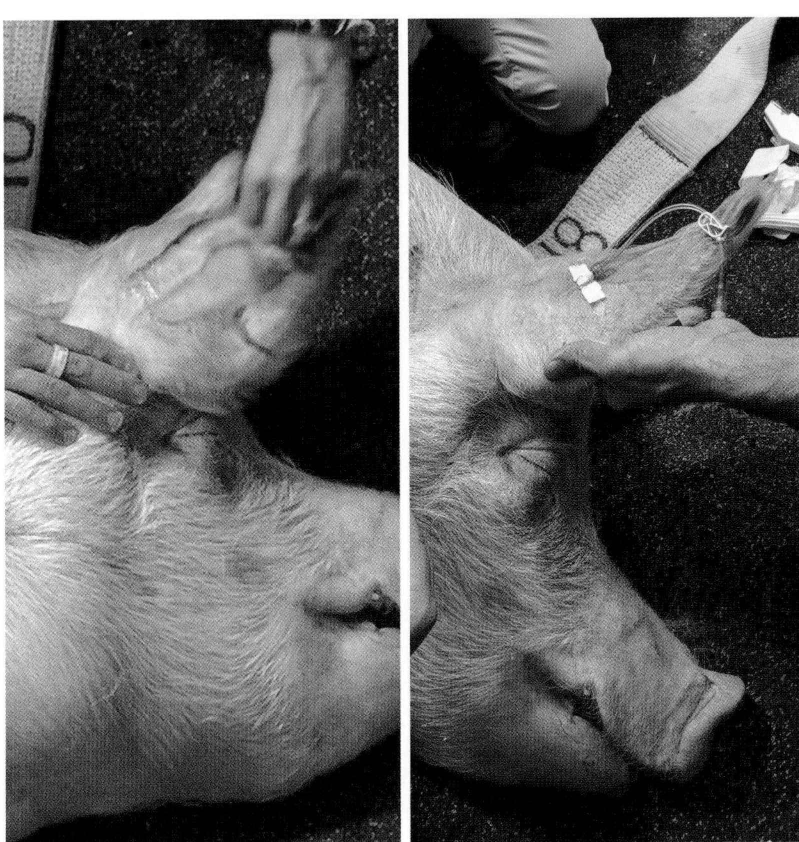

Figure 6.4 Intravenous catheter placement in the auricular vein of a large pig.

Box 6.2 Heparinized Saline IVC Flush Solution

Heparin 50 IU/ml
Saline 3 ml

TECHNICIAN TIP 6.3: In regard to quantities 1 ml = 1 cc.

Patency and placement of the catheter should be confirmed prior to administration of any drugs or fluids by drawing back on a syringe of 0.9% sterile saline to look for a flash of blood in the catheter extension and then flushing the catheter. The catheter should always be flushed after drug administration, including between drugs being given consecutively (see Box 6.2 for Heparinized Saline recipe). Failure to flush between drugs may result in drug precipitation within the catheter and/or catheter extension. Even when no drugs are scheduled to be given, catheters should be flushed every 6 hr to help maintain patency. If the catheter is covered with a bandage, it should be visually inspected underneath the bandage daily, or more often if concerns arise.

TECHNICIAN TIP 6.4: Patients that try to rub their catheter should have a neck wrap or collar placed to prevent catheter damage.

Long-Term Catheters

Long-term catheters used in large animals are generally over-the-wire, made of polyurethane to reduce the risk of thromboembolism, and intended for use over a period of days to weeks. The most common indication for this type of catheter is a neonate that requires parenteral nutrition in addition to fluids and medications (multi-lumen catheter), but long catheters are also used in situations where monitoring central pressure (i.e. near the level of the heart) is desirable, or in patients considered more susceptible to venous thrombosis. These catheters are available in a variety of sizes, from 14-gauge to 19-gauge, in lengths up to 25 cm (10 in). These are usually placed in the jugular vein. The same preparation and aseptic technique should be used for the placement of these catheters as described for short catheters (described previously). It may be useful to have an assistant in sterile gloves available to keep the various pieces of the catheter kit organized during placement. After preparation of the site, a short needle is inserted into the vessel with one hand while holding off the vein. Correct placement is verified by blood exiting the hub of the needle. With the vein still held off to prevent air entering

Box 6.3 Heparin Lock

1) Determine the total priming volume of the catheter (and extension set).
2) Divide total priming volume in half.
3) Draw up half the volume using hep/saline.
4) Draw up half the volume using 1000 units of heparin to create a one-to-one solution.

i.e. take 1.5 cc of 1000 units heparin and mix it with 1.5 cc of hep/Saline solution for a total volume of 3 cc priming volume.

Take that heparin lock solution mixture and push it into the catheter. Lock the catheter without flushing it further.

Label the catheter port "hep lock" and note on the medical record. Change hep lock every 24 hr.

To remove the heparin lock, aspirate the priming volume out of the catheter and then flush with normal hep/saline solution. This is particularly important with small patients. Note that some Veterinarians are OK with adult horses having heplock flushed in, if they do not have any problem that could be worsened when given heparin.

through the needle, the guide wire is threaded through the needle into the vessel. The wire is passed for a distance of several centimeters (generally marked on the wire) before removing the needle, leaving the wire in place. It is very important to maintain control of the end of the wire so that it remains sterile and is also not inadvertently released entirely into the vein. The catheter is then threaded over-the-wire and guided into the vessel, through the hole in the skin left by the larger needle. Placement of the catheter within the vein is verified by holding off the vein and seeing blood exit the hub, then the wire is carefully removed. An extension set is attached, and the catheter secured in place as described previously for short catheters. Patency and placement of the catheter should be confirmed prior to administration of any drugs or fluids by drawing back on a syringe of 0.9% sterile saline to look for a flash of blood in the catheter extension and then flushing the catheter.

Complications

While mild localized swelling around the catheter site can be innocuous, especially if it is not hot or painful, it may be an indicator of a more serious complication. Inflammation and formation of a clot within a vein, referred to as thrombophlebitis, may be caused by excessive vessel trauma, turbulent blood flow at the catheter tip, infection due to contamination during or after catheter placement, or leaving a catheter in for too long. Catheter kinks can also cause irritation and obstruct catheter function. (Figure 6.5) Certain medical conditions, including endotoxemia, hypoproteinemia, sepsis, and other systemic illnesses may also predispose patients to thrombophlebitis, even if proper catheter care is followed. Thrombophlebitis is generally accompanied by pain at the catheter site as well as swelling/edema. The vein is often firm to hard upon palpation in the region of the catheter, although depending on the severity of the condition, it can extend for some distance distally. Affected patients often have a fever and may show other nonspecific signs of malaise. Presence of a thrombus in the vein can be confirmed by ultrasound examination.

The most important treatment for thrombophlebitis is immediate removal of the catheter. Hot packing the site will help with swelling and edema, and superficial abscesses should be drained and flushed. The catheter site or catheter itself should be cultured. Until the bacteria involved in the infection are identified, broad-spectrum systemic antibiotics should be initiated or continued, although the drug regimen may need to be altered based on the bacterial antibiotic susceptibility profile. Strict aseptic technique during catheter placement and frequent checks of the catheter site, including regular catheter flushing, as well as a timely removal of short-term catheters will reduce the risk of thrombophlebitis. In general, any catheter that is questionable should be removed or replaced.

Other complications that can occur include catheter breakage, extravasation of fluids into the subcutaneous space, and hemorrhage. When a catheter breaks, it is most likely to occur at the junction between the hub and the shaft. The body of the catheter can remain within the superficial vein or migrate toward the heart. If the body of the catheter is missing at the time of removal, an ultrasound examination may be used to try to locate it. Fortunately, this complication is rare, although retrieval of broken catheters has been reported. Hemorrhage from a catheter site is generally associated with accidental loss of the injection port or disconnection of a fluid line and is usually not serious if noticed and addressed in a timely manner. If extravasation of fluids is noted, the catheter has almost certainly become dislodged and should be removed. Introduction of an air embolism is another potentially serious, but uncommon complication that may be due to operator error (direct injection of air into a catheter), an uncapped catheter, or pressure being forced through an empty fluid bottle or bag (i.e. from an automated pump without a safety shutoff). Air embolism has been reported to result in cyanosis, collapse, and death.

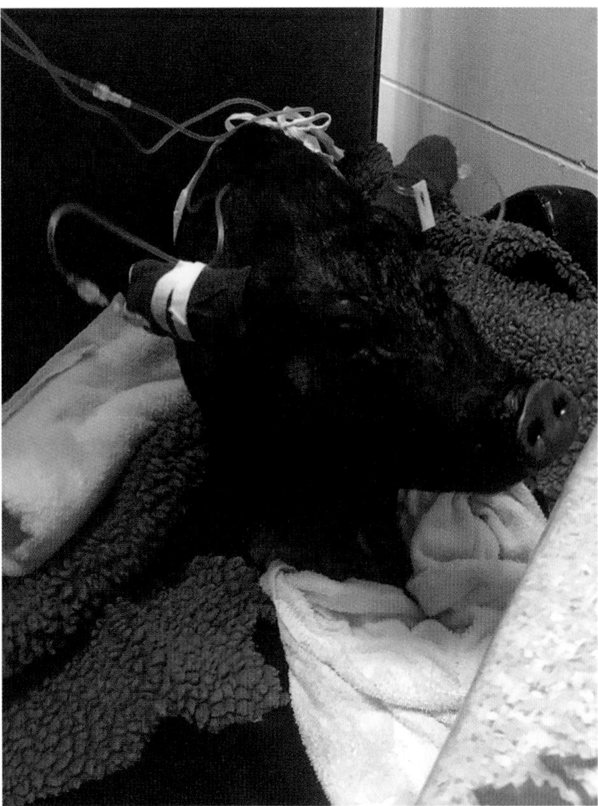

Figure 6.6 Pet Pig with IVs in both ear veins. It can be so tricky to place these catheters, that securing them is critical for patency and security. In some cases, it may help to place a rolled-up gauze on the inside of the ear flap to help avoid bending the catheter.

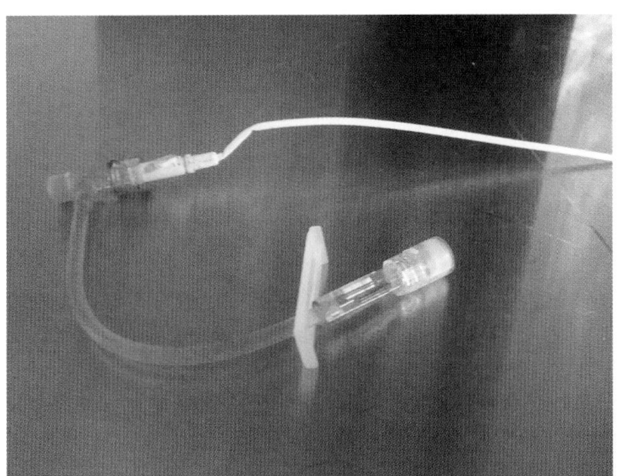

Figure 6.5 Short-term polyurethane 5″ catheter kinked.

Arterial Catheterization

The primary indication for arterial catheterization is ongoing monitoring of arterial blood pressure during

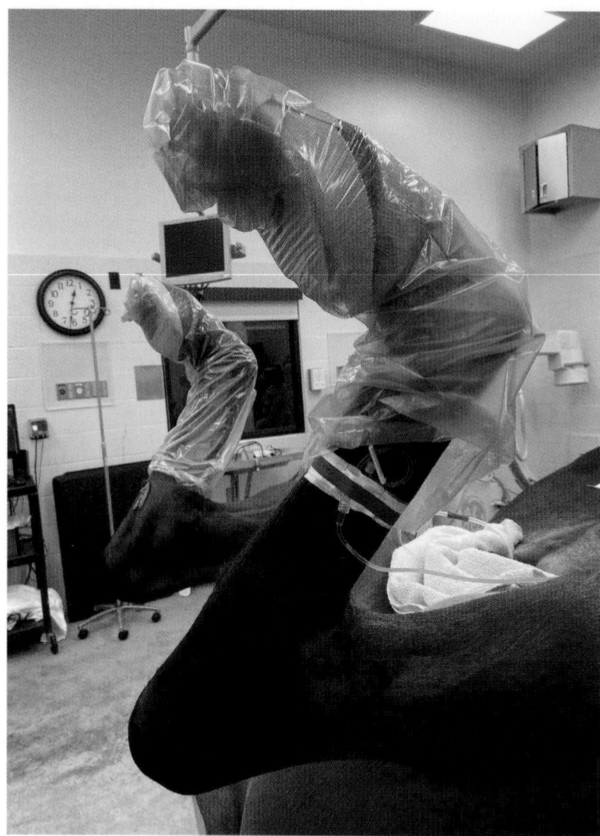

Figure 6.7 Arterial line placed in the hind leg of a horse during an anesthetic procedure. (*Source:* Courtesy of Shana Lemmenes)

anesthesia, and these catheters are rarely maintained past cessation of the anesthetic period. The choice of artery is largely based on convenience and accessibility. For most procedures, the transverse facial artery, located caudal and ventral to the eye, or the facial artery ventral to the mandible, are useful. If the head is in the surgical field, the lateral dorsal metatarsal artery can be used (Figure 6.7). In smaller animals, such as camelids, the femoral artery may be easiest to access. The auricular artery is also an option in certain cases.

Palpation of a pulse is the primary guide for differentiating an artery from an adjacent vein. Light pressure during palpation is preferred, as firm pressure may result in occlusion of the vessel and cessation of the pulsatile flow of blood under the fingers. Once the artery has been located, the surrounding skin should be clipped, and aseptically prepared and sterile gloves should be worn for catheter placement. A short 18- or 20-gauge over-the-needle catheter is mostly used. Digital stabilization of the artery during stylet insertion may help to keep the thick-walled vessel from rolling to the side. The stylet should be inserted for a short distance into the artery before slipping the catheter over it to prevent a burr, bend, or kink in the catheter. Blood will flow freely from the catheter hub as soon as the stylet is removed; thus, placement of several gauze sponges beneath the hub is recommended to keep the skin dry. After attachment of the catheter to the manometer or pressure transducer, it can be secured in place with the use of cyanoacrylate tissue glue or suture. When properly placed in an artery, a pulse will be visible in the fluid line adjacent to the catheter hub. If this blood reaches the manometer or the pressure transducer, it can damage them; thus, regular flushing of the catheter is required. This is facilitated by placement of a three-way stopcock in the fluid line connecting the catheter to the manometer or pressure transducer.

Complications

The most common complication associated with short-term arterial catheters is the formation of a hematoma at the insertion site, either related to a failed insertion attempt or removal of the catheter. Firm digital pressure for 3 min at the catheter site after removal will help to prevent this complication. Long-term arterial catheters have similar risks to venous catheters, including catheter-site infections and loss of patency. Regular flushing, more frequent than for venous catheters, and regular inspection of the catheter and all attachments will help to reduce the instance of complications. Automated continuous flushing devices are commercially available.

Urinary Catheterization

Placement of a urinary catheter is primarily performed to empty the bladder for diagnostic, therapeutic, or surgical purposes. Specific indications include:

1) obtaining an uncontaminated urine sample
2) emptying the bladder of a patient unable to urinate on their own
3) preparing for surgery of the bladder or penis
4) emptying the bladder during general anesthesia to prevent surgical site contamination or prior to anesthetic recovery (as some practitioners feel that a longer quiet period in recovery is possible if the patient's bladder is empty).

Urinary catheters can be placed in a standing animal or under general anesthesia (Figure 6.8). If the procedure is performed while standing, the patient should ideally be in a set of stocks, and sedation is recommended. Acepromazine is often used as part of the sedation protocol for this procedure in males because it promotes relaxation of the penis. However, caution should be used, especially with stallions,

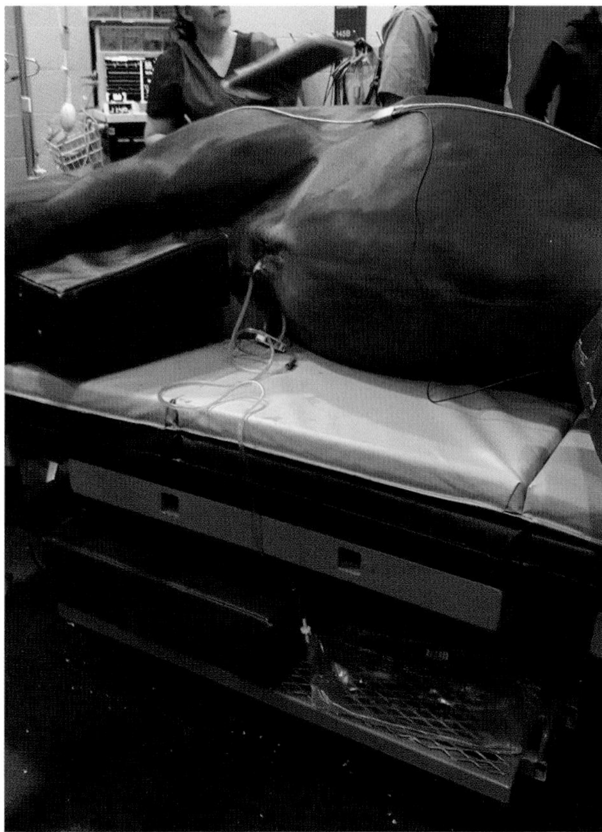

Figure 6.8 Urinary catheter placed in a gelding during a myelogram procedure.

as penile paralysis is an uncommon but recognized potential side effect of this medication. After the bladder has been emptied, or at the end of the surgical procedure, the urinary catheter should be removed. Placement of a urinary catheter is associated with a small risk of iatrogenic bladder infection. This risk increases if the catheter is maintained in place for a long period of time. Adhering to aseptic technique minimizes risk of infection.

Males

The penis and sheath should be cleaned to remove gross debris using warm water and mild soap. The penis should then be aseptically prepared with alternating dilute povidone-iodine or chlorhexidine and water, working outward from the end of the urethra. Sterile gloves should be used to handle the sterile urinary catheter, avoiding touching the tip. A second gloved assistant is useful to hold the penis extended during the procedure. The end of the catheter should be lubricated with a small amount of sterile K-Y® Jelly. The end of the penis should be stabilized as the catheter is gently inserted into the urethral opening. Advance the catheter slowly until urine flows.

If the catheter has been advanced to the level of the bladder (50–70 cm in an adult equid or bovid) and no urine is seen, the catheter tip may be against the bladder wall and moving it slightly may correct this. If urine still does not flow, a sterile 60 ml catheter tip syringe can be attached to the end of the catheter and gently aspirated. A small amount of air or local anesthetic can be injected through the catheter if needed to aid passage through the urethral sphincter. If firm resistance is encountered as the catheter is passed, do not force it, especially if urethral obstruction is suspected. Forceful passage of a catheter through an obstructed urethra will traumatize the tissue and may even lead to urethral rupture.

Females

The mare's tail should be wrapped and held or tied to one side. Always tie to the mare, never to the stocks. The perineum should first be cleaned with a mild soap and water to remove gross debris, then aseptically prepared with alternating dilute povidone-iodine or chlorhexidine and water, working outward from the vagina (Figure 6.9). Sterile gloves should be used to handle the sterile urinary catheter, avoiding touching the tip. A gloved hand is inserted into the vagina to locate the urethral opening on the vaginal floor; one finger is inserted into the opening. The end of the catheter should be lubricated with a small amount of sterile K-Y Jelly, and then guided into the urethra. Advance the catheter slowly until urine flows. If the catheter has been advanced to the level of the bladder (10 cm) and no urine is seen, a sterile 60 ml catheter tip syringe can be attached to the end of the catheter and gently aspirated. Although urethral obstruction in females is rare, the catheter should never be forced against firm resistance during placement to prevent mucosal damage.

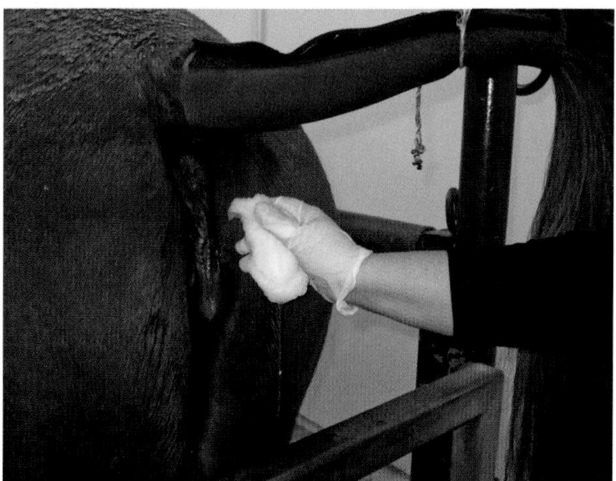

Figure 6.9 Preparation of a mare's vulva for urinary catheter placement.

Box 6.4 Common Supplies Used for Tracheostomy Placement

- sedation or appropriate restraint
- clippers with #40 surgical blades
- surgical preparation solutions (iodine or chlorhexidine based)
- local anesthetic (2% lidocaine or similar)
- sterile gloves
- scissors
- hemostats (curved and straight)
- j-type silicon tube with cuff relative to the size of the patient's airway
- self-retaining tracheostomy tube
- sterile dry gauze sponges
- petroleum jelly
- suture material

Tracheostomy

Indication

A patient may need a temporary or permanent tracheostomy if their natural airway is compromised along the head and upper neck region. Common causes of upper airway obstruction can include trauma, anaphylactic reactions, choke, arytenoid chondritis, or strangles in horses. A tracheostomy will not be helpful to the patient if the distal trachea or lower airway is compromised with disease. See Box 6.4 for supplies list.

Patient Preparation

A sterile prep should be performed prior to this procedure, however, in emergent situations, where the animal has a severely compromised airway and is in severe respiratory distress, preparation can be bypassed. Secondary infections of the tracheostomy site or airway related to lack of preparation can be treated later. Ideally, the patient's hair or fiber is clipped with a #40 surgical blade, allowing a margin of 2–3 in around the intended site of entry. Thorough skin prep would then follow.

Procedure

This procedure is mostly performed with the patient standing. If the procedure is not being performed under duress, local anesthetic can be infiltrated along the line of the intended incision site.

A midline longitudinal incision 8–10 cm in length is made at the junctions of the proximal and middle third of the neck above the "V" created by the sternothyrohyoideus muscles (Figure 6.10). The sternothyrohyoideus muscles are separated to expose the trachea using curved hemostats. A transverse incision is made between two rings of the trachea avoiding the cartilage portion. This incision allows the operator to insert the temporary j-tube directly into the opening with the tube's lumen facing downward toward the lungs. Once the patient is stable enough and able to get a satisfactory oxygen supply, a self-retaining tracheostomy tube can be placed. Depending on the type of tube used and the species of patient, it may be necessary to secure the tube in place with suture material (Figure 6.11).

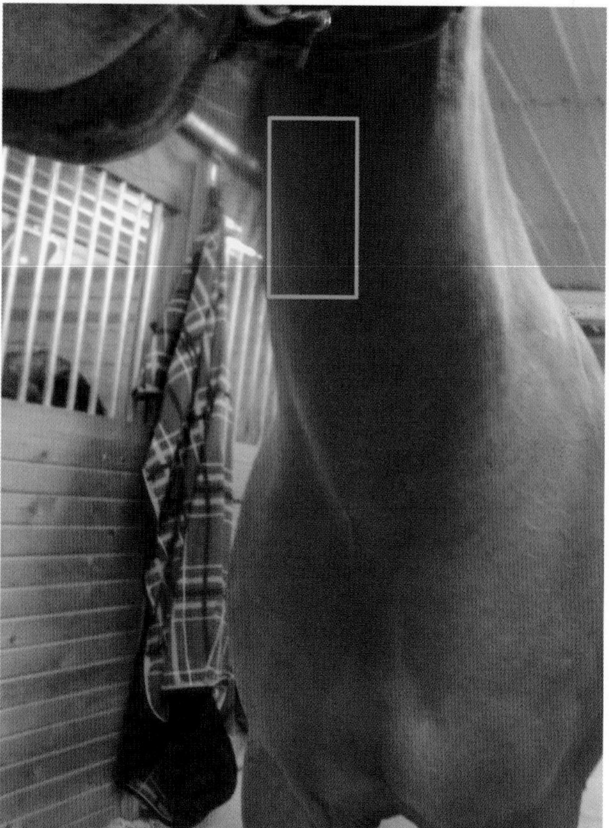

Figure 6.10 Location for tracheotomy on a horse.

TECHNICIAN TIP 6.5: Aseptic technique in tracheostomy placement should be overridden in critical cases where moments without an airway could be devastating.

Considerations

Patients will need to be monitored hourly or more often to ensure the temporary airway remains patent and functional.

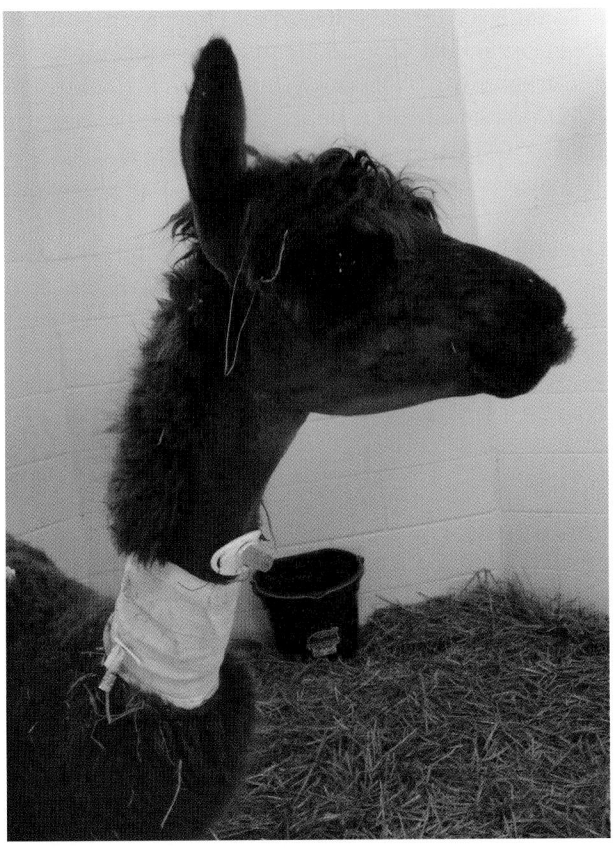

Figure 6.11 Alpaca with a temporary tracheostomy tube. This must be monitored for patency hourly.

The tracheostomy tube should be cleaned twice daily or more often if needed to prevent obstructive secretions accumulating. In some cases, the patient may be stable enough to allow the tube to be removed, cleaned, and replaced, while in other patients, it may be warranted to change the tube daily as to facilitate a faster exchange and continuously patent airway. The tube should be cleaned in an effective antiseptic solution such as chlorhexidine solution. It is important to rinse the equipment prior to replacement in the patient to avoid chemical tissue irritation. The skin around the tracheostomy site should also be cleaned of exudates daily. Petroleum jelly should be applied around the incision after cleaning to prevent skin irritation from exudate and drainage (Figure 6.12).

Before permanent removal of the tube, the clinician will often decide to occlude the opening for a period and monitor the patient to see if they can tolerate permanent removal. If the patient's airway is recovered, they should be able to breathe comfortably through their nostrils after occlusion of the tracheostomy tube or tracheostomy site. After tube removal, the wound is left to heal by secondary intention. Air may continue to pass through the site for several days as the wound starts to heal but this rarely impedes the healing process or the ability of the patient to breathe normally. The site should continue to be cleaned daily for 10–14 days or until no more drainage is produced.

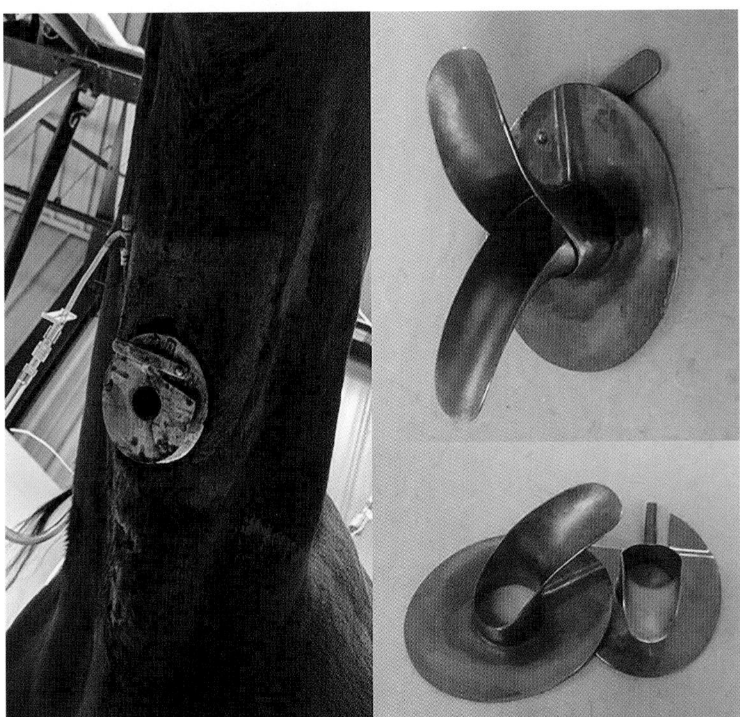

Figure 6.12 A removable trach both in a horse and separated into two pieces.

Blood Products and Administration

Blood and blood products are less commonly used in large animals than are crystalloids and other colloids, but there are a variety of indications for their use in both adults and neonates. Plasma and artificial blood products are commercially available and may be kept "on hand" for use as needed. Whole blood is generally not banked ahead of time, so one or more donors should be identified and available if the need arises (Figure 6.13). To reduce the risk of a transfusion reaction, a blood donor should be a healthy vaccinated gelding (a stallion or a mare that has never been pregnant may also be used) weighing at least 450 kg (~1000 lb). If screening is available, the donor should be negative for Aa and Qa blood antigens as well as negative for alloantibodies. Even if this screening is not available, the donor and recipient's blood can be rapidly crossmatched by mixing donor serum with recipient red blood cells and looking for agglutination (clumping) of the cells. Up to 8–10 l of blood (33% of their blood volume) can be collected from a 450 kg donor at one time and can be used as whole blood product or separated into its components, depending on the need of the recipient(s). Ideally, the donor receives equal volume back in isotonic fluids after donation to balance the fluid volume.

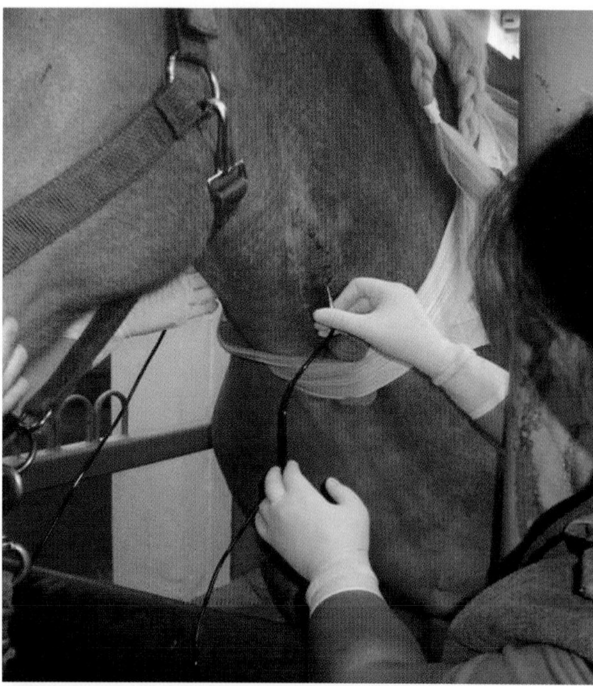

Figure 6.13 Collection of whole blood from a donor horse. Both jugular veins are occluded and used for collection simultaneously.

Donor blood can be collected into commercially available collection bags containing the anticoagulant acid citrate dextrose (ACD) or citrate-phosphate-dextrose-adenine (CPDA). It can also be collected into glass bottles to which ACD or CPDA is added immediately prior to collection. The glass bottles will inactivate platelets, so bags are preferred for thrombocytopenic patients. Collected blood can be stored in the refrigerator at 4 °C (40 °F) for up to 3 weeks. Blood products can be administered through the same catheter as other fluids and medications, although they should not be given through any line dedicated to parenteral nutrition. A special blood delivery set that includes a filter should be used rather than a regular fluid drip set (Figure 6.14).

Whole Blood

Whole blood may be used to expand circulatory volume, to temporarily enhance oxygen-carrying capacity by providing red blood cells, and to replace serum proteins and coagulation factors. It may be utilized in cases of severe acute blood loss (i.e. injury, surgery, guttural pouch mycosis) or to address chronic blood loss or red cell destruction (i.e. parasitism, neonatal isoerythrolysis, hemolytic anemia).

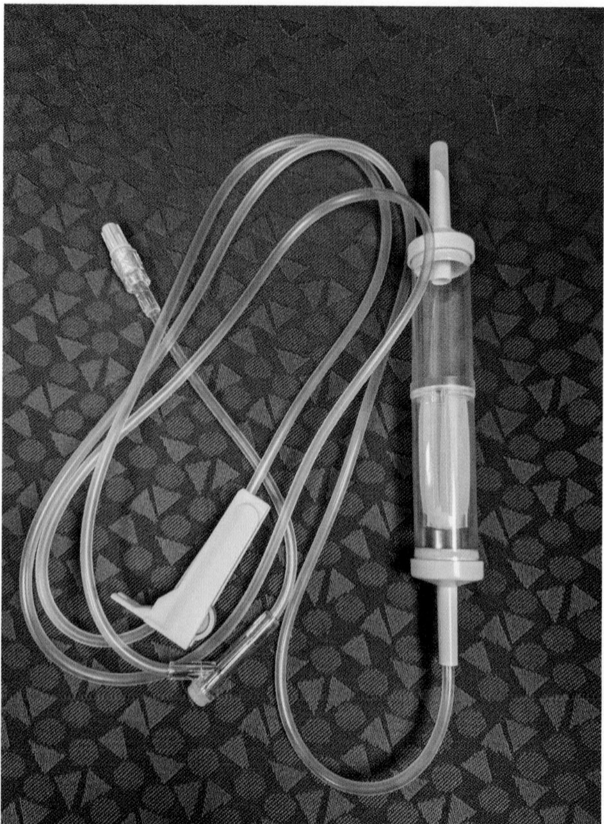

Figure 6.14 Delivery set with a filter for whole blood or plasma.

A blood transfusion is generally indicated in acute blood loss if one-third or more of the circulating blood volume has been lost or if the packed cell volume (PCV) falls below 15%. Normal blood volume is ~8–9% of BW, or ~36–40 l in a 450 kg (1000 lb) horse. It should be noted, however, that PCV is not a good indicator of blood loss in cases of acute hemorrhage due to the release of large numbers of red blood cells from splenic contraction and will in fact lag by 12–24 hr. Total protein (TP) will fall more rapidly. However, a rapidly falling PCV/TP may therefore be a better indicator of the need for a blood transfusion than the absolute value of those parameters, and other supporting evidence for the need for transfusion includes tachycardia, weakness, pale mucous membranes, and low venous or arterial oxygen values. Patients that are experiencing significant hemorrhage will generally need rapid volume expansion to avoid circulatory shock and should be given hypertonic saline followed by bolus intravenous isotonic fluids in addition to whole blood. In cases of chronic blood loss, the body has time to gradually become used to a state of anemia, and PCV may fall as low as 8% before a blood transfusion is necessary.

When determining the volume of blood to be transfused, the following formula should be used:

$$\text{Volume to be infused}(\text{L}) = \frac{(\text{desired PCV} - \text{recipient PCV})}{\text{donor PCV}} \times (\text{bodyweight}[\text{kg}] \times 0.08) \quad (6.1)$$

The primary concern when giving whole blood is transfusion reactions. For this reason, the temperature, pulse, and respiratory rate of recipients should be monitored closely throughout the transfusion process. Although blood transfusions can be administered rapidly in an emergency, it is preferable to start at a slow drip rate (0.1 ml/kg) for the first 10–15 min. If there are no changes in the recipient's vital signs during this time, then the drip rate can be increased to 15–30 ml/kg/h. If at any time the heart, respiratory rate, or temperature increase, or if trembling or hives develop, the transfusion should be stopped. Some practitioners favor pretreatment with flunixin meglumine or diphenhydramine. The risk of a transfusion reaction is greater with repeated transfusions from the same donor, especially if they are administered more than one week apart. This is because the recipient may develop antibodies against the donor's red blood cells. A mild transfusion reaction can generally be treated with flunixin meglumine while a severe reaction may require epinephrine, which should be readily available any time a transfusion is planned.

Plasma

Plasma is used in neonatal animals suffering from failure of passive transfer (FPT), patients with protein losing enteropathies, and things like snake bites. While the preferred treatment for neonates is colostrum administered via nasogastric or orogastric tube to these individuals, the window during which immunoglobulins can be effectively absorbed through the gastrointestinal tract is short. Therefore, if FPT is diagnosed in a neonate older than 12 hr, plasma is generally recommended, even if colostrum is also given (Figure 6.15).

Normal and hyperimmune plasma is available commercially for horses, cattle, and camelids. Alternatively, plasma may be collected from a healthy donor, including the dam, if there are no concerns about incompatibility. Frozen plasma may be stored at −4 °C (25 °F) for up to one year.

TECHNICIAN TIP 6.6: Frozen plasma should always be thawed slowly in warm water, not in the microwave.

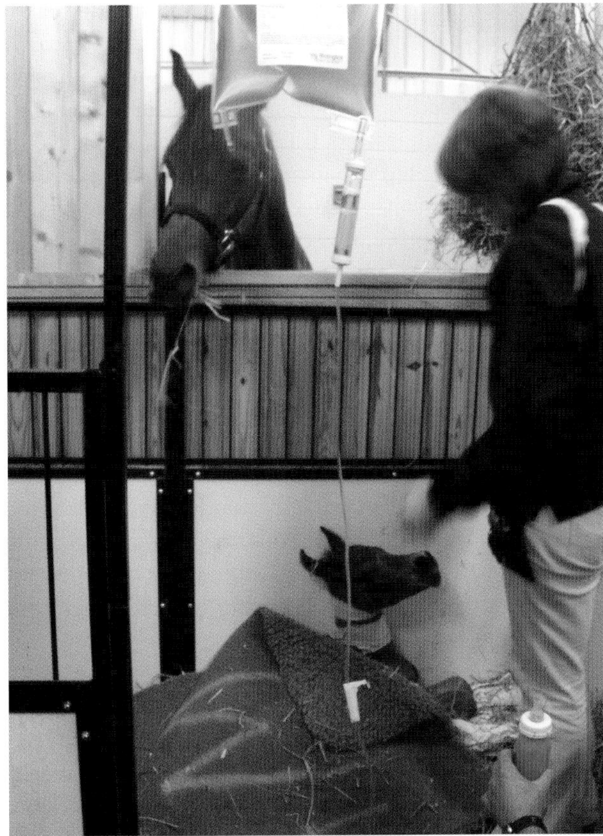

Figure 6.15 Foal receiving a plasma transfusion.

Plasma immunoglobulin G (IgG) concentration will vary between donors; thus, serial monitoring of the blood IgG of the recipient is recommended to determine how much plasma should be administered. For otherwise healthy neonatal foals and calves with partial FPT, a single 1 l transfusion may be sufficient, and for neonatal crias, one unit (~300 ml) may be sufficient. However, for ill neonates, or those with total FPT, two or more plasma transfusions over several days may be required to boost plasma IgG concentrations to desired level. IgG should be measured 4–12 hr after plasma administration for the most accurate result.

As is true for whole blood transfusion, transfusion reaction is of concern during plasma administration. Pulse, respiratory rate, and temperature should be monitored closely throughout the transfusion process. The first 50 ml of the transfusion should be given slowly. If there are no changes in the recipient's vital signs during this time, then the drip rate can be increased. One liter of plasma can be given safely over 20–30 min to an otherwise healthy equine neonate. The rate of administration should be slower for septic patients. If at any time the heart, respiratory rate, or temperature increase, or if trembling or hives develop, the transfusion should be stopped (Figure 6.16). Signs of a mild transfusion reaction generally subside once the transfusion is stopped, but a severe reaction may require treatment with epinephrine, which should be readily available any time a transfusion is planned.

Use of commercially available hyperimmune plasma against *Rhodococcus equi* in neonatal foals is popular among some farm owners who have a high incidence of this disease in their population. Research on the effectiveness of this product has produced mixed results, suggesting that it does not prevent disease, although it may reduce severity of clinical signs. Regardless, the same method of administration is used, and the same precautions should be observed as for other plasma products.

Artificial Blood Products

Oxyglobin® is a commercial purified bovine hemoglobin product that is stable at room temperature for up to three years. It also has the advantage of being non-immunogenic because it is a cell-free product. Although it is labeled for use in dogs, this product has been used in some critically ill neonates to temporarily improve oxygen-carrying capacity. A blood transfusion is usually required subsequent to treatment with this product because of the extremely short half-life of the hemoglobin. When monitoring a foal, it is important to remember that the PCV/TP will not increase and may in fact decrease due to the volume-expanding effects of the product related to increased oncotic pressure from the large molecules.

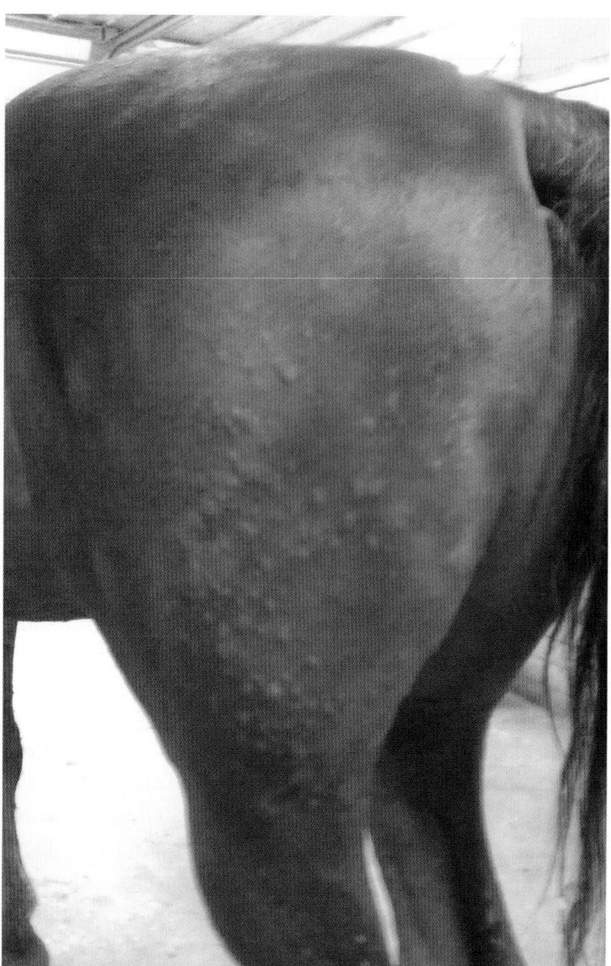

Figure 6.16 A horse with hives or wheals. This is a common reaction noted in plasma or whole blood transfusion.

Medication Administration

Administration of medication is a routine procedure performed for hospitalized patients yet represents a significant risk for errors. Observation of appropriate dose, dose frequency, and route of administration of all medications is important, as serious complications can result if any of these are incorrect. It is the responsibility of all personnel to make sure that medical records are complete, and instructions double-checked before any drug is administered. Complete medical records should always include:

1) drug name (generic name, rather than brand name, is generally preferred)
2) drug strength
3) drug dosage in milligrams, grams, or other appropriate weight measure, *never* as a volume measure such as milliliters
4) dose frequency
5) route of administration.

Medications are often administered enterally or parenterally, although other routes may be encountered in a clinical setting (intraosseous, epidural). Some drugs may be available in various formulations that allow them to be administered by more than one route, so it is important to read the manufacturer's package label or insert prior to administration.

Enteral Administration

Enteral administration of medications includes delivery via oral, gastric, and per rectum methods. Oral administration is commonly used in the clinic and is preferred for medications that need to be given at home by the owner due to ease of administration and low risk for administration-related complications. Oral administration is contraindicated for a patient that is dysphagic or has gastric reflux, and it is not appropriate for animals with significant neurological disease. Some animals are quite resistant to oral drug administration and may be difficult to handle especially for less experienced personnel. In such cases, another route of drug delivery may be preferred.

For drugs that are available as tablets, the most common way to prepare an oral dose is to crush and mix them in a large (60 ml) dosing syringe with a small amount of water and a sticky substance such as molasses or corn syrup (Figures 6.17–6.20). This not only thickens the solution but also makes it more palatable. The dosing syringe can then be placed in the mouth at the commissure of the lips with the head restrained by use of a halter and lead rope. For animals that are highly resistant to having the dosing syringe placed in their mouth, the powdered drug and molasses/corn syrup mixture can be added to a small amount of feed. This latter option is not appropriate if the animal is group-housed or if observation of consumption of the treated feed is impossible.

TECHNICIAN TIP 6.7: When administering a large dose of oral medications via a dosing syringe, try administering 20–30 ml at a time and then wait until you see or hear a swallow to give the next portion of the dose.

Enteral medications can also be administered via nasogastric or orogastric intubation. It is crucial that proper placement of the tube in the stomach is confirmed before the medication is administered (see the section titled "Nasogastric and Orogastric Intubation" later in this chapter). Tablets may be pulverized and mixed with water to facilitate this method of administration, while liquid drugs may be given directly. Due to the length of the tube, it is advisable to follow the drug with a volume of plain water to assure that the entire dose has reached the stomach prior to tube removal. It is important to remember that this route of administration is not appropriate for horses that have a nasogastric tube in place due to ongoing gastric reflux.

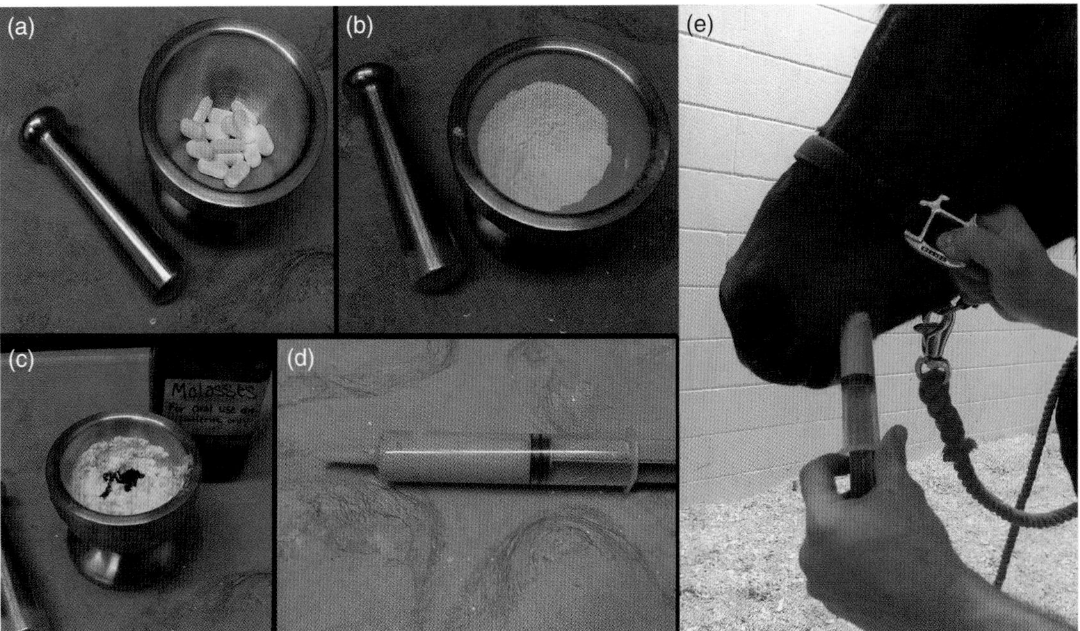

Figure 6.17 (a) Sucralfate tablets ready to be crushed with a mortar and pestle. (b) Tablets in a powder form after crushing. (c) Powder is then mixed with water and molasses to form a paste. (d) Paste in a catheter tip syringe. (e) Administration of oral medication paste.

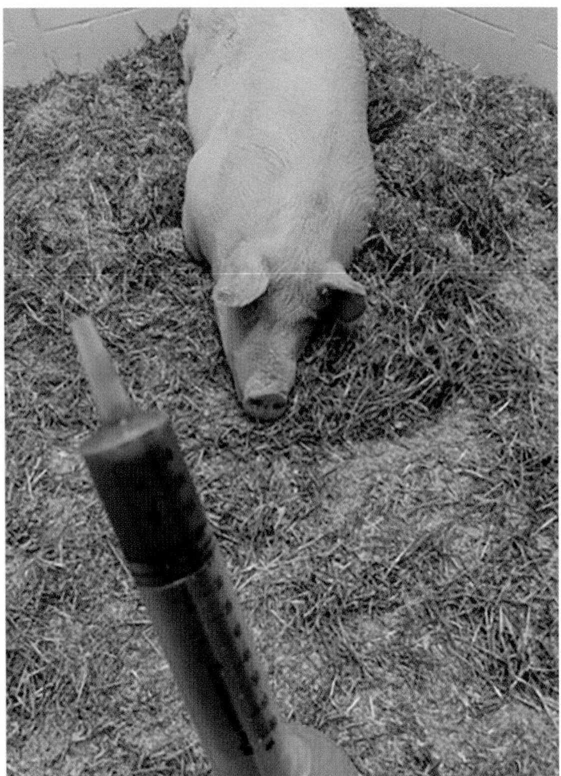

Figure 6.18 Oral meds in pigs can be tricky. The safest option is going to be to hide medication in food.

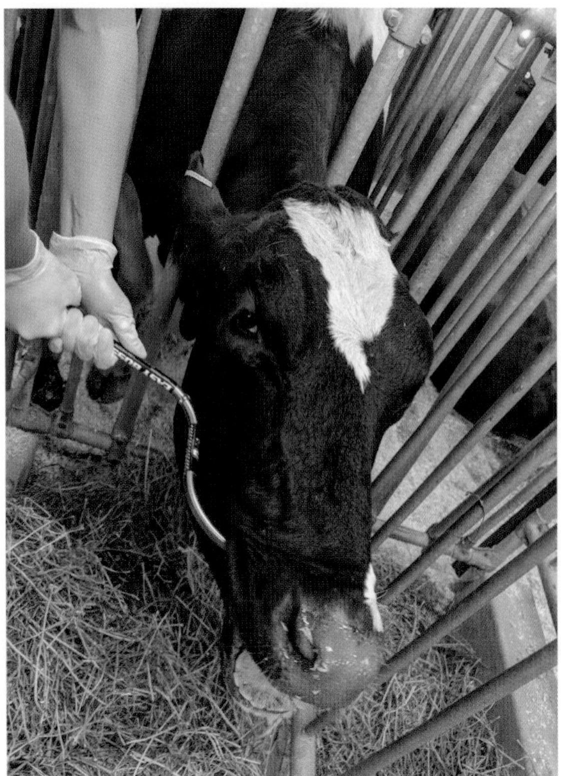

Figure 6.19 A Schoupe mouth speculum in a cow.

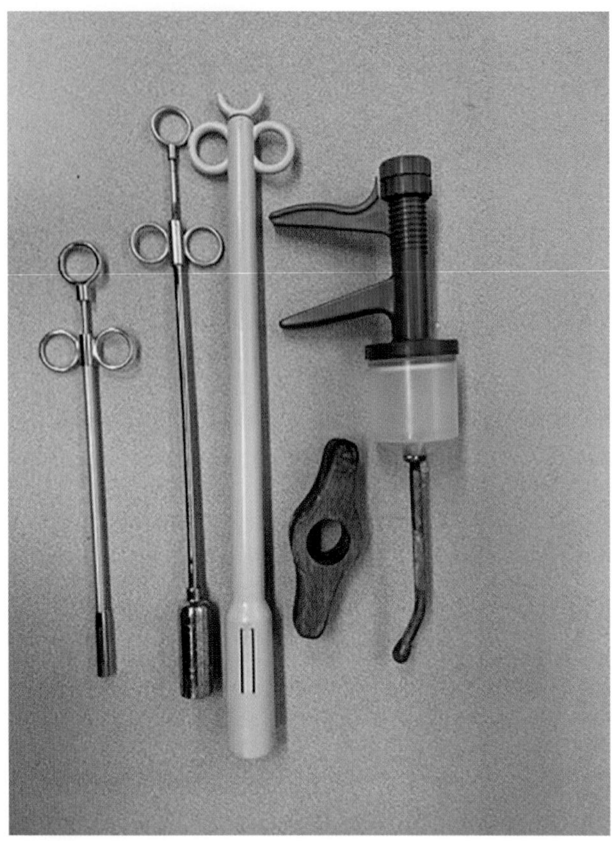

Figure 6.20 A bolus gun for large tablet administration.

Parenteral Administration

Parenteral drug administration is indicated for any patient with a nonfunctioning gastrointestinal tract or those under anesthesia and is recommended for animals with abnormal neurologic states. It may be preferred when possible for animals that are difficult to handle for enteral drug administration. The primary routes of parenteral administration in large animals are intravenous, intramuscular, and subcutaneous.

Intravenous (IV)

Drugs may be administered IV either directly into the vein or through an indwelling venous catheter (see Venous Catheterization earlier in this chapter). Typically, small volumes of drug given as either a single dose or with a small number of repeated doses are given directly by direct venipuncture, while large doses or those that must be repeated on a regular schedule are more safely given via a catheter. Certain drugs that are highly irritating if given perivascular should ideally be administered through a catheter to reduce the risk of skin sloughing from improper administration (Figure 6.21). Crystalloid and colloid fluids, as well as blood products, are usually also given using an intravenous catheter, though crystalloids can also be provided through nasogastric or orogastric tube, and colloids such as plasma are occasionally administered via other routes (oral, intraperitoneal) to very young neonates.

In large animals the jugular vein is the most common site of IV administration of fluids, colloids, and medications. If the jugular veins are unavailable, any superficial vein may be used. Prior to any IV injection, the site should be cleaned of any gross debris and then wiped with an alcohol-soaked gauze pad. When administering drugs into the jugular vein, care must be taken not to place the needle in the carotid artery, as intra-arterial injection can result in seizures, other neurologic deficits, and even death. To reduce this risk, the proximal one-third of the jugular vein should be used for IV injections, as this is the region in which it is the most superficial. An IV injection given at the thoracic inlet carries a much higher risk of intra-arterial administration, as the jugular vein and carotid artery are in closer proximity at this location. When using an 18-gauge 1.5-in needle, blood will drip slowly from the hub if it is properly placed in the jugular vein.

If the needle is in the carotid artery, bright red blood will spurt from the hub in a pulsatile fashion. If this is seen, the needle should be partially withdrawn and redirected more superficially. The needle may be placed with the tip aimed proximally or distally, but in either case should be buried to the hub prior to injection to prevent advancing the tip more deeply while depressing the syringe. If the needle tip is aimed distally and inserted while unattached to a syringe, the jugular vein should be held off distal to the needle tip to prevent aspiration of air through the needle. In cattle, a larger bore needle may be used to administer a single large fluid bolus. In this case, blood will often flow freely from the hub even when properly placed but there will be no pulsatile rhythm.

When using an intravenous catheter for IV drug administration, it should be checked for patency and flushed prior to giving the drug (Figure 6.21). This can be accomplished by drawing back on a syringe of 0.9% sterile saline to look for a "flash" of blood in the catheter extension or in the syringe itself. Then flush 10–20 ml of saline through the catheter. The catheter should always be flushed before, between, and after drug administration. Failure to flush between drugs may result in drug precipitation within the catheter and/or catheter extension. Even if no drugs are scheduled to be given, catheters should be flushed every 6 hr to help maintain patency. Smaller flush volumes should be applied in small neonates such as crias and lambs. If no drugs are to be given for 24 hr or more, a heparin lock may be placed in the IV catheter (see Box 6.3 for heparin lock information).

In certain patients, drugs may be continuously administered via the intravenous route, which is referred to as a continuous rate infusion (CRI) (Figure 6.22). Drug dosages for this route of administration are generally calculated on a mg/kg/min or mg/kg/h basis. Drugs are frequently added

Box 6.5 Common Supplies Used for Regional Limb Perfusion

- sedation
- surgical preparation solutions (iodine or chlorhexidine based and isopropyl alcohol)
- clipper with #40 surgical blades
- sterile gloves
- local anesthetic (lidocaine or mepivacaine)
- tourniquet
- 20–22 g butterfly catheter or small Jelco short-term catheter with extension set
- 20–60 ml 0.9% Saline
- bandage material for a small pressure bandage

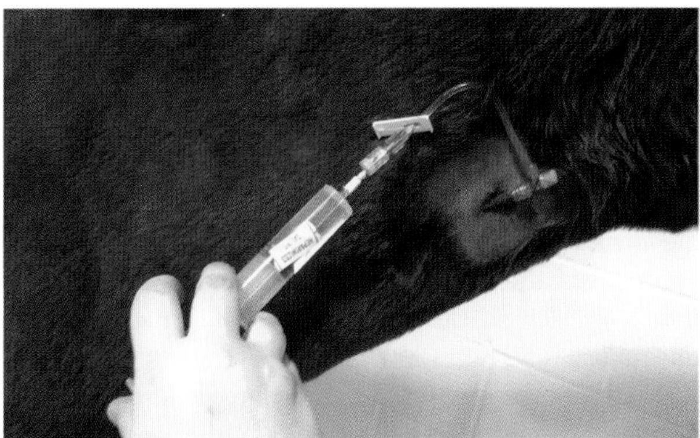

Figure 6.21 IVC catheter being flushed with heparin/saline following medication administration.

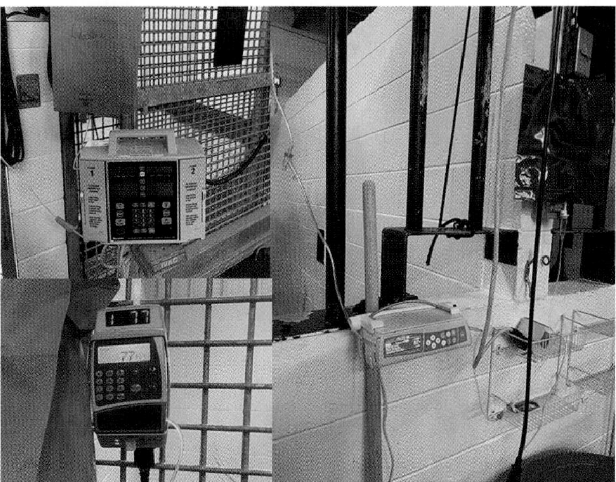

Figure 6.22 A variety of IV pumps used for constant rate infusion.

to a larger fluid volume (1–5 l) for CRI. Drug administration rates may be precisely regulated using an infusion pump or may be approximated by setting an appropriate drip rate from a bag of fluids. Catheter care is identical for CRI as for intermittent IV drug administration, with the exception that regular flushing of the catheter is generally not required due to the constant flow of fluid through the catheter. The catheter should be flushed with 0.9% sterile saline after a CRI has been discontinued and every 6 hr if the catheter is to be maintained after CRI is ceased.

Regional IV drug administration or intravenous regional limb perfusion (IVRLP) is often used for animals with infection localized to a bone and/or joint of the distal limb. It is often used with systemic intravenous antibiotics, although care must be taken not to exceed the total daily systemic dose of any drug when considering the combination of both administration methods. This is of special concern in small ruminants, camelids, foals, and calves. The principle behind IVRLP is that regional sequestration of an antibiotic will result in local levels of the drug that far exceed the minimum therapeutic concentration required to eliminate bacterial infection. A crucial factor in successful IVRLP is the placement of an effective tourniquet proximal to the site of infection. Therefore, this technique is not recommended for infections above the carpus or the hock. Several types of tourniquets are available in clinical practice, including narrow rubber tourniquets, wide rubber tourniquets, and pneumatic tourniquets (Figure 6.23). It has been demonstrated that for IVRLP in the proximal limb, the use of a pneumatic tourniquet resulted in the highest levels of antibiotic in the synovial fluid when compared to the rubber tourniquets. It has been further reported that the narrow rubber tourniquet was completely ineffective in this location and should not be used, although the wide rubber tourniquet was adequate. Narrow rubber tubing is commonly used as a tourniquet in the distal limb but its effectiveness in this location has not been objectively evaluated.

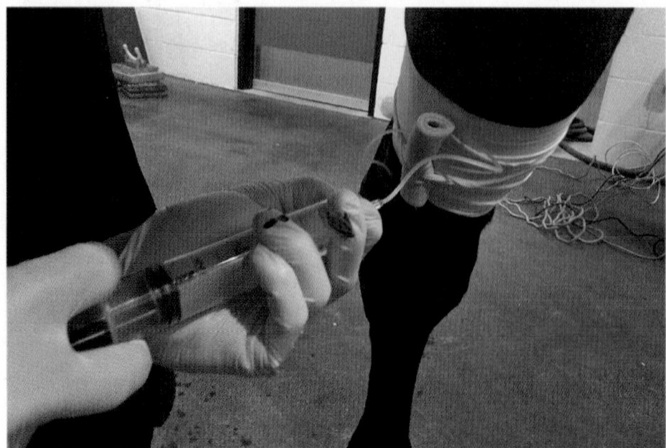

Figure 6.23 Regional limb perfusion being performed on the medial aspect of an equine tarsus.

When a tourniquet is placed around superficial tendons, such as the mid-metacarpal/metatarsal region, padding should be placed on either side of the tendons. This allows for more even compression around the entire circumference of the limb and thus a more effective tourniquet and prevents uneven tension on the tendons. Most animals object to the placement of the tourniquet even under sedation; it is recommended that initial antiseptic preparation of the IV injection site be carried out prior to this event, with only a final alcohol rinse afterward. The site does not need to be clipped unless it makes visualization of the vein easier. Aseptic preparation is not required, but since the injection is in the distal limb, there may be significant gross contamination that must be removed. A 20- or 22-gauge butterfly catheter filled with 0.9% sterile saline is placed into the appropriate peripheral vein (most commonly, the palmar/plantar digital vein, cephalic vein, or saphenous vein) without the syringe attached. This reduces the risk of the needle becoming dislodged if the patient reacts to insertion. A small Jelco short-term catheter can also be used in conjunction with an extension set. A flash of blood in the tubing adjacent to the needle (generally accompanied by dripping of the saline out the end of the tubing) confirms correct placement. The syringe can then be attached, and the drug slowly injected over 3–5 min. Drugs given by IVRLP are commonly diluted in 20–60 ml of 0.9% saline, which allows sufficient volume to perfuse the regional vasculature. Once the total volume has been administered, digital pressure is applied over the injection site prior to needle removal, followed by application of a small pressure bandage to help prevent fluid extravasation. The tourniquet should remain in place for a minimum of 20–30 min to allow adequate tissue penetration of the drug.

Intramuscular (IM)

Intramuscular (IM) administration is appropriate for many drugs and vaccines and tends to be the second most common choice for medications that must be given at home, as the proper technique is easy to teach owners. Risks associated with IM administration are accidental IV administration and abscess formation at the injection site. Proper IM injection placement and technique will reduce the risk of the former and minimize the impact of the latter should it occur. Medications not specifically labeled for IM administration in each species should never be administered via this route.

Drugs are best given IM into large muscle groups. Primary sites of administration are the neck, gluteal muscles, and semimembranosus/semitendinosus muscles, and the pectoral muscles are also occasionally used

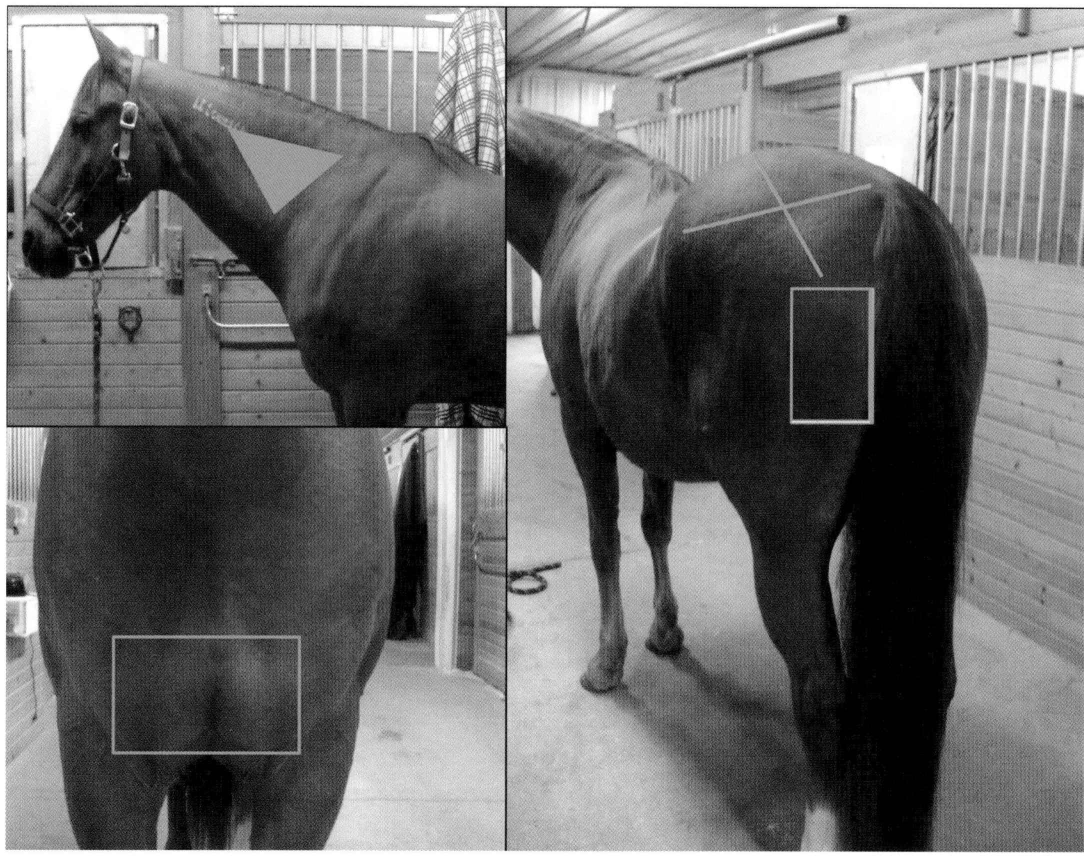

Figure 6.24 Common locations for IM drug administration in the horse are highlighted, including the neck, gluteals, semimembranosus/semitendinosus, and pectorals.

(Figure 6.24). The proper location for IM administration in the neck is within the region outlined by the cervical spine ventrally, the nuchal ligament dorsally, and the scapula caudally.

In animals intended for human consumption, the neck is the primary and preferred location for injection. Injection in any other location can result in significant tissue damage and partial or complete carcass condemnation. While the gluteal muscles in the horse present a large target for injection, they are the most difficult location for which to establish drainage should an abscess form and present the risk of personnel being injured by a kick while giving an injection. The semimembranosus/semitendinosus muscles are much easier to drain if needed, but like the gluteal muscles they carry a higher risk of injury to the person administering the drug. Pectoral muscles provide the best drainage for an abscess but are generally overlooked in favor of the neck due to location. In pet pigs, the epaxial muscles present an alternative IM injection location that may be easier to reach than the other sites and require minimal restraint.

Prior to injection, the site should be cleaned of any gross debris and wiped with an alcohol-soaked gauze pad. An 18-gauge, 1- to 1.5-in needle is mostly used for IM drug administration and should be inserted perpendicular to the skin surface directly into the muscle belly. The needle should ideally be inserted to the hub without the syringe attached. This allows the animal to react to the needle without the risk of dislodging the needle due to drag from a filled syringe. After attaching the syringe to the needle hub, draw back on the syringe to make sure that the tip of the needle is not in a blood vessel. Accidental IV administration of drugs intended only for IM use can result in serious complications, including seizures and death. For large volumes of drugs greater than 20–30 ml, it is recommended that the dose be split into two or more locations. This can be easily accomplished by partially withdrawing the needle and redirecting its tip. Each time the needle is redirected, draw back on the syringe to check needle placement. If a large volume must be given repeatedly, or if multiple IM drugs must be given simultaneously, change the injection location for each dose whenever possible. Alternate injection sites between the left and right sides of the neck. The location of each IM injection should be recorded in the medical record so that if complications arise, appropriate measures can be taken.

Subcutaneous (SC or SQ)

The subcutaneous (SC or SQ) route is less commonly used in large animals than in small animals but may still be of use in certain situations. It is best to use a relatively loose flap of skin for this route and thus the most chosen sites tend to be in front of the shoulder or behind the elbow. Prior to injection, the site should be cleaned of any gross debris and then wiped down with an alcohol-soaked gauze pad. The skin should be firmly grasped and tented up prior to slipping the needle beneath the skin, buried to the hub. Aspirate prior to injecting the drug to make sure that the needle tip is not within a blood vessel. A 20-gauge, 1.5-in needle is often sufficient for drugs administered SQ depending on the total volume.

Other Administration Routes

Transdermal/Topical

Certain analgesics are available in preparations that require topical application, such as transdermal patches or creams/ointments. When administering these drugs, it is important to wear gloves to avoid accidental exposure, as the carrier that allows penetration through the patient's skin will just as readily transfer a drug across human skin. For creams/ointments, the skin surface should be clean and dry prior to administration. For drugs administered repeatedly, this includes cleaning off the remnants of past applications. In the case of transdermal patches, hair or fiber should be clipped from the site of application first. Transdermal patches should be secured in place using tissue glue and/or elastic tape and should be closely monitored to make sure that the patient does not dislodge them. While the method of attachment has not been shown to affect drug transfer, the location of the patch may make a difference in how quickly the drug reaches steady state and the total amount of drug transferred. After removal, patches must be appropriately disposed of, as residual drug content could lead to toxicity from accidental ingestion or skin exposure by other animals or people. This is especially crucial for patches that contain regulated drugs.

Wound management also commonly requires the use of topical medications. Typically, these are antimicrobial creams/ointments that are either applied directly to the wound or on a bandage. As with other topical medications, the site of application should be clean of gross debris and dried as much as possible prior to application.

Intraocular

Patients with ophthalmologic diseases often require the administration of one or more drugs directly on the surface of the eye. These drugs are typically formulated as ointments or liquid drops. In the case of an ointment, direct

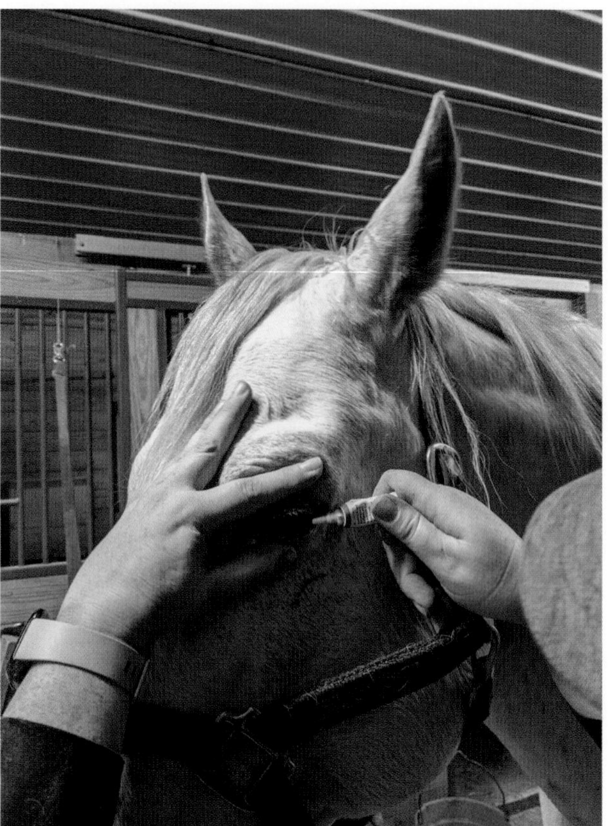

Figure 6.25 Two-handed technique for eye medication administration.

application from the tube of medication to the eye surface is typically the only option. Hands should be thoroughly washed prior to administration of these drugs and gloves may be worn. A one-handed or two-handed technique may be employed (Figure 6.25). For the former, hold the tube between the thumb and index finger and use the middle or ring finger to lift the upper lid or depress the lower lid, placing the ointment directly on the corneal surface without allowing the applicator tip to touch. Release the lid and massage the ointment beneath the lid across the entire surface. The two-handed technique is generally easier for the novice, as it allows the non-dominant hand to hold open both lids while the dominant hand administers the drug. Excellent restraint is generally required for both techniques unless the patient is exceptionally compliant.

Liquid medication may be applied directly to the eye as described previously. When animals receive multiple drugs and/or repeated doses throughout the day, a subpalpebral lavage system greatly reduces the stress for both patient and personnel, since drugs can be administered without manipulating the eye (Figure 6.26). Both commercial and homemade systems are available, and placement is easily accomplished under local anesthesia or sedation. The most reported side effects are mild and include minor eyelid

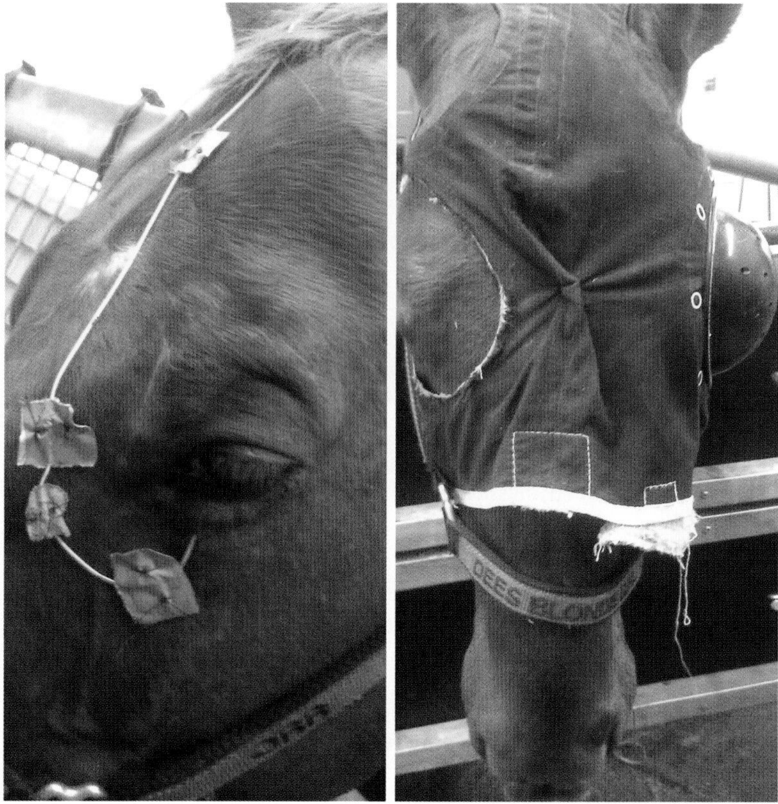

Figure 6.26 Patient with a subpalpebral lavage system indwelling. A protective eye mask can protect the apparatus.

swelling, tearing of the tubing, and loss of injection caps. More severe complications of corneal ulceration can occur. Patients with subpalpebral lavage systems are typically receiving medication often enough that additional flushing of the tubing is not required, but the system should be closely monitored to make sure it is patent and intact. Some patients can be quite reactive to ocular medication administration even with a lavage system in place, so medications should always be given slowly and carefully, with positive reinforcement as needed.

TECHNICIAN TIP 6.8: It is advised, when utilizing an SPL, to use an eye mask to avoid the patient rubbing out the apparatus.

Epidural

The two most common indications for epidural administration of drugs are: (i) long-acting analgesia, and (ii) regional nerve blocks for procedures involving caudal structures, including the tail, rectum, vagina, and perineum. Single drug doses may be given through direct injection with an 18- or 20-gauge, 2.5-in spinal needle. For patients requiring repeated doses of analgesia an epidural catheter is generally placed. The preferred location for epidural injections or catheter placement is the first intercoccygeal space, which can be palpated on midline by repeatedly moving the tail dorso-ventrally. The hair should be clipped from this area allowing for 2-in margins or greater and the skin aseptically prepared. Both the person performing the injection and any assistants should always wear sterile gloves during epidural injections, and drugs should be drawn up aseptically. For catheter placement, small surgical drapes are generally used to maintain a sterile field. After the catheter is in place, it is secured using a tape butterfly sutured or stapled to the skin and covered with a sterile bandage.

Close monitoring of epidural catheters is crucial. The catheter should be inspected and the skin around the catheter insertion site cleaned daily. The injection cap will need to be replaced on a regular basis depending on the frequency of injections. Prior to injecting any drug, the injection cap should be wiped with alcohol and the catheter should be checked for the presence of blood, which suggests that the catheter tip may be in a blood vessel. After each drug is injected, the catheter should be flushed with sterile 0.9% saline. If an epidural catheter is maintained without regular drug administration, it should be flushed at least daily with sterile 0.9% saline. When administering drugs through an epidural catheter, mild resistance is to be expected, especially if the volume is large (10–20 ml). If severe resistance is encountered, fluid should not be forced through the catheter; the catheter most likely has become dislodged or clogged and needs to be replaced. The proper force for injection can be judged by creating a small air bubble in the syringe between the plunger and the medication. During injection, this air bubble should not be compressed by the force exerted on the plunger. Use caution, however, and stop injecting once the last of the medication has gone into the catheter. Never inject air into an epidural catheter.

Intra-Articular

Intra-articular medications are administered for both diagnostic and therapeutic purposes. Aseptic preparation of intra-articular injection sites is crucial to reduce the risk of complications, most notably joint infection. There is some debate over the necessity of clipping the injection site prior to scrubbing. It has been reported that bacterial load was effectively reduced with antiseptic scrubbing on both clipped and unclipped skin and suggested that clipping was unnecessary prior to arthrocentesis. However, hair transfer during arthrocentesis has been demonstrated to occur under certain conditions. In most practices today, the decision to clip or not remains largely on a reflection of veterinarian and owner preference.

Respiratory Treatments

Horses that suffer from recurrent airway obstruction or inflammatory airway diseases, or even disease process such as pneumonia, often benefit from medications that can be administered directly to the respiratory tract in addition to systemic therapies. Similar treatments can be used in other large animal species, although it is less common in part due to the athletic usage of horses in comparison to ruminants.

Nebulization

Nebulization is like vaporization and involves a piece of equipment called a nebulizer. The nebulizer creates a mist of fine fluid droplets, which are small enough to penetrate down into the lung to treat lower airway disease. It is used to moisten lower airway secretions and may carry antibiotics with it, thus providing an additional source of moisture and antibiotic for the sick lung therefore deeply treating the infection.

With a little patience and training, horses can be taught to tolerate wearing a mask that adapts and connects to traditional nebulizers. Several commercial made products, such as AeroMask® or Era®mask, can be easily purchased for patients that may need long-term treatment with owners at home (Figure 6.27). Nebulizing treatments vary in length, but average 30 min or more. It is important that the horse is being lightly restrained and closely monitored during the treatment process, as the connections generally do not allow for free movement of the patient during treatment.

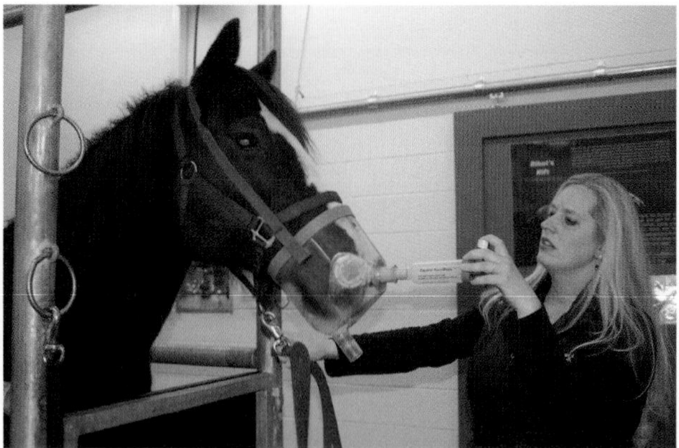

Figure 6.27 Horse wearing the AeroMask®, which can be used for nebulization or metered dosing sprays. *Source:* Reproduced with permission of Sue Kirchoff.

Metered Dose Inhalers

One of the main advantages of using metered dose inhalers for the administration of respiratory therapies is that it is a considerably shorter treatment time than nebulizing.

The function of using a small inhaler on a full-sized equine patient does have its own complications. Equine adapters are commercially (AeroHippus®) made and available, or one may choose to use the previously mentioned masks (Figure 6.28). The most important key to remember when treating with inhalant metered dose medications is to hold the mask or nasal cover in place for multiple breaths following the metered sprays. It may be necessary to train

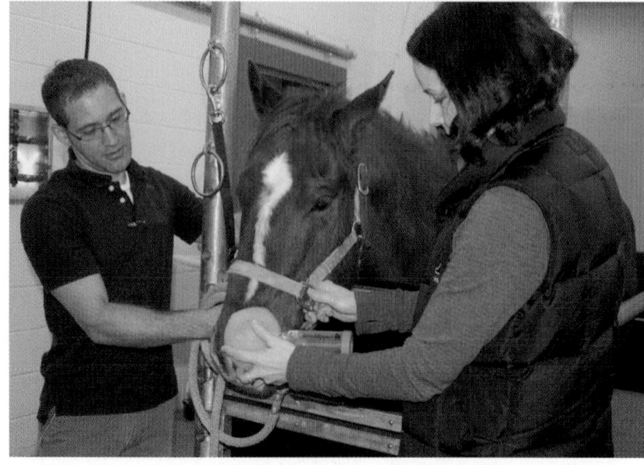

Figure 6.28 Horse being administered a metered dose spray via the Aerohippos®. *Source:* Courtesy of Sue Kirchoff, University of Minnesota.

the patient to be comfortable with the sound of the metered sprayer, but most patients are tolerant of the procedure after a period of adjustment and some repetition.

Fluid Administration

Fluid therapy for maintenance or volume replacement is commonly performed in large animal patients. In general, when determining a fluid plan, the following questions should be answered:

- What type of fluid is needed?
- What volume of fluid is needed?
- What route of administration should be used?
- What rate of administration should be used?

Fluids may be administered orally (see the section titled "Nasogastric and Orogastric Intubation" later in this chapter) or intravenously, although the latter is preferred in any situation where rapid expansion of circulating volume is required. The two categories of fluids most commonly used for volume expansion are crystalloids and colloids, which may include plasma and whole blood depending on patient need. Often a combination of crystalloids and colloids are used.

When determining the amount of fluid to administer to a patient, three factors should be taken into account:

- existing fluid deficit
- ongoing fluid losses
- maintenance fluid requirements.

Fluid deficit can be estimated by the percent dehydration of the patient:

$$\text{Patient size in kg} \times \%\ \text{dehydrated} = \text{of liters needed for return to hydration} \tag{6.2}$$

Ongoing fluid losses must be estimated based on clinical assessment. The easiest situation to quantify is in a horse with gastric reflux that is being measured every few hours, but other losses may result from diarrhea or third-spacing of fluids into the pleural or peritoneal space. Maintenance requirements are estimated to be 60 ml/kg/day for adults and 100 ml/kg/day for neonates.

TECHNICIAN TIP 6.9: Approximately half of the replacement volume of an intravenous fluid plan should be given as a rapid bolus, then the remainder can be given more slowly. The patient's response to a fluid plan should be reassessed after the first 6–12 hr and the plan adjusted as needed.

In adult horses and cattle, volume overload is rarely a concern, even if fluids are administered as rapidly as possible via a large diameter jugular catheter. However, in small ruminants and neonates of all species, care should be taken not to exceed a fluid administration rate of 10–20 ml/kg/h except in cases of severe shock. When calculating the rate at which the fluids are to be administered, it is important to know the number of drops per ml for the specific fluid administration set being used. This can range from 10 to 60 drops/ml, with the latter being used in cases when finer control of the drip rate is required, such as for neonates (Figure 6.29). Fluid pumps are strongly recommended for small neonates in which fluid overload is a potential risk (i.e. crias, young pot belly pigs, lambs, etc.).

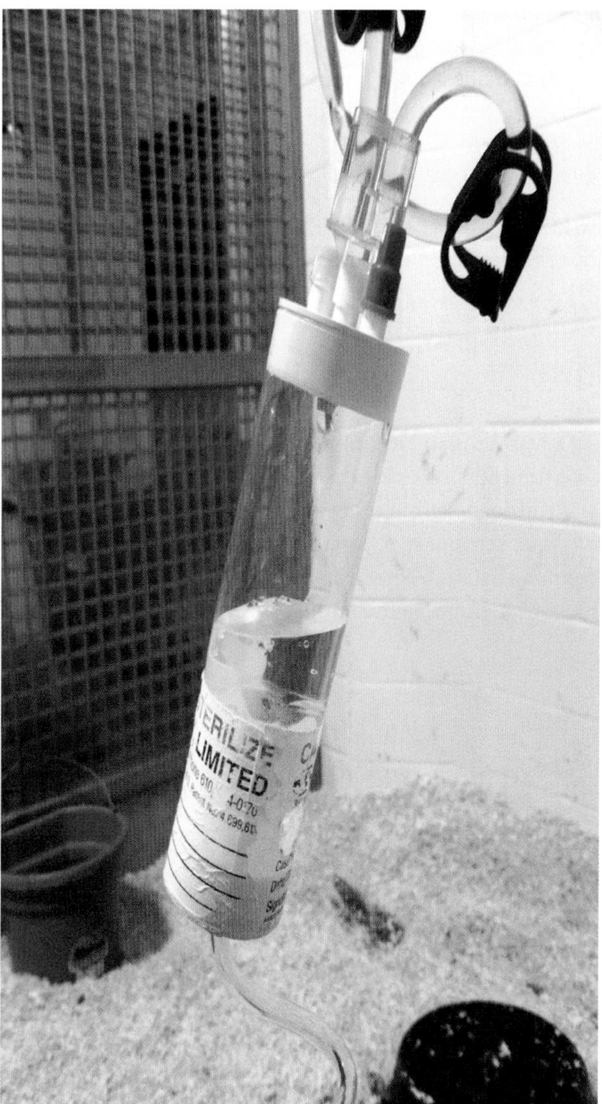

Figure 6.29 Drip chamber from a large 10 drop/ml set commonly used for administration in large animals.

$$\frac{\text{Total \# ml}}{\text{Total \# of minutes}} \times \frac{\text{drip factor}}{\text{total \# of seconds}} = \text{drip / second} \quad (6.3)$$

Example doctor orders: Administer 1 l/h. Administration set is 15 drop/S.

$$\frac{1000\,\text{ml}}{60\,\text{min}} \times \frac{15\,\text{drip factor}}{60\,\text{s}} = 4.2\,\text{drip / s} \quad (6.4)$$

A long-coiled extension set should be used when giving fluids to large animal patients, especially those that are ambulatory or that get up and down a lot. It helps to secure the line to a mane, to help prevent accidental disconnection of the fluid line from the catheter (Figure 6.30). For patients that are difficult to manage, blousing fluids is an alternative. Goats and sheep like to chew on dangling IV lines and may benefit from blousing fluids rather than trying to manage a CRI (Figure 6.31). Bolusing fluids to foals and crias that are being housed with their mother can also be considered.

TECHNICIAN TIP 6.10: Make a simple braid in the patient's mane and then run a re-closable zip tie through the hair. Use the zip tie to tether the fluid line, which can then easily be detached and reattached as needed.

Dehydration in large animals may be secondary to excessive fluid loss or inadequate fluid uptake. In adult horses and ruminants, fluid sequestration within the gastrointestinal tract secondary to intestinal impaction or volvulus is a common cause. Dehydration can be assessed by skin turgor, mucous membrane moisture level, and capillary refill time.

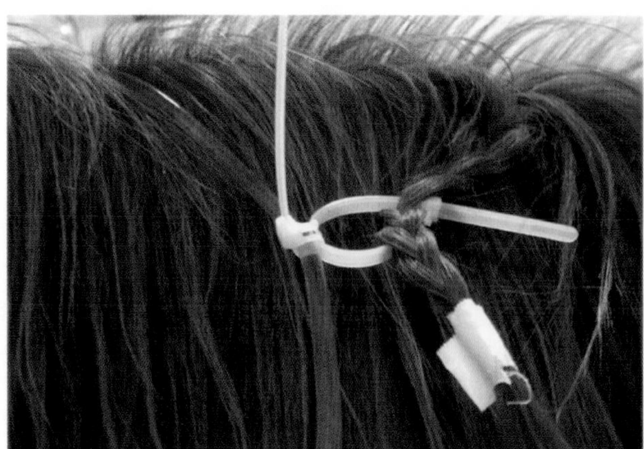

Figure 6.30 Mane braid and zip tie to anchor an IV fluid line.

PCV and TP will also increase as dehydration worsens, although these parameters should be interpreted in context with other clinical signs as they can be affected by other conditions. Depending on the cause(s) of dehydration, acid-base and electrolyte imbalances may exist in the patient. These can be evaluated using a serum chemistry profile or arterial blood gas and should be considered when formulating a fluid plan. A serum chemistry profile will also give creatinine and blood urea nitrogen (BUN) levels, which are indicators of renal perfusion; these are generally increased in dehydrated patients (prerenal azotemia).

The changing hydration status of an individual on fluids should be closely monitored. Clinical signs, including heart rate, pulse quality, capillary refill time, and mucous membrane moisture level, should be interpreted in combination with serial PCV/TP. Serum chemistry profiles and/or arterial blood gas analysis should also be repeated, especially if correction of derangements in acid-base balance and electrolyte levels is a goal of fluid therapy. Urine output and specific gravity should also be monitored. Urine specific gravity in dehydrated patients often exceeds 1.045 but usually responds rapidly with IV fluid administration. Failure to see improvement of this parameter despite therapy suggests that the fluid plan is inadequate and should be reassessed.

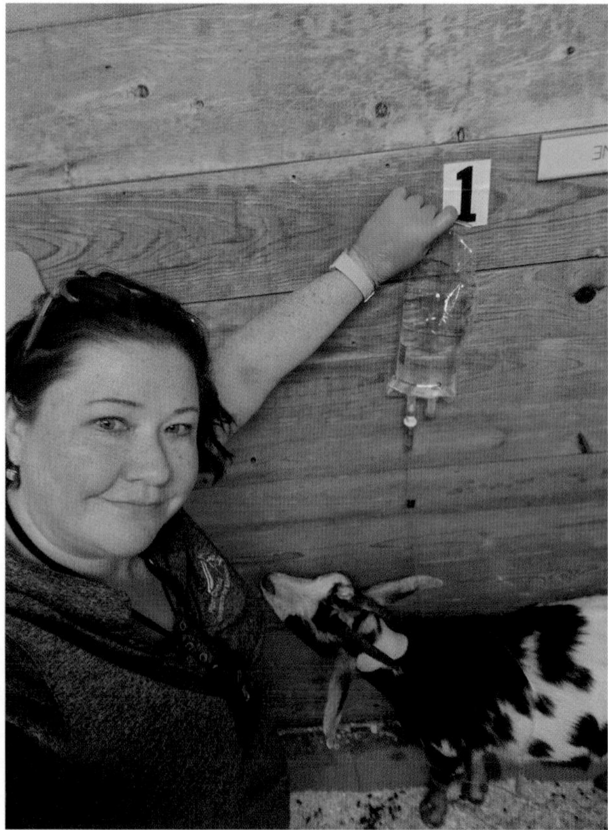

Figure 6.31 Delivering a fluid bolus to a goat.

Box 6.6 Dehydration Chart

Amount Dehydrated	% Dehydrated	Other	CRT
Mild	5%	Slightly prolonged skin tent test	1–3 S
Moderate	7–8%	Delayed skin tent	3–4 S
Marked	10–12%	Eyes may have a sunken appearance and peripheral pulses may become weak or absent	4–5 S

Crystalloids

Crystalloid fluids used for replacement can be categorized by electrolyte content as saline or balanced electrolyte solutions. Several balanced electrolyte solutions are commercially available and contain varying concentrations of sodium, chloride, potassium, calcium, and magnesium in addition to a buffer (a bicarbonate precursor) (Figure 6.32). Each is designed to approximate the makeup of extracellular fluid, which is high in sodium and low in potassium. Balanced electrolyte solutions are more commonly used for rehydration or maintenance than saline, except in situations where sodium concentration is very low (<125 mEq/l) or potassium is very high. Despite the name "balanced electrolyte solution," long-term therapy with these fluids alone in a patient that is not eating will result in low serum potassium, calcium, and magnesium, and therefore these are frequently supplemented in the fluids. Other additives that may be used include potassium chloride, bicarbonate, and dextrose (Figure 6.33). Serum chemistry profiles should be monitored to determine if supplementation should be continued, although ionized calcium from a blood gas profile is a more accurate measure of calcium status than total calcium concentration, especially if the patient is hypoalbuminemic, acidotic, or alkalotic.

Normal saline (0.9%) and balanced electrolyte solutions are isotonic fluids. They have the same effective osmotic pressure as extracellular fluid and therefore stay in the extracellular space. Since blood volume is approximately one-third of the total extracellular fluid space, crystalloids rapidly redistribute across the entire extracellular fluid volume. This means that approximately three times the volume of crystalloids must be administered to achieve the desired circulating volume expansion. If a more rapid expansion of circulating volume is required, then hypertonic saline may be administered. The high osmotic pressure exerted by hypertonic saline pulls fluid from the

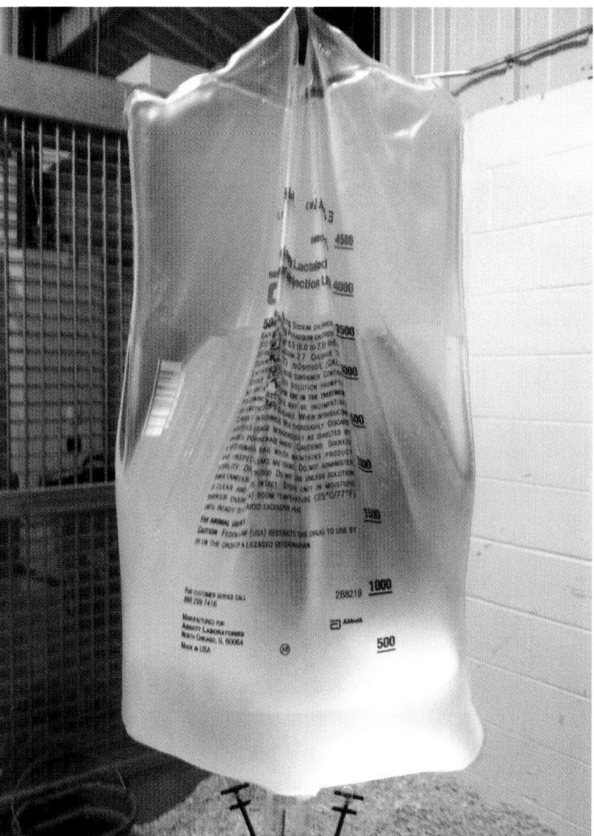

Figure 6.32 A 5 l bag of lactated ringers solution with 3 l remaining.

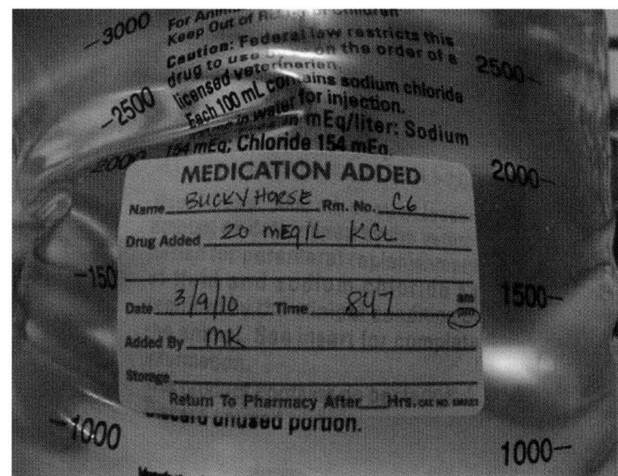

Figure 6.33 Example of a fluid bag label after additional supplementation has been added.

intracellular space into the extracellular space immediately expanding vascular volume. Administering a liter of hypertonic saline does little to correct volume depletion over the long term, so large volumes of isotonic crystalloids should subsequently be given.

Isotonic crystalloids that are less commonly used include 5% dextrose and 2.5% dextrose in 0.45% saline. Any time intravenous dextrose is given, blood glucose levels should be monitored to avoid hyperglycemia.

Colloids

Colloids contain large molecules that exert oncotic pressure and draw fluid into the vascular space from the interstitium. Although the molecules do eventually redistribute out of the vasculature, this occurs slowly, and thus the effect on circulating volume expansion is much longer than that of hypertonic saline.

The most commonly used colloid in large animals is plasma, but there are other options commercially available such as hetastarch. One liter of hetastarch will expand vascular volume by 2l, and its effect can last for up to 120hr in relatively healthy horses. Using only colloids for volume expansion is cost-prohibitive in large animals, and they are generally only used in cases of severe hypoproteinemia or to treat shock in neonates. Colloids can be successfully used in combination with hypertonic saline with isotonic crystalloids administered for sustained volume expansion. In fact, hypertonic saline and hetastarch at 4mg/kg each is reportedly more beneficial than hetastarch alone at 10mg/kg.

Intraosseous Administration

Intraosseous administration is an alternative to IVRLP for patients with an infection affecting a bone and/or joint in the distal limb, or to provide fluid therapy when intravascular access is challenging. Intraosseous medication administration is effectively absorbed systemically just like medication given IV. As with IVRLP, an effective tourniquet is the key for achieving high levels of antibiotics locally. Intraosseous administration of antibiotics may be preferred over the IV route for patients with osteomyelitis and for patients in whom the distal limb vasculature is difficult to access due to size (such as young foals, calves, and camelids), edema, or repeated IVRLP procedures. Care must be taken to not exceed the total body dose for any drug given intraosseously, especially if it is being used in combination with systemic antibiotics.

The initial drilling procedure for intraosseous administration is generally performed under short-acting anesthesia and the site should be routinely clipped, aseptically prepared, and draped. A 4-mm drill bit is used, which is the same size as the male adaptor of a standard IV extension set. An initial perfusion is generally performed at the time of drilling. The site should be maintained under a sterile bandage. Subsequent perfusions may be carried out under short-acting anesthesia, especially in young animals, or under sedation. The site should be aseptically prepared prior to each perfusion, and sterile gloves and a new extension set should be used each time. Needle holders may be needed to securely wedge the end of the extension set in the drilled hole. Similar to IVRLP, the drug to be administered is typically diluted in 60ml of saline and is administered over 5–10min to avoid excessive intramedullary pressure.

Complications associated with intraosseous administration are typically mild and include localized and temporary pain and swelling. Careful, regular monitoring of the condition of the administration site and the level of patient lameness should allow for early intervention should complications arise.

Nasogastric and Orogastric Intubation

Nasogastric Intubation

Prior to the wide availability of oral medications formulated as pastes, nasogastric intubation was routinely used as a method of drug administration in horses, especially for anthelmintics. While some practitioners may still choose this route of administration for specific purposes, such as assurance of ingestion of a complete dose of medication, it has largely fallen out of favor. Today, nasogastric intubation is most often used as a diagnostic and therapeutic tool for horses with colic or for administration of large volumes of oral fluids.

Passing a nasogastric tube can be somewhat intimidating at first, especially because many horses are highly resistant to having the procedure performed. To protect involved personnel adequate physical and/or chemical restraint should be addressed prior to attempting intubation. The horse should be placed in a set of sturdy stocks if available. A snug halter and nonelastic lead rope should be used. Additional physical restraint such as a twitch may also be required. The person passing the tube should not be holding the lead rope and/or twitch but should place the hand not holding the tube on the bridge of the patient's nose so that there is some additional control of the head. Care must be taken not to occlude the nares. The decision of whether or not to use sedation as a form of restraint should be addressed on a case-by-case basis.

Sedation can be beneficial in cases where physical restraint is inadequate, but it dulls the swallow reflex making intubation more difficult. Keep in mind that even sedated horses can react suddenly when a tube is placed in their nose, so chemical restraint should never be used as a substitute for physical restraint and all involved personnel should remain alert. Horses that are quite ill and/or that are very compliant may be intubated with minimal restraint, but it is unwise to assume that a horse will not resist the procedure.

Nasogastric tubes are available in a range of diameters and stiffness. In general, the larger bore tubes are stiffer and are somewhat easier to pass because they do not kink as easily. Smaller bore tubes may be easier to pass through the horse's nose and cause less irritation. Selection of a tube often comes down to personal preference and availability, but for most cases in which the tube will only be passed once, the largest diameter tube that can reasonably be used, given the size of the patient, is the best choice. For horses that require frequent repeated intubation, an indwelling nasogastric tube may be used for 12–48 hr. For these cases, a smaller diameter, softer tube may be preferred.

Prior to passing the nasogastric tube, determine the approximate lengths that will be needed to reach the pharynx and the stomach (Figures 6.34 and 6.35). This will help when judging if the tube has been placed appropriately. For inexperienced personnel, this length should be marked on the tube with permanent marker. The end of the tube should be lubricated with K-Y Jelly or water prior to insertion into the nares. The tube can be passed up either nostril; if the left nostril is used, the right hand should be placed on the bridge of the nose to help control the head and guide the tip of the tube into the ventral nasal meatus. The left hand is used to push the tube forward. The role of the hands is switched if the right nostril is chosen.

Do not force the tube if firm resistance is encountered, especially in the first few inches. Touching the ethmoid turbinates in the dorsal caudal aspect of the nose with the tube will cause bleeding, often profuse. If bleeding is encountered while passing the tube, it is generally best to try passing up the opposite nostril to avoid getting blood in the tube. Nosebleeds generally stop on their own within a few minutes without additional treatment.

Once the tube reaches the level of the pharynx it is helpful to flex the horse's neck. This facilitates passage into the esophagus rather than the trachea. The tube should pass into the esophagus as the horse swallows. Gentle stimulation of the esophageal opening with the tip of the tube may facilitate swallowing but patience at this step is important. If properly placed in the esophagus, the tube can be passed with minimal resistance and is generally visible and palpable on the left side of the neck near the jugular furrow. If

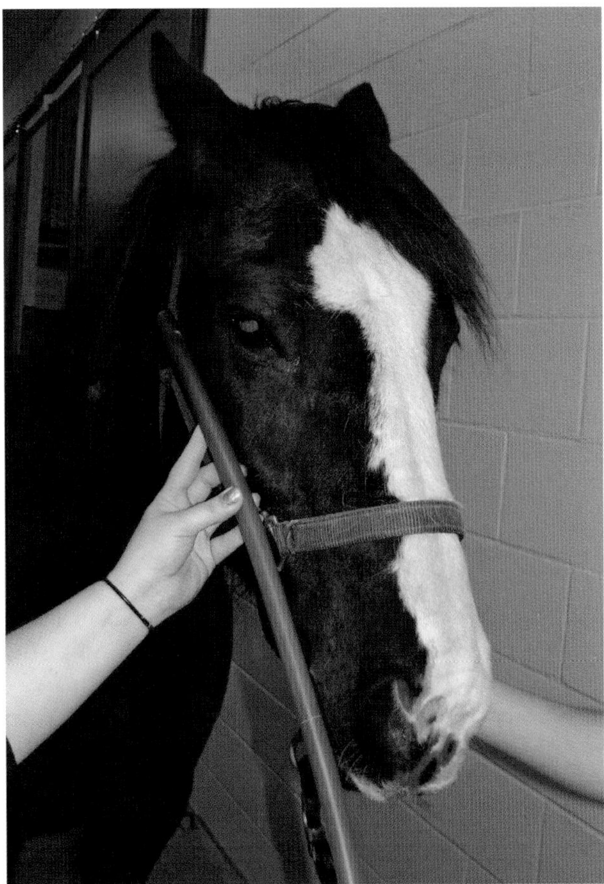

Figure 6.34 Measuring the length of tube needed to reach the pharynx.

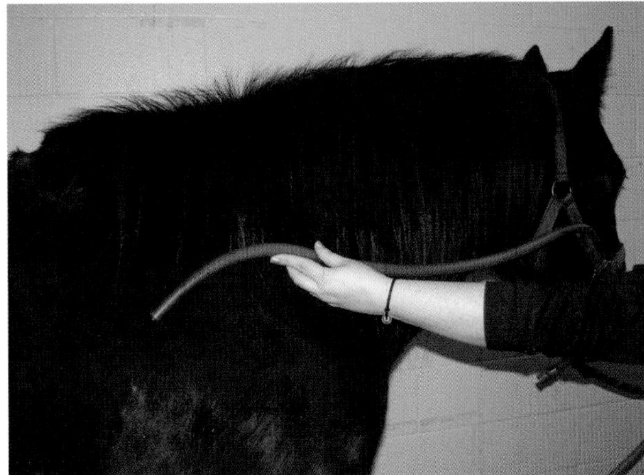

Figure 6.35 Measuring the length of tube needed to reach the stomach.

the tube is placed in the trachea instead, the horse may or may not cough. There will be no resistance to passage and the tube will rattle against the sides if the trachea is moved back and forth. If this occurs the tube should be backed out to the level of the pharynx and another attempt made. Some people like to suck back on the tube to check whether positioned in the esophagus. If the tube is in the esophagus, it will feel like sucking through a straw with a finger over the end, but if it is in the trachea, there will be no resistance. Be aware that there is a risk of aspirating gastric contents with this method and many people avoid it for that biosecurity reason.

The time during which the end of the nasogastric tube is in the nostril is when a horse is most likely to react strongly, most commonly by tossing or shaking its head. Once the end of the tube is in the oropharynx, it is often helpful to stop momentarily before trying to pass it into the esophagus to allow the patient to calm down. The tube should be held in place against the medial aspect of the nostril using the fingers of whichever hand is placed on the bridge of the nose to keep the horse from dislodging the tube while moving its head. This assures the tube stays in the oropharynx and does not enter the respiratory tract. Once calm again, the horse is much less likely to object to the rest of the procedure.

Once in the stomach, an odor ranging from sweet to fetid can often be detected through the tube. Blowing air into the tube will cause bubbling in the stomach that can be ausculted on the left side between the 8th and 14th ribs. Tube placement should be verified by one or more of the methods mentioned prior to administering any fluids, feed, or drugs through the tube. Serious complications, often fatal, can occur if these are accidentally administered into the lungs rather than the stomach.

Horses with a lot of gastric contents may spontaneously reflux as soon as the tube is placed (Figure 6.36). If this does not occur, a siphon should be established to check for gastric reflux by pumping a small amount of water through the tube, removing the tube from the pump, then lowering the end of the tube below the level of the stomach. In horses without pathological reflux, several liters may have to be pumped in prior to getting any flow back. Pump in 1–2 L at a time but no more than 8 L total if none of the administered volume has come back through the tube. Gastric contents can almost always be obtained with patience and repeated attempts.

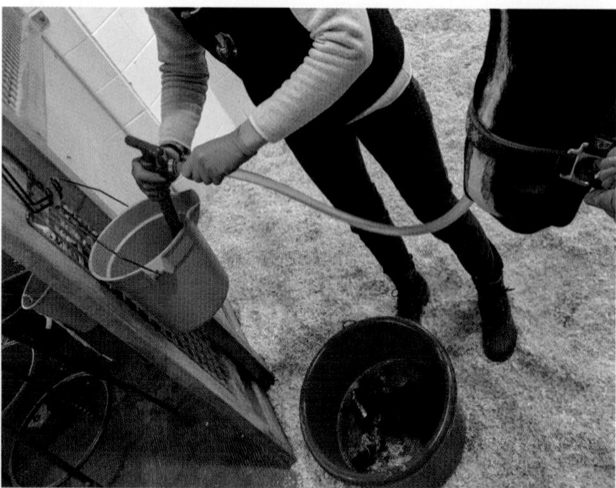

Figure 6.36 Refluxing via a nasogastric tube in a horse.

Before removing the nasogastric tube, the end must be kinked to prevent aspiration of fluid into the lungs. The tube should be pulled out smoothly and relatively slowly especially as the distal end reaches the nostril. The hand on the bridge of the nose should be used to keep the tube ventral within the nostril as it is being removed. If the end of the tube flicks upward as it passes through the nasal cavity, it can touch the ethmoid turbinates and cause epistaxis.

TECHNICIAN TIP 6.11: If the end of the nasogastric tube flicks upward as it passes through the nasal cavity during removal, it can cause a nosebleed.

If the nasogastric tube is going to be left in for repeated use, "indwelling," then the end should be capped with an appropriately sized empty syringe case and the tube secured to the halter in at least two locations to help prevent accidental removal (Figure 6.37). The placement of the tube within the stomach must be verified each time it is used, as tubes that were initially placed correctly can migrate out of the stomach. Care should be taken when leaving in a nasogastric tube for any significant duration of time as the risk of mucosal irritation and pharyngitis increases the longer a tube is in. Lubrication of the portion of the tube that is in contact with the nasal mucosa prior to each use will help with the irritation, but mild bleeding is not uncommon in these cases.

A special use of indwelling nasogastric tubes is to feed horses that cannot acquire food and/or swallow normally but have a functional gastrointestinal tract. This technique is mostly used in foals that cannot nurse for some reason. Enteral feeding in these foals is performed through a small diameter, soft tube. The method of placement of the tube is like that described earlier, and it should be secured to a halter and/or the forelock and mane to avoid accidental removal. Colostrum, milk, or milk replacer can be administered via nasogastric tube in foals and should be gravity fed rather than pumped through the tube. The foal should always be checked for gastric reflux prior to each feeding.

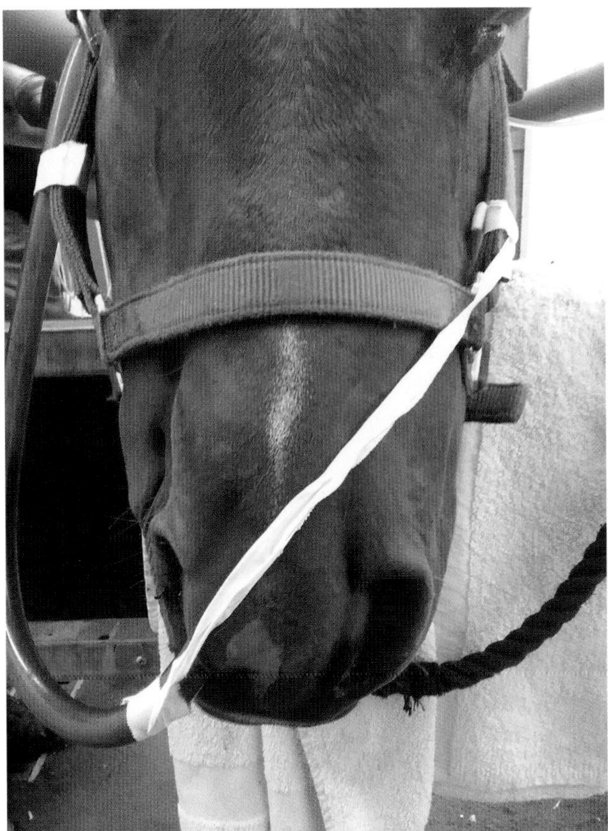

Figure 6.37 Indwelling nasogastric tube. Note it is secured on both sides to the halter.

Orogastric Intubation

Orogastric intubation is mostly used in ruminants, especially cattle, for administration of a fluid bolus. Due to the large capacity of the rumen, several gallons of fluid can be administered to adult cattle via this method without concern of rupture. Physical restraint, including a head gate and rope halter, is typically sufficient to perform this procedure in adult cattle. The cow's halter should be tied snugly to one side if possible, to minimize the range of head movement during tube passage. The tube can be passed while standing next to the side of the head facing the same direction as the cow. The arm closest to the head is placed on top of the nose to provide more control of head movement and that hand is used to hold the Frick speculum in place against the dental pad. The Frick speculum is placed over the tongue and passed back to the level of the pharynx to prevent the tube from being chewed while in the mouth (Figure 6.38). With the speculum in place, the opposite hand is used to pass the tube through the speculum and into the esophagus as the cow swallows. Maintaining the neck in slight flexion will facilitate passage of the tube into the esophagus rather than the trachea. If properly placed in the esophagus, the tube can be passed with minimal resistance and may be visible and palpable on the left side of the neck near the jugular furrow. If the tube is placed in the trachea instead, most cattle will cough. There would be no resistance to passage, and the tube will rattle against the sides if the trachea is moved back and forth. If this occurs, the tube should be backed out to the level of the pharynx and another attempt made.

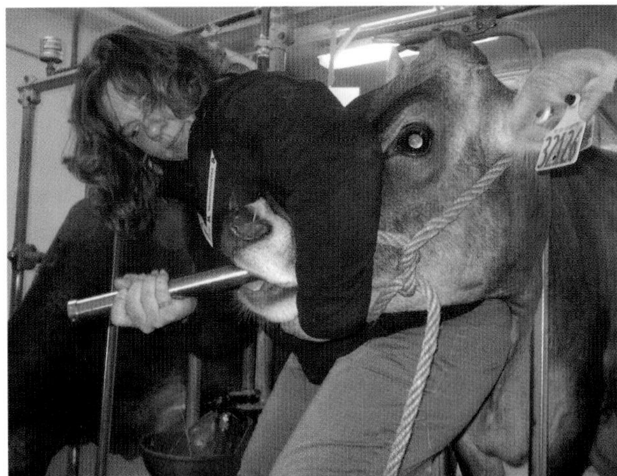

Figure 6.38 Frick speculum placed in an adult cow.

Once in the rumen, rumen gas can be detected by smelling the end of the tube. Blowing air into the tube will cause bubbling in the rumen that can be ausculted in the left paralumbar fossa. Cattle with rumen pathology may spontaneously reflux as soon as the tube is placed. If this does not occur, a siphon should be established to check for gastric reflux by pumping a small amount of water through the tube, disconnecting the tube from the pump, and then lowering the end of the tube below the level of the rumen. Tube placement should be verified by one or more methods prior to administering any fluids, feed, or drugs via the tube. Serious complications, often fatal, can occur if medications are accidentally administered into the lungs rather than the stomach. This is of especial concern in neonatal calves, which frequently have colostrum administered via orogastric tube. In these calves, there will be no rumen odor or rumen contents as the rumen is not fully developed, so care must be taken to verify placement by observation and palpation. Esophageal feeding bags for calves have reduced the incidence of accidental tracheal intubation, as the distal end of the feeding tube has a large ball that can be easily palpated in the esophagus when correctly placed.

Before removing any orogastric tube, the end must be kinked to prevent aspiration of fluid into the lungs. The tube should be pulled out in one smooth motion.

Transfaunation

The procedure of transfaunation is used to reintroduce normal flora to the gastrointestinal system of a sick patient. It can be performed in any species, although it is most commonly performed on ruminants and occasionally in equids.

Ruminant Transfaunation

Transfaunation in ruminants is often prescribed for patients that have been acidotic, anorexic for three to five days, or have had prolonged diarrhea. It involves the collection of rumen fluid from a known healthy host and delivering it to a patient to provide and encourage normal rumen flora presence. Normal healthy rumen fluid contains ruminal bacteria, protozoa, and many useful fermentation factors.

Collection of healthy rumen fluid is most easily and conveniently done through the port of a rumen canulated cow. It can also be collected through a stomach tube using a pump or siphon. Rumen fluid is most generally collected from cattle for administration to any of the ruminant species (Figures 6.39 and 6.40). Cattle can provide the necessary quantity and quality that any ruminant species needs.

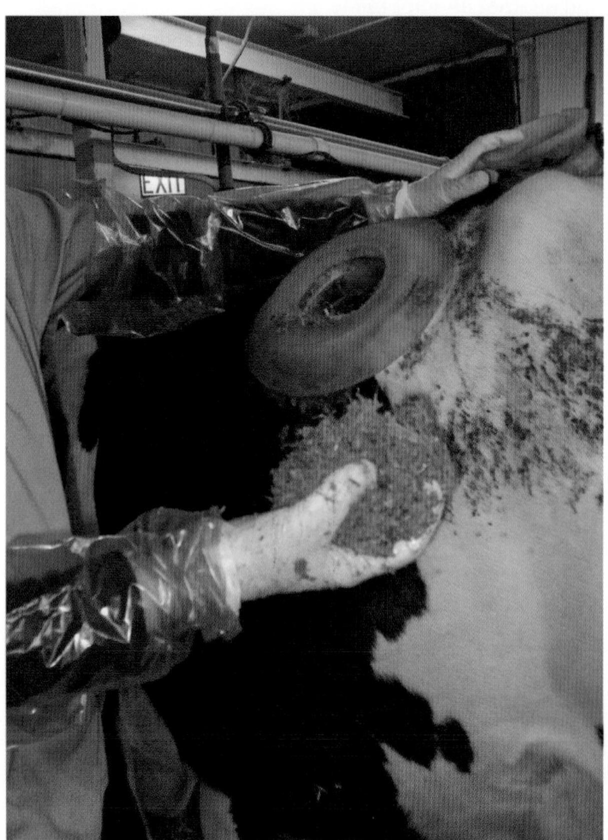

Figure 6.39 Collection of rumen fluid via a canulated cow's rumen.

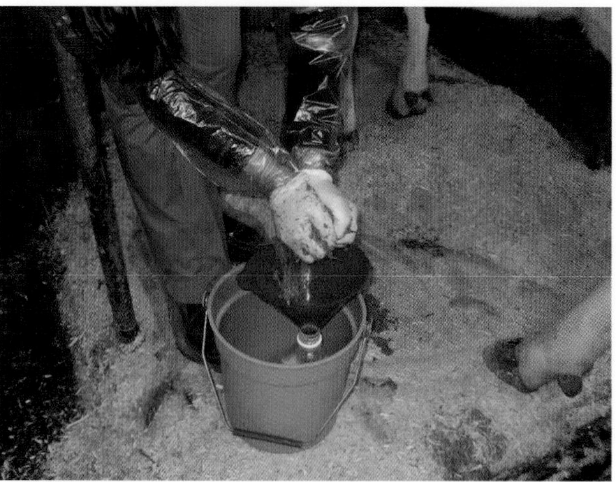

Figure 6.40 Funneling transfaunate after collection.

Camelids and other small ruminants respond well to bovine rumen fluid, which is generally easier to collect in significant quantity.

It is important for the ongoing health of the host to track the amount and frequency of rumen fluid collection. It should be closely monitored, and overdrawing should be avoided, as it may create new pathophysiological concerns for an otherwise healthy host.

Sheep, goats, and camelids generally should receive 0.5–1 l of strained rumen fluid, while adult cattle should receive 3–10 l. The process is usually repeated once daily for several days until a response has been seen. Typical response in camelids that are off-feed and then transfaunated is to see appetite return as soon as 1 h post administration.

The fluid is best administered through an orogastric administration or stomach tube, or it can be instilled during the performing of a rumenotomy. Rumen fluid should be administered soon after collection to avoid damaging the anerobic microbes.

Transfaunation can also be performed in foals and adult horses, using fresh manure collected via a rectal exam from a healthy donor horse on a regular deworming schedule. Manure is mixed with some warm water and then strained before administration via NG tube.

> **Technician Tip 6.12:** Rumen fluid should be administered soon after collection to avoid damaging the anerobic microbes.

Collection Considerations

Pathological status of the host must always be considered before collection of fluid. The time of day for collection of rumen fluid is ideally 2 hr postprandial, when the host's rumen is at the peak of function.

Time between fluid collection and delivery to the patient is critical in the success of the procedure. Ideally, the time between collection and administration should be under 30 min. Delay on the administration will result in degradation of the sample and potentially the successful outcome of the procedure. If administration cannot be performed within 2 hr of collection, a new dose should be collected.

Equine

The practice of transfaunation in equine medicine is not nearly as common as it is with ruminants. It may be considered as a treatment in relation to patients suffering from ongoing colitis, colic, or endotoxemia, and who have not responded to more traditional treatments, including probiotic administration.

Fresh cecal contents or fecal extracts are collected from a healthy equine host. The contents are then diluted with regular water and filtered through a strainer before administration via a nasogastric tube. The fluid is rich in normal intestinal organisms and can be an important part of getting a sick patient's gastrointestinal track back to normal function. The procedure of transfaunation is typically repeated daily for several days to be effective. Additional items to record are appetite, if food is being offered, and fecal and urinary output.

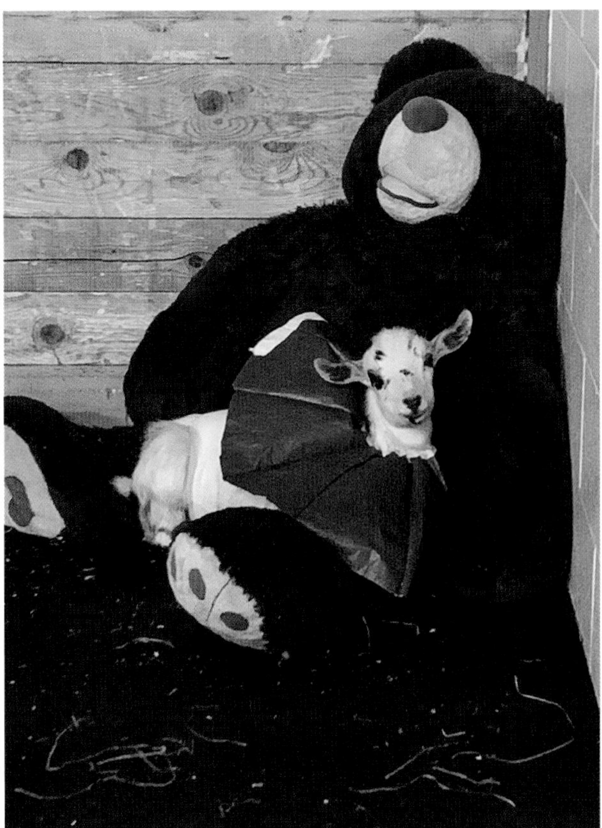

Figure 6.41 A small patient that found comfort in an unlikely companion.

Ongoing Monitoring

The most important ongoing monitoring procedure for hospitalized patients is a complete physical examination on a regular basis. Depending on patient status, this exam should be completed at least every 6–12 hr with more frequent walk-by monitoring during which the general attitude of the patient should be noted. Additional items to record are appetite, if food is being offered, and fecal and urinary output.

Additional components to the physical exam should be included as appropriate and may include checking catheters and bandages as well as palpation for heat and swelling associated with injuries or surgical sites. Physical examination findings should be recorded in the patient's medical record along with relevant clinician parameters. These may include an increased heart rate, respiratory rate, or temperature. See Figures 6.41–6.46 for examples of monitoring considerations.

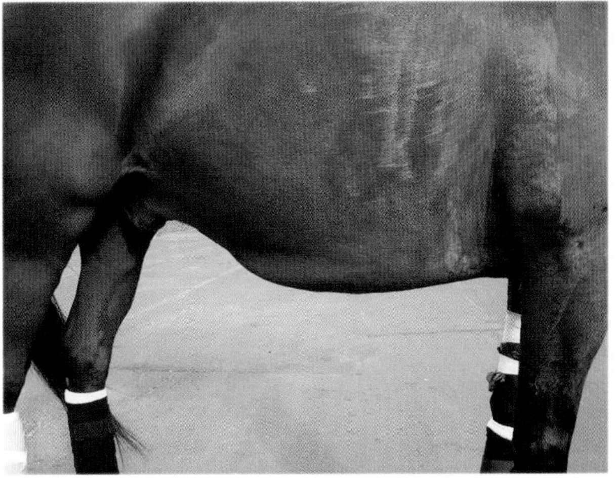

Figure 6.42 Patient that developed ventral edema during the course of treatment.

Continuous instrumented monitoring of large animal patients is relatively rare, especially if they are ambulatory. Serial monitoring is frequently utilized to obtain a picture of how the patient is responding over time to a disease and/or a course of treatment. This monitoring may include repeated laboratory analyses, stall-side tests such as urine chemistry or blood glucose, diagnostic imaging such as radiographs or ultrasound, or instrumented exams such as electrocardiography. Test results must be recorded in the patient's record so trends can be recognized, and sudden changes rapidly addressed. If images cannot be directly

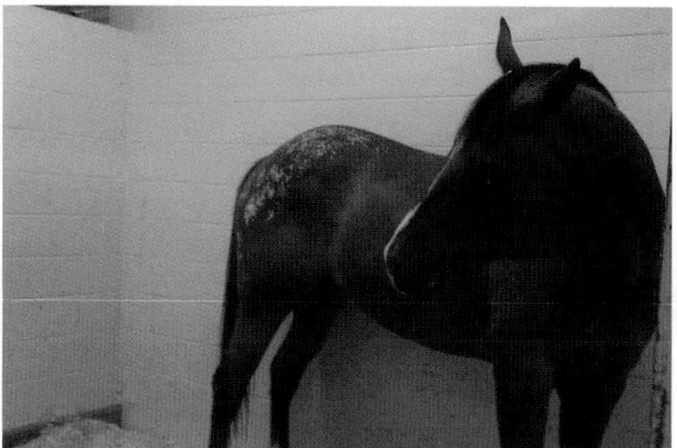

Figure 6.43 Flank watching behavior in horses can be an indication of a medical problem.

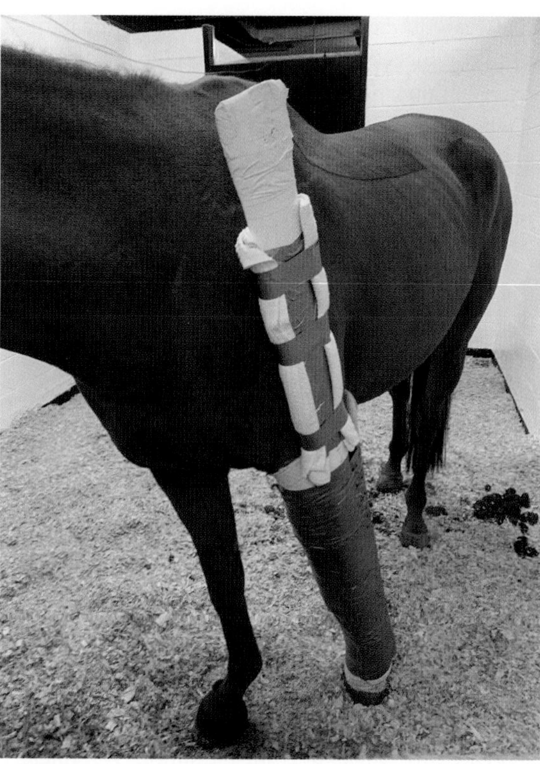

Figure 6.45 Patients wearing a splint should be monitored for slippage, chewing at the bandages, and ability to ambulate.

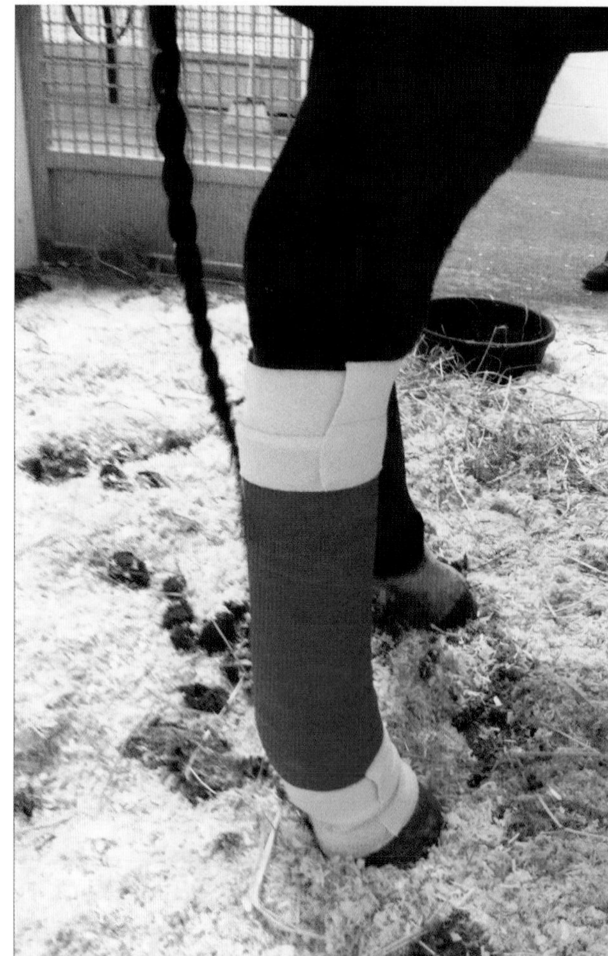

Figure 6.44 Bandaged leg of a horse should be monitored for slipping.

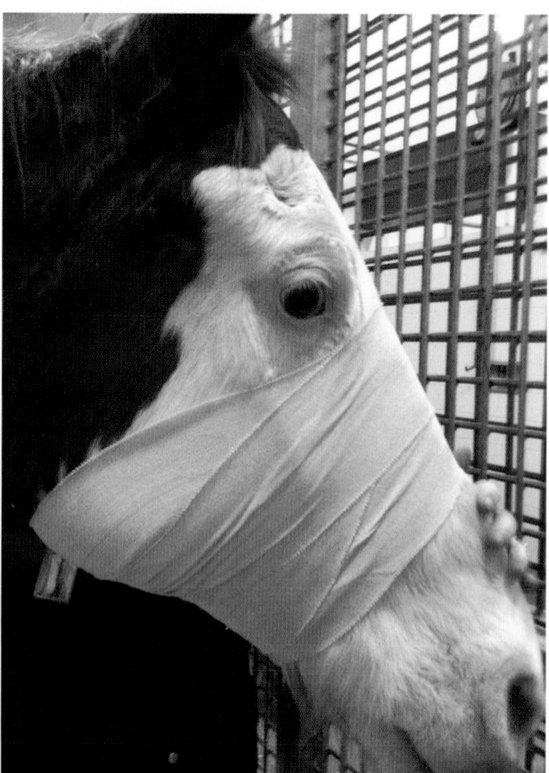

Figure 6.46 Horse with a bandaged face. It is important to note its location and monitor for changes.

included in the record, findings should be described in detail.

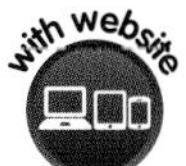

Test your knowledge with extra patient situations in our online chapter resource!

Nursing Care for the Recumbent Patient

Recumbent large animal patients can come in all sizes with all sorts of disease processes. In general, recumbency is a sign of serious disease and is usually associated with a poor prognosis depending on the size of the patient and the cause of recumbency. One thing is clear, excellent nursing care can make a substantial difference to patient outcome by preventing potentially disastrous complications and significantly reducing distress and pain.

Although these principles are fairly intuitive to the compassionate and experienced caregiver, it is very easy to overlook one or more in the hectic and complicated setting where personnel care for recumbent patients. It may be helpful to consider posting a concise "cheat sheet" or standard operating procedure (SOP) in appropriate locations in the clinic to remind team members of the significant number of things that require attention during care of recumbent patients. Two specific SOPs can be drawn up for neonatal and neurologic patients, since these are the two most common types of patients that present with recumbency.

Thermoregulation

Maintenance of an appropriate body temperature enhances patient comfort and reduces caloric requirements. Suboptimal body temperatures can impair digestive processes and immune function in critically ill patients and can delay wound healing in post-operative patients. Conversely, aggressive, or careless heating can create complications including hyperthermia and cutaneous burns. Hyperthermia can be falsely mistaken for true fever. In general, recumbent neonates require the most attention to thermoregulation, but this is also important in adult horses with cachexia, malnutrition, or with significant anemia or hemorrhage, since hypothermia will increase caloric requirements and oxygen deprivation, respectively.

Adult animals can usually achieve acceptable body temperatures through blanketing unless significantly hypothermic, but neonates often require active warming. Techniques for active warming include application of warm blankets; hot water bottles; bags or pads; warm air applicators, such as the Bair Hugger®; application of heat lamps; and administration of actively warmed intravenous fluids if fluids are prescribed. Heat lamps should never be placed close to an immobile patient to avoid hyperthermia and cutaneous burns (Figure 6.47).

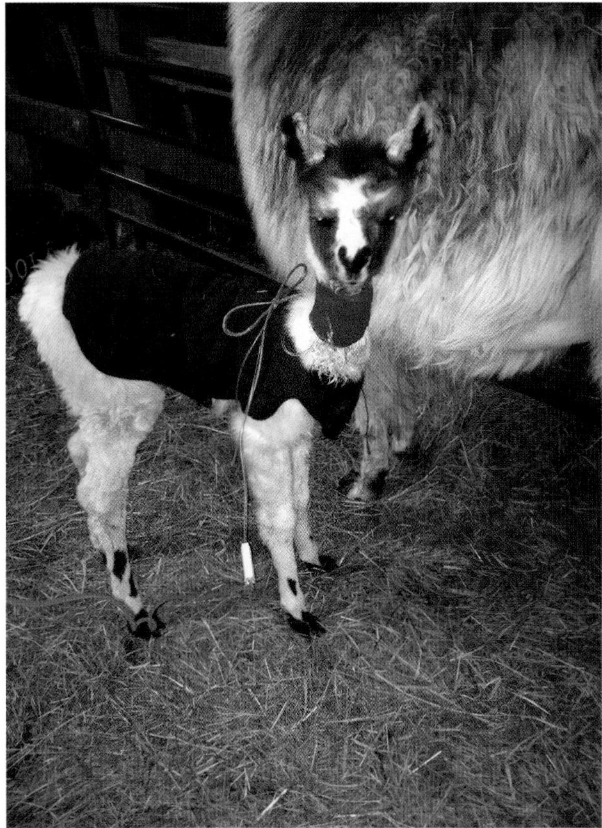

Figure 6.47 Coats and blankets can help little animals stay warm like this cria in a coat.

Protection from Trauma

It is much easier to prevent than to treat traumatic injuries. Recumbent patients can be injured in many ways, including externally inflicted injury to foals from careless or aggressive dams, unintentional injury from incorrect handling by caregivers, and self-inflicted injury from thrashing and struggling. Trauma prevention should be tailored for each patient based on the probable risks.

Preventing Head Trauma

Horses and camelids that are thrashing or seizing can easily damage their heads and should have a padded head protector securely applied, in addition to a deep soft bedding to help prevent contact with a solid surface. Sedation is often helpful. For recumbent neonates, ensure pillows surround the head, especially if the patient is placed next to a wall as they commonly flop their heads about.

Preventing Eye Trauma

Recumbent patients frequently traumatize their eyes through foreign substance abrasion, blunt trauma during thrashing, or from reduced blinking activity creating drying of the cornea. Ideally, lubricant ointment should be applied to the eyes of a recumbent patient every 4–6 hr and the eyes flushed of foreign material as needed. Fluorescein staining should be performed daily as corneal ulcers can form and progress rapidly. Clinical indications of corneal ulceration are often more subtle or likely to be missed in recumbent patients.

Preventing Limb Trauma

Thrashing can lead to significant abrasive and blunt limb trauma in recumbent adult large animal patients. Stimulus to thrashing should be reduced by keeping the surrounding area quiet, avoiding transit of other animals nearby, or administering sedation. In horses, the distal regions of all four legs should be wrapped in protective bandages containing a padding layer. Stack wraps should be applied to the hind limbs if significant hock trauma is occurring. Ideally, shoes should be removed from equine patients or taped with Elasticon®, since they are a common source of injury during thrashing or attempts to stand.

Dams should be separated from their offspring by at least a low fence so that they do not step on them but are close enough not to become distressed by separation. Aggressive dams could potentially be sedated and separated by more substantial fencing to protect caregivers from injury.

Both neonates and adults are prone to the formation of decubital sores, which can form in as little as 48 hr of recumbency. Susceptible areas include the bony prominences of the hip, hock, and shoulder. Decubital sores form as a result of pressure, abrasion, and moistness, so each of these factors must be controlled. Sustained pressure can be reduced through frequent rotation every 2 hr for neonates and four to six times a day for adults. Other measures include appropriate soft bedding and padding and application of pressure relieving bandages to regions of bony prominence. Wrapping limbs and controlling thrashing will reduce abrasive motion.

Using permeable bedding to avoid urine pooling controls moisture. Dirty bedding or blankets should be periodically removed. Careful drying of the skin and application of talcum powder to susceptible areas and application of silver sulfadiazine to abraded areas also helps to prevent decubital ulcers.

Preventing Muscle and Joint Trauma

Forced recumbency can quickly result in significant muscle damage (myopathy) and nerve damage (neuropathy) in large patients as a result of impaired blood flow and venous drainage in the dependent musculature. Ideally, patients should be kept in recumbent positions most natural to them or rotated periodically from side to side as frequently as every 2 hr depending on the degree of associated difficulty in achieving the position. For large patients, deep soft bedding should be provided and cleaned as effectively as possible twice daily. For small patients, large pads can be used. Waterbed mattresses have also been successfully used for both neonates and adults. Neonatal patients that are able should be assisted to stand periodically by placing a towel under the sternum and holding the tail or stifles. Premature neonates with significantly immature bones in the carpus and tarsus, if allowed to stand, may require additional limb support with bandages or splints to prevent damage to maturing joints.

Maintenance of Urinary Passage

Recumbent patients should be constantly assessed for their ability to urinate and to pass adequate urine volume (about 30 ml/kg/day in adults, 140 ml/kg/day for neonates). Repeated severe distension of the bladder can be very problematic, facilitating the development of patent urachus or ruptured bladder in foals, and reduced bladder function and rupture in adults. Lifting a neonate by the abdomen also promotes urinary tract complications. If urinary frequency and volume in the appropriately hydrated patient are inadequate, placement of urinary catheter may be considered if an enlarged bladder is identified. Recumbent neonates should have the umbilicus dipped in dilute iodine or chlorhexidine every 6 hr and permeable bedding should be used to avoid pooling of urine that promotes umbilical infection and decubital ulcers.

Maintenance of Fecal Passage

To maintain fecal passage, recumbent adults can be provided laxative substances, such as bran mashes, and neonates can receive mineral oil once a day via tube feeding. Oil should never be mixed into bottle-fed milk due to the risk of aspiration. A warm soapy enema should be provided to neonates if needed, although repeated enemas should be avoided since they can cause rectal irritation and straining that promotes patent urachus. Feces of all patients should be checked for abnormalities such as mucus, blood, or diarrhea. Adult horses with herpes myelitis frequently require periodic manual evacuation of the rectum to avoid obstruction and colic.

Respiratory Support

Appropriate respiratory system monitoring and support is a critical part of reducing morbidity in recumbent patients and preventing complications such as pneumonia, particularly in patients already struggling with suboptimal lung function such as premature neonates. Body position is one of the most important influences on respiratory function. Patients should be kept in sternal recumbency to allow equivalent inflation of both lungs. Sternal recumbency can be achieved in recumbent large animals through positioning straw bales or partial sling support and in neonates using pillows and "V pads." Intermittent assistance to allow neonates to stand will help reinflate lungs and stimulate respiration. Unfortunately for recumbent adults, slings compromise rather than help respiratory function. Animals that insist on lying in lateral recumbency should at least be rotated periodically to relieve the dependent lung. Daily monitoring of the respiratory system including auscultation can be critical for early detection of respiratory disease, but caregivers should be aware that recumbency could lead to substantial abnormalities of the lung sounds in the absence of serious disease such as pneumonia. Likewise, abnormal noise may be minimal even in diseased lungs so monitoring for changes in respiratory rate and rectal temperature are often more helpful. In patients receiving oxygen, the nasal catheter should be placed to the level of the medial canthus of the eye and taped or sutured in place. Oxygen flow rates should be appropriate for the patient in question and humidified to reduce irritation of the respiratory tract. Coupage is useful to evacuate respiratory secretions in recumbent patients and is performed by gently thumping the thorax with a slightly cupped hand to generate a wave of air. Small particle bedding should be avoided in recumbent patients to avoid risk of aspiration and ophthalmic complications.

Physical Therapy

Physical therapy may be overlooked due to the time demands in a busy hospital but can be critical in preventing trauma and assisting return to full function. In addition, it forces closer inspection of the patient and may identify early complications when changes in sensation, mobility, or appearance of limbs or the patient are noted. Basic physical therapy consists of passive mobilization of the limbs. It is performed on the upside limbs of a laterally recumbent patient with subsequent rotation of the patient for access to the down limbs. More intensive physical therapy includes massaging large muscle groups, assisting a patient to stand periodically, or assisting attempts to walk and suckle. For recumbent camelids and cows, float tanks can be a great way to relieve weight bearing while encouraging the animal to move its limbs around (Figure 6.48). Animals can be left in float tanks for hours as long as food and water are available to them. Severe infections are possible in patients that have intravenous catheters in place or open wounds so extreme caution should be applied in floating such patients.

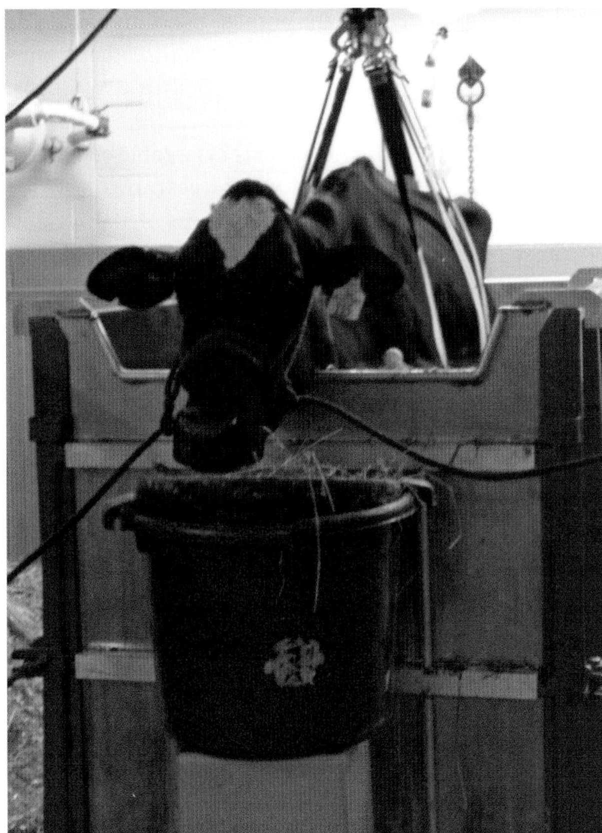

Figure 6.48 Cow hoisted by the Large Animal Lift® (LAL) in order to get it into the float tank. Once floating in the tank, the sling remains in place but is not acting as a support.

Slinging the Recumbent Patient

Slinging, even for short periods at a time, gives relief to dependent muscles and enhances limb mobility. There are a large variety of slings available for large animal patients and selection should be made carefully. General principles to follow when selecting a sling include the size of the intended patients, the intended use (quick lifting device versus sustained slinging), price, and reliability of the manufacturing company. For prolonged slinging, the selected sling should provide broad-based body support focused on appropriate regions (sternum not abdomen), safely contain the patient (front and rear sash to avoid malposition of the sling), be relatively easy to apply to the recumbent animal, and should not have a focal point of lift above the animal (side bars, end bars, or a long central bar should be present). Slings are truly useful for large patients that retain some ability to stand since the purpose of a sling should be to assist such patients to stand, to stabilize them once standing, and to provide some support of their BW (ideally, no more than 25%).

Slings can be used for brief periods in less able patients to check for ability to stand and weight bear or to provide short periods of relief by removing most of the weight-bearing load for a short time. Prolonged periods of substantial weight bearing via sling are dangerous due to the risk of compromising respiration in the heavily supported patient.

Patients should be carefully assessed for their behavioral response to the sling when it is first introduced, as some patients can become frantic and dangerous when lifted. There is potential for spine or limb fractures when struggling. The Anderson® sling is the most highly regarded sling for equine patients and is even used for air transport. It can be left on the horse when it is recumbent so frequent positioning is not needed (Figures 6.49 and 6.50).

Other advantages is the support this sling provides via the skeletal system rather than the body, and this sling also

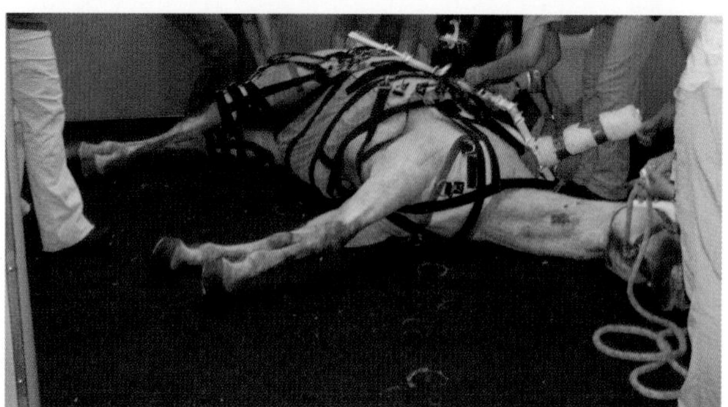

Figure 6.49 Horse under heavy sedation being placed into the Anderson Sling.

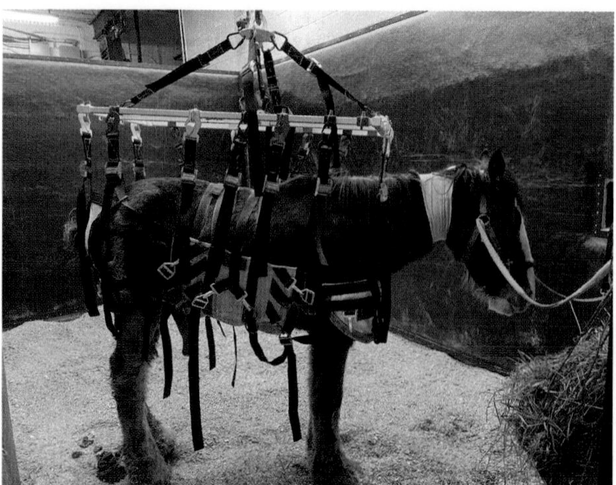

Figure 6.50 Horse standing in the Anderson Sling.

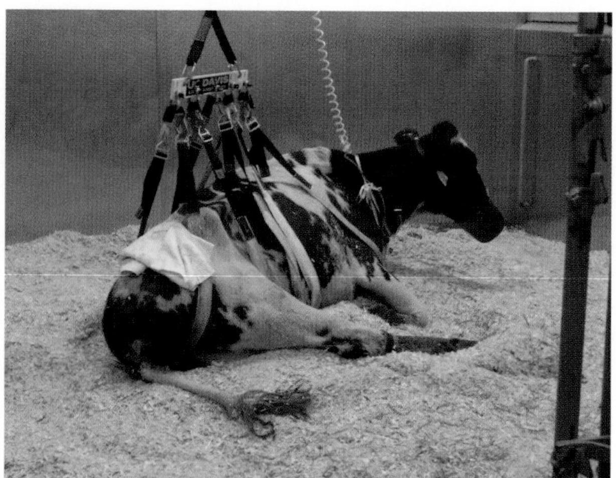

Figure 6.51 Cow resting in the large animal lift sling.

has a head restraint system and can be easily manipulated to reduce weight bearing on specific limbs if required. It is expensive and somewhat complicated to apply. The Liftex® sling is also a good equine sling and is considerably less expensive and easier to apply.

There are a variety of slings made specifically for smaller camelids and larger ruminants. One must pay special attention to udder support in milk-producing dairy cattle when selecting a sling. Some multispecies slings can cause blood vessel occlusion or undue stress on a cow's mammary gland, especially if she is in heavy milk. The LAL is a good multipurpose sling that fits several different species, though is not as ideal for long-term support. It may be helpful to add additional padding wherever signs of rubbing, wear, or stress begin to appear (Figure 6.51).

Safety Considerations

In general, recumbent adult patients should be placed in the largest stall possible to provide more clearance for lunging attempts to rise and to give caregivers more room to work safely. Ideally, there should be more than one exit to the stall and the walls should be padded. An overhead hoist is essential, and staff must be aware of its rated weight capacity and it should have annual maintenance (Figure 6.52). The stall should be organized ahead of patient arrival so there are no delays in transferring the patient to its safest location as soon as it arrives. Safe transfer can be challenging in itself, and frequently recumbent horses are best moved by placing an intravenous catheter in the trailer, then sedating or anesthetizing the horse before wrapping its limbs and moving it by rescue slide or cart into the hospital. Other methods can be used to move smaller patients, such as sliding or lifting on a tarp or blanket, frequently with manual restraint.

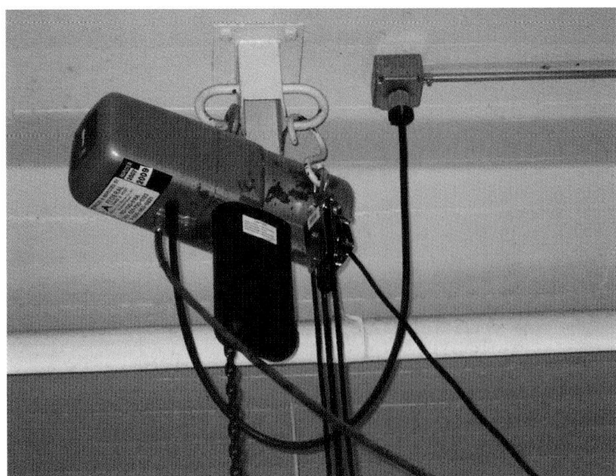

Figure 6.52 Electrical hoist used for slinging large animal patients.

TECHNICIAN TIP 6.13: Have all hoists and support gear inspected annually to mitigate potential safety concerns.

Managing recumbent patients is labor-intensive and requires considerable effort, time, and compassion to perform at a high standard. Good nursing skills are a valuable part of patient care that can contribute substantially to a successful outcome. Constructing volunteer teams to contribute to the care of a recumbent patient can be very valuable. Involving owners themselves or friends of the client can be helpful but frequently results in more complications than benefit due to vested interests, intense concern, and liability. Helpful teams can be constructed from veterinary, pre veterinary, and technician student clubs, and even from external volunteers with an animal interest. An advantage of this approach is that greater numbers of personnel are available, which helps reduce wear on the volunteer staff and technicians. A disadvantage is reduced continuity of care, since the attentive, experienced, and frequently present caregiver is more likely to note small changes in condition that can be harbingers of serious problems. Volunteer teams are usually best applied to neonatal care, since the recumbent adult horse presents a substantial risk to inexperienced helpers. Any volunteer should be thoroughly versed in the specifics of each particular patient before they embark on care services.

Dentistry

Dental procedures are among the most performed in equine practice. For other large animal species, dental procedures are mostly limited to addressing disease and routine dental floating is not performed. The exception to this is camelids in which malocclusion of the incisors is relatively common; this is generally addressed by grinding down overgrown teeth with a Dremel® tool. The remainder of this section will focus on dentistry procedures in horses, though most of the general concepts can be applied to any species.

The practice of equine dentistry has been the subject of much legislative debate in recent years. As a result, practice law varies from state to state, with some states allowing lay dentists to perform procedures under the supervision of a licensed veterinarian while others restrict dentistry to veterinarians only. Regardless of this distinction, the safety of all personnel is of primary importance during routine dentistry. The most important component to this is adequate restraint of the patient, which involves a combination of appropriate sedation and continuous control of the head. Controlling the head is of particular importance once a dental speculum is in place, as this can easily become a dangerous weapon for even an appropriately sedated horse, leading to serious injury.

A thorough physical examination should precede administration of a sedative to identify potential complicating conditions. During this examination, the head should be examined visually and by palpation for any areas of soft or hard swelling. The nostrils should be checked for malodorous discharge. If possible, the horse should be observed while chewing and swallowing, as oral pain may result in dropped boluses of partially chewed food, a phenomenon referred to as "quidding." (see Nutrition chapter for picture). Cheek teeth can be palpated through the cheeks for sharp points or obvious malocclusions. The lips can be separated to check for incisor alignment. Manual manipulation of the mandible while holding the maxilla steady allows evaluation of lateral movement of the jaw and can be performed in cooperative patients without sedation. Examination of the interior of the mouth should not be performed prior to placement of a mouth speculum, which is generally done after the horse has been sedated. The horse's mouth should be rinsed out with water prior to administering sedation to remove food and other gross debris (Figure 6.53).

The sedation protocol of choice for many practitioners uses an α_2-agonist with or without the addition of an adjunct drug such as butorphanol. Detomidine is usually favored over xylazine because of its longer duration of action. Profound rather than light sedation should be induced to reduce the risk of the horse jerking its head during the procedure. Procedures should not commence for several minutes after administration of sedative agents to allow for maximal effect and to let a period of mild ataxia pass. The horse's head should rest on a padded chin rest or

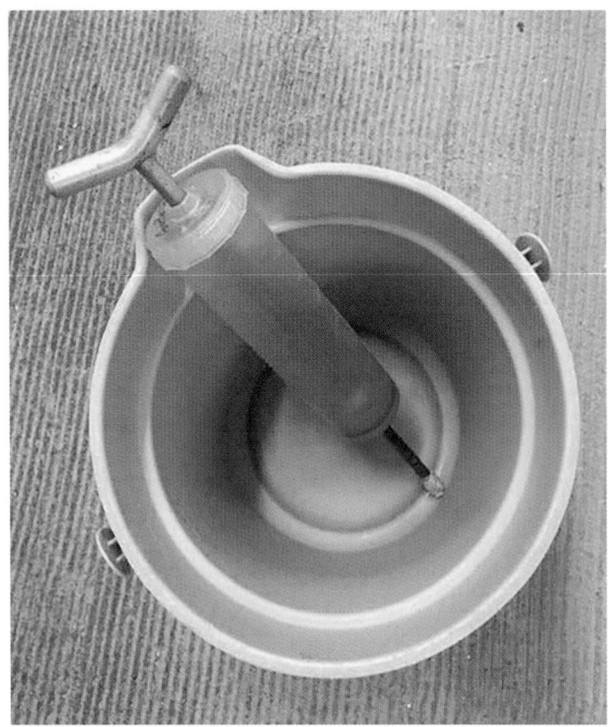

Figure 6.53 Bucket and dosing syringe are helpful for a routine dental examination.

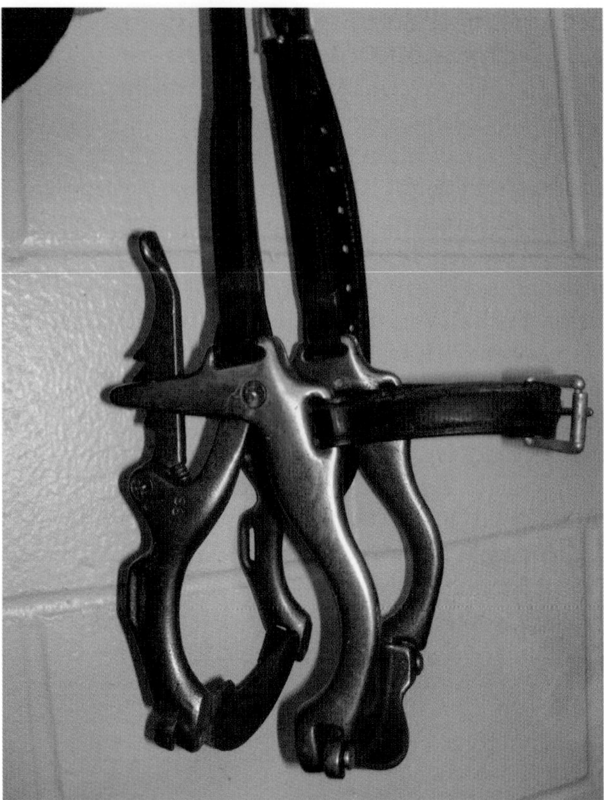

Figure 6.54 McPherson (Hausman) dental speculum.

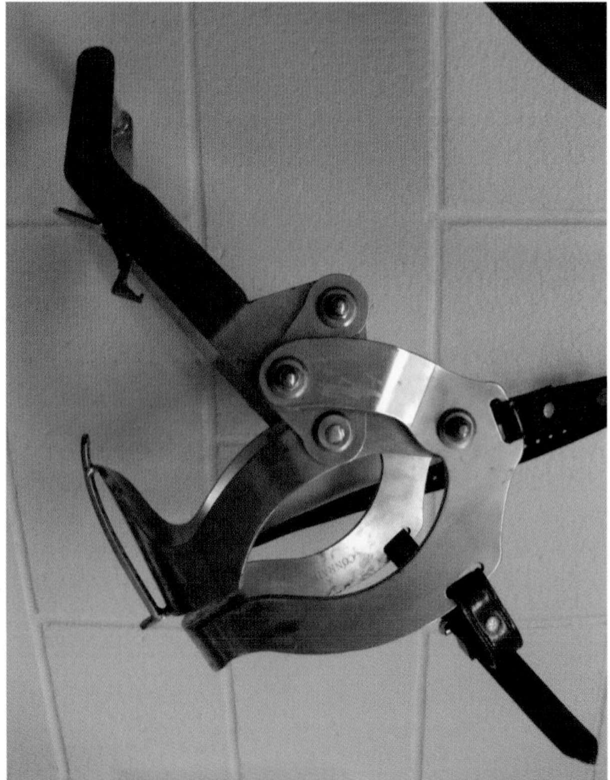

Figure 6.55 Conrad dental speculum.

be suspended using a halter depending on the available setup. Resting the horse's head on an assistant's shoulder should be avoided if possible.

Ideally, two people should place the oral speculum, one on each side of the horse's head. There are a variety of mouth speculum styles available, the most popular being the Mcpherson style and may be referred to by different names (Figures 6.54–6.57). The speculum is placed between the incisors in the closed position and the head straps are tightened before opening the speculum slowly one "click" at a time, preferably with both sides widened simultaneously. Once the speculum is open as wide as possible, the patient's mouth can be rinsed and an intraoral exam should be performed (Figure 6.54).

A headlamp greatly aids visual inspection of the caudal cheek teeth, but palpation should also be utilized to identify sharp points, food pocketing, and other abnormalities. The tongue and buccal mucosa may have visible abrasions or lacerations inflicted by sharp points. The use of gloves during this exam is a matter of personal preference but if the examiner has any open wounds on their hands, gloves are highly recommended. Smelling the hand or glove used for palpation may reveal the presence of an abscess. The use of a dental mirror may also be useful for visualizing the caudal teeth. Failure to identify premolar and molar fractures and partial fractures can cause problems down the road. The tongue of the patient should be pulled to the

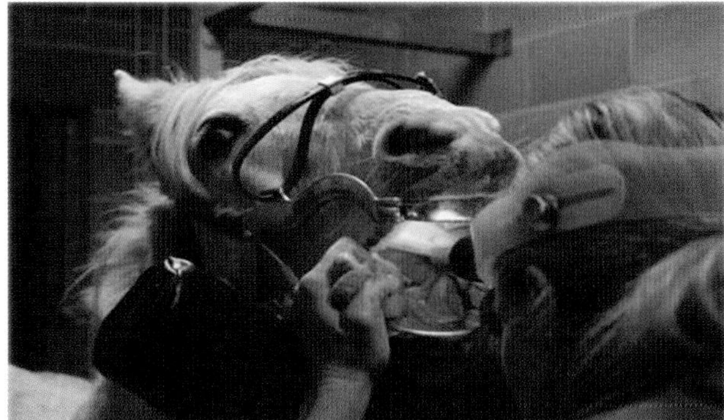

Figure 6.56 Dental speculum placed for examination.

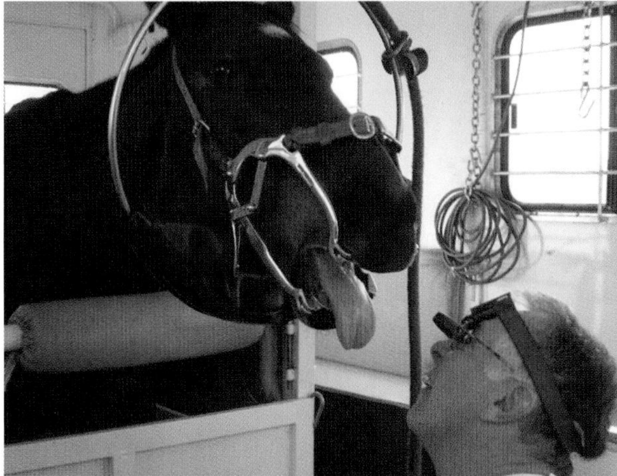

Figure 6.57 McPherson (Hausman) dental speculum and use of a suspended chin rest.

opposite side of the mouth for better visualization during the exam. Even under sedation, many horses will move their tongues, so keeping the tongue out of the way during dental procedures will also help prevent accidental abrasion or laceration of the tongue with dental tools. The assistant holding on to the speculum can do this. Use of gauze around the tongue can help to improve grip.

When recording abnormal findings in the patient's medical record, the Modified Triadan system should be used (Figure 6.58). Use of a standardized system makes it easier to track changes in oral health from visit to visit and to share information with others involved in the patient's care.

Hand floats for routine dentistry have largely been supplanted using motorized instruments. Motorized instruments allow for rapid completion of routine dental floating. Caution must be exercised to avoid removing excessive amounts of tooth material (Figure 6.59). Periodic palpation of the teeth to feel for progressive removal of sharp points and hooks will help to guide appropriate use (Figure 6.60). Floats of either type should be thoroughly cleaned and

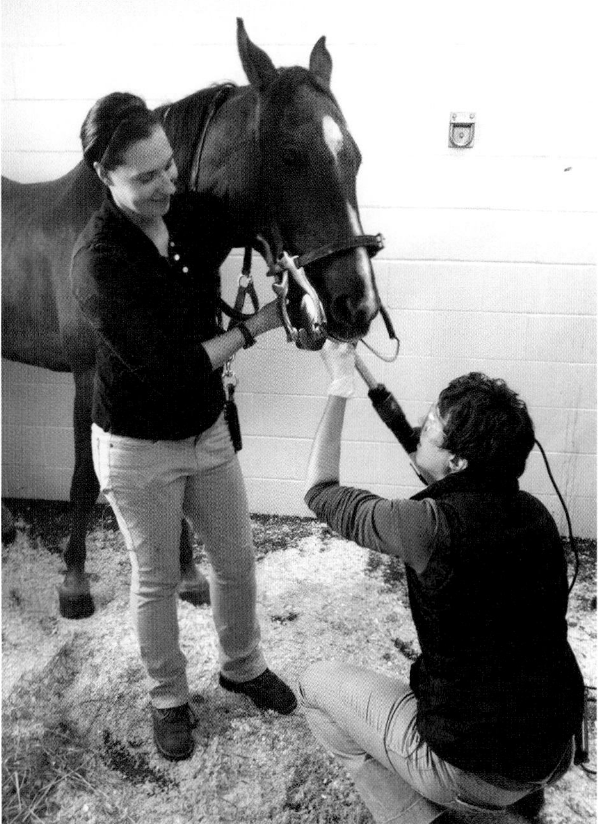

Figure 6.58 A routine dental float being performed with a power float.

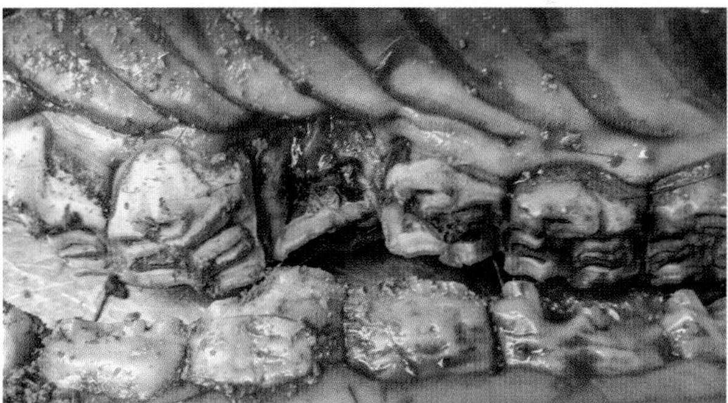

Figure 6.59 Example of an overgrowth of one tooth from the lower arcade due to a partial fracture space on the upper arcade.

disinfected in dilute chlorhexidine between uses. Built-up debris should be removed as needed during each procedure by rinsing. If motorized equipment is used, eye, hearing, and respiratory protection are strongly recommended for all personnel. A surgical mask is not adequate protection against aerosolized tooth dust; a mask or respirator should be used. Some practitioners prefer the use of a full plastic face mask, especially if extensive work with a Dremel will be performed.

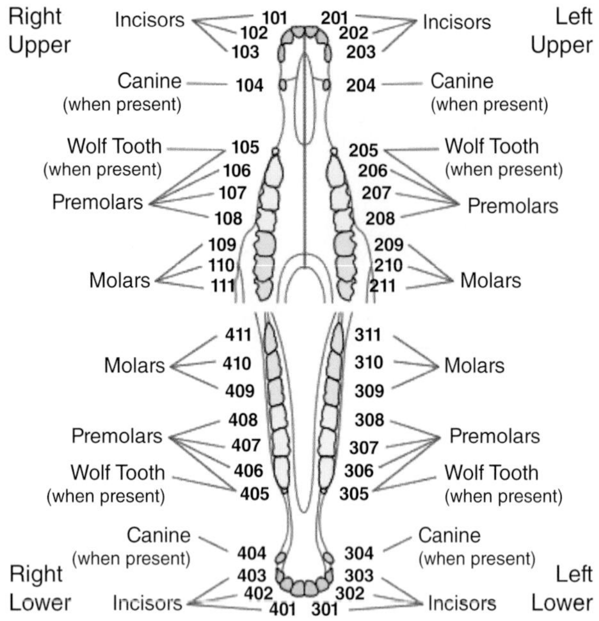

Figure 6.60 Nomenclature of equine teeth. Upper right arcade are 100s, upper left arcade are 200s, lower left arcade are 300s, and lower right arcade are 400s.

> **TECHNICIAN TIP 6.14:** If motorized equipment is used, eye, hearing, and respiratory protection are strongly recommended for all personnel.

At the completion of the dental procedure, the speculum should be carefully closed and removed from the horse's mouth. The mouth should be rinsed out with dilute chlorhexidine and water. The horse may need to stand with its head supported until some degree of sedation has worn off. They should be placed in a stall with food withheld until completely recovered from sedation to reduce the risk of esophageal obstruction. One or more doses of a nonsteroidal anti-inflammatory drug may be administered, especially if iatrogenic damage to the soft tissues of the mouth occurred. Prophylactic antibiotics are not required for routine dentistry procedures. Bleeding from minor wounds will generally stop on its own without treatment, although repeated flushing of the mouth with an antiseptic solution may be recommended for several days. If a tooth was extracted, a plug of dental wax or acrylic should be placed in the empty socket prior to removing the speculum to prevent feed packing into the cavity and to reduce the risk of an infection and/or sinus fistula formation. As the space fills with granulation tissue during healing, this plug will fall out and should not need to be replaced. Routine dental floating can generally be completed in the field or clinic with a single dose of sedation. Indeed, some practitioners may decide to reverse α_2-agonist sedation with tolazaline or yohimbine at the end of a float procedure.

More involved procedures, however, such as standing tooth extraction, may require repeated doses of sedation or a CRI of sedation. Instruments used for probing, examination, and some extractions can be quite specialized (Figures 6.61 and 6.62). Most come in stainless surgical steal but can be hard to grip, using a long piece of soft rubber, such as an inner tube tire, works well to provide grip.

Procedures involving the incisors are best done using an incisor gag which allows for access to the front teeth while also maintaining a slightly open mouth to avoid biting (Figure 6.63). The incisor teeth in horses were overlooked for many years but more recently have been recognized for

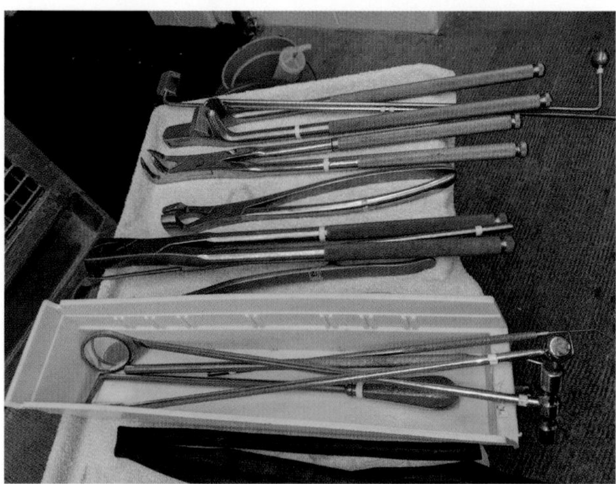

Figure 6.61 An array of equine dental instruments.

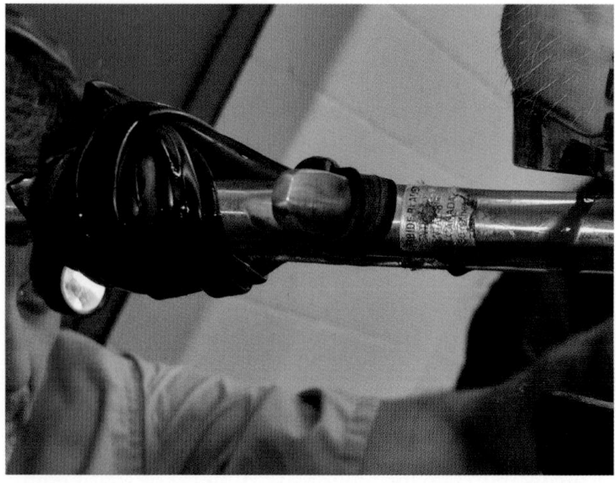

Figure 6.62 Long dental instrument using a piece of long rubber to secure the handle during use.

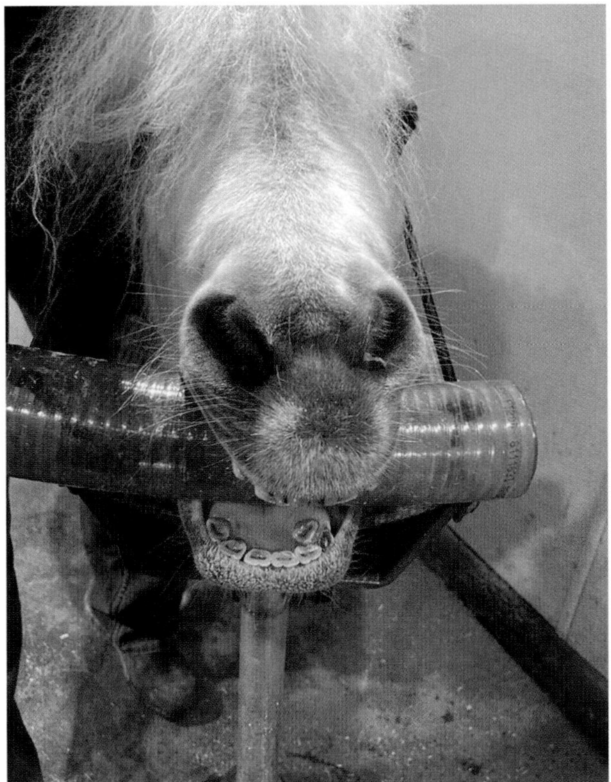

Figure 6.63 Horse with an incisor gag.

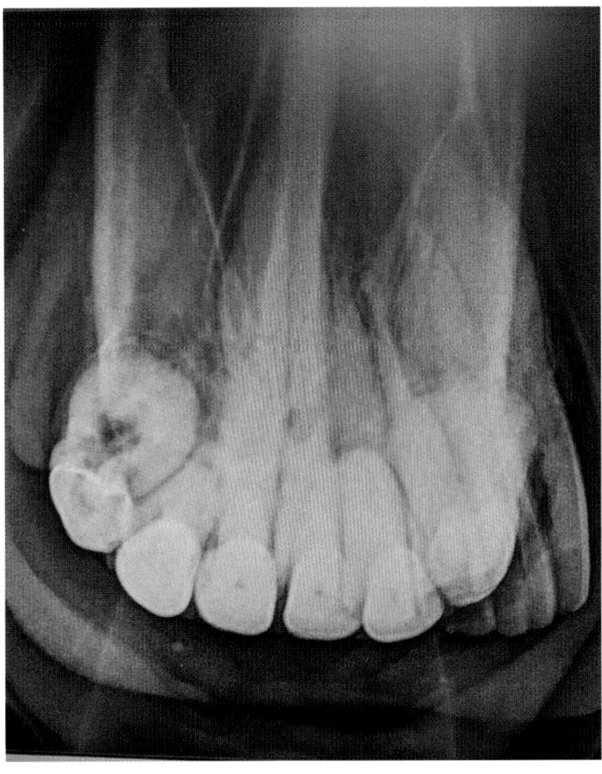

Figure 6.64 X-ray of equine incisors afflicted with equine odontoclastic tooth resorption and hypercementosis.

problems of chronic pain such as equine odontoclastic tooth resorption and hypercementosis (EOTRH) (Figure 6.64). This disease primarily affects one or more incisors and canines. It is progressive, where resorptive lesions cause destruction of the tooth roots. It is commonly identified through radiographs revealing bulbus root changes. Removal of the affected tooth (teeth) is common practice to avoid fractures and ongoing pain. Horses do quite well with no incisors!

Some procedures, such as sinus trephination and tooth repulsion, are mostly performed in a hospital setting, either standing using a CRI or under general anesthesia. See the surgery chapter for more on dental surgical procedures.

> **TECHNICIAN TIP 6.15:** Using a long piece of soft rubber, such as an inner tube from a tire, works well to provide grip on long dental instruments.

References

Adams, S.B., Moore, G.E., Elrashidy, M. et al. (2010). Effect of needle size and type, reuse of needles, insertion speed, and removal of hair on contamination of joints with tissue debris and hair after arthrocentesis. *Veterinary Surgery* 39 (6): 667–673. https://doi.org/10.1111/j.1532-950x.2010.00649.x.

Bradbury, L.A., Archer, D.C., Dugdale, A.H. et al. (2005). Suspected venous air embolism in a horse. *Veterinary Record* 156 (4): 109–111. https://doi.org/10.1136/vr.156.4.109.

Burnett, K.M. (2005). Equine dentistry: safety considerations for practitioners. *Clinical Techniques in Equine Practice* 4 (2): 120–123. https://doi.org/10.1053/j. ctep.2005.04.003.

Caston, S.S., McClure, S.R., Martens, R.J. et al. (2006). Effect of hyperimmune plasma on the severity of pneumonia caused by *Rhodococcus equi* in experimentally infected foals. *Veterinary Therapeutics* 7 (4): 361–375.

Corley, K. and Stephen, J. (eds.) (2008). *The Equine Hospital Manual*. (pp. 61, 468–470). West Sussex, UK: Blackwell Publishing.

Culp, W.T., Weisse, C., Berent, A.C. et al. (2008). Percutaneous endovascular retrieval of an intravascular foreign body in five dogs, a goat, and a horse. *Journal of the American Veterinary Medical Association* 232 (12): 1850–1856.

Giguère, S., Gaskin, J.M., Miller, C., and Bowman, J.L. (2002). Evaluation of a commercially available hyperimmune plasma product for prevention of naturally acquired pneumonia caused by *Rhodococcus equi* in foals. *Journal of the American Veterinary Medical Association* 220 (1): 59–63.

Hague, B.A., Honnas, C.M., Simpson, R.B., and Peloso, J.G. (1997). Evaluation of skin bacterial flora before and after aseptic preparation of clipped and nonclipped arthrocentesis sites in horses. *Veterinary Surgery* 26 (2): 121–125. https://doi.org/10.1111/j.1532-950x.1997.tb01474.x.

Hardy, J. (2006). Fluids, electrolytes, and acid-base therapy. In: *Equine Surgery*, 3e (eds. J.A. Auer and J.A. Stick), 29. St. Louis, MO: Saunders Elsevier.

Haskel, S.R. (2008). *Blackwell's Five-Minute Consult: Ruminant* (pp. 800, 884–885). Ames, IA: Wiley Blackwell.

Holbrook, T.C., Dechant, J.E., and Crowson, C.L. (2007). Suspected air embolism associated with post-anesthetic pulmonary edema and neurologic sequelae in a horse. *Veterinary Anaesthesia and Analgesia* 34 (3): 217–222. https://doi.org/10.1111/j.1467-2995.2006.00317.x.

Lees, M.J., Read, R.A., Klein, K.T. et al. (1989). Surgical retrieval of a broken jugular catheter from the right ventricle of a foal. *Equine Veterinary Journal* 21 (5): 384–387.

Levine, D.G., Epstein, K.L., Ahern, B.J., and Richardson, D.W. (2010). Efficacy of three tourniquet types for intravenous antimicrobial regional limb perfusion in standing horses. *Veterinary Surgery* 39 (8): 1021–1024. https://doi.org/10.1111/j.1532-950x.2010.00732.x.

Little, D., Keene, B.W., Bruton, C. et al. (2002). Percutaneous retrieval of a jugular catheter fragment from the pulmonary artery of a foal. *Journal of the American Veterinary Medical Association* 220 (2): 212–214.

Mills, P.C. and Cross, S.E. (2007). Regional differences in transdermal penetration of fentanyl through equine skin. *Research in Veterinary Science* 82 (2): 252–256.

Parker, R.A., Bladon, B.M., McGovern, K., and Smith, K.C. (2010). Osteomyelitis and osteonecrosis after intraosseous perfusion with gentamicin. *Veterinary Surgery* 39 (5): 644–648. https://doi.org/10.1111/j.1532-950x.2010.00685.x.

Reed, S.M., Warwick, B.M., and Sellon, D.C. (2010). *Equine Internal Medicine*, 3e, pp. 256, 276–277, 322. St. Louis, MO: Elsevier.

Reed, F., Burrow, R., Poels, K.L.C. et al. (2011). Evaluation of transdermal fentanyl patch attachment in dogs and analysis of residual fentanyl content following removal. *Veterinary Anaesthesia and Analgesia* 38 (4): 407–412. https://doi.org/10.1111/j.1467-2995.2011.00628.x.

Rush, B.R., Davis, E.G., and McCue, M. (2004). Equine recumbency: complications and slinging. *Compendium on Continuing Education for the Practicing Veterinarian* 26 (4): 256–265.

Sweeney, C.R. and Russell, G.E. (1997). Complications associated with use of a one-hole subpalpebral lavage system in horses: 150 cases (1977–1996). *Journal of the American Veterinary Medical Association* 211 (10): 1271–1274.

Clinical Case Resolution 6.1

The signalment, history, and presentation of this patient are strongly suggestive of a small intestinal obstruction. A nasogastric tube should be passed immediately to relieve pressure that may be built up in the stomach from excess fluid and to reduce the risk of gastric rupture. This procedure is both diagnostic (allows quantification of reflux) and therapeutic (remember, horses cannot vomit). The nasogastric tube may be left in place if a large amount of reflux is obtained. A second important procedure is placement of a venous (jugular) catheter that can be used to administer drugs (i.e. analgesia, presurgical antibiotics) and fluids. Bolused intravenous fluids should be started as soon as a catheter is placed to address hypovolemia/dehydration. Assuming that this horse's lesion is surgically corrected, repeated passage of a nasogastric tube to manage ongoing reflux and administration of intravenous fluids (and drugs) is likely to be needed for several days. Fluids will need to be supplemented with potassium, magnesium, calcium, and dextrose for as long as the horse is unable to eat. Catheter management may be especially challenging if endotoxemia develops, as this will increase the risk of thrombophlebitis. Frequent physical exams and repeated blood work (i.e. serum chemistry profile, complete blood count) should be performed to stay abreast of any changes in the patient's condition.

Activities

Multiple Choice Questions

(Answers can be found in the back of the book.)

1. Which of the following would be the most appropriate catheter choice for an adult horse that will be on fluids for several days following colic surgery?
- **A** 18-gauge, 6.25-cm (2.5-in), polyurethane, over-the-needle
- **B** 14-gauge, 13-cm (5.25-in), polypropylene, through-the-needle
- **C** 19-gauge, 25-cm (10-in), polyurethane, over-the-wire
- **D** 14-gauge, 13-cm (5.25-in), polyurethane, over-the-needle

2. Which of the following is not a sign of a possible transfusion reaction?
- **A** urticaria (hives)
- **B** increased heart rate
- **C** increased urination
- **D** collapse

3. Which of these patients should not have PO medication administered?
- **A** a foal that is being fed enterally through a nasogastric tube
- **B** an adult gelding recovering from arthroscopic surgery of the stifle
- **C** an adult mare with 4 l of gastric reflux every 4 hr
- **D** a foal with clostridial diarrhea

4. Which of the following statements about plasma is true?
- **A** Frozen plasma can safely be stored at −4 °C for 1 year.
- **B** There is no risk of a transfusion reaction with plasma administration because there are no red blood cells present.
- **C** Immunoglobulin (IgG) concentration of the recipient will increase 200 mg/dl for each liter of plasma administered.
- **D** Plasma is the primary treatment of choice for failure of passive transfer in neonates less than 12 hr old.

5. Which of these routes of administration would be least appropriate for antibiotic treatment of a patient with an infected metacarpophalangeal joint (fetlock)?
- **A** intravenous regional limb perfusion
- **B** intraosseous
- **C** intravenous (systemic)
- **D** topical/transdermal

6. Which of the following anatomic structures is not encountered during proper passage of a nasogastric tube?
- **A** lower esophageal sphincter
- **B** ethmoid turbinates
- **C** ventral nasal meatus
- **D** pharynx

7. Which location is most appropriate for intramuscular administration of drugs in a beef cow?
- **A** neck muscles
- **B** gluteal muscles
- **C** pectoral muscles
- **D** epaxial muscles

8. What is the approximate fluid deficit for a 550-lb pony estimated to be 8% dehydrated?
- **A** 10 l
- **B** 20 l
- **C** 35 l
- **D** 45 l

9. Which of the following is not an important safety precaution to take when performing routine dentistry in horses?
- **A** resting the horse's head on an assistantns shoulder to reduce movement
- **B** use of chemical restraint for the patient
- **C** wearing a mask or face shield
- **D** maintaining control of the dental speculum

10. Which of the following fluids will increase osmotic pressure in the vasculature?
- **A** 0.9% saline
- **B** lactated ringers solution
- **C** 7.2% saline
- **D** 5% dextrose in water

Test Your Learning

1. List four ways in which proper placement of a nasogastric tube in the stomach can be confirmed.
2. Calculate the approximate amount of fluids to be given in the first 12–24 hr for an adult Quarter Horse mare weighing 950 lb, estimated to be 7% dehydrated on presentation, and producing 4 l of gastric reflux every 4 hr.
3. A yearling Thoroughbred weighing 454 kg is presented with a severe laceration to the axillary region that occurred the night before. PCV is 14%. How much whole blood would be needed to raise the PCV to 22% in this individual? Would a single donor with weighing 550 kg with a PCV of 40% be sufficient to provide this volume?
4. What are major risk factors for the development of thrombophlebitis?
5. Compare and contrast crystalloid and colloid fluids, and explain why a combination of the two might be useful in a fluid plan.
6. Describe physical exam findings that might be suggestive of pathology related to the teeth.

Answers can be found in the back of the book.

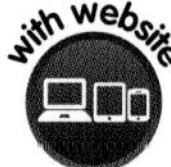

Extra review questions, case studies, and a breed ID image bank can be found online at www.wiley.com/go/loly/veterinary.

Chapter 7

Diagnostic Procedures

Sue Loly, LVT, VTS (EVN), JoAnn Slack, DVM, MS, DACVIM (LAIM), Laura Lien, MS, CVT, VTS (LAIM), Rolf B. Modesto, VMD, and Sheryl Ferguson, CVT, VTS (LAIM)

Learning Objectives

- Understand the indications for various diagnostic procedures.
- Identify equipment needed for diagnostic procedures.
- Identify sample collection containers and when they are needed.
- Describe indications for sterile endoscope preparation.
- Understand anatomical entry points for thoracocentesis, abdominocentesis, and liver biopsy.
- Differentiate indications for bronchoalveolar lavage (BAL) and tracheal wash (TW).
- Know the appropriate volume of fluid to be infused during transtracheal wash (TTW) and bronchoalveolar lavage.
- Describe safety measures that should be taken for all routine diagnostic procedures.
- Describe the indications for performing an electrocardiogram (ECG or EKG).
- Describe or demonstrate electrode placement and obtain standard lead configurations.
- Describe paper speed and gain adjustments and recognize common artifacts in an ECG or EKG.
- Recognize normal sinus rhythm, common physiologic arrhythmias, and common pathologic arrhythmias.
- Recognize life-threatening arrhythmias and understand when immediate intervention is required.

Key Terms

Arrhythmia
Carina
Costochondral
Cystoscopy
Depolarization
Enterocentesis
Gastroscopy
Holter monitor
Hysteroscopy
Paroxysmal
Peritonitis
Repolarization
Retroflex
Surfactant
Rhythm strip
Telemetry

Clinical Case Problem 7.1

An irregular cardiac rhythm develops in a horse being treated for diarrhea. Describe the lead system and electrode placement used to obtain a rhythm strip in a horse. What is your rhythm diagnosis? Is this a life-threatening arrhythmia? What further diagnostics might you consider in this case relative to determining the cause of the arrhythmia?

See Clinical Case Resolution 7.1 at the end of this chapter.

Large Animal Medicine for Veterinary Technicians, Second Edition. Edited by Sue Loly and Heather Hopkinson.

Companion website: www.wiley.com/go/loly/veterinary

Introduction

Diagnostic procedures are performed to collect samples and information from a patient in order to determine the causes of illness and severity, and sometimes to monitor the response to a treatment.

Sedation or restraint may be needed to safely perform the procedure, depending on the species involved. The doses and types of sedatives are often selected based on species, potency, and side effects of each medication. Bovine, small ruminants, and equine oftentimes tolerate the procedure without sedation, as long as some form of physical restraint (nose tongs or twitch respectively) is applied. The use of exam stocks (open sides) can greatly enhance restraint and movement during the procedure. On the other hand, camelids need to be sedated in order to execute the procedure and minimize complications. Butorphanol tartrate is often the drug of choice, due to its analgesic and sedative properties. A single intramuscular dose of 0.04–0.08 mg/kg (0.02–0.04 mg/lb) can provide adequate sedation and analgesia, with less risk of recumbency. The use of stocks with camelids is recommended. If any animal, independently of the species, is nervous during handling, sedation should be considered.

Abdominocentesis

Indication

Analysis of peritoneal fluid obtained by abdominocentesis is a useful diagnostic and prognostic aid to assess pathological conditions involving the abdominal cavity. Several disorders within the abdominal cavity, including gastrointestinal disease, uterine disease, bacterial infection, splenic or hepatic torsion, urinary tract leakage, and neoplasia, have been diagnosed with peritoneal fluid analysis in conjunction with other tests. Though repeated abdominocentesis may be indicated to monitor changes in the abdominal fluid, studies have shown that repeating at 24-h intervals has no effect on peritoneal fluid constituents in the horse. Different Veterinarians have different preferences for supplies used for an abdominocentesis (Box 7.1).

> **TECHNICIAN TIP 7.1:** Different Veterinarians have different preferences for supplies used for an abdominocentesis.

Box 7.1 Supplies for Abdominocentesis

- sedation/restraint
- clippers with #40 surgical blades
- surgical preparation solutions (iodine or chlorhexidine based) and isopropyl alcohol
- sterile gloves
- syringe (10 ml)
- needles (18-gauge)
- teat cannula
- collection tubes (plain tube, potassium-EDTA tube)
- #15 scalpel blade
- local anesthetic (lidocaine/mepivacaine)

Patient Prep

Several sites are available for performing abdominocentesis, depending on the species, and either a blind or an ultrasound-guided technique can be utilized. Transabdominal ultrasound helps to identify free fluid accumulations, and the proximity of any relevant anatomical structure, which may improve safety margins. Due to the unique anatomy of camelids and ruminants, transabdominal ultrasound is extremely helpful to consistently collect a high-quality sample.

Equine

In the equine, abdominocentesis can be easily performed at the most dependent part of the abdomen, 10–15 cm caudal to the xyphoid, at or 4–5 cm to the right of midline to avoid the spleen. Some veterinarians will prefer using an 18 g needle, while others will prefer a blunt tip teat cannula, which can be inserted after a stab incision is made.

Large Ruminants

Clinically significant peritoneal fluid collection in ruminants can become a challenge due to the unique anatomy: a large rumen, which occupies a significant amount of the abdominal cavity, extensive omentum, and a high propensity for fibrin deposition. The ideal site for abdominocentesis is near the disease process, under ultrasonographic guidance. If a specific disease site is not evident, four standard sites are available. The two caudal sites are 3–6 cm to the right and/or left of the caudal midline, 3–6 cm cranial to the mammary gland in the female or 3–6 cm caudal to the prepucial opening of the male. The two cranial sites are 3–6 cm to the right and/or left of the cranial midline at the most dependent site of the abdomen, around 5–6 cm caudal to the xiphoid process. In calves, peritoneal fluid can be collected along the ventral midline, 4 cm cranial to the umbilicus.

Small Ruminants

Abdominocentesis in small ruminants can be performed at four different sites, similar to large ruminants. The cranial sites are just caudal to the xiphoid and 2–5 cm to the right and/or left of midline. The caudal sites are just cranial to the mammary gland or scrotum, also 2–5 cm to the right and/or left of midline. The two caudal sites are more frequently used for diagnosis of uroperitoneum, which is the most common use of peritoneal fluid analysis in small ruminants.

Camelids

Similar to large ruminants, abdominocentesis in New World camelids is performed in the cranioventral region of the abdomen, and it bares the risk of gastrointestinal puncture, omental interference, and sample contamination. The modified paracostal approach is the most common and the safest technique for abdominocentesis in camelids. The abdominocentesis site in alpacas is around 1 cm dorsal and 3 cm caudal to the costochondral junction of the last rib, while in llamas it is around 2 cm dorsal and 5 cm caudal to the costochondral junction of the last rib.

Procedure

- Clip and sterile prep the site of choice.
- Once the site is appropriately cleaned and scrubbed, one of two techniques for abdominocentesis can be utilized: (i) using an 18- to 20-gauge needle, (ii) using a teat cannula. The second technique requires a local block (1–3 ml of local anesthetic subcutaneous and intramuscularly with a 25-gauge needle), and a skin stab incision, which is made with a #15 scalpel blade. While the first technique offers a higher risk of enterocentesis, the second increases the risk of blood contamination of the sample. One way to decrease the risk of blood contamination with the second technique is to place the teat cannula through a single sterile gauze before entering the body wall. This step will avoid blood from the skin incision dripping into the collection tubes.
- Once either the needle or cannula is through the body wall, fluid may be observed at the hub if not draining (Figure 7.1).
- If fluid is not evident, a small amount of air can be injected to remove a possible tissue plug or a slight rotation of the needle/cannula may facilitate fluid drainage. Collect fluid via gravity flow into sterile tubes (serum and with EDTA) Attempts to aspirate the fluid with a syringe are usually unsuccessful because either omentum or peritoneal fat end up plugging the needle/cannula.
- Once a sample is obtained, the teat cannula/needle is then withdrawn, and the skin incision left to heal by second intention.

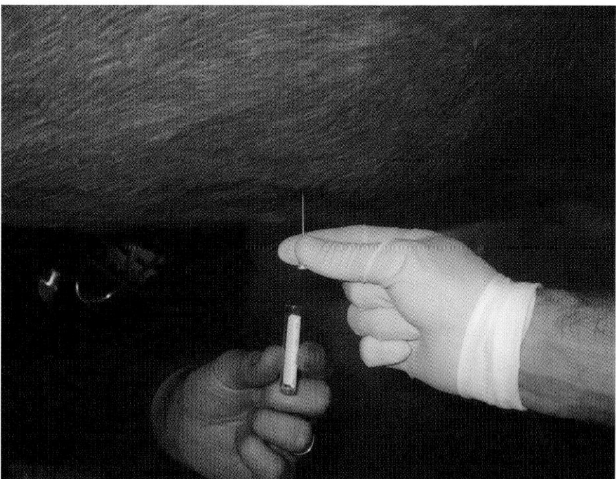

Figure 7.1 Abdominocentesis on a horse.

> **TECHNICIAN TIP 7.2:** Shake out the EDTA from the tube before collection in order to have a more accurate sample to EDTA ratio.

Post-procedure

Given that abdominocentesis is frequently performed in animals with distended viscera, care should be taken to avoid enterocentesis. The presence of ingesta in the abdominal fluid suggests either a ruptured viscous or accidental enterocentesis. In the event of an accidental enterocentesis, the needle should be immediately removed, and the patient monitored closely for any signs of peritonitis. However, if after repeated abdominocentesis ingesta remains present in the fluid, it usually indicates a ruptured viscous, which carries a grave prognosis.

Pregnant mares sustain the risk of amniocentesis. If pure blood is collected during abdominocentesis, spleen puncture should be suspected. In this case, a packed cell volume of the collected fluid will be like a packed cell volume of the patient's whole blood. Blood contamination of the sample can easily change the gross appearance of the fluid. If specimen is uniformly bloody or discolored throughout collection, and at different sites, hemoabdomen is likely. If the peritoneal fluid is normal, the fluid can be centrifugated and a small sediment of red blood cell will collect at the bottom of the tube, leaving a normal peritoneal fluid on top.

Evaluation

Abdominal fluid should be evaluated grossly for clarity, color, opacity, and odor. Normal equine peritoneal fluid has a clear, colorless to light yellow appearance. The total protein of normal abdominal fluid in horses is <2–2.5 g/dl, but it can increase with gastrointestinal disease. Total nucleated cell count is typically less than 10 000/μl, and often below 5000/μl in mature or aged horses. In addition, several other parameters, such as fibrinogen, lactate, phosphate, glucose, and pH, can be measured from abdominal fluid.

Normal peritoneal fluid for ruminants should be clear and colorless to straw-colored. Even though there is a wide range in cattle, it is considered normal when the total protein is less than 3.0 g/dl and a total nucleated cell count is less than 5000 cell/μl.

In healthy camelids, normal abdominal fluid typically contains a low cell count and protein concentration, with similar electrolyte levels when compared to venous blood. A large amount of fluid, or a high cell count (>3000 nucleated cells/ml) and protein concentration (>2.5 g/dl), likely indicates the presence of gastrointestinal disease.

Arthrocentesis

Indication

This procedure is used to collect and evaluate synovial fluid, the viscous lubricant from a joint capsule. A similar technique can be used to also flush a joint or instill a medication. Collection of synovial fluid is used to help identify inflammation and/or sepsis of a region.

Patient Prep

Provide adequate restraint appropriate for the patient and the area being sampled. Sedation is often not required; however, it will depend mostly on the type of patient, area being tapped, and demure of the patient. See Box 7.2 for supplies list. Horses will often stand for a fetlock joint sampling or injection, but an adult cow with a painful septic joint likely will require some chemical sedation and restraint.

- clip selected areas with #40 clipper blades, allowing for 1–2-in area around the estimated target entry spot
- surgical sterile scrub sample location

Box 7.2 Supplies for Arthrocentesis

- sedation/restraint
- clippers with #40 surgical blades
- surgical preparation solutions (iodine or chlorhexidine based and isopropyl alcohol)
- sterile gloves
- syringes (3–10 ml)
- collection tubes (plain sterile or red top tube, potassium-EDTA tube)
- 20 g 1-in needles (ideal for distal limb joints that are superficial)
- 6–10-in spinal needle (for deep joints like sacroiliac, coxofemoral, scapular bursa)
- optional: ultrasound for deep landmarks

Procedure

Arthrocentesis procedure will vary significantly according to the anatomical location area of interest. Needle insertion for most distal limb joints will be approximately 0.5 cm or less. In most circumstances and unless otherwise indicated, large adult patients should be sampled while fully weight bearing. Smaller patients, including neonates, may need to be restrained in lateral recumbency.

Coffin and Pastern Joint Taps

Coffin and pastern joint taps are ideally done while weight bearing. A dorsal or lateral approach is considered ideal for sampling and for the safety of the operator.

Fetlock Arthrocentesis

Fetlock arthrocentesis is again ideally performed with the patient weight bearing. A choice of three entry points can be made between the proximal-palmar/plantar, distal palmar/plantar, or dorsal aspects of the joint.

Carpal Joints

Carpal joints are generally easy to tap with the limb in a flexed position and entering with a dorsal approach to the radiocarpal or middle carpal joint.

Tarsal Joints

Tarsal joints can be tapped with a dorsal approach to the tibiotarsal joint, 2–4 cm below the medial malleolus. A plantarolateral approach to the tarsometatarsal joint can also be effective and both may be necessary since tarsal joint communication varies between patients (Figures 7.2 and 7.3).

Sacroiliac

Sacroiliac arthrocentesis may be performed based on anatomical boney landmarks or may be ultrasound-guided. A stab incision is made at the entry site of the needle, 2-cm cranial to the cranial aspect of the contralateral tuber sacral (TS) to reduce skin resistance during needle advancement. A 10-in, 15-gauge curved or bent needle is then advanced along the medial aspect of the iliac wing to the dorsal surface of the sacrum.

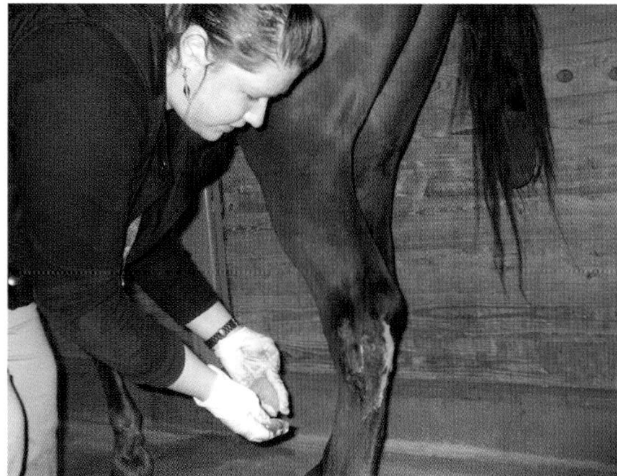

Figure 7.2 Preparing a tarsus joint for sampling.

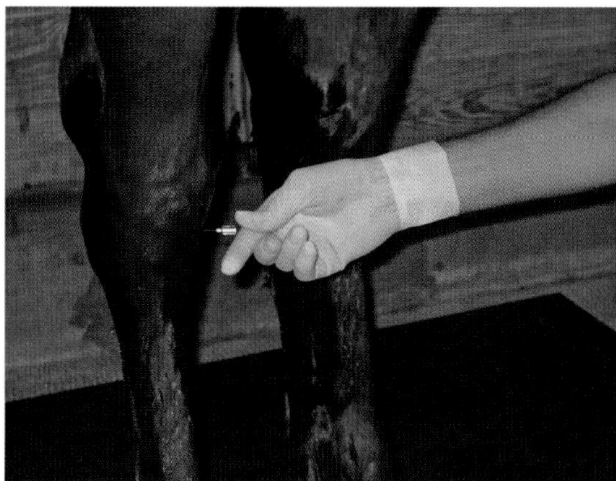

Figure 7.3 Arthrocentesis of the tibiotarsal joint in an adult horse.

Coxofemoral Joint

A Coxofemoral joint can be located and penetrated at the craniodorsolateral aspect under ultrasonographic guidance using a 10-in, 15-gauge spinal needle.

Evaluation

Regardless of the species being evaluated, normal synovial fluid should appear pale yellow, clear, and viscous.

Nucleated cell counts should be less than 500/μl. Total solids should be less than 2 g/dl. Synovial fluid glucose and lactate levels are also considered helpful in determining sepsis or other diseases. Lactate is considered a more useful piece of information related to acute conditions. Normal synovial lactate is considered 1.2–2.7 mmol/l and increases greater than 3–4 mmol/l could be indicative of a disease process. Synovial glucose levels should be equal to systemic blood values. A decreased value could be indicative of sepsis or other articular disease.

In addition, samples may be submitted for bacterial culture, cytology, electrolyte levels, and Gram stain.

Bronchoalveolar Lavage (BAL)

Indication

The bronchoalveolar lavage, or BAL, is one of the most useful diagnostic procedures used for respiratory workups. It allows for sampling of cells in the lower airway for diagnostic purposes. It can also be used for the collection of healthy pleural cells or surfactant for administration to a patient in need of pleural lipids and proteins. If multiple diagnostics are being used to gather information, the BAL procedure should be performed after completion of a TTW. There are two common techniques for performing a BAL, the blinded technique is described in this section, and the guided endoscopic technique is described later in this chapter under endoscopic techniques. See Box 7.3 for supplies list.

Patient Prep

Essentially, no special patient preparation is required for this procedure beyond sedation of the patient and the use of proper restraint. Sedation is recommended for this procedure to reduce the amount of coughing and movement from the patient during collection. It is advisable to clean the patient's nares prior to beginning.

Procedure

The BAL catheter is an open-end silicone heavy wall catheter for the lavage of selected segments of the lung fields (Figure 7.4). For this procedure, it is advisable to have one person restraining the animal, one person to pass and hold

Box 7.3 Supplies for BAL

- sedation/restraint
- 10 ml local anesthetic (2% lidocaine or similar) diluted into a 60 ml syringe of sterile saline
- 500 ml sterile saline
- 5–6, 60 ml luer syringes containing sterile buffered saline
- BAL catheter (clean or preferably sterilize)
- 6 ml empty syringe
- three-way stopcock
- sterile gloves
- sodium heparin or EDTA anticoagulant vacutainer
- empty sterile sample container(s) or red top tubes
- sterile culture tube (aerobic and anaerobic)

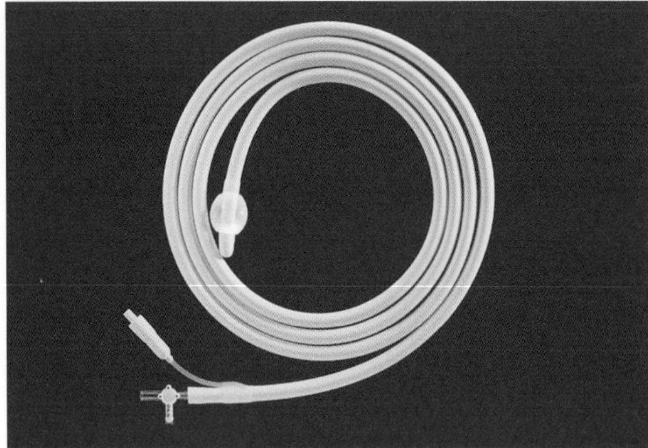

Figure 7.4 Bronchoalveolar lavage catheter.
Source: Reproduced with permission of MILA International, Inc.

the BAL catheter in place, and a third person to flush and withdraw samples (Figure 7.5).

- Pass lavage tube through one of the nares, through the sinus, and toward the trachea.
- Advance the tube blindly down the patient's airway, past the bifurcation of the primary bronchi until resistance is felt and the tube is wedged.

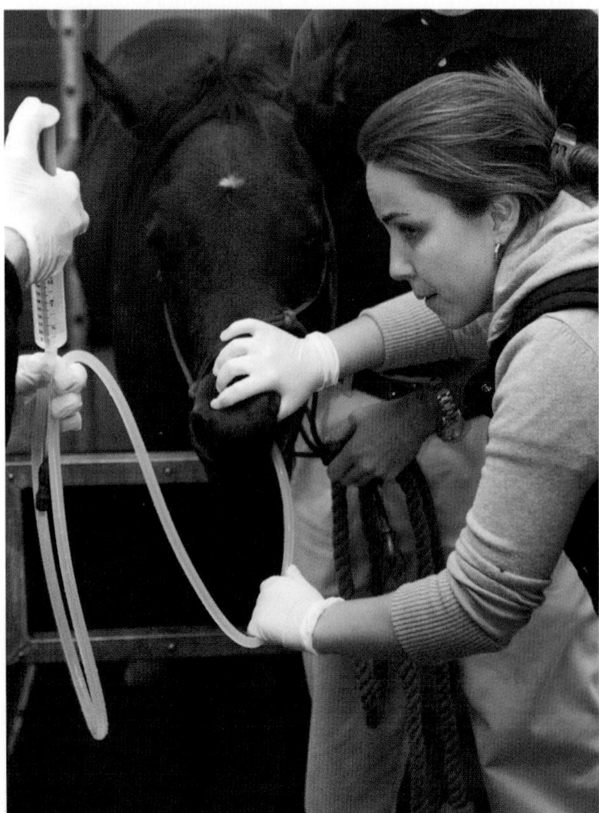

Figure 7.5 Bronchoalveolar lavage syringe being performed on a sedated horse. *Source:* Courtesy of Dr. Christie Ward.

- Inflate the distal balloon with approximately 5 ml of air to prevent retrograde fluid flow. At this time, some clinicians will choose to instill 30–60 ml of lidocaine, while others will prefer to move forward with the procedure in a timely manner.
- Push 150–500 ml of sterile saline is through the catheter into the dead space of the lung field that is beyond the wedged catheter. Some patients may begin coughing as this occurs. The goal is to instill as little fluid as possible and to yield 30–50 ml of sample volume.
- As soon as the saline has been administered, the process should be reversed, and suction of the fluid begins. With a negative pressure on the syringe, the operator should draw back fluid until no more is easily retrieved. The initial part of the sample typically looks much like the saline that was put in, but the end of the sample, also known as surfactant, should appear foamy.
- When the fluid is collected, it brings with it the alveolar compounds like emulsifiers that reduce surface tension between a gas and a liquid and allow the transfer of oxygen into the bloodstream. This sample is also referred to as surfactant (Figure 7.6). This may take two or three 60 ml syringes to accomplish. Once the sample has been collected, the catheter's balloon can be deflated, and the tube can be removed from the airway.

Some BAL catheters have proximal two-way fitting, which allows simultaneous connection for both irrigation and aspiration. If it does not, some operators prefer to use a three-way stopcock at the end of the BAL tube. This is optional and up to the particular operator's discretion.

> **TECHNICIAN TIP 7.3:** The goal of the BAL is to instill as little fluid as possible and to yield 30–50 ml of sample volume.

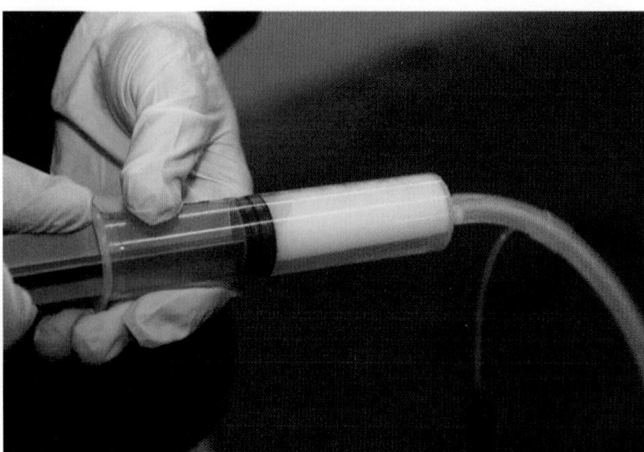

Figure 7.6 Bronchoalveolar lavage syringe with surfactant sample. *Source:* Courtesy of Dr. Christie Ward.

Evaluation

Samples should be submitted to the lab for cytology and cell evaluation. Sample centrifugation is often required for cytology evaluation because of low cellularity of BAL samples. There should be minimal to no mucous found. Common cellular findings are columnar epithelia cells, macrophages, and lymphocytes, and occasional eosinophils or mast cells (<2%), neutrophils (<5%).

Precautions

BAL procedures should not be performed on patients that are in severe respiratory distress, tachycardia, or pulmonary hypertension.

Blood Sampling

Blood sampling and the supplies needed for large animals varies between species and size of the patient. Being prepared with the correct supplies and restraint are keys to success. Patients can easily become distressed during restrain procedure, their well-being must always be considered and monitored. Give the animal a break if it appears distressed or shows signed of respiratory compromise. If the blood vessel has been punctured, be sure to hold off appropriately to avoid bleeding. The initial entry through the skin is usually the most irritating part of the procedure, having to repeat entry through the skin multiple times will generally cause the animal to become irritated. In many cases, it can be easier to get the needle through the skin, sticking with the patient if they move or react, and then proceeding with redirection to enter the vessel.

Equipment for blood sampling from a blood vessel can be the drawer's preference of either a vacutainer system or needle and syringe. Smaller patient like lambs, crias, and small foals warrant smaller gauge 25–22 g needles (Figure 7.7). Adult camelid, and horse blood sampling typically use 22, 20, or 18 g needle size, and large ruminants with thick skin can require 18, 16 g, or even 14 g needles depending on the anatomical location and approximate size of the blood vessel. In other words, a smaller gauge needle should be used for a cow's coccygeal (tail) vein than for its jugular. It is important to consider alternate sites for sampling, particularly when the patient has an indwelling catheter, hematoma, sepsis, localized cellulitis, or just for patient procedure tolerance.

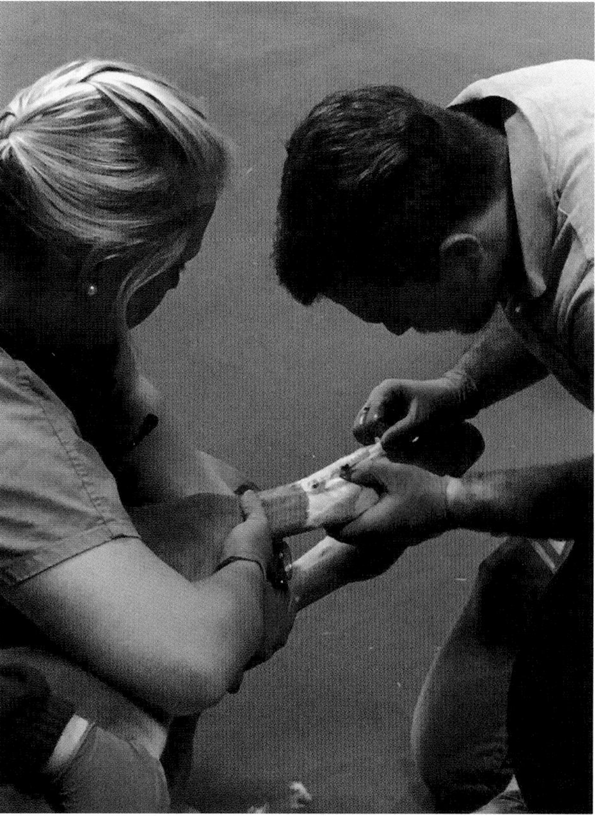

Figure 7.7 Sampling from the palmar digital vein in the hind leg of a foal.

Anterior Vena Cava

The anterior vena cava is a blood sampling location used only in swine. Large swine can remain standing, snared for restraint, and therefore are much more tolerant than some other options. The needle is inserted along the front of the breastbone, directed inward and upward slightly toward the spine (Figure 7.8). One must use caution if redirecting the needle in order to avoid acerating the jugular, causing hemorrhage. Needle gauge varies according to the size of the animal, from 20 g 1″ in piglets to 16 g 4″ in a large boar.

Auricular (Ear) Vein

The auricular or marginal ear vein may be suitable for blood sampling or placement of an intravenous catheter in some swine. Most swine, industrial or pet, are not likely to favor restraint and sampling from the ear. Restraint can also be stressful, hard on both the staff and the patient. Swine can also be quite loud when they object; therefore, staff should consider wearing hearing protection. An intramuscular injection of chemical restraint should also be considered for this procedure. An assistant can occlude the vein or a rubber band can be placed at the base of the ear.

Coccygeal (Tail) Vein

The coccygeal vein is a popular option for blood sampling in cattle and some swine but poorly tolerated in horses. The

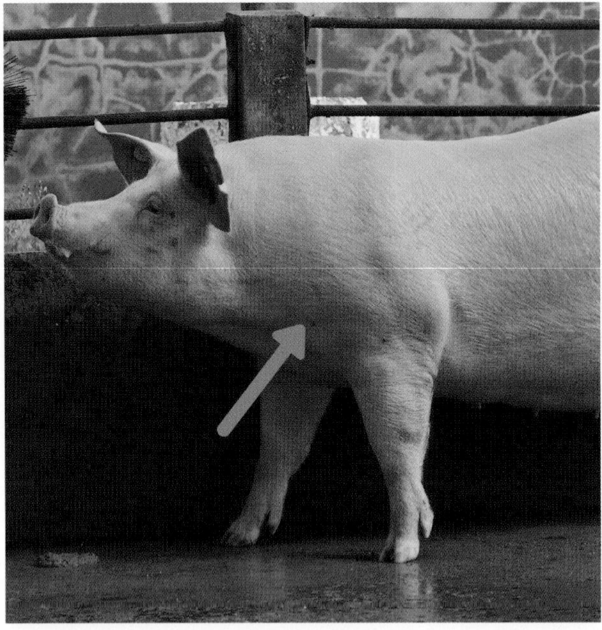

Figure 7.8 Angle of the needle/syringe for blood sampling of the anterior vena cava of a pig.

underside of the animal's tail is most often hairless. The animal should be well-restrained and the tail should be cleaned of any feces or debris prior to sampling. Hold the tail approximately 1/3 away from the base. Access the ventral surface by raising the tail vertically until it is horizontal with the ground (Figure 7.9). Palpate to locate the space between two coccygeal vertebrae and the underlying groove in the midline of the tail in the proximal ¼ of the tail base. Insert the needle at a perpendicular angle to the surface of the skin and advance a few millimeters deep to the vessel. Either a needle and syringe or a vacutainer system can be used for collection, depending on the amount of sample required.

Femoral Vein

The femoral vein is more often utilized in smaller patients that can be restrained in a lateral recumbency, much like sampling in a dog or cat. The restrainer can both control the animal and hold off the vein and the base of the limb. This technique works well for crias, foals, lambs, and kids provided the animal does not struggle excessive or show signs of significant respiratory distress.

Jugular Vein

The jugular vein is the most common place to draw blood from in adult horses, llama, and alpacas (Figure 7.10). Occlude the jugular vein 2–3 in below the desired sampling area by applying pressure in the jugular groove. When possible with large ruminants, use a halter to control and secure their head, tie to the side if possible, exposing the jugular vein. In small ruminants, they can be positioned much like a large dog, with the handler bracing behind them and extending the head upward, exposing the jugular veins for the drawer sitting in front of them.

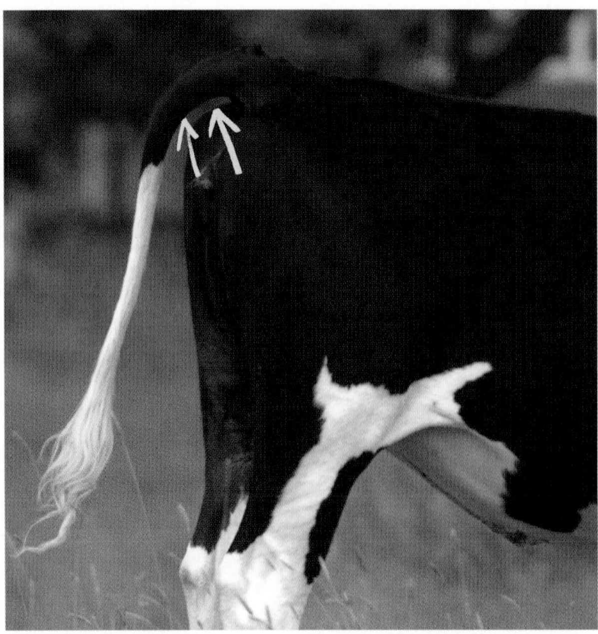

Figure 7.9 Location for sampling from the coccygeal vein of a cow.

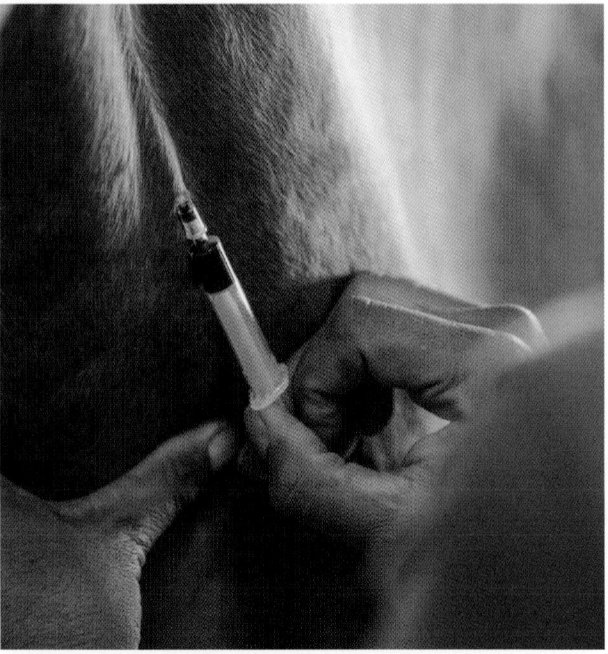

Figure 7.10 Blood draw from the jugular of a horse.

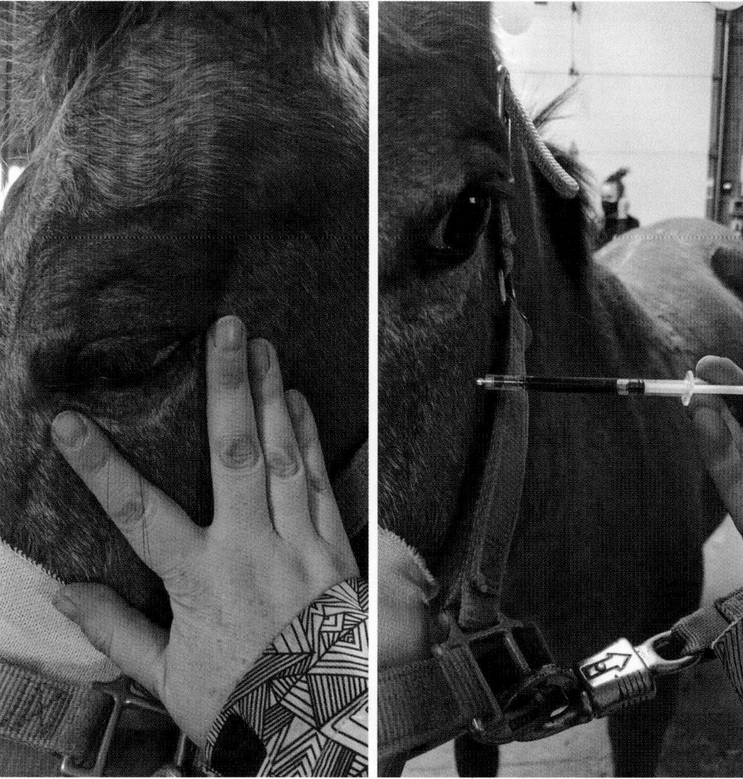

Figure 7.11 Blood draw from the facial sinus of a horse.

Transverse Facial Venous Sinus

Horses generally tolerate blood sampling of the transverse facial venous sinus quite well. It is located a couple of inches below the eye where the transverse facial vein dilates. It is relatively easy to locate by placing your index finger at the medial canthus of the eye and your thumb at the lateral canthus, the point of the hand that forms the bottom of the "V," which should be below the facial crest, is the point of the venipuncture site (Figure 7.11). A 1″ 20 or 22 g needle can be inserted at a 60–90° angle through the skin all the way down to the bone, aiming toward the base of the facial crest. If no blood flows, rotate the needle and aspirate or redirect until a blood flash appears. Backing out just slightly can also help. The operator may feel a slight crepitus from connective tissue during the procedure.

Other

Cephalic and saphenous veins are more commonly used in smaller sized large animals like lambs and crias. They can be held and restrained similar to a dog or cat with the handler holding off the vein from the base of the limb. Use of the cephalic vein of sampling purposes is rarely done in adult horses and cattle. Lateral thoracic veins are also seldom used in blood sampling.

Sampling through a venous or arterial catheter is another way to obtain a blood sample for testing and it avoids sticking the patient. This is commonly done during anesthetic procedures for monitoring patient blood values but can be done at other times as well. It is critical to ensure that an adequate, undiluted sample is obtained. One must keep in mind that blood catheter is flushed with hep/saline before clamping, so the first part of anew sample could be diluted; therefore, 1–2 ml of blood should be removed before taking the sample. For small patients such as neonates, they can become anemic if blood samples are taken frequently. This is an occasion to perform a three-syringe technique (Box 7.4 and Figure 7.12).

First draw a volume of 5 ml blood from the catheter using the syringe with 1 ml of heparin. Mix the sample within the syringe. Next draw the blood sample needed for testing in the second syringe. Return the first syringe of blood and heparin to the patient via the catheter, ensuring first that clotting has not occurred. Then flush the catheter with the hep/saline solution and clamp closed.

Box 7.4 Three-Syringe Technique

1 – 6 cc syringe with 1 ml of hep saline
1 – syringe, sized appropriate for blood sampling
1 – 6 cc syringe with flush

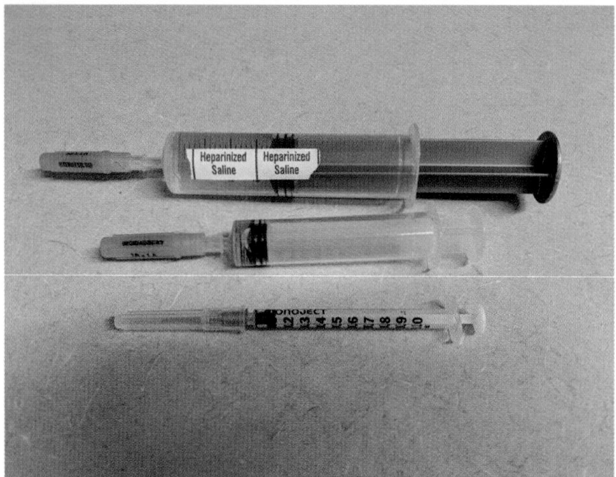

Figure 7.12 Syringes ready for the three-syringe technique.

Biopsies

Bone Marrow Biopsy

Indication

The primary function of bone marrow is the production of erythrocytes, leukocytes, and platelets. Bone marrow biopsy may be indicated to provide diagnostic or prognostic evaluation in patients with anemia, lethargy, weight loss, or neoplastic cells identified on CBC. See Box 7.5 for supplies list.

Patient Prep

- Prepare supplies and Sedate patient (Box 7.5).
- Palpate the sternum from the point between the forelimbs caudally (approximately 16 cm) to identify the caudal most aspect of the sternum.

Box 7.5 Supplies for Bone Marrow Biopsy

- sedation
- clippers with #40 surgical blades
- surgical preparation solutions (iodine or chlorhexidine based)
- local anesthetic (2% lidocaine or similar)
- #15 scalpel blade
- 11-gauge 4-in bone marrow biopsy needle or EZ-IO® Intraosseous Infusion System
- 60 ml luer syringe
- sterile gloves
- sodium heparin, EDTA, or sodium citrate anticoagulant solution
- sterile dry gauze sponges
- glass slides
- EDTA and red top vacutainer tubes
- skin staples or suture material

- Clip and aseptically prepare an area directly between the forelegs and extending at least 8–10 cm caudally and 2 cm laterally of the sternal midline.
- Block an area approximately 8 cm cranial to the caudal most aspect of the ilium with approximately 6 ml of local anesthetic. Local anesthetic should affect subcutaneous tissues as well as the deep muscle and periosteal layers of the sternum.

Procedure

- The sampler must be familiar with the function of the bone marrow needle or EZ-IO tool prior to sample collection (Figures 7.13 and 7.14).
- Make a stab incision through the skin and deeper subcutaneous tissue with the scalpel blade to the point of the sternum.
- Insert the needle through the incision approximately 2 cm cranial to the ventral sternum, carefully angled cranially.

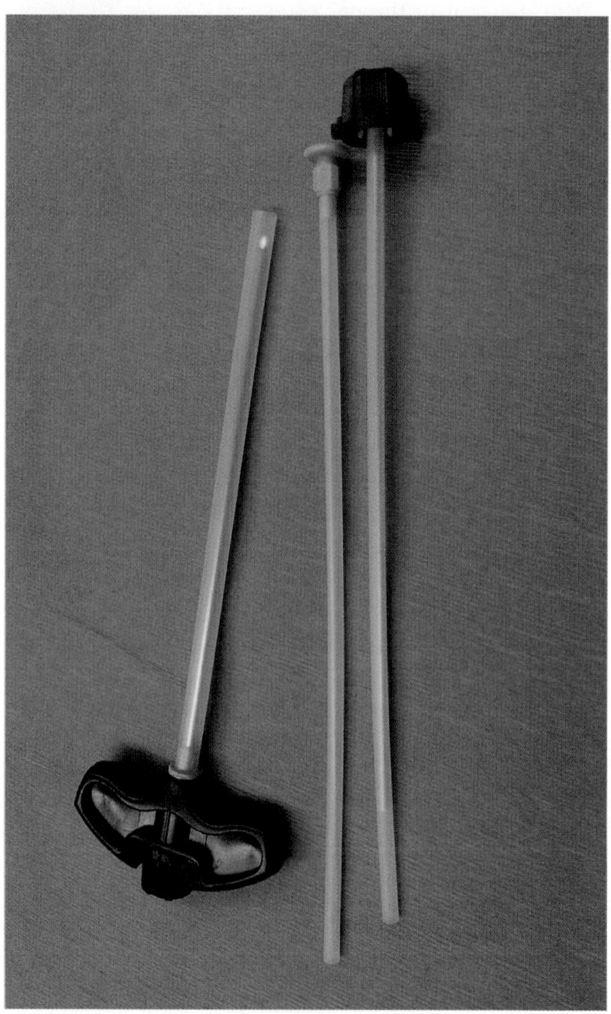

Figure 7.13 Common bone marrow biopsy needle with stylet.

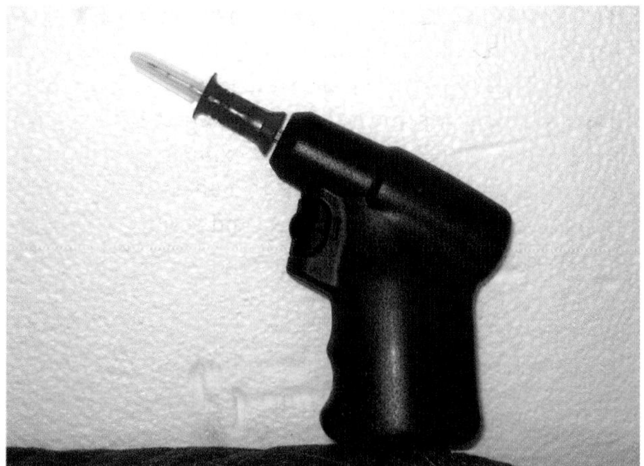

Figure 7.14 EZ-IO® driver used for bone marrow biopsy. *Source:* Reproduced with permission from Vidacare®.

- Once direct sternal contact has been confirmed, gently rotate the needle using mild, controlled force until the needle extends approximately 3 cm into the sternum. To avoid puncturing through the dorsal sternum, it is important that the needle not be inserted more than 3 cm.
- Remove the obturator and attach a 60 ml syringe preloaded with anticoagulant solution directly to the needle.
- Obtain 5–7 ml of bone marrow aspirate. To create sufficient negative pressure for aspiration of the thick bone marrow, withdraw the plunger the length of the syringe. It may take 1–2 min of constant pressure to begin to retrieve the aspirate sample.
- Remove the needle and apply pressure for several minutes with dry sterile gauze sponges.
- Close incision with skin staples or suture(s).

Sample Handling

Smears can be made immediately using a slide-to-slide smearing technique. The remaining sample should be divided among EDTA and red top vacutainer tubes so that lab personnel may create new slides or for other lab processes.

Precautions

Potential complications of sternal bone marrow collection may include cardiac puncture, infection, or hemorrhage.

Submissions

A sample of systemic blood in EDTA should be obtained and CBC evaluated at the same time a bone marrow biopsy is submitted for evaluation and comparison.

> **TECHNICIAN TIP 7.4:** Do not use an extension set as its use tends to result in significant clotting and a lower volume sample.

Liver Biopsy

Indication

Patients with significantly abnormal liver blood chemistry values may benefit from a liver biopsy sampling to yield diagnostic, prognostic, and therapeutic information. This can be done using a choice of biopsies (Box 7.6, Figures 7.15 and 7.16). Potential diagnosis may include mineral concentrations, including copper analysis, acute hepatitis, toxic hepatopathy, hyperammonemia, icterus, or secondary photosensitization.

Patient Prep

Equine: Clip a 10 × 10 cm area at the patient's right side between the 12th and 14th intercostal spaces where a line drawn from the tuber coxae to the elbow intersects the selected intercostals space. Bovine: Clip a 10 × 10 cm area at the patient's right side at the 10th intercostal space where it intersects an imaginary line from the tuber coxa to the olecranon. Prepare skin for an aseptic procedure. Infiltrate

Box 7.6 Supplies for Liver Biopsy

- local anesthetic (2% lidocaine or similar)
- #11 scalpel blade (or similar)
- clippers with #40 surgical blades
- surgical preparation solutions (iodine or chlorhexidine based)
- sterile dry cotton gauze 8 × 8 cm^2 (or similar)
- sterile gloves
- small sterile drape for working surface (tray, table, or similar)
- non-sterile working surface (tray, table, or similar)
- liver biopsy instrument (14-gauge Tru-CutTM or Monopty biopsy needle, or similar)
- sterile sample container(s)
- buffered neutral formalin (for histopathology)

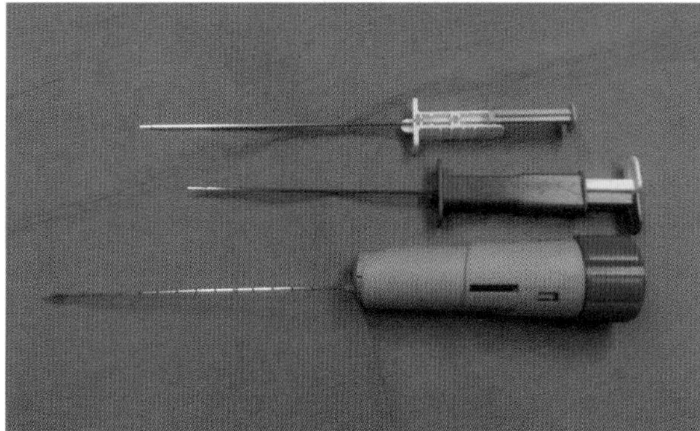

Figure 7.15 Tru-CutTM versus Monopty® biopsy instruments.

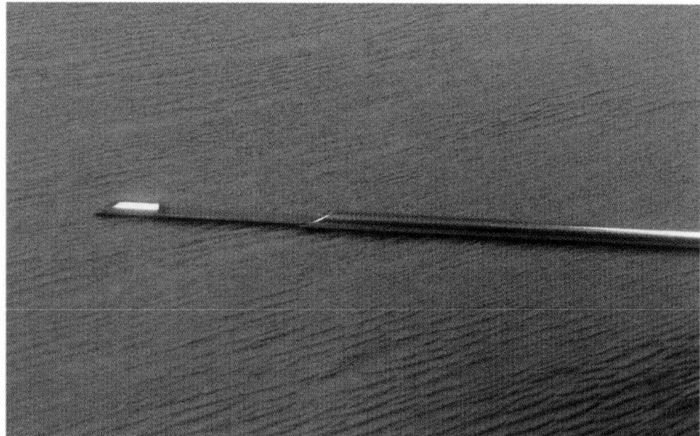

Figure 7.16 Tip of a liver biopsy instrument.

2–5 ml of lidocaine or other local anesthetic subcutaneously and deep into the intercostal muscles.

Procedure

- Ultrasound-guided biopsy will ensure accurate placement. Test the sampling instrument prior to use to ensure its proper function. Wearing sterile gloves, create a stab incision through the skin at the biopsy site.
- Insert the instrument through the stab incision and direct toward the left elbow. Increased resistance is felt as the needle enters the liver (Figure 7.17). Open and close the biopsy needle rapidly to obtain a sample. Withdraw the needle and check to ensure an adequate sample is obtained. Multiple samples may be safely obtained from the liver using the same instrument and stab incision and repeating the procedure.

Sample Handling

Take extreme care when reopening the biopsy instrument so the sample is not dropped or lost accidentally. Samples may be removed from the biopsy instrument using a sterile hypodermic needle and placed in plain sample containers or formalin for histopathology, then media is transported for microbiology evaluation.

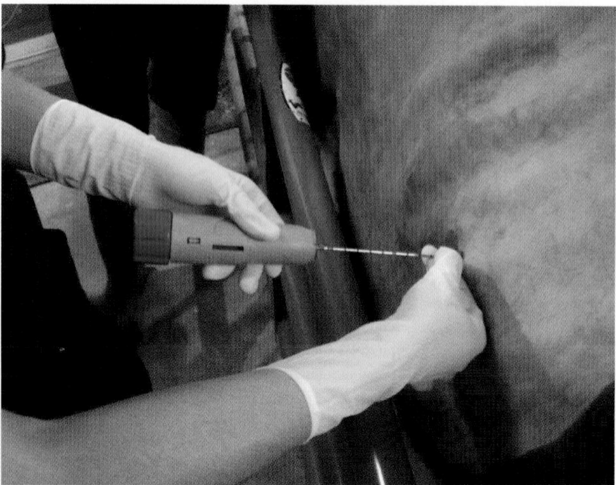

Figure 7.17 Liver biopsy on an adult cow using the Monopty instrument.

Post-procedure

Potential post-procedure complications include hemorrhage, spread of infectious hepatitis, peritonitis, or pneumothorax.

Submissions

Herd evaluation should include testing of at least seven animals per feeding group. At least 15 mg of sample is required for mineral analysis.

> **TECHNICIAN TIP 7.5:** A coagulation panel is recommended prior to a liver biopsy procedure.

Muscle Biopsy

Indication

Muscle biopsy can be indicated for various reasons, including diagnosis of Exertional Myopathies (including chronic exertional rhabdomyolysis syndrome [ER], polysaccharide storage myopathy [PSSM], or equine polysaccharide storage myopathy [EPSM]), equine motor neuron disease (EMND), immune-mediated myositis (IMM), or white muscle disease.

Patient Prep

Select the appropriate muscle for biopsy in order to get an accurate diagnosis.

ER and PSSM: biopsies of the semi-membranous and tendinous muscle

EMND: sacrocaudalis dorsalis coccygeus

IMM: semi-membranous and epaxial muscles

- prepare the supplies (Box 7.7)
- clip selected areas with #40 clipper blades
- surgical sterile scrub sample locations

Box 7.7 Supplies for Muscle Biopsy

- biopsy needle, modified Bergström 6 mm
- standard laceration pack including needle drivers, scalpel handle, thumb forceps
- suturing materials (for wedge and excision biopsies)
- local anesthetic (2% lidocaine or similar)
- #11 scalpel blade (or similar)
- animal clippers with #40 surgical blades
- surgical preparation solutions (iodine or chlorhexidine based and isopropyl alcohol)
- buffered neutral formalin

Procedure

- Tranquilize the patient.
- Wrap the tail if sampling on the hindquarters.
- Lidocaine is injected under the skin but not into the muscle belly.
- For a wedge biopsy (Figures 7.18 and 7.19):
  - A one-and-one-half-inch incision is made through the skin and subcutaneous fat and fascia.
  - Parallel longitudinal incisions are made in the muscle one-quarter inch apart.
  - The cranial aspect of the muscle is grasped with forceps and the muscle is dissected out one-quarter-inch deep and one-half-inch long.
  - Close dead space with subcutaneous layers.
  - Close skin with intradermal sutures or staples.
- For a biopsy using Bergström (Figure 7.20):
  - Make a stab incision at the skin's surface.
  - Insert the biopsy needle to the depth of the handle.
  - Open and close the instrument quickly and repeat 4–6 times.
  - Remove the instrument and reopen carefully over a sterile surface to capture the sample.

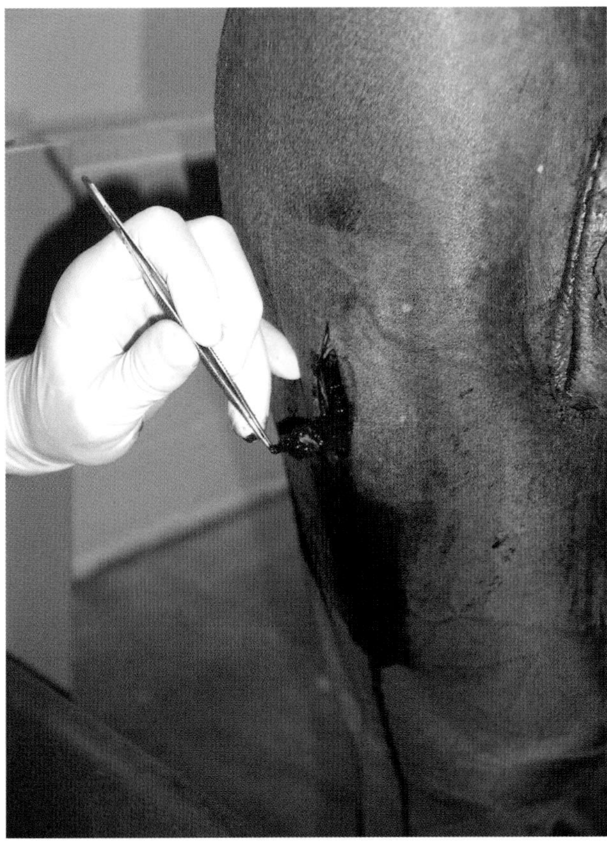

Figure 7.18 Muscle biopsy using a wedge technique from the semimembranosus/semitendinosus. *Source:* Reproduced with permission of Dr. Stephanie Valberg.

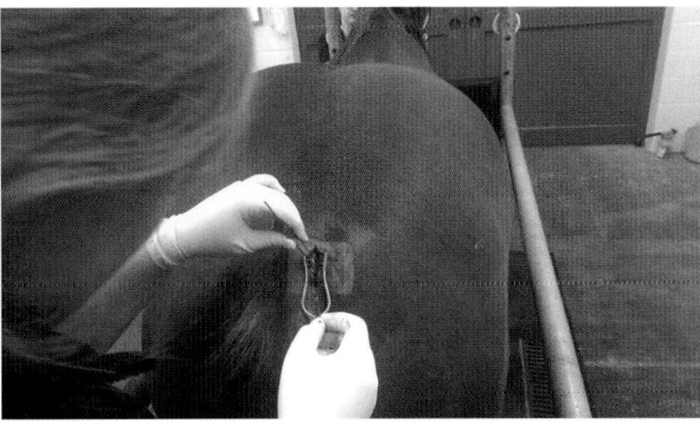

Figure 7.19 Muscle biopsy using a wedge technique from the sacrocaudalis dorsalis.

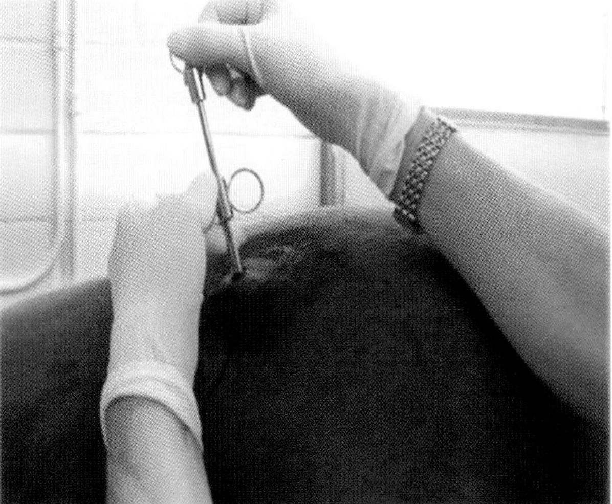

Figure 7.20 Muscle biopsy using a Bergström needle. *Source:* Reproduced with permission of Dr. Stephanie Valberg.

Sample Handling

- Avoid crushing, squeezing, or squishing the muscle sample, as that can damage cells.
- Fresh samples are best, frozen muscle samples require special processing to prevent ice crystals from forming vacuoles in the tissue.
- Fresh muscle should be wrapped in saline moistened gauze, placed in a hard, watertight container for protection, and shipped overnight on icepacks.
- Formalin fixed sample should sit in the air for 5 min before placing in formalin to prevent contraction bands from forming.

Post-procedure

Surgeons often recommend stall rest until the skin sutures are removed at 10–14 days after procedure, however, stall rest may not be ideal given the patient's neuromuscular condition. Typically, the sample location is not problematic for post-procedure complications.

Submissions

Muscle samples from EPSM/PSSM suspect horses are processed by the laboratory both for a routine stain and also with a special stain for glycogen.

US laboratories that accept fresh muscle samples include The Veterinary Pathology Laboratory at Oregon State University or The Neuromuscular Laboratory of the University of Michigan and University of Minnesota Equine Genetics and Genomics Laboratory.

Rectal Mucosal Biopsy

Indication

Rectal mucosal tissue sampling is a simple procedure to perform for evaluation of focal or diffuse inflammatory infiltration. It is thought to be indicative of intestinal function further proximal and may help evaluate inflammatory disorders including eosinophilic enterocolitis, granulomatous enteritis, or lymphocytic enterocolitis. See Box 7.8 for supplies list.

Patient Prep

- Patient's tail is wrapped and may be tied to one side dependent on the collector's preference.
- Since the sample is collected directly from the rectum, this procedure is not considered sterile; therefore, no further patient preparation is required.
- Patient may be given Butylscopolamine (Buscopan®) to aid in smooth muscle relaxation during the procedure.

Sampling

- The operator wears an obstetric sleeve and begins with manual evacuation of feces from the rectum, similar to preparing for rectal palpation.
- A sleeved hand then leads the biopsy instrument, with jaws closed, approximately 8 in into the rectum.
- Once in place, the instrument jaws can be opened and guided to one side for sampling.
- The instrument's jaws are closed to grab a sample of tissue and the instrument can be removed from the rectum.

Box 7.8 Supplies for Rectal Mucosal Biopsy

- an alligator-type biopsy rod is used to obtain the specimen, which should be at least 5 × 12 mm in diameter and preferably a basket approximately 3.5 × 2 cm (Figure 7.21).
- obstetric sleeve
- lubricant for rectal palpation
- 10% formalin and specimen cup

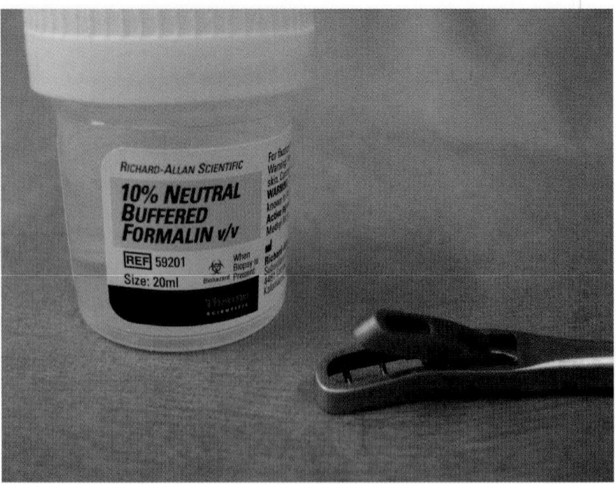

Figure 7.21 Alligator forceps with biopsy basket, commonly used for rectal mucosal and uterine biopsies.

- Lift sample from the basket with a 25 g sterile needle or forceps and place into solution.
- Collect multiple samples to ensure a good sample has been collected for evaluation.

Sample Handling

The specimens are placed in 10% formalin for at least 24 hr before proceeding with evaluation.

Post-Procedure

No suturing or patient care is required following this procedure. The patient's peritoneum should be cleansed following the procedure for hygiene and to prevent contamination of the mare's vulva.

Submissions

Once appropriately fixed in buffered formalin, samples can be transferred to a pathologist for cytological evaluation.

Uterine Biopsy

Indication

Endometrial uterine biopsies may be indicated as a part of a prepurchase, breeding soundness exam being performed for infertility concerns, or other abnormal clinical findings such as vaginal discharge or chronic uterine infections. A uterine biopsy is also warranted in mares over 12 years of age who have not had a foal within the last year.

Patient Prep

Samples are ideally obtained during diestrus or estrus. Diestral samples are preferred due to reduced physiological changes to the endometrium; however, it is easiest during

Box 7.9 Supplies for Uterine Biopsy

- An alligator-type biopsy rod is used to obtain the specimen, which should be at least 5 × 12 mm in diameter and preferably have a basket approximately 3.5 × 2 cm.
- sterile obstetric sleeve
- sterile lubricant
- cotton wash and mild soap
- Bouin's fixative or 10% formalin

estrus when the cervix is relaxed, and immune function is highest. See supply list in Box 7.9.

- Wrap the tail and tie to the side.
- Wash the perineum and lips of the vulva.

Sampling

- A sterile obstetric sleeved hand leads the biopsy instrument with jaws closed through the cervix and into the uterus.
- Once passed into the uterine lumen 2–3 cm, the instrument jaws can be opened, then advanced an additional 1–2 cm and to one side and cranial to be near the bifurcation.
- The instrument's jaws are closed to grab a sample of tissue and the instrument can be removed from the cervix.
- The endometrial sample is then gently lifted from the basket with a 25 g sterile needle or forceps and placed into solution.
- A retro-vaginal technique is also possible, first introducing the instrument into the uterine lumen as previously described, but then the operator withdraws the guiding hand, reintroducing it to guide per rectum. This style of collection is discouraged, as it is difficult to quickly return for an additional sample if needed (patient would need another full prep).
- Culture and cytology samples may also be collected at this time.

Sample Handling

Samples placed in Bouin's fixative should be transferred to 70% ethanol or 10% formalin after 3–4 h of fixation to prevent hardening of the tissue, which results in poor staining. Samples placed directly in a 10% buffered formalin solution should rest for 24 hr prior to further processing or evaluation.

Post-procedure

No suturing or patient care is required following this procedure. The mare's peritoneum should be cleansed to prevent contamination and for good measure.

Submissions

Samples are recommended to be evaluated by clinical pathologist or board certified theriogenologist with experience.

Skin Biopsy

Indication

A collection of one or more small samples is taken of full thickness integumentary, from a generalized or widespread lesion, for evaluating hair follicles, adrexal structures, and inflammation. Results can reveal potential autoimmune skin diseases, hair follicle disorders, deep infections, and cancer. Often, the skin biopsy is performed after a skin scrapping procedure and will allow the dermatologist to exclude several serious skin diseases if a specific cause cannot be identified.

Patient Prep

- Prepare supplies in advance. See Box 7.10 and Figure 7.22.
- Clipping of the hair may be warranted if the coat is long, but the surface of the skin should not be compromised for testing.
- No skin preparation, such as scrubbing, should be performed prior to sampling.

Box 7.10 Supplies for Skin Biopsy

- #15 scalpel blade and/or Keyes biopsy punch
- sterile sample containers
- local anesthetic
- buffered neutral formalin (for histopathology)
- suturing materials (for wedge and excision biopsies)
- may require sedation
- sterile gloves

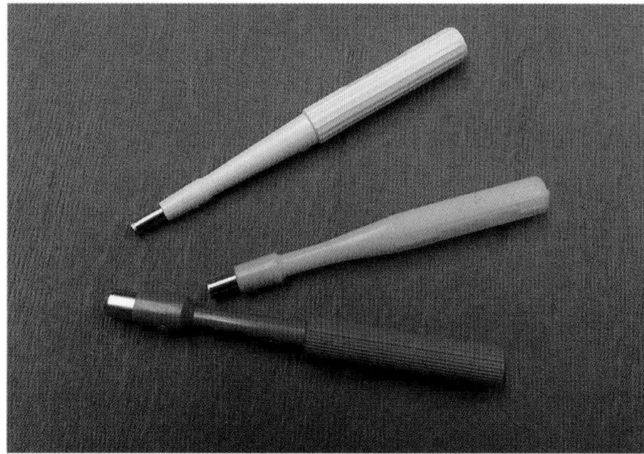

Figure 7.22 Punch biopsies in various sizes, commonly used for small skin biopsies.

- Superficial crusts can be removed if they are a hindrance.
- Local sedation should be avoided as not to compromise the integrity of the cells and structures being sampled.

Procedure

- Sedate patient to relieve anxiety related to sampling and any potential discomfort.
- Sampler should wear sterile gloves to avoid introducing anything additional to the sample during handling.
- Using a keyes biopsy tool: at a 90° angle to the skin, rotate the cylindrical blade while pressing into the skin to cut a full thickness sample.
- Using a scalpel blade: a wedge-shaped piece of full thickness skin should be created by the operator.
- Depending on the size of the biopsy, a small dissolvable suture or removable staple can be placed over the biopsy site to aid in healing.
- Take multiple samples and place into various mediums for transport. Care must be taken to ensure that no sample dries out during transport. If no transport medium is chosen, such as formaldehyde, and so forth, place the sample on a gauze square dampened with sterile water and in a secure container.

Post-procedure

Biopsy sites should be kept clean and dry for at least seven days. Suture or staple removal should occur at 10–14 days post-procedure.

Precautions

- Sample handling: Samples that are very small (<4 mm) are subject to crushing and distortion. Handle very carefully.
- Distortion and crushing of samples can occur due to stretching of skin during biopsy or crushing of tissue with scissors or large forceps.
- Inadequate fixing of large samples should be avoided by ensuring proper ratios are used.

Submissions

After sample collection, send the tissue to a dermatopathologist (pathologist who specializes in skin disease) for processing, microscopic evaluation, and interpretation. This process generally takes 7–10 days.

Cerebrospinal Fluid (CSF)

Indication

This procedure is a valuable tool, as the analysis of the fluid can determine if there is inflammation, infection, or neoplasia in the spinal canal of a patient exhibiting neurologic symptoms. Spinal fluid may be collected from either the atlantooccipital, Cervical 1–2 intervertebral space or lumbosacral spaces. Collection from the atlantooccipital space requires anesthesia, while the lumbosacral space is usually collected while under standing sedation, preferably in a set of stocks to help keep the patient from excessive swaying. After collection, it may be analyzed using a variety of tests, such as total protein, total cell count, differential cell count, and bacterial culture.

Patient Prep

Prepare the supplies in advance (see Box 7.11 and Figure 7.23). The patient should be held off-feed for a

Box 7.11 Supplies for CSF Tap

- injectable or inhalant anesthesia for atlantooccipital or sedation for C1–C2 or lumbosacral spaces
- clippers with #40 surgical blades
- surgical preparation solutions (iodine or chlorhexidine based)
- sterile dry cotton gauze 8 × 8 cm^2 (or similar)
- sterile gloves
- small sterile drape for working surface (tray, table, or similar)
- spinal needle, 18-gauge × 3-in for atlantooccipital location in the equine patient or for lumbosacral space in the ruminant; spinal needle, 18-gauge × 6-in for lumbosacral space in the equine
- 12 cc syringe(s)
- EDTA tubes and serum sample tubes
- transport media for microbiology evaluation

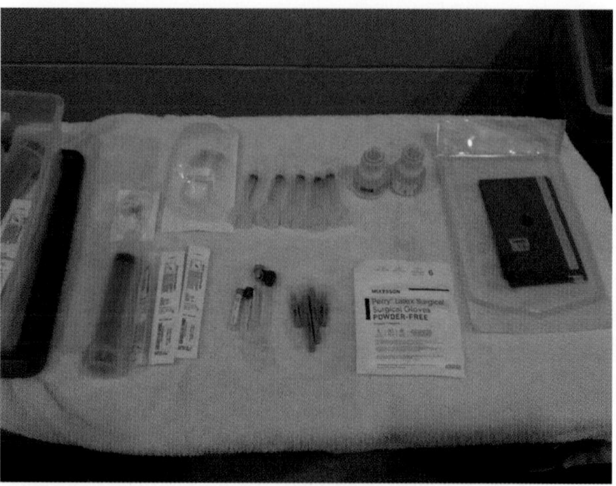

Figure 7.23 Supplies set up for a CSF tap.

minimum of 12 hr if undergoing general anesthesia. A 10 × 10 in square is clipped at the appropriate sampling site and then surgically scrubbed. For the atlantooccipital location, this is the area just caudal to the poll, on midline, at the level of the wings of the atlas. For lumbosacral, this is the area on the dorsal midline, at the level of the wings of the ilium. Landmarks for the lumbosacral site are the intersection of the imaginary lines joining the caudal borders of the tuber coxae along the midline or at the high point of the gluteal region of the horse.

Procedure

> **TECHNICIAN TIP 7.6:** Occlusion of the jugular veins can cause a concomitant increase in the CSF pressure, which may help facilitate the collection of the fluid.

- A sterile prep should be performed to the appropriate area.
- Infiltrate 2–5 ml of lidocaine or other local anesthetic subcutaneously and deep into the muscles.
- Perform another sterile prep.
- The clinician will advance the needle into the subarachnoid space. The patient may indicate discomfort when the needle is advanced into the space. The patient may exhibit discomfort by flagging their tail or hunching up the hindquarters. Less frequent but of special note is a violent reaction to the needle being advanced into the dura mater. Precautions should be taken not to endanger the clinician or the patient. Fluid may flow freely but more common of the lumbosacral tap is that it will need to be gently aspirated via a sterile syringe. Occluding both jugular veins may help to increase the amount of fluid collected.
- The fluid is placed in EDTA and serum tubes for submission to the lab, and the appropriate transport media is prepared. The clinician may choose to draw several syringes of fluid if they feel that the fluid in the first syringe may be contaminated with red blood cells due to a traumatic tap.

Atlantooccipital

General anesthesia is induced with either injectable or inhalant agents. Recovery is a concern with general anesthesia, as this procedure is performed on an already ataxic patient, and there is a greater risk of patient injury. The patient is placed in lateral recumbency with the patient's head flexed at the poll so that the median axis of the head is at a right angle to the median axis of the cervical vertebrae. This flexion allows the atlantooccipital space to open up and assists in fluid collection (Figure 7.24).

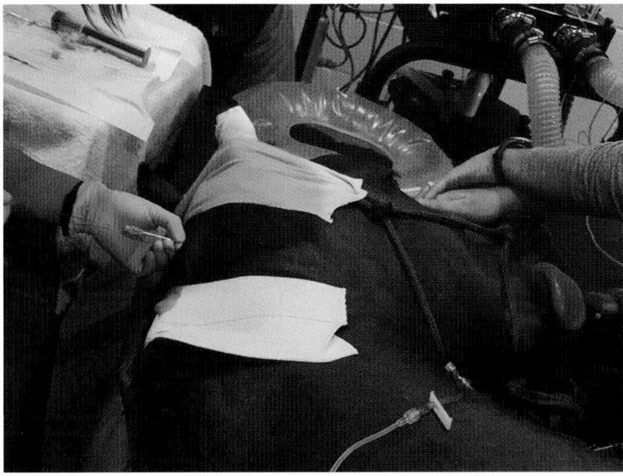

Figure 7.24 Atlantooccipital tap prior to a myelogram procedure on an adult horse.

Cervical 1–2

Ultrasound-guided cervical centesis is becoming more popular for CSF sampling. Sedate patient using titration techniques, as heavy sedation is contraindicated in ataxic patients. It may help to use a head stand to support the head and avoid motion during the sampling. An ultrasound is used to locate the intervertebral space and advance the needle into the space from a lateral approach (Figure 7.25).

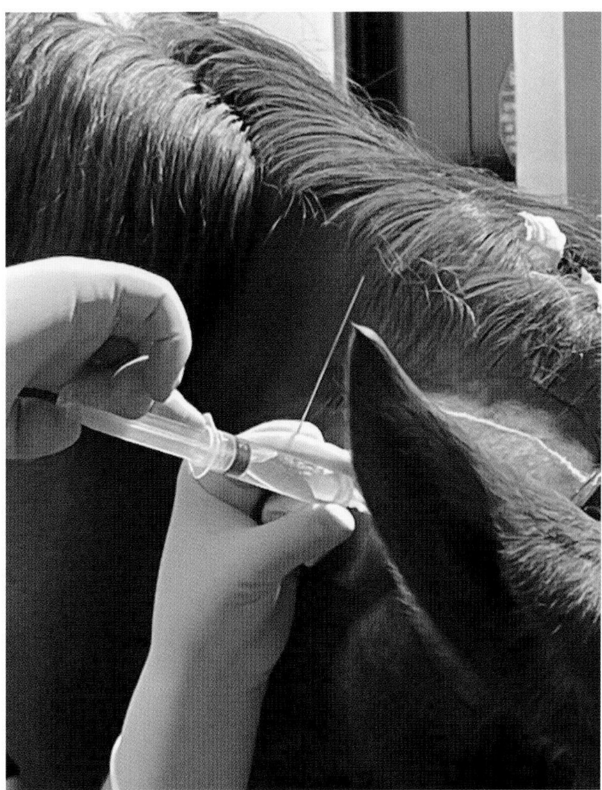

Figure 7.25 Ultrasound-guided lateral approach C1–C2 spinal tap.

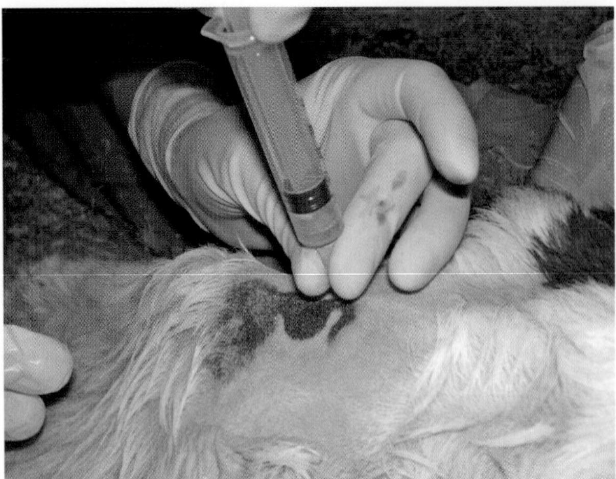

Figure 7.26 CSF Lumbosacral tap performed on a calf.

Lumbosacral

Sedate patient using titration techniques, as heavy sedation is contraindicated in ataxic patients. The patient must stand as squarely as possible with their weight evenly distributed on all four limbs. Excessive sedation will result in the patient swaying, which makes collection difficult, if not impossible, to complete. The depth of the lumbosacral space makes collection of the fluid more difficult than collection at the atlantooccipital space (Figure 7.26).

Post-procedure

Post-procedure complications may result in an infection, but it is uncommon. Clean collection area of any blood. Antibiotic ointment may be applied if desired.

Submissions

Normal CSF is clear, odorless, and colorless (Figure 7.27). The clinician will direct the veterinary technician as to which tests should be ordered. Submissions may include:

- total protein
- total cell count
- microscopic evaluations of cytology or Gram stain
- serology
- microbial culture and sensitivity

Coagulation Studies

Activated Clotting Time (ACT)

Indication

Activated clotting time (ACT) is a rapid, inexpensive test for clinically significant factors except factor VII. Prolonged times will not occur until 95% of factors are depleted. Activated partial thromboplastin time (APTT) will be prolonged when 70% of factors are depleted. See Box 7.12 for supplies list.

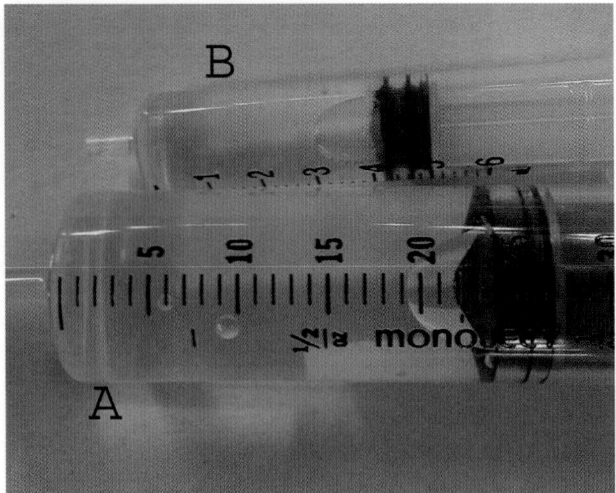

Figure 7.27 (a) Normal CSF fluid compared. (b) xanthochromia CSF fluid.

Procedure

Tubes should be pre-warmed to 37 °C. Jugular venipuncture should be performed per clinic protocol. The vein selected should reflect possible thrombolytic changes in the blood sample. Draw a 2 ml blood sample, transferring the blood to the tube, inverting the tube several times to mix. Timing begins. Tube is returned to the heat source and allowed to sit 60 S. At 60 S and every 5 S afterward, slightly tilt the tube to observe for clotting. Return the tube to the heat source between each observation. Results are recorded to the nearest 5-S increment when an unmistakable clot is observed.

Lab Results

Cow <145 S
Horse <40 S

Normals can be determined for the lab by testing 5–10 normal individuals.

Box 7.12 Coagulation Supplies

- non-vacuum diatomaceous earth blood tubes (Vetlab Supply, Inc.) (Figure 7.28)
- syringe and needle in size appropriate for patient
- blood sample ~2 ml
- 37 °C environment: water bath or heat block
- thermometer
- stopwatch

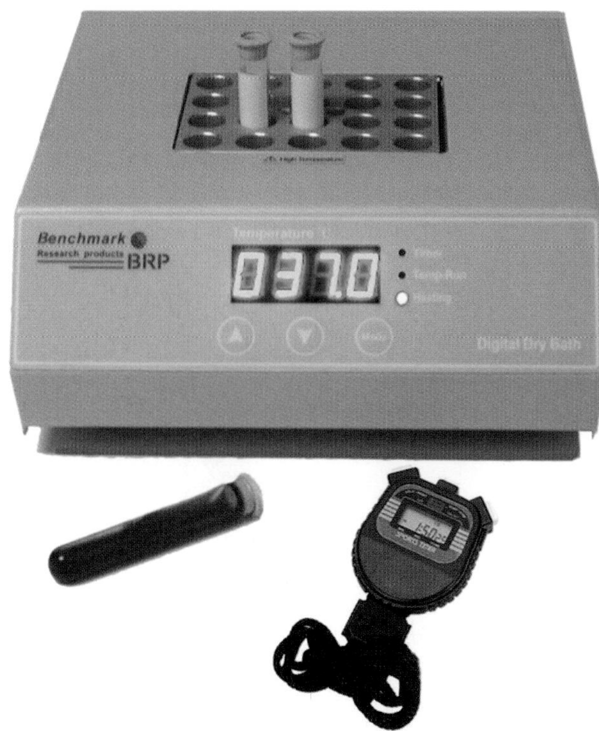

Figure 7.28 ACT system. *Source:* Courtesy of Vetlab Supply, Inc.

Aftercare

Normal hemostatic procedures of the venipuncture site should be performed and observed.

Adapted from Vetlab Supply, Inc.

Coombs' Test

Indication

Direct antiglobulin test is used to detect sensitization of erythrocytes by host antibody. The patient's RBCs, which are coated with anti-erythrocyte autoantibody *in vivo*, are collected, washed, and incubated *in vitro* with species-specific Coombs' reagents. The Coombs' reagents cross-link the surface antibodies and/or complement and lead to micro or macroscopic agglutination of the patient's RBCs (Box 7.13).

Box 7.13 Coombs' Test Supplies

- 1–12 × 75 mm glass disposable culture tubes
- adjustable p200 pipette and tips
- phosphate-buffered saline (PBS)
- u-bottom plastic microtiter plate and adhesive plate cover
- 37 °C incubator
- MP Biomedicals Coombs' reagent, specific for species
- cellwasher
- permanent marker

A minimum of 150 μl of nonhemolyzed EDTA whole blood (more if the animal has a very low PCV) is needed. Samples less than 24 hr old are ideal but may be up to 3 days old if no hemolysis has occurred. Red cells may be acquired by teasing a small amount off the clot and washing before testing, though 60 μl is required using this method.

Procedure

- Wash patient RBCs twice. Add 200–400 μl of EDTA whole blood to disposable culture tube. Wash RBCs in cellwasher according to manufacturer instructions.
- Resuspend cells in PBS to a concentration of 1–2% for all species except horses, which require a 3–4% suspension (Figure 7.29).
- Use the u-bottom microtiter plate to set up the Coombs reaction. Only species-specific polyclonal antisera will be tested; therefore, cut off 1 row of 12 wells from the microtiter plate. Using a permanent marker, draw a line in front of the last well (well 12) to use as a control well.
- Add 50 μl of PBS to each well in the row. Add 50 ml of polyvalent Coombs antiglobulin reagent to the first well in the row. Dispense the sample and mix carefully by drawing the sample up and expelling it back into the well. With the same tip, aspirate 50 μl and repeat in well 2. Continue to serially dilute the antisera through the remaining wells up to well 12, the control well. Mix the dilution in well 11, withdraw 50 μl, and discard with tip. Do not put antisera in well 12, as well 12 is used as the negative control containing only the PBS and patient RBC suspension.
- Add 50 μl of appropriate patient RBC suspension to each row of 12 wells, respectively.
- Cover plate using adhesive clear plate cover. Gently mix plate by taping against a finger for approximately 15 S. Place plate in incubator for 20–30 min.
- Remove plate from incubator and leave sitting on bench at room temperature for 20–30 min (approximately 25 °C incubation). The test is ready to read after this step.

Quality Control

A known commercial Coombs' positive product is run with each new lot number of Coombs' reagent. This must be positive before the reagent is aliquoted for use. Every Coombs' test that is set up includes a negative (saline and cells) control.

Species	% RBC Suspension	Volume packed, washed RBCs	Volume PBS
Equine	3–4 %	60 μl	2940 μl
Other Species	1–2 %	20 μl	900 μl

Figure 7.29 RBC suspension preparation.

Result Reporting

- The microtiter plate is read for hemagglutination. To check this, raise plate to eye level and tip, with a light source immediately behind plate. Non-agglutinated cells (negative) will "tear-drop" down each well. Agglutinated (positive) cells form a smooth cell surface covering the bottom of each well. These cells adhere to each other and will not tear-drop.
- Examine the negative control well (well 12) for agglutination. The negative control well needs to show no agglutination to report test results. If agglutination is present in control well, do not report the results for the antisera tested. Add a comment to the reported results that test could not be interpreted due to patient RBC autoagglutination.
- If there is no agglutination present in the control well, proceed with reading the rest of the wells. Examine each well for agglutination for each antisera tested. The last well to show agglutination is the titer for the antisera tested.
- A negative result (less than 2) shows no agglutination in all wells. Record and report titer as <2.
- Record polyclonal antisera results. The titer is the reciprocal of the dilution, that is, dilution of 1:2 is a titer of 2, dilution of 1:4 is a titer of 4, and so forth.

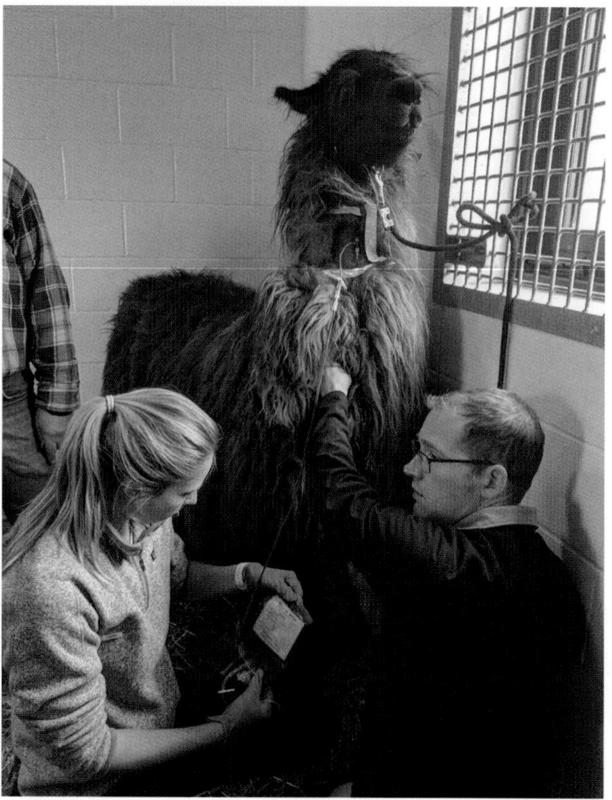

Figure 7.30 A llama donating whole blood.

Crossmatch

Indications

Blood typing of high value bulls and certain breeds of horses is practiced to reduce the incidence of hemolytic disease in offspring. Blood transfusions for most large animal species thankfully occur infrequently, but this need in an already compromised individual necessitates caution (Figure 7.30). While a single blood transfusion event usually occurs without hemolytic incident, subsequent transfusions may not. Crossmatch testing, therefore, is necessary to reduce the incidence of transfusion reactions and negative outcomes of treatment. Major crossmatch will detect antibodies present in the recipient's plasma when introduced to the donor's transfused RBCs but will not detect possible developing sensitization. Minor crossmatch will show possible problems when the recipient's RBCs are combined with the donor's plasma. See Box 7.14 for supplies list.

Box 7.14 Crossmatch Supplies

- EDTA blood from recipient and donor
- serum samples from recipient and donor
- 0.9% saline
- clean plastic tubes
- pipettes

Procedure

Major Crossmatch

- Centrifuge samples for 5 min.
- Remove plasma and serum from each sample into clean, labeled plastic tubes.
- Wash donor RBCs three times suspending the RBCs with 0.9% saline.
- Make a 4% RBC suspension in saline with the washed cells.
- Combine equal volumes, approximately 0.1 ml, of donor RBC suspension and recipient plasma.
- Create a control tube containing the recipients 4% RBC suspension and plasma. Incubate all tubes at 37 °C for 15 min and centrifuge at 1000 g for 15 S.
- Evaluate the supernatant for hemolysis by comparing the color with the control sample.
- Resuspend the cells again comparing any clumping observed to the control sample.
- Test results are negative if all cells resuspend with no clumping observed. Test results are positive if any hemolysis and/or hemagglutination are observed. Microscopic examination should be completed with horse samples due to equine RBC normal tendency to produce rouleaux.

Minor Crossmatch

Perform the above procedure instead using the recipient RBCs with donor plasma. Minor crossmatch is important for formally transfused or pregnant mares.

Dermatology

Allergy Testing

Indication

Intradermal testing (IDT) or allergy skin testing is a tool that aids the dermatologist in the selection of environmental allergens, pollens (plants, bushes, and trees), molds, grasses, weeds, dust mites, insects, and farm plants, for subsequent immunotherapy (allergen specific allergy serum). Importantly, this test is used for environmental allergies (atopic dermatitis), not food-related allergies. Intradermal allergy testing is best performed after other possibilities for the itchy skin disease have been excluded. See Box 7.15 for supplies list.

Patient Prep

- The horse should be pulled off medications (steroids or antihistamines) 10–30 days prior to testing.
- A 15×8-in rectangle is clipped on both sides of the lateral aspect of the neck or chest.
- Draw grid with permanent marker within the clipped area on each side of the neck consisting of 10 squares across and 3 squares down. (Some clinicians will choose to bypass the grid marks.)
- With permanent marker or Wite-Out, place small dots in a linear array on the shaved skin to know where to place each injection.

Procedure

- Sedate patient as needed.
- Intradermal skin test injections (30/side; 60 total) are performed on both sides of the neck with a panel of allergens (~0.1 ml/site).
- Evaluation of the sites should occur at 15–30 min, 4 hr, and 24 hr post-injection (Figure 7.31).

Box 7.15 Testing Supplies

- sedation
- clippers with #40 surgical blades
- permanent marker or Wite-Out®
- panel of allergens in tuberculin syringes, including a negative and positive control
- standard ruler

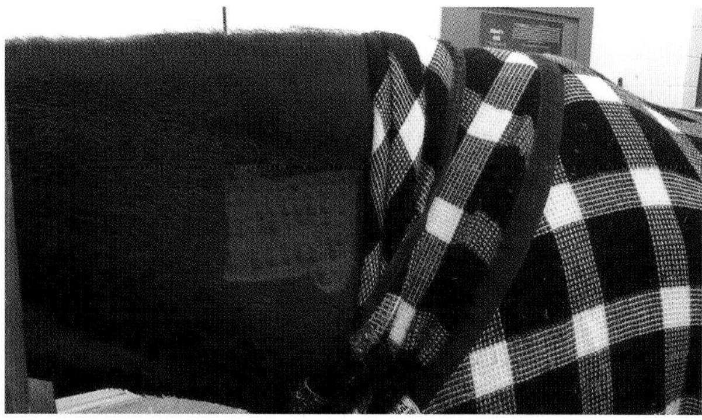

Figure 7.31 Allergy testing being performed on an equine patient.

- Measure wheal or hive diameter in millimeters.
- The test sites are compared with the negative (0) and positive (4+) control wheals, and all reactions that are greater than or equal to a set standard (i.e. 2+) are considered potential causative antigens.

Post-procedure

Patient care post-procedure can include steroid or histamine treatment to aid in control of wheals that have developed from the testing.

Test results can be used to direct clients to avoid specific allergens or to create a tailor-made allergen serum specific injectable.

Submissions

None required, procedure is performed and interpreted within a short period of time.

Cytology

Indication

To collect tissue cells as well as any microorganisms, such as bacteria, yeast, or parasites, from the superficial epidermis. See Box 7.16 for supplies list.

Patient Prep

Surface of epidermis should not be altered with cleaning or preparation prior to sampling.

Box 7.16 Cytology Supplies

- exam gloves
- #10 scalpel blade
- glass slides
- cotton swabs
- scotch-tape

Procedure Options

- #1 option: rub a glass slide directly on topical lesion (sore).
- #2 option: repeatedly press clear acetate tape on a lesion, then affix the tape to a slide for evaluation.
- #3 option: a cotton swab can be rolled on the epidermis surface to pick up cells. Roll collected contents on a glass slide for examination.
- Multiple samplings are recommended and may include more than one of these techniques.

Post-procedure

This procedure is noninvasive and does not require post-procedure patient care related to the collection procedure.

Submissions

Samples on slides can be examined unaltered or can be stained with Wright's stain and/or with a Gram stain procedure. Wright's stain will aid in the identification of yeast or bacteria, but not which type of bacteria. A Gram stain on a separate slide sample will identify gram-positive or gram-negative bacteria. Parasites can often be identified without staining.

Skin Scraping

Indication

Sampling of superficial or deep layer of epidermis used to identify suspected parasitic skin mites, bacterial infections, or yeast infections. See Box 7.17 and Figure 7.32 for supplies list.

Patient Prep

The clipping of the hair or fur prior to sampling is not required.

Procedure

- Sedation of the patient may be required to keep patient quiet and comfortable to obtain a good sample.
- Apply a small amount of mineral oil to the surface that will be sampled. This is especially helpful with dry scaly lesions.
- Scrape the surface of the skin with a #15 scalpel blade held at a 90° angle to the skin, while holding the skin taut, until the stratum corneum is removed.

Box 7.17 Skin Scrape Supplies

- exam gloves
- microscope with 10× and 20× objectives
- scalpel blade (size 22)
- glass microscope slides
- coverslips
- mineral oil/potassium hydroxide

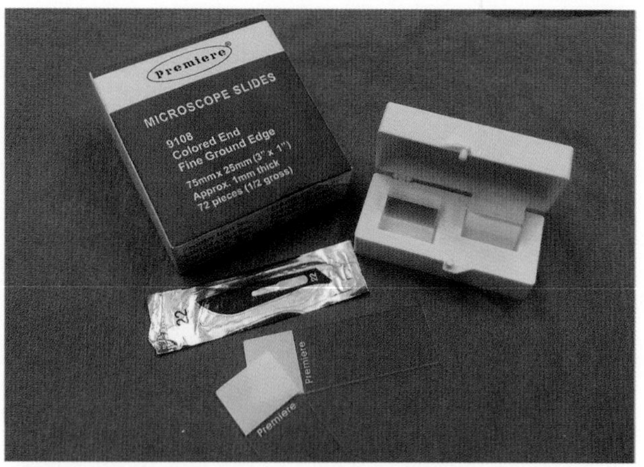

Figure 7.32 Supplies used for skin scraping.

- A small amount of fresh blood may be produced or seen. Significant bleeding is an indication of having scraped too deep.
- Sampling of more than one site is recommended.
- Add a drop of mineral oil to the examination slide and carefully spread the collected cells from the scalpel blade onto the slide.

Sample Handling

Take caution not to squish or damage cells while transferring onto the examination slide. Scraping to an inadequate depth may result in a false negative result.

Post-procedure

The sampled area will appear as an abrasion, which should heal over within a few days. No suturing or topical solutions are required unless prescribed.

Diagnosis

Potential diagnosis may include the following parasites: *Chorioptes* spp, *Sarcoptes* spp., *Psoropte* spp., *Demodex* spp., Dermatophytes.

Submissions

No formal submission required. This procedure is performed and interpreted within a short period of time and can be evaluated under the microscope, first at 4× power, and up to 50× power.

Electrocardiogram

The ECG or EKG is used in large animal patients primarily for determination of abnormalities of heart rate and rhythm. Because of the unique arrangement of the Purkinje system in large animals, the ECG is not used to determine abnormalities in heart size. To master electrocardiography, a veterinary technician must understand the indications for performing an ECG, the techniques for obtaining a diagnostic tracing, and the electrical pathways of the heart.

Electrocardiography is an important part of many facets of veterinary medicine, including anesthesia, cardiology, emergency and critical care medicine, sports medicine, and internal medicine.

Indications

Indications for performing an ECG are numerous but most commonly include auscultation of an arrhythmia during a physical examination and the presence of structural heart disease. Electrocardiography is also indicated in the workup of veterinary patients with a history of collapse with or without loss of consciousness and those presenting for poor athletic performance. As a monitoring tool, continuous electrocardiography is very valuable for monitoring patients under anesthesia as well as those with ongoing occult blood loss (internal hemorrhage), pain, blunt chest trauma, and/ or exposure to a cardiotoxin, such as monensin. ECG analysis should also be strongly considered in patients with elevated heart rates that cannot be explained by excitement or pain, even if the rhythm is regular. This is because sustained ventricular tachycardia (VT) is a rapid, regular rhythm that can be easily misdiagnosed as a sinus tachycardia based on auscultation alone, if the inappropriate heart rate is not taken into consideration.

Procedures

Specific techniques for obtaining an ECG will depend on whether a single short recording (rhythm strip) is required; whether multiple leads are necessary to make a diagnosis; or whether continuous electrocardiographic monitoring is needed. The standard resting ECG is usually obtained with the patient in a standing position, whether lightly restrained by the handler (equine, small ruminant, camelid), restrained in stocks (equine, bovine), or restrained in a head catch or chute (bovine, small ruminants). Sedation should be avoided if possible and care should be taken to minimize stress to the patient, as increased sympathetic tone will affect the rate and possibly the rhythm. Modifications to restraint may be needed for neonates, who are in lateral recumbency, and camelids, who may kush (lay in sternal recumbency) during the procedure. Positioning under anesthesia will be dictated by the procedure being performed.

A rhythm strip can be obtained by attaching the electrodes in a variety of configurations. The "base-apex" configuration is commonly used as it typically produces a diagnostic strip and is generally well-tolerated by most large animal patients. Standard electrode placement for the base-apex lead system is described in Figure 7.33.

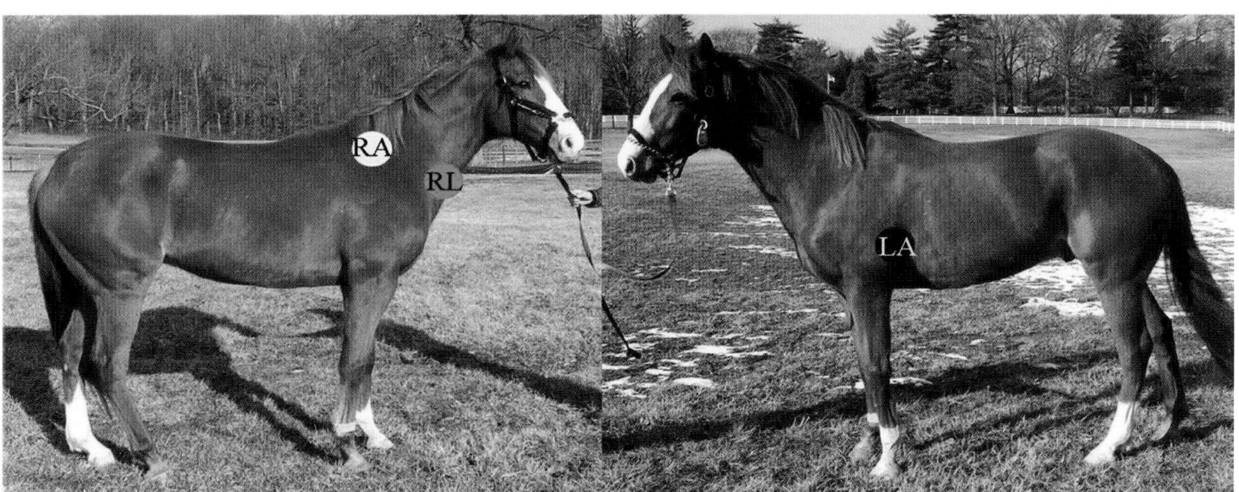

(as shown, the electrocardiograph should be set to read in lead I)

Possible base apex configurations:

RA at top of right scapula, LA over left heart apex, RL over right jugular groove: read in lead I
RA at top of scapula, LL over left heart apex, RL over right jugular groove: read in lead II
LA at top of scapula, LL over left heart apex, RL over right jugular groove; read in lead III

For all configurations, the RL acts as a ground and can be placed anywhere remote from the heart or the other electrodes.

Figure 7.33 Standard placement for base-apex lead system.

For patients under anesthesia, modifications to the standard lead placement may be necessary due to patient positioning. A 12-lead system has also been described for large animals. This is rarely needed but can be performed when the rhythm diagnosis is not clear on a base-apex tracing.

Electrodes are usually attached to the patient by means of alligator clips or electrode patches. Electrode patches typically have an adhesive backing, which requires the hair to be removed. In some cases, it may be necessary to suture or glue the patches to the skin in addition to the hair removal. Electrodes are then either snapped onto the patches or attached to the patches via alligator clips. This is mostly done in animals undergoing general anesthesia. Equine and camelid owners may object to removal of the hair or fiber, and alligator clips attached directly to the skin is often the preferred method for electrode attachment in the awake animal. A coupling agent such as isopropyl alcohol or coupling gel is then applied to the electrodes and skin.

> **TECHNICIAN TIP 7.7:** Equine and camelid owners may object to removal of the hair or fiber, and alligator clips attached directly to the skin is often the preferred method for electrode attachment in the awake animal.

Once electrodes are correctly placed, the settings on the ECG machine (electrocardiograph) must be adjusted and optimized. First, note that there is no "base-apex" lead option. The correct lead is chosen based on electrode placement (see Figure 7.33 Base-apex). Second, the paper speed should be adjusted. The method for doing this will vary from machine to machine and a technician must become familiar with the equipment they are using. For large animals, most ECGs are obtained at a paper speed of 25 mm/S. However, if significant tachycardia is present, it may be useful to run a portion of the recording at 50 mm/s paper speed, as this will spread out the complexes and make certain diagnoses easier to see (see Figure 7.34). Lastly, gain settings need to be optimized. Most standard recordings are performed at 10 mm/mV. If the complexes are very small (such as occurs with pericardial and pleural effusions, obesity, or a very large patient) increasing the gain will make the complexes easier to see. In VT, the complexes may be so large that decreasing the gain is helpful. Lastly, basic troubleshooting skills are necessary. A tracing that is unreadable or appears as a flat line should alert the technician to the possibility that an electrode has become disconnected or that more coupling gel or isopropyl alcohol is needed. A patient that is shivering, fasciculating, or moving excessively will cause undulations and other artifacts in the baseline of the recording. Motion should be minimized and shivering or muscle fasciculations should be noted on the recording.

> **TECHNICIAN TIP 7.8:** Failure to optimize the ECG settings is a common reason for rhythm misdiagnoses.

In addition to the standard ECG, other devices including Holter monitors (Figure 7.35) telemetry (Figure 7.36), handheld devicesand internal cardiac recorders are used in large animal clinical practice. Continuously recording Holter monitors are particularly useful for identifying and quantifying cardiac arrhythmias over a 24- to 48-h time period. Digital Holter devices designed for human patients can be readily adapted for large animal patients. Application

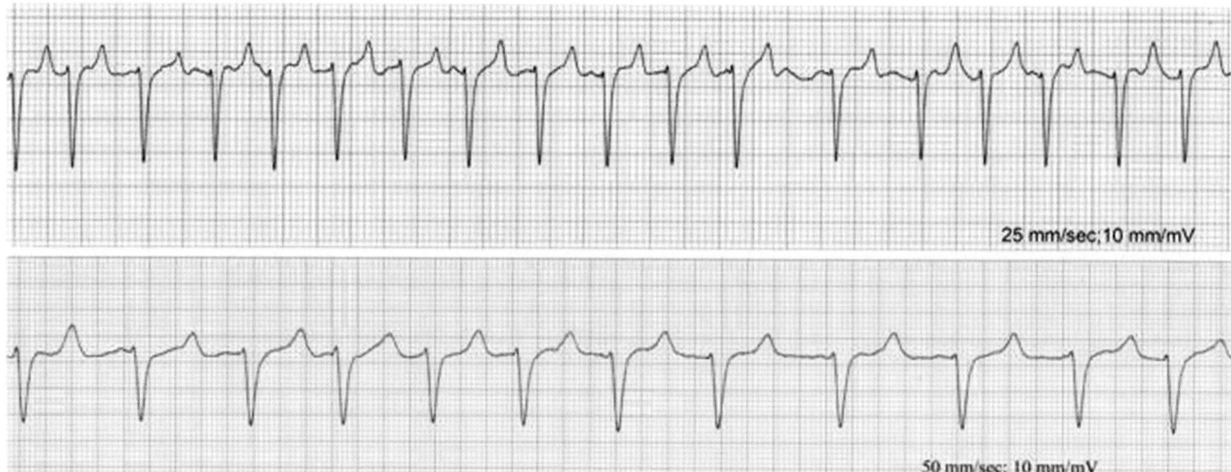

Figure 7.34 Atrial fibrillation at different paper speeds.

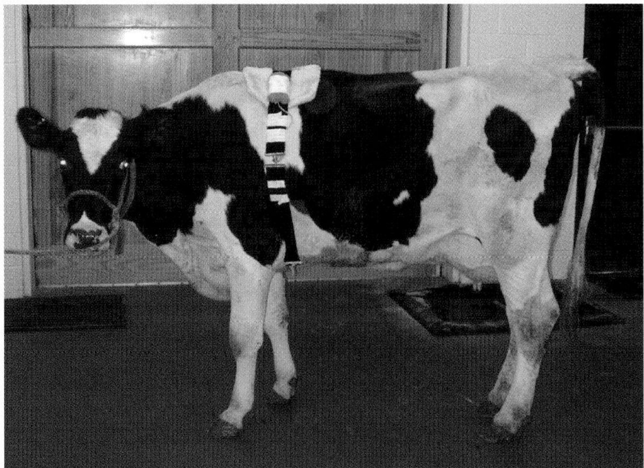

Figure 7.35 Holter monitor on an adult cow.

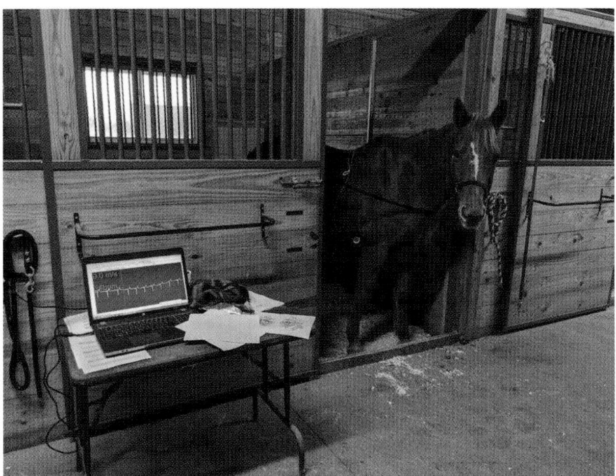

Figure 7.36 Televet monitor on a horse.

of the Holter device is well-tolerated in most large animal patients and, when properly applied, the recordings are of excellent quality. With Holter monitors, the ECG is not read or monitored in real time. Instead, the device records the ECG onto a secure digital (SD) card. The digital information is then imported into a specialized software program that permits viewing and editing of the tracing.

> **TECHNICIAN TIP 7.9:** The diagnosis of infrequent cardiac arrhythmias requires longer recordings than those obtained with a standard ECG. Holter monitors are designed specifically for this purpose.

Telemetric ECG devices are often employed in intensive care and cardiac units when real-time monitoring of a patient's heart rate and rhythm is critical. Telemetric ECG devices are also useful in the setting of equine sports medicine when an exercising ECG is indicated. The electrodes can be securely applied to the girth area and fit well underneath most tack. Careful application is required to limit the motion artifact created by footfall and chest excursions. Real-time viewing of telemetric recordings permits precise coordination of performance problems with cardiac rhythm events and can be combined with GPS (global positioning system) information regarding exercise speed and distance. Both radiotelemetric and Blue-tooth® enabled telemetric devices exist for this purpose. The advantages of the computer-based programs are convenient ECG storage and retrieval, as well as transmission of data to remote locations, via remote viewing software.

> **TECHNICIAN TIP 7.10:** Telemetric ECGs can be used in veterinary patients to monitor heart rate as an indicator of pain. This is particularly useful in stoic animals that do not outwardly demonstrate pain.

Wireless handheld ECG devices are convenient for rapid rhythm diagnosis, especially in the setting of large animal ambulatory medicine (Figure 7.37). Short ECG recordings are obtained by holding the device against the patient's chest wall. Digital recording devices, such as the one developed for use with an iPhone®, permit rapid sharing of the recording if consultation is necessary.

While not commonly applied, ECG recordings can be obtained from specialized catheters placed within heart. The most common clinical application of this procedure is for the electrical cardioversion of atrial fibrillation in horses. Programmable, implantable ECG recorders are also available for recording data over long periods of time (months to years). The device is implanted in the subcutaneous tissues of the pectoral region (equine). The ECG information can be retrieved while the device is in situ or once it is removed. This device is mainly applied in the workup of horses with infrequent collapse.

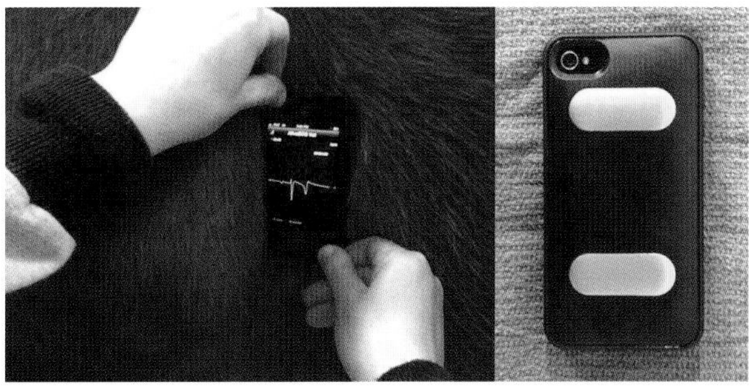

Figure 7.37 Wireless ECG. Digital recording devices such as the one developed for use with an iPhone permit rapid sharing of the recording if consultation is necessary.

Electrical Pathways in the Heart

The information recorded on an ECG represents the heart's electrical activity, not its mechanical activity. Electrical activity precedes mechanical activity but does not guarantee it. Heart muscle cells become electrically excited by a process that involves the movement of ions (primarily, potassium, sodium, and calcium) into and out of the heart muscle cells. When the net effect of ion movement is to make the cells more positively charged, the process is called depolarization. When the net effect is for the cell to return to its resting state (become less positive), the process is called repolarization.

In the normal healthy heart, all electrical activity is initiated in the sinus node. The sinus node is a group of specialized cells located within the right atrium. The sinus node is the dominant pacemaker of the heart and has the quality of automaticity, which means it depolarizes spontaneously without the need for some other stimulus. The rate at which the sinus node depolarizes is affected by the autonomic nervous system, increasing its rate in response to sympathetic stimulus and decreasing in response to parasympathetic (vagal) stimulus. Depolarization (and subsequent repolarization) of the sinus node cannot be seen on the ECG.

Once the sinus node has depolarized, the electrical activity spreads throughout the right and left atria resulting in a P wave on the ECG. Said another way, the P wave represents atrial depolarization. Atrial repolarization is not typically seen on the ECG. The electrical activity then reaches the atrioventricular (AV) node where electrical conduction is delayed. This period of conduction delay corresponds to the PR interval on the ECG. (The delay is important as it permits sequential rather than simultaneous contraction of the atria and ventricles.) Following this brief delay, electrical activity is conducted along the His-Purkinje system of the ventricles (the ventricles are depolarized) resulting in a QRS complex on the ECG. Repolarization of the ventricles is represented by a T wave. The time between the QRS and the T wave is called the ST segment and represents time during which the ventricles are refractory (resistant) to another electrical stimulus. The area between the end of the T wave and the next P wave is referred to as the baseline. Deflections above the baseline are called positive deflections and those below the baseline are called negative deflections.

ECG Interpretation

Mastering ECG interpretation takes practice. Understanding basic electrophysiology and recognizing the common arrhythmias is the first step toward this goal. While a complete description of all possible dysrhythmias is beyond the scope of this section, the most common and straightforward diagnoses are described later in this chapter.

Calculating Heart Rate

The first step of analyzing an ECG is to calculate the heart rate. To do this, one needs to know the paper speed of the tracing and to understand the layout of the graph paper. ECG tracings are laid out such that time in seconds is on the x-axis and amplitude in millivolts (mV) is on the y-axis (figure graph paper). The smallest of the boxes on the graph paper is a 1 × 1 mm box. For paper speeds of 25 mm/S, each small 1 mm box equals 0.04 S, five 1 mm boxes equal 0.20 S, and twenty-five 1 mm boxes equal 1 S (hence 25 mm/s). Since it is difficult for the eye to focus on the smallest boxes, each group of 5 × 5 boxes (equaling 0.20 S) is typically highlighted on the graph paper. This makes it easier to calculate out a 1-S interval by counting five of these larger boxes. Some graph paper comes with tic marks at 1-S or 3-S intervals.

After understanding the graph paper layout, one can easily calculate heart rate. Count the number of QRS complexes in 6 S (30 larger boxes) and multiply by 10 to get beats per minute. What if paper speed is 50 mm/s? Then each small 1 × 1 mm box is only 0.02 S and five small boxes are 0.10 S long. That would mean you need to count 60 larger boxes to get 6 S. An easier approach is to count out 30 boxes but instead multiply the number of QRS complexes by 20 instead of 10 to calculate beats per minute.

The focus on counting 30 larger boxes is due to the fact that the average writing pen is 30 boxes long. Rather than causing eyestrain by counting boxes, simply place a pen on the ECG tracing and count the number of complexes along the length of the pen (see Figure 7.38). Multiplying by 10 (25 m/s paper speed) or 20 (50 mm/s paper speed) gives a good approximation of the heart rate. This is handy in emergency situations where the exact heart rate is not as critical as determining a good estimate.

Normal Resting ECG: Normal Sinus Rhythm

Atrial depolarization (P wave), ventricular depolarization (QRS complex), and ventricular repolarization (T wave) can be recognized on all normal ECGs in large animal patients (Figure 7.39). On rare occasions, atrial repolarization (Ta) can be seen (Figure 7.40), particularly in equine tracings. The P wave on a normal equine ECG trace can be "notched or bifid." This is because the large atrial mass and slower heart rate compared to other species allows depolarization of the right atrium and then the left atrium to be inscribed on the ECG. This finding can also be normal in cattle with low normal heart rates or bradycardia. P waves

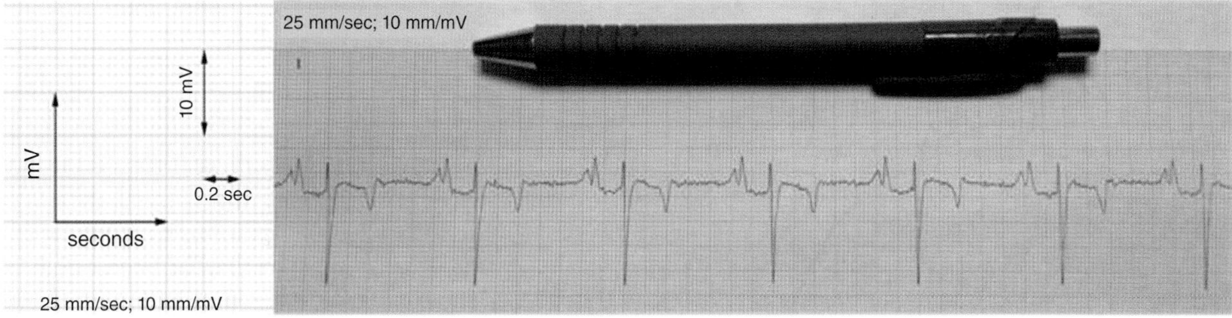

Figure 7.38 ECG graph paper and pen. Count the number of complexes along the length of the pen.

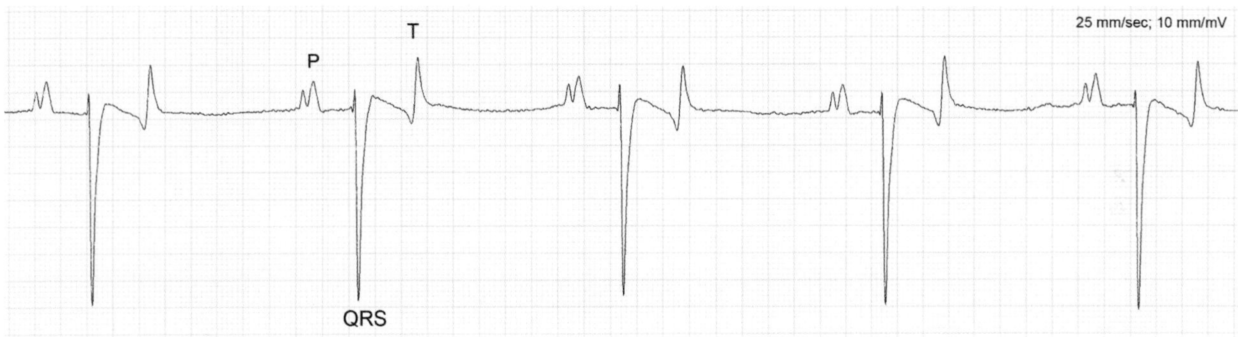

Figure 7.39 Normal equine complexes.

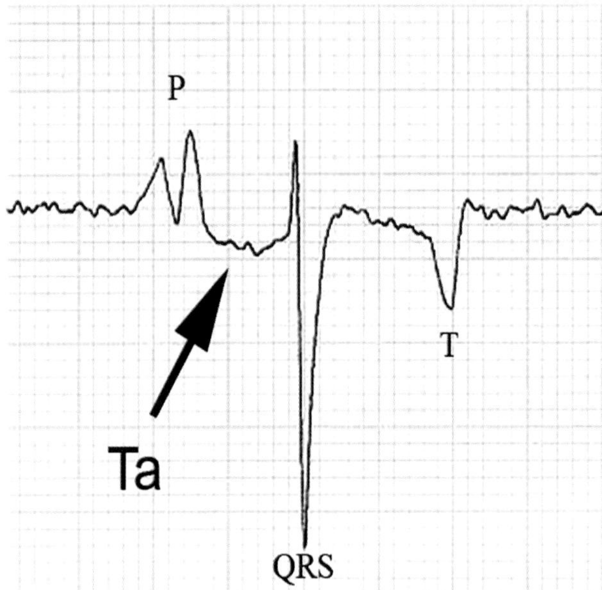

Figure 7.40 Ta wave. Atrial repolarization.

should be positive in the base-apex lead. The major deflection of the QRS complex should be negative in the base-apex lead. T waves can be quite variable (positive, negative, or biphasic) and T wave size is not a reliable indicator of serum potassium levels in large animal patients.

Arrhythmias

Cardiac arrhythmias can be classified as physiologic, occurring secondary to normal processes such as changes in autonomic tone or respiratory patterns, or pathologic, due to heart disease or systemic disease. While the veterinarian is ultimately responsible for making an electrocardiographic diagnosis, the veterinary technician must be able to distinguish normal from abnormal and recognize the common rhythm disturbances that are potentially life threatening.

Common Physiologic Arrhythmias

Sinus Tachycardia

Sinus tachycardia happens secondary to increased sympathetic tone as may occur with exercise, pain, excitement, or parasympatholytic or sympathomimetic drugs. ECG criteria include a rapid regular rhythm with normal P, QRS, and T waves. The heart rate is above the resting upper limit of normal for that species (Figure 7.41). At very high heart rates, such as those that occur with exercise, the P wave is difficult if not impossible to identify, the ST segment can become raised or slurred, and the T waves can become as large as the QRS complexes. It is important to use calipers to be sure that the rhythm is regular. "Eyeballing" an ECG when the heart rate is high can lead to misdiagnoses.

> **TECHNICIAN TIP 7.11:** Calipers are handy tools for determining if a rhythm is regular or not. Using calipers is critical at higher heart rates when it is more difficult for the eye to discern small differences in R-to-R intervals.

Sinus Bradycardia

Sinus bradycardia occurs secondary to increased vagal (parasympathetic) tone. Anorexia (in ruminants) and administration of alpha-adrenergic agonists are common causes. ECG criteria include a slow regular rhythm with normal P, QRS, and T waves. The heart rate is below the lower limit of normal for that species. It is not unusual to have other vagally mediated rhythms present at the same time, such as sinus arrhythmia, second-degree AV block, or sinus block.

Sinus Arrhythmia

Sinus arrhythmia is quite common in resting large animals, particularly small ruminants and camelids. It is not always linked to the respiratory cycle. In horses, the rhythm is frequently seen in the first 1–2 min following intense exercise but also occurs commonly alongside physiologic second-degree AV block. Sinus arrhythmia occurs alongside sinus bradycardia in food-deprived cattle. ECG criteria include an irregular sinus rhythm, variable P-to-P intervals, normal P, QRS and T waves, and normal P-R intervals.

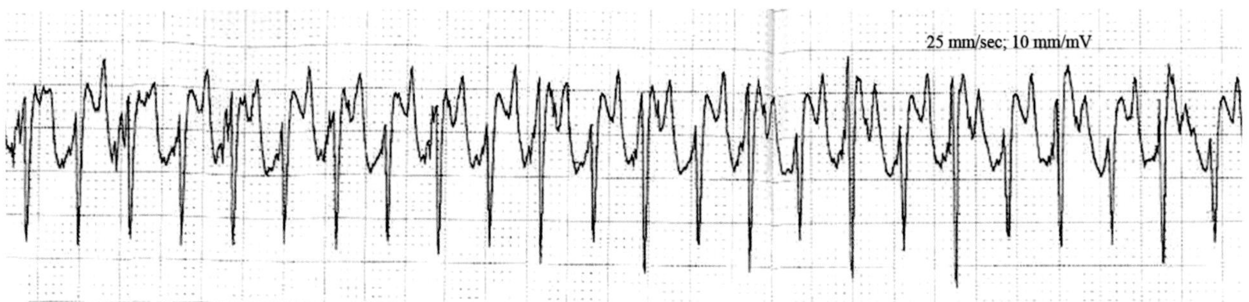

Figure 7.41 Sinus tachycardia in an exercising horse.

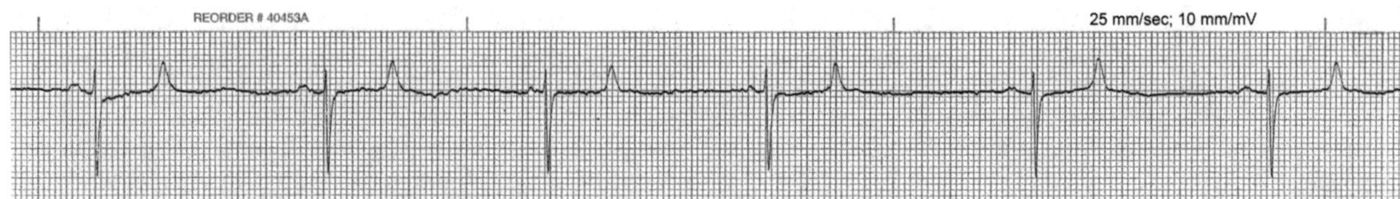

Figure 7.42 Sinus bradycardia with slight sinus arrhythmia in an alpaca.

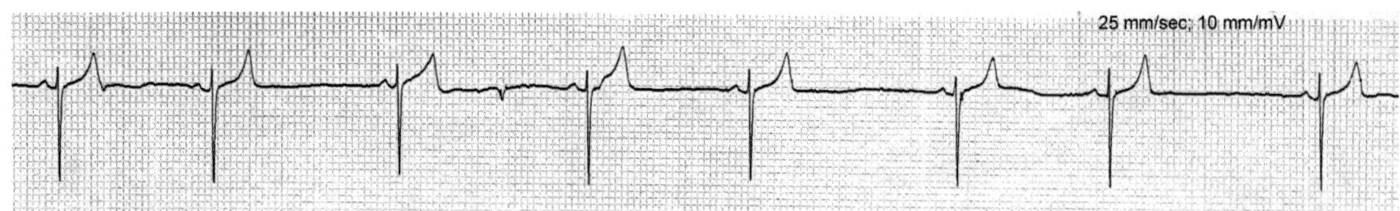

Figure 7.43 Sinus arrhythmia in an alpaca.

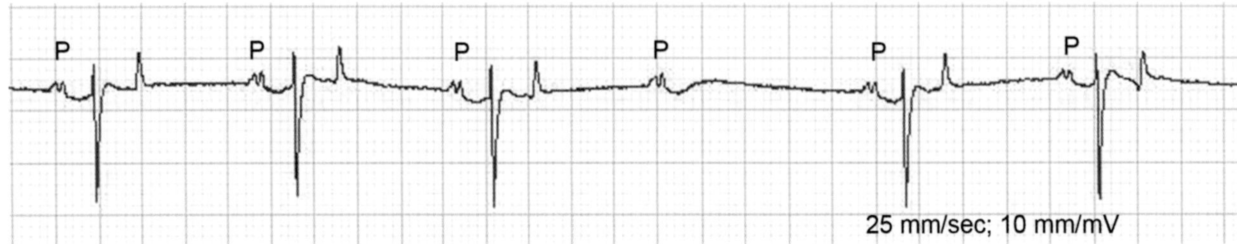

Figure 7.44 Second-degree AVB in an equine patient.

Second-Degree Atrioventricular (AV) Block

Second-degree AV block can be divided into type I/physiologic AV block and type II/advanced AV block. Type I is by far the most common arrhythmia to encounter, especially in horses. It is less common to encounter second-degree AV block (either type) in ruminants and camelids. High vagal tone is the most common cause of this rhythm. The ECG criteria for type I AV block include a regular underlying rhythm with an occasional P wave not followed by a QRS complex (a "blocked" P wave). The blocked P wave is on time (being neither premature nor late) and the P-to-P intervals are regular. The P, QRS, and T waves all have normal morphology. Usually, only one P wave is blocked; rarely two in a row are blocked. More than two blocked P waves in a row should raise suspicion for advanced/type II second-degree AV block (Figure 7.44).

> **TECHNICIAN TIP 7.12:** Physiologic/type I AV block should disappear when vagal tone is reduced, such as with exercise or administration of vagolytic drugs (atropine or glycopyrrolate).

Common Pathologic Arrhythmias

Supraventricular Premature Complexes (SPCs) (Figure 7.45)

Supraventricular premature complexes (SPCs) arise from ectopic foci within the supraventricular (atrial or junctional) tissues. The ECG shows an early P′ wave (P prime wave) that is a different morphology than normal sinus P waves. Most commonly, the P′ wave is followed by a normal QRS and T at a normal P-R interval. However, on occasion, the P′ wave is so early that it is "blocked" at the AV node and therefore not followed by a QRS and T. In these cases, the P′ wave may be between the QRS and T of the previous beat or buried in the previous T wave (Figure 7.46 Non-conducted SPC). P′ waves can also be followed by a slightly abnormal QRS complex if conduction through the ventricles occurs early enough that parts of the ventricle are still refractory to depolarization. This is called an aberrantly conducted SPC. It can be distinguished from a VPC (ventricular premature complex) by the normal P′-R interval.

Ventricular Premature Complexes (VPCs) (Figure 7.47)

VPCs arise from ectopic foci within the ventricular myocardium. The ECG shows an early QRS-T complex that is different in morphology from the normal QRS-T complexes. The early QRS-T is not associated with a P wave, although P waves are present, and the P-P intervals are regular.

Atrial Fibrillation (A-fib)

Atrial fibrillation is the most common arrhythmia to affect athletic performance in horses and is commonly encountered in ruminants with gastrointestinal disease. ECG characteristics include the absence of P waves, irregular R-to-R intervals, the presence of fibrillation or "f" waves, and normal QRS-T complexes. Fibrillation or "f" waves are undulations in the baseline that can be confused with motion artifact. The undulations can be "coarse" and easy to recognize or "fine" and difficult to see. At higher heart

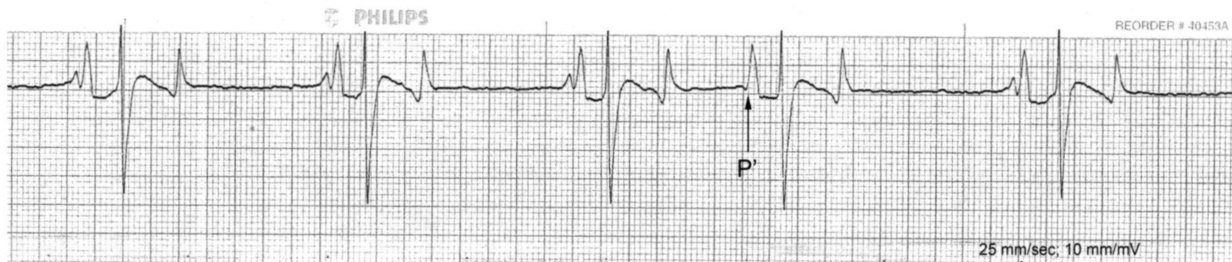

Figure 7.45 Supraventricular premature complex (SPC).

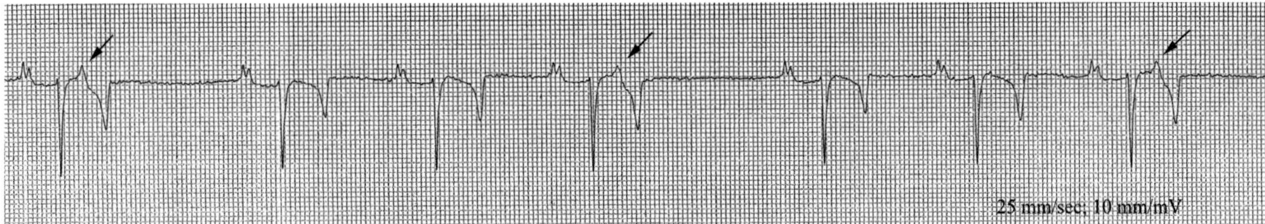

Figure 7.46 Non-conducted supraventricular premature complex (SPC).

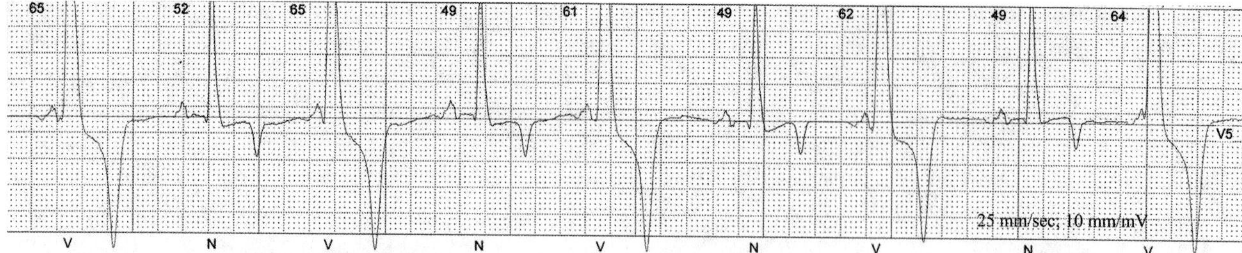

Figure 7.47 VPCs or ventricular premature complexes.

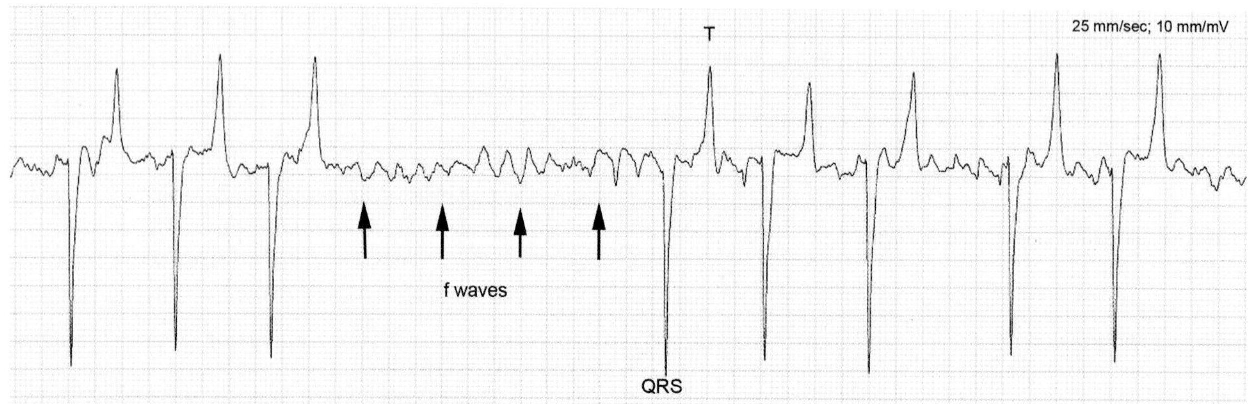

Figure 7.48 Atrial fibrillation in an equine patient.

rates, atrial fibrillation can be easily overlooked unless calipers are used to evaluate the R-to-R intervals.

Ventricular Tachycardia (VT) (Figures 7.49–7.51)

VT is a potentially life-threatening arrhythmia that needs to be immediately recognized. ECG characteristics depend on whether the rhythm is paroxysmal or sustained, and whether the VPCs are unifocal or multifocal. More than three VPCs in a row is considered VT. The most common presentation is sustained unifocal VT, where the ECG characteristics include a rapid, regular rhythm, abnormal QRS-T morphology, and dissociation of the P waves and QRS-T complexes. The P waves are present and the P-to-P intervals are regular but may be difficult to see, as they can be buried in the abnormal QRS-T complexes. With multifocal VT, the rhythm is irregular, and there are at least two different abnormal QRS-T morphologies.

> **TECHNICIAN TIP 7.13:** Atrial fibrillation is always an irregularly irregular rhythm regardless of the heart rate. Sustained unifocal ventricular tachycardia is a regular rhythm.

Medical intervention may be necessary for VT. Reasons include evidence of cardiovascular compromise (low blood pressure, evidence of poor tissue perfusion, abnormal mentation, collapse), heart rates sustained above 120–130 bpm in horses and cattle, ECG evidence of R on T phenomenon, or sustained multiform VT. While horses and cattle can often maintain adequate cardiac output with heart rates of 120–130 at rest, they will eventually go into heart failure from myocardial exhaustion.

> **TECHNICIAN TIP 7.14:** R on T phenomenon and multiform VT increase the risk for ventricular fibrillation and death.

Third-Degree (Complete) Atrioventricular (AV) Block (Figure 7.52)

Complete heart block is an uncommon cardiac arrhythmia in large animal patients. It is caused by inflammation or fibrosis of the AV node and is occasionally seen in septic large animal neonates. ECG characteristics include normal P waves that usually occur at a rate slightly higher than the normal resting sinus heart rate. The ventricular rate is slow, and the QRS complexes are abnormal in morphology. These abnormal looking QRS complexes are not VPCs. They are "escape" complexes originating from secondary pacemakers located in junctional or ventricular tissues. Treatment with anti-inflammatory is rarely successful. Definitive treatment requires a pacemaker. Animals with complete heart block are at risk for sudden death.

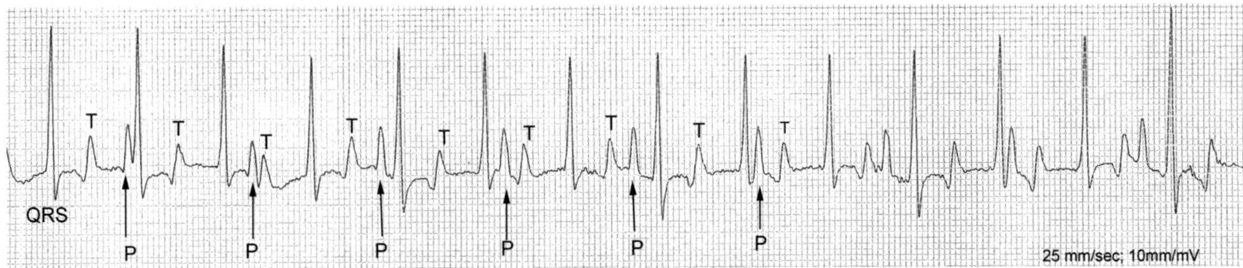

Figure 7.49 Ventricular tachycardia at a rate only slightly faster than the sinus rate.

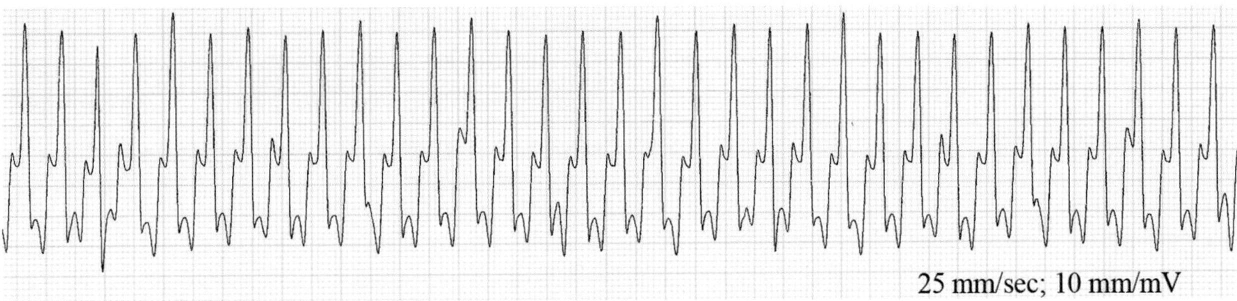

Figure 7.50 Rapid ventricular tachycardia.

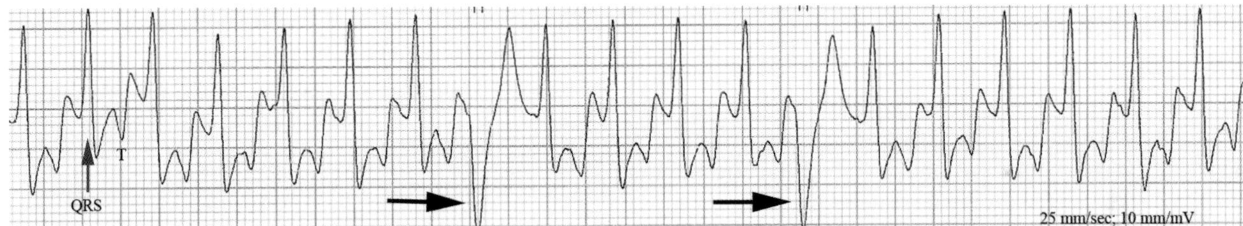

Figure 7.51 Multiform ventricular tachycardia.

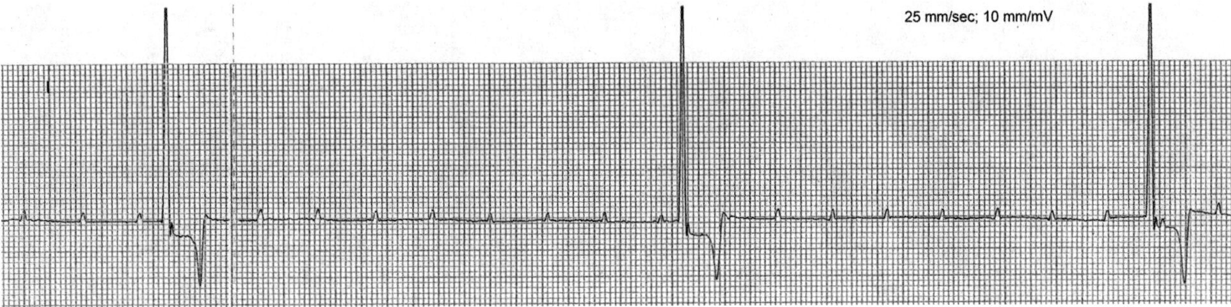

Figure 7.52 Complete heart block in an alpaca.

Endoscopy

Indication

Endoscopy provides a relatively noninvasive view into body systems via access through body orifices. For other procedures, sampling may be the primary reason for utilizing a flexible endoscope. Endoscopes are primarily operated by two individuals, one to drive the direction left/right/up/down and to operate the water, air, and suction functions, while the other individual passes or controls the inward and outward movement.

Supplies

- flexible endoscope in specific length and width to enter through the patient's nares, oral cavity, vulva, penis, rectum, or surgically prepared opening

- lubricant specific to the body system being examined
- sampling items that may include polypropylene tubing, basket, or biopsy forceps
- suction to remove instilled air/water from the body cavity
- sterile gloves dependent on body system explored
- surgical preparation solutions (iodine or chlorhexidine based) for skin prep in sterile procedures
- non-sterile or sterile working surface (tray, table, or similar)
- sterile sample container(s)
- syringes containing sterile saline for sterile procedures
- syringes containing tap water for non-sterile procedures
- three-way stopcocks
- buffered neutral formalin (for histopathology)
- solutions for disinfection or sterilization of equipment

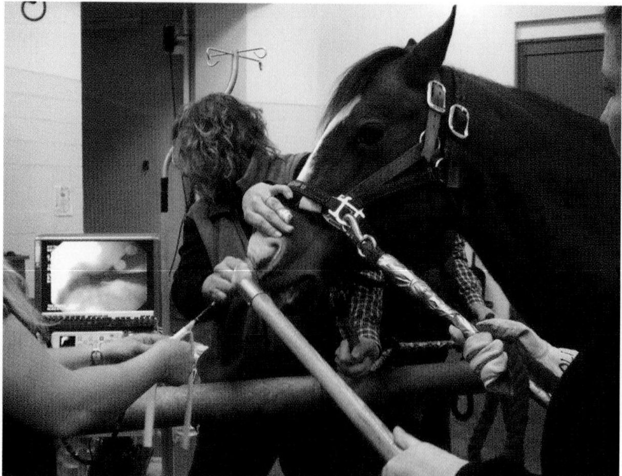

Figure 7.53 Endoscopic exam of a horse in motion utilizing an over-ground high-speed treadmill.

Patient Prep

Dependent on body system explored or need for sedation, the patient may be held off-feed or the orifice sterilely prepped.

Instrument Prep

When performing a general endoscopic examination, the endoscope should be routinely cleaned and disinfected between patients and hung up to air-dry. Placing the endoscope in storage with distal and proximal lengths fully extended, without loops, provides one of the best preventions to nosocomial infections.

> **TECHNICIAN TIP 7.15:** Placing the endoscope in storage with distal and proximal lengths fully extended, without loops, provides one of the best preventions to nosocomial infections.

When performing an endoscopic TW, cystoscopy, or hysteroscopy, the endoscope requires high-level disinfection or sterilization immediately before the procedure. After disinfection/sterilization, the scope should be placed within sterile drapes or towels to reduce incidence of environmental contamination before the procedure. If a cold sterile solution is used for disinfection, be sure to thoroughly rinse the endoscope with sterile water before beginning the procedure.

Procedure

Upper Respiratory

Upper respiratory exploration evaluates the structures or the larynx, nasopharynx, epiglottis and arytenoids. Evaluating the upper respiratory area is best done without sedatives whenever possible, as medications can affect the function and can skew results. During the exam, a veterinarian may request that a slap test be performed. The slap test evaluates the adductor function of the arytenoids by gently slapping the upper right chest near the withers with an open hand. Additionally, dynamic abnormalities or problems that only occur during exercise may require an examination while the patient is in motion. This has traditionally been accomplished by training a horse to work on a high-speed treadmill and then performing an endoscopy exam in motion (Figure 7.53). Advances in technology now allow for dynamic scoping to occur more easily. There are systems that can mount to a headstall or bridle. Some record the image to be played back and others can be monitored in real time by the clinician using remote monitors (Figure 7.54).

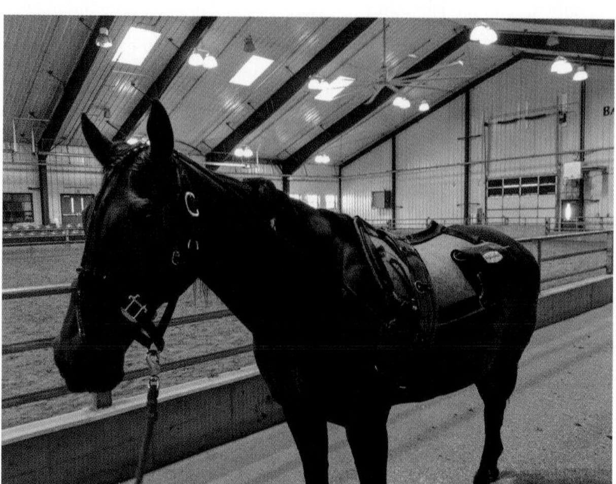

Figure 7.54 Dynamic endoscopic exam.

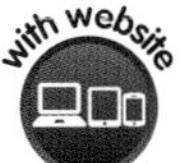

Check out the online resources for additional images and abnormal examples.

Guttural Pouches

For evaluation of equine guttural pouches, the scope is advanced to the nasopharyngeal area to start. A regular or biopsy probe is advanced in front of the scope and passed into one of the guttural pouch openings (Figure 7.55). Once it has passed through, the scope is then advanced to follow it with a gentle twisting motion at the same time. Patients that swallow at this time can easily bump the scope out of the pouch and the operator must start the approach again. Evaluation of the guttural pouches will not be affected by sedatives. Once inside the guttural pouch, evaluation and treatment of conditions such as guttural pouch mycosis, purulent discharge, or chondroids related to bacterial infections such as *Streptococcus equi* be executed (Figure 7.56).

Tracheal Wash and Evaluation through the Scope

During endoscopic TW, the scope is advanced through the nares into the trachea toward the carina. Polypropylene tubing is threaded into the biopsy port. When the carina is reached, the tubing is advanced into the trachea. Sterile saline is instilled then quickly aspirated back into the syringe. Samples are usually tested for cellularity and culture/sensitivity. See TTW later in this chapter for more interpretation information (Figures 7.57 and 7.58).

Gastroscopy

The patient is restrained in head catch or stocks. Sedation is administered and endoscope advanced through the nares. Careful advancement is required so the patient readily swallows the endoscope for passage into the esophagus. When passage is difficult or in dysphagic patients extreme caution must be used, as due to its flexible nature the endoscope may retroflex and advance into the oral cavity. Severe damage to the endoscope may occur and make removal of the scope difficult to impossible. Air is instilled to expand the stomach to easily view the entire stomach wall surface. In the equine patient, the margo plicatus should be clearly visible (Figure 7.59). With practice, a long enough scope

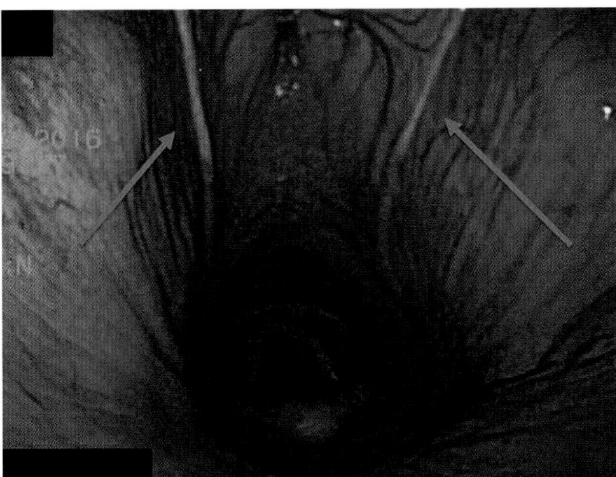

Figure 7.55 Endoscopic view of an adult equine upper airway. Guttural pouch openings indicated with blue arrows.

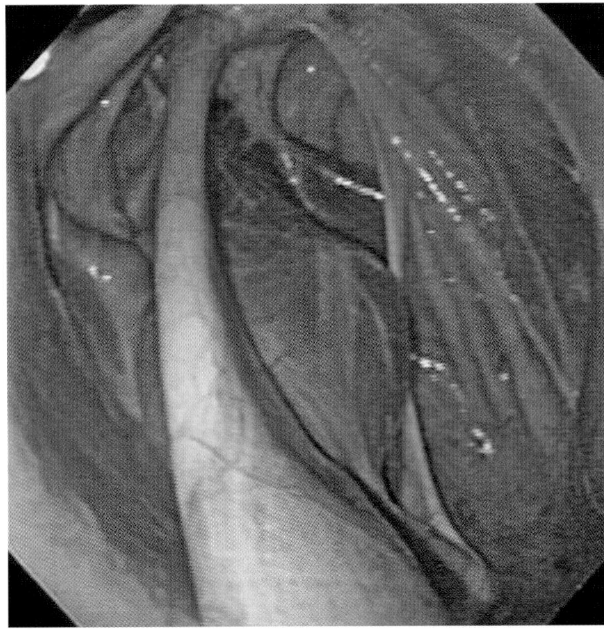

Figure 7.56 Endoscopic view of an adult equine guttural pouch. The styloid hyoid can be visualized in the middle.

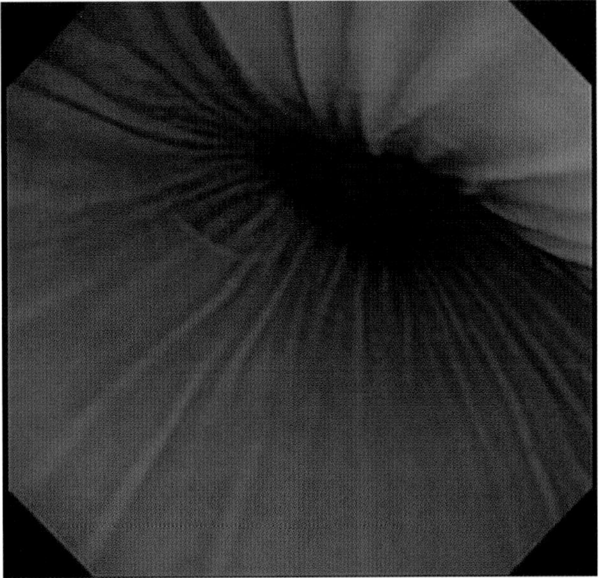

Figure 7.57 Normal esophagus of an adult equine patient. Note the scabbing in several locations as a result of a choke incidence.

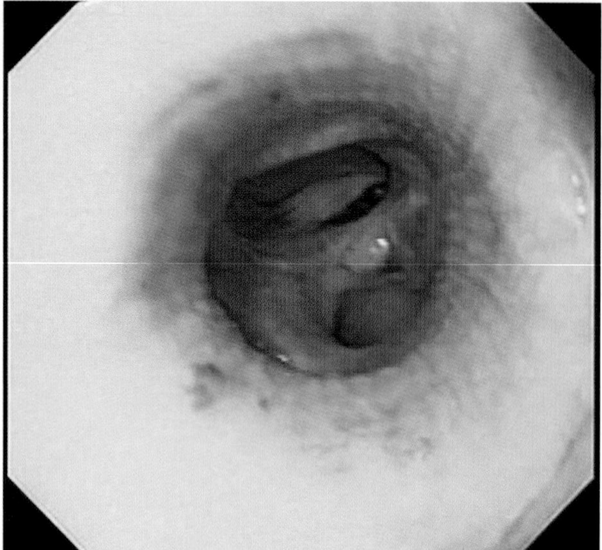

Figure 7.58 Endoscopic view of an adult equine at the bifurcation of the primary bronchi.

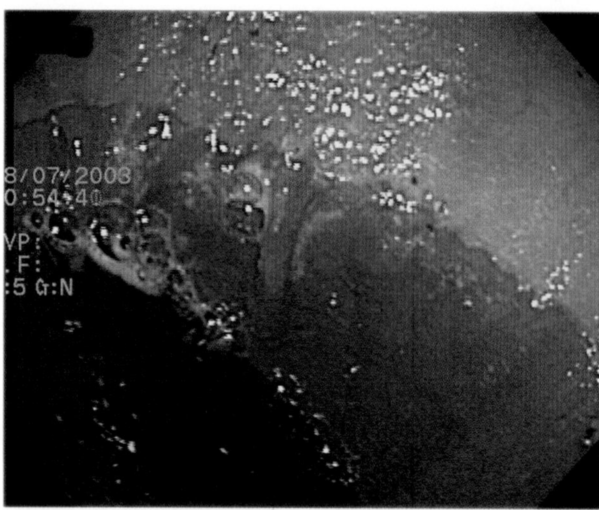

Figure 7.59 Endoscopic view of margo plicatus in an adult horse. This junction is the transition between the glandular and non-glandular portions of the stomach.

and the patient is sufficiently held off-feed, the operator may be able to view the pylorus (Figure 7.60). When removing the endoscope from the stomach, air should be suctioned out to reduce incidence of colic. The esophagus is routinely examined during removal of the endoscope. See Box 7.18 for the grading scale of equine gastric ulcers syndrome (EGUS).

> **TECHNICIAN TIP 7.16:** Caution should be taken to avoid suction of stomach content, which could easily lodge and obstruct the channel of the endoscope.

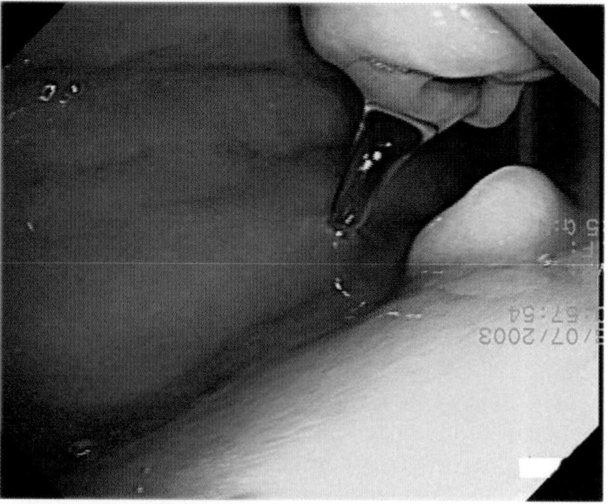

Figure 7.60 Endoscopic view of the duodenum opening.

Box 7.18 Grading Scale for Equine Gastric Ulcers

Grade	Description
0	The mucous membrane does not appear red (hyperemic) or yellow (hyperkeratotic) and the epithelium is intact.
1	Presence of regions of redness or yellow, the mucous membrane is intact.
2	Shallow lesions in the mucous membranes. May be isolated or multifocal.
3	Severe lesions, showing redness and or minor bleeding. May be isolated, multifocal, or widespread.
4	Lesion areas of deep ulceration, typically widespread. May be signs of bleeding or perforation.

Hysteroscopy

The patient must be sterilely prepped for hysteroscopy. Sterile gloved hands guide the sterile endoscope through the vulva and vagina into the uterus. Warm sterile saline is used to expand the uterus for visualization. Instilling excessive amounts of saline may cause colic.

Cystoscopy

Cystoscopy requires sterile patient prep and cold sterilization of the endoscope. Sterile gloved hands handle both the passing of the scope and prepped orifice while another person manages the endoscope mechanics. Air is used to visualize the urinary bladder. Removal of air before removing the scopes is optional. Sterile tubing may be passed through the endoscope channel and may be directed and used to collect urine samples directly from each ureter.

Sample Handling

Dependent on sample type, it may be submitted for cytology, histopathology, or culture/sensitivity. Follow the laboratory's requirements for submission.

Post-procedure

Potential post-procedure complications include hemorrhage, colic, or nosocomial infection. Consider sterilizing the endoscope following guttural pouch examination when strangles is a differential.

Milk Cultures

Indication

Some mastitis can be asymptomatic and/or transmitted via the environment and, therefore, difficult to track. Producers may choose to perform random milk culture sampling throughout the herd as well as testing all quarters of any individual herd member that shows clinical signs. See Box 7.19 for supplies.

Dairy producing animals with new cases of high somatic cell counts (SCC) on the DHIA (Dairy Herd Improvement Association) monthly test report should have a California Mastitis Test (CMT) scored and all quarters cultured.

Note: Bulk tank cultures are never substitutes for quarter milk samples.

Patient Prep

- Wash teats with individual paper towels; pre-dip can be used for this.
- It is very important to scrub the teats farthest away from you first then scrub the closer teats.
- Dry teats with individual paper towels.
- Wipe each teat end with an alcohol-soaked cotton ball or swab.

Procedure

- When taking the milk samples, start sampling the closest teats first, followed by the teats farthest away last.

Box 7.19 Supplies for Milk Culture

- sterile culture tubes or containers
- pre- and post-teat dip
- paper towels
- teat wash
- teat dip
- alcohol swabs
- non-sterile gloves

- When taking milk from each teat, discard the first two squirts then put the next two to four streams into a culture vial.
- Only a small amount of milk is needed.
- Securely cap the vial closed.
- Be sure to record proper cow number or name on the lid of the vial, along with the teat location, farm name, and date.
- Any doubt of a contaminated sample necessitates throwing the sample away and repeating with a new vial. Common sources of contamination are straw, dirt, or manure falling from the base of the udder into the vial.
- For screening for *Mycoplasma* or *Staph aureus*, milk from all four teats can go in the same vial.

Sample Handling

The best results occur when samples are cooled immediately after being obtained. Freeze milk samples if they are not going to be delivered to the laboratory the same day they are taken. The freezing of the samples will not affect the culture results.

Post-procedure

Proceed with routine milking followed by teat dip and/or udder treatment (Figure 7.61).

Submissions

Milk samples should be sent to a diagnostic laboratory for special culture techniques required to identify the organism, unless laboratory supplies and trained personnel are readily available. Large producers may have a lab of their own.

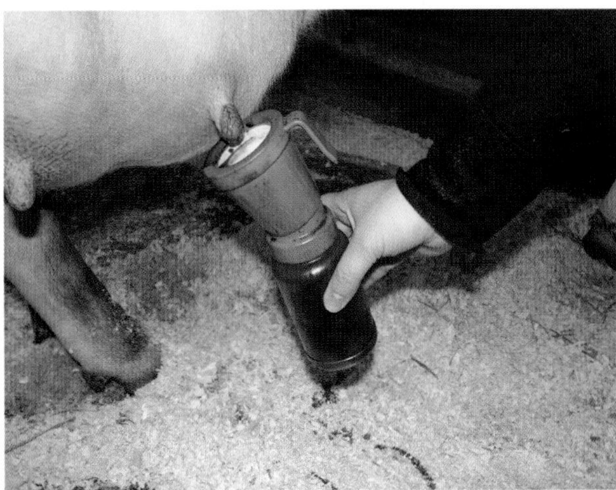

Figure 7.61 Teat dipping a cow udder.

> **TECHNICIAN TIP 7.17:** DO NOT hold the vial directly under the udder. Hold the vial horizontally and direct milk flow into the vial to avoid foreign particles falling in and contaminating the sample.

Thoracocentesis

Indications and Considerations

Analysis of pleural fluid obtained by thoracocentesis is a useful diagnostic and therapeutic aid to assess alterations in the thoracic cavity. Pleural fluid accumulation occurs in cases of pleuropneumonia, penetrating wounds to the thorax, thoracic neoplasia, and hydatic cyst, among other pathologies. When indicated, the pleural space content, usually air or fluid, can be drained to facilitate lung expansion. The aspirated fluid should be submitted for cytology, aerobic and anaerobic culture, and antimicrobial sensitivity testing. Based on the results of these tests, appropriate antimicrobial therapy can be instituted, especially in cases of hemothorax secondary to traumatic wounds due to the high risk of contamination and infection. See Box 7.20 for supplies list.

> **TECHNICIAN TIP 7.18:** A three-way stop cock is very useful in a thoracocentesis.

Patient Prep

Sedation or restraint may be needed to safely perform the procedure, depending on the species involved and the temperament of the animal. In many cases, sedation is unnecessary due to minimal discomfort caused by the procedure. If any animal, independent of the species, is nervous during handling, sedation should be considered for the procedure. The doses and types of sedatives are often selected based on species, potency, and side effects of each medication.

Box 7.20 Supplies for Thoracocentesis

- sedation/restraint
- animal clippers with #40 surgical blades
- surgical preparation solutions (iodine or chlorhexidine based) and isopropyl alcohol
- variety of syringes (35–60 ml)
- extension set
- three-way stopcock
- catheter (14-gauge 3-in)
- teat cannula/chest tube with Heimlich valve
- collection tubes (plain and EDTA tube)
- culture media (aerobe and anaerobe)
- #15 scalpel blade
- local anesthetic (lidocaine/mepivacaine)
- sterile gloves

Multiple sampling locations are available in large animals, depending on the species. The ideal sites should be determined by the physical and/or thoracic ultrasound examination. The most ventral site(s) should be determined for effective drainage of fluid, as well as the position of the heart, diaphragm, loculation, or pleural adhesion, and any other thoracic abnormality such as neoplasia.

Ultrasound imaging also helps determine the thickness of the body wall and minimizes the risk of penetration of surrounding viscera. In cases of acute pneumothorax, after sealing off the wound, the negative intrathoracic pressure should be reestablished. The thoracocentesis is performed on the most dorso-caudal aspect of the thoracic cavity, just below the epaxial muscles.

Equine

In the horse, ultrasound examination usually locates the best sites, based on where the fluid is located. The sixth or seventh intercostal space in the left hemithorax or the seventh to eighth intercostal space in the left hemithorax, 10 cm dorsal to the olecranon and above the lateral thoracic vein, are the most common sites for thoracocentesis. Bilateral thoracocentesis in horses is frequently indicated, despite communication between the left and right hemithorax through the mediastinum. The opening between the two sides of the thoracic cavity is relatively small, and is often occluded with fibrin when inflammatory processes, such as septic pleuritis, are present. Once fluid has been removed from one side of the thorax, ultrasound can be helpful to reevaluate and monitor fluid distribution within the thoracic cavity.

Large Ruminants

In large ruminants, the distal fifth intercostal space is the most commonly used site, as it is in the most ventral aspect of the pleural cavity accessible for this procedure. If ultrasound is not available, the sixth and seventh intercostal space, within the ventral border of the lung field, is recommended for decreased risk of puncturing the heart.

Small Ruminants

In small ruminants, the best location for thoracocentesis is in the cranioventral portion of the chest, in the most dependent part of the thorax. Caution should be taken to avoid puncture of viscera, and the use of ultrasound is indicated.

Camelids

Thoracocentesis in New World Camelids is performed preferably at the sixth or seventh intercostal space, 10–15 cm dorsal to the ventral aspect of the sternum, or 2–4 cm dorsal to the costochondral junction of the ribs.

Procedure

Once the site is selected, clipped, and aseptically prepared, a local block of the skin and intercostal soft tissues should be performed with local anesthetic. In order to prevent a hematoma, the local block should be performed just cranial to the rib, to avoid trauma to the intercostal nerves and vessels. Even though the use of a sterile 14-gauge catheter for thoracocentesis has been described in the literature, the use of a teat cannula or bitch catheter is recommended due to the decreased risk of pleural damage. Despite increased safety to the pleura, the side holes of the teat cannula can predispose it to bending or breaking during the procedure. The size and length of the cannula needs to be adjusted to the size of the animal and thickness of the thoracic wall. The teat cannula or catheter is attached to an extension set and three-way stopcock, using sterile technique, prior to the start of the procedure. In order to avoid pneumothorax, the three-way stopcock should be in the off position to the patient.

- make a stab skin incision is made with a #15 scalpel blade, on the cranial aspect of the rib, at the desired site. It is important to recognize that a stab incision of the intercostal soft tissues facilitates penetration of the blunt tipped of the teat cannula.
- Carefully introduce the teat cannula is carefully through the stab incision, perpendicular to the skin, along the cranial border of the rib.
- once through the musculature, a "pop," or sudden loss of force required to advance, will be felt, which will indicate entrance of the pleural cavity.
- aspiration should be attempted at this point, through the three-way stopcock. Ultrasound, using sterile technique, can also be performed to confirm appropriate location of the cannula.
- the orientation of the cannula can be adjusted to promote maximal collection and drainage. If a large amount of fluid is drained or expected, the tubing can be extended to a bucket on the ground for gravity drainage, or a suction pump can also be used.
- the patient should be closely monitored throughout drainage, and, when that drainage stops, the stopcock should be immediately closed to the patient.
- a purse-string nonabsorbable suture should be placed around the cannula and tightened as it is removed.

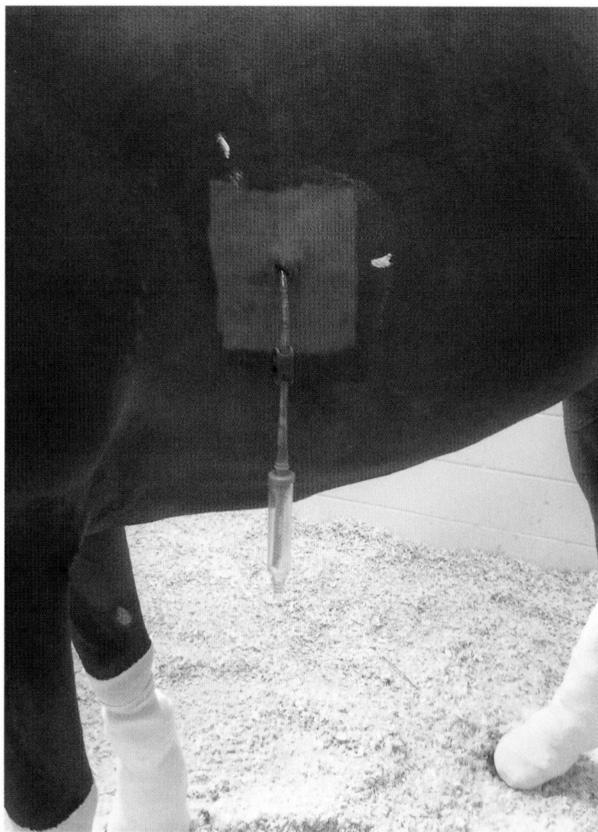

Figure 7.62 Equine patient with a chest tube placed for pleural drainage.

If large amount of fluid is expected, or continued fluid accumulation is expected, a chest tube can be placed instead of a teat cannula. The placement technique is similar, keeping in mind the size difference and the presence of a trocar. Since the chest tube is frequently kept in place to enable drainage over a period of time, a Chinese finger trap pattern with nonabsorbable suture material and a Heimlich valve should be placed, to secure the tube in place and prevent aspiration of air into the thoracic cavity. When a chest tube is used to remove thoracic fluid, the animal should be monitored closely for signs of distress, and the fluid should be removed slowly (Figure 7.62). Drainage of large volumes of fluid can cause disturbances to the cardiovascular system, such as hypotension, due to third space loss. Intravenous fluid therapy during thoracocentesis is indicated during removal of large quantities of pleural fluid. In the case of pneumothorax, air may be removed rather than fluid (Figure 7.63).

Complications

The most common complications of thoracocentesis are pneumothorax and cellulitis around the indwelling chest

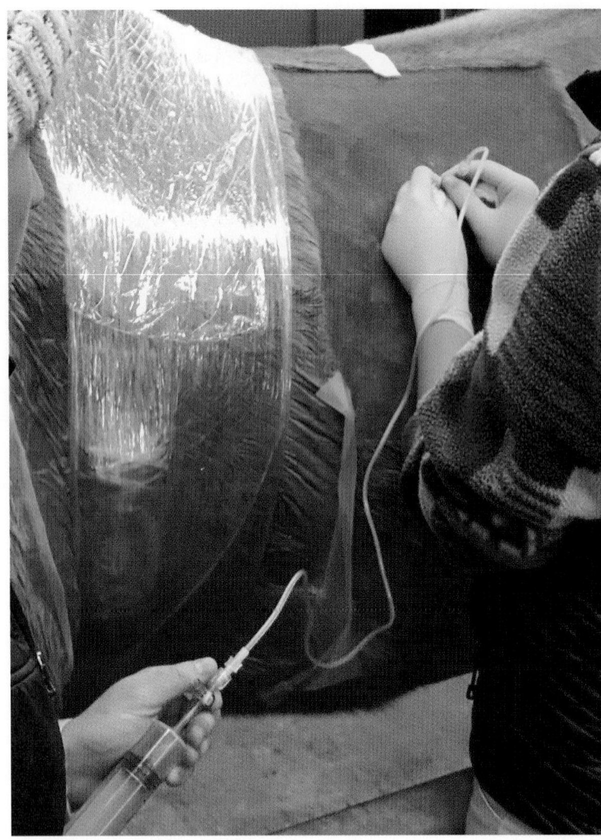

Figure 7.63 Thoracocentesis on a horse to remove air from the chest for treatment of pneumothorax.

tube. Iatrogenic pneumothorax is usually self-limiting and cellulitis usually improves once the tube is removed. Major complications such as cardiac puncture, cardiac arrhythmias, pulmonary laceration, diaphragmatic laceration, and damage to liver can occur, but are much less frequent.

Interpretation

The sample should be evaluated for appearance, odor, volume, and turbidity, in addition to being submitted for bacterial culture, cytology, and Gram stain. The presence of a foul odor oftentimes suggests an anaerobic infection and indicates a more guarded prognosis.

Equine

Normal pleural fluid in the horse contains less than 1000 cells/μl and less than 2.5 g/dl of protein. Biochemical test can also assist to differentiate septic from neoplastic effusions. Glucose, pH, and lactate dehydrogenase are the most reliable tests. Cytology evaluation of the sample might reveal presence of neoplastic cells.

Serosanguinous pleural fluid has been correlated with necrotizing pneumonia, pleural infarction, and thoracic cavity neoplasia. Large volumes of clear, yellow pleural fluid with no odor and minimal turbidity is oftentimes consistent with neoplastic effusion.

Camelids

Pleural fluid of healthy llamas is usually pink-red, and hazy or opaque. Nucleated cell count ranges from 200–1500/μl with the majority of cells being lymphocytes and monocytoid cells, and total protein less than 2.7 g/dl. Normal glucose and lactate concentration are 126–144 mg/dl and 1.6–4.2 mg/dl respectively.

Transtracheal Wash

Indication

Diagnostic evaluation of the lower airway is relatively easy to obtain through TTW and BAL. Information from this procedure can be used to diagnose or rule out acute or chronic inflammation, recurrent airway obstruction (RAO) (Heaves, chronic obstructive pulmonary disease [COPD]), exercise-induced pulmonary hemorrhage (EIPH), hypersensitivity, and more. See Figure 7.64 and Box 7.21 for supplies list.

Potential complications of this procedure include subcutaneous emphysema, local cellulites at the tracheal puncture site, damage to the tracheal cartilage, or development of pneumonia.

Patient Prep

A $5 \times 5\,cm^2$ area immediately overlying the mid-cervical trachea above the strap muscles is clipped and then aseptically prepared. An infiltration of 2–3 ml local anesthetic can be placed subcutaneously at the intended insertion site. Most patients will tolerate the procedure best under standing sedation.

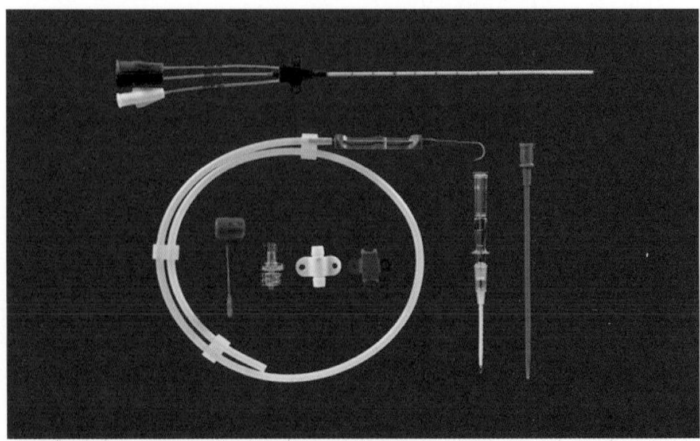

Figure 7.64 Transtracheal wash kit. *Source:* Reproduced with permission of MILA International, Inc.

Box 7.21 Supplies for TTW

- sedation/restraint
- clippers with #40 surgical blades
- surgical preparation solutions (iodine or chlorhexidine based) and isopropyl alcohol
- 3–4 ml local anesthetic (2% lidocaine or similar)
- sterile gloves
- sterile polyurethane guarded aspiration catheter (12-gauge × 28-in) or commercially prepared TTW kit
- 10-gauge needle or sterile catheter or cannula
- 30–40 ml sterile buffered saline in a 60 ml syringe
- sterile culture tube (aerobic only)
- sodium heparin or EDTA anticoagulant vacutainer
- empty sterile sample container(s) or red top tubes

Procedure

A percutaneous technique begins as a sterile technique to pass a large bore needle or sterile catheter or cannula into the trachea lumen. At this point, some clinicians may choose to instill 3–5 ml of local anesthesia to reduce patient irritation and reactive coughing from the procedure. The guarded aspiration catheter or sterile polyurethane catheter is then passed through the bore and advanced downward through the lumen of the trachea to the thoracic inlet. An amount of 30–40 ml of sterile saline is instilled in the tracheal lumen at the thoracic inlet and then aspirated back to acquire a sample. The catheter may need to be readjusted slightly if fluid is not readily collected. On occasion, a second instillation of sterile saline may need to be provided to gather enough of a sample for testing. Bandaging of the tracheal entry site is optional and up to clinician discretion.

See endoscopy section previously in this chapter for TTW through the scope technique.

Interpretation

Transtracheal fluid should appear cloudy or flocculent. Samples should be evaluated for cytology and bacterial and fungal cultures. Normal samples have a wide range of cell types, similar to a BAL sample.

Samples submitted for culturing should only be for aerobic bacteria because of the anatomical location and natural air access, it would be virtually impossible for an anaerobic bacterium to proliferate.

Inflammatory cells could indicate parasitic infections such as lung worm. Cell counts are rarely performed because fluid infused will skew results.

Squamous cells could indicate contamination from skin or oropharynx.

References

References for Abdominocentesis

Anderson, D.E., Cornwell, D., Anderson, L.S. et al. (1995). Comparative analyses of peritoneal fluid from calves and adult cattle. *American Journal of Veterinary Research* 56 (8): 973–976.

Bickers, R.J., Templer, A., Cebra, C.K. et al. (2000). Diagnosis and treatment of torsion of the spiral colon in an alpaca. *Journal of the American Veterinary Medical Association* 216 (3): 380–382.

Butters, A. (2008). Medical and surgical management of uroperitoneum in a foal. *The Canadian Veterinary Journal* 49 (4): 401–403.

Cebra, C.K., Cebra, M.L., Garry, F.B. et al. (1998). Acute gastrointestinal disease in 27 New World camelids: clinical and surgical findings. *Veterinary Surgery* 27 (2): 112–121.

Cebra, C.K., Heidel, J.R., Cebra, M.L. et al. (2000). Pathogenesis of *Streptococcus zooepidemicus* infection after intratracheal inoculation in llamas. *American Journal of Veterinary Research* 61 (12): 1525–1529.

Cebra, C.K., Tornquist, S.J., and Reed, S.K. (2008). Collection and analysis of peritoneal fluid from healthy llamas and alpacas. *Journal of the American Veterinary Medical Association* 232 (9): 1357–1361.

Costarella, C.E. and Anderson, D.E. (1999). Ileocecocolic intussusception in a one-month-old llama. *Journal of the American Veterinary Medical Association* 214 (11): 1672–1673. 1640.

DeHeer, H.L., Parry, B.W., and Grindem, C.B. (2002). Peritoneal fluid. In: *Cytology and Hematology of the Horse*, 2e (eds. R.L. Cowell and R.D. Tyler), 127–162. St. Louis, MO: Mosby.

Javsicas, L.H., Giguere, S., Freeman, D.E. et al. (2010). Comparison of surgical and medical treatment of 49 postpartum mares with presumptive or confirmed uterine tears. *Veterinary Surgery* 39 (2): 254–260.

Jones, M., Miesner, M.D., Baird, A.N. et al. (2012). Disease of the urinary system. In: *Sheep and Goat Medicine*, 2e (eds. D.G. Pugh and A.N. Baird), 325–334. Maryland Heights, MO: Elsevier Saunders.

Juzwiak, J.S., Ragle, C.A., Brown, C.M. et al. (1991). The effect of repeated abdominocentesis on peritoneal fluid constituents in the horse. *Veterinary Research Communications* 15 (3): 177–180.

Milne, E. (2004). Peritoneal fluid analysis for the differentiation of medical and surgical colics in horses. *In Practice* 26 (8): 444.

Newman, K.D. and Anderson, D.E. (2009). Gastrointestinal surgery in alpacas and llamas. *The Veterinary Clinics of North America. Food Animal Practice* 25 (2): 495–506.

Schumacher, J., Spano, J.S., and Moll, H.D. (1985). Effects of enterocentesis on peritoneal fluid constituents in the horse. *Journal of the American Veterinary Medical Association* 186 (12): 1301–1303.

Smith, J.J. and Dallap, B.L. (2005). Splenic torsion in an alpaca. *Veterinary Surgery* 34 (1): 1–4.

Stockham, S.L. and Scott, M.A. (2008). Cavity effusion. In: *Fundamentals of Veterinary Clinical Pathology*, 2e (eds. S.L. Stockham and M.A. Scott), 831–868. Ames, IA: Blackwell.

Taylor, S.D., Pusterla, N., Vaughan, B. et al. (2006). Intestinal neoplasia in horses. *Journal of Veterinary Internal Medicine* 20 (6): 1429–1436.

Trent, A. (2004). Surgery and the peritoneum. In: *Farm Animal Surgery* (eds. S.L. Fubini and N.G. Ducharme), 267–282. St Louis, MO: Saunders.

References for Arthrocentesis

Corley, K. and Stephen, J. (2008). *The Equine Hospital Manual* (pp. 576, 579. Oxford, UK: Blackwell Publishing.

Dechant, J.E., Symm, W.A., and Nieto, J.E. (2011). Comparison of pH, lactate, and glucose analysis of equine synovial fluid using a portable clinical analyzer with a bench-top blood gas analyzer. *Veterinary Surgery* 40: 811–816. https://doi.org/10.1111/j.1532950X.2011.00854.x.

Engeli, E., Haussler, K.K., and Erb, H.N. (2002). How to inject the sacroiliac joint region in horses. *Proceedings of the Annual Convention of the AAEP 2002* 48: 257–260.

Tennent-Brown, B.S. (2012). Interpreting lactate measurements in critically ill horses: diagnosis, treatment, and prognosis. *Compendium* 4 (1): E1–E5.

References for BAL

Corley, K. and Stephen, J. (2008). *The Equine Hospital Manual* (pp. 70–71, 471–472. Oxford, UK: Blackwell Publishing.

Lavoie, J.P. and Hinchcliff, K.W. (2008). *Blackwell's Five-Minute Veterinary Consult Equine*, 2e, pp. 213, 219, 412. Ames, IA: Wiley-Blackwell.

Reed, S.M., Warwick, B.M., and Sellon, D.C. (2010). *Equine Internal Medicine*, 3e, 295. St. Louis, MO: Elsevier.

References for Bone Marrow Biopsy

Corley, K. and Stephen, J. (2008). *The Equine Hospital Manual*, 89–91. Oxford, UK: Blackwell Publishing.

Reed, S.M., Warwick, B.M., and Sellon, D.C. (2010). *Equine Internal Medicine*, 3e, 734. St. Louis, MO: Elsevier.

Sellon, D.C. (2006). How to obtain a diagnostic bone marrow sample from the sternum of an adult horse. *AAEP Proceedings* 52: 621–625.

References for CFS Taps

Hanie, E.A. (2005). *Large Animal Clinical Procedures for Veterinary Technicians*, 100–103. St. Louis, MO: Elsevier Mosby.

McCurnin, D.M. and Bassert, J.M. (2006). *Clinical Textbook for Veterinary Technicians*, 6e, 927–928. St. Louis, MO: Elsevier Saunders.

Reed, S.M., Warwick, B.M., and Sillon, D.C. (2004). *Equine Internal Medicine*, 2e, 542–544. St. Louis, MO: Saunders.

References for Coombs

Courtesy University of Wisconsin, School of Veterinary Medical Teaching Hospital, Clinical Pathology Department. Adapted from AABB Technical Manual and Manual of Clinical Laboratory Immunology Rose, Conway deMacario, et al.

References for ECG

Ferasin, L., Ogden, D., Davies, S. et al. (2005). Electrocardiographic parameters of normal alpacas (lama pacos). *Veterinary Record* 157 (12): 341–343.

Lyle, C. and Keen, J. (2010). Episodic collapse in the horse. *Equine Veterinary Education* 22 (11): 576–586.

Marr, C. and Bowen, I. (2010). *Cardiology of the Horse.* Kidlington, Oxford, UK: Elsevier Limited.

Mcguirk, S., Bednarski, R., and Clayton, M. (1990). Bradycardia in cattle deprived of food. *Journal of the American Veterinary Association* 196 (6): 894–896.

McGuirrin, M., Physick-Sheard, P., and Kenney, D. (2005). How to perform transvenous electrical cardioversion in horses with atrial fibrillation. *Journal of Veterinary Cardiology* 7 (2): 109–119.

Scheffer, C., Robben, J., and Sloet van Oldruitenborgh-Oosterbaan, M. (1995). Continuous monitoring of ECG in horses at rest and during exercise. *Veterinary Record* 137 (15): 371–374.

References for Endoscopy

Birks, E.K., Durando, M.M., and Martin, B.B. (2004). Clinical exercise testing: evaluation of the poor performing athlete. In: *Equine Sports Medicine and Surgery* (eds. K.W. Hinchcliff, A.J. Kaneps and R.J. Geor), 9–18. St. Louis, MO: Saunders Elsevier.

Lindegaard, C. et al. (2007). Sedation with detomidine and acepromazine influences the endoscopic evaluation of laryngeal function in horses. *Equine Veterinary Journal* 39 (6): 553–556.

Parente, E.J. and Derksen, F.J. (2006). Diagnostic techniques in equine upper respiratory tract disease. In: *Equine Surgery*, 3e (eds. J.A. Auer and J.A. Stick), 522–533. St. Louis, MO: Saunders Elsevier.

Robertson, J.T. (1991). Pharynx and larynx. In: *Equine Respiratory Disorders* (ed. J. Beech), 346. Philadelphia, PA: Lea and Febiger.

Sykes, B.W., Hewetson, M., Hepburn, R.J. et al. (2015). European College of Equine Internal Medicine Consensus Statement--Equine Gastric Ulcer Syndrome in Adult Horses. *Journal of Veterinary Internal Medicine* 29 (5): 1288–1299. https://doi.org/10.1111/jvim.13578.

Workshop on Equine Recurrent Neuropathy. (2003). Havemeyer Foundation Monograph Series No. 11, 96.

References for Liver Biopsy

Corley, K. and Stephen, J. (2008). *The Equine Hospital Manual*, 26–28. Oxford, UK: Blackwell Publishing.

Reed, S.M., Warwick, B.M., and Sellon, D.C. (2010). *Equine Internal Medicine*, 3e, pp. 956, 968. St. Louis, MO: Elsevier.

Reference for Milk Cultures

Sterner, K. E. (2007). On-farm milk culturing and mastitis. *Michigan Dairy Review*, January 2007, 1–4.

References for Muscle Biopsy

Corley, K. and Stephen, J. (2008). *The Equine Hospital Manual*, 112–114. Oxford, UK: Blackwell Publishing.

Knottenbelt, D.C. (2006). *Saunders Equine Formulary*, 376. St. Louis, MO: Elsevier.

Reed, S.M., Warwick, B.M., and Sellon, D.C. (2010). *Equine Internal Medicine*, 3e, 496. St. Louis, MO: Elsevier.

References for Rectal Mucosal Biopsy

Corley, K. and Stephen, J. (2008). *The Equine Hospital Manual*, 25–26. Oxford, UK: Blackwell Publishing.

Lindberg, R., Nygren, A., and Persson, S.G. (1996). Rectal biopsy diagnosis in horses with clinical signs of intestinal disorders: a retrospective study of 116 cases. *Equine Veterinary Journal* 28: 275–284.

Reed, S.M., Warwick, B.M., and Sellon, D.C. (2010). *Equine Internal Medicine*, 3e, 850. St. Louis, MO: Elsevier.

References for Skin Biopsy, Cytology, Scraping, and Allergy Testing

Phillips, T.J. and Dixon, P.M. (2000). *Veterinary Clinical Examination and Diagnosis* (eds. O.M. Radostits, I.G. Joe Mayhew and D.M. Houston). W. B. Saunders ISBN: 0-7020-2476-7.

Reed, S.M., Warwick, B.M., and Sellon, D.C. (2010). *Equine Internal Medicine*, 3e, 566. St. Louis, MO: Elsevier.

Wong, D. (2005). Equine skin: structure, immunologic function, and methods of diagnosing disease. *Compendium* 2005: 463–473.

References for Thoracocentesis

Axon, J.E., Russell, C.M., Begg, A.P. et al. (2008). Erythrocytosis and pleural effusion associated with a hepatoblastoma in a Thoroughbred yearling. *Australian Veterinary Journal* 86 (8): 329–333.

Bueno, A.C., Watrous, B.J., Parker, J.E. et al. (2000). Ultrasonographic diagnosis: cranial vena cava thrombosis in a cow. *Veterinary Radiology & Ultrasound* 41 (6): 551–553.

Collins, M.B., Hodgson, D.R., and Hutchins, D.R. (1994). Pleural effusion associated with acute and chronic pleuropneumonia and pleuritis secondary to thoracic wounds in horses: 43 cases (1982–1992). *Journal of the American Veterinary Medical Association* 205 (12): 1753–1758.

Foreman, J.H., Weidner, J.P., Parry, B.W. et al. (1990). Pleural effusion secondary to thoracic metastatic mammary adenocarcinoma in a mare. *Journal of the American Veterinary Medical Association* 197 (9): 1193–1195.

Fowler, M.E. (2010). Clinical diagnosis: examination and procedures. In: *Medicine and Surgery of Camelids*, 3e (ed. M.E. Fowler), 89–109. Ames, IA: Willey Blackwell.

Gerros, T.C. and Andreasen, C.B. (1999). Analysis of transtracheal aspirates and pleural fluid from clinically healthy llamas (*Llama glama*). *Veterinary Clinical Pathology* 28 (1): 29–32.

Jackson, P. and Cockcroft, P. (2002). Clinical examination of the respiratory system. In: *Clinical Examination of Farm Animals*, 1e (eds. P. Jackson and P. Cockcroft), 65–80. Ames, IA: Blackwell Science.

Jorgensen, J.S., Geoly, F.J., Berry, C.R. et al. (1997). Lameness and pleural effusion associated with an aggressive fibrosarcoma in a horse. *Journal of the American Veterinary Medical Association* 210 (9): 1328–1331.

Meuten, D.J., Price, S.M., Seiler, R.M. et al. (1978). Gastric carcinoma with pseudohyperparathyroidism in a horse. *The Cornell Veterinarian* 68 (2): 179–195.

Morris, D.D., Acland, H.M., and Hodge, T.G. (1985). Pleural effusion secondary to metastasis of an ovarian adenocarcinoma in a horse. *Journal of the American Veterinary Medical Association* 187 (3): 272–274.

Plummer, P.J., Plummer, C.L., and Still, K.M. (2012). Disease of the respiratory system. In: *Sheep and Goat Medicine*, 2e (eds. D.G. Pugh and A.N. Baird), 126–149. Maryland Heights, MO: Elsevier Saunders.

Rendle, D.I., Hewetson, M., Barron, R. et al. (2006). Tachypnoea and pleural effusion in a mare with metastatic pancreatic adenocarcinoma. *The Veterinary Record* 159 (11): 356–359.

Rush, B. and Mair, T. (2004). Technique for infectious respiratory disease. In: *Equine Respiratory Disease*, 1e (eds. B. Rush and T. Mair), 291–303. Ames, IA: Blackwell Science.

Toribio, R.E., Kohn, C.W., Lawrence, A.E. et al. (1999). Thoracic and abdominal blastomycosis in a horse. *Journal of the American Veterinary Medical Association* 214 (9) 1335: 1357–1360.

Wrigley, R.H., Gay, C.C., Lording, P. et al. (1981). Pleural effusion associated with squamous cell carcinoma of the stomach of a horse. *Equine Veterinary Journal* 13 (2): 99–102.

References for Transtracheal Wash

Corley, K. and Stephen, J. (2008). *The Equine Hospital Manual* (pp. 69–70, 458–459, 681. Oxford, UK: Blackwell Publishing.

Lavoie, J.P. and Hinchcliff, K.W. (2008). *Blackwell's Five-Minute Veterinary Consult Equine*, 2e, 220–221. Ames, IA: Wiley-Blackwell.

Reed, S.M., Warwick, B.M., and Sellon, D.C. (2010). *Equine Internal Medicine*, 3e, 124–126. St. Louis, MO: Elsevier.

References for Uterine Biopsy

Lavoie, J.P. and Hinchcliff, K.W. (2008). *Blackwell's Five-Minute Veterinary Consult Equine*, 2e, 274–275. Ames, IA: Wiley-Blackwell.

Reed, S.M., Warwick, B.M., and Sellon, D.C. (2010). *Equine Internal Medicine*, 3e, pp. 1014–1015, 1019–1020. St. Louis, MO: Elsevier.

Reeder, D. and Zimmel, D. (2009). *AAEVT's Equine Manual for Veterinary Technicians*, 121–123. Ames, IA: Wiley-Blackwell.

Clinical Case Resolution 7.1

The base-apex lead is commonly used to obtain a rhythm strip in large animal patients. The electrodes are placed as follows: LA over the left heart, just behind the triceps muscle; RA at the top of the right scapula; RL over the right jugular grove. The machine would be set to read in lead I. The rhythm diagnosis is atrial fibrillation and is not a life-threatening arrhythmia. Checking serum or plasma electrolytes and a venous blood gas would be reasonable next steps in a patient with diarrhea and atrial fibrillation. Atrial fibrillation can be caused by derangements of acid–base and electrolyte balance.

Activities

Multiple Choice Questions

(Answers can be found in the back of the book.)

1. Aseptic preparation should be used for each of the following procedures except:
A liver biopsy
B uterine biopsy
C bone marrow biopsy
D skin biopsy

2. Which specialized tool could be used for a muscle biopsy?
A Monopty
B Tru-Cut
C EZ-IO
D Bergström

3. Which cycle is the most preferred during the sampling for a uterine biopsy?
   A diestrus
   B anestrus
   C estrus
   D proestrus

4. Mineral deficiencies, acute hepatitis, or icterus may warrant which of the following tests:
   A liver biopsy
   B muscle biopsy
   C bone marrow biopsy
   D rectal biopsy

5. Normal activated clotting time for a cow is:
   A 30 S
   B 90 S
   C 145 S
   D 300 S

6. Which cardiac abnormality is commonly found in athletic horses?
   A atrial fibrillation
   B ventricular tachycardia
   C third-degree atrioventricular block
   D ventricular premature complexes (VPCs)
   E sinus bradycardia

7. Besides checking total protein levels and cell counts, peritoneal fluid may also be tested for:
   A PCV, glucose, and bacterial cultures
   B opacity, total solids, and sensitivity
   C fibrinogen, BUN, and AST
   D glucose, lactate, and pH

8. Which cerebrospinal fluid location will be more likely to yield a large sample?
   A atlantooccipital space
   B lumbosacral space
   C thoracolumbar junction
   D sacral vertebral space

9. How many times should RBCs be washed for a Coomb's test?
   A once
   B twice
   C three times
   D none at all

10. Which of the following crossmatches should be performed for a pregnant mare or previously transfused patient?
    A major crossmatch
    B minor crossmatch
    C both A and B
    D none of the above

Test Your Learning

1. Describe three diagnostic procedures that may be performed on a patient with an airway disease.
2. Describe the different sites that can be used for abdominocentesis in a small ruminant patient.
3. Describe the process for culturing a milk sample.
4. Name two key functions of bone marrow and list two locations that may be commonly used for the collection of bone marrow.
5. Describe each of the following and what they represent in an ECG tracing: P wave, PR interval, QRS complex, T wave, ST segment, baseline.

Answers can be found in the back of the book.

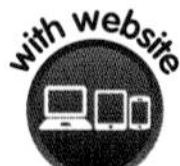

Extra review questions, case studies, and a breed ID image bank can be found online at www.wiley.com/go/loly/veterinary.

Chapter 8

Medical Imaging

Myra F. Barrett, DVM, MS, DACVR, Kurt Selberg, MS, DVM, DACVR, Sheryl Ferguson, CVT, VTS (LAIM), JoAnn Slack, DVM, MS, DACVIM (LAIM), and Sue Loly, LVT, VTS (EVN)

Learning Objectives

- List the three basic principles of radiation safety.
- Describe the minimum patient information and labeling that should be included for an imaging study.
- Summarize standard radiographic views of the equine foot and joints.
- Explain ultrasound settings that are commonly manipulated during an exam.
- Compare advantages and disadvantages of radiography, nuclear scintigraphy, and ultrasound.

Clinical Case Problem 8.1

A four-year-old Thoroughbred gelding used for racing is brought into the clinic for a lameness evaluation. The assessment shows 2/5 right front lameness, and the horse is resistant to carpal flexion. The middle joint of the right carpus is effusive (increased fluid in the joint). Radiographs of the carpus are acquired to further evaluate these findings, as it is one of the tools in the equine diagnostic imaging tool chest. Understanding the advantages and disadvantages of the various imaging modalities and how they work is the key to knowing when to utilize them. When correctly utilized, imaging can play a crucial role in the diagnostic workup and therapeutic plan.

See Clinical Case Resolution 8.1 at the end of this chapter.

Key Terms

Artifact
C-arm
Computed tomography (CT)
Distance
Doppler
Gantry
Gauss
Hounsfield scale
Kilovoltage (kVp)
Magnetic resonance imaging (MRI)
Milliampere (mA)
Milliampere-seconds (mAs)
Nuclear scintigraphy
Radiation safety
Radiography
Shielding
Tesla
Time
Transducer
Ultrasonography

Introduction

Diagnostic imaging is an essential tool in veterinary practice, including for lameness evaluation, internal medicine workups, and neonatal care. The value of diagnostic imaging is directly related to the quality of the images that are obtained. Poor-quality imaging leads to little useful information and possible misdiagnosis, and wastes both time and money. As in many realms of veterinary practice, the veterinary technician plays an essential role in ensuring the patient

Large Animal Medicine for Veterinary Technicians, Second Edition. Edited by Sue Loly and Heather Hopkinson.

Companion website: www.wiley.com/go/loly/veterinary

receives the best possible care and aids veterinarians to achieve this goal.

TECHNICIAN TIPS 8.1: Poor-quality imaging leads to little useful information and possible misdiagnosis, and wastes both time and money.

By understanding the choice of modalities, having a good working knowledge of imaging equipment and anatomy, and striving to obtain high-quality images, the veterinary technician becomes an invaluable member of the diagnostic imaging team.

The goal of this chapter is to provide a fundamental overview of radiography, ultrasonography, nuclear scintigraphy, and advanced imaging modalities, including computed tomography (CT) and magnetic resonance imaging (MRI). Guidelines for patient preparation, pre-acquisition planning, obtaining images, and evaluating image quality are included, as well as a discussion of common errors and pitfalls.

Safety and Quality

The primary goal of imaging is to obtain high-quality diagnostic images that increase our knowledge about a particular patient and a disease process. Attention must be given to quality control. This means keeping equipment in good operating condition, upgrading software and hardware when needed, proper patient preparation, and adhering to image acquisition principles as discussed in this chapter.

As important as it is to obtain high-quality images, imaging should not be performed at the sacrifice of safety. Safety of personnel and patient must come first. If an image cannot be obtained without endangering personnel or patient, then the environment should be reevaluated, approached in a different fashion, or abandoned completely. For example, a flexed view of the stifle may not be possible in a horse that kicks when the foot is lifted. This patient may need physical or chemical restraint or additional personnel to increase safety.

Safety should not be sacrificed for the sake of speed. Working without proper shielding, such as wearing lead aprons, is not an appropriate way of saving time. Workflow or patient load may increase pressure to hurry and complete the process, but this must not be done by sacrificing personnel safety.

TECHNICIAN TIPS 8.2: The need for taking radiographs quickly should never affect safety.

Radiography

Radiography is a mainstay of imaging in an equine practice. It is commonly performed for lameness evaluation, prepurchase examinations, trauma, and dental disease. At hospitals with large in-house generators, thoracic and abdominal studies are also performed. In some practices, veterinary technicians acquire all of the radiographic studies, while in others, their role is to assist the veterinarian. Regardless of their role, technicians are often responsible for helping maintain quality and managing equipment.

Radiation Safety

Unfortunately, radiation safety may fall to the wayside in the veterinary practice. This may be because people are in a hurry, have not invested in the proper safety equipment, or do not believe that radiation is a real threat; however, excessive exposure to ionizing radiation should be avoided as much as possible. While there are many facets to radiation safety that are beyond the scope of this chapter, some basic principles are discussed in the following sections. The mantra of radiation safety is:

- Time
- Distance
- Shielding

Time

Time refers to the amount of time an individual is exposed to radiation. Minimizing the amount of time exposed to radiation can be challenging, especially in a small veterinary practice with fewer personnel. In cases where the same people are regularly acquiring radiographs, rotating who holds the cassette, who holds the horse, and who holds the X-ray machine can be helpful. The person holding the cassette generally receives the highest dose of scatter radiation; therefore, it is ideal to share this job among several individuals whenever possible.

Reducing the number of images acquired can also minimize exposure. Taking time for proper patient preparation and radiographic technique can improve image quality and decrease the number of repeat images required.

Distance

Increasing the distance between personnel and the radiation source helps decrease exposure to radiation. The inverse-square law ($1/x^2$) explains the principle. For example, by stepping 2 ft away, the amount of radiation exposure is decreased by one-fourth. In practice, this can be applied in multiple ways. Leaning the body away from the beam when holding the limb or cassette and using long cassette handles are some examples. People who are not directly involved in obtaining the radiographs should always leave the room.

Shielding

Lead aprons, thyroid shields, and lead gloves help minimize exposure. Although they are often hot and can be uncomfortable, lead aprons must be considered an essential part of the procedure. Lead aprons come in multiple sizes and can come with supportive back bands that improve comfort and ease of motion. Lead gloves protect hands and should be used, particularly if a cassette holder is not available. All personnel should have individual dosimeters that record radiation exposure.

General Imaging Technique

Technique settings vary with the type of equipment and type of study. Most systems, both digital and screen film, will have a recommended technique chart. The technique chart may be provided by the X-ray machine manufacturer or has been developed at the practice for the individual machine. Technique charts provide a guide for peak kilovoltage (kVp), milliampere (mA), and time in seconds (s) for a particular study. You may also encounter the term mAs, which represents a combined measure of radiation produced over a set time. These settings may need to be modified. For example, settings may need to be increased if radiographing a draft horse leg and decreased for a foal. The film focal distance, which is the distance between the X-ray machine and the cassette, is generally 60 cm with a portable system but should follow manufacturer recommendations. The gradient of tissue density in radiology is referred to as a Hounsfield scale or unit (Figure 8.1).

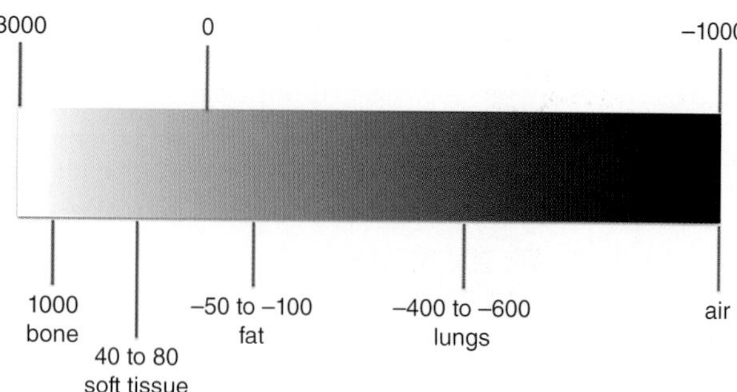

Figure 8.1 Hounsfield scale.

Standard Radiographic Studies

Within this section, common equine radiographic views and techniques are discussed. Radiographic views for equine can be applied to other large animal species with a few setting and positioning changes based on anatomic differences between species. For example, reticular views for cattle are helpful for diagnosing hardware disease, and uroliths can be imaged via views of the urinary system in small ruminants. Some references for other species are included within this chapter and more are available on the online resources.

Foot

Feet are one of the most commonly radiographed anatomical regions and also require the most preparation. Ideally, shoes should be removed prior to radiography. Unfortunately, this is often not clinically practical, and studies are often acquired with the shoes on despite the limitations visualizing some parts of the foot.

Prior to radiography, the foot should be thoroughly cleaned to remove dirt and debris. A wire brush and hoof pick may be used to remove debris from the sole, frog sulcus, and hoof wall. Excessive horny tissue should be removed. A moderate amount of packing material (usually, Play-Doh®) should be pressed firmly into the sulci of the frog to help eliminate gas artifacts.

The standard radiographic views included in a foot series include:

- lateral medial (lateral)
- horizontal dorso-palmar or dorso-plantar (DP)
- dorsal60 proximal-palmar distal oblique (D60P)
- palmaroproximal-palmar distal oblique (skyline view of the navicular bone)

Dorsolateral-palmaromedial oblique (DLPMO) and dorsomedial-palmarolateral oblique (DMPLO) radiographs are not often included but can be utilized for better evaluation of the distal phalanx, particularly if shoes are left on. For the lateral and DP images, the patient's feet should be placed on two wooden blocks of equal height. This elevates the foot from the ground to allow for adequate assessment of the sole. It is important to place both (fore or hind) feet on blocks, even if only one foot is being imaged, because otherwise the uneven footing can falsely alter the appearance of the joint space.

> **TECHNICIAN TIPS 8.3:** Placing the patient's feet on blocks of equal height allows for adequate assessment of the sole for the lateral and DP images.

A high-quality lateral view will show a distinct radiolucent line through the distal interphalangeal joint space with no evidence of superimposition of bone due to obliquity. The lateral view is taken with a beam horizontal to the animal as seen in Figures 8.2–8.4. The palmar cortex of the navicular bone should be a single, distinct line. This view is important for assessing the joint spaces and alignment of the phalanges. Note that this view is much more challenging in ruminant species that have two digits such as camelids, bovine sp., ovine, caprine, and swine. The lateral view results in imposition of the two digits (lateral and medial) consisting of P1, P2, P3 (Figure 8.5). Furthermore, the interdigital space should be cleaned to avoid any dirt-type artifacts that will further complicate the radiographic interpretation.

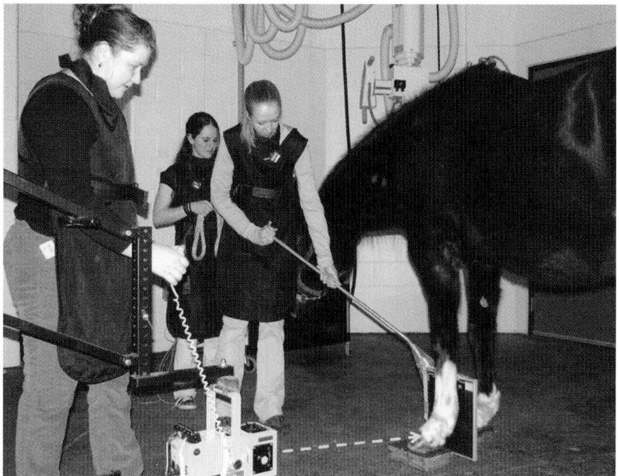

Figure 8.2 Lateral foot is shot with beam horizontal.

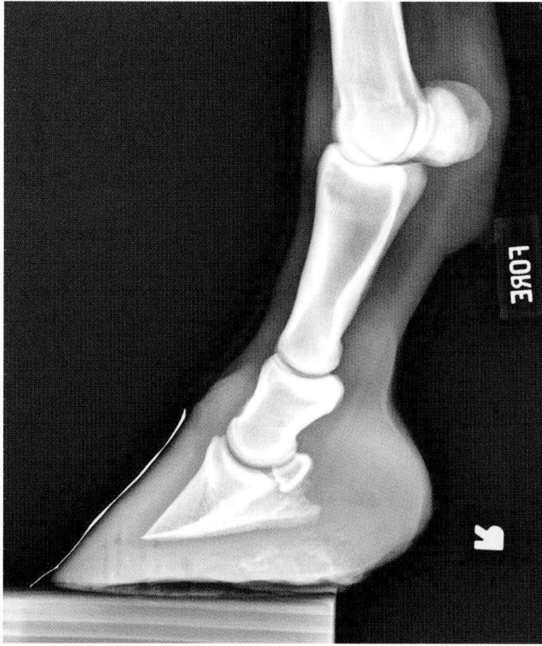

Figure 8.3 Well-positioned lateral view of the distal interphalangeal joint. There is a single line of the palmar surface of the navicular bone and radiolucent joint space. Note the obliquity of the fetlock joint. Due to conformational variability, it is common that a true lateral to the distal interphalangeal joint will not be a true lateral to the fetlock joint, underscoring the need for each joint to be imaged individually.

Website Be sure to check out the online resource for this chapter to see additional images of abnormalities.

The horizontal DP is also important for evaluation of the joint spaces. For this view to be accurate, the patient must be standing as straight and square as possible. Abduction of the limb can falsely create the impression of medial-lateral imbalance (Figures 8.6 and 8.7).

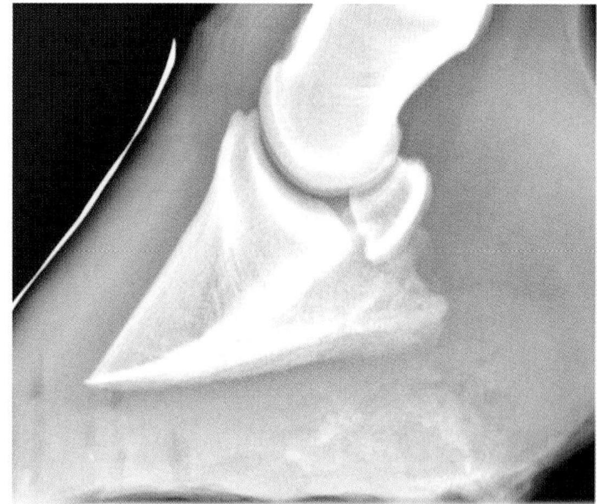

Figure 8.4 Zoomed-in image of Figure 8.3.

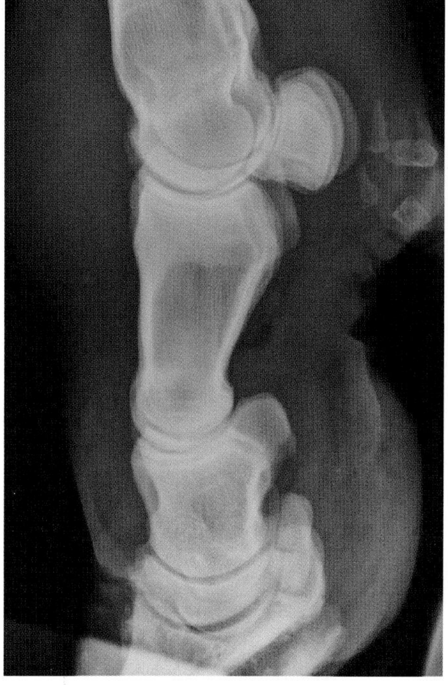

Figure 8.5 Lateral view of the digits of a bovine foot with superimposition of the digits.

The D60P view can be acquired in several ways. The foot can be placed on a cassette tunnel, with the cassette inside (Figure 8.8). The X-ray machine is aimed at the cassette at a 60° angle, and the beam is centered on the coronary band. The advantage of this technique is that horses are usually compliant for standing on the tunnel. The tunnel is also used for the navicular skyline view, so no extra equipment is needed. The disadvantage of this approach is that it introduces some distortion artifact, as the beam is not perpendicular to the cassette. Another approach is for the horse's foot to be placed on a block at an upright angle, with the cassette placed behind the foot and the beam directed

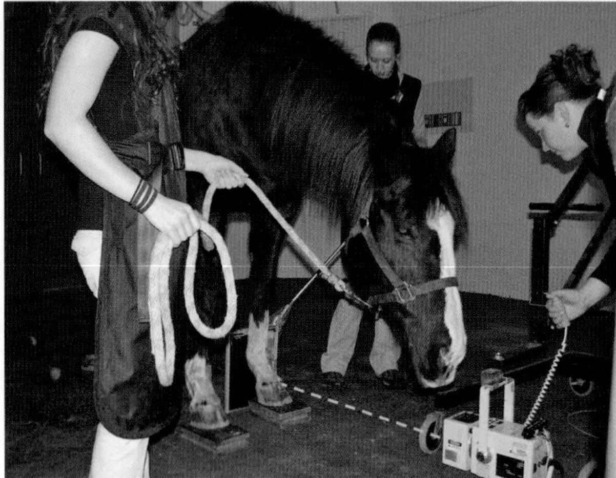

Figure 8.6 The DP Foot is radiographed on tunnel with the beam horizontal.

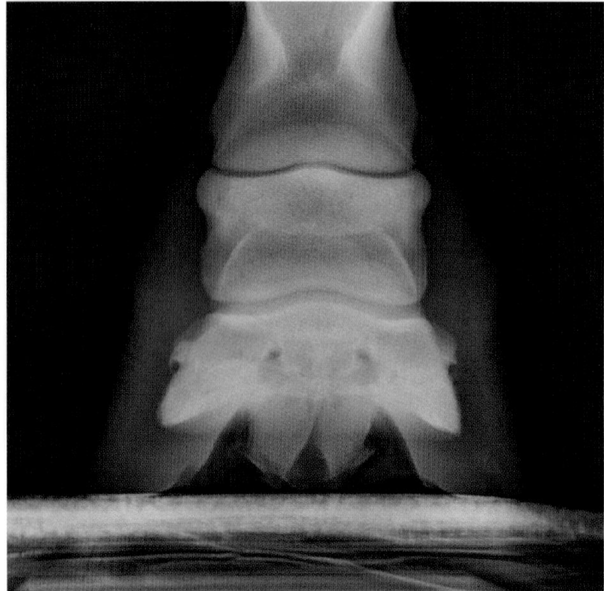

Figure 8.7 DP Foot.

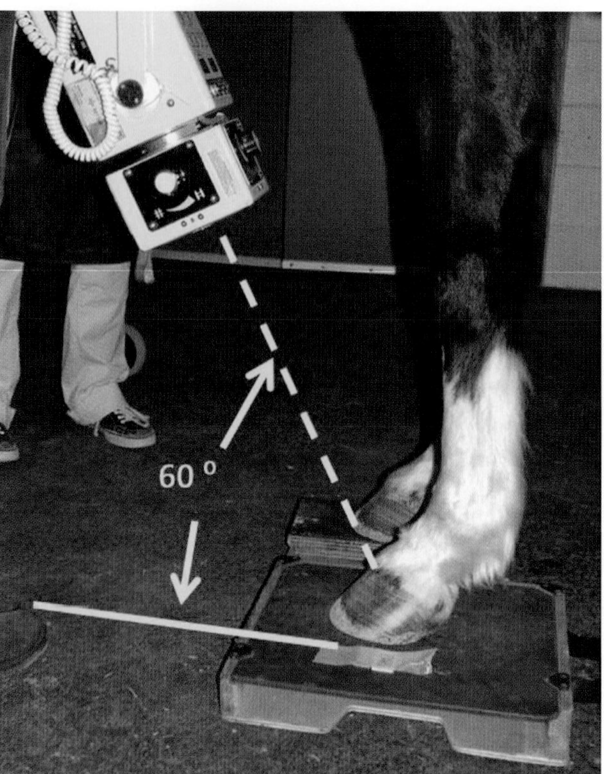

Figure 8.8 D60P on tunnel.

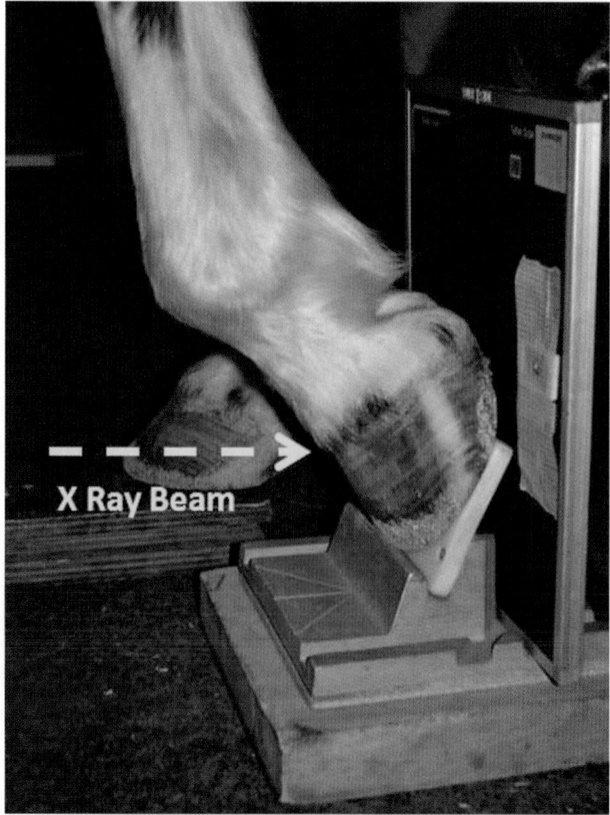

Figure 8.9 D60P on block at an upright angle.

perpendicularly to the cassette (Figure 8.9). Debris and gas artifact can seriously affect image interpretation in this view, and may create mock fracture lines; therefore, having the foot clean and well-packed is essential (Figure 8.10).

> **TECHNICIAN TIPS 8.4:** To help eliminate gas artifacts, packing material should be pressed firmly into the sulci of the frog.

The navicular skyline view is an essential view for evaluating the palmar cortex of the navicular bone, which is a frequent site of pathologic change. The skyline is obtained by extending the leg caudally behind the contralateral

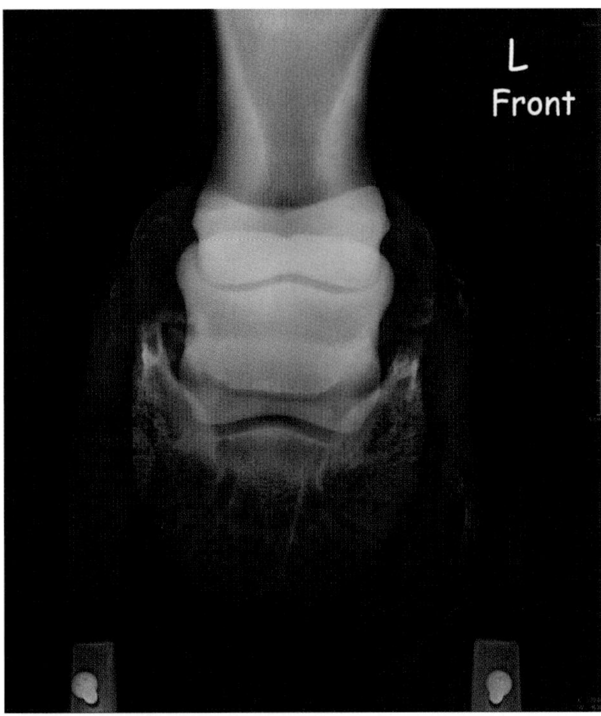

Figure 8.10 D60P image on X-ray.

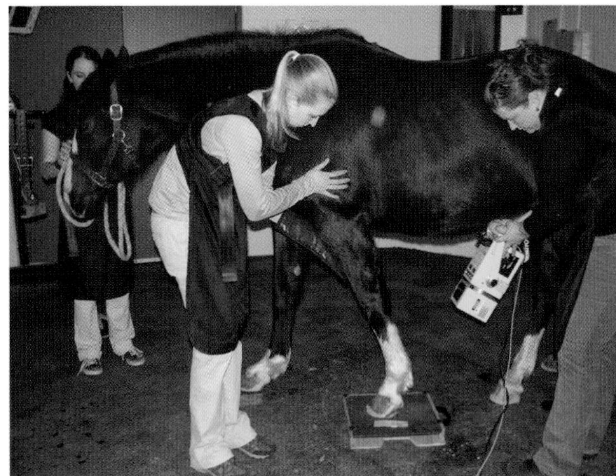

Figure 8.11 Navicular skyline.

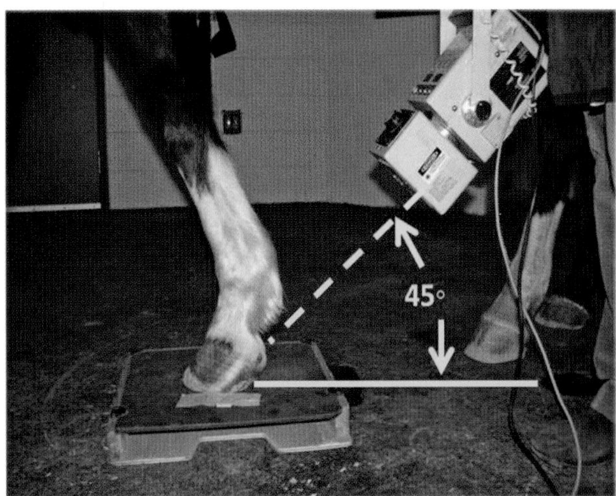

Figure 8.12 Zoom-in of navicular skyline.

limb, keeping the heel flat (Figures 8.11 and 8.12). The X-ray machine is placed below the thorax, and the beam is centered between the heel bulbs at a 45° angle. In a well-positioned skyline image, the articulation of dorsal aspect of the navicular bone and the palmar aspect of the middle phalanx is well-defined and the entire medullary cavity of the navicular bone is visualized (Figure 8.13 to 8.15).

TECHNICIAN TIPS 8.5: A frequent site of pathologic change in the foot is the palmar cortex of the navicular bone.

Generally, if the articulation of the navicular bone and middle phalanx is indistinct, it means that the beam was angled too shallowly, or the foot was not placed sufficiently caudal. This can result in an artifactual appearance of navicular medullary sclerosis.

Fetlock

The standard radiographic views included in a fetlock series include:

- lateromedial (lateral)
- dorso 15–30 proximal-palmar/plantar distal oblique (DP)
- flexed lateromedial (f-LM)
- dorso 15–20 proximal 45 lateral-palmaromedial oblique (DLPMO)
- dorso 15–20 proximal 45 medial-palmarolateral oblique (DMPLO)

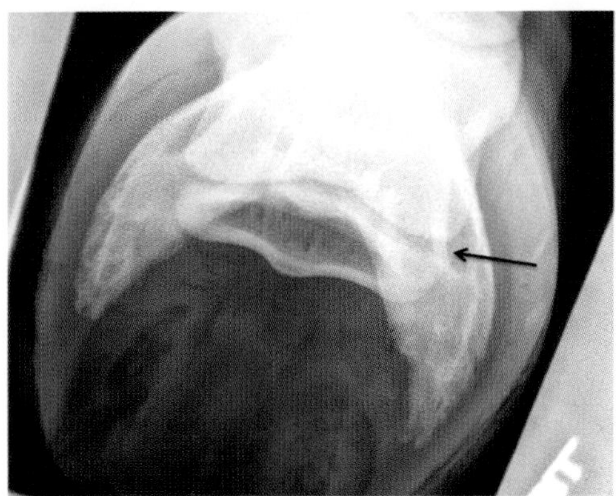

Figure 8.13 A well-positioned navicular skyline view. There is a distinct radiolucent line at the articulation of the navicular bone and middle phalanx (black arrow). The cortex and medulla of the navicular bone are well-defined, and there is no superimposition of debris or gas artifact. A laterality marker is in place.

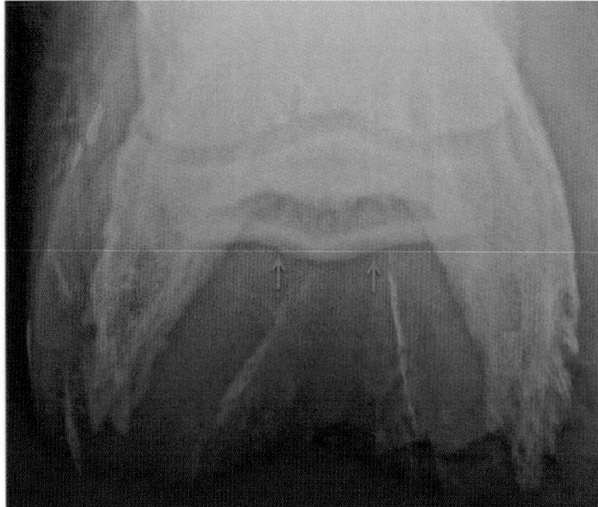

Figure 8.14 A poorly prepared and positioned navicular skyline radiograph. There is poor corticomedullary distinction; the spongiosa appears sclerotic. There is debris in the sulci. Lucent areas are seen on the palmar cortex of the navicular bone (arrows). With this radiograph, it is difficult to distinguish true pathologic change (sclerosis and possible cortical lysis) from artifact.

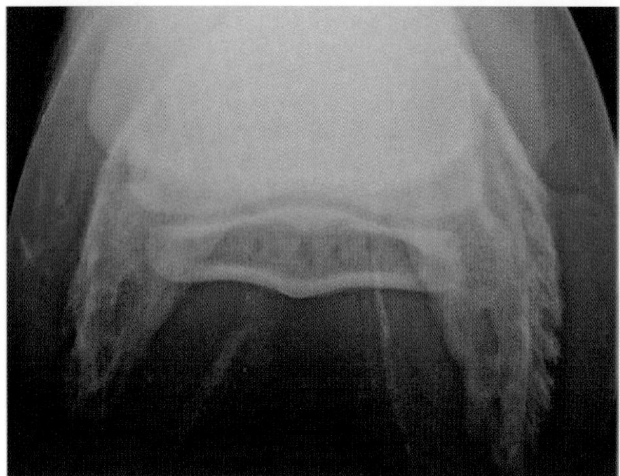

Figure 8.15 Repeat navicular skyline radiograph on the same horse. There is good corticomedullary distinction and no evidence of cortical lysis. The synovial invagination is mildly dilated with mild surrounding sclerosis. Debris remains in the sulcus of the frog; however, this is a much better-quality diagnostic radiograph when compared to Figure 8.13.

The lateromedial view is obtained with the foot on the ground. The X-ray cassette is also placed on the ground along the medial surface of the distal limb. The X-ray beam is centered at the fetlock (Figure 8.16). When assessing correct positioning, it is often helpful to align the X-ray parallel with the heels and ground. The hind limb often requires a slight 5° upward angle to superimpose the condyles. A properly positioned lateromedial radiograph should have the condyles of the metacarpus/tarsus and proximal sesamoid bones perfectly superimposed (Figure 8.17).

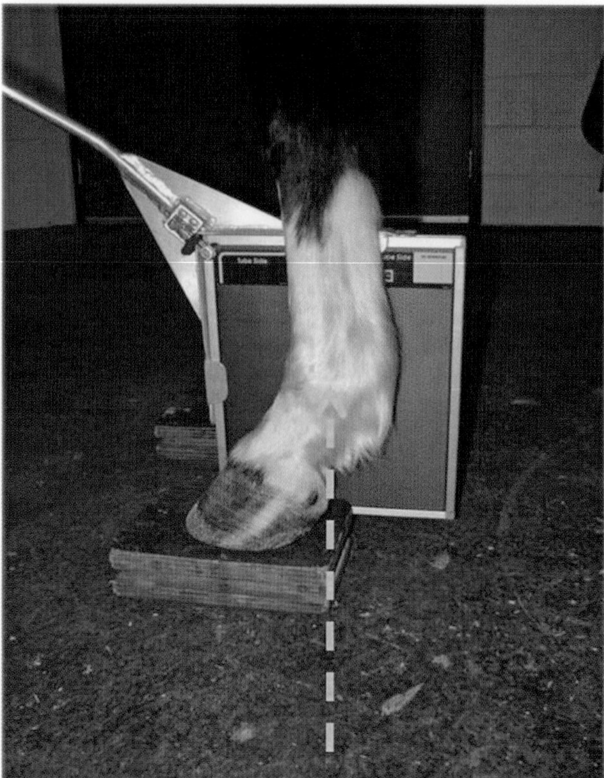

Figure 8.16 Lateromedial fetlock with beam centered on the fetlock.

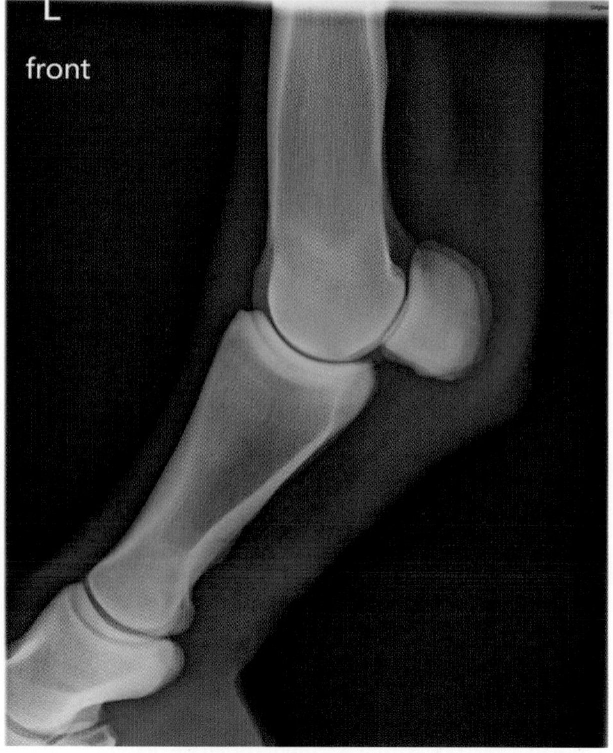

Figure 8.17 Lateromedial fetlock.

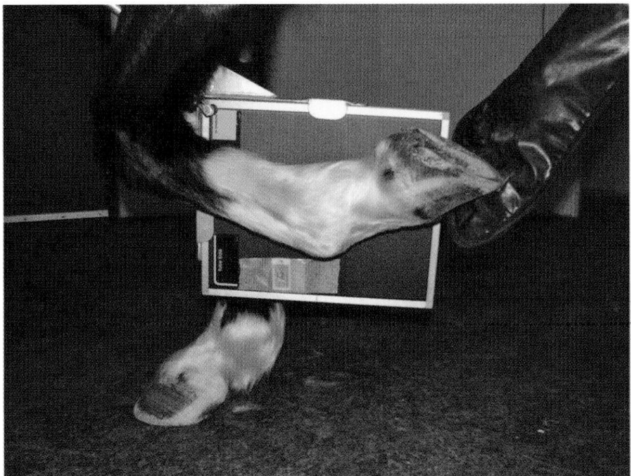

Figure 8.18 Flexed lateral fetlock.

TECHNICIAN TIPS 8.6: It is often helpful to align the X-ray parallel with the heels and ground when assessing correct positioning of the lateromedial fetlock.

The flexed lateromedial image is obtained in a non-weight-bearing position. The X-ray machine and cassette are positioned similar to that of the standing lateromedial radiograph. The flexion permits better evaluation of the dorsal aspect of the sagittal ridge, condylar surfaces, and periarticular surface of the sesamoid bones (Figures 8.18 and 8.19).

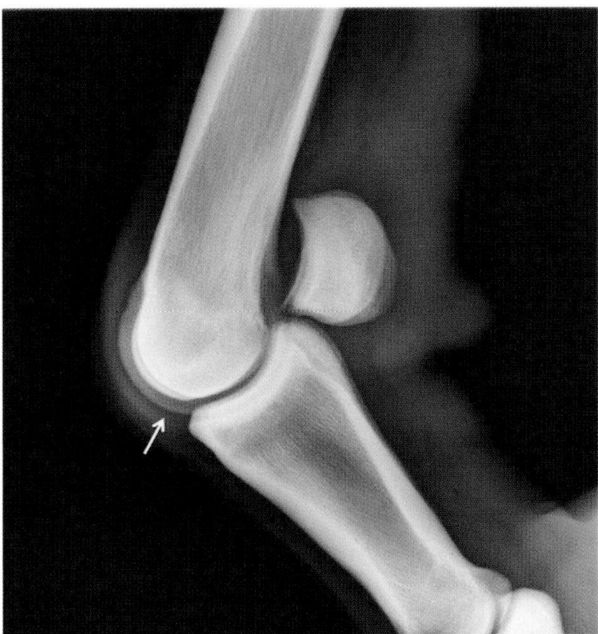

Figure 8.19 A perfectly positioned flexed lateral radiograph of the fetlock allows for evaluation of the sagittal ridge of the third metacarpal bone, free from superimposition. The arrow denotes a common site of pathologic change on the sagittal ridge, which can often only be seen with this projection.

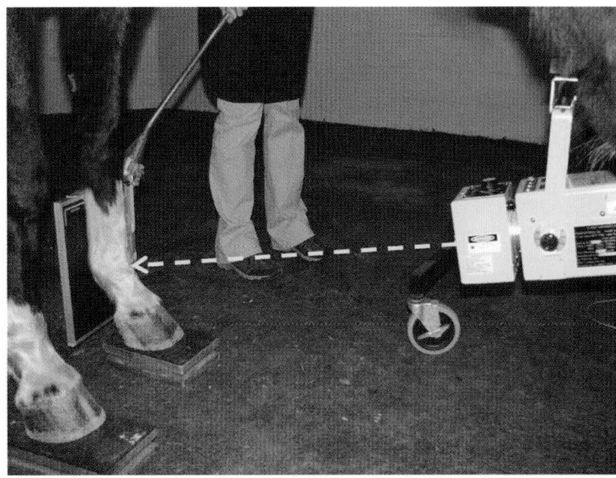

Figure 8.20 The DP fetlock angles downward 15–30°.

A DP of the fetlock is obtained with the X-ray machine positioned dorsally angling down 15–30°. The cassette is positioned along the palmar/plantar surface of the fetlock and perpendicular to the X-ray beam. This angulation to the X-ray beam results in the proximal sesamoids being projected proximal to the joint, allowing for better evaluation of the joint space and underlying bone (Figures 8.20 and 8.21).

Oblique radiographs of the fetlock are obtained with the X-ray machine positioned 45° dorsal medial/lateral to the sagittal plane of the fetlock, angling down 15–20°. The light should be centered on the fetlock. The cassette is positioned

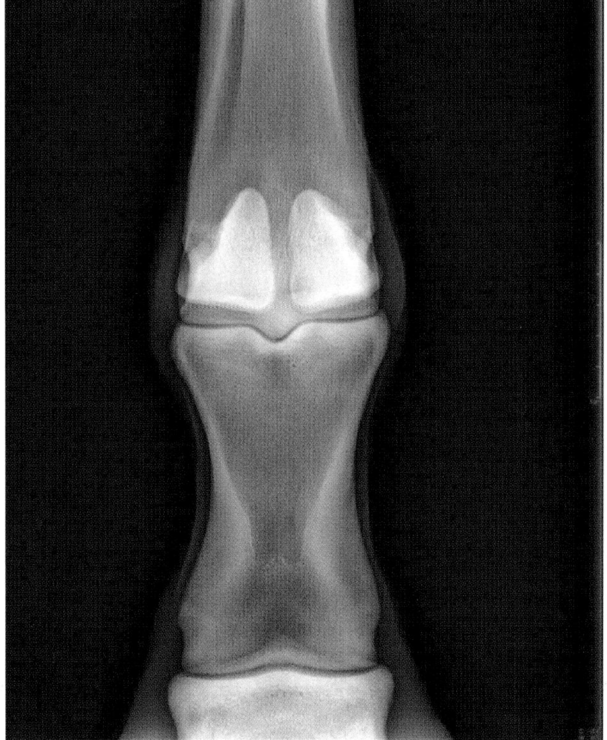

Figure 8.21 DP fetlock.

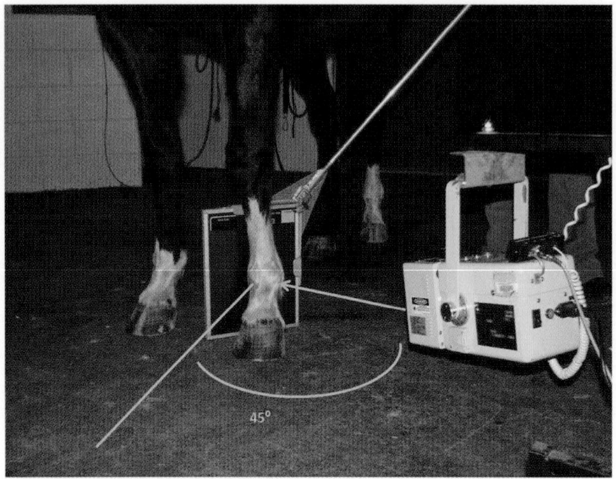

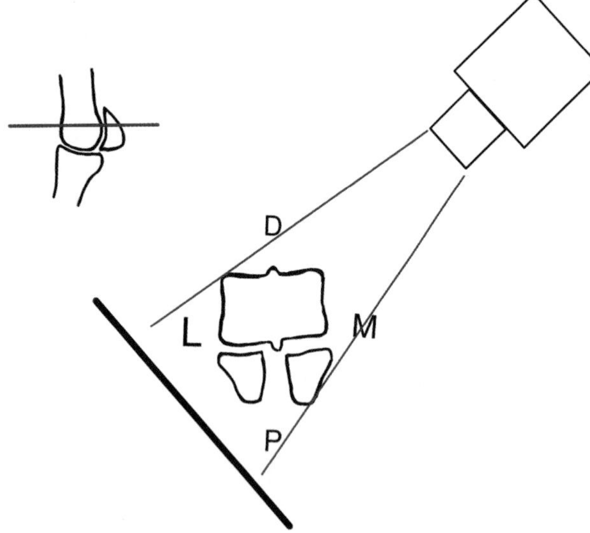

Figure 8.22 (a) Schematic of DLPMO fetlock is 45° off of dorsal. (b) DLPMO fetlock is 45° off of dorsal, angled down 15–20°.

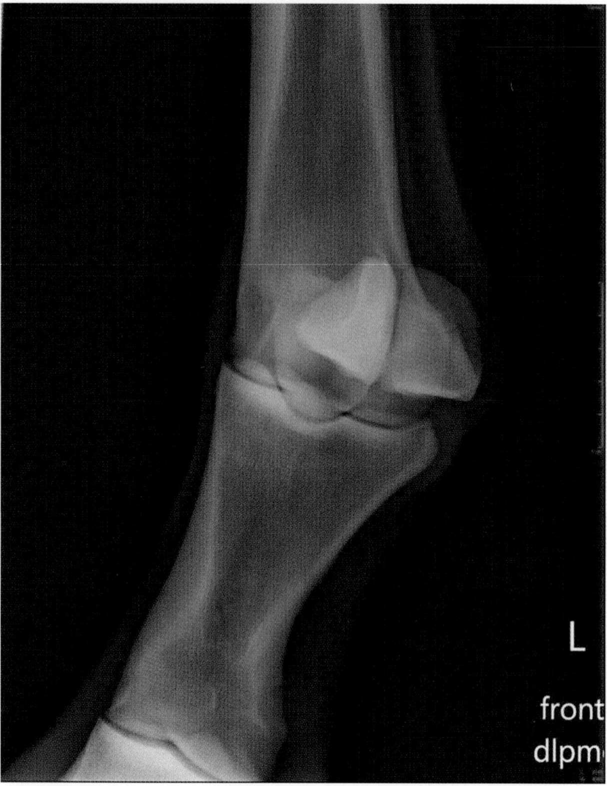

Figure 8.23 DLPMO fetlock.

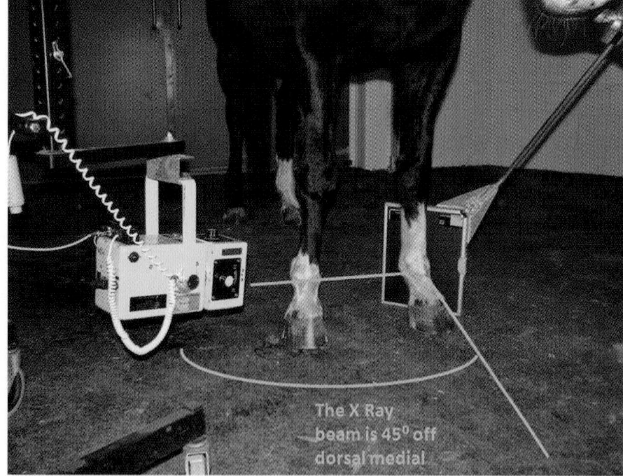

Figure 8.24 DMPLO fetlock is positioned at a 45° off dorsal medial/lateral to the sagittal plane of the fetlock, angling down 15–20°.

against the palmar (plantar) medial or lateral aspect of the fetlock. The resultant image should eliminate superimposition of the sesamoid bone on each other and the palmar (plantar) aspect of the joint. The obliquity of the radiograph defines the surfaces that are highlighted. When obtaining a DLPM-oblique radiograph, the dorsomedial surface and palmarolateral surfaces are projected (Figures 8.22–8.25).

Carpus

The five standard radiographic views included in a carpus series are:

- lateromedial (lateral)
- flexed lateromedial (f-LM)
- dorso-palmar (DP)
- dorso 45–60° lateral-palmaromedial oblique (DLPMO)
- dorso 60–70° medial-palmarolateral oblique (DMPLO)

A lateral view is performed with the horse bearing weight. There should be superimposition of the dorsal surfaces of the radial and intermediate carpal bones. The joint spaces should be seen as distinct radiolucent lines. If there is proximal-distal obliquity of the radiograph, the joint spaces will be superimposed and cannot be adequately assessed (Figures 8.26 and 8.27).

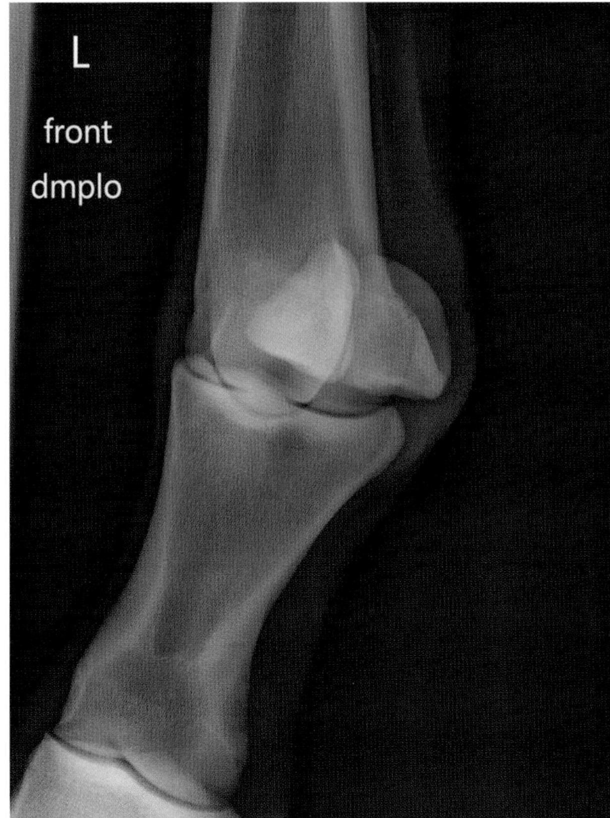

Figure 8.25 DMPLO fetlock.

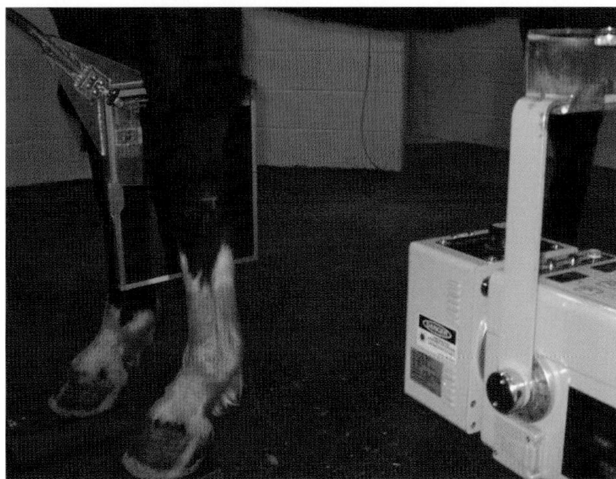

Figure 8.26 Lateral carpus is weight bearing.

The flexed lateral view is an essential view for the equine carpus and should not be excluded from a series. The carpus is flexed approximately 60° by an assistant holding the foot distal to the elbow and pushing the carpus cranially (Figure 8.28). The limb should not be rotated or abducted. When positioned properly, there will be good separation of the cuboidal bones of the carpus, with the intermediate

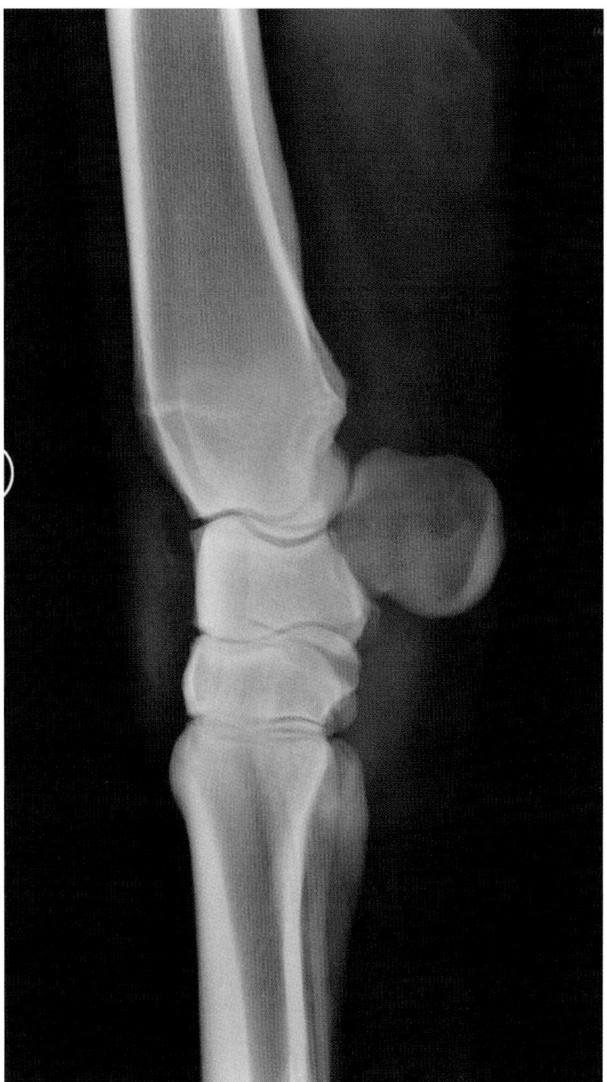

Figure 8.27 Lateral carpus.

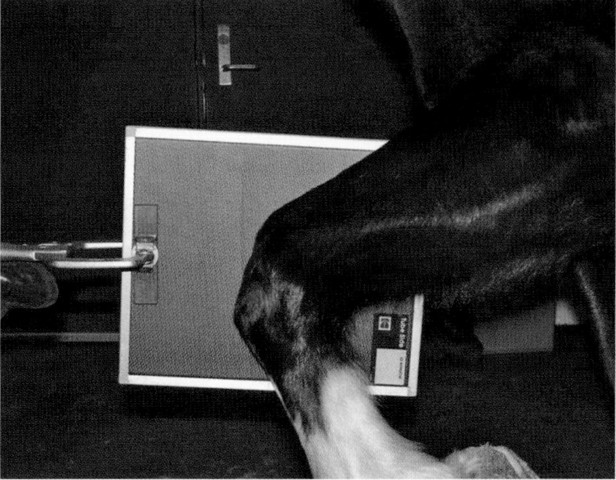

Figure 8.28 Flexed carpus is flexed 60°, pushing the carpus cranially. No rotation or abduction should occur.

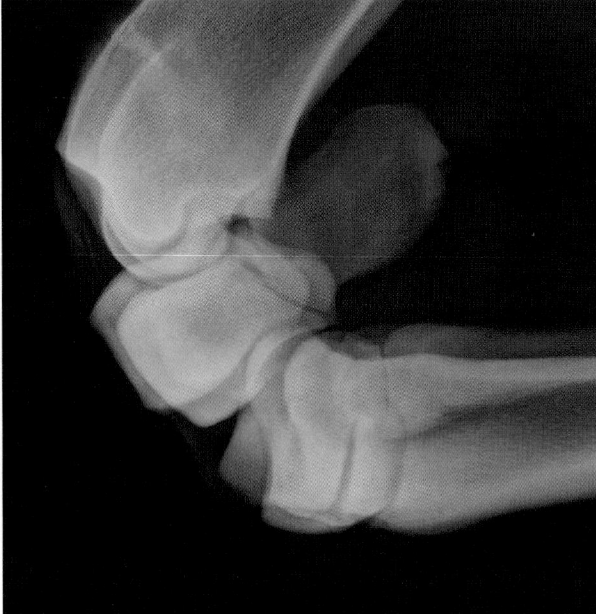

Figure 8.29 A well-positioned flexed lateral view of the carpus. Note the separation of the radial and intermediate carpal bones, which is necessary for complete evaluation of common areas of pathologic change.

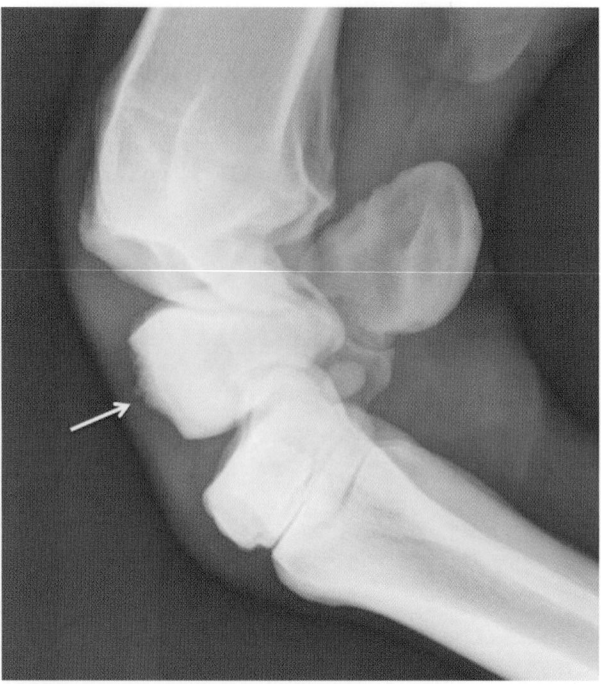

Figure 8.30 A poorly positioned flexed lateral view. Inadequate flexion does not allow for separation of the cuboidal bones. There is dorsal osseous remodeling (arrow), but due to the superimposition, it is not possible to tell if it is on the radial or intermediate carpal bone (or both). Mild motion artifact is also present.

and fourth carpal bones projected proximally, which allows for better evaluation of individual bone surfaces and common areas of injury (Figures 8.29 and 8.30).

TECHNICIAN TIPS 8.7: The limb should not be rotated or abducted when taking a flexed lateral carpus view.

A DP carpus view is obtained with the limb positioned squarely and the beam aimed horizontally from dorsal to palmar. If positioning of the cassette, X-ray machine, and joint are not a true DP, proximal to distal obliquity will occur, disallowing adequate evaluation of the joint spaces (Figures 8.31 and 8.32).

Oblique views are obtained in a weight-bearing position as well. A common mistake is to make the DMPLO view a 45° oblique, when ideally it should be at approximately 60°. This means that the view is taken closer to a lateral projection than oblique views in some other joints (Figures 8.33 and 8.34). The reason for this is that pathologic changes commonly affect the dorsomedial surface of the intermediate carpal bone and if the view is too oblique, this surface will not be highlighted. If this view is positioned properly, the accessory carpal bone will be bisected by the caudal margin of the radius. When obtaining a DLPMO view, a way to determine whether the radiograph is properly positioned is to visualize that the fourth metacarpal bone (medial splint) is superimposed

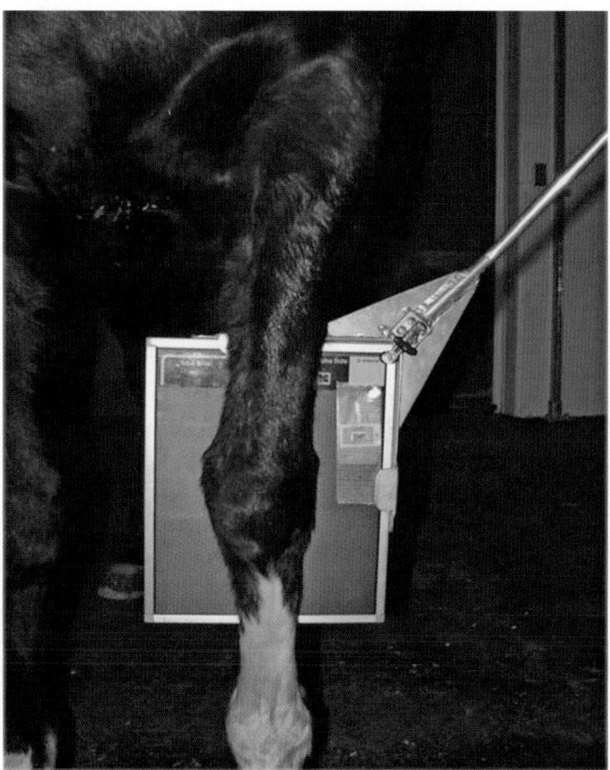

Figure 8.31 DP carpus with horse standing squarely. Avoid being narrow or wide based.

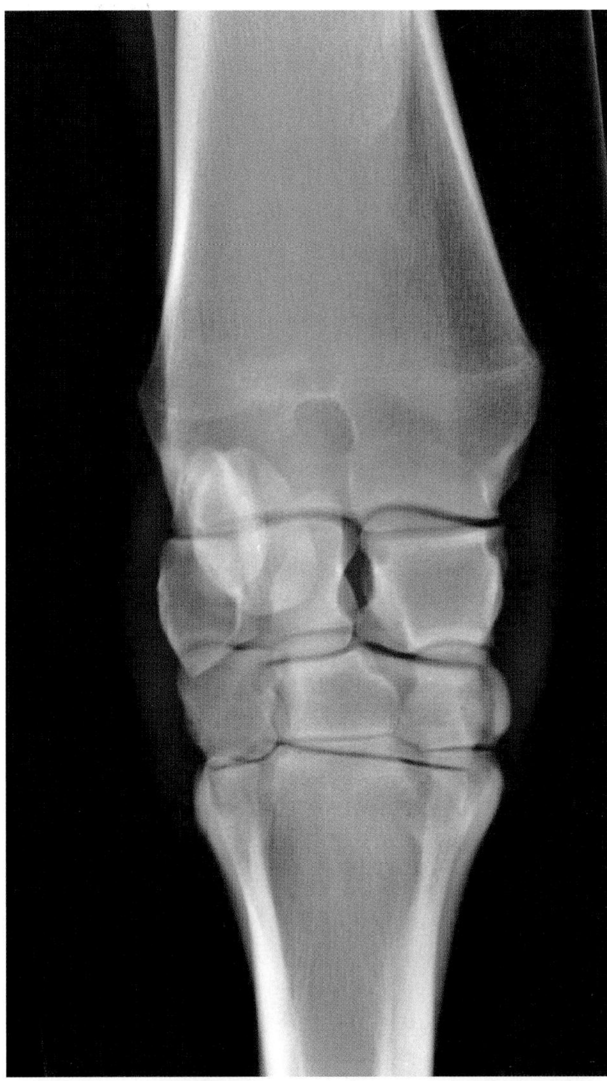

Figure 8.32 DP carpus is taken with beam horizontal.

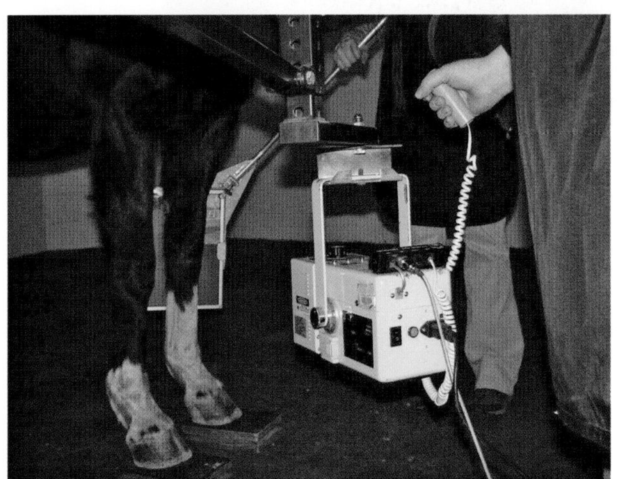

Figure 8.33 DMPLO carpus approximately 60° – this means that the view is taken closer to a lateral projection than oblique views in some other joints.

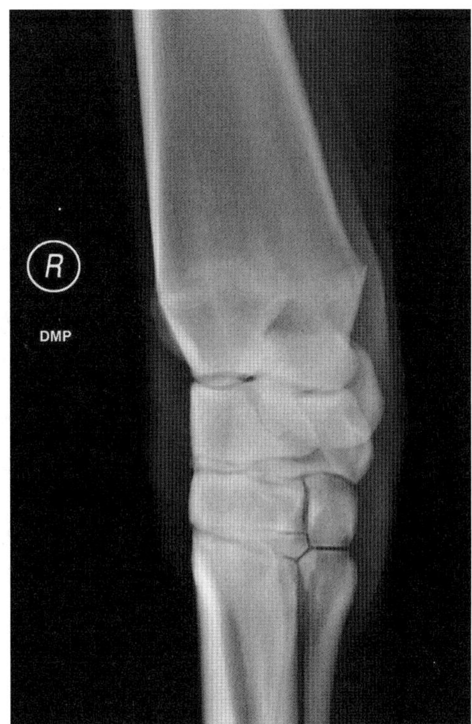

Figure 8.34 DMPLO carpus.

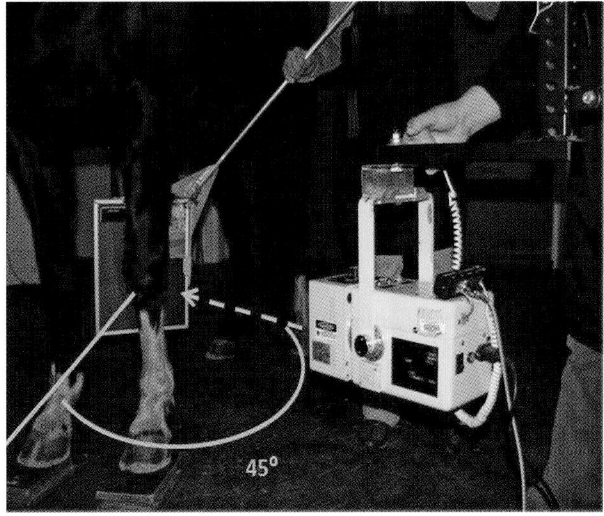

Figure 8.35 DLPMO carpus is taken 45° off dorsal.

over the medullary cavity of the third metacarpal bone (Figures 8.35 and 8.36).

TECHNICIAN TIPS 8.8: Ideally, the carpus DMPLO should be images at approximately 60° of obliquity.

Flexed dorsoproximal-dorsodistal oblique (skyline) views of the carpus can also be obtained. These views help

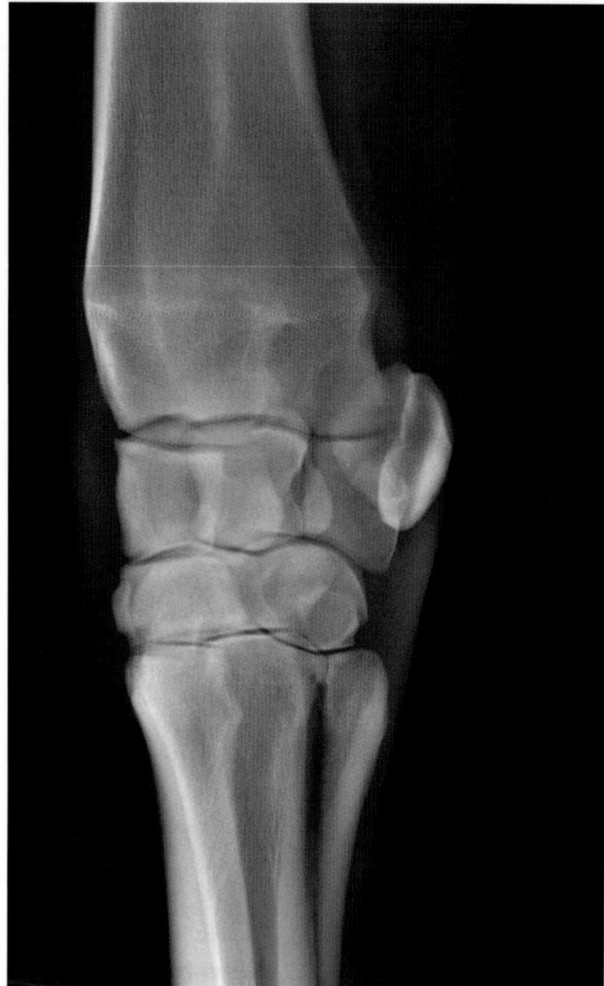

Figure 8.36 DLPMO carpus.

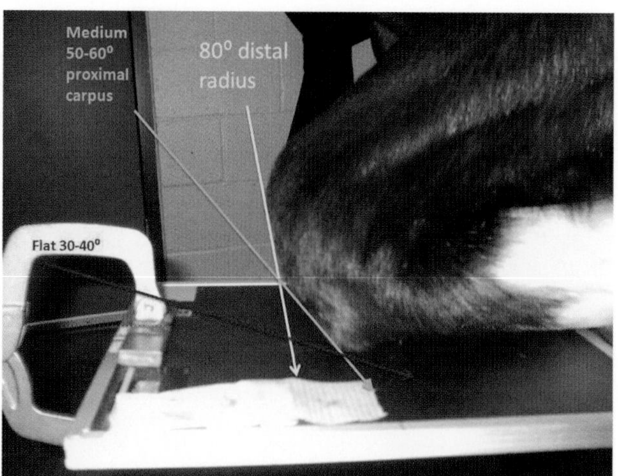

Figure 8.37 The limb is flexed and pushed cranially; the cassette is placed parallel to the floor. An 80° angle will highlight the distal radius, a medium angle of 50–60° highlights the proximal row of carpal bones, and a flat angle 30–40° will show the distal row of carpal bones.

to examine the dorsal surfaces of the carpus. The limb is flexed and pushed cranially by the holder and the cassette placed parallel to the floor, below the carpus. The degree of angulation will vary with the area to be examined. The steepest angle (approximately 80°) will highlight the distal radius, a medium angle (50–60°) will highlight the proximal row of carpal bones, and a flat angle (30–40°) will show the distal row of carpal bones. The latter is the most commonly used of these projections as sclerosis and damage to the third carpal bone is best assessed with this view (Figures 8.37 and 8.38a,b).

(a)

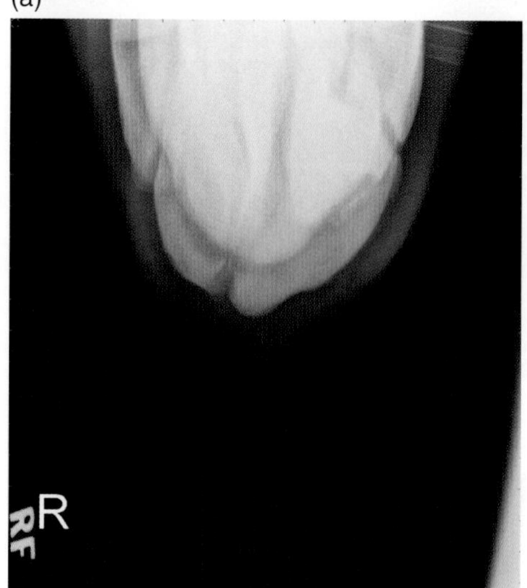

(b)

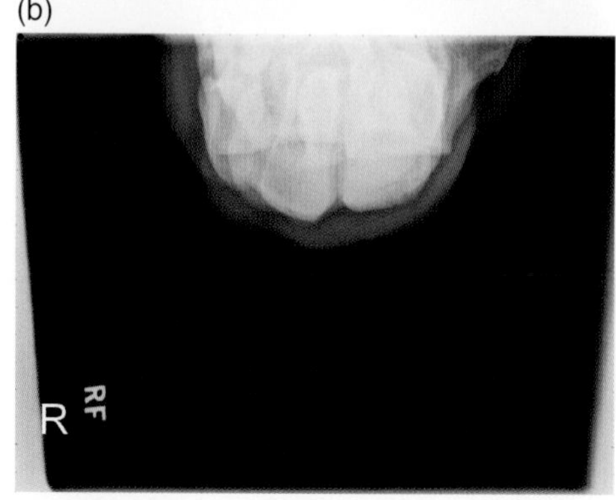

Figure 8.38 (a) Flexed (skyline) carpus proximal. (b) Flexed (skyline) carpus distal.

Elbow

The standard radiographic views of the elbow include:

- mediolateral
- craniocaudal

Radiographs of the elbow can be technically challenging. For the medial-lateral view, the limb is lifted and extended, pulling the elbow joint of interest cranially to minimize

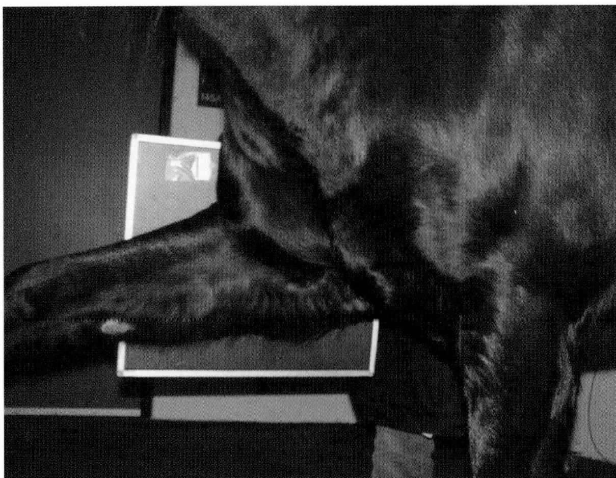

Figure 8.39 Elbow is lifted and pulled cranially; the view is taken with beam medial to lateral.

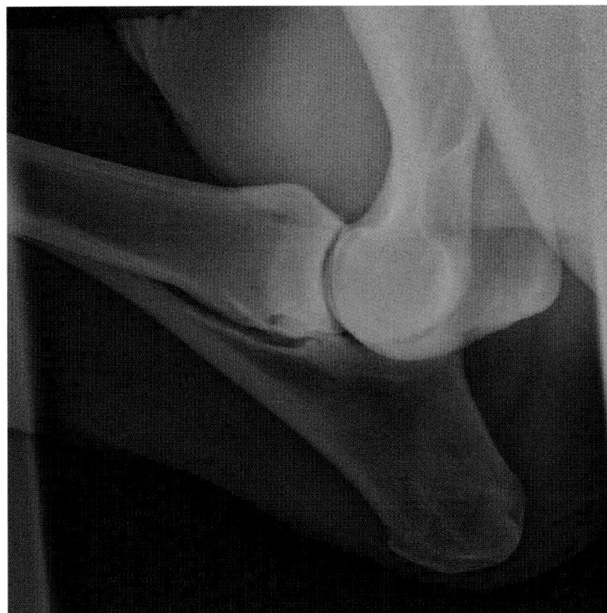

Figure 8.40 Mediolateral elbow.

superimposition. The X-ray machine is positioned on the medial aspect of the elbow and the cassette on the lateral aspect (Figures 8.39 and 8.40).

> **TECHNICIAN TIPS 8.9:** Rotate the plate 90° so that it is diamond shaped when taking the craniocaudal view of the elbow.

The craniocaudal view of the elbow is generally positioned with limb in a weight-bearing position. The cassette is positioned caudal to the elbow and is pressed closely against the patient's thorax. Rotating the cassette 90°, so

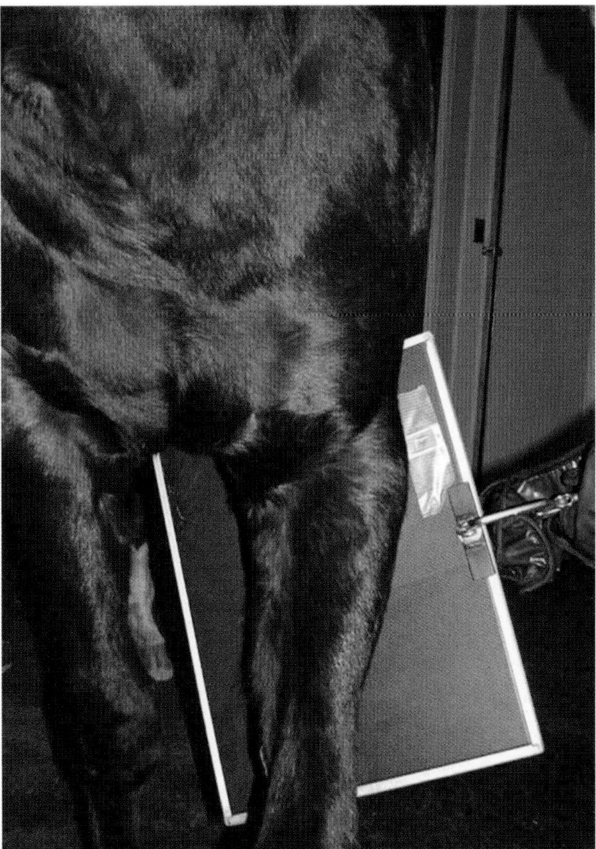

Figure 8.41 Craniocaudal elbow-limb is weight bearing.

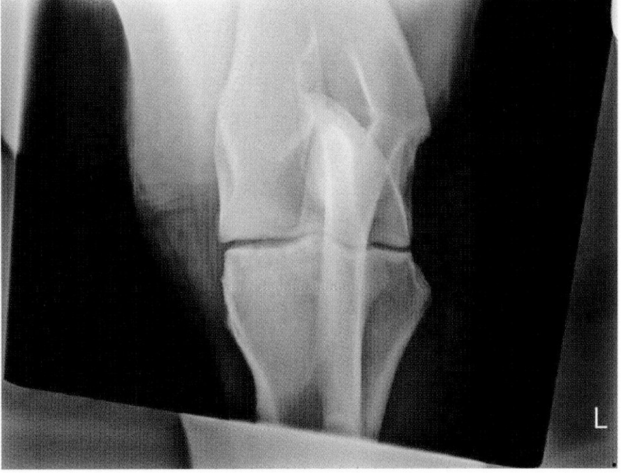

Figure 8.42 Craniocaudal elbow.

that it is in a diamond position, can help it conform better to the thorax and for better contact (Figures 8.41 and 8.42).

Shoulder

Similar to the elbow, the mediolateral view of the shoulder is obtained with the limb lifted and extended. The X-ray

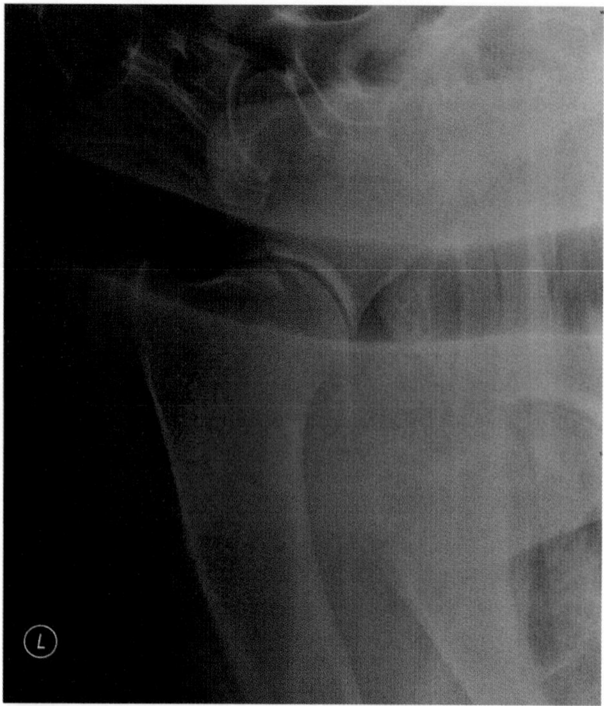

Figure 8.43 Mediolateral shoulder with joint space superimposed over the trachea.

machine is positioned on the medial aspect of the limb, cranial to the pectoral muscles, and the cassette on the lateral aspect of the limb. It can be helpful to try to align the image so that the more lucent gas in the trachea helps allow better definition of the joint. Oblique views can be obtained if needed for further evaluation, but are often not included in a standard exam (Figure 8.43).

> **TECHNICIAN TIPS 8.10:** Superimposing the shoulder joint space over the trachea helps allow for better definition of the joint.

Tarsus

The standard radiographic views included in a tarsus series include:

- lateromedial (lateral)
- dorso-plantar (DP)
- dorso 45° lateral-plantaromedial oblique (DLPMO)
- dorso 45° medial-plantarolateral oblique (DMPLO)

The most common challenge in obtaining high-quality tarsal radiographs is to avoid proximal-distal obliquity. Because the joint spaces of the tarsus are thin, small amounts of obliquity can artifactually create the appearance of joint space narrowing or ankylosis. This obliquity typically results because the horse stands somewhat base-wide (especially, if sedated), resulting in angulation of the limb and obliquity of the lateral and oblique views. Also, if the horse is not standing squarely for the DP view, it can create the appearance of joint narrowing if the angulation of the limb is not accounted for by the angle of the X-ray machine.

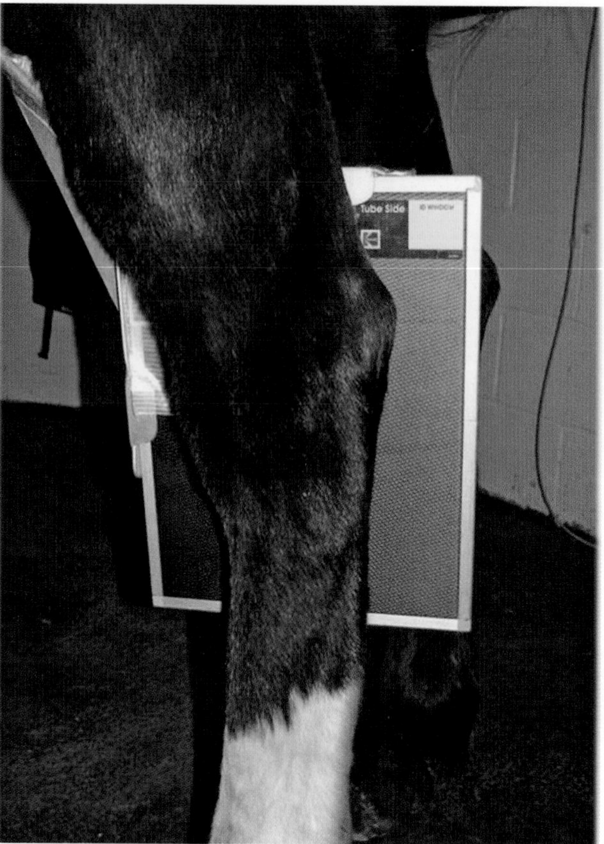

Figure 8.44 Lateromedial tarsus (lateral).

> **TECHNICIAN TIPS 8.11:** Be sure that the horse is standing square and not standing wide or narrow based when radiographing the tarsus.

In all views, when positioned correctly, the joint spaces of the distal tarsal joints are seen as thin, single lucent lines, without overlap of the proximal and distal row of cuboidal bones. In a properly positioned lateral view, the medial and lateral trochlear ridges will be superimposed (Figures 8.44 and 8.45).

The DP view can be modified to a dorso 10–15° lateral-plantaromedial oblique. This slight degree of obliquity allows for better evaluation of the medial malleolus of the tibia, which is a site that can be affected with osteochondrosis lesions (Figures 8.44–8.48).

Similar to the DLMPO view of the carpus, a hint for checking the degree of obliquity of the oblique views of the

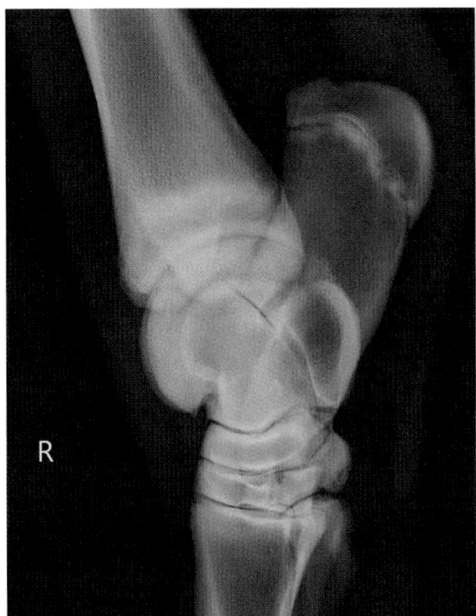

Figure 8.45 Lateromedial tarsus (lateral). This particular view shows a fragment off the distal intermediate ridge of the tibia.

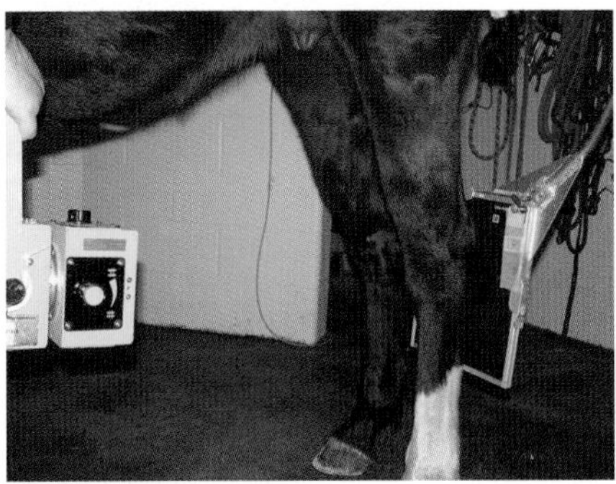

Figure 8.46 Dorso-plantar (DP) tarsus.

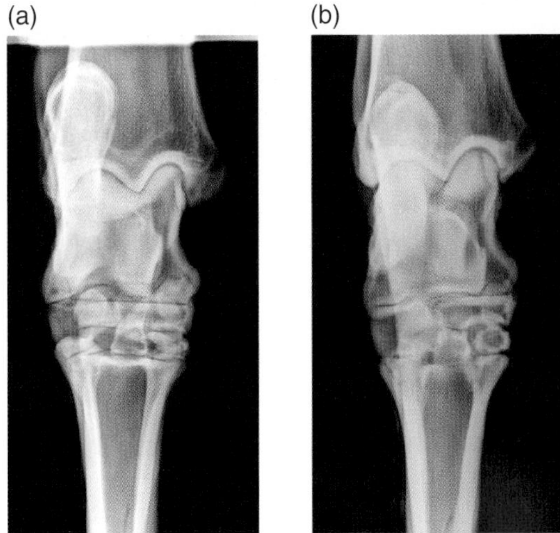

Figure 8.47 (a) and (b) show a well-positioned and a poorly positioned DP view of the tarsus. The proximal-distal obliquity of image B does not allow for adequate evaluation of the distal tarsal joints and can create an artifactual appearance of joint space narrowing.

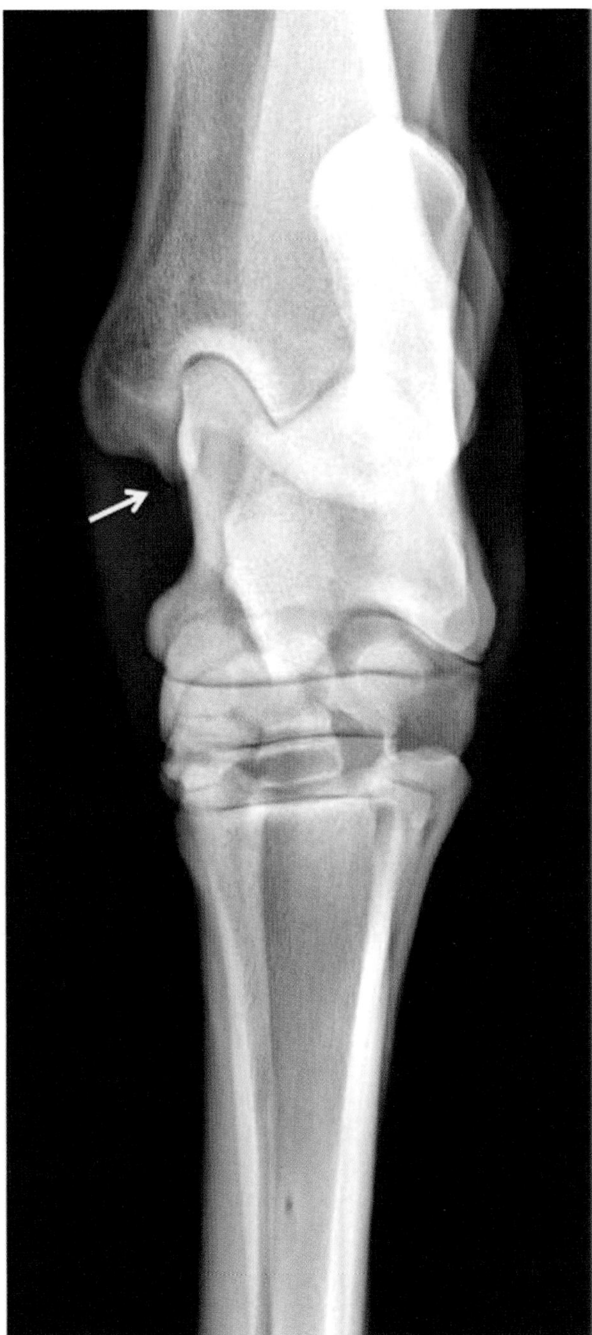

Figure 8.48 Shows a mild obliquity to DP view, which allows for better evaluation of the medial malleolus (arrow).

tarsus is that the more dorsally projected splint bone is superimposed over the medullary cavity of the third metatarsal bone (Figures 8.49–8.52).

Stifle

The standard radiographic views of the stifle include:

- lateromedial (lateral)
- lateral oblique (oblique)

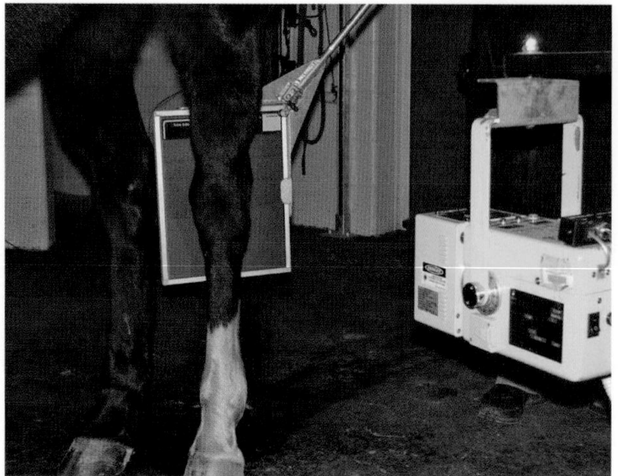

Figure 8.49 DLPMO tarsus is radiographed at a 45° angle off lateral.

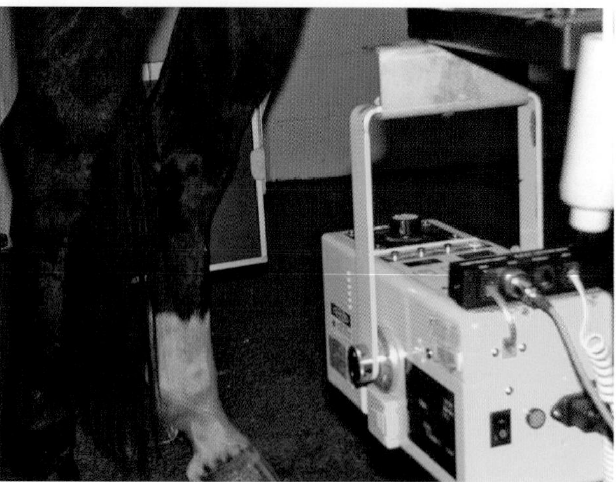

Figure 8.51 DMPLO tarsus is positioned at a 45° off dorsal medial/lateral to the sagittal plane of the tarsus.

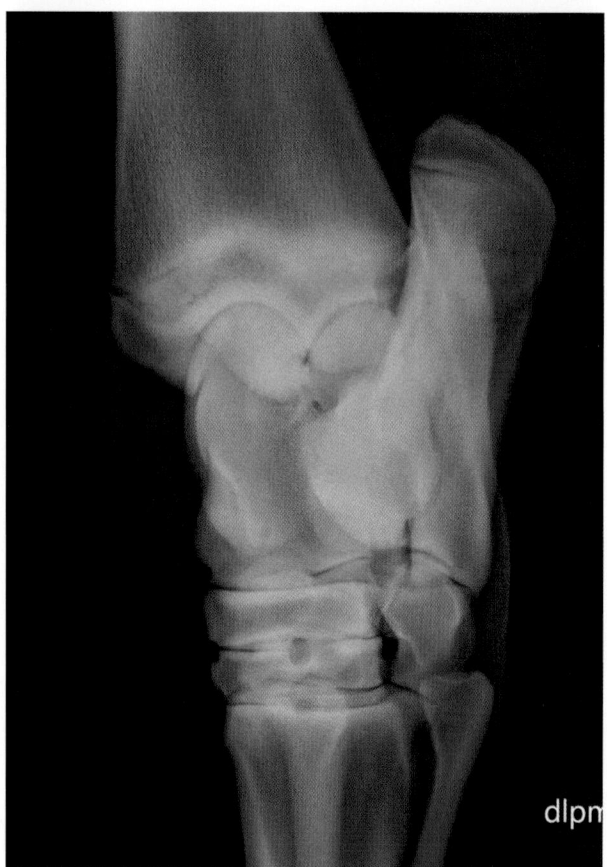

Figure 8.50 DLPMO tarsus.

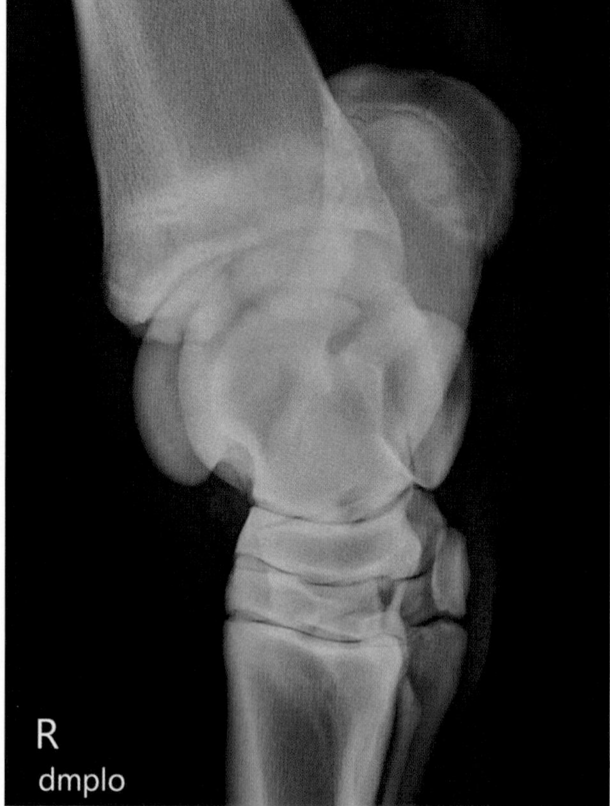

Figure 8.52 DMPLO tarsus. This horse shows a fragment off the distal intermediate ridge of the tibia.

- caudo-cranial (CC)
- caudo 45° lateral-craniomedial oblique (CLCMO)

Stifle radiographs require a higher radiographic technique than radiographs of the distal limb, particularly the CC view. When acquiring the lateral view, the cassette must be placed high on the inside of the horse's leg (Figure 8.53). Some horses resent this and will kick out, but most horses will be compliant, especially if the cassette is introduced slowly. As with all studies, administering light sedation can often facilitate a faster and higher-quality exam.

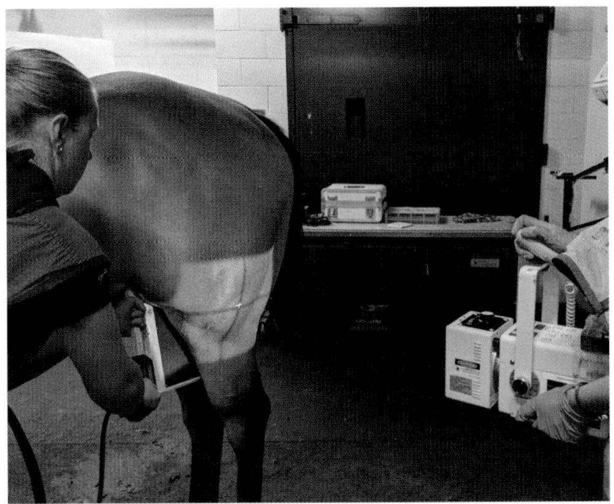

Figure 8.53 Lateromedial stifle (lateral).

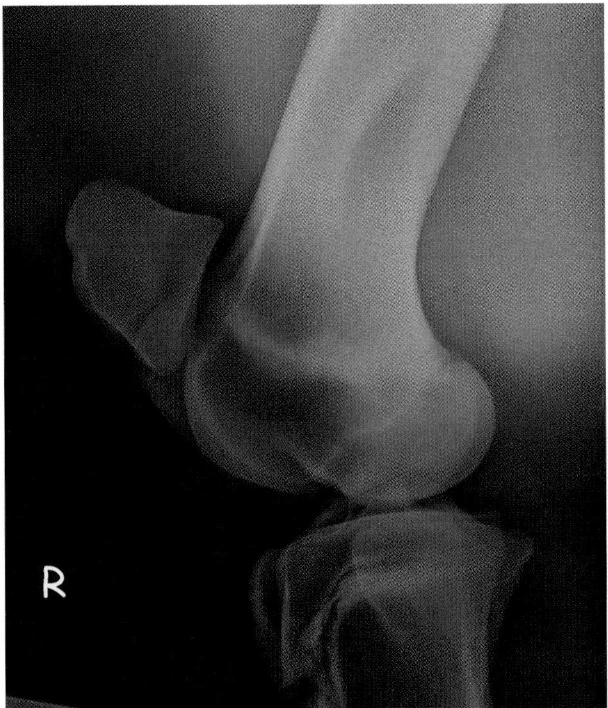

Figure 8.54 Lateromedial stifle (lateral).

A correctly positioned lateral view will have superimposition of the medial and lateral femoral condyles and trochlear ridges (Figure 8.54).

> **TECHNICIAN TIPS 8.12:** Caution should be taken when shooting views of the stifle, as the horse may kick.

The CC view is taken with X-ray machine directly behind the horse's stifle. It is best if the limb is extending slightly behind the horse, and the X-ray machine is directed cranially

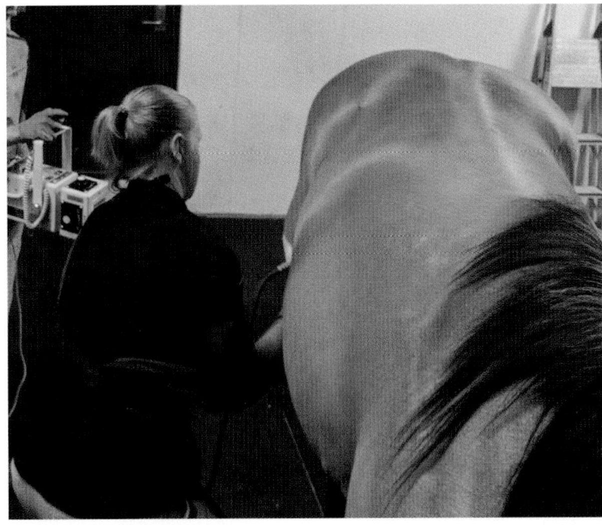

Figure 8.55 Oblique stifle.

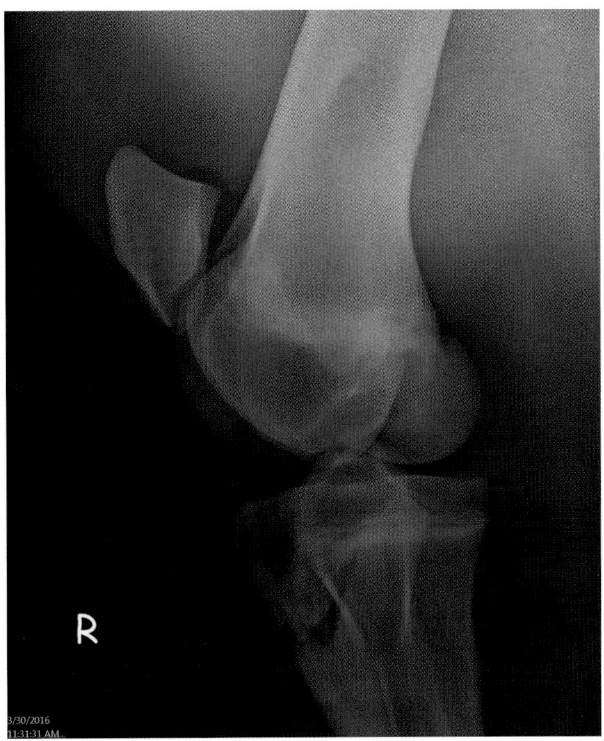

Figure 8.56 Oblique stifle.

and slightly distally (aiming down) (Figure 8.55). This will facilitate accurate evaluation of the joint space (Figure 8.56). Obliquity in positioning can create the false appearance of a narrowed joint space. If this occurs, the radiograph should be repeated, as joint space narrowing can be a very significant finding and must be differentiated from artifact.

> **TECHNICIAN TIP+S 8.13:** Joint space narrowing is a significant finding.

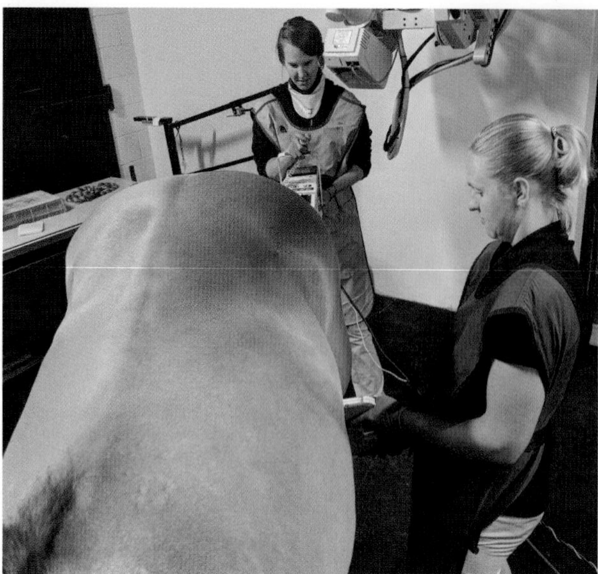

Figure 8.57 Caudo-cranial (CC) stifle – limb is slightly extended; beam should be shot cranially and slightly distally (aiming down).

The CLCMO view is primarily used to highlight the medial femoral condyle and lateral trochlear ridge. A common positioning mistake is to have insufficient obliquity, resulting in the medial femoral condyle being superimposed with the tibial eminence, masking a common area of pathologic change (Figures 8.57 and 8.58).

Another useful view that is often not commonly included, but one that the authors feel should be frequently utilized, is the cranio 5° disto 10° lateralcaudoproximomedial oblique (flexed lateral oblique) view. The technique for this view has been described in detail elsewhere. While this view requires extra personnel and can take some time to master, it is an excellent view for assessing the medial femoral condyle, which is a common area of pathologic change in the stifle (Figure 8.59).

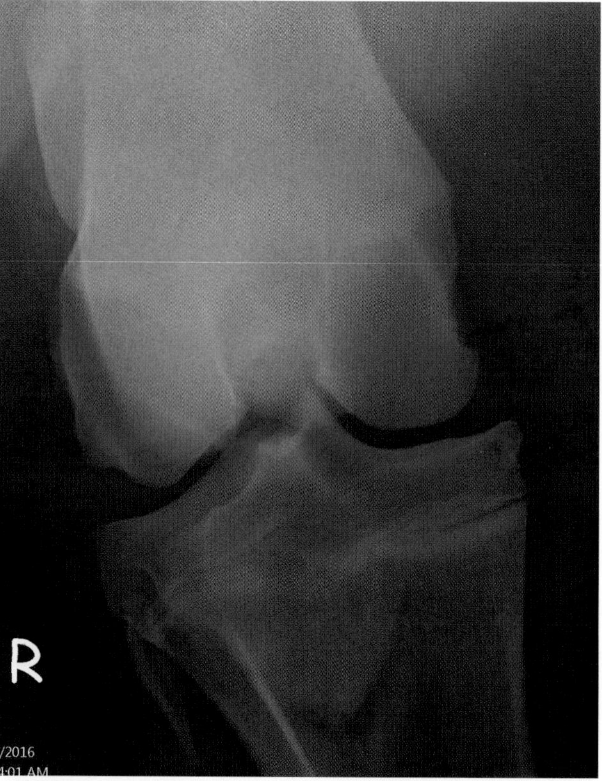

Figure 8.58 CC stifle.

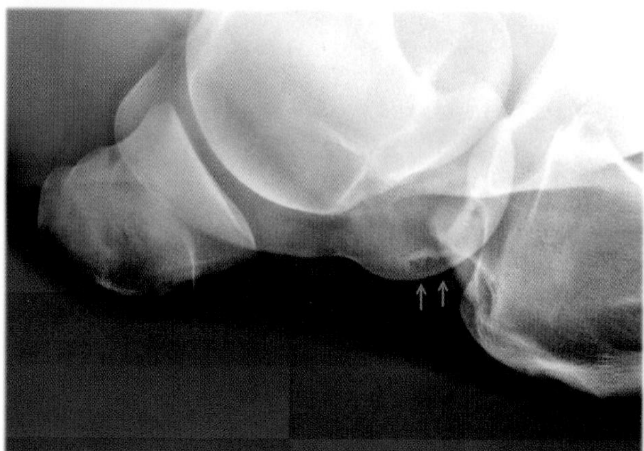

Figure 8.59 A flexed lateral oblique view of the stifle. The arrows indicate a subchondral bone defect on the medial femoral condyle.

Cervical Spine

In the typical adult horse, standard views of the cervical spine are limited to lateral views, although including oblique views can often be useful as well. To prepare for lateral views of the cervical spine, a rope halter without metal pieces should be placed on the patient, to limit superimposition. Generally, it is best for the patient to be sedated, which will cause them to drop their head, making it easier to radiograph the cranial cervical vertebrae. It is important to keep in mind that C3, C4, and C5 are identical in appearance and cannot be distinguished radiographically, except when seen adjacent to C2 (the axis) or C6 (which has a shorter vertebral body and wider transverse processes than C3–5). It is helpful to mark the neck in a way that indicates the level of the cervical spine at which the image was acquired. One way in which this can be done is to fix tape with metallic markers to the skin. It is also helpful to hold the cassette lengthwise to the neck, to try to include as many vertebrae as possible per image. Redundancy in the images is helpful. In other words, one view may be of C2–4 and the next of C4–6, including C4 in both images (Figure 8.60). The number of vertebrae that

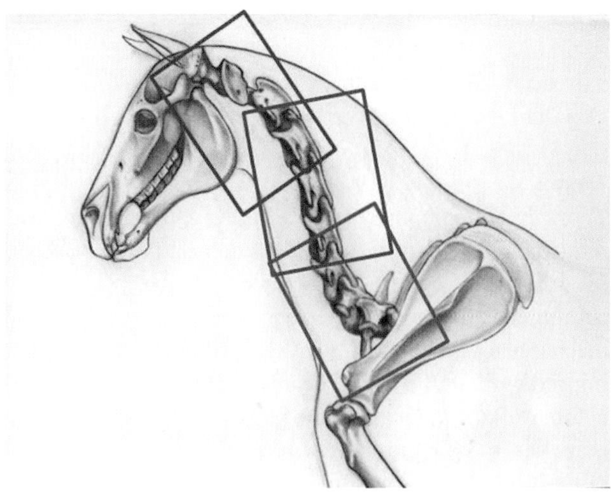

Figure 8.60 Cervical spine positioning. *Source:* Photo courtesy of Mary Michele Pico.

can be included is typically between two and three, depending on both the size of the horse and the cassette. The last cervical vertebrae, C7, lies in an area of heavy density within the horse's shoulders and can be difficult to image well (Figure 8.61).

> **TECHNICIAN TIPS 8.14:** A rope halter without metal pieces should be placed on the patient in preparation of radiographing the cervical spine.
>
> **TECHNICIAN TIPS 8.15:** Overlapping the images of the cervical spine is helpful for evaluation.

Lining up cervical radiographs can be challenging when using a portable X-ray machine, as the person holding the machine cannot see cassette location on the other side of the neck. The person holding the horse's head can help by determining if the cassette and X-ray machine are

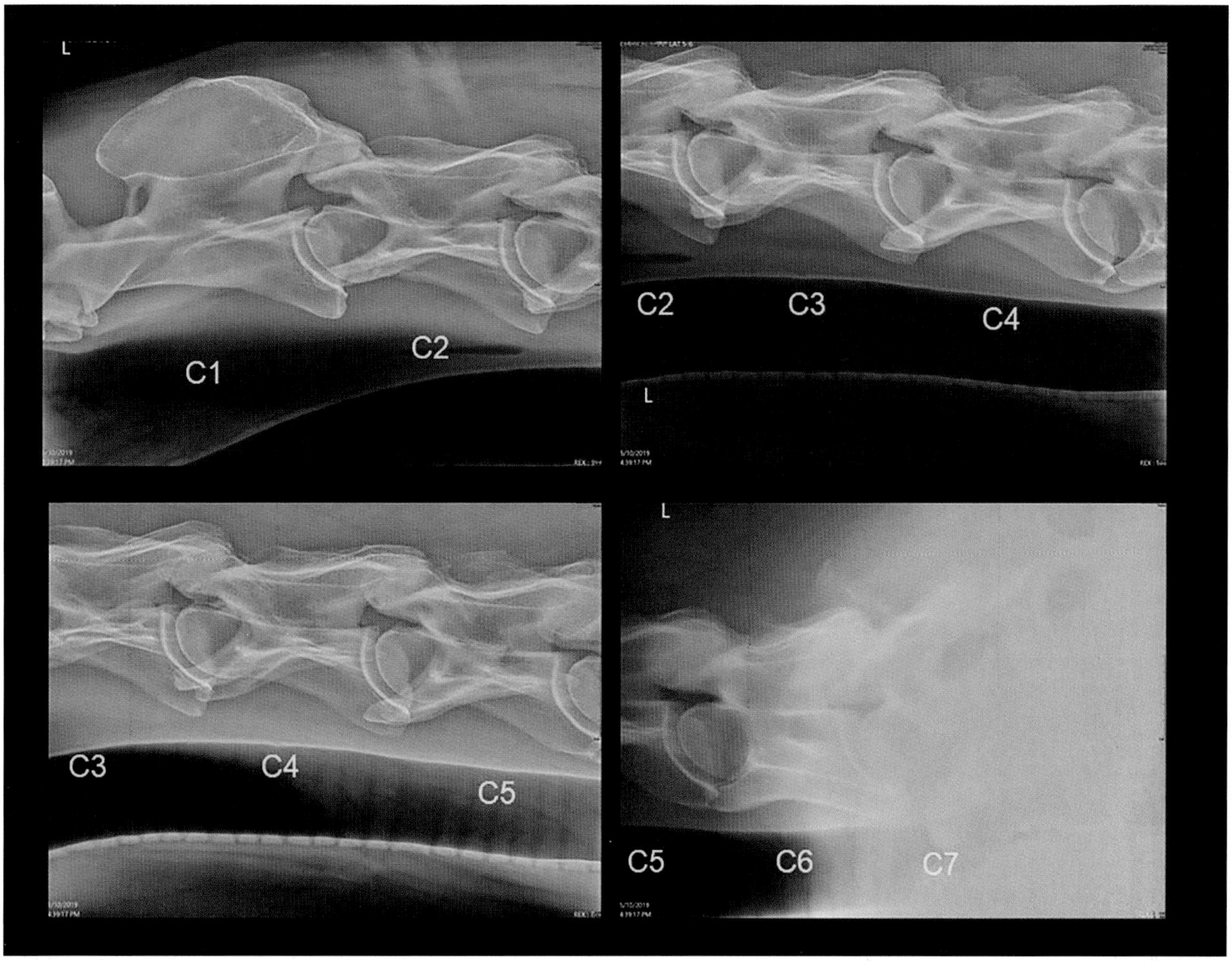

Figure 8.61 C-spine series.

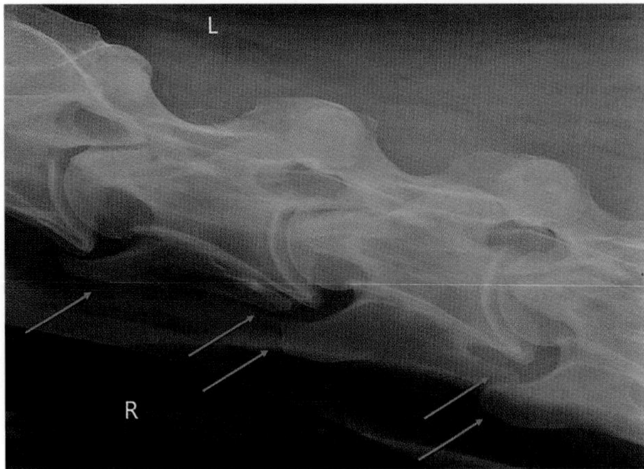

Figure 8.62 C-Spine oblique.

aligned. It is important to remember that the cervical spine runs in the ventral part of the neck; care should be taken to not position the beam too dorsally. When positioned properly, the medial and lateral transverse processes will be superimposed and the intervertebral disk spaces will be radiolucent. Obliques of the cervical spine may also be requested. The oblique images allow for viewing the tips of each of the facet more clearly (noted by blue arrows in Figure 8.62).

TECHNICIAN TIPS 8.16: Keep in mind that C3, C4, and C5 are identical in appearance and cannot be distinguished radiographically, except when seen adjacent to C2 (the axis) or C6.

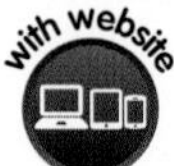

Check the website for images of a c-spine myelogram.

Thorax and Lumbar Vertebrae

The vertebral bodies of 8–9 thoracic vertebrae are well hidden in the density of the chest, similar to C7 of the cervical vertebrae. The spinous processes begin to extend above the ridge of the scapula around T3–T4 and can be imaged quite well along the rest of the thoracic vertebrae. The technique for spinous processes is less than that needed for the vertebral bodies. Abnormalities can occur in either area, so it is prudent to evaluate both. The tips of the spinous processes are susceptible to trauma and fractures as well as overriding dorsal spinous processes or kissing spine. In the horse, the underside of the vertebral bodies of the thoracic and lumbar vertebrae can also develop spondylosis deformans or boney spurs and calcification. It is important to remember that the sacral vertebrae 1–5 are fused. Lumbar vertebra L5, L6, and the sacral bodies are again in a location and density difficult to image. The caudal vertebrae image well though and require much less kVp than the proximal vertebrae.

Thorax

Thoracic radiographs require a higher radiographic technique, and a grid must be used. Centering of the beam on the cassette is a must, and a linkage between the X-ray equipment and the cassette will allow this. If a standing mechanical cassette holder with a built-in grid is used, it is important that the X-ray beam is centered on the grid before walking the patient into position. The exposure time is higher and should be executed at the peak of the animal's inspiration. The suspected "normal" side of the thorax should be closest to the beam with the suspected diseased side placed closest to the grid. The size of the patient limits the ability to take views other than lateral in the adult patient.

In smaller patients, such as a foal or calf, it may be possible to obtain a ventro-dorsal view by rolling them on their back. The patient should be positioned with the front legs extended cranially, as much as the patient will allow, avoiding any superimposition over the cranial aspect of the heart (Figure 8.66). The beam should be perpendicular to the grid. In the standing patient, the person holding the patient can help verify the grid position so that it is as close to the thorax as possible, without actually touching the patient. The size of the patient determines the number of images that will need to be taken. In the adult patient, four overlapping views is the standard (Figures 8.63–8.68).

The standard radiographic images include:

- dorso-cranial
- dorso-caudal
- ventro-cranial
- ventro-caudal

Abdomen

Similar to thoracic radiographs, abdominal radiographs in a full-sized horse, cow, or wider small ruminants require a higher radiographic technique and a grid must be used. Centering the beam on the cassette is a must. Ideally, a system that links the X-ray equipment and the cassette is used. If a standing mechanical cassette holder with a built-in grid is used, it is important that the X-ray beam is centered before the patient is placed in position. Abdominal radiographs may be used to diagnose enteroliths, presence of sand, urinary calculi, and bowel obstructions. The number of images that need to be taken varies

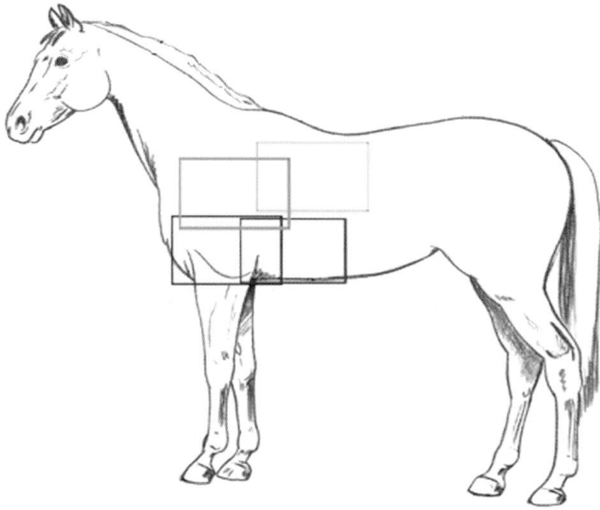

Figure 8.63 Thoracic radiograph positioning.

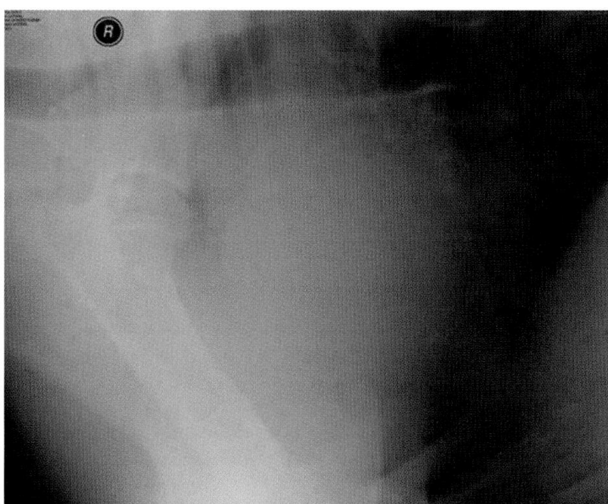

Figure 8.64 Ventro-cranial thorax.

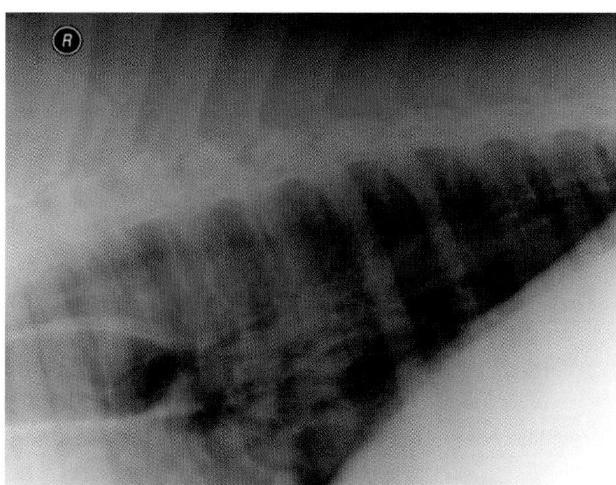

Figure 8.65 Dorso-caudal thorax.

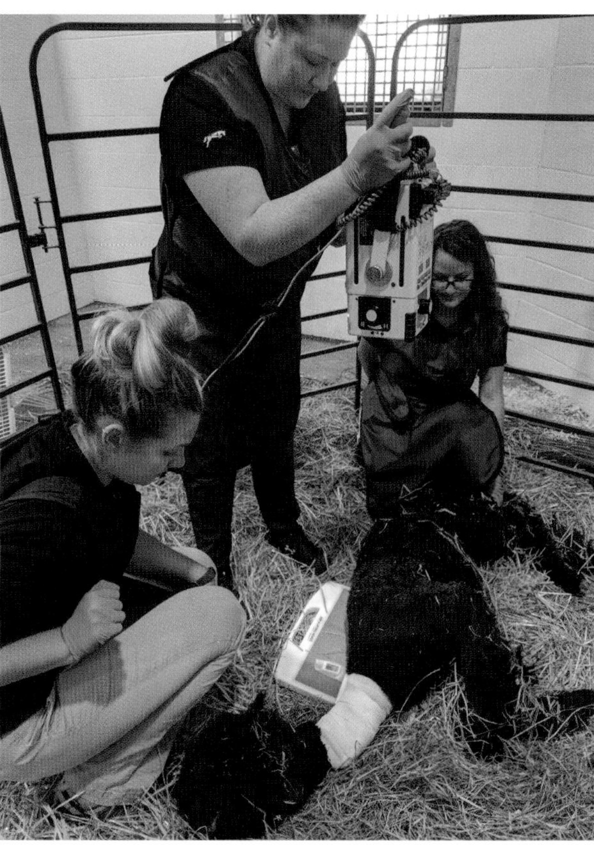

Figure 8.66 Stall-side thoracic radiograph of an alpaca in lateral recumbency.

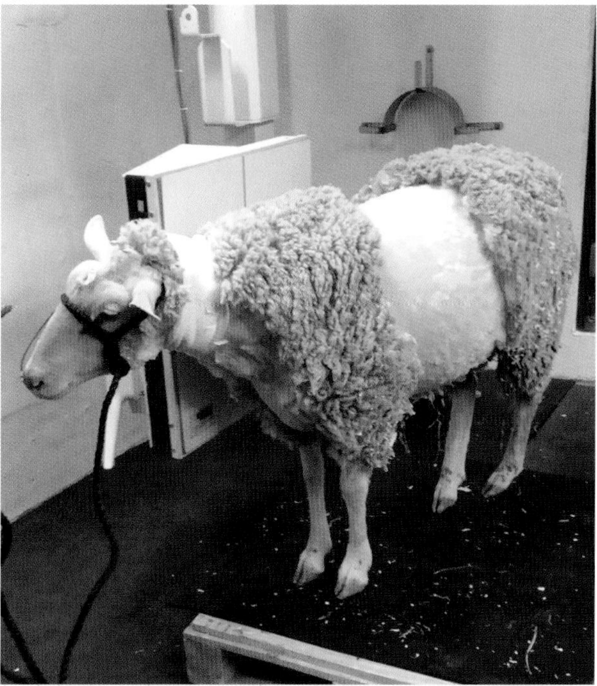

Figure 8.67 Thoracic radiograph of a sheep. Due to the limitations of the tube, a pallet is used to raise the animal up slightly.

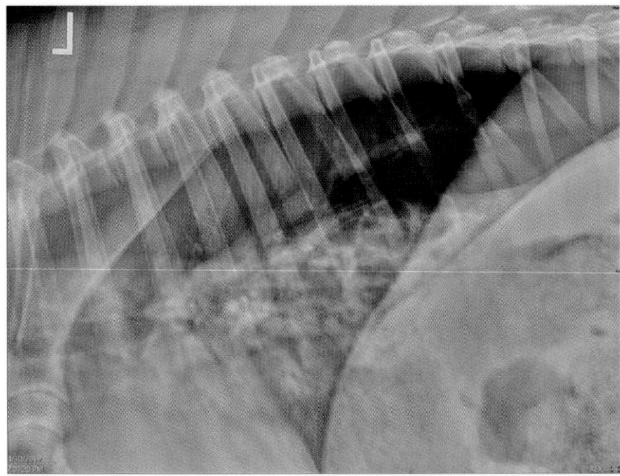

Figure 8.68 Thoracic radiograph of a sheep with marked alveolar pattern (often noted with pneumonia).

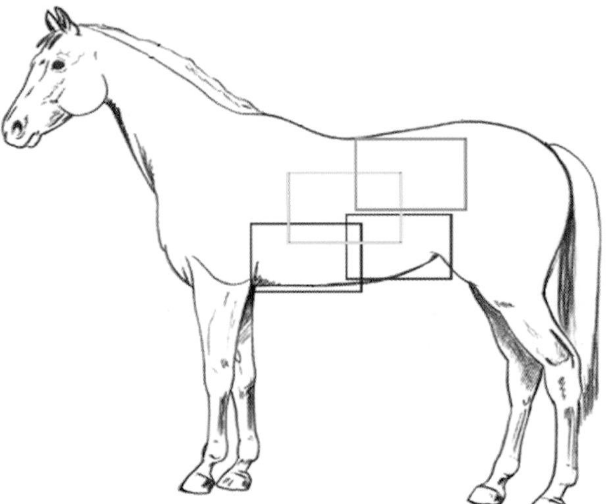

Figure 8.69 Abdominal radiograph positioning for an adult horse.

dependent on patient size, with the average patient needing three. Overlapping views are obtained starting cranioventral and extending caudo-dorsal (Figure 8.69). Imaging the abdomen is possible but limited in the denser areas. The ventral abdomen often reveals the best images and concurrently, heavy materials like magnets used to treat hardware disease, and sand accumulation will occur in this area (Figures 8.70–8.72).

Skull

Similar to patient prep for cervical radiographs, a rope halter without metal pieces should be placed on the patient to limit superimposition (Figure 8.73). Sedation is helpful, which will cause them to drop their head, making it easier to radiograph (Figure 8.74). Clinical signs help direct the area and views that need to be taken, and may focus on the dental arcades, mandible or maxillary regions, frontal

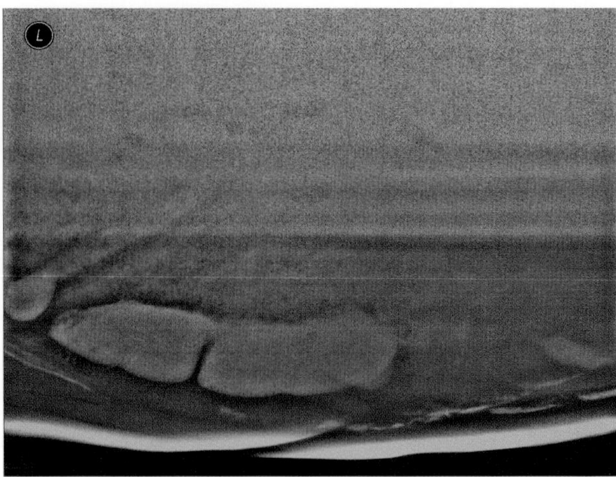

Figure 8.70 The presence of sand in the ventral abdomen of a horse.

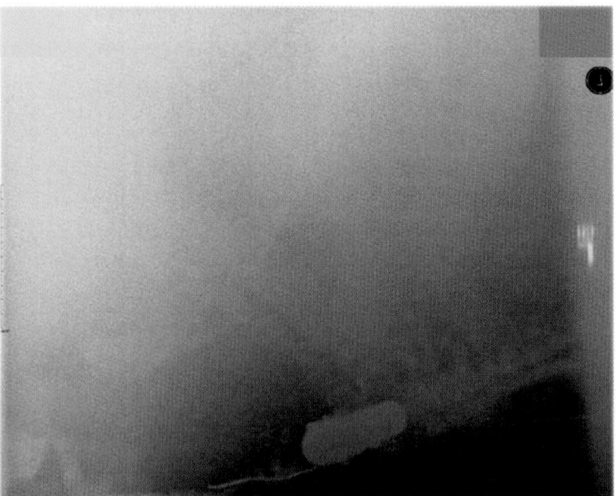

Figure 8.71 The presence of hardware and magnet in the reticulum of a bovine.

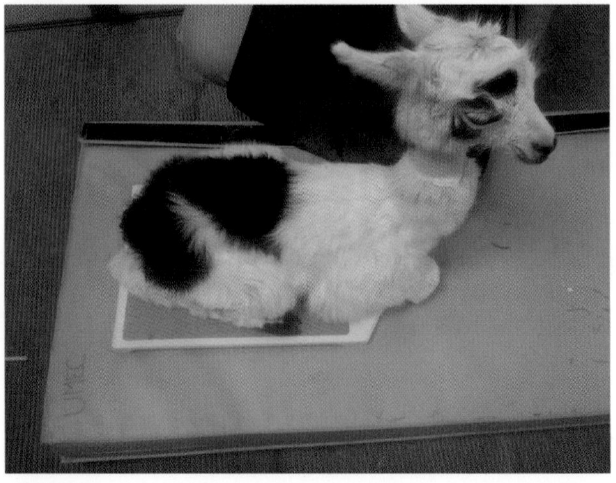

Figure 8.72 Dorsoventral abdominal radiograph of a small cria in kush.

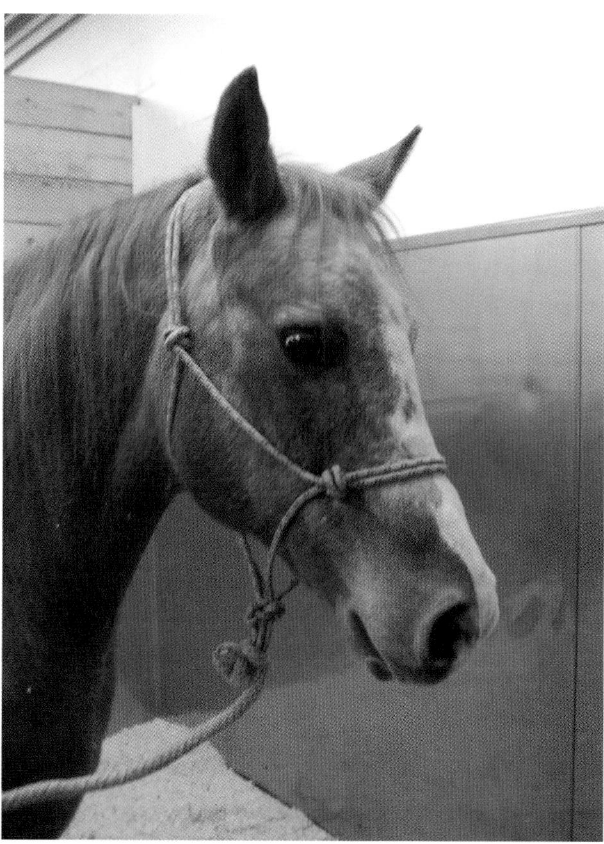

Figure 8.73 A rope halter on horse.

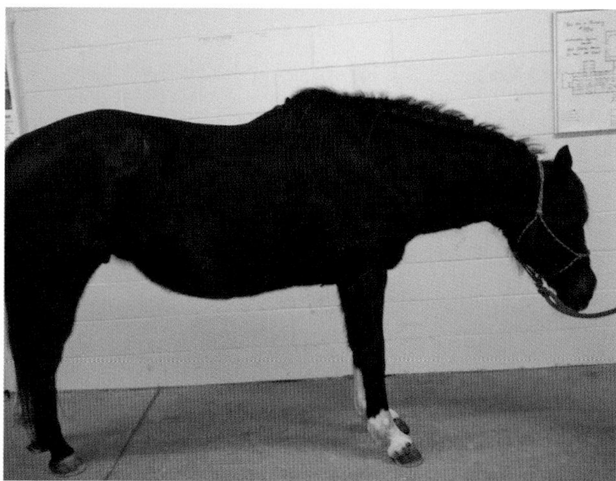

Figure 8.74 A sedated horse.

region or the guttural pouch, pharynx, and larynx. The standard radiographic images include:

- lateral
- dorsoventral
- obliques

The lateral view is taken with the horse standing in normal position. The side with the suspected pathology should be placed closest to the cassette with the normal side closest to the beam. The beam should be perpendicular to the cassette. If the guttural pouch, larynx, and pharynx are the area of interest, the cassette should be placed with the beam centered caudal to the vertical ramus of the mandible (Figures 8.75–8.78).

A dorsoventral view has the horse's head lowered as much as possible. The cassette is placed under the mandible, with the beam positioned over the horse's head. The beam is directed perpendicular to the cassette, on midline, just rostral to the orbits (Figures 8.79–8.82).

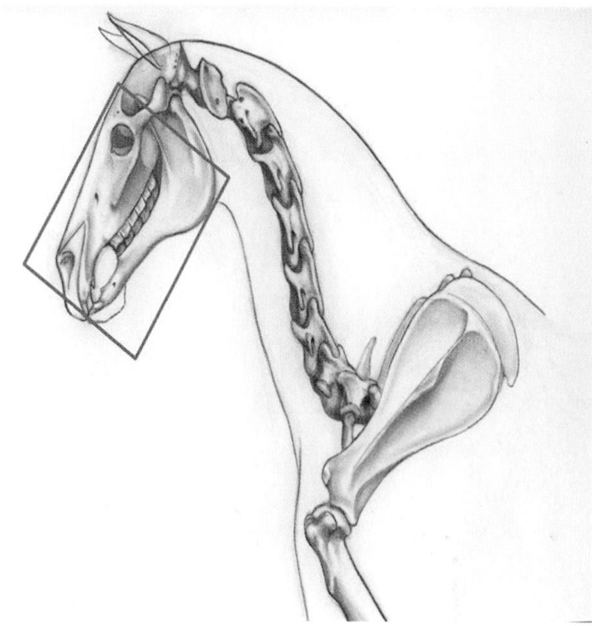

Figure 8.75 Positioning the cassette for lateral skull with focus on teeth. *Source:* Photo courtesy of Mary Michele Pico.

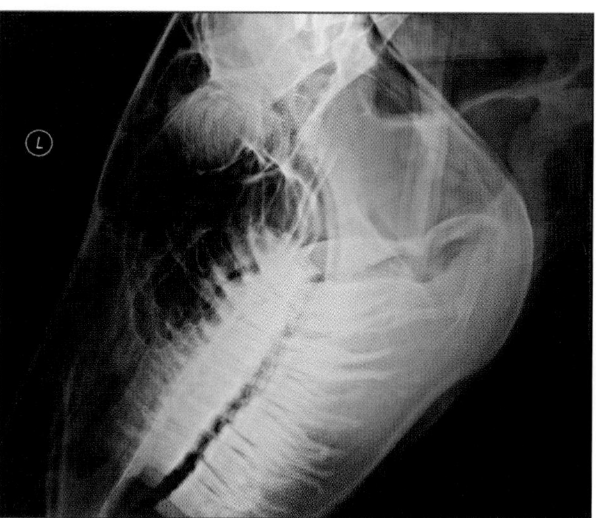

Figure 8.76 Lateral skull-teeth.

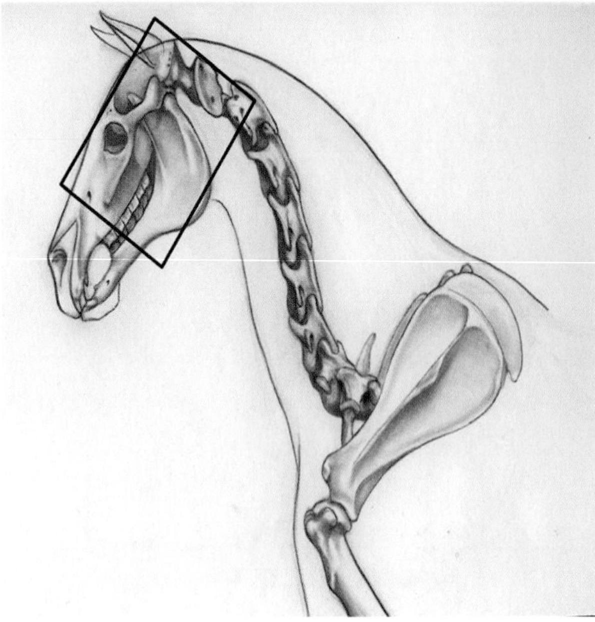

Figure 8.77 Positioning the cassette for lateral skull with focus on guttural pouch. *Source:* Photo courtesy of Mary Michele Pico.

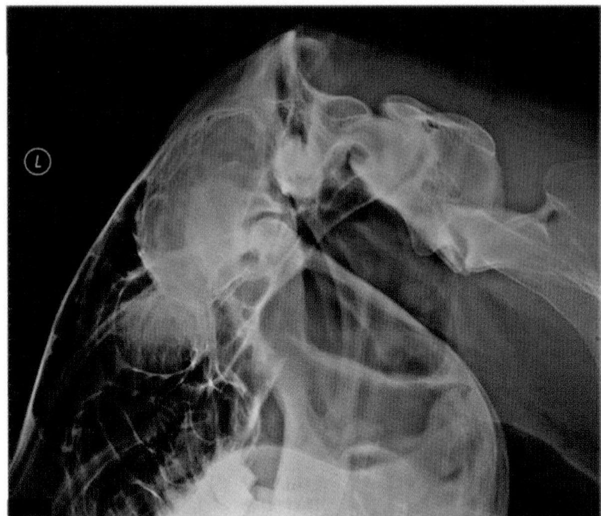

Figure 8.78 Lateral skull-guttural pouch.

Oblique views are important, as skull structures such as the cheek teeth may be hard to visualize as superimposed. Oblique views help to isolate the area of interest. It is important to take both oblique views. For visualizing the maxillary arcade, the beam is directed upward or approximately 45° down from parallel. For visualization of the mandible, the beam is placed over the horse's head, shooting downward at approximately 30° up from parallel. The degree of obliquity may need to be altered to highlight the interested area of pathologic change, particularly in the case of fractures (Figures 8.83–8.85).

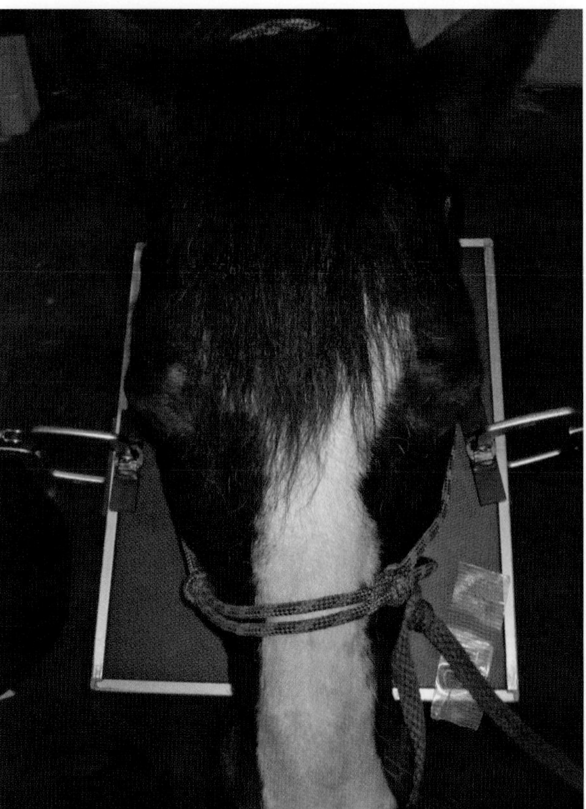

Figure 8.79 A DV skull with horse's head positioned low, emphasis on guttural pouch.

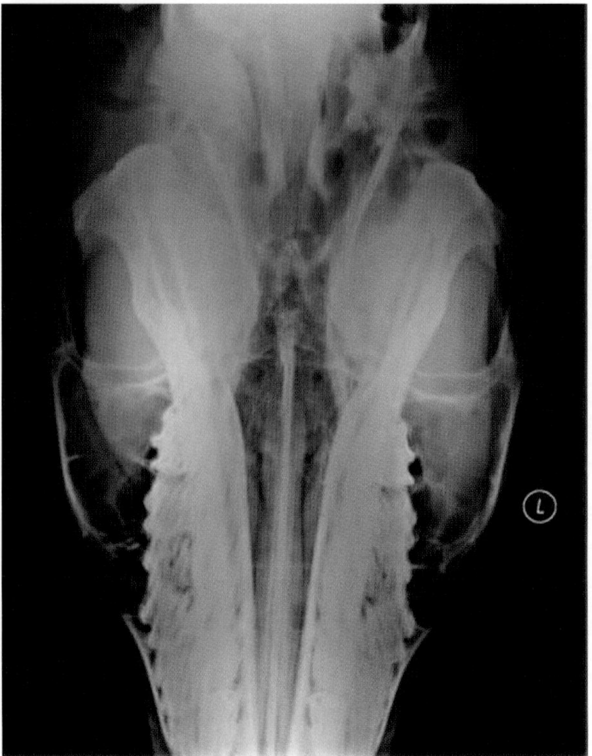

Figure 8.80 DV skull positioned over guttural pouch.

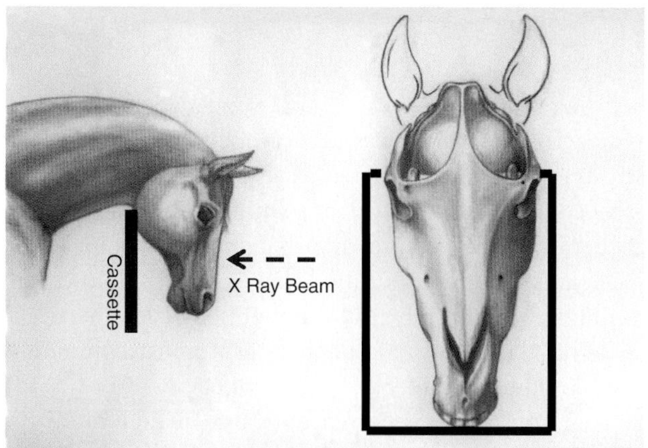

Figure 8.81 DV skull with emphasis on cheek teeth. *Source:* Photo courtesy of Mary Michele Pico.

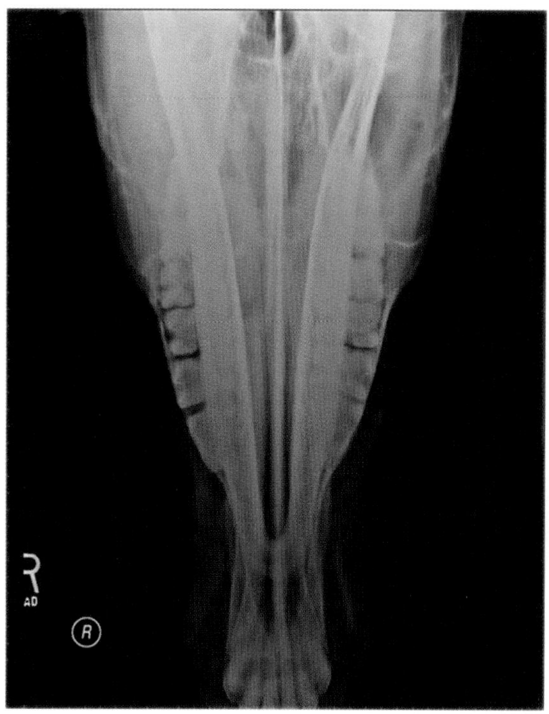

Figure 8.82 DV skull positioned rostral.

(a)

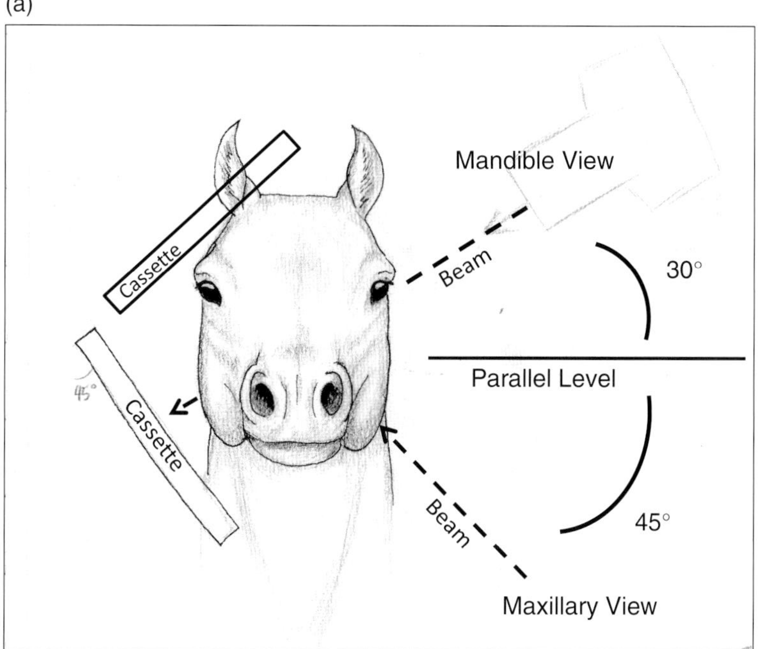

(b)

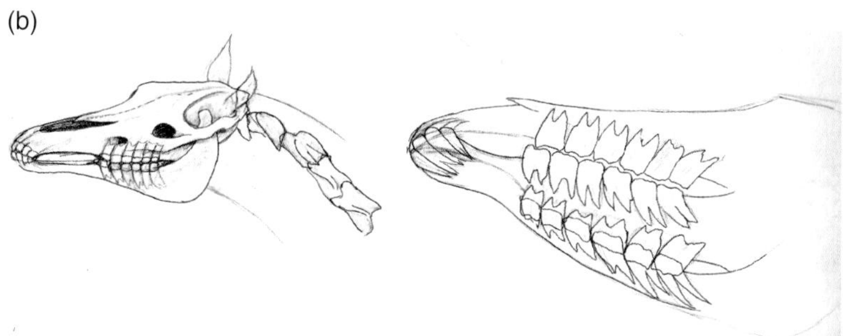

Figure 8.83 (a) For visualizing the maxillary arcade, direct the beam upward 45°; for visualizing the mandible, the beam is directed downward 30° up from parallel. *Source:* Photo courtesy of Lisa Haviland (b) Oblique skull. *Source:* Photo courtesy of Lisa Haviland.

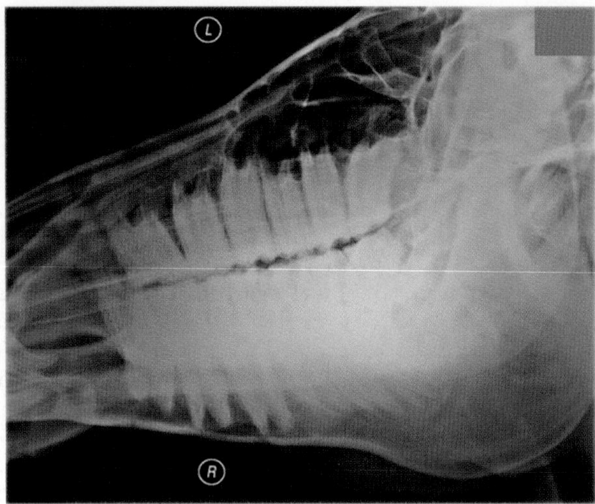

Figure 8.84 Oblique skull emphasizing the maxillary arcade.

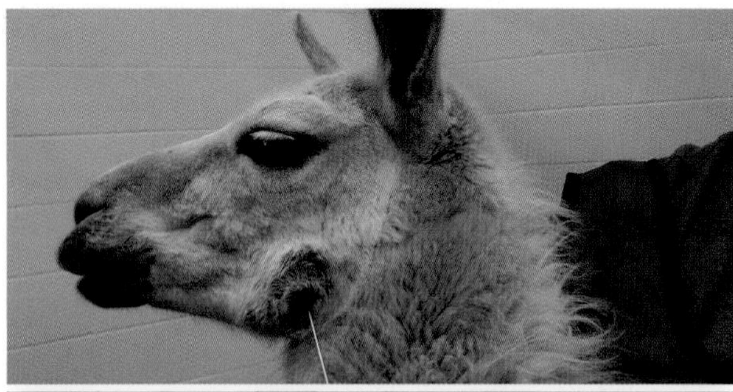

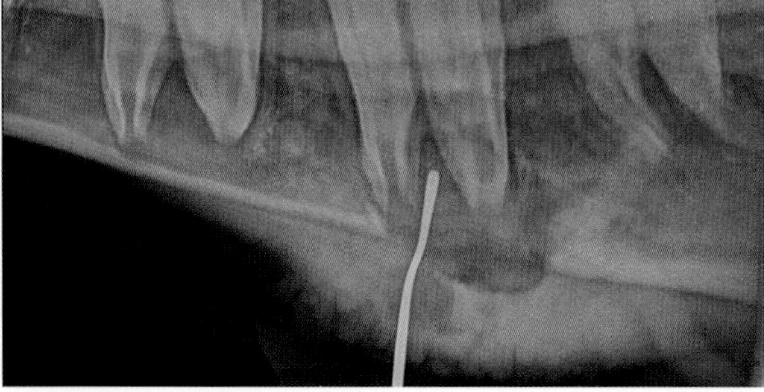

Figure 8.85 Camelid presenting with a draining track. A malleable probe was inserted into the track before the oblique radiograph was taken.

Nuclear Scintigraphy

Nuclear scintigraphy, specifically bone scintigraphy, has preserved its relevance in the imaging of acute and chronic trauma, and athletic injuries in particular, in spite of cross-sectional imaging modalities such as MRI. In the first part of the twentieth century, the relationship between musculoskeletal disorders and accumulation of radioactive substance was first recognized. Now, nuclear scintigraphy has widespread use and availability. The most common use for nuclear scintigraphy in the horse is as a diagnostic tool to aid in lameness diagnosis 5. Nuclear scintigraphy's advantage is that it allows for evaluation of physiological function; however, there is a trade-off with anatomic detail 6. The most commonly used radionuclide in horses is technetium 99 m (^{99m}Tc) labeled to tracers (pharmaceuticals), which binds to bone. The most commonly used bone tracers are methylene diphosphonate (MDP) and hydroxymethylene diphosphonate (HDP). While both formulations will allow for lesion detection, HDP may have better bone uptake. A bone scan consists of three phases after intravenous injection of radiopharmaceutical (Table 8.1). The vascular phase (flow phase) occurs within 30 S after injection; in the soft tissue phase (pool phase) the region of interest is imaged 3–5 min after injection; and, in the bone phase (delayed phase), the images are obtained 2 or more hours after injection. Two-dimensional images, called planar images, are obtained.

> **TECHNICIAN TIPS 8.17:** The advantage of nuclear scintigraphy is that it allows for evaluation of physiological function.

Bone scintigraphy gives veterinary medicine the ability to image the entire skeleton (Figure 8.86), which makes it an appealing imaging choice for horses to detect sites of trauma that may not be recognized in other modalities such as radiography. Indications for a nuclear scintigraphic scan include:

- acute or chronic lameness
- obscure or multi-limb lameness
- poor performance
- lameness that is localized to a specific region where other imaging fails to reveal abnormalities
- anatomic regions that are difficult to evaluate with other imaging modalities.

> **TECHNICIAN TIPS 8.18:** Bone scintigraphy allows for the entire skeleton, which makes it an appealing choice for diagnosing sites of trauma that may not be recognized in other imaging modalities.

Quality Control

Nuclear scintigraphy uses a gamma camera to take the images. To ensure quality images, as well as ensuring the gamma camera is functioning properly, a series of preliminary tests should be performed. The operating procedure for these tests may be different dependent on the system available and should be obtained from the systems' manufacturer. Technetium 99 is utilized, and the gamma emission of technetium is 140 KeV (kiloelectron volt). To ensure the proper sensitivity of the gamma camera, a peak and uniformity of the camera should be checked monthly and weekly, respectively. Generally, this may be done with a radioactive source similar to what is being used for the procedure, such as Technetium or Gallium. The source is typically suspended over the center of the face of the camera without a collimator on the camera. This is also referred to as a "flood." The peak should be within four numbers of 140 KeV. After peaking the camera, a new energy table and uniformity table should be completed. These procedures are often outlined by the gamma camera manufacturer in a standard operating procedure.

Table 8.1 The three phases of a bone scan after intravenous injection.

Phase	Time after Injection
Vascular	30 S
Pool (soft tissue)	three to five min
Delayed (bone)	2 hr

Patient Preparation

Placement of an indwelling intravenous catheter in the external jugular vein facilitates radioisotope administration as well as the chemical sedation necessary for a smooth imaging procedure. The catheter will decrease occurrence of perivascular injection of the isotope. The feet should be

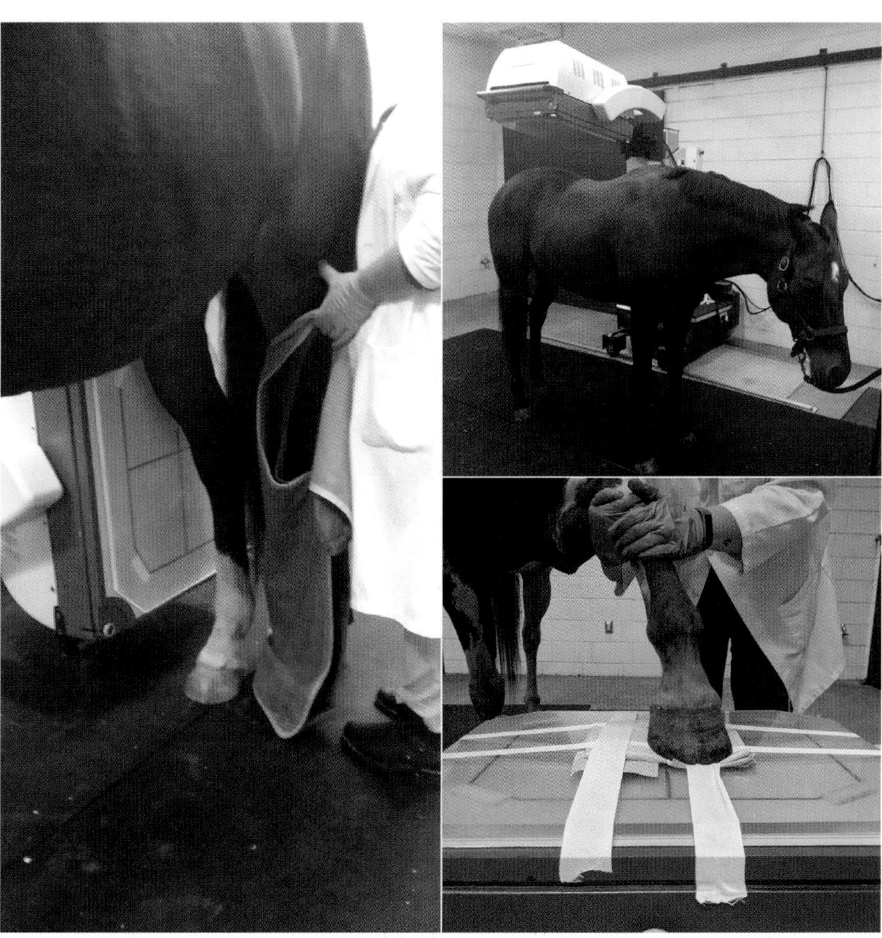

Figure 8.86 Various sequences of a bone scintigraphy being performed.

wrapped before injection and removed during the exam, as foot wraps reduce radioactive urine contamination on the feet creating false lesions and masking true lesions. The radiopharmaceutical is administered at a dose of 7 – 11 MBq/kg (0.2 – 0.3) mCi/kg.

Image Acquisition

Acquisition parameters used in scintigraphic imaging varies based on phase and body part imaged. Typically, extremities are imaged in a static frame mode. The static acquisition consists of using a 256 × 256 matrix. Images may be acquired in a count-limited (75 000–150 000 counts for distal extremity up to 300 000 counts for pelvis and axial skeleton) or a time-limited (60 S) acquisition. Images are often compared for symmetry. This requires similar scan time or similar count number. Due to decay and time between extremity acquisitions, the time-limited acquisition may create more variation between images. The counts-limited acquisition provides more uniformity between images.

Dynamic images are obtained during vascular studies and often in the axial skeleton. Images of the axial spine often incorporate motion software. Motion correction improves image quality in examinations of the standing sedated horse. This process obtains "stacked" images at 1–2 S intervals and outlying images with excessive motion are rejected. The images within the same spatial registration are superimposed on one another, creating an image with better resolution when compared to single, static acquisitions when motion is a factor. Dynamic (motion correction) acquisition parameters for axial spine are generally set at 256 × 256 matrix with image acquisition every second. Vascular studies are generally set at 128 × 128 matrix with image acquisition every second for 120 S to acquire images at the time of injection.

Institutions vary on the minimum amount of images for a whole body bone scan. An example of properly positioned images from a basic whole body bone scan is illustrated in Figure 8.87. Images are displayed from the camera view. For example, lateral images acquired on the left side of the patient are viewed so that cranial is to the left, and for dorsal and cranial images, the left lateral aspect of the patient is to the right of the image. When possible, orthogonal images should be obtained. Nuclear scintigraphy scans should not be limited to whole body bone scan. Focused exams are particularly useful for examination of skull and localized lameness.

Ultrasonography

Ultrasonography plays a vital role in many large animal practices. Advantages of ultrasound include that it is relatively inexpensive, can be performed almost anywhere, and is readily available. Ultrasound is most widely applied in the areas of reproduction and equine sports medicine. However, it is also very valuable for the assessment of thoracic, abdominal, urinary tract, and ophthalmic diseases; abnormalities of the bovine teat and udder; wounds; and various lumps, bumps, and swellings.

> **TECHNICIAN TIPS 8.19:** The advantage of ultrasound is that it can be performed almost anywhere, is readily available, and is relatively inexpensive.

One of the greatest disadvantages of ultrasound is that it is very operator dependent, and without experience and sufficient training, the usefulness of ultrasound suffers. A strong understanding of anatomy is a prerequisite for all diagnostic imaging, and ultrasound is no exception. In addition, a full understanding of the settings and functions of the ultrasound machine will make an enormous difference in the quality of the images obtained. While different brands and types of ultrasound machines vary greatly in their image quality, at least some of this can be overcome by applying the proper machine settings and knowing how to manipulate the images. It is in this realm in particular that many technicians can truly shine. Many veterinarians do not take the time to properly learn the equipment, and an educated technician can be of great help in manipulating the machine settings to provide the best possible image quality.

> **TECHNICIAN TIPS 8.20:** Understanding the settings and functions of an ultrasound makes a difference in obtaining quality images.

Exam Location

A thorough ultrasound exam takes time. The better the environment in which to scan, the easier it is to take the time to perform a good-quality scan. Ideally, the patient should be in a quiet, dimly lit area. In ambulatory situations, sometimes the best situation is a wash rack or within a stall, to minimize the amount of ambient light. Too much light hinders visualization of the screen and to compensate images tend to be acquired on too bright a setting. If ultrasound is frequently performed in a practice, it is helpful to get a light on a dimmer switch so as to be able to control the amount of light needed.

> **TECHNICIAN TIPS 8.21:** A wash rack or stall may be a good option for performing an ultrasound to help minimize the amount of light.

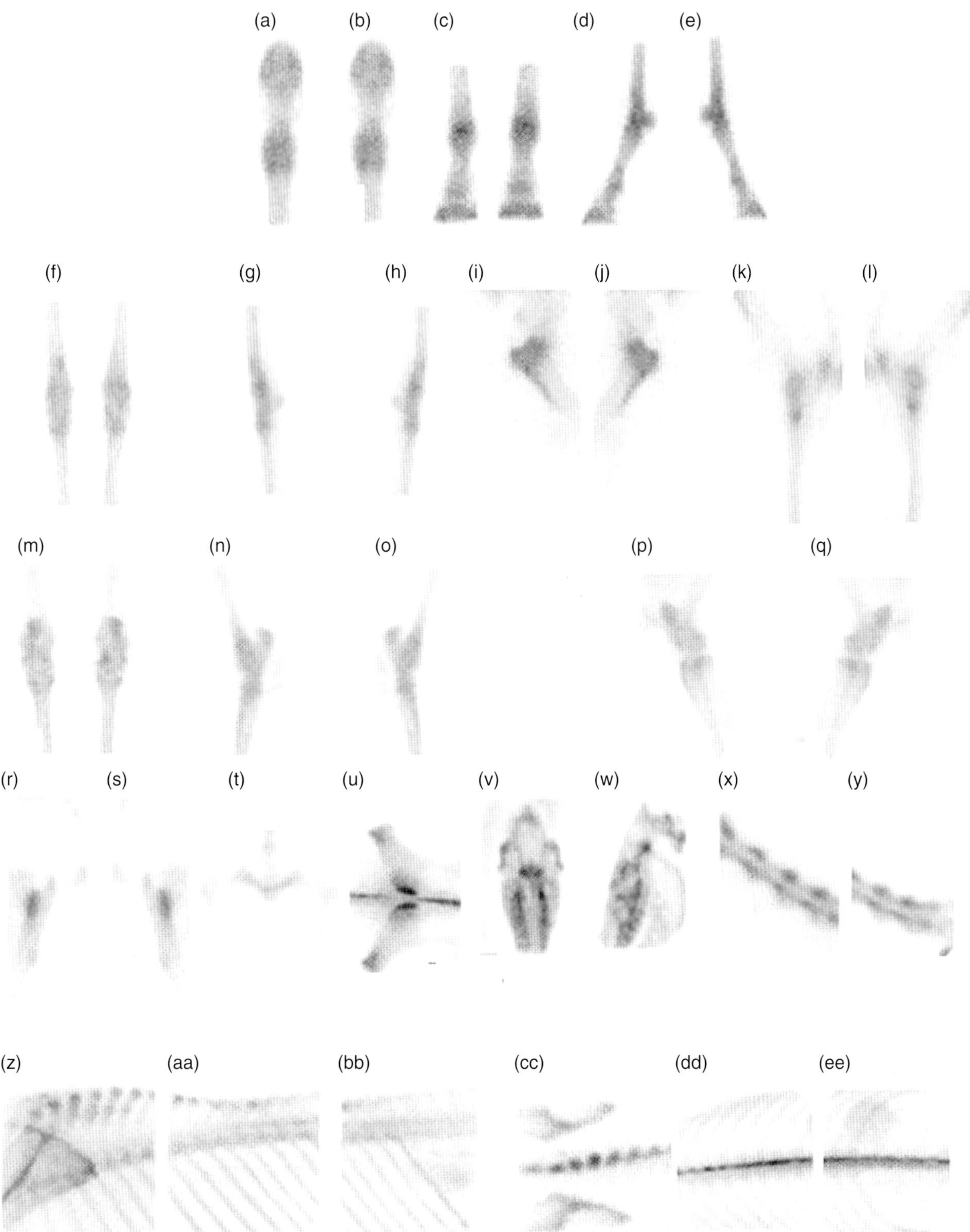

Figure 8.87 Foot: (a and b) palmar feet; (c) dorsal fetlock; (d) lateral left front fetlock; (e) lateral right front fetlock. Carpus: (f) dorsal carpus; (g) lateral left carpus; (h) lateral right carpus. Elbow and shoulder: (i) lateral left shoulder; (j) lateral right shoulder; (k) lateral left elbow; (l) lateral right elbow. Tarsus: (m) plantar tarsus; (n) lateral left tarsus; (o) lateral right tarsus. Stifle: (p) lateral left stifle; (q) lateral right stifle. Hip and pelvis: (r) lateral left hip; (s) lateral right hip; (t) caudal pelvis; (u) dorsal pelvis. Skull and spine: (v) dorsal skull; (w) left lateral skull; (x) left lateral cranial cervical spine; (y) left lateral caudal cervical spine. Spine: (z) left lateral cranial thoracic spine; (aa) left lateral mid-thoracic spine; (bb) left lateral caudal thoracic spine. Spine: (cc) dorsal cranial thoracic spine; (dd) dorsal mid-thoracic spine; (ee) dorsal caudal thoracic spine.

Additionally, it is important that the person acquiring the images be in a safe and comfortable position. A low stool is very helpful for examining the distal limb. Stocks are often helpful and can improve safety. The ultrasound machine should be within easy reach so that the settings can be constantly manipulated and images properly labeled.

Patient Preparation

Gas is the enemy of ultrasound. Gas is very reflective, and when the ultrasound beam encounters air, most of the sound beam is reflected back to the probe rather than continuing through the tissue. This principle comes into play when considering patient preparation. When air is trapped between the probe and the skin surface, which happens within hair, image quality will suffer. That is why, whenever possible, the patient should be closely clipped with a 40 blade to remove as much hair as possible. Once clipped, the area to be imaged should be washed with soap, rinsed thoroughly, and gel applied. In some places, such as the distal fetlock, where hair tends to be coarse, or pastern, where there is a central linear "cowlick," shaving with a razor can be very helpful.

TECHNICIAN TIPS 8.22: The patient should be closely clipped with a 40 blade to remove as much hair as possible for performing an ultrasound.

In some cases, such as with show animals or fiber animals (camelids), clipping is not possible. In those cases, the region to be imaged should be soaked with water and gel applied over the water. Alternatively, isopropyl alcohol can be applied to the haircoat or fibers. Combining alcohol and gel can cause the gel to slide off the area where alcohol is applied. Some transducers are sensitive to the drying effects of alcohol and may need to be covered with a glove or transducer sheath if alcohol is used. Especially, in dry climates, the longer the skin has time to soak in moisture from gel and water, the better the image quality.

TECHNICIAN TIPS 8.23: The longer the skin has time to soak in moisture from gel and water, the better the image quality of the ultrasound.

Restraint techniques will vary by species, age, and temperament of the individual patient. In some cases, it is to the patient's and ultrasonographer's benefit to sedate the patient prior to scanning. Scans are faster and easier if the animal is quietly restrained. However, if an abdominal scan is to be performed, the effects of the sedation on certain ultrasound findings must be weighed against the benefits of sedation-induced restraint. Even light sedation will induce some animals (camelids and small ruminants) to lie down or kush. This can be an inconvenience if the abdomen is the area of interest.

Image Labeling and Storage

Proper labeling of images is mandatory for a responsible and useful medical record. Prior to starting the study, the patient's and owner's names, at a minimum, should be entered into patient menu. If the patient has a medical record number, this too should be entered.

Once the study begins, every image should have labels that include the part of the body being scanned and the specific structure being imaged. When appropriate, additional markers, such as medial or lateral, cranial or caudal, left or right, should be included. For the distal limb, the location can be recorded using a zone system or via measurements in centimeters distal to the accessory carpal bone (DACB) or calcaneal tuberosity (DCT). For example, a scan of the right fore medial suspensory branch would be labeled "RF MED SLB 34 cm DACB." For the thorax and abdomen, intercostal spaces (ICS) can be used as a localizer. A scan of the equine stomach on the left side of the abdomen may read "Lt and stomach ICS 14." Without adequate labeling, it is impossible to accurately review images at a later date or send them to someone else for review.

At the end of a scan, images should be stored in a secure location. This may include backing up to an external hard drive, burning to a CD, or transferring to a PACS (picture archiving and communication system) or cloud storage. Images are an important part of the medical record and should be accessible for review. In the United States, veterinary technicians need to become familiar with their state's laws regarding storage of digital veterinary medical images.

TECHNICIAN TIPS 8.24: Veterinary technicians should know their state's laws regarding proper storage of digital veterinary medical images.

Ultrasound Machine Settings

Most modern ultrasound machines have a seemingly overwhelming number of buttons and settings. While they are not all used routinely in every scan, there are certain functions that are essential to know and use. The knob locations and labels will vary from machine to machine; therefore, it is important to learn how the individual machine is being used.

Presets: Presets are settings that have been created by the manufacturer for certain types of study (e.g. tendon, abdomen). Presets include idealized settings for the "average" exam and can be customized by species, body part, and the preferences of individual imagers. Selecting the appropriate preset at the beginning of a study will save time with image manipulation during the study.

TECHNICIAN TIPS 8.25: To avoid wasting time during the study, appropriate presets should be selected at the beginning of the study.

Transducer selection: Transducer types are generally described as linear, curved, or curvilinear. Linear transducers produce a rectangular-shaped image whereas the curved and curvilinear transducers create pie-shaped or fan-like images that are narrow in the near field (closest to the transducer) and wider in the far field (farthest from the transducer) (Figure 8.88). The scanning surface (the part that touches the patient) is called the footprint. The shape and size of the footprint together with the transducer frequency limit where on the body the transducer can be effectively used.

Frequency settings determine the depth of penetration of the ultrasound beam and the resolution of the image. Most ultrasound transducers are capable of operating over multiple frequencies but usually within a narrow range. Therefore, it may be necessary to use multiple transducers of varying frequencies to perform a complete examination, particularly when examining the abdomen. Higher frequency transducers have a limited depth of penetration but the best resolution. Lower frequency transducers offer better depth of penetration but less resolution. There is always a trade-off between depth of penetration and resolution, and an individual should always use the highest frequency setting that permits adequate penetration.

Linear transducers are typically the highest frequency transducers and may be used for musculoskeletal examinations, transrectal examinations of the reproductive tract, superficial scans of the thorax and abdomen, examination of bovine teats, and ophthalmic examinations. Microconvex transducers have midrange frequency capabilities and have the advantage of small, curved footprints that fit into small spaces and conform to curved surfaces. Microconvex transducers may be used for musculoskeletal examinations (stifle, cervical facets, imaging equine foot between heel bulbs), abdominal exams on neonates as well as adult small ruminants and camelids, thoracic examinations, and retrobulbar ophthalmic examinations. Microconvex transducers can also be used transrectally as they have the advantage of additional depth of penetration and a wider field of view over a standard transrectal linear transducer. Macroconvex transducers are the lowest frequency transducers and are used for abdominal and thoracic imaging, as well as for imaging deeper skeletal structures such as the hip and back. Phased array transducers are specifically designed for cardiac ultrasound. They are mid-to-low frequency transducers with small footprints that fit easily between the ribs. This makes them ideally suited for echocardiography (ultrasound of the heart). Three-dimensional (3-D) ultrasound imaging requires a specific 3-D transducer and an ultrasound machine with 3-D capability. This type of ultrasound has not yet gained widespread application in large animal practice.

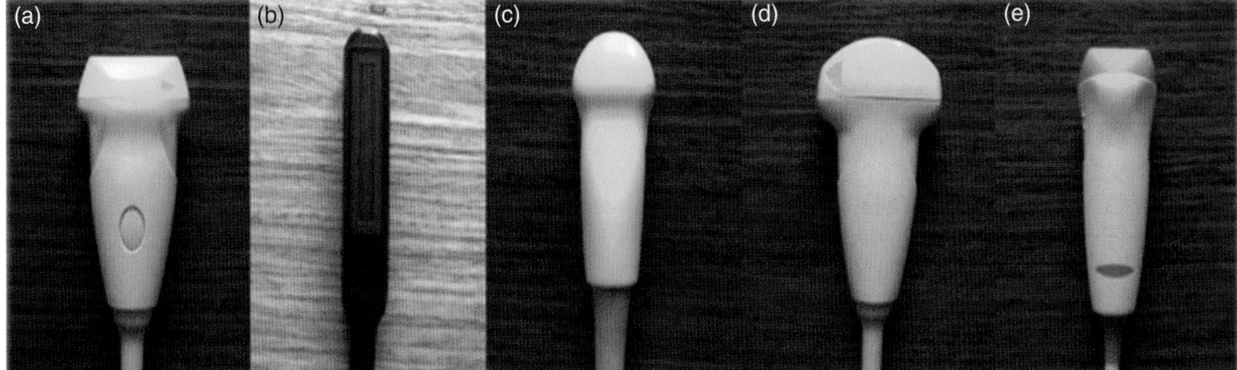

Figure 8.88 Ultrasound transducer types: (a) Linear transducer often called a "tendon probe" because of its frequent application in equine musculoskeletal imaging; (b) Linear transducer often called a "rectal probe" because of its application in reproductive sonography; (c) Microconvex transducer; note the small footprint compared to the macroconvex transducer. This transducer often has mid-frequency range capabilities and is excellent for large animal neonatal exams and small ruminant or camelid abdomens. This transducer can also be used transrectally; (d) Macroconvex transducer; this is most often used for transcutaneous examinations of the abdomen, but also the hip and back; and (e) Phased array transducer often called a "cardiac probe." This transducer has a mid-to-low frequency range, fits between the ribs, and can be rotated within that space to obtain images in two mutually perpendicular planes.

- Depth: It is common for many individuals to scan with too much depth. Ideally, the area of interest should be centered in the image, and there should be little extra in the far field. For example, when scanning a metacarpus, the correct depth setting is typically about 4–6 cm of depth, depending on the specific structure being imaged. If the machine is set at 8 cm of depth, there is too much empty space in the far field, and it hinders evaluation of the important structures. Depth controls are typically dials or toggle buttons.
- Gain/Time Gain Compensation: The gain controls the overall brightness of the image. Increasing the gain will make the entire image brighter; decreasing the gain makes the entire image darker.

A common mistake is to scan with too much gain, resulting in images that are too bright. This is particularly common when a scan is performed in a well-lit area. The time gain compensation (TGC) control is usually a row of slider knobs, although on some ultrasound machines, it is a part of touch screen controls. The TGC allows for more localized control of the gain, and sliding the knob(s) right or left can alter the gain at a specific depth. If the TGC is set inappropriately, it can result in a bright or dark band across the image. Focal zones control the width of the ultrasound beam. The ultrasound beam narrows at the level of the focal zone. The narrowest part of the ultrasound beam is where there will be the best resolution.

Therefore, the focal zone should be centered on the area of interest (Figure 8.89). The placement of the focal zone should be altered throughout the course of an exam, depending on the area imaged. Returning to our example of imaging the metacarpus, the focal zone should be placed in the near field for evaluation of the flexor tendons and in the far field for evaluation of the suspensory and distal check ligaments.

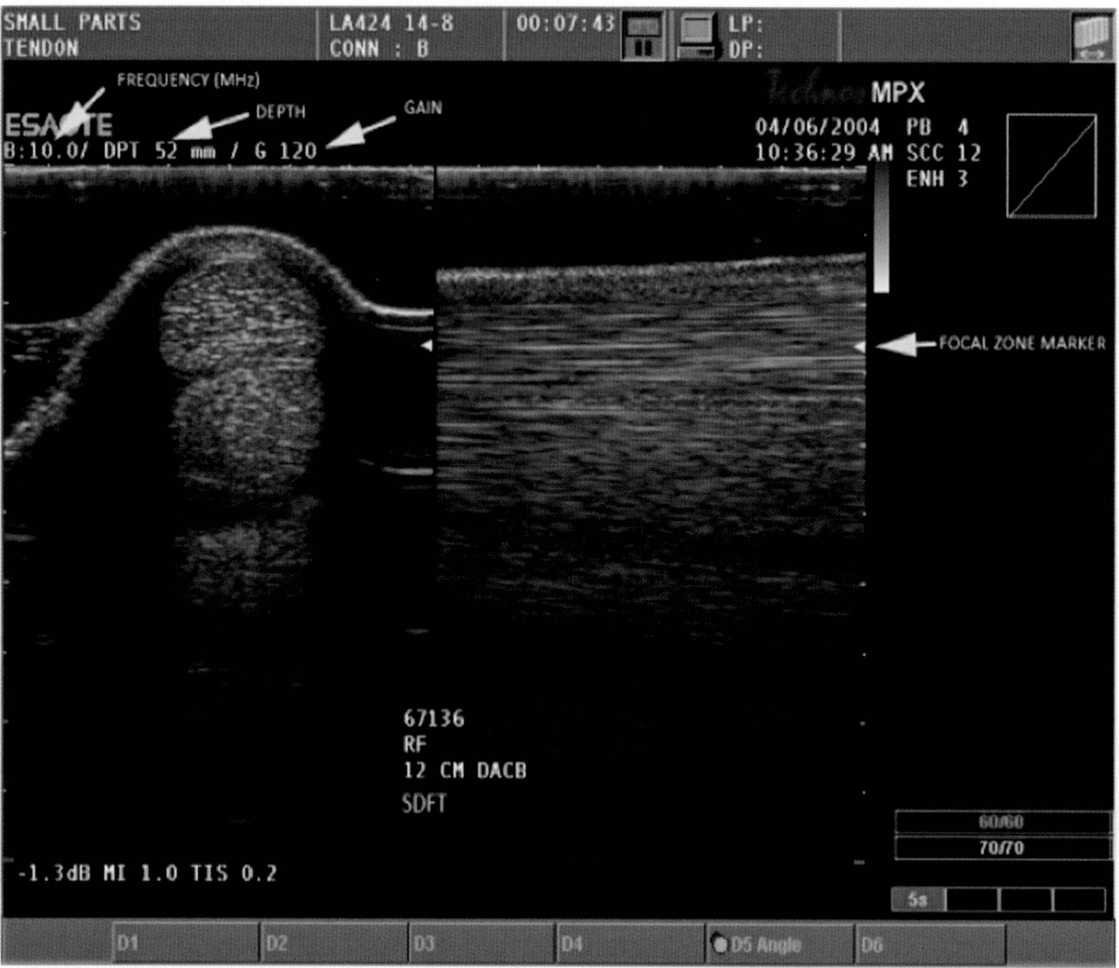

Figure 8.89 Focal zone and other settings; the focal zone marker is often an arrow. When properly adjusted, it should point to the structure of interest. In this image, the focal zone is set for evaluating the superficial digital flexor tendon. The frequency, depth, and gain settings are displayed at the top of the screen. Note that the image is labeled with the medical record number, "RF" for right forelimb, distance from the accessory carpal bone, and structure of interest (SDFT).

> **TECHNICIAN TIPS 8.26:** The narrowest part of the ultrasound beam is where there will be the best resolution. Therefore, the focal zone should be centered on the area of interest.

- Freeze/Store: How an image is saved and stored. Most machines now will also allow the user to scroll back multiple frames after freezing in order to save and store the best image.
- Labeling: Many machines allow for a customizable menu of labels or they can be typed out each time.
- Measuring: This may be a linear measurement (e.g. length of a lesion) or a cross-sectional area. This is often used to measure the size of tendons and dimensions of lesions. Keeping accurate measurements is helpful for recheck examinations.

There are many other controls and settings that can help advance or fine tune image quality. Spending time with a company representative or experienced ultrasonographer can be very helpful in learning the advanced settings.

Understanding Image Orientation

Standard image orientation consists of the transducer surface at the top of the screen (in the near field) with deeper tissues displayed in the far field. Whether the left and right sides represent medial and lateral, cranial and caudal, or dorsal and ventral depends on how the sonographer is holding the ultrasound transducer (Figure 8.90). Every ultrasound transducer has a marker (either on the scan head or handle, sometimes both) that corresponds to the orientation marker on the ultrasound image. For example, if the transducer is held such that the marker is on the lateral side of the structure being imaged, then the side of the screen with the orientation marker represents lateral and the opposite side of the screen represents medial. It should be noted that an individual can alter the side of the screen on which the orientation marker is displayed. Sometimes, side-by-side images are displayed on a single screen, a so-called split screen view. This has the advantage of displaying a structure in two imaging planes and is most commonly applied to equine tendon ultrasounds. Commonly, the short axis (transverse) image is displayed on the left and the long axis (longitudinal) image is displayed on the right side of the screen.

Cardiac-Specific "Knobology"

When echocardiography is part of the large animal ultrasound practice, a few additional "standard" knobs need to be learned. These mostly relate to acquisition of M-mode images, color-flow Doppler, and spectral Doppler.

M-mode: Standard ultrasound images are performed in B-mode (brightness-mode). B-mode produces a two-dimensional ultrasound image composed of "bright dots" that represent ultrasound echoes. M-mode (motion-mode) produces one-dimensional ultrasound images that are displayed over time. Time is displayed on the x-axis, depth is displayed on the y-axis, and a simultaneous ECG recording is displayed over the top of the M-mode image. The simultaneous ECG permits precise measurements of the heart during specific parts of the cardiac cycle. M-mode images are obtained by first scanning in B-mode and obtaining standard echocardiographic views then selecting for M-mode (Figure 8.91). Many ultrasound machines will simultaneously display the M-mode and the B-mode image, permitting easier optimization.

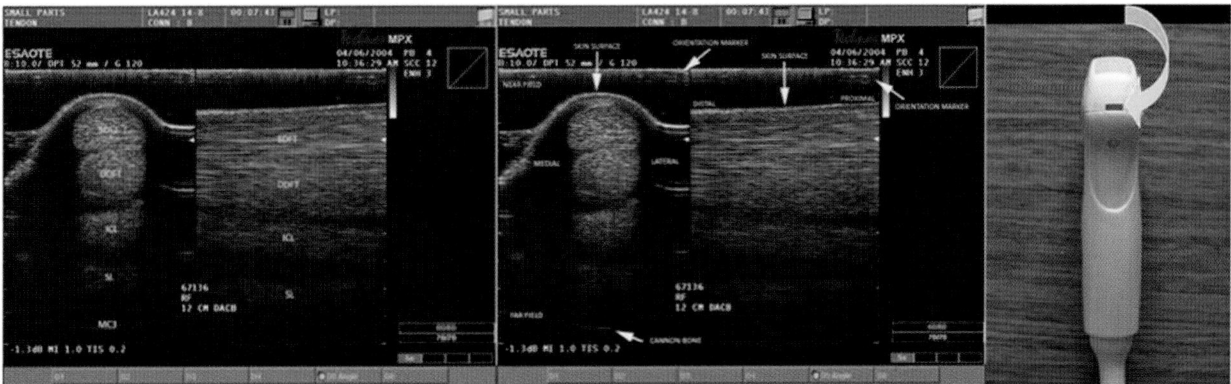

Figure 8.90 Transducer and image orientation; images a and b show how the structures of the palmar metacarpal region of the horse are displayed when the transducer is applied to the limb with the transducer marker held either laterally (left-sided image of a and b) or proximally (right-sided image of a and b). The side-by-side display of two images on the same screen is called a "split screen" view. The yellow arrow in image c is pointing to the transducer marker, in this case a green light. This marker corresponds to the orientation marker in images a and b.

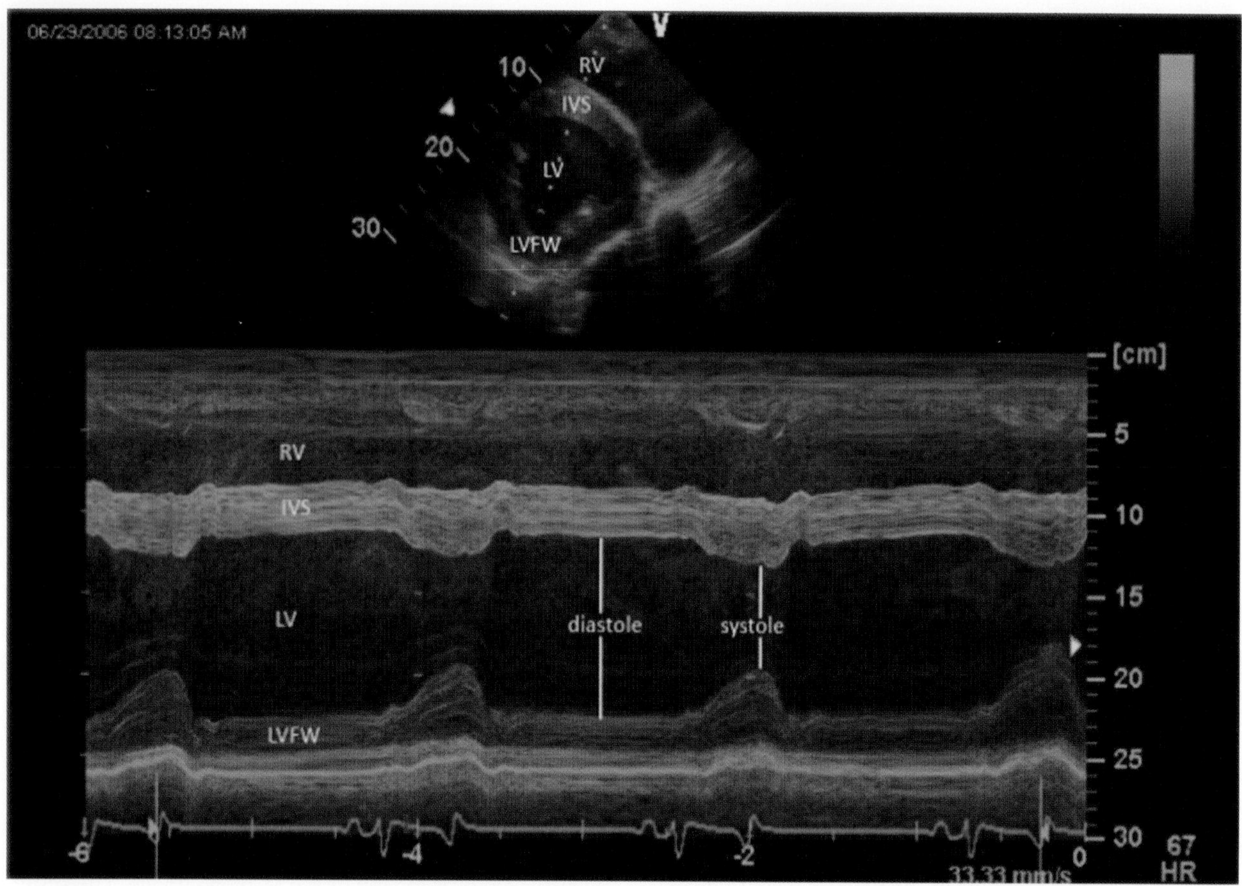

Figure 8.91 M-mode of heart. The image at the top of the screen is a two-dimensional B-mode image of the left ventricle in short axis. The dotted line running through the middle of the image is the M-mode cursor. The location of the cursor corresponds to the image slice that is displayed as a one-dimensional M-mode image at the bottom of the screen. Time is on the x-axis and depth is on the y-axis. RV: right ventricle; LV: left ventricle; LVFW: left ventricular free wall.

Doppler: Doppler echocardiography is a method for evaluating blood flow within the heart. The best Doppler signals are produced by low frequency transducers and by aligning the imaging plane as parallel to blood flow as possible (Figure 8.92). Color-flow Doppler produces a color picture of blood flow superimposed on top of the B-mode or M-mode image. Blood flow velocity, direction, and turbulence are displayed with different color maps. Color-flow Doppler is most often used to identify regurgitant jets ("leaky valves") and/or flow through congenital or acquired defects. Spectral Doppler includes both pulsed wave and continuous wave Doppler. Pulsed wave Doppler is used to localize flow to a specific area but cannot resolve velocities >1.5–2 m/S. Continuous wave Doppler is used to determine blood flow velocities >2 m/S, important for calculating pressure differences across a valve or shunt (Figure 8.93).

Echocardiography is a very specialized field of ultrasound. While the general principles described for B-mode ultrasound still apply, there are several specialized exams in addition to the ones just described. Expertise in echocardiography usually requires focused training beyond that for general ultrasound.

Acquiring the Images

In large animal practice, most ultrasound scanning is performed by the veterinarian. However, some practices have begun to utilize technicians for image acquisition (similar to the human field). In these situations, it is very important to have a standard set of images that are acquired in each case. Cine loops (short digital ultrasound movies) can also be useful, as they allow for more complete review of the study. Hand position and probe angle can dramatically affect the appearance of structures and may produce artifactual lesions; images must be acquired with great care to avoid such artifacts. The standard image acquisition for ultrasound studies is beyond the scope of this text. Technicians that are looking to pursue knowledge of ultrasound imaging are recommended to attend ultrasound courses and make use of the available imaging textbooks and journal articles.

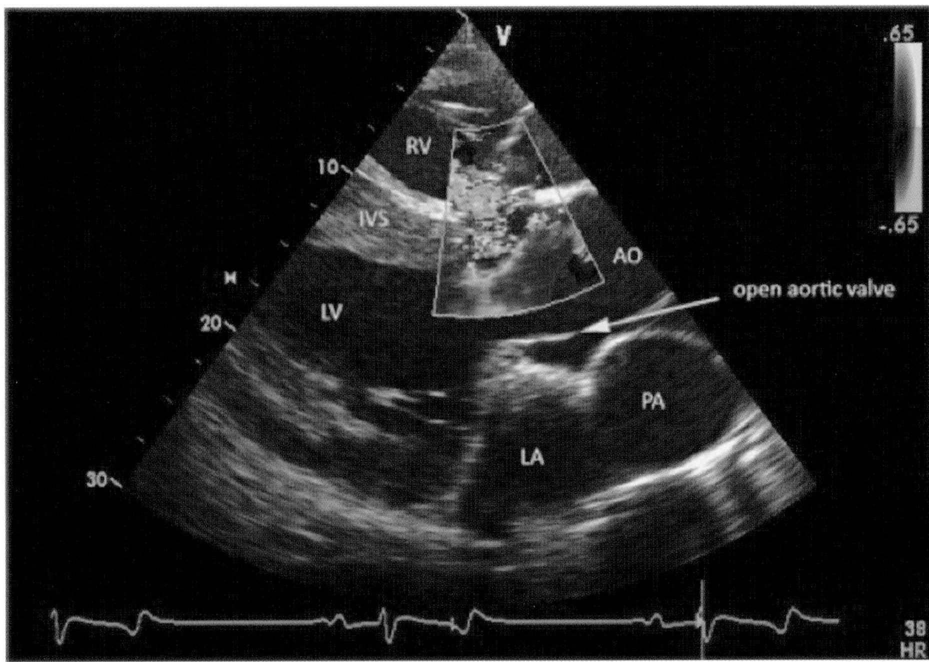

Figure 8.92 Color Doppler image of a horse with a congenital heart defect (ventricular septal defect or VSD). The color Doppler window is placed over the interventricular septum (IVS) in the area of the aorta (AO). The color red represents normal blood flowing from the left ventricle out the aorta during systole. The green/yellow/turquoise color represents turbulent flow across the VSD. RV: right ventricle; LV: left ventricle; LA: left atrium.

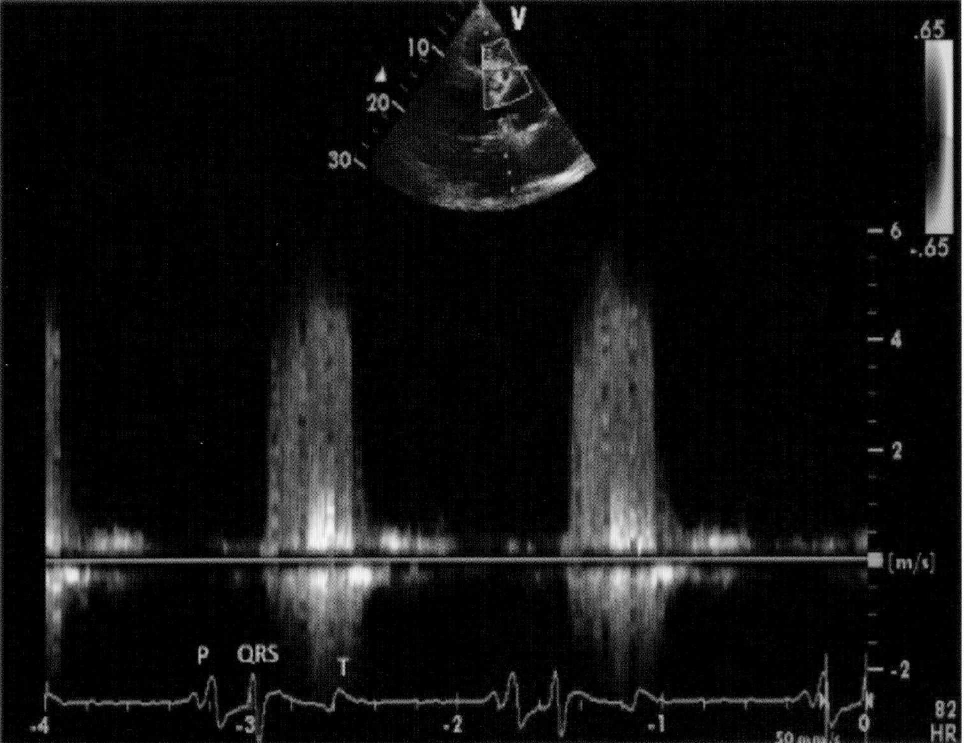

Figure 8.93 Continuous wave Doppler display from horse with a ventricular septal defect (VSD). The image at the top of the screen is the B-mode image of the heart with color Doppler superimposed over the VSD (see Figure 8.5). The continuous wave Doppler tracing is displayed with time on the x-axis and velocity in m/s on the y-axis. A simultaneous ECG is superimposed for timing. During systole (between the QRS and T or the ECG), there is a large positive deflection that peaks at just over 5 m/s. This is the velocity of blood as it crosses the VSD. The high velocity is consistent with a small defect.

Magnetic Resonance Imaging

The technology of MRI and CT, in the human and animal world is one that is rapidly changing and advancing, to the point that texts such as these have a hard time remaining relevant for very long.

Magnetic resonance imaging, commonly called MRI, is a noninvasive procedure that produces very detailed pictures of body soft tissue, bone, and organs without using ionizing radiation, as with other diagnostic imaging procedures such as X-ray, computed tomography (CT), and C-arm. The modality uses a very large magnet, radio waves, complex computer, and software technology to scan the patient's body and produce two- or three-dimensional cross-section images.

When exposed to the magnetic field of an MRI unit, the nuclei line up in parallel formation, like rows of a tiny magnet. Nearly, two-thirds of a veterinary patient's body is hydrogen atoms, found in water and fat molecules. When the nuclei are subjected to a strong pulse of radio waves from an MRI unit, they are knocked out of their parallel alignment. As they fall back into alignment, they produce a readable radio signal. The signal is recorded by the machine and transferred to a computer. The computer uses these signals to create an image.

The strength of an MRI, originally measured in "gauss," is now measured in "Tesla." Low-field MRIs are typically less than 1 T but high-field MRIs vary anywhere from 2 to 5 or more teslas. In veterinary medicine, a common high-field MRI is around 3 T (in 2020). The term gauss is still utilized, particularly in mapping out safety distance from an MRI unit (Figure 8.94).

TECHNICIAN TIPS 8.27: There are 10 000 gauss in one tesla.

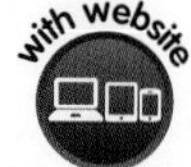

Check out our website for a chart of common MRI terminology!

All types of MRI require specific safety precautions to avoid injury of personal and patient. One of the biggest concerns when working around an MRI is the permanent magnetic field, which is always on. Due to the powerful magnetic field created by MRI machines, they must be carefully operated under close supervision, and certain precautions according to the manufacturer must be taken to prevent injury. Non-conductive monitoring equipment and oxygen tanks, placing the arterial line prior to entering the active magnetic space, need to be considered. Five gauss and below are considered safe for the general public. Cardiac pacemakers, aneurysm clips, and other implanted electronic or metal devices may be interfered with under five gauss. Additionally, the presence of even a tiny metallic fragment can produce significant artifact (Figure 8.95).

MRI scanners used for clinical interpretation fall into two categories: high-field scanners and low-field scanners (See Table 8.2). The high-field MRIs have better image

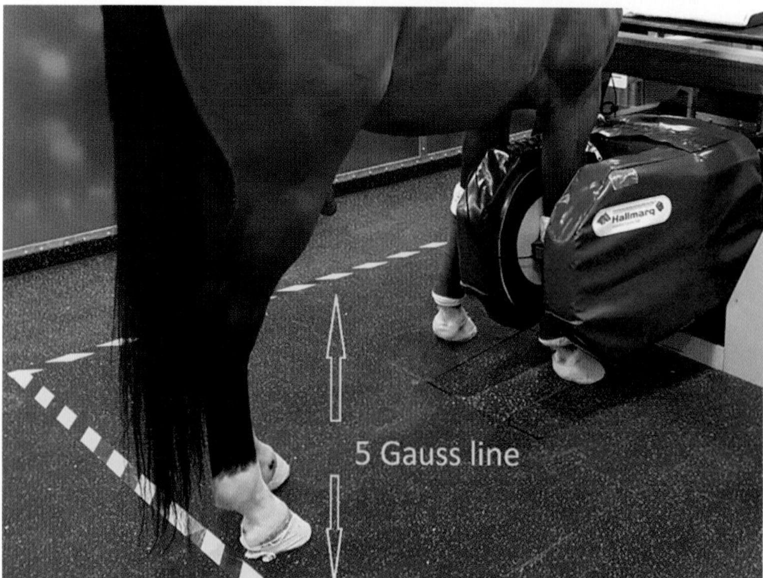

Figure 8.94 Note the tape around the magnet that represents the point at which stray magnetic field is five gauss.

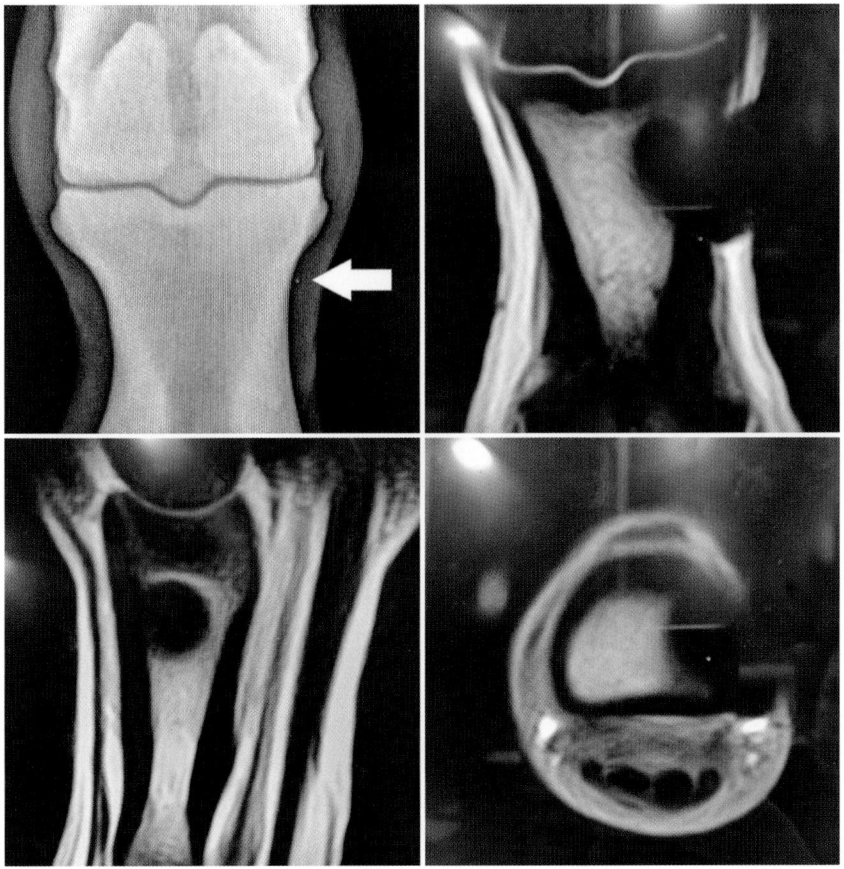

Figure 8.95 Example of a needle fragment interfering with MRI image from three different perspectives.

quality, have a limited bore opening (gantry), and thus far require general anesthesia in order to perform. The low-field MRIs have a grainier image quality, in a c-shape with an opening and some have been adapted to be used in a standing position under a mild sedation. An analogy is comparing a Polaroid picture to a digital picture. Both pictures will demonstrate an object; however, the resolution and quality will differ between the two. In clinical practice, MRI is used to distinguish pathologic tissue (such as tumors, suspensory, tendon, or ligament tears) from normal tissue. This can oftentimes be accomplished using a low-field MRI; while the image is grainier, it can still be diagnostic provided good technique, and good interpretation is used (Figures 8.96–8.98).

Table 8.2 Low-field MRI vs. high-field MRI.

Low-field MRI	High-field MRI
~ 0.5–1 T	2–5 T
Quiet function, but still loud enough to bother an animal	Loud sound during operation, requires hearing protection for the patient and any personnel in the area
Patient under standing sedation	Patient must be under general anesthesia
Patient may remain standing	Lateral recumbency
Anatomy	Anatomy that can be scanned is limited to the size and position due to the gantry size
Low-quality image, grainy	Higher-quality image

Each scan series takes approximately 30–90 min, depending on the protocol and how many sequences are run. Different sequences will highlight tissues differently and allow different pathology to stand out. The two main factors that can be altered to create different image sequences are "time to echo" (TE) and "repetition time" (TR). The most common sequences are called T1, using shorter TE and TR times and T2 or T2-weighted sequences using longer TE and TR times. A third type of sequence called a "STIR" (short-TI Inversion recovery) is one that creates a fat suppression image, great for highlighting joint fluid. In horses, stirs are particularly challenging to sequence, especially in the standing patient that is subject to motion (Table 8.3).

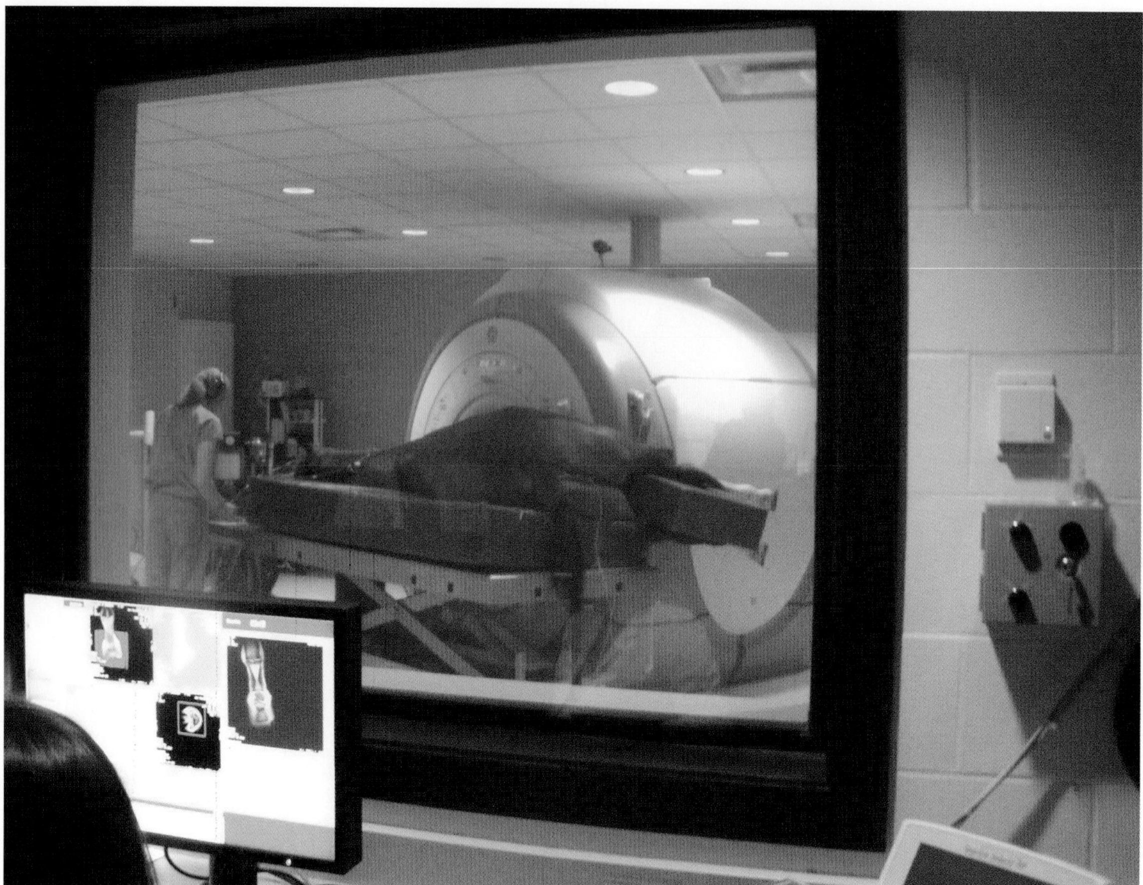

Figure 8.96 3T MRI unit.

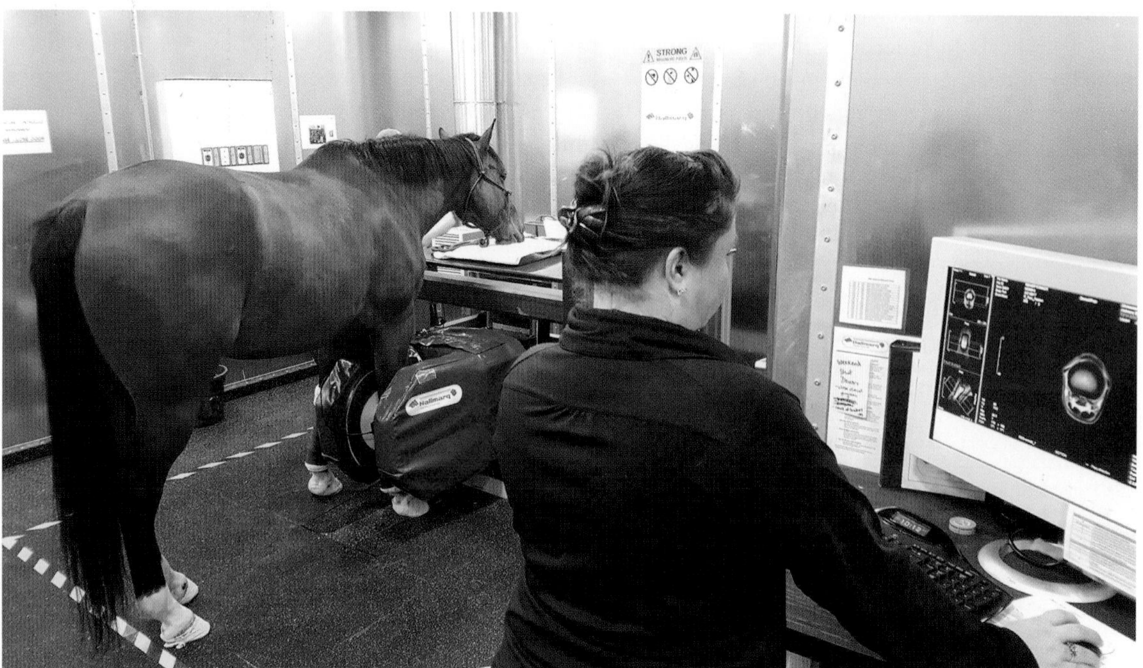

Figure 8.97 Hallmarq MRI unit. *Source:* Courtesy of the University of Minnesota Leatherdale Equine Center.

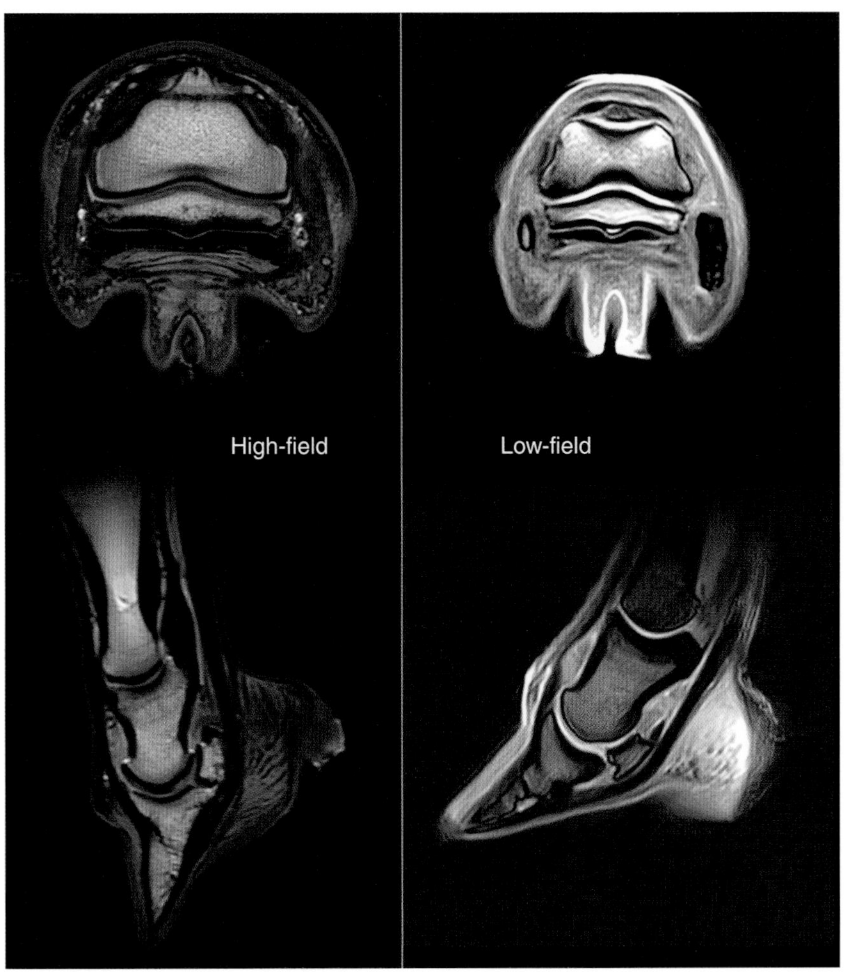

Figure 8.98 Comparison of an equine foot in a low-field vs high-field MRI.

Table 8.3 Common MRI terminology.

MRI abbreviation	Terminology
RF	Radio frequency – a frequency band in the electromagnetic spectrum with frequencies in the millions of cycles per second.
TE	Time to echo – the time in an imaging sequence between the initial RF pulse and the maximum in the echo.
TR	Repetition time – the time between repetitions of the basic sequence in an imaging sequence.
SE	Spin Echo – a multiple echo spin-echo sequence, which records different regions of k-space with different echoes.
GE	Gradient Echo – a form of MR signal from the refocusing of transverse magnetization caused by the application of a specific magnetic field gradient.
IR	Inversion recovery – IR pulse sequences are a type of MRI sequence used to selectively null the signal for certain tissues (fat or fluid).
Isocenter	A location in an imaging magnet assigned the most centered coordinates.

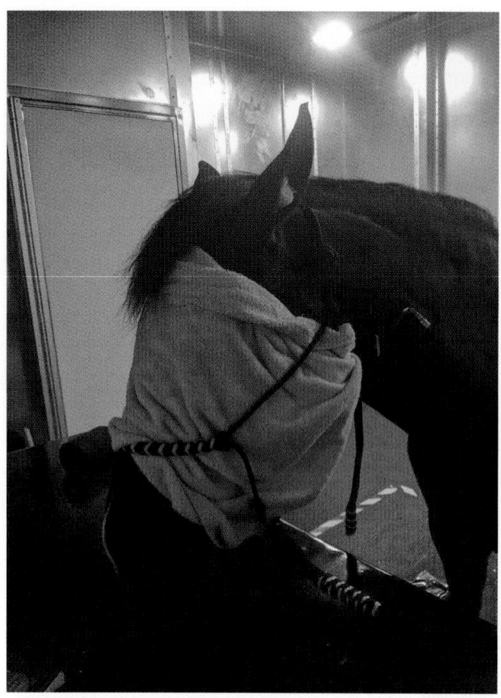

Figure 8.99 A horse blindfolded with a towel in a standing MRI.

In horses, high-field MRIs are generally limited to the foot, fetlock, and pastern regions due to the limitations of the gantry's bore and the bulkiness of the horse's hindquarters or shoulders as well as the length of the limb. The low-field MRIs have different limiting capabilities than those of the high-field MRIs. Low-field open bore MRIs such as the Hallmarq unit have the capability to image proximal suspensory ligaments, carpus, and tarsus. Extremely, large patients such as drafts can be problematic due to their size, even for a foot scan.

TECHNICIAN TIPS 8.28: Blinkers, blindfolds, and ear plugs can help to avoid distraction and motion of the patient during standing MRI and CTs (Figure 8.99).

Computed Tomography

Computed tomography (CT), also known as computerized axial tomography (CAT) or CT scan. CT combines a series of X-ray views taken from different angles and processed by a computer to create cross-sectional images of bones and soft tissue structures inside the body (Figure 8.100). The images created by a CT scan are dependent on the density of specific tissue. This is a very different principle than used with MRI. Hounsfield unit is the term given for each specific density within the body that is measured.

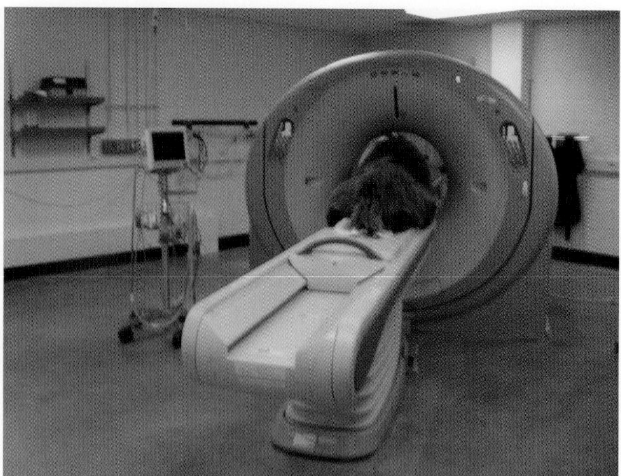

Figure 8.100 CT views; (a) transverse (b) sagittal (c) dorsal.

A CT unit has a circular gantry, which moves in and out during imaging (or the patient moves). The gantry stores electrical equipment, an X-ray tube, and multiple detectors, much like a baggage scanner at an airport. The detectors measure the strength and number of X-rays that pass through a patient around 360°, so that a cross-sectional map can be made through the anatomy being imaged. The newest technology allows us to image in a helical (fast) fashion obtaining multiple slices of information. In older, single slice scanners, the system needed time to reset after each rotation of the X-ray tube. Helical CT scanners can produce a series of images through a part of a large animal's body in less than 1 min. The bore size of the gantry, like MRI, is the limiting factor to what body parts can be imaged. In an adult horse that is typically limited to head, some neck and lower extremities but a full body of smaller animals like a foal, goat, or pig can often fit.

CT units adapted from human medicine around 2000–2010 required large animal patients to be positioned in dorsal or lateral recumbency under heavy sedation or general anesthesia (Figure 8.101). Then some CT models began to emerge into the industry that allowed for scanning of the skull while standing under light sedation. The same units could also be used to scan limbs but require general anesthesia and lateral positioning. In 2019, the first standing CT machine by Asto CT (Figure 8.102) was developed for large animals, allowing for standing scans of bilateral front or hinds as well as rotating to allow for head scans. Depending on the patient's size and confirmation, it has been possible to scan just over the tarsus or carpus, completing a full limb scan in under 1 min using only a sedative protocol.

CT is excellent for imaging bone structures and is very beneficial in trauma patients to survey the extent of all types of injury in a very short amount of time. Additionally, software technology now allows for 3D reconstruction using the acquired images (Figures 8.103 and 8.104). The

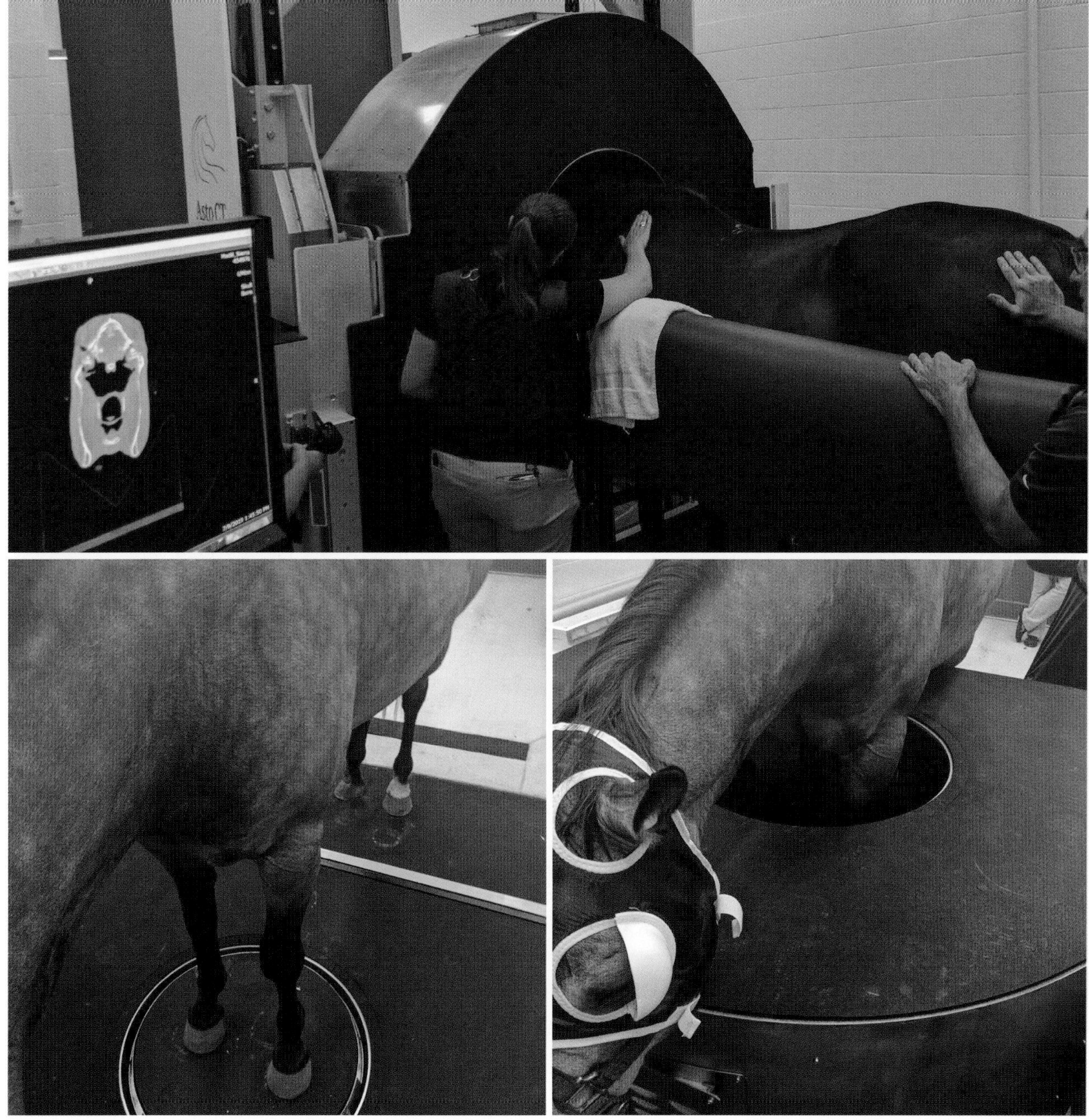

Figure 8.101 Asto CT Unit, capable of performing standing limb or head CTs.

advantages of CT over MRI are reduced costs and quick scan times; however, soft tissue details still lack currently, making MRI ideal for certain cases.

> **TECHNICIAN TIPS 8.29:** CT is excellent for imaging bone structures.

C-arm

A C-arm is a type of fluoroscope; similar to an X-ray, this medical imaging device uses radiation. It is named for the "C" shape of the machine which combines the X-ray source and detector. It can capture images in real time and is most commonly used in orthopedic and vascular procedures.

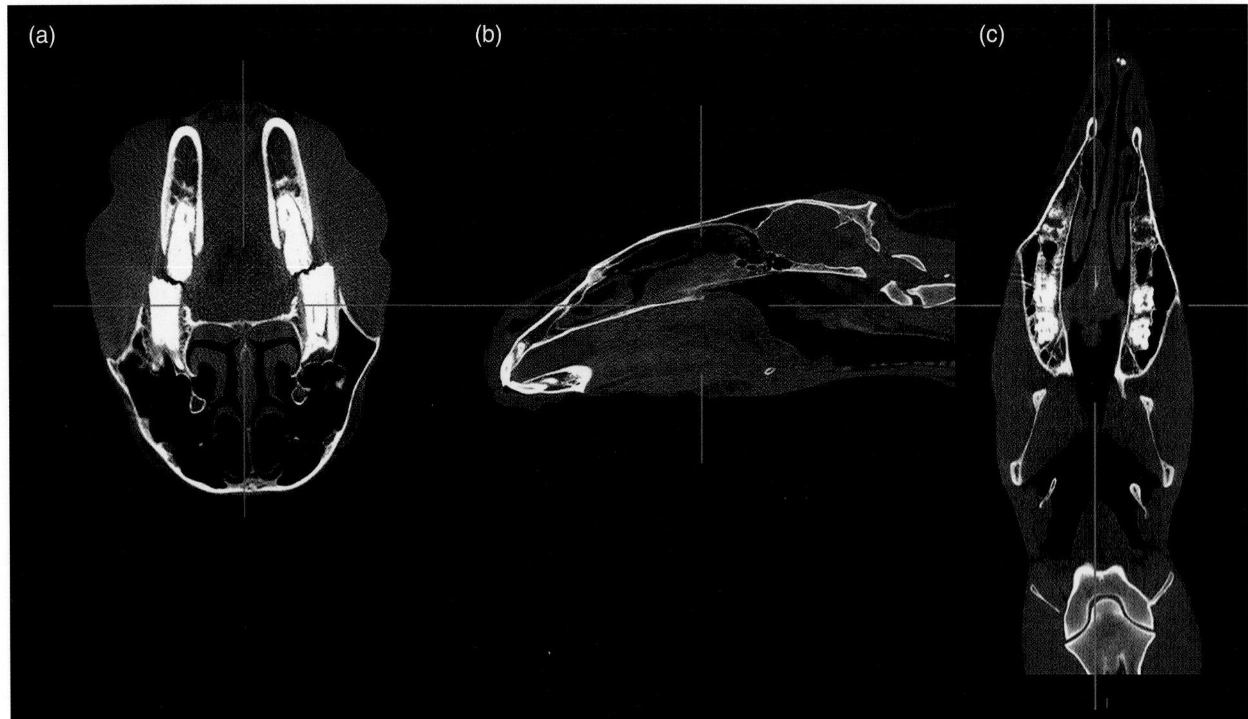

Figure 8.102 CT views a. transverse b. sagittal c. dorsal.

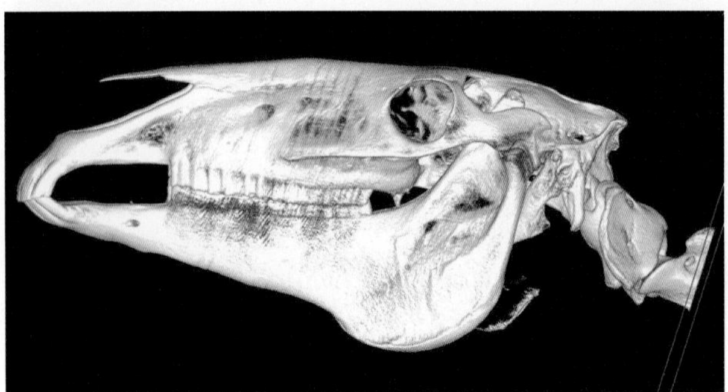

Figure 8.103 A 3D view of equine CT skull.

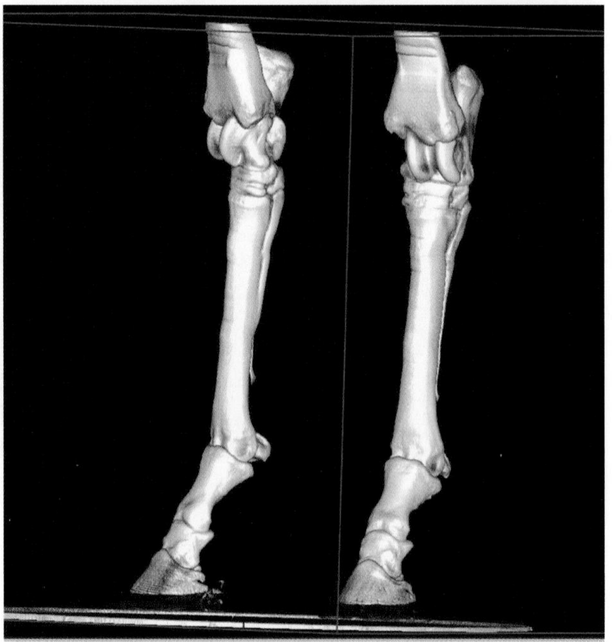

Figure 8.104 A 3D reconstruction view of CT bilateral equine hind limbs (standing).

The flexibility of the C-arm allows for it to be used at almost any angle. It can be operated by a surgeon with a hands-free foot pedal, therefore, eliminating the need to stop to perform X-rays and have X-ray equipment in the surgical field. Real-time fluoroscopy is especially helpful for procedures such as screw placement, where the distance of advancement can be monitored closely (Figures 8.105 and 8.106).

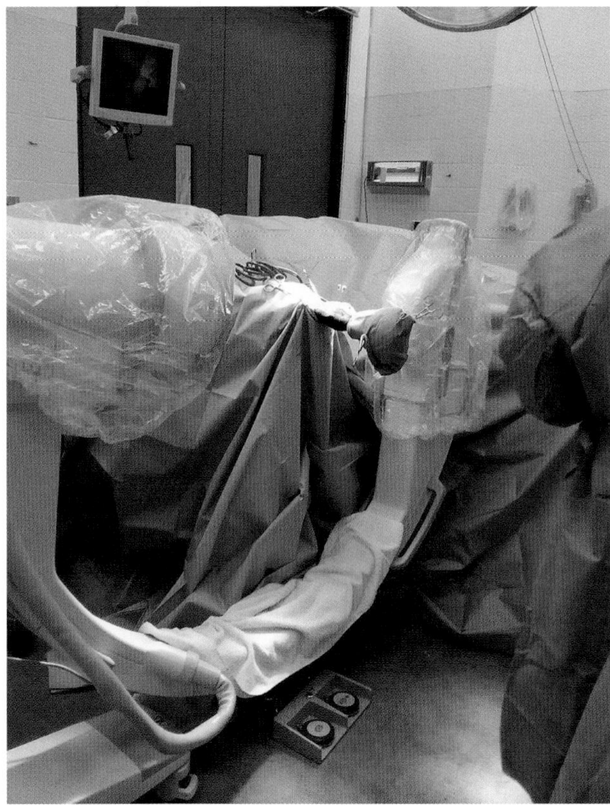

Figure 8.105 A C-arm set up for an equine distal limb screw placement.

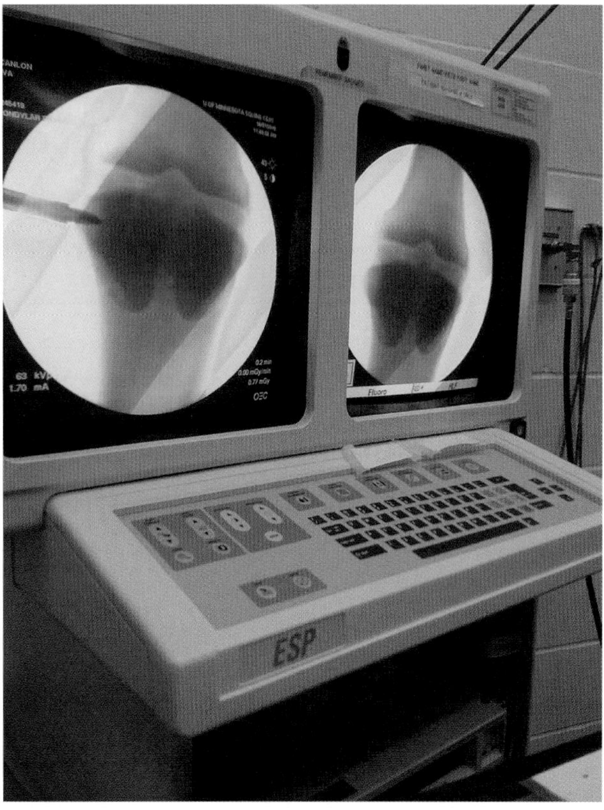

Figure 8.106 A C-arm console displaying an image.

References

Archer, D., Boswell, J., Voute, L., and Clegg, P. (2007). Skeletal scintigraphy in the horse: current indications and validity as a diagnostic test. *Vet. J.* 173 (1): 31–44. PubMed PMID: 16359891.

Barrett, M. & Selberg, K. (2012). How to obtain flexed lateral oblique radiographs of the equine stifle. *AAEP Proceedings*, 58.

Baxter, G. and Adams, O. (2011). *Adams and Stashak's Lameness in Horses*. Chichester, West Sussex; Ames, Iowa: Wiley Blackwell.

Blum, T. (1924). Osteomyelitis of the mandible and maxilla. *J. Am. Dent. Assoc.* 11: 802–805.

Bushberg, J. (ed.) (2002). *The Essential Physics of Medical Imaging*. Philadelphia, PA: Lippincott Williams & Wilkins.

Butler, J. (ed.) (2008). *Clinical Radiology of the Horse*. Ames, IA: Wiley Blackwell.

Contino, E., Barrett, M., & Werpy, N. (2012). Joint balance as evaluated on dorsopalmar radiographs. *AAEP Proceedings*, 58.

Hornak, J. P. (2020). The basics of MRI. Retrieved January 14, 2021, from https://www.cis.rit.edu/htbooks/mri/gloss.htm

Lamb, C. and Koblik, P. (1988). Scintigraphic evaluation of skeletal disease and its application to the horse. *Vet. Radiol.* 29 (1): 16–27.

Lavin, L. (1994). *Radiography in Veterinary Technology*. Philadelphia, PA: Saunders.

Levine, D., Ross, B., Ross, M. et al. (2007). Decreased radiopharmaceutical uptake (photopenia) in delayed phase scintigraphic images in three horses. *Vet. Radiol. Ultrasound* 48 (5): 467–470. PubMed PMID: 17899984.

Martland, A. (1929). Osteogenic sarcoma in dial painters using luminous paint. *Arch Pathol.* 17: 40–417.

Mendenhall, A. and Cantwell, H. (1998). *Equine Radiographic Procedures*. Philadelphia, PA: Lea & Febiger.

Morgan, P. and Silverman, S. (1984). *Techniques of Veterinary Radiology*, 4e. Ames, IA: Iowa State University Press.

Reef, V. (1998). *Equine diagnostic ultrasound*. Philadelphia, PA: W. B. Saunders.

Thrall, D. (ed.) (2013). *Textbook of Veterinary Diagnostic Radiology*. St. Louis, MO: Saunders Elsevier.

Weaver, M. (1995). Twenty years of equine scintigraphy—a coming of age? *Equine Vet. J.* 27 (3): 163–165. PubMed PMID: 7556041.

Clinical Case Resolution 8.1

The carpal radiographs of the racehorse described at the beginning of the chapter demonstrated multiple osseous fragments (chip fractures) within the middle carpal joint. The best visualization was on the flexed lateral view. Carpal chip fragments are a common condition in racehorses, and are readily diagnosed radiographically. Often the source of lameness needs to be localized with diagnostic blocking prior to radiography. However, in cases such as this where the signalment and physical exam findings indicate a likely location of pathology, radiographs can be a practical next diagnostic procedure. This horse underwent arthroscopic surgery and recovered successfully.

Activities

Multiple Choice Questions

(Answers can be found in the back of the book.)

1. Which of the following is not a principle of radiation safety?
A time
B power
C distance
D shielding

2. A racehorse presents with a hot, swollen, and thick superficial digital flexor tendon (bowed tendon). Which is the best imaging modality to use to examine this?
A radiography
B soft tissue phase nuclear scintigraphy
C ultrasonography
D This is not an injury that needs imaging.

3. How does increasing the gain change an ultrasound image?
A makes it darker
B increases the contrast
C makes it brighter
D decreases the contrast

4. Which of the following is not considered a standard radiographic view of the tarsus?
A flexed lateral
B dorso-plantar
C lateral
D dorsolateral-palmaromedial oblique (DLPMO)

5. Which of the following is not an indication to perform a nuclear scintigraphy bone scan?
A a stress fracture is suspected
B a patient has a multi-limb lameness
C to better evaluate back pain
D to accurately evaluate the extent of a fracture line for surgical planning

6. When making radiographs of the foot, you see a thin radiolucent line extending across the navicular bone on the D60P view. What do you do next?
A Consider it likely that the patient has a fractured navicular bone.
B Nothing. This is an artifact and does not mean anything.
C This could be a gas artifact from packing, but it would be significant if it were a real fracture line. It is important to know the difference. Repack the sole and repeat the view.
D Take a radiograph of the other foot to compare.

7. To perform a suspensory ligament ultrasound, what would be the ideal ultrasound transducer to use?
A a low frequency macroconvex probe
B a mid-to-high frequency linear array probe
C a mid-frequency curvilinear probe
D a mid-frequency rectal probe

8. Which of the following is the minimum amount of information that should be included with a patient's musculoskeletal ultrasound exam?
A the patient's and owner's names and the specific structure being imaged
B the patient's name and the date
C the specific body part being imaged and the name of the veterinarian in charge of the case
D the owner's name and the limb that is being imaged

9. Why is radiography the mainstay of equine imaging?
   - **A** It is widely available, affordable, and gives good bone and soft tissue detail.
   - **B** It is widely available, requires minimal user expertise, and provides good soft tissue detail.
   - **C** It is widely available, requires minimal user expertise, and provides good bone detail.
   - **D** It is widely available, affordable, and gives good bone detail.

10. Which of the following does not degrade the quality of an equine bone scan?
    - **A** patient motion
    - **B** too high a dose of ^{99m}Tc
    - **C** urine contamination
    - **D** imaging 8 hr after administration of the radiopharmaceutical

Test Your Learning

1. Explain the importance of properly preparing a horse for an ultrasound exam.
2. Why is nuclear scintigraphy useful in cases of multi-limb lameness?
3. Give three examples of how to put the principle of time, distance, and shielding to use.
4. Why is it important to have a full radiographic study of an affected joint?
5. Describe some of the limitations of ultrasonography.

Answers can be found in the back of the book.

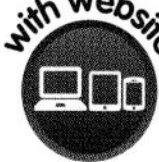

Extra review questions, case studies, and a breed ID image bank can be found online at www.wiley.com/go/loly/veterinary.

Chapter 9

Reproduction

Harry Momont, DVM, PhD, Dipl ACT, Celina M. Checura, DVM, MS, PhD, Dipl ACT, Zach Loppnow, DVM, and Sue Loly, LVT, VTS (EVN)

Learning Objectives

- Explain reproduction basics as they apply to large animal species.
- List comparative anatomy and physiology for various species.
- Describe how anatomy and physiology similarities and differences affect the approach to disease diagnosis and treatment of disease.
- Describe management and control of reproduction in the normal animal.

Clinical Case Problem 9.1

A 12-year-old mare presents to the veterinary hospital with failure to conceive. What parts of a patient history are pertinent to record when the mare arrives?

See Clinical Case Resolution 9.1 at the end of this chapter.

Key Terms

Artificial insemination (AI)
Breeding soundness exam
Bright-field microscopy
Colostrum
Corpus luteum
Cryoprotectant
Cryptorchidism
DAMNIT system
Diestrus
Differential interference contrast microscope
Embryo transfer
Endometrial cytology
Estradiol
Estrogen
Estrous
Estrus
Feedback mechanism
Fetotomy
Flushing
Follicle-stimulating hormone (FSH)
Gametes
Gonadotropin-releasing hormone (GnRH)
Gonads
Haploid
Hemocytometer
Hormone
Inhibin
Luteinizing hormone (LH)
Morphology
Open
Oviducts

(continued)

Large Animal Medicine for Veterinary Technicians, Second Edition. Edited by Sue Loly and Heather Hopkinson.

Companion website: www.wiley.com/go/loly/veterinary

KeyTerms (*continued*)

Oxytocin
Phase-contrast microscopy
Proestrus
Prostaglandin F2 alpha (PGF_2 alpha)
Sertoli cells
Sigmoid flexure
Spectrophotometry
Spermatogenesis
Superovulation
Transrectal ultrasonography
Utrecht guidelines
Vaginoscopy

Introduction

Survival of a species over the long run is dependent on its ability to adapt. The reproductive system provides a mechanism for that adaptation to occur by reshuffling the genetic deck every time a new generation of offspring is produced. Man has learned to manipulate this system in domestic animals to rapidly and dramatically alter the form, function, and productivity of companion animals and livestock.

"Theriogenology" is the name applied to the discipline of veterinary reproductive medicine and surgery. Theriogenology is a fertile field for expanding the capabilities and utilization of veterinary technicians in veterinary practice and livestock production systems. This chapter is intended to serve only as an introduction to the topic. Ultimately, clinical expertise can only be achieved by hands-on training with each individual species.

To make the content manageable, this chapter focuses on the major species of large animals of veterinary interest, namely, cattle, pigs, sheep, goats, horses, and camelids.

After introductory anatomy, physiology, and endocrinology, this chapter describes the general approaches to the examination and assessment of the male and female reproductive systems. Next follows a broad overview of reproductive disorders that provides some examples of important diseases with which veterinary technicians should be familiar. Finally, this chapter discusses the reproductive management of normal animals from breeding through delivery of their young.

Anatomy and Physiology of Reproduction

The basic aspects of reproductive anatomy and physiology are quite similar in all domestic mammals. Control of the reproductive processes in both sexes is a complex interaction between the brain, the pituitary gland, and the reproductive tract.

> **TECHNICIAN TIP 9.1:** Controlling reproduction is a complex interaction between the brain, pituitary gland, and reproductive tract.

Both sexes possess paired gonads (testes in the male and ovaries in the female) that are responsible for producing the haploid gametes (sperm and ova) that will combine at fertilization to produce the new individual (a diploid zygote). The gonads also have an endocrine function and produce the hormones that are critical for control of the reproductive processes.

Mammalian sex is determined by the chromosomal makeup of the embryo. The male (XY) embryo produces a compound that causes development of the testes and the mesonephric (Wolffian) duct system that will become the epididymis and ductus deferens. The female (XX) embryo develops ovaries and the paramesonephric (Müllerian) duct system that will become the oviducts, uterus, cervix, and vagina. This tubular component of the genital system in each sex is responsible for the delivery of the respective gametes to the copulatory organs (penis and vagina). In addition, the tubular genitalia in the female provide the environment that allows for fertilization, gestation, and delivery of the offspring.

Beyond these generalities, many of the reproductive details vary significantly between species. A thorough understanding of these details is necessary before you can offer effective reproductive services for client animals.

General Endocrinology of Reproduction

An endocrine gland is one that produces a product, called a hormone, which is secreted directly into the blood rather than locally through a duct. The hormone is capable of interacting with target cells that may be quite some distance from the organ where the hormone was produced. The common reproductive hormones, along with their chemical composition, primary source, and major reproductive functions, are listed in Table 9.1. At its most basic, reproductive endocrinology is a feedback loop that is controlled by the brain through its regulation of the hypothalamic releasing factor, gonadotropin-releasing hormone (GnRH). GnRH is transported from the hypothalamus to the pituitary gland at the base of the brain through a specialized portal vascular system. Here it causes the release of the pituitary gonadotropins, luteinizing hormone (LH), and follicle-stimulating hormone (FSH). LH is responsible for stimulating the production of the gonadal steroid hormones, progesterone in the female, and testosterone in the male. FSH plays a critical role in development of the ovarian follicle in the female and spermatogenesis in the male, and is, therefore, the primary hormone responsible for regulating gamete production. The action of reproductive hormones on their target tissues listed in Table 9.1 is a critical control point for reproductive processes. Equally important is the complex interaction of the hormones themselves through feedback mechanisms, where one hormone will regulate the rate of production or secretion of other hormones. Knowledge of the hormonal actions and feedback mechanisms is essential to understanding disease, but also allows for recommending hormonal therapy to control reproductive activity or manage breeding programs.

TECHNICIAN TIP 9.2: Endocrine glands produce hormones that are secreted directly into the blood rather than through a duct.

TECHNICIAN TIP 9.3: Feedback mechanisms regulate the rate of production or secretion of other hormones.

The information in Table 9.1 shows most common hormones are also available as therapeutic agents. In addition, laboratory tests are available to measure almost all of these substances in blood, milk, or tissue. Measurement of these hormones can play a vital role in the diagnosis of reproductive disorders as well as the management of breeding programs.

TECHNICIAN TIP 9.4: Measuring hormone levels plays a vital role in the diagnosis of reproductive disorders and breeding program management.

Anatomy and Physiology of Reproduction in the Male

A schematic illustration of the bovine testis is shown in Figure 9.1. Figure 9.2 is a photograph of the excised bovine testis from approximately the same orientation as Figure 9.1. The paired testes of the male are located in the scrotum. The location of the testes outside the body wall provides a mechanism for cooling the testes that is essential for normal sperm production. In most domestic animals, the abdominal testicles descend into the scrotum prior to or shortly after birth. Table 9.2 provides an overview of male reproductive anatomy.

TECHNICIAN TIP 9.5: In most domestic animals, the abdominal testicles descend into the scrotum prior to or shortly after birth.

Table 9.1 Name, chemical composition, source, and action of the major reproductive hormones in male (M) and female (F) animals.

Hormone	Chemical composition	Source hypothalamus	Action
Gonadotropin-releasing hormone (GnRH)[a]	Small (deca) peptide		Stimulates FSH and LH release from the anterior pituitary
Follicle-stimulating hormone (FSH)[a]	Glycoprotein	Anterior pituitary	Follicle growth and estrogen production (F); spermiogenesis (M)
Luteinizing hormone (LH)[a]	Glycoprotein	Anterior pituitary	Follicular maturation, ovulation, luteinization, and progesterone production (F); testosterone production (M)
Estradiol (E_2)[a]	Steroid (estrogen)	Large ovarian follicles	Mating behavior, secondary sex characteristics, mammary growth (ductular) (F)
Progesterone (P_4)[a]	Steroid (progestin)	Ovarian corpus luteum	Maintenance of pregnancy, mammary growth (alveolar) (F)
Testosterone[a]	Steroid (androgen)	Interstitial (Leydig) cells of the testis	Mating behavior, spermatocytogenesis, accessory gland function, secondary sex characteristics (M)
Prostaglandin F2 alpha (PGF_2)[a]	Fatty acid	Endometrium of the uterus	Luteolysis, smooth muscle contraction (uterine, epididymal) (F)
Inhibin	Protein	Ovarian granulosa cells and testis sustentacular (Sertoli) cells	Block FSH release (M&F)
Oxytocin[a]	Small (nona) peptide	Neurohypophysis and corpus luteum	Smooth muscle contraction (uterine, mammary, F; epididymal, M)

[a] Hormone or its functional equivalent is commercially available for use in veterinary practice.

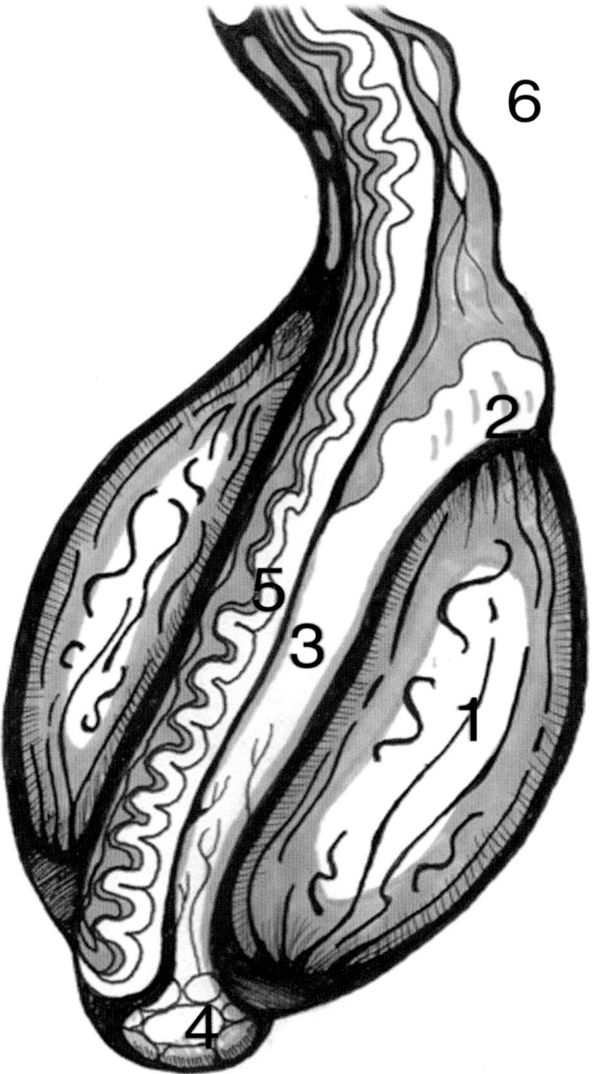

Figure 9.1 Caudomedial view of the right testes of a bull (schematic). Key: testis (1), head of the epididymis (2), body of the epididymis (3), tail of the epididymis (4), ductus deferens (5), spermatic cord (6).

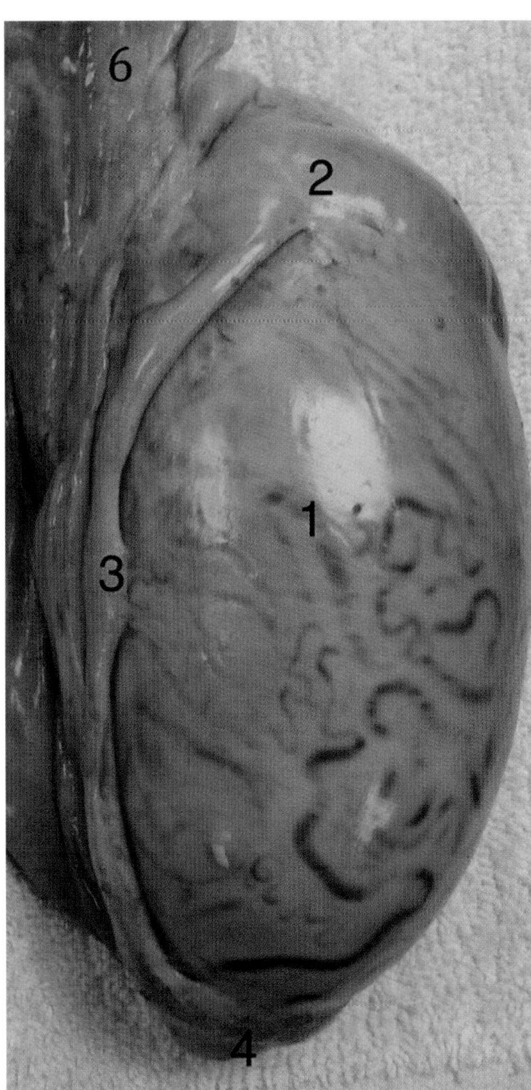

Figure 9.2 Caudal view of the right testes of a bull (photograph). The key is same as for Figure 9.1; however, the ductus deferens is obscured by the mesorchium in this photograph.

Sperm are produced in the convoluted germinal tubules that occupy most of the testes parenchyma. Unlike the situation in the female ovary, sperm production in the testes of domestic animals is not cyclical but rather goes on nearly continuously after puberty. Depending on the species, millions or even billions of sperm cells are produced every day. Sperm precursor cells (spermatogonia) line the convoluted tubule and undergo meiotic division to form the haploid sperm cells. The process of spermatogenesis is supported within the tubules by Sertoli cells that are also responsible for isolating the sperm cells from the immune system. Because sperm cells are first produced at puberty, they are recognized by the immune system as a foreign substance and will elicit an autoimmune reaction if this protective barrier breaks down.

> **TECHNICIAN TIP 9.6:** Sperm cells are first produced at puberty and would be recognized by the immune system as a foreign substance if not for the protective barrier of Sertoli cells.

Interstitial cells are found between the tubules in the testes. LH from the pituitary gland stimulates the interstitial cells to produce testosterone that is required for normal sperm production. As testosterone levels rise, they trigger a negative feedback mechanism that decreases the release of GnRH from the hypothalamus. Lower GnRH levels result in a decrease in the amount of LH released from the pituitary gland, thus lowering testosterone production from the

Table 9.2 Selected anatomical features of male animals.

Species	Timing of testicular descent	Penis type[a]	Accessory sex organs[b]	Specialized penile adaptation	Sigmoid flexure and frenulum
Bull	Fetal	FE	P, SV, BU	Counter-clockwise spiral of glans when erect	Yes
Boar	Fetal	FE	P, SV, BU	As for bull	Yes
Ram	Fetal	FE	P, SV, BU	Filiform urethral process extends beyond the end of the glans penis	Yes
Buck	Fetal	FE	P, SV, BU	As for ram	Yes
Alpaca	Fetal	FE	P, BU	Terminal cartilaginous process	Yes
Stallion	At or shortly after birth	MC	P, SV, BU	Urethral sinus	No

[a]FE = fibroelastic; MC = musculocavernous.
[b]P = prostate; SV = seminal vesicle; BU = bulbourethral gland.

interstitial cells. As the testosterone concentration in the blood subsequently declines, the suppression of GnRH release is ended, and the system returns to a stimulatory mode. In this way, testosterone is maintained at the level required for optimal production of sperm. The proximity of the interstitial cells and the germinal tubules in the testes allows for testosterone concentrations in the testes that are dramatically higher than those in the peripheral circulation. This is why treating male animals with testosterone generally leads to a paradoxical decrease in sperm production and atrophy of the testes. The exogenous testosterone maintains high concentrations in the peripheral circulation and effectively blocks GnRH and the pituitary release of LH, suppressing interstitial cell production of testosterone. The result is an inadequate level of testosterone within the testes.

After Sertoli cells release sperm, they are collected in a central channel that exits the testis and becomes the epididymal duct that flows through the head, body, and tail of the epididymis. Sperm undergo a further maturation process and become motile as they progress through the epididymis. The process of sperm production in the testes parenchyma can take 35–60 days depending on the species. Epididymal transport time is an additional 10–12 days.

> **TECHNICIAN TIP 9.7:** Sperm production in the testes parenchyma can take 35–60 days depending on the species.

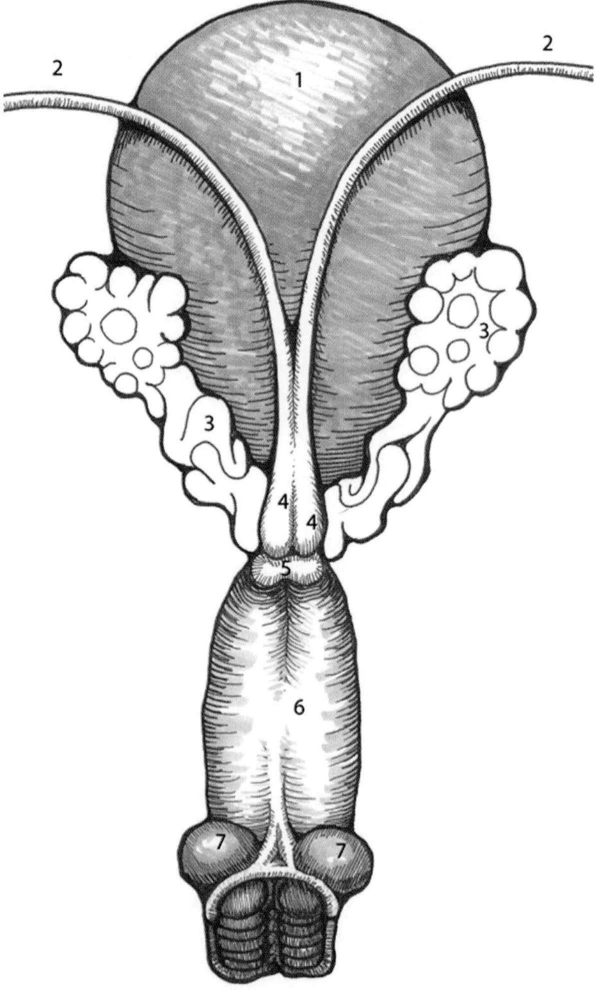

Figure 9.3 Dorsal view of the pelvic urogenital organs of the bull. The top of the image is cranial and bottom caudal. Key: bladder (1), ductus deferens (2), seminal vesicles (3), ampullae (4), prostate (5), urethralis and disseminated prostate (6), bulbourethral glands (7).

The epididymal duct becomes the ductus deferens as it exits the scrotum and enters the abdomen through the inguinal ring. These paired ducts enter the pelvic urethra at the colliculus seminalis. Pelvic accessory sex organs (see

Figure 9.3) secrete additional chemical and fluid components. The combination of sperm and accessory gland fluid forms the ejaculated semen that is deposited in the female reproductive tract.

The male copulatory organ is the penis. Ruminants, swine, and camelids have a fibroelastic penis with a sigmoid flexure. This type of penis has relatively more connective tissue than erectile tissue and as a consequence does not dramatically increase in size when erect. The elongation necessary for copulation comes primarily from extension of the sigmoid flexure. By contrast, horses have a musculocavernous penis that contains relatively more erectile tissue, which is responsible for the increase in size during sexual activity. The prepuce functions to protect the non-erect penis and to provide the excess tissue necessary for penile extension during erection.

TECHNICIAN TIP 9.8: Ruminants, swine, and camelids have a fibroelastic penis with a sigmoid flexure, whereas stallions have a musculocavernous penis with more erectile tissue.

Another feature of the fibroelastic penis is the presence of a penile frenulum that attaches the penis to the prepuce before the onset of puberty and prevents extrusion of the penis from the prepuce. This frenulum breaks down as testosterone levels rise near puberty. Failure of this process results in a persistent frenulum that requires surgical correction if normal mating is to occur.

Anatomy and Physiology of Reproduction in the Female

The paired ovaries are found within the abdominal cavity. Follicles and the corpus luteum are the functional elements of the ovary (see Figure 9.4). The follicles initially contain only a few cell layers surrounding the immature oocyte. After puberty, these primordial follicles grow in size in response to increasing levels of FSH and develop a fluid-filled antrum. As the follicle(s) continue to grow, they produce increasing amounts of estradiol and inhibin. The inhibin is responsible for suppressing FSH levels and limiting the number of ovulatory follicles to an appropriate level for each species. The increase in estradiol eventually results in a surge of LH that will cause ovulation and luteinization of the mature follicle(s). Thus, LH is responsible for both the release of mature ova that will be fertilized as well as the formation of the corpus luteum that will produce the progesterone that is needed to support the ensuing pregnancy. A corpus luteum forms at the site of each ovulation.

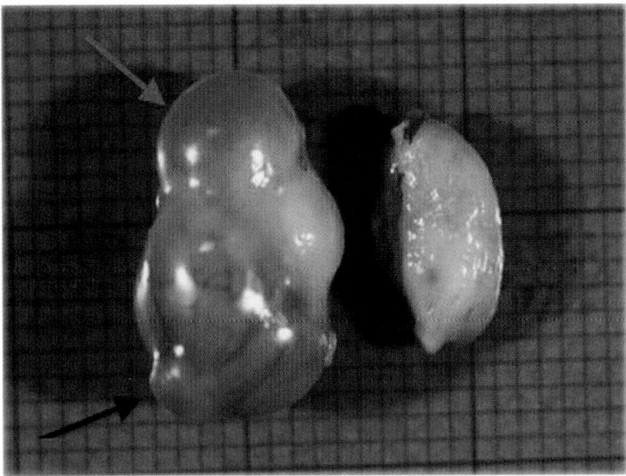

Figure 9.4 Excised bovine ovaries. The ovary on the left contains a 1.5 cm diameter follicle (red arrow) and a mature corpus luteum (black arrow). The ovary on the right contains no significant structures.

TECHNICIAN TIP 9.9: Inhibin is responsible for suppressing FSH levels and limiting the number of developing ovulatory follicles.

The oviducts (uterine tubes) are specially adapted tubules that gather the ova released from the ovary at the time of ovulation, provide the site for fertilization, and deliver the resulting embryo to the uterus. The uterus is composed of two distinct horns joined by a body of variable size (see Figure 9.5). The uterine body is separated from the vagina by the cervix. The cervix opens and relaxes during estrus to allow sperm to enter and again at parturition to allow for delivery of the fetus. At all other times, the cervix must be tightly closed to maintain a sterile uterine environment.

The vagina serves as the copulatory organ in the female. It is the site of semen deposition in ruminants. In horses, pigs, and camelids, the cervix or the uterus is the site of semen deposition. The most caudal aspect of the female tubular tract is the vestibule. The vestibule is formed by an invagination of the ectoderm in the embryo and must meet and fuse with the developing vagina. Failure of this fusion can lead to strictures, tissue bands, or even complete obstruction at the juncture of the vestibule and vagina.

TECHNICIAN TIP 9.10: The vagina is the site of semen deposition in ruminants whereas the cervix or the uterus is the site in horses, pigs, and camelids.

Reproductive activity in female animals is cyclical. The cycles of domestic animals are defined by their receptive or estrous behavior and are called estrous cycles. Some of the

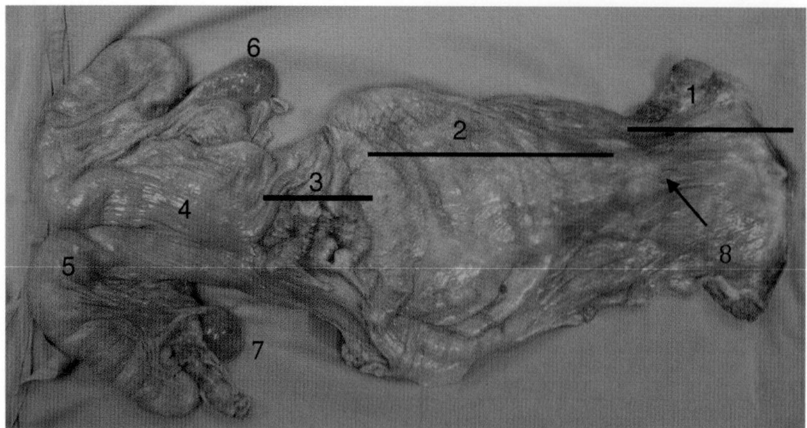

Figure 9.5 Dorsal view of the excised bovine reproductive tract. The dorsal aspect of the vestibule, vagina, and cervix has been opened to expose the lumen of these three areas. Note the complex interdigitating folds in the cervix. Key: vestibule (1), vagina (2), cervix (3), right uterine horn (4), left uterine horn (5), right ovary (6), left ovary (7), urethral opening into vestibule (8). For scale, the cervix (bar 3) is 9 cm in length.

important temporal features of the cycles of domestic animals can be found in Table 9.3.

Seasonal influences on reproduction are evolutionary adaptations that allow for the birth of young at a time of year that increases the likelihood of survival. The mare is an example of a seasonal species that begins to cycle in response to increasing day-length in the spring. Ewes and goat does begin to cycle in the late summer or fall in response to decreasing amounts of daylight.

TECHNICIAN TIP 9.11: Seasonal influences on reproduction are evolutionary adaptations allowing for the birth of young at a time of year that increases the likelihood of survival.

The estrous cycle is typically divided into functional components. Proestrus is the period of follicular development and increasing estrogen production leading up to estrus. Typically, females in proestrus begin to show interest in the male but will not allow mating. Estrus follows proestrus and is the period of sexual receptivity and maximum fertility. Growing follicles produce increasing levels of estrogen. An estrogen-induced surge in LH release from the pituitary coincides with the onset of estrus in ruminants and the sow. Diestrus is the luteal phase that follows estrus and ovulation. During diestrus, the corpus luteum matures and progesterone production increases to prepare the uterus for pregnancy. The female is not receptive to mating at this time. If conception occurs, a pregnancy-recognition signal is produced, and the life span of the corpus luteum is prolonged.

Most animals ovulate spontaneously during or shortly after estrus. A corpus luteum forms at the site of each ovulated follicle and diestrus begins even if the females were not bred. In these animals, as well as in those females that

Table 9.3 Estrus cycles of domestic animals.

Species	Age at puberty	Cycle type	Cycle length	Duration of estrus	Duration of diestrus (or luteal phase)
Cow	10–12 months	True polyestrous	21 days	18 hr	16 days
Sow (pig)	Four to nine months	True polyestrous	21 days	One to four days	16 days
Ewe (sheep)	Six to eight months	Seasonally polyestrous	16 days	36 hr	11 days
Doe (goat)	Five to seven months	Seasonally polyestrous	21 days	12–24 hr	16 days
Alpaca	12–18 months	Induced ovulator (non-seasonal)	Not applicable	Not applicable	10–12 days (Induced)
Mare	One to two years	Seasonally polyestrous	21 days	Five to seven days	14 days

are bred and fail to conceive, there is no pregnancy and the corpus luteum subsequently regresses allowing the female to recycle through another proestrus and estrus. Prostaglandin F2 alpha (PGF_2 alpha) is the luteolytic hormone that causes regression of the corpus luteum at the end of diestrus and pregnancy.

TECHNICIAN TIP 9.12: PGF_2 alpha is the luteolytic hormone that causes regression of the corpus luteum at the end of diestrus and pregnancy.

In contrast to spontaneous ovulating species, camelids (the alpaca, for example) are induced ovulators. In these animals, there is no GnRH-induced surge of LH unless mating occurs. In the alpaca, ovulation occurs in response to a chemical compound contained in the seminal fluid of the male alpaca.

TECHNICIAN TIP 9.13: Camelids are induced ovulators.

Pregnancy is maintained by continued production of progesterone from the ovarian corpus luteum, the placenta, or both. Progesterone causes endometrial gland proliferation and maintains the uterine musculature in a relaxed state. Some important features of pregnancy and parturition in domestic animals are summarized in Table 9.4. A complex interaction of maternal and fetoplacental hormones occurs at the end of pregnancy to signal fetal readiness for life outside the uterus. In response to elevated levels of fetal cortisol, progesterone levels decline, freeing the uterus from their inhibitory effects on contraction. During stage one of labor, increasing levels of estrogen and relaxing cause the cervix to relax and open while uterine contractions position the fetus for delivery. Finally, the fetus enters the vagina causing a reflex release of oxytocin from the pituitary gland resulting in powerful uterine and abdominal wall contractions that define the second stage of labor. In the normal animal, this process coincides with the presence of colostrum in the mammary glands and the onset of lactation. Second-stage labor ends with the birth of the fetus. The third stage of labor involves the passage of the placenta and the initial involution or repair of the uterus in preparation for the next pregnancy.

Clinical Examination of the Male and Female for Breeding Soundness

Every clinical examination begins with a thorough history. This should include the age and sex of the animal as well as its intended use. The method, timing, and outcome of previous mating attempts are critical pieces of information as well. A history of delivering live young and the ability to support them to weaning age is also vitally important. Once a complete history is obtained, the next step in the evaluation process is a general physical examination. As a general rule, only healthy, normal animals should be considered as candidates for breeding. The breeding soundness examination (BSE) is the final step in the evaluation process.

Breeding Soundness Examination of the Male (Male BSE)

Reproductive success of male animals requires three things:

- the desire to mate (libido)
- the physical ability to mate
- adequate semen quantity and quality for fertility

The male BSE focuses on the third component, the production of sufficient numbers of normal sperm for fertility. First, confirm the presence of two normal testes in the scrotum. Retention of one or both testes in the abdomen is called cryptorchidism. Retained testes cannot produce sperm but they do produce testosterone, so bilaterally cryptorchid animals usually have normal libido but they are sterile. Cryptorchid animals should not be used for breeding.

Table 9.4 Selected features of pregnancy and parturition in domestic animals.

Species	Gestation length	Progesterone source(s)	Placentation type	Duration of stage 2 labor
Cow	Nine months	Corpus luteum; placenta>150 days	Cotyledonary	1–2 hr
Sow (Pig)	114 days	Corpus luteum	Diffuse	2–12 hr
Ewe (Sheep)	150 days	Corpus luteum; placenta>50 days	Cotyledonary	½–2 hr
Doe (Goat)	150 days	Corpus luteum	Cotyledonary	½–2 hr
Alpaca	11 months	Corpus luteum	Diffuse microcotyledonary	½–1 h
Mare	11 months	Corpus luteum; placenta>90 days	Diffuse	½ h

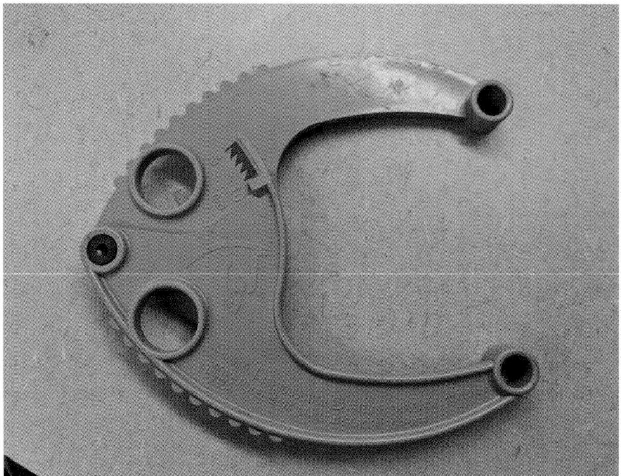

Figure 9.6 Equine Caliper Tool used to measure the circumference of a stallion's testicles.

In bulls and rams, testicular size is considered in the breeding soundness exam. The testicles are measured using a caliper or measure tape and then compared to breed standards. An animal can potentially fail a BSE based on scrotal size, before a sample is even collected. In horses, scrotal size is a consideration but may not result in BSE failure. Scrotal size is often cross referenced with age and then correlated with ejaculate volume and future breeding success rates.

The next step is the collection and assessment of a semen sample. Semen collection can be done in a variety of ways. The ideal collection system mimics the stimuli of a natural mating situation, in both a psychic and physical sense. This method generally requires a female in estrus and some degree of training for the sperm donor. Once trained, the male can often be collected without a female present. Typically, the semen sample is collected into an artificial vagina that mimics the temperature and physical sensation of natural mating. An equine artificial vagina is shown in Figures 9.7 and 9.8. Boars can be collected by a manual technique that requires only the exertion of pressure on the distal glans penis and a collection container for the ejaculate. For males that cannot be trained to provide a sample by these methods, electroejaculation is an option. The bull and ram are frequently collected by electroejaculation for clinical evaluation of semen quality. An example of the necessary equipment is shown in Figure 9.9. Electroejaculation in other species generally requires that the semen donor be anesthetized before attempting a collection. It is not recommended for the stallion.

> **TECHNICIAN TIP 9.14:** Bulls and rams are frequently collected by electroejaculation.

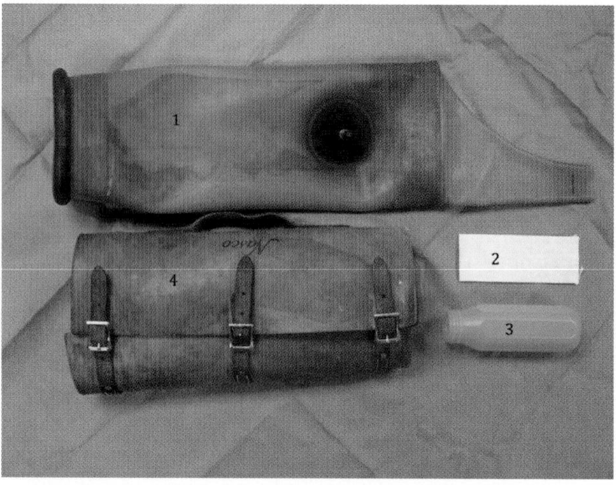

Figure 9.7 Missouri model equine artificial vagina (AV) for collection of semen from the stallion (unassembled). Key: double-walled latex AV (1), in-line filter to remove gel (2), semen receptacle (3), leather AV holder (4).

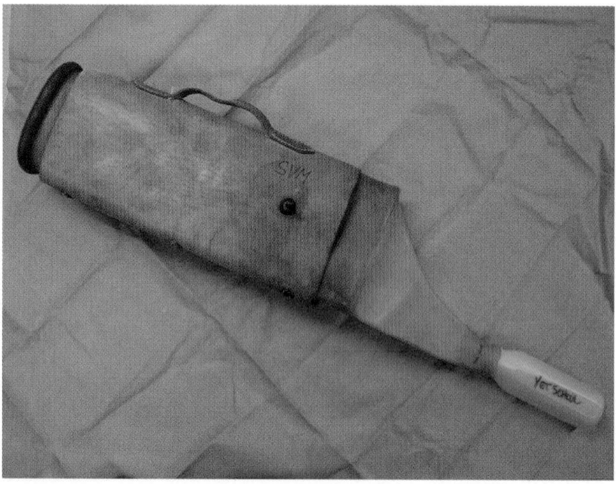

Figure 9.8 Missouri model equine artificial vagina (assembled).

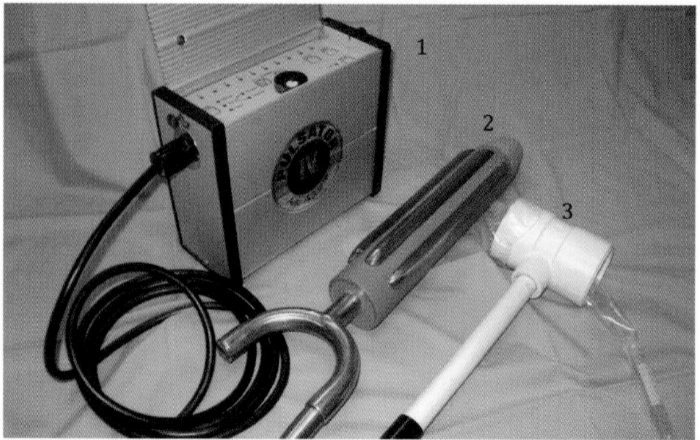

Figure 9.9 Electroejaculator for semen collection from the bull. Key: battery-operated power supply (1), intra-rectal probe (2), collection handle, cone, and tube (3).

A semen evaluation should be done every time semen is collected for insemination. It is an important part of the male BSE and should always be conducted as part of the investigation of suspected subfertility of a male. A stallion is used as our example for semen evaluation.

TECHNICIAN TIP 9.15: A semen evaluation should be done every time semen is collected for insemination.

After the semen is collected, care should be taken to avoid abrupt changes in temperature of the sample. First, slowly disconnect the semen receptacle from the artificial vagina as the gel may be delaying the entrance of semen into the receptacle. The gel portion of the ejaculate is separated from the sperm rich fraction either by an in-line filter inside the artificial vagina (recommended), or separated in the laboratory by filtration or by aspiration of the gel fraction with a syringe. Filtration is preferred as it also removes large debris and hair from the sample.

The color of the ejaculate should be inspected; normal color should be off-white to cream or light gray. Color changes may indicate problems; for example, pink to red indicates possible blood contamination while yellow indicates a possible urine contamination.

TECHNICIAN TIP 9.16: Ejaculate color should be off-white to cream or light gray. Other colors may indicate a problem.

The volume of the sample should be recorded, as it is important for the calculation of the total number of sperm per ejaculate. Volumes are highly variable but tend to be constant for an animal collected under the same conditions. If a collection results in a very low volume, it could be due to an incomplete ejaculation, while a very large volume may indicate excessive teasing, urine, or water contamination.

If the semen is going to be processed for artificial insemination (AI), a small subsample of raw semen should be taken for further analysis. The rest should be mixed with extender to at least a 1 : 1 dilution to maintain viability until the final dilution is calculated and the sample is processed. Semen should be gently but thoroughly mixed every time a subsample is taken for evaluation.

Sperm motility generally reflects the viability of a sperm population. Good motility does not necessarily mean good fertilizing capacity, but very low motility is indicative of a problem. Sperm motility is better assessed when the semen is diluted in semen extender at a 1 : 20 ratio. The sample should be allowed to equilibrate for a few minutes and all items should be kept at body temperature to obtain an accurate estimate. A small drop of extended semen is placed on a warm slide, taking care to avoid air bubbles when placing the cover slip. Total sperm motility (percentage of sperm that are moving) and progressive sperm motility (percentage of sperm that cross the field rapidly and in a relatively straight line) are estimated as an average of five fields at 200× magnification using a phase-contrast microscope. Motility of raw semen can be estimated, but it is mainly used in species other than the horse or as a baseline to test the possible detrimental effects of the extender on sperm motility. This visual assessment of sperm motility is not objective and, therefore, it is subjected to operator error and differences between operators. Computerized analysis of motility provides a more objective assessment of sperm motility and provides a series of motion characteristics, allowing a more in-depth analysis of the sample.

TECHNICIAN TIP 9.17: Sperm motility is best assessed when the semen is diluted with extender at a 1 : 20 ratio.

Sperm concentration could be determined by a direct method (counting spermatozoa under the microscope) or by indirect methods, of which the most common is spectrophotometry. For the direct method, a hemocytometer chamber is filled on both sides with a 1 : 100 semen: buffer dilution. After waiting a few minutes to allow the spermatozoa to settle, all 25 squares of the center area of the chamber should be counted to obtain the number of sperm cells per milliliter of ejaculate. Calculating the average of both sides of the chamber may decrease counting errors, and if the counts vary more than 10% between the sides, the entire process should be repeated. This methodology is fairly accurate and inexpensive, and allows for estimation of concentration in samples that are extended or contaminated with other cells, but it is time-consuming.

The most common indirect method for determining sperm concentration in a sample is spectrophotometry (Figure 9.10). The number of spermatozoa in the sample will affect its optical density and, therefore, it could be estimated based on comparison to a standard curve. A disadvantage of this method is that any other particles that affect optical density, such as other cells or debris, will affect the accuracy of the sperm count. By the same principle, samples that have been diluted in an opaque seminal extender cannot be counted by this method.

Several companies offer spectrophotometers that are pre-calibrated for a given species, making the determination of

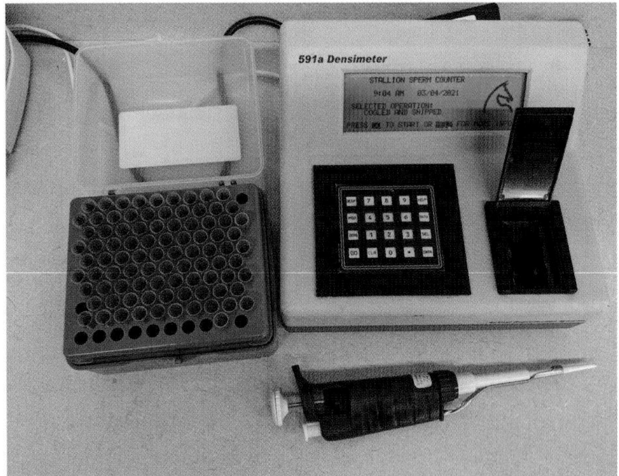

Figure 9.10 Spectrophotometer.

sperm concentration in raw semen quick and fairly accurate. In addition, some of these instruments have software that will calculate the dilution rate needed for further processing of the sample.

> **TECHNICIAN TIP 9.18:** Spectrophotometry is the most common indirect method of determining sperm concentration.

Newer instruments are entering the market every day. One such system uses a fluorescent dye to stain sperm nuclei and is more accurate than spectrophotometers. Some computer-assisted sperm analysis systems use a chamber with a known volume and therefore can estimate concentration based on the number of sperm it detects per field.

Once the concentration of the sample has been estimated, the total sperm number for the ejaculate should be calculated as the product of sperm concentration and semen volume. Total sperm number should be a function of testicular size and, therefore, is useful for estimating a stallion's fertility when the daily sperm output (DSO) is calculated. Mature stallions typically produce 4–12 billion sperm per ejaculate. Total sperm number for a given individual will be high when sexually rested and lower in winter than during the breeding season; age also affects DSO. In practice, two collections 1 h apart are used to partially deplete sperm reserves and provide an indicator of the sperm production capacity of the stallion. Determination of DSO usually requires semen collection once daily for 7–10 days; an average of the total sperm number of the last three collections is then used to estimate DSO.

Evaluation of sperm morphology consists of microscopically evaluating the shape and structure of fixed spermatozoa. As with motility, sperm morphology alone cannot be used to estimate fertilizing capacity of an ejaculate, but when a high proportion of spermatozoa present abnormalities, poor fertilizing capacity is expected. The two most common techniques are the use of an eosin-nigrosin stain followed by an evaluation under bright-field microscopy, and fixation in buffered formol-saline and evaluation of a wet mount slide with a phase-contrast or differential interference contrast microscope. A minimum of 100 spermatozoa should be evaluated at 1000×, preferably in each of two slides, and the average used to estimate the number of normal sperm and those presenting specific defects.

> **TECHNICIAN TIP 9.19:** An eosin-nigrosin stain with bright-field microscopy and buffered formol-saline fixation is used for evaluating morphology.

> **TECHNICIAN TIP 9.20:** At least 100 spermatozoa should be evaluated at 1000x to estimate the number of normal sperm and those showing specific defects.

To prepare a sample with eosin-nigrosin, roughly equal-sized droplets of stain and semen should be made on one end of a pre-warmed glass slide. After mixing the drops, a second glass slide is used to smear the sample (similar to the preparation of a slide for blood cytology). Nigrosin provides a dark background allowing the visualization and classification of the light spermatozoa. In addition, eosin does not penetrate cells with intact membranes; therefore, white sperm have intact membranes and are considered live, and those stained pink are considered dead. The percentage of morphologically normal spermatozoa should be recorded as well as the abnormalities found. There are different notation and classification systems for the abnormal spermatozoa; some record each abnormality in a chart, others will group the abnormalities as primary or secondary depending on the position and severity of the defect. Examples of several sperm abnormalities are shown in Figures 9.9–9.11.

Cytologic evaluation of the semen sample is useful to determine the presence of cells other than spermatozoa in the ejaculate. Round germ cells, white blood cells, red blood cells, epithelial cells, bacteria, and so forth are easier to observe in a smear of semen stained with Romanowsky stain than in the eosin-nigrosine preparation. In addition, some of the defects found in the morphological evaluation could be confirmed, thus ruling out abnormalities induced by problems with the eosin-nigrosin technique.

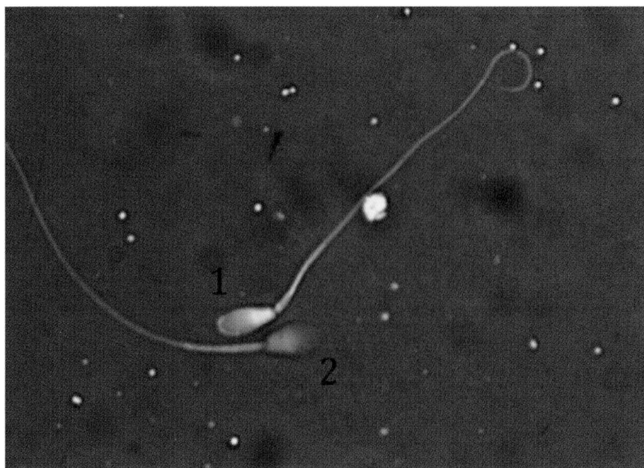

Figure 9.11 Eosin-nigrosin stained stallion semen. Key: normal live cell (1), normal dead cell (2). note the uptake of pink (eosin) stain by the dead sperm.

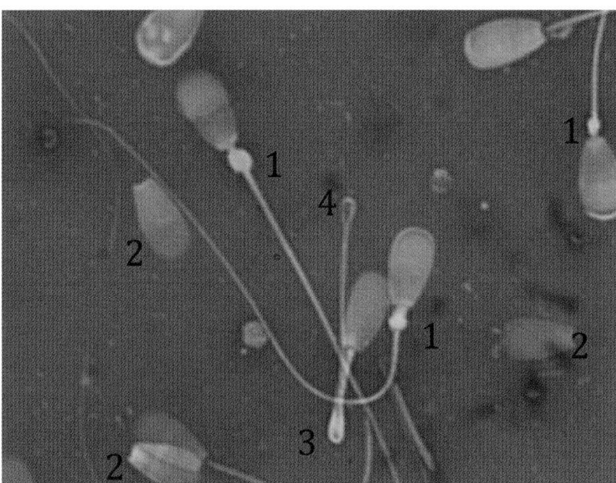

Figure 9.12 Eosin-nigrosin stained bull semen. Key: proximal droplet (1), detached head (2), distal droplet with bent midpiece (3), bent tail (4).

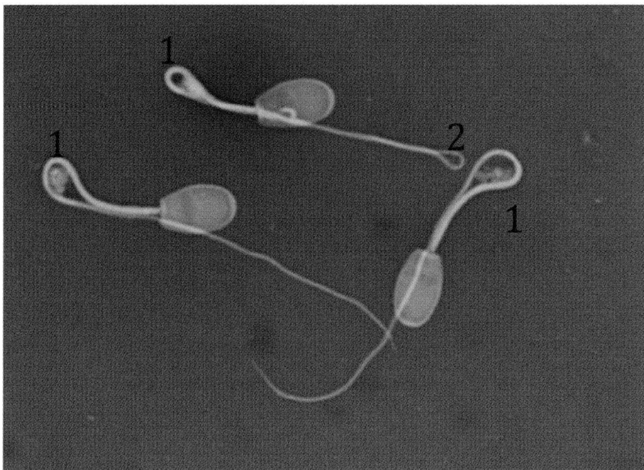

Figure 9.13 Eosin-nigrosin stained ram semen. Key: distal droplet with bent midpiece (1), bent tail (2).

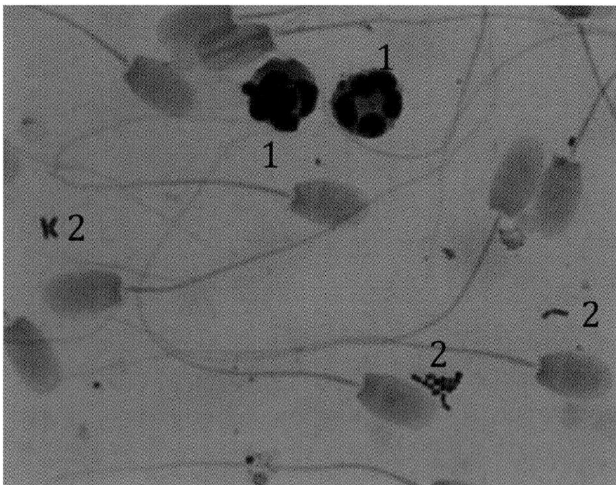

Figure 9.14 Romanowsky stained ram semen. Key: white blood cell (1), bacteria (2). Note the many faintly stained normal sperm cells.

TECHNICIAN TIP 9.21: A Romanowsky stain should be used to evaluate the presence of other cells in ejaculate.

Using the information from the history, physical examination, and the BSE, a decision is made regarding the potential suitability of the male animal as a sire. This evaluation is only a predictor of the male's potential fertility. The only true test of fertility is the ability to produce viable offspring.

Female BSE

Using a cow as an example for a female BSE, a complete history and general physical examination is completed. The genital examination of the cow begins with a careful visual inspection of the udder and perineum. The vulva should be nearly vertical and located mostly ventral to the floor of the pelvis. Tilting and dorso-cranial displacement of the vulva predispose the cow (or horse) to vaginal contamination with air or feces. That can affect fertility as well as potentially cause ascending placentitis during pregnancy. The next step is to manually palpate the tubular tract and ovaries through the rectal wall to check for abnormalities of size, symmetry, and consistency. The presence of functional ovarian structures (follicles and corpus luteum) can be assessed by palpation, but transrectal ultrasonography provides a more accurate diagnosis. The pregnancy status of the cow is also determined at this time. If the cow is not pregnant, a more complete and invasive examination can be conducted. This may include vaginoscopy and transcervical sampling for endometrial cytology, culture, or biopsy.

TECHNICIAN TIP 9.22: Tilting and dorso-cranial displacement of the vulva predispose the horse/cow to vaginal contamination with air or feces (Figure 9.15).

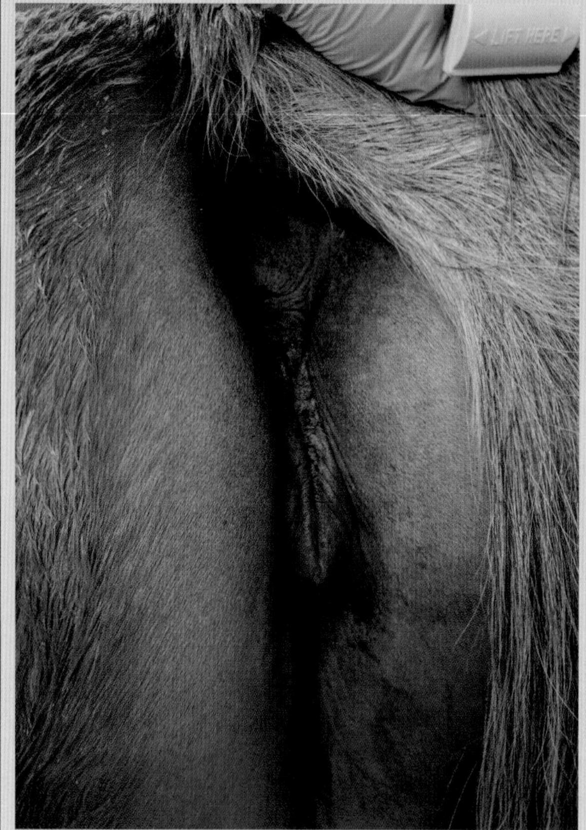

Figure 9.15 Tilting and dorso-cranial displacement of the vulva in a mare.

The approach to the female BSE is similar in the mare, but palpation per rectum is not possible in small ruminants and is seldom done in pigs. Camelids may be palpated if the examiner's hand is not too large, but many prefer to use a rigid extension for the ultrasound probe that allows the uterus and ovaries to be examined without inserting the operator's arm into the rectum (Figure 9.16).

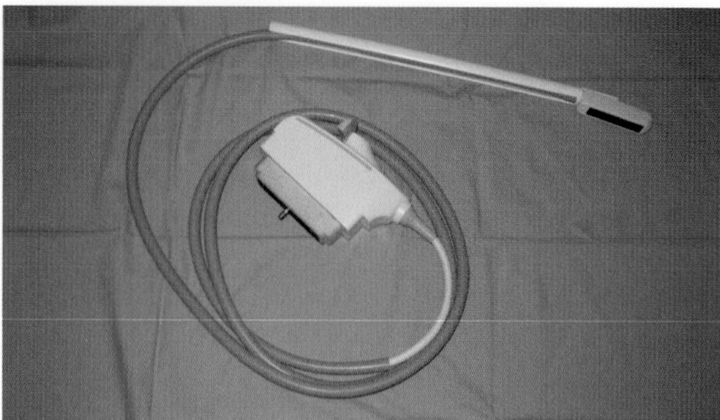

Figure 9.16 A linear array, transrectal ultrasound probe fitted with a rigid extension for use in alpacas and miniature mares. During use, the probe is taped securely to the extension, being careful not to cover the transmitting surface.

Reproductive Disorders

The topic of reproductive diseases is vast and complex. This chapter is limited to a general overview of the topic. The immense number of potential diseases and causative agents requires the veterinary professional to organize the approach to disease investigations. A thorough history and physical examination is essential. For herd or flock problems, an understanding of epidemiology is required. Veterinary technicians should be prepared to obtain appropriate samples for submission to a diagnostic laboratory. Laboratory personnel are often the best resource for information about local diseases of concern, as well as the specific samples needed and the best way to preserve and transport them.

Classification of reproductive disease can be used to help arrive at a specific diagnosis needed to formulate treatment and prevention plans. Veterinarians often divide diseases into infectious and noninfectious categories. Venereal disease is a class of infectious diseases of particular concern when looking at problems with reproduction. These are diseases that are spread primarily by sexual contact. Some examples are bovine trichomoniasis and contagious equine metritis. Other disease classification systems focus on the type of disease (e.g. the DAMNIT system), the timing of the disease in the reproductive process, or the localization of the disease within the genital tract. By combining a systematic evaluation of the individual animals affected by the disease with an epidemiological assessment of the problem, veterinarians can use various disease classification systems, along with their own clinical expertise, to arrive at a list of potential diagnoses. This process will allow preliminary treatment and preventative measures while waiting for laboratory confirmation of the diagnosis.

TECHNICIAN TIP 9.23: Venereal disease is a class of infectious diseases of particular concern with reproduction problems.

Reproductive Management

Humans choose to manage reproduction in animal populations for a variety of reasons. One is to control the number and types of mating for each animal involved on the assumption of improving the quality of the resulting offspring. This is primarily a genetic selection motivation. The validity of this notion is evidenced by the incredible advances in milk production that have occurred since the adoption of AI in the dairy industry. Producers have used this same basic approach to improve carcass quality in beef cattle and fiber quality in sheep and alpacas.

Fertility is defined as the ability to produce offspring. A sow that produces one piglet in the course of her lifetime is, by definition, fertile. It is obvious that producers require more than fertility in animals used for breeding. *Fecundity* is defined as the ability to rapidly and efficiently reproduce. This level of reproductive efficiency should be the goal when selecting animals for breeding programs.

Natural Service

Natural service, or mating, is the term for those systems where the male is allowed to physically mate with individual female animals. Most beef cattle, sheep, and goats are bred by this method. In pasture mating situations, commonly used for beef cattle and sheep, the males are turned out with the females and pretty much left to their own devices. A male BSE is recommended for all animals used in this system. Consideration must also be given to the number of males needed to efficiently breed the herd or flock of female animals.

> **TECHNICIAN TIP 9.24:** Natural service, or mating, is allowing the male to physically mate with individual female animals.

For horses and alpacas, farm managers often control access of the males to the females. In many instances, both the male and female will be haltered and on lead ropes. This is referred to as *hand-mating*. This method provides an additional level of safety for the animals involved and assures that mating actually occurs. Camelids, such as llamas and alpacas, breed in a kush position where the male mounts and sits behind the female (Figure 9.17). A female is considered receptive when she drops to the ground for breeding.

> **TECHNICIAN TIP 9.25:** For horses and alpacas, farm managers often control access of the males to the females and use hand-mating.

> **TECHNICIAN TIP 9.26:** Hand breeding stallions is safest when wearing head protection to prevent head injuries.

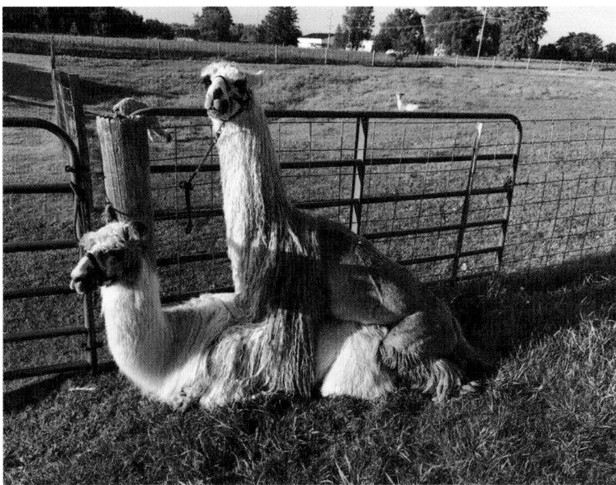

Figure 9.17 Llama breeding occurs in a kush position.

Advanced Reproductive Technology

Many of the advanced reproductive technologies in use today were first developed in domestic animals. AI was first used extensively for cattle breeding. The first successfully cloned animal was a sheep named Dolly.

Artificial Insemination

AI is a common alternative to natural mating. Most dairy cattle and pigs are bred using AI. AI may be done using fresh, chilled, or frozen semen. Semen to be held more than a few minutes after collection should always be extended with a solution that buffers, nourishes, and stabilizes the sperm. Semen that is to be frozen requires the addition of a specific cryoprotectant agent that allows the sperm to survive the freezing and thawing process.

Assuming that both the male and female are normal, fertile animals, and that the semen is carefully collected and processed, the most critical remaining elements of AI are the timing of the insemination and the deposition of semen at the correct site. Generally, the best fertility is obtained if the semen is deposited in the uterus within 12–24 hr prior to ovulation.

Proper timing of AI relies on accurate detection of estrus in the female to be bred. Timing of AI in the mare is complicated by the relatively lengthy estrus and the fact that mares ovulate one to two days before the end of estrus. The technique for intrauterine deposition of semen varies with species and ranges from relatively easy (mare and sow), to moderately difficult (cow and alpaca), to very difficult (ewe and doe).

While most breed registries readily recognize offspring produced by AI, this is not universally true. Thoroughbred horses to be used for racing can only be produced by natural mating, as the Jockey Club does not allow registration of foals produced by AI. At present, the principal alpaca registry in North America also does not allow AI. Furthermore, collection of camelid semen for shipment is fairly difficult and unpracticed due to the registry limitations. It is important that veterinary technicians be aware of any restrictions or additional requirements that might be attached to the use of reproductive technologies such as AI before breeding a client's animals.

> **TECHNICIAN TIP 9.27:** Most, but not all, breed registries recognize offspring produced by AI.

Embryo Transfer

Embryo transfer (ET) can be used to produce offspring in most large animal species. ET is significantly more expensive than AI and is usually reserved for propagating very valuable animals. In cattle, the donor cows are usually treated with FSH before breeding in order to increase the number of ovulated follicles. This is referred to as *superovulation*. The donor cow is bred at estrus and the embryos are flushed from the uterus seven days later. The recovered embryos are either transferred immediately to synchronized recipients or frozen for future transfer. ET is commonly done in horses as well, but the donor mare is not super-ovulated, and the embryos are generally transferred immediately and not frozen. ET is less commonly done in small ruminants and alpacas, and rarely used for swine reproduction.

> **TECHNICIAN TIP 9.28:** ET is significantly more expensive than AI and is usually reserved for propagating very valuable animals.

In Vitro Fertilization

In vitro fertilization (IVF) requires the collection of unfertilized ova from the female, either surgically or by ultrasound-guided follicular aspiration. The ova are then mixed with sperm in the laboratory, incubated, and the resulting embryos transferred to recipient animals. While significantly more costly than ET, this procedure is commonly used for reproducing very valuable cattle. It can be used to produce calves from cows that cannot conceive but are still producing viable ova.

> **TECHNICIAN TIP 9.29:** *in vitro* fertilization (IVF) requires collection of unfertilized ova from the female, either surgically or by ultrasound-guided follicular aspiration.

Pregnancy Diagnosis

The diagnosis of pregnancy is a critical aspect of breeding management. The primary reason for pregnancy examination is to identify animals that have failed to conceive and target them for re-insemination. Pregnancy diagnostic methods can be classified as indirect or direct. Indirect methods do not rely on the detection of a positive sign of pregnancy but rather are based on detection of signs consistent with the non-pregnant state. This is usually some aspect of the return to estrus after an unsuccessful breeding. Direct methods rely on the detection of a physical or laboratory finding that confirms the presence of an embryo or fetus. Direct methods are generally more reliable than indirect tests but may be more costly and often require more time to pass after breeding before they can be used.

> **TECHNICIAN TIP 9.30:** Pregnancy diagnostic methods can be classified as direct or indirect.

The classic indirect method is to carefully monitor for estrus approximately one estrus cycle after mating occurs. Animals that return to estrus are assumed to be "open" (not pregnant). Animals that do not return to estrus are assumed to be pregnant. Measuring progesterone in milk or serum at this same time is another indirect method for pregnancy diagnosis. For example, cows that have a high level of progesterone 21 days after breeding are assumed to be pregnant, while those with low progesterone are probably returning to estrus and are not pregnant.

Most veterinary clinics prefer to use direct methods for pregnancy diagnosis. These include palpation per rectum, ultrasonography, and laboratory assay of pregnancy-specific substances. The method and timing of pregnancy diagnosis in common large animal species is summarized in Table 9.5.

> **TECHNICIAN TIP 9.31:** Most veterinary clinics prefer to use direct methods for pregnancy diagnosis.

Bovine Pregnancy and Parturition

The final element of reproductive management is to assure the safe delivery of live young at the end of gestation. Eutocia, or normal birth, requires the presence of an appropriately sized fetus, a normal maternal pelvis, expulsive capability, and normal fetal presentation in the birth canal. Parturition is usually divided into three stages. First-stage labor begins with uterine contractions that position the fetus(es) for delivery and is complete when the cervix is dilated and the fetus enters the vagina. It generally lasts

Table 9.5 Timing and methodology of direct methods for pregnancy diagnosis in cattle, horses, and alpacas.

Species	Transrectal palpation	Transrectal ultrasound	Laboratory assay (blood sample)
Cow	After 35 days	After 25 days	Pregnancy associated glycoprotein assay after 29 days
Alpaca	Not applicable	After 20 days	Progesterone assay after 17 days
Mare	After 30 days	After 12 days	Equine chorionic gonadotropin assay after 45 days

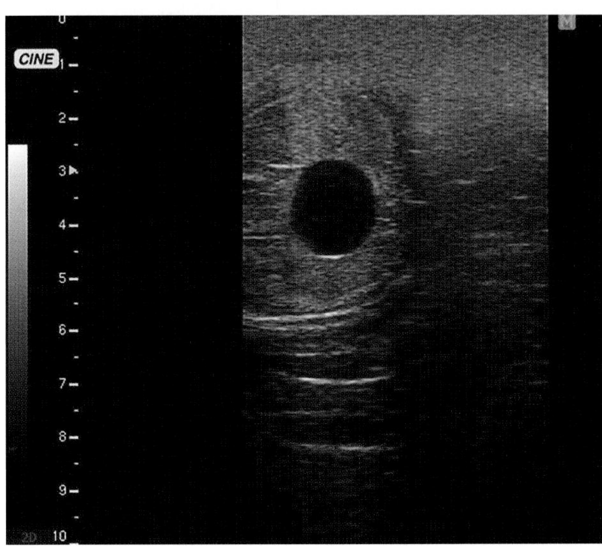

Figure 9.18 Ultrasound showing a 14-day-old equine embryo.

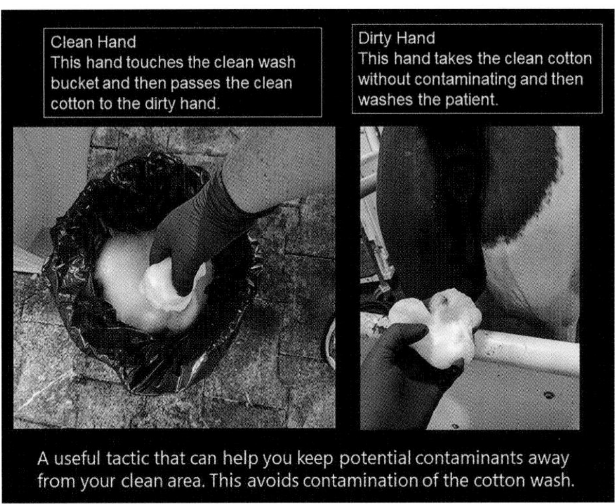

Figure 9.19 Clean hand, dirty hand technique.

2–6 hr but can be longer and more apparent in younger dams. Animals in first-stage labor will isolate themselves from the herd or group, they may appear restless and show signs of abdominal discomfort. In older dams, external signs of first-stage labor are often more subtle. The presence of fetal parts in the vagina induces the abdominal press and the onset of second-stage labor. This stage is characterized by the release of allantoic fluid and the onset of forceful abdominal straining. Second-stage labor typically lasts less than 4 hr in cattle but can be much longer in litter bearing species. The second stage in equines is much more time sensitive and should result in expulsion in 20–30 min. Third-stage labor is the detachment and expulsion of the placenta and the initiation of uterine involution. The time of the third stage can vary, ruminants can complete this stage in as little as 20 min or as long as 12 hr.

> **TECHNICIAN TIP 9.32:** External signs of first-stage labor are often more subtle in older dams.

A clean, dry delivery area is essential. It should have good footing to minimize the chances of injury to the dam. Adequate dimensions will reduce the likelihood of the dam pushing the fetus against a wall and also provides room to assist the delivery if that becomes necessary.

> **TECHNICIAN TIP 9.33:** A clean, dry area with good footing and adequate dimensions is crucial for a successful delivery.

Dystocia, or difficult birth, is any condition where the delivery of the fetus is significantly delayed or would be impossible without assistance. Of the common domestic animals, dystocia occurs most frequently in cattle, especially dairy cattle. This discussion will use the cow as an example for obstetrical procedures, with other species-specific information later in the chapter.

Fetal-maternal disproportion is the most common cause of dystocia in cattle. The relative mismatch in fetal and maternal size can be influenced by age of the dam, nutrition, fetal sex, and genetics. Dystocia is more common in heifers delivering their first calf than in older cattle. Either nutritional extreme can lead to dystocia by limiting the size of the heifer in cases of starvation or by increasing the size of the fetus and the amount of pelvic fat deposition in cows that are fed excessively. Bull calves are generally larger than heifer calves and more prone to causing dystocia.

TECHNICIAN TIP 9.34: Fetal-maternal disproportion is the most common cause of dystocia in cattle.

Other types of dystocia are classified as having either a maternal or fetal cause. Examples of dystocias due to maternal causes include immature heifers, uterine inertia, deficient abdominal press, failure of the cervix to dilate, pelvic abnormalities, uterine torsion, and hydrallantois. Fetal causes include errors in positioning for birth; fetal anomalies or fetal monsters; hydramnios; prolonged gestation; twins; and IVF or embryo culture.

Criteria for intervention in a calving include first-stage labor lasting more than 6 hr; second-stage labor lasting more than 2–3 hr; excessive hemorrhage; abnormal odor or appearance of the calf or fetal membranes; and excessive straining for more than 30 min with no visible progress. Diagnosis of dystocia is based on the history and physical examination. The history should include the number and outcome of previous calvings, breeding dates, and any efforts that have been made to relieve this dystocia. Palpation per rectum is performed to assess cervical dilation and fetal viability, although these functions are usually more accurately assessed during the vaginal examination. The diagnosis of a uterine torsion is most readily made during the rectal examination. After the perineum is cleaned, a manual vaginal examination is done to confirm cervical dilation, to assess fetal viability, and to diagnose problems with fetal positioning or anomalies. The vagina, cervix, and uterus should also be carefully examined at this time for evidence of preexisting trauma. Care should be taken to use adequate lubrication and to be as clean as possible during the obstetrical procedure. If necessary, straining can be controlled by use of epidural anesthesia.

Assisted vaginal delivery of the fetus is the first choice of most veterinary clinicians. In most cases, a calf may be delivered vaginally if its shoulders or hips can fit within the pelvis of the dam, as these represent the largest parts of the calf. This reasoning forms the basis for the Utrecht guidelines for forced extraction. To apply the guidelines, the calf must first be correctly oriented. This may require rotating the calf or extending a flexed neck or limb. Once this is accomplished, obstetrical chains are place around the pastern with an assistant pulling on each chain. Ideally, the test is done with the cow in lateral recumbency, but it can be accomplished with the cow standing, provided the assistants have the strength to raise the calf out of the cow's abdomen. In anterior presentation, the calf can usually be delivered vaginally if the fetlocks can be extracted about 10 cm beyond the vulvar opening. In posterior presentation, the hips of the calf can be assumed to have entered the maternal pelvis if the hocks of the calf are presented at the

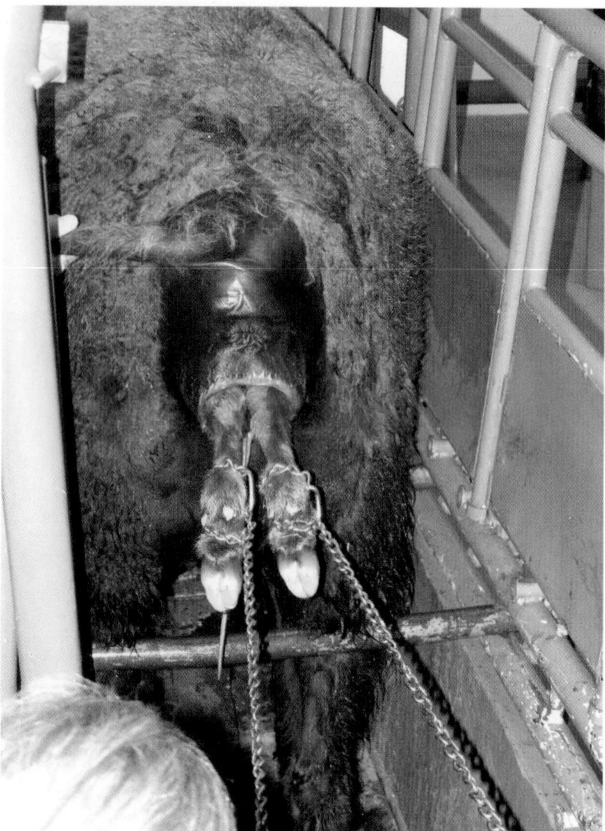

Figure 9.20 Assisted vaginal delivery of a Bison dystocia using repositioning technique and chains to assist the delivery.

vulva. Because the biggest fixed dimension of the calf is the distance from one greater trochanter of the femur to the other, the calf should always be rotated 90° prior to pulling its hips into the maternal pelvis to avoid locking the hips of the calf in the pelvis of the cow. The calf may now be safely extracted without undue risk of injury to the calf or cow.

TECHNICIAN TIP 9.35: Excessive straining for more than 30 min with no visible progress should be reported to a veterinarian immediately.

TECHNICIAN TIP 9.36: Fetotomy should be reserved for situations in which the fetus is dead.

If vaginal delivery is not possible, a fetotomy or cesarean section should be considered. Fetotomy should usually be reserved for situations in which the fetus is dead. It is also imperative that there be adequate room and lubrication to safely perform the procedure. A fetotome is used for this procedure. Complete fetotomies are extremely laborious and should only be attempted with proper equipment and skilled assistance. Cesarean section is the method of choice

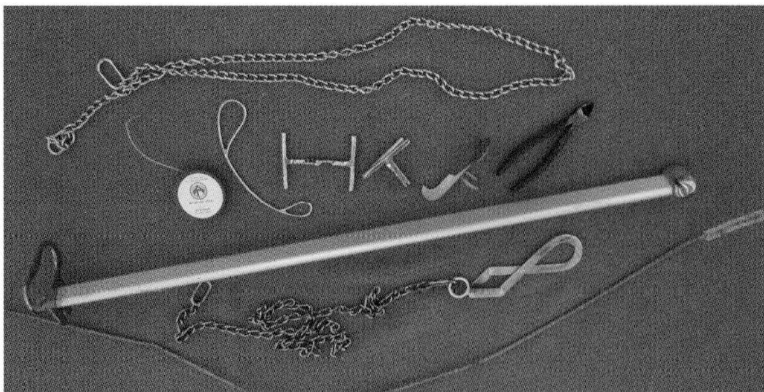

Figure 9.21 Large animal fetotomy equipment.

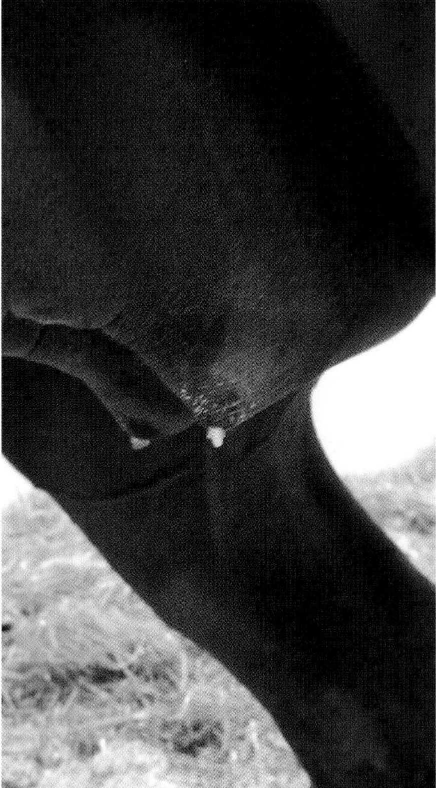

Figure 9.22 Mammary development and waxing in a mare.

for delivery of a live calf when vaginal delivery is not possible.

Equine Parturition

Equine first stage of labor is similar to that described of bovines; they can be quite variable depending on whether they are a seasoned broodmare or maiden. In the days prior to parturition, a mare may show similar physical symptoms such as mammary development, relaxation of the vulva and pelvic ligaments around the tailhead, and the development of died secretions on the tip of her teats known as wax or waxing.

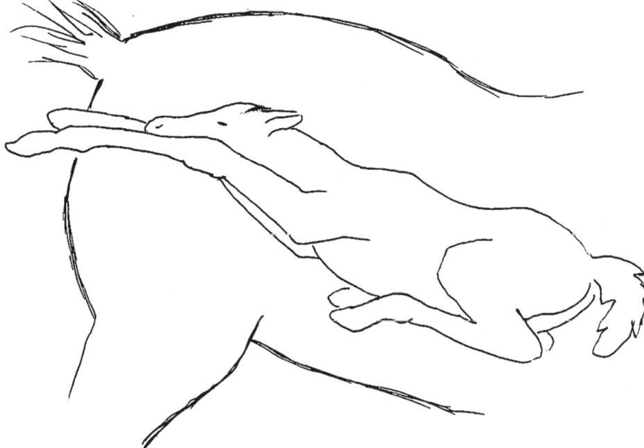

Figure 9.23 Normal presentation for most large animal species.

In horses it can last anywhere from 30 min to 6 hr. However, second stage of equine labor should normally last in 15–30 min. The mare is most often in a lateral recumbency with all four legs extended. Normal presentation should include front limbs extended forward and facing downward with head and neck following facing forward (Figure 9.23). One of the foals' feet may be slightly ahead of the other (15–20 cm). Some mares will push the fetus out partway, to the point of the pelvis, take a break for a minute or two, and then finish.

The foal is normally born covered in the fetal membranes and umbilical cord still intact. This is normal and intervention is not generally needed. While the cord is still intact, the foal has an oxygen supply. One may gently open the sac around the foal's face and clear the membranes and mucous, as long as it is not disturbing to the mare in any way. A mare's temperament may change with foaling, a once quiet and gentle mare may suddenly become aggressive toward people, always be prepared for the unexpected. Some mares will remain down in a dorsal or lateral position for 10–15 min after delivery; this is normal and she should not be rushed to stand, even if the foal is moving about. This is a critical time for instinctive bonding and imprinting. A mare will lick her foal, which both stimulates the foal's breathing and activity and contributes to their bonding.

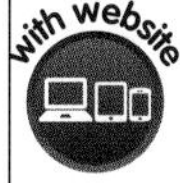

Website check out our online resource for step by step pictures of foaling.

Foaling 1, 2, 3

1. The foal should stand within one hour of delivery.
2. Nurse within two hours.
3. Placenta should pass within three hours.

Figure 9.24 Proper foaling sequence.

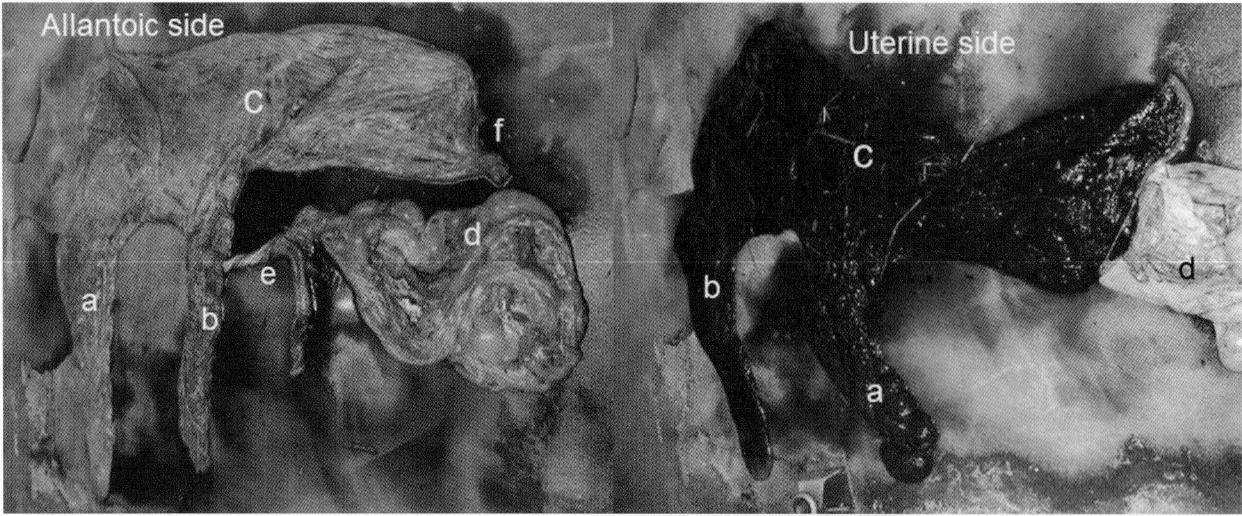

Figure 9.25 "F" configuration of an equine placenta. The allantoic side which faces the foal and chorion side which is attached to the lining of the uterus. a. pregnant horn b. non-pregnant horn c. body d. fetal membranes e. umbilical vessels f. cervical star.

The third stage of labor should occur within 3 hr of delivery. Failure to pass the fetal membranes within that time frame generally requires intervention. It is a good recommendation to examine the fetal membranes after delivery. Examining the fetal membranes can help warn of potential problems with the foal including sign of sepsis before clinical presentation. They should be the mirror image of the mare's uterus body and horns. Many times in the delivery process, the placenta may be inverted. The surface of both sides should be examined (Figure 9.25). The allantoic side, which is smooth, shiny, and pale, is closer to the foal and can tear normally in delivery. The chorion side which has a velvety soft villus surface that attaches to the uterine lining should be fully intact. The umbilical cord should have a few twists. The hippomanes is an 8–10 cm olive to pale brown, liver-like textured, oval disk which is a collection of allantoic cellular debris (Figure 9.26).

Signs of abnormality in the fetal membranes may include excessive twists/torsion of the cord, endometrial cysts in the chorion, placental edema, hemorrhage, bruising, meconium staining, or signs of placentitis (Figure 9.27).

TECHNICIAN TIP 9.37: Equine fetal membranes should weigh approximately 11% of the foal's BW at birth.

Placentitis

Placentitis, or inflammation of the placenta, occurs in less than 10% of equine pregnancies. Of those affected, the majority are a result of bacteria entering the vagina and

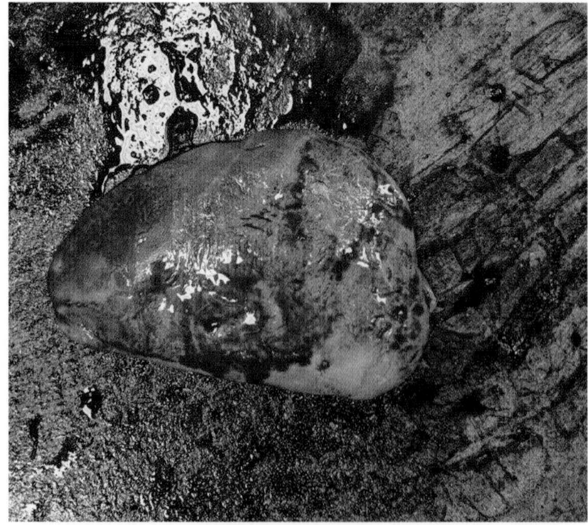

Figure 9.26 A hippomane.

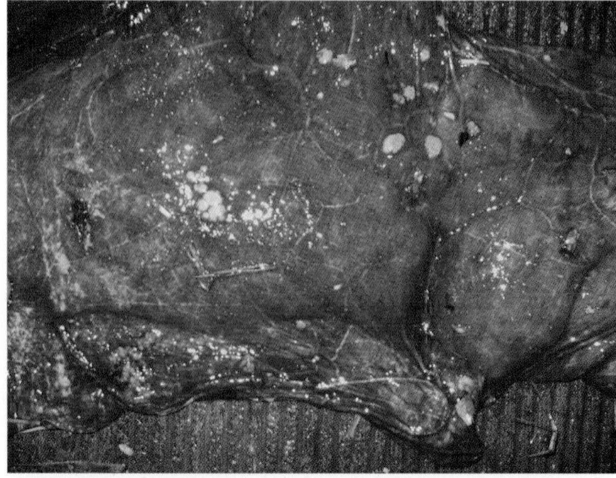

Figure 9.27 Example of abnormal placental surface, seen by the lighter colored lesions.

traveling up the reproduction tract, also known as an ascending cervical infection. Fescue toxicity as well as other fungal or viral infections, such as Equine Herpes Virus, may also initiate placentitis. It can go unnoticed, sometimes the entire pregnancy, but foals born from this will likely decline rapidly after delivery.

Signs of placentitis:

- vaginal or vulvar discharge
- thickened fetal membranes
- thickened placenta
- premature separation of the placenta
- abortion
- premature udder development or lactation
- lesions found on the placenta during evaluation

If caught prior to parturition, broad-spectrum antibiotics and anti-inflammatories can be used for bacterial placentitis. Post-parturition, a uterine culture should be performed to determine the best treatment plan.

TECHNICIAN TIP 9.38: Any vulvar discharge in the pregnant mare should be addressed in a timely manner.

TECHNICIAN TIP 9.39: With placentitis, the foal often deteriorates quickly after birth.

Equine Dystocias

Equine dystocias can occur for a wide variety of reasons including improper presentation, fetal-maternal disproportion, uterine inertia, premature placental separation, prepubic ligament tears/ruptures or uterine torsion. These are true emergencies, and time is of the essence. Failure to act quickly can result in losing the foal and possibly the mare as well.

Improper fetal position may be identified as the fetus begins to emerge through the vaginal canal or from a lack of progression during the second stage of labor (Figure 9.28).

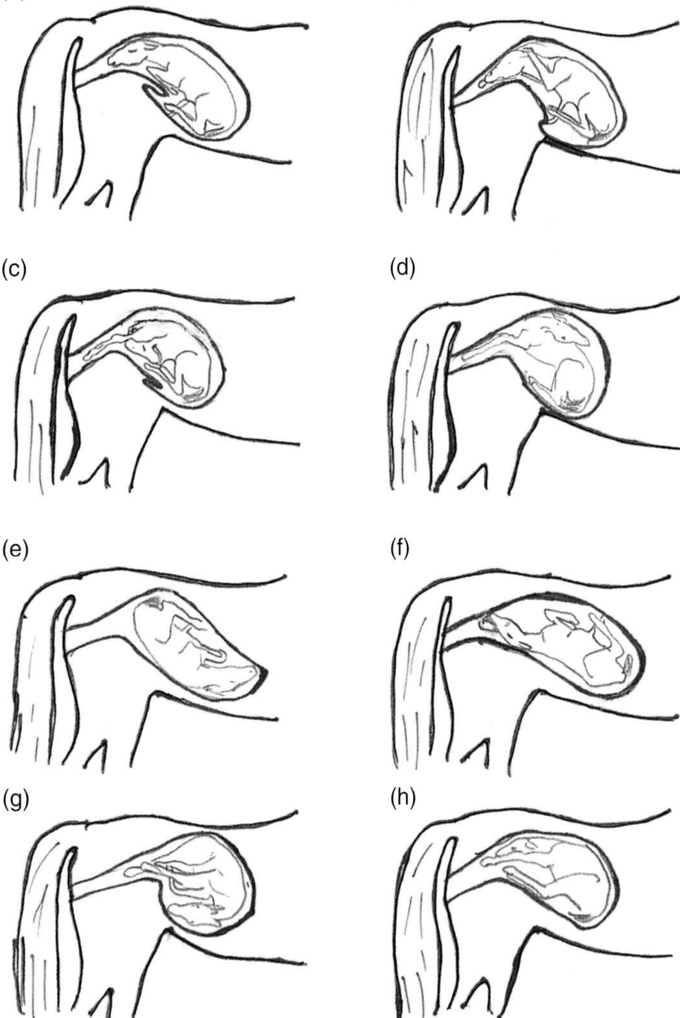

Figure 9.28 Example of improper fetal presentations; (a) carpal flex (b) foot nape (c) ventral retroflexion (d) cranial presentation, upward deviation of head (e) caudal presentation with back down (f) cranial presentation with back down (g) all feet presented (h) ventral transverse.

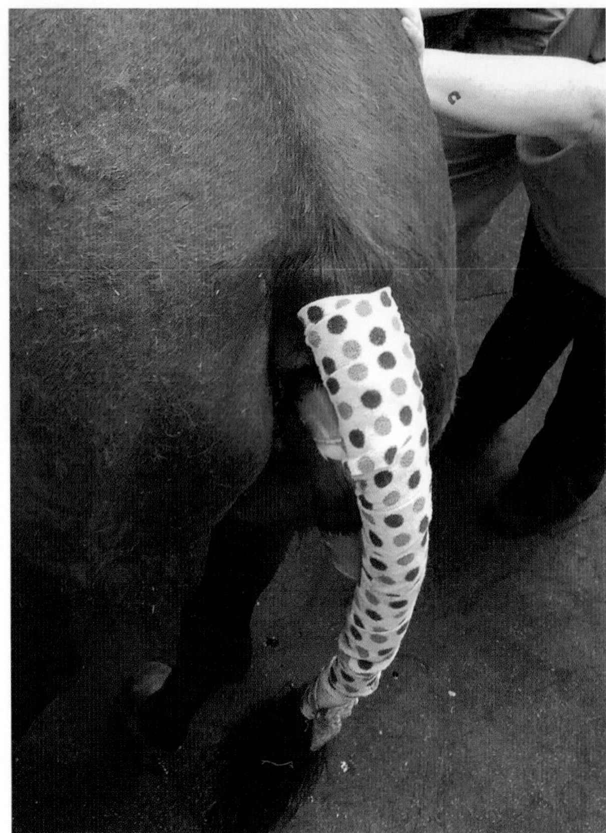

Figure 9.29 A mare in dystocia with being anesthetized for a C-section.

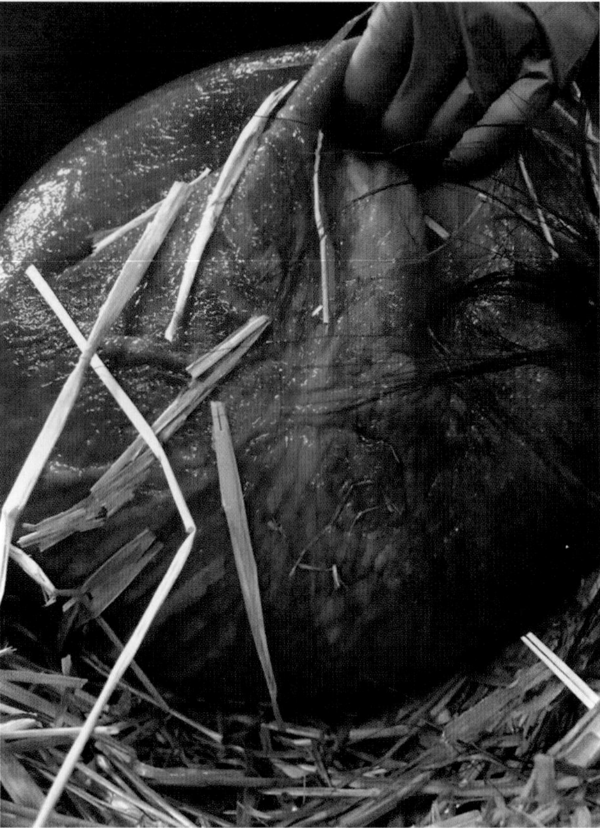

Figure 9.30 Red Bag presentation. *Source:* Courtesy of Andrea Whittle.

In normal presentation, like a diving position, the foal's front feet should emerge first with the soles facing downward. Presentation of the headfirst or the soles of the feet facing sideways or upward will indicate malpositioning. Presentation of just one foot can indicate a trapped shoulder or having one leg backward. Occasionally, owners may not be aware of twinning; the addition of a second fetus can also affect presentation.

Fetal-maternal disproportion and uterine inertia is rare in mares. If there is poor or no progression in second-stage labor, a physical and uterine exam can quickly help determine if there is disproportion, in other words, the fetus is too large to pass through the pelvic canal. In such cases, fetal status should next be confirmed as well as discussing the viability and future breeding prognosis with the owner. Either a C-section or a fetotomy will be required to resolve (Figure 9.29).

Premature placental separation, also commonly referred to as a "Reg Bag" delivery is an urgent risk for the foal. In normal delivery, the pale fetal membranes will appear, followed by the foal's front feet and head. In a red bag delivery, the placenta has prematurely separated from the uterine lining and is exteriorized first. This is identified by a velvety red sac rather than the pale shiny amniotic sac and it leaves the fetus without an oxygen source due to the detachment. The red placenta must be quickly but carefully cut open to access the foal. At times, a veterinarian may instruct the client to do this over the phone to avoid any time delay. After delivery, the foal should be watched for signs of dummy foal syndrome, or hypoxic ischemic encephalopathy.

TECHNICIAN TIP 9.40: A red bad delivery is a critical emergency.

Prepubic ligament tear or ruptures and/or ventral abdominal muscles is not common but can be seen in late stage heavily pregnant mares (Figure 9.32). Twinning, excessive edema, increased uterine weight, hydrops, or trauma may contribute, or there may be no predisposing factors. Hydrops is categorized as excessive fluid, either allanotic or amniotic in nature, the cause is unknown but is a great risk to the mare and the foal (Figure 9.31). Diagnosis is primarily made through physical exam, and treatment is limited to abdomen support such as belly bands and wraps; in the case of hydrops, drainage may be

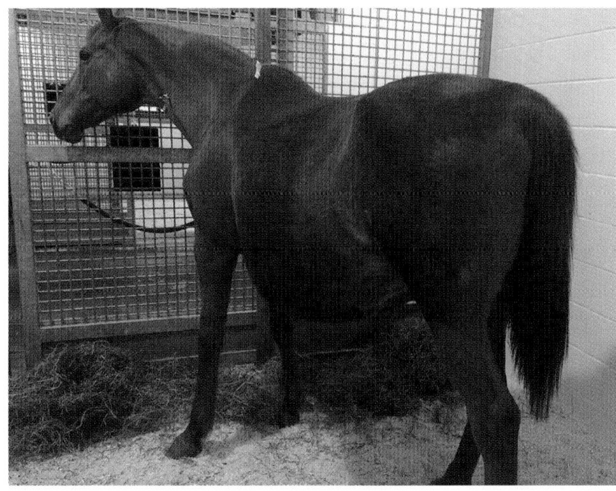

Figure 9.31 A mare with hydrops.

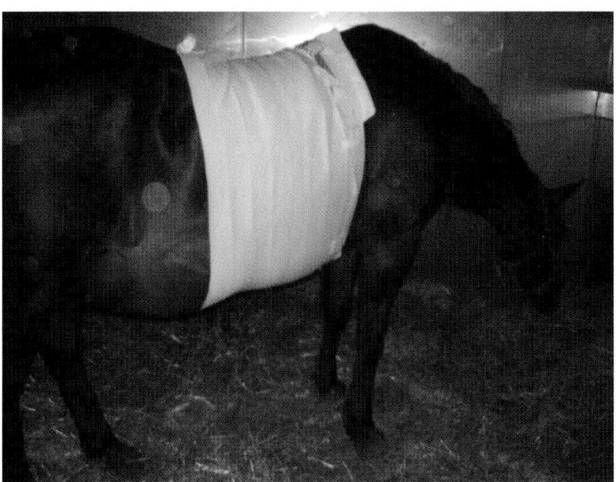

Figure 9.32 A mare with a prepubic ligament tear in supportive bandaging.

elected. Delivery assistance is often necessary, due to the damaged abdominal musculature. It is not advised to re-breed such a mare unless ET is planned.

A uterine torsion is a rotation of the uterus, typically more than 45°. It can occur in any animal at any stage of gestation. The success rate of recovery from uterine torsion is directly correlated to the stage of gestation. Prior to 320 days, the success rate is quite good but after that time, the prognosis decreases for both mare and foal as the increased size of the fetus adds to the complications. Typical signs of a uterine torsion in a mare resembles signs of colic.

Options for correction of uterine torsion are limited to either a surgical correction via a flank or ventral midline incision or using a plank roll technique. With the rolling technique, the animal is anesthetized under general anesthesia, and the animal is then rolled over while using a plank to stabilize the uterus. This technique is sometimes referred

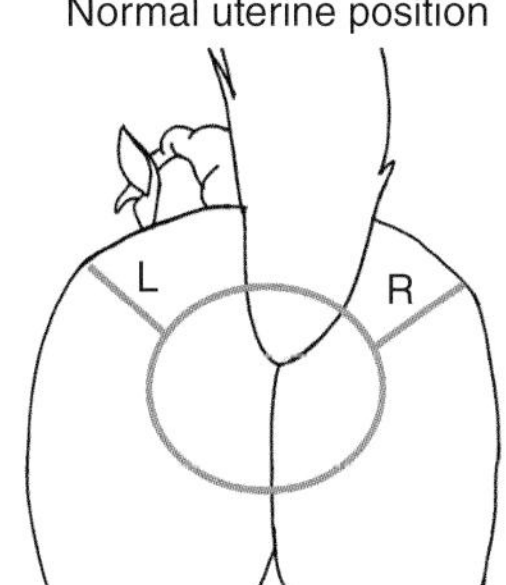

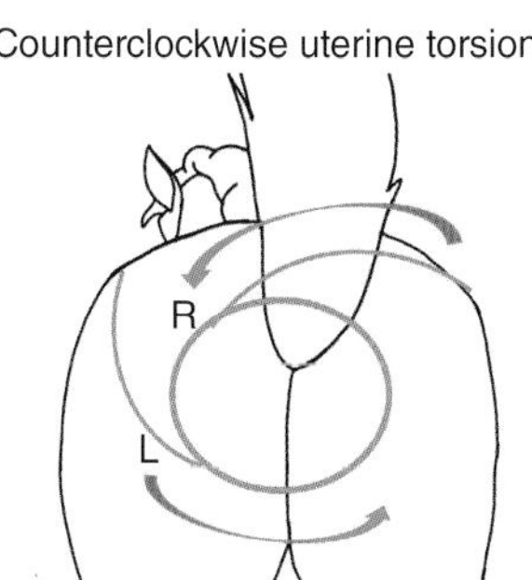

Figure 9.33 Illustration representing uterus gravity in a normal and torsed uterus.

to as a modified Schaffer's method and may be used in various species, not just the horse. Manual pressure may work without a plank in smaller ruminants and small camelids.

Retained Placenta

The mare should pass the fetal membranes within 3 hr of delivery. Horses with retained fetal membranes are often very crampy and uncomfortable, this can cause the mare to avoid caring and feeding the foal sometimes, this should be monitored closely. When the situation is prolonged, it will initiate an inflammatory reaction resulting in septicemia, metritis, or even peritonitis. Secondary to infection, the risk of developing laminitis from a toxic event may also occur. Typically, a veterinarian will perform a vaginal exam in addition to administering oxytocin (5 U, IM, every 2–3 hr) to encourage the body to release and expel the membranes. If the membranes are still intact, knots may be tied in the amino and umbilical cord, above the hocks, to utilize the aid of gravity and to help avoid the mare stepping on them (Figure 9.34). It is generally not recommended to forcefully remove any tissue as it can increase the risk of tearing or fragments being left behind as well as potential for uterine prolapse. Some Veterinarians may opt to perform a large volume uterine lavage technique to promote separation and remove debris and bacteria. It can take several lavage attempts to succeed. Generally, an antimicrobial regime is also initiated to help manage developing infection.

TECHNICIAN TIP 9.41: Equine fetal membranes should not be forcefully removed.

Camelid Parturition

South American camelids typically deliver in the late morning to afternoon. Delivering in the evening or overnight can be an indication of an abnormality. Normal

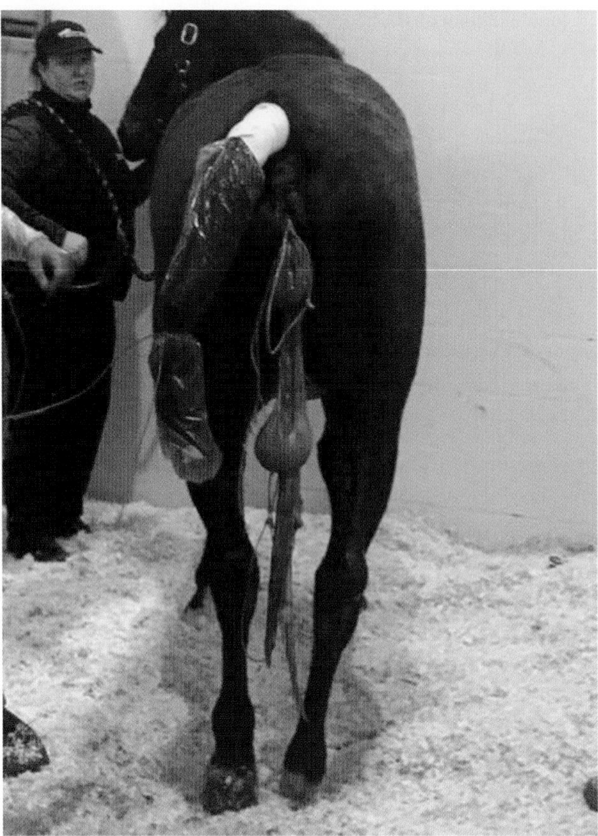

Figure 9.34 Mare with retained fetal membranes tied up and being prepared for a uterine lavage.

presentation is similar to other mammalian species previously discussed, in a diving position with front feet first with head following.

A llama or alpaca is considered in dystocia if stage one of labor lasts more than 6 hr or if there is no fetal progression within 10 min of the allantochorion sac ruptures. Fetal-maternal disproportion is rarely a concern in camelids. Malpositioning is the most common cause of dystocia in camelids. Larger camelids such as llamas may be able to be manually palpated via the vaginal canal, and the fetus may be able to be repositioned. In smaller alpacas, however, vaginal canal limitations similar to other small ruminants may warrant a C-section. Uterine torsion is also a possibility in a camelid dystocia. A modified Schaffer's method may be used to assist in the delivery. The female or dam may be positioned with her hips and pelvis over a bale of straw to help utilize gravity in the repositioning of the fetus or torsed uterus.

Small Ruminant Pregnancy and Parturition

First time Does and Ewes will often only have 1–2 offspring. Thereafter, provided being well fed, triplets and quadruplets are not uncommon. A farmer may increase nutrition around the time of breeding particularly to increase ovulation, conception, and embryo implantation rates, this is referred to as "Flushing" and can work in ovine, caprine, and porcine.

Incidence of dystocia in sheep and goats is minimal. If there is no progression within 30 min of active labor, intervention should be initiated. Kids and lambs should normally present in the diving position like foals and calves. Dystocia can be a matter of maternal-fetal disproportion and/or mal-presentations. More commonly, dystocia is seen in twins, triplets, and quadruplets, including size disproportion of one fetus compared to the others or one blocking the other. Dystocia in ovine and caprines can be difficult to manage depending on the size of the animal. Pigmy goats, for example, are often too small for vaginal evaluation or manipulation but a mature goat or ewe may be possible to manage depending on the hand size of the Veterinarian. It may be helpful to consider an abdominal X-ray to get a count of the number of feti. A placenta is considered retained 12 hr after parturition.

Pregnancy toxemia in sheep and goats, also referred to as lambing-sickness, twin lab disease or pregnancy ketosis, is more common of an issue in ovine and caprine gestation than in equine and bovine. It is commonly linked to stress including bad weather or nutritional deficiencies (over and underweight).

Vaginal prolapse may occur toward the end of gestation or at the time of parturition. It is more common in cattle and sheep than in other large animal species. The recurrence of vaginal prolapse is significant and owners should consider culling or ceasing to rebreed that animal. Temporary resolution can be achieved using a Buhner stitch or using a commercial made vaginal retention device known as a bearing retainer or permanent fixation using the Johnson button technique.

Hypocalcemia, also known as milk fever or parturient paresis. Unlike paresis in dairy cattle which occurs three to four days after parturition, it is more commonly seen in ewes before parturition. Signs of tachycardia, muscle weakness and muscle tremors are some of the symptoms that may be noted. See the disease chapter for more on hypocalcemia.

Porcine Pregnancy and Parturition

The majority of swine breeding in today's production facilities is done through AI. This is quite different than the reproduction techniques of hobby-farm-type pet pigs. Typical farms will have a few "teaser" boars on hand to check for the beginning of standing estrus in the females. The entire swine heat cycle is usually 21 days, with 14 days in diestrus followed by five to seven days of estrus or "standing heat." The estrus phase in swine is identified by a gradual increase in a willingness to be mounted by the male, ultimately resulting in a completely rigid posture and a drawing back of the ears by the female in the presence of the male. This rigid posture typically occurs during the period around ovulation. Once this "standing heat" has occurred, most insemination is done on a timed basis. Gilts are typically inseminated at 12 and 24 hr after full estrus has begun. Sows are typically inseminated at 24 and 36 hr after the start of full estrus due to a delayed ovulation in multiparous swine. During insemination, a pipette is advanced into the vagina until it is locked into the cervix. Due to the anatomy of swine penis, the pipettes must mimic the "corkscrew" like grooves that allow the cervix of the female to lock on to the pipette and create an appropriate seal that will not allow semen to backflow out of the uterus. Once the pipette is locked into the cervix, fresh-cooled semen is pushed quickly into the uterus. Once completely in, the pipette is sealed, and allowed to remain in place while the female relaxes the cervix and allows the pipette to be removed. Typical AI fresh-cooled semen doses range from 50 to 100 ml and contain between 2 and 4 billion progressively motile sperm, and each female is bred with two doses.

The female reproductive anatomy in swine is somewhat unique, especially as it relates to parturition. The swine uterus has very little true body, and instead has two large uterine horns. These horns are where the embryos attach and grow during gestation. The multiple embryos can move freely between each horn until they finally do implant. During parturition, these uterine horns may contract and empty at the same time, or one at a time. Swine gestation takes approximately 114 days, or in lay terminology "3 months, 3 weeks, 3 days." Pregnant females are moved from gestation facilities to a farrowing barn between 7 and 10 days prior to their due date. They are housed in "farrowing crates" that has plenty of room for the female to move around in and lay down, but not to turn around. Additionally, there are two areas on each side of the crate that are enclosed for the piglets that she will have to move around in without risk of their mother crushing them when she lays down. Farrowing begins with a few telltale signs including nesting behavior, restlessness, and the development of milk excretion from her mammary glands, beginning in the front teats and eventually extending through her whole udder. A female can exhibit all, some, or none of these signs prior to the beginning of parturition.

Once parturition begins, the female will spend a large majority of her time in a recumbent position. The farrowing manager may notice a relaxing of the vulva and exterior genitalia, streaming of milk from the udder with the oxytocin release, and some vaginal discharge as the cervix relaxes. Eventually, contractions will begin, and it will be easy to see the female attempting to push with each contraction. Once the first piglet is passed, some managers will elect to give a dose of oxytocin intramuscularly to increase the contractility of the uterus and ensure swift delivery of the litter. Many females are able to have their litter without complications. Average litter size in swine has increased through the years due to selective breeding and herd improvement programs, and currently sits at around 11 piglets. Litter size can vary from as little as 4 piglets, to as many as 20.

Complications can and often do occur during parturition in swine. Dystocia is the most common complication often relating to fetal orientation in the birth canal or due to a fetus that is too large to pass easily through the birth canal. Most breeding managers may have to assist the female by manual extraction or re-orientation of the fetuses. This can be done with just the manager's own arm and hand, or through the use of specialized forceps to minimize the damage done in repeated manipulations with a rough arm or hand. Other complications include still births, piglets born with their amnion still intact, which can asphyxiate the piglet if the manager does not intervene, piglets born hypoxemic resulting in some neurologic deficits, mummified fetuses that had died prior to parturition, or a number of other rare genetic malformations like hydrocephalus or hydro-abdomen. On the rare case where a dystocia is unable to be resolved by the breeding manager, if a litter is valuable enough, a C-section may be attempted. C-sections are best done under general anesthesia with veterinarian, but when a veterinarian is unavailable, a breeding manager may attempt a euthanasia C-section. Piglets that are recovered after the euthanasia C-section are fostered off onto other mothers in the farrowing barn with active litters. If a litter is not considered valuable enough to attempt a veterinary C-section, or the farm does not want to do a euthanasia C-section, re-absorption of the litter will attempt to be facilitated. This will be done through a combination of antibiotic administration, supportive care, and daily movement to help the body try to break down and reabsorb the litter inside the female. This is no small task and can result in the death of the female as well, so it should only be undertaken as a salvage procedure, with the expectation that if the female recovers, she is sent to market after fully healing.

Once a parturition is complete, the female will expel the placenta and afterbirth, and very rarely has any issues with a retained placenta. Most piglets are able to stand and nurse within 30 min after being born. There is very little aftercare that is needed for the mother as swine are adept at involuting their uterus and resetting their reproductive environment for the next litter. A sow will nurse her litter for three to four weeks, and once weaned, be returned to the breeding shed to begin monitoring her estrous cycles again.

With pet pig breeding, it can resemble to dog breeding, where the female may spend weeks or even a few months at the breeder's. Pig can be aggressive breeders and there is a good chance that the female will be scratched and bitten during breeding. Prior to parturition, owners may set up a farrowing box for the gilt. Farrowing has the same sequence in pigs, regardless of being in production or private ownership. Pot belly piglets average 6–12 oz in weight at birth. They are generally weaned between five and six weeks of age. It is not uncommon to have 1–2 runts or poor-doers in a litter. Owners need to consider supplementing milk for them, away from their mother.

TECHNICIAN TIP 9.42: Retained placentas in swine is rare and usually an indication that not all piglets have been born.

Poultry Reproduction

Poultry Reproduction is really in a class of its own. Though many urban farmers and homesteaders will raise birds.

Brooding

There are a few ways that backyard chicken owners may develop new chicks. The first is by accident from not collecting eggs daily while also having a rooster present. Having a fertilized egg requires a viable male for fertilization, if no rooster is present, then fertilized eggs cannot occur. Hens can store semen in their reproduction track for up to two to three weeks so be aware that fertilization can occur in the period after male is removed. Clients may also purchase eggs to hatch out or order newly hatched chicks (one-day old) to be delivered. There are several companies that specialize in selling and shipping newly hatched chicks, which allows clients to try a variety of different breeds.

Embryonic development takes place over 21 days, at which point the egg hatches. Success of egg hatching begins with good nutrition for the hen prior to egg production. Other factors that affect fertilization and hatching success include environment (temp and moisture), genetics, and age of parents as well as egg damage.

A decision needs to be made before starting whether to use a hen to brood or an incubator (Figure 9.35). Eggs should be turned two to four times daily until 18 days and maintained at adequate temp and humidity. A hen will take care of most of this, but clients should be prepared for the commitment of using an incubator. Also, note that a brooding hen will not resume egg production until her chicks are grown (Figure 9.36).

TECHNICIAN TIP 9.43: Egg shells are permeable and an important part of air and gas exchange for the developing embryo.

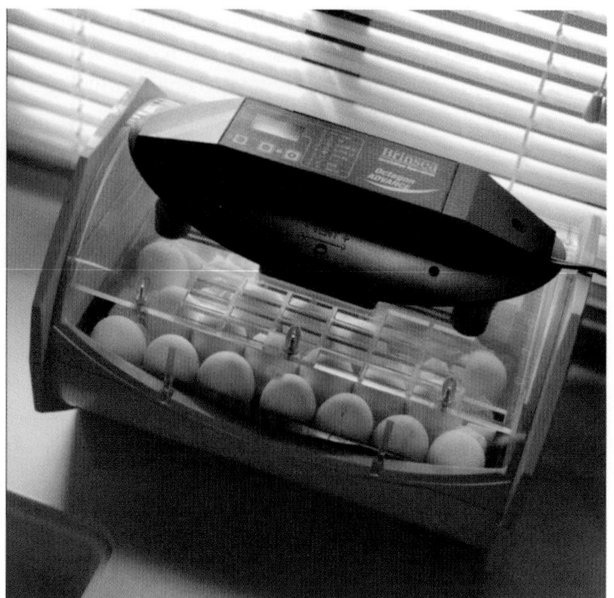

Figure 9.35 Homestead-type incubator.

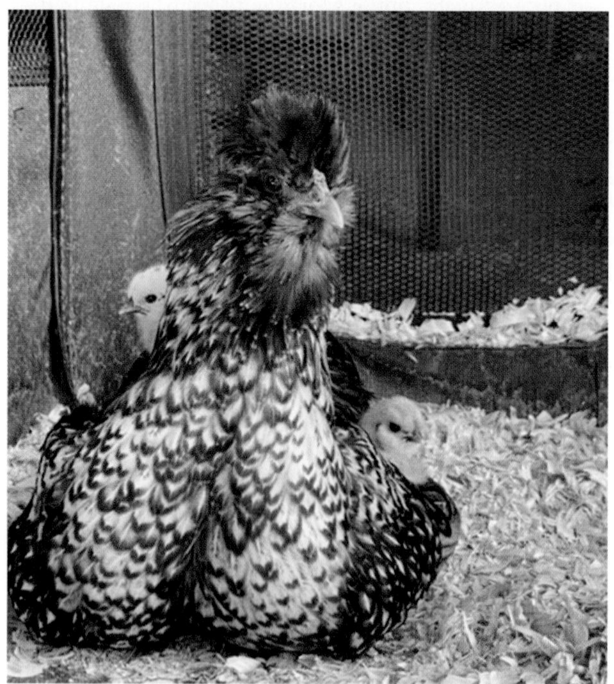

Figure 9.36 Brooding hen.

Environment for Egg Development

Do not wash or soak eggs if possible. Egg shells are permeable and an important part of air and gas exchange for the developing embryo. Eggs should be stored with the large end up and at a slant of 30–45%. Failure to turn eggs could result in development of adhesions and poor embryo development, among other things. Incubator temperature should be 97–102 °F, ideally 99–100 °F. Beyond that range there is a high likelihood of embryonic death. Optimum humidity for egg development is 60% with an increase to 70% the last three days before hatching. Ventilation should be around 20%. Failure to have any ventilation will affect the embryo/shell to environment gas exchange which is critical to success.

Chicks should not need assistance hatching; they may begin to crack on day 20 and hatch on day 21. Chicks can remain in the incubator for 6–12 hr post hatch. Chicks are precocial, meaning they are hatched in a state ready to feed themselves; therefore they do not need hen or human assistance for feeding in their early days.

Hatchling Management

Newly hatched chicks should be housed brooder pen, whether they are being reared by a hen or by humans. The bedding should be 2–4″ deep, highly absorbent, non-toxic, and reduce thermal conductivity. Things like wood shavings, pine sawdust, or paper by-products are the most common but additional options include chopped straw, ground corn cobs, sand, or leaves. Avoid cardboard, plastics, and free of contaminants. The bedding should be kept clean and dry in order to avoid caking.

Supplemental heat should be provided until the birds are fully feathered, approximately four to six weeks of age. Depending on climate and season, heat may need to be provided for longer. The ideal temperature for chicks during the first week should be around 90 °F–95 °F and can generally be reduced by 5 °F weekly. A heat lamp, hanging approximately 18–24″ above the bedding is recommended. Use a 100-watt bulb for small brooders and 250-watt for larger brooders. A red bulb reduces the chance of the birds pecking each other. Use a lamp with a ceramic socket to avoid melting plastic from the heat. One must watch the bird's behavior and positioning around the heat source to get an indication of its effectiveness. If it is too warm, the chicks will be scattered away from the source and if it is too cool, the chicks will cluster together as close to the heat source as possible. Extreme conditions for chicks can quickly result in death.

Food and water should not be too far from the heat source, nor should it be too deep where the chicks could drown. When first introduced to the environment, one can dip the beak of each chick into the water, so that they learn where the source is. In terms of lighting, it should meet the biological requirements of the bird, which will vary according to life stage and type of production. Intensity duration and quality of the lighting all matter.

TECHNICIAN TIP 9.44: The ideal temperature for chicks during the first week should be around 90–95 °F and can generally be reduced by 5 °F weekly.

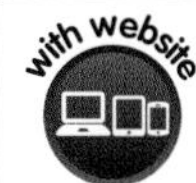

See the online Poultry Breed resource for bred varieties and coup designs.

References

Carlton, C. (2011). *Blackwell's Five-Minute Veterinary Consult Clinical Companion: Equine Theriogenology*. Ames, IA: Wiley Blackwell.

Embertson, R. (1992). The indications and surgical techniques for caesarean section in the mare. *Equine Vet. Educ.* 4 (1): 31–36. https://doi.org/10.1111/j.2042-3292.1992.tb01543.x.

Lawhorn, D., DVM, MS, By, Lawhorn, D., & Last full review/revision Jul 2020 | Content last modified Jul 2020. (2020, July). Breeding and reproduction of potbellied pigs – all other pets. D. Bruce Lawhorn. Retrieved January 14, 2021, from https://www.msdvetmanual.com/all-other-pets/potbellied-pigs/breeding-and-reproduction-of-potbellied-pigs

Pregnancy Toxemia in Ewes and Does (Twin lamb disease, By, Menzies, P., & Last full review/revision Jun 2015 | Content last modified Jun 2015. (2015, June). Pregnancy toxemia in ewes and does – metabolic disorders. Retrieved March 2, 2021, from https://www.merckvetmanual.com/metabolic-disorders/hepatic-lipidosis/pregnancy-toxemia-in-ewes-and-does

Samper, J. C., & Plough, T. A. (2012). How to Deal with Dystocia and Retained Placenta in the Field. Retrieved January 6, 2021, from https://aaep.org/sites/default/files/issues/proceedings-12proceedings-How_to_Manage_the_Subfertile_Mare-Samper_-_How_to_Deal_with_Dystocia.pdf

Sertich By Patricia L. Sertich, P. L., MS, VMD, DACT, By, Sertich, P., & Last full review/revision Oct 2014 | Content last modified Nov 2014. (2014, November). Parturition in Horses – Management and Nutrition. Retrieved December 28, 2020, from https://www.merckvetmanual.com/management-and-nutrition/management-of-reproduction-horses/parturition-in-horses

Slovis, N. M., Lu, K. G., Wolfsdorf, K. E., & Zent, W. W. (2013). How to Manage Hydrops Allantois/Hydrops Amnion in a Mare. Retrieved February 11, 2021, from https://aaep.org/sites/default/files/issues/AmbulatorySlovis.pdf

Sturtz, R. and Asprea, L. (2012). *Anatomy and Physiology for Veterinary Technicians and Nurses: A Clinical Approach*. Ames, IA: Wiley-Blackwell.

Thompson, D.L. Jr., Pickett, B.W., Squires, E.L., and Amann, R.P. (1979). Testicular measurements and reproductive characteristics in stallions. *J. Reprod. Fertil. Suppl.* 27: 13–17. PMID: 289781.

Yorke, E.H., Caldwell, F.J., and Johnson, A.K. (2012 Dec). Uterine torsion in mares. *Compend Contin. Educ. Vet.* 34 (12): E2. PMID: 23532880.

Youngquist, R. and Threlfall, W. (2007). *Current Therapy in Large Animal Theriogenology*. Philadelphia, PA: W. B. Saunders https://www.merckvetmanual.com/exotic-and-laboratory-animals/potbellied-pigs/reproduction-of-potbellied-pigs#:~:text=Dystocia%20is%20of%20special%20concern,the%20vaginal%20canal%20is%20patent.

Clinical Case Resolution 9.1

Recording a thorough history is vital to resolution of patient problems. Items that must be recorded are:

- number of breedings this season;
- breeding method used;
- intervention or therapy used thus far;
- amount and frequency of exercise or training;
- number of live offspring produced;
- type and number of breedings used to produce live offspring;
- any instances of dystocia;
- other health problems;
- diet;
- housing;
- any history of travel; and
- immunizations.

Activities

Multiple Choice Questions

(Answers can be found in the back of the book.)

1. The hormone that causes the release of FSH and LH is:
   A GnRH
   B inhibin
   C estradiol
   D estrogen

2. The hormone that causes the destruction of the CL is:
   A GnRH
   B inhibin
   C estrogen
   D luteinizing hormone

3. Specially adapted tubule that gathers the ova release from the ovary is:
   A vagina
   B oviduct
   C ovary
   D cervix

4. A BSE concentrates on:
   A the physical ability to mate
   B the desire to mate
   C libido
   D adequate quantity and quality of semen

5. The instrument used to manually count sperm in a quantity of ejaculate is:
   A spectrophotometer
   B hemocytometer
   C sphygmomanometer
   D dosimeter

6. Which of the following species is a seasonal breeder that responds to decreasing day-length?
   A bovine
   B ovine
   C equine
   D porcine

7. The part of the estrous cycle where follicular development and increasing estrogen leads to demonstration of sexual characteristics is called:
   A diestrus
   B proestrus
   C anestrus
   D estrus

8. The species that possesses a musculocavernous penis is:
   A ovine
   B porcine
   C camelids
   D equine

9. The stage of labor where the cervix relaxes and the fetus is positioned for delivery is:
   A stage 1
   B stage 2
   C stage 3
   D stage 4

10. The stage of labor where the placenta is passed is:
   A stage 1
   B stage 2
   C stage 3
   D stage 4

Test Your Learning

1. A male porcine patient must have a semen evaluation. What procedures must be accomplished during a BSE? What species-specific concerns should a veterinary technician be aware of?
2. When collecting a stallion for semen evaluation, is there any collection method that cannot be used on this species?
3. You are asked to perform a semen evaluation. List the areas of concern when performing the laboratory portion of the evaluation?
4. A cow visits the hospital for a BSE. What items would need to be assembled to assist the veterinarian to perform the evaluation?
5. You are attending to a dystocia at a cattle ranch. The cow is in the pasture with a dead fetus. The veterinarian needs to perform a fetotomy. What concerns are there for this procedure?

Answers can be found in the back of the book.

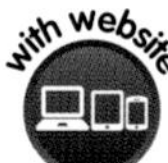

Extra review questions, case studies, and a breed ID image bank can be found online at www.wiley.com/go/loly/veterinary.

Chapter 10

Anesthesia and Surgery

Shana Lemmenes, CVT, VTS (EVN), Jennifer Halleran, DVM, DACVIM (LAIM), and Meagan Smith, RVT, VTS (Anesthesia and Analgesia)

Learning Objectives

- Describe the importance of post-operative care.
- List the drugs that may be used for sedation/anesthesia for each species.
- List the precautions to take when intubating each species.
- List indications of each surgery.
- Describe the food animal considerations when it comes to surgery.

Clinical Case Problem 10.1

A 15-year-old Paint horse presents to the hospital with 6-h history of colic. What indications will make this patient a surgical candidate? What are post-operative concerns if this patient does go to surgery?

See Clinical Case Resolution 10.1 at the end of this chapter.

Key Terms

Agonist
Analgesia
Antagonist
Auricular vein
Bicornuate uterus
Buccotomy
Central nervous system (CNS)
Demand valve
Diastema
Hypercapnia
Hypoxemia
Laryngoscope
Minimal alveolar concentration (MAC)
Neuroleptanalgesia
Normovolemic
Postsynaptic
Presynaptic
Respiratory acidosis
Respiratory depression
Rut
Scur
Thalamocortical
Total intravenous anesthesia (TIVA)
Vasoconstriction
Vasodilation

Large Animal Medicine for Veterinary Technicians, Second Edition. Edited by Sue Loly and Heather Hopkinson.

Companion website: www.wiley.com/go/loly/veterinary

Introduction

Large animal surgery and anesthesia requires considerable forethought and planning. Knowing your drugs could be life and death. The drugs may be the same but the amount and route that you give them varies across species. And since we are dealing with multiple species, it is important to realize a surgical procedure on one species may not be the same as another species. For example, you can do a cesarean section on cow standing but for a horse it is much more complicated and done under general anesthesia. The veterinary technician is responsible for all aspects of surgery and anesthesia including sterile prep, intubation through recovery, and surgical assistant.

Large Animal Surgery Considerations

Prior to the start of any surgical procedure, certain considerations need to be pondered, discussed, and decisions need to be made. First, all patients need to have a thorough history collected and a physical examination conducted. For the physical examination, at least, a temperature, heart rate, respiratory rate, and rumen contraction need to be evaluated. Respiratory pattern, abdominal distention and a rectal examination are also warranted. Under certain emergency situations, this limited physical examination would be all that can be performed; however, if the situation is not emergent, a complete and thorough physical examination should be conducted to ensure the patient is deemed healthy and fit and for surgery and anesthesia.

For patients undergoing general anesthesia, relevant clinical diagnostics are warranted. These would include a packed cell volume (PCV) and total solids (TS), a complete blood count (CBC) and a biochemistry profile. This minimum database would allow the clinicians, technicians, and anesthesia to ensure the patient is healthy for general anesthesia, what complications may be expected, or what problems need to be dealt with prior to general anesthesia induction. Based on the underlying pathophysiology, the clinical tests may help decide appropriate fluid therapy, electrolyte supplementation, or the potential for blood loss. In some situations, imaging, such as radiographs or ultrasound, or even advanced imaging, CT, or MRI, would be warranted.

Large Animal Sedation and Anesthesia

Sedation and Analgesia

Sedation plays a crucial role in safely handling all species in the veterinary community. It not only increases the safety of the handler but for the animal as well. Handling animals can be extremely stressful for the animal itself, especially when placed in a new environment or having to endure travel. All prey species have a flight response when frightened and can be difficult to calm down once startled; these animals will also require higher drug dosages or additional medications to achieve a sedative effect.

While individual drugs can be effective, some drug can provide a synergistic effect allowing sedation and analgesia to be achieved. Route of administration is important to consider when choosing a protocol for sedation as some species will be harder to gain venous access.

If possible, procedures in large animals should be done standing with sedation or local blocks to avoid the risks of anesthesia and recovery. In ruminants, anesthesia with a protected airway is best due to risk of regurgitation.

> **TECHNICIAN TIP 10.1:** Regurgitation is a risk when doing anesthesia on ruminants.

In this section, we will discuss the commonly used drugs for sedation and analgesia of equine, porcine, ruminants, and camelids.

Alpha-2 Agonists

Alpha-2-adrenergic agonists (α_2 agonists) work on α_2 receptors in the central nervous system (CNS) and periphery. Depending on the formulation, the α_2 used will also affect the α_1 receptors as well. By activating the presynaptic and postsynaptic receptors in the CNS, a sedation effect and analgesic effect is achieved. However, this effect is not without side effects.

Respiratory depression occurs, which can further lead to hypoxemia and hypercapnia, resulting in a respiratory acidosis. In small ruminants, particularly sheep, α_2 agonists can cause pulmonary edema. The cardiovascular system is also heavily affected: peripheral vasoconstriction causes a profound decrease in heart rate, which significantly decreases cardiac output.

Caution must be exercised when using α_2 agonists in ruminants as there are subject to more profound sedation and side effects, especially with xylazine.

Alpha$_2$ agonists combined with opioids can provide effective sedation for standing procedures and adequate premedication prior to anesthesia. The effect is known as neuroleptanalgesia. This combination will also reduce the minimal alveolar concentration (MAC) required for anesthesia. Additionally, a dexmedetomidine constant rate infusion will decrease the MAC and provide analgesia during surgery. The average equine dexmedetomidine rate is 1–2 mcg/kg/hr.

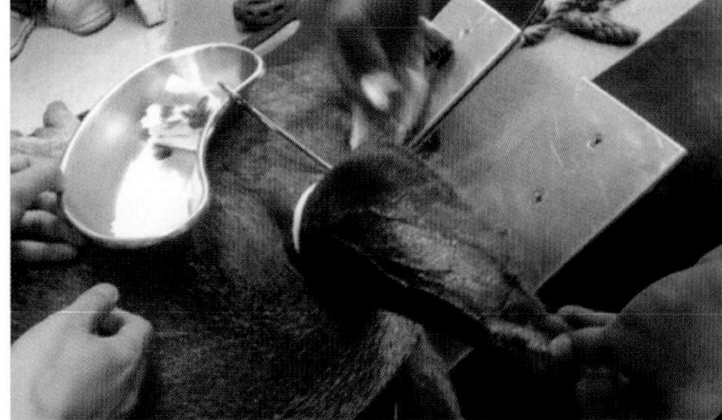

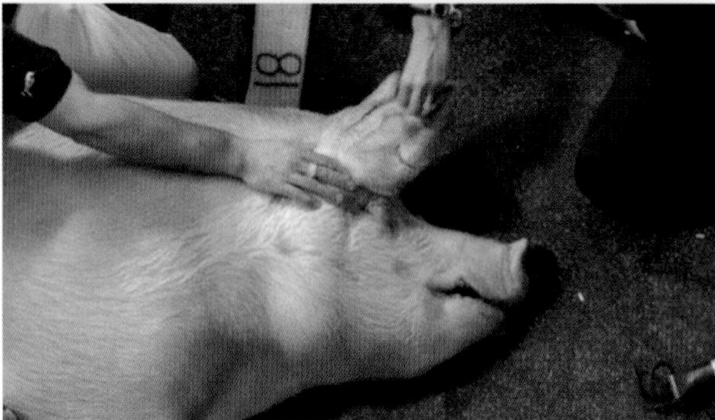

Figure 10.1 Venous access is obtained by using the pig's auricular vein.

In pigs, dexmedetomidine combined with ketamine provides moderate to deep sedation. This will allow for some minor procedures or catheter placement in the auricular vein for induction and maintenance of general anesthesia (Figure 10.1).

The most commonly used α_2 agonists are romifidine, xylazine, detomidine, and dexmedetomidine.

Alpha$_2$ agonists can be reversed. There are three antagonists available: yohimbine, tolazoline, and atipamezole.

Phenothiazines

Acepromazine maleate works on the CNS to provide sedation and is a potent α_1 antagonist that causes sedation via the anti-dopaminergic effect. Primarily used for its neuroleptic effects, this drug provides no analgesia. Due to its effect on the α_1 receptor, acepromazine causes profound vasodilation and should be only used in patients with normovolemic status. This drug can cause profound hypotension, myocardial depression, and tachycardia. Acepromazine relaxes the lower esophageal sphincter and increases the risk of regurgitation; therefore, it is not commonly used in ruminants, as risk of regurgitation is already high. Caution must be exercised when using in farm production animals, as this product takes 7 days to clear from meat and 48 hr to clear from milk of cattle.

> **TECHNICIAN TIP 10.2:** Use caution when using acepromazine in intact males due to the possibility of penile prolapse.

Additionally, caution must be used in stallions, geldings, and bulls as the relaxation effect causes penile prolapse, which can cause injury and require treatment or amputation.

Benzodiazepines

Benzodiazepines work in the CNS by effecting the gamma-aminobutyric acid A (GABA$_A$) receptor. This produces several affects, including muscle relaxation, sedation, and anticonvulsant properties. They have little to no effect on the cardiovascular and respiratory systems. The two drugs in this category are diazepam and midazolam. Diazepam is made with propylene glycol and alcohol and is therefore not water soluble. This means that diazepam should not be given intramuscularly and can cause phlebitis and thrombosis with repeated administration intravascularly.

Midazolam, combined with an opioid, ketamine, or α_2 agonists, can be greatly beneficial in sedation or premedication of ruminants, camelids, and pigs. In pigs, midazolam can be given intranasally to create sedation rapidly, allowing additional medications to be given intramuscularly in the non-compliant patient.

As a co-induction agent, midazolam or diazepam can aid in smooth inductions and intubations of horses; however, it is suggested that for short procedures, benzodiazepines can create rough recoveries with profound ataxia.

Benzodiazepines can be reversed with flumazenil IV.

Dissociative Agents

Ketamine is a n-methyl-D-aspartate (NMDA) antagonist. By binding at these sites, ketamine becomes a dissociative agent that causes a state of catalepsy by inhibiting the thalamocortical pathways. It also works as a potent analgesic by reducing the activity of neurons in the spinal cord and stopping transference. Many patients receiving ketamine can maintain ocular, laryngeal, pharyngeal, pinna, and pedal reflexes in addition to having increased muscle tone. Therefore, it is always given with other injectable agents.

In horses, extreme excitability and tonic–clonic muscle activity is noted when given as a sole agent, which can lead to injury of the horse, handler, or both. Ketamine constant rate infusions can reduce the mean alveolar concentrations of inhalants by up to 25%, though prolonged infusions can cause a buildup of norketamine leading to excitable patients during recovery.

Telazol or tiletamine zolazepam is a combination of a dissociative agent and a benzodiazepine in a single bottle. This combination works similarly to a ketamine/diazepam or midazolam combination, the benefit typically being a smaller volume. Studies in horses, swine, and llamas have shown that it can produce adequate inductions and tranquilization. However, elimination and poor recoveries can vary among species.

Opioids

TECHNICIAN TIP 10.3: All opioids are considered a controlled substance and, therefore, need to be logged when used.

A combination of an opioid such as butorphanol and an α_2 agonists work well for sedation and pre-medication in large animal and ruminant species. Side effects from mu opioid use in these species severely limit the selection for analgesia. Rough recoveries, gastrointestinal stasis, excitation, and hypoventilation outweigh the risk of use.

Morphine is a pure mu agonist that in low doses can be used as an analgesic but still has the same side effects. While horses given morphine can show excitatory behavior and experience post-operative colic signs after recovery, morphine can be used as an intra-articular injection without behavioral side effects and has been shown to reduce lameness.

Butorphanol is a kappa agonists and mu antagonists that functions as a sedative and analgesic. Due to its high affinity for the kappa receptor, making it a decent analgesic. However, at high doses or if given prior to a sedative, excitation can still occur in horses.

Opioids can be reversed with naloxone IV.

Nonsteroidal Anti-Inflammatory Drugs

Nonsteroidal anti-inflammatory drugs (NSAIDs) are used to control pain and inflammation by inhibiting cyclooxygenase (COX) enzymes and further inhibiting the production of prostaglandins. This is all a part of the arachidonic acid cycle. By inhibiting prostaglandins, side effects like kidney and gastrointestinal injury occur. Additionally, NSAIDs can be irritating to the gastric mucosa, which can further develop into ulcerations. Animals receiving anti-inflammatory agents should be monitored closely for side effects.

While many NSAIDs are on the market, only a few can be used in horses and even fewer in food production animals, especially in the United States, due to the withdrawal times and research available.

TECHNICIAN TIP 10.4: The use of NSAIDS (especially the overuse) can be a cause of right dorsal colitis in horses.

Local Blocks

All local anesthetics work by inhibiting sodium channels in nerve cell membranes. This leads to cessation of generation and propagation of action potentials in the nerve fiber. These drugs do not have an affinity for motor or sensory nerves and can cause an effect on either.

Generally, the most commonly used agents in veterinary medicine are chloroprocaine, lidocaine, mepivacaine, bupivacaine, and ropivacaine. However, lidocaine tends to be more commonly used for ruminants due to its price, rapid onset, and volume for coverage.

Overall, these drugs are relatively safe, but it is always important to keep in mind the toxic dose for the medication being used as well as how safe it is for accidental intravenous injection or rapid systemic uptake. More systemically friendly medications like lidocaine or ropivacaine are advisable whenever possible for this reason. Another consideration must be withdrawal times for meat and milk when working with food animals.

Choice of Drugs

When preparing local nerve blocks, considerations need to be made for type of block to be used, length of procedure, size of patient, and what the mobility needs of the patient may be following the procedure (Table 10.1). These can have major impacts on choice of medication as well as the feasibility of certain blocks.

Testicular Blocks

For this block, the longer acting local anesthetic the better (e.g. bupivacaine or ropivacaine.) Draw up 0.1–0.2 ml/kg/testicle. Isolate the testicle in non-dominant hand and insert a 22 g 1–1.5 in needle distal to proximal, using caution

Table 10.1 Duration of action.

Local anesthetic	Duration of action
Lidocaine	1–2 hr
Mepivacaine	1–3 hr
Bupivacaine	4–6 hr
Ropivacaine	4–6 hr

to prevent penetrating the epididymis. Without moving the location of the needle, gently aspirate the syringe to check for blood in the needle hub or syringe. If blood is noted, the needle is likely to be intravascular and should be redirected. If no blood on aspiration, the local anesthetic solution is injected until testicle feels firm/turgid. The process is repeated for the second testicle. If the block is successful, blockade of the genital branch of the genitofemoral, cremaster, and sympathetic nerve fibers should be observed.

Dehorning of Ruminants

Disbudding/dehorning of ruminants is a routine procedure performed to prevent injury to herd mates or the people working with the animals. Typically, it is performed in younger animals prior to development of the horns. While many professional farmers may perform this task on their own, this is not ideal. While the horn itself does not have innervation, the horn bud and the surrounding tissues that are removed in the dehorning process do, and as such, it is important to provide sedation and analgesia to the patients to make the patient as comfortable as possible for the procedure.

As a word of caution, always aspirate the syringe prior to injection. This will help to prevent accidental systemic injection of the local anesthetic of choice. Due to patient size and the vascular nature of the region being blocked, the local anesthetic can be systemically absorbed rapidly leading to a systemic overdose in kid goats.

Dehorning of Cattle

The cornual branch of the zygomaticotemporal nerve runs along the temporal ridge, approximately halfway between the lateral canthus of the eye and the base of the horn. It is in this region where the nerve that the most success can be had by performing a regional nerve block. The cornual branch of the infratrochlear nerve passes over the orbital rim close to, but dorsal to, the medial canthus of the eye. The cutaneous branches of C2 may be blocked by the local anesthetic at the dorsal midline level with the base of the ear. In rare instances, some cattle have innervation of the horns with branches of the frontal nerve. Unfortunately, due to location deep within the temporal fossa or within the horn, it is not possible to perform a nerve block on this branch. In older cattle, the addition of a ring block around well-developed horns may also be beneficial.

Dehorning of Sheep/Goats

The cornual branch of the lacrimal nerve is blocked close to the supraorbital process. A needle depth of approximately 1.5 cm is needed to perform this block as close to the root of the supraorbital process as possible.

The cornual branch of the infratrochlear nerve can be palpated at the dorsomedial rim of the orbit. A needle depth of approximately 0.5 cm is needed to adequately block this nerve bundle and is inserted halfway between the medial canthus and horn.

Flank Anesthesia

Given the nature of ruminant anatomy and pathology, it is necessary (and beneficial) to perform some procedures standing. In order to achieve this, standing sedation and proper local blockade are necessary.

Inverted L/Reverse 7 Block

This block is used to provide anesthesia to most of the flank and is often used for surgical correction of displaced abomasum (DA) in cattle. It is relatively simple to perform but requires large volumes of local anesthetic (most often, lidocaine) and multiple injection sites. While performing this block, keep in mind the maximum dose of local anesthetic (Lidocaine- 5 mg/kg small ruminants or 10 mg/kg in cattle) to prevent toxicity. When using lidocaine, there is approximately 1 h of analgesia to the region covered by the block. One disadvantage of this block is incomplete analgesia and muscle relaxation to the deeper layers of the abdominal wall. However, the local anesthetic is far enough from the incision site to not cause complications such as hematoma, seroma, tissue edema, and possible delayed wound healing.

Starting in the flank, ventral to L7, an 18g needle is inserted through the skin and muscle layers until approximately to the depth of, but not piercing, the peritoneum. The syringe is aspirated to prevent intravenous injection and the local anesthetic is injected through the layers as the needle is withdrawn. This pattern continues in a cranial direction in the flank at approximately 1 cm intervals until reaching the caudal border of the last rib. The pattern is then continued in a ventral direction on the caudal aspect of the rib. Total volume typically used for this block in cattle is 60 ml and is divided among all the injection sites. This block can also be performed on sheep and goats with appropriately lower volumes of local anesthetics.

TECHNICIAN TIP 10.5: The inverted L and line block can be used on cows for standing C-sections.

Line Block

This is the simplest technique for incisional local anesthetic. It is performed directly where the incision will be made at a dosage of 1 ml/cm for small ruminants and 2 ml/cm in large animals. The planned incision site should be

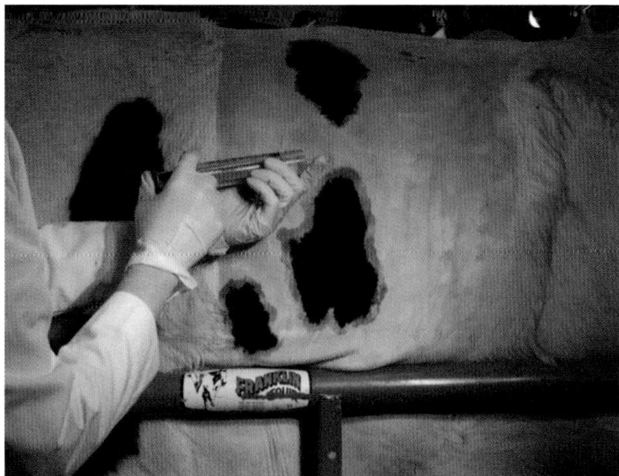

Figure 10.2 Line block performed on cow. *Source:* Courtesy of Jennifer Halleran, DVM, DACVIM (LAIM).

marked, and the needle inserted approximately 1 cm dorsal. Just as with the inverted L, the needle will be directed toward, but not through, the peritoneum. Aspirate the syringe to avoid intravascular injection and begin injecting as the needle is withdrawn. Repeat this every 1 cm ventrally along the incision line until 1 cm ventral to the end of the incision (Figure 10.2). Like the inverted L, this block can be less effective for deeper tissues. There is also the possibility for delayed wound healing should vasculature be disturbed from the volume of local anesthetic or with the addition of epinephrine to prolong the effects of the block.

Extremities

Bier Block

This block is most effectively used for the anesthesia of distal limbs and can be beneficial for digit amputations or any other surgical procedure below the level of the tourniquet. Planning prior to catheter placement can help to decrease the odds of block failure. An IV catheter should be placed in the distal limb and held secure. Identify an arterial pulse distal to the area where the tourniquet will be placed and make note of this area for later palpation.

When using a pneumatic cuff as a tourniquet, it is important to assess the minimal pressure needed to occlude the arterial blood flow. The cuff should be inflated until the arterial pulse is no longer palpable. For the duration of the procedure, the cuff will need to be kept well above this pressure (approximately 100 mmHg higher) to prevent any arterial blood from entering the exsanguinated region due to spikes in blood pressure.

To exsanguinate the limb, it is held higher than the elevation of the heart and an elastic bandage is applied distal to proximal in tight concentric circles. Be mindful of the placement of the catheter when reaching that point of the limb. Following exsanguination, the tourniquet should be placed just proximal to the top of the wrap. Pneumatic cuffs should be inflated to a pressure higher than previously noted to occlude the arterial blood flow.

If using a non-pneumatic/rubber tourniquet, it should be placed above the top of the bandage. In order to prevent leakage of the arterial flow past the tourniquet, a roll of gauze or cling can be placed over the artery and under the tourniquet. This will apply more pressure to the artery and provide better control of leakage. Once the tourniquet is placed, the planned procedure should be completed within 90 min to prevent permanent damage from prolonged ischemia to the distal limb as well as region under the tourniquet.

Following secure tourniquet placement, begin removing the elastic bandage, beginning distal to proximal. Using the previous mark, palpate for arterial pulse. If a pulse is noted, repeat the procedure beginning with the exsanguination process until the pulse is no longer palpable. Inject the local anesthetic (lidocaine 2–5 mg/kg) over the next 2–3 min. Observe for signs of systemic administration that could include toxicity (e.g. cardiac complications, neurologic signs). If no complications are noted, remove the IV catheter and begin the procedure.

Once the procedure has been completed, slowly begin to remove the tourniquet and again observe for signs of toxicity or complications that could be related to either the local anesthetic or due to the release of by-products from ischemic reperfusion injury.

Epidural

In cattle, sheep, and goats, the spinal cord ends at the level of the last lumbar vertebrae. However, the meningeal sac continues into the sacral region. For this reason, epidural anesthesia should be performed between the first and second coccygeal vertebra (Figure 10.3). This can be found by lifting and lowering the tail of the animal. The point where the tail pivots is the joint between Co1 and Co2. This region is shaved and sterilely prepared. A 20 g 1.5 in needle is inserted into the space between the vertebra and several "pops" are noted. Typically, 5–10 ml 2% lidocaine is injected and should begin to take effect within 2 min.

TECHNICIAN TIP 10.6: An indwelling epidural catheter must be kept sterile at the insertion site (Figure 10.4).

The animal will show no signs of ataxia or paralysis of the limbs; however, the tail will be paralyzed. This should allow for surgery of tail as well as the perineum. Additional volume will cause the block to proceed cranially. With the injection of 100–150 ml of 2% lidocaine, the hind limbs, mammary tissue, flanks, and abdominal wall will be anesthetized, but the animal will no longer be able to stand. The same technique can be used in sheep and goats. In addition to the caudal epidural, sheep and goats can benefit from lumbosacral epidurals. They may be recumbent following the injection, but it is less of a problem due to their size. Caution must be taken to prevent subarachnoid injection.

General Anesthesia

Prior to general anesthesia, sedation should be achieved with a pre-medication. The anesthesia machine with ventilator and monitor should be prepped and ready as well as supplies for induction depending on species. If not being placed on inhalant or if a machine is unavailable, oxygen supplementation must be provided. A demand valve fitted to oxygen line can be used for assisted breathing and supplementation (Figure 10.5).

For horses and cows, use a mouth gag with appropriate size endotracheal tubes and arterial line supplies. For ruminants and swine, a laryngoscope and endotracheal tubes with ties should be made available as well as catheter supplies, arterial line supplies, and blood pressure cuffs. Recovery stalls should be prepared with any supplies

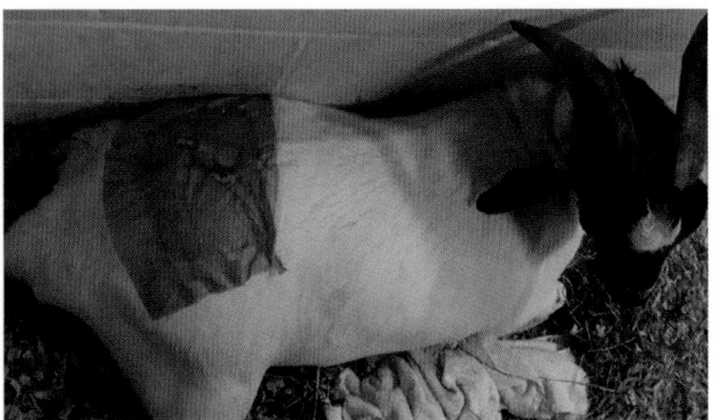

Figure 10.3 Epidural catheter placed in a goat. *Source:* Courtesy of Meagan Smith, RVT, VTS (Anesthesia).

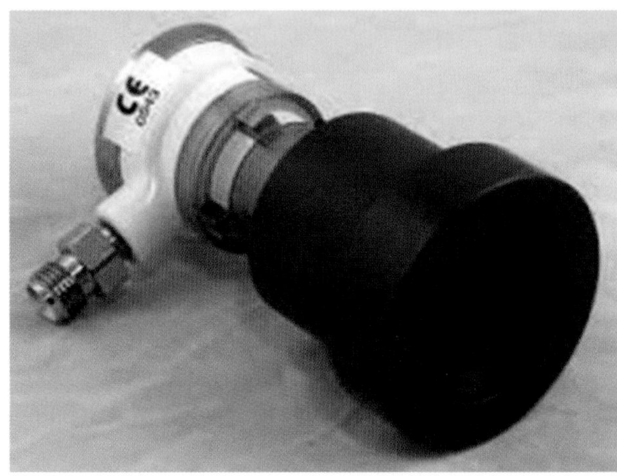

Figure 10.5 A demand valve is used to assist in breathing during recovery of anesthesia. Source: Courtesy of Meagan Smith, RVT, VTS (Anesthesia).

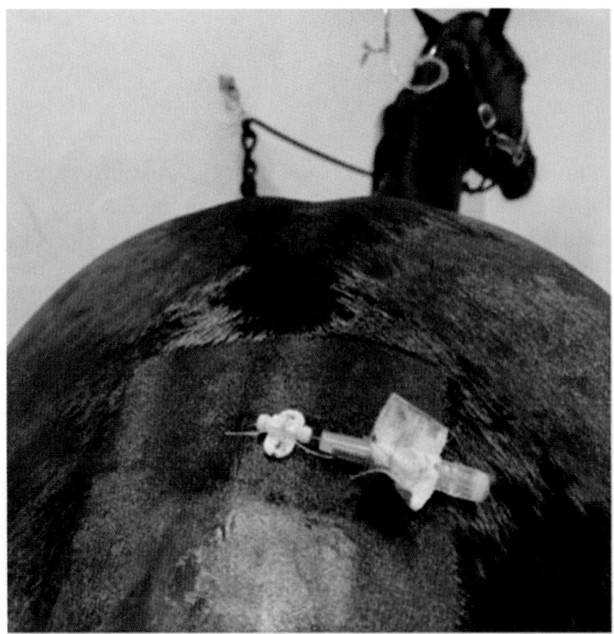

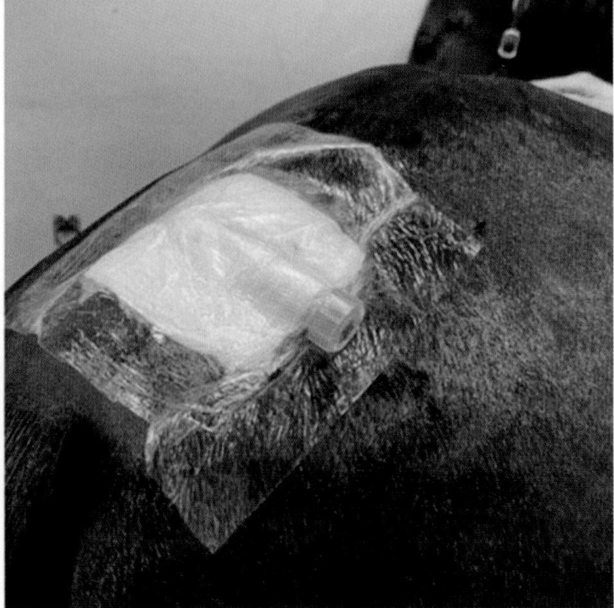

Figure 10.4 Epidural catheter placed in a horse. Source: Courtesy of Weston Davis Equine Surgery.

needed, including padding, oxygen demand valve, hobbles, ropes, bumpers, halters, nasal tracheal tubes for larger species, and an emergency crash box should be nearby. All horses, cows, and ruminants should have their mouths rinsed after sedation to remove any lingering feed that could enter the airway during intubation.

TECHNICIAN TIP 10.7: Occasionally, horses may be induced with a nasogastric tube in place to prevent gastric rupture.

Patients should be fasted prior to anesthetic events to decrease the risk of regurgitation and aspiration. Gastric emptying time varies between different species; therefore, fasting times will vary.

For induction, the common drug of choice is ketamine combined with another agent like propofol. Propofol is a fast-acting $GABA_A$ agonist and when combined with ketamine or midazolam/diazepam produces a smooth induction that allows adequate time for intubation (Figure 10.6). However, it is rapidly metabolized and has dose-dependent effects. Propofol causes apnea and decreased cardiac output, so patient co-morbidities should be considered when choosing induction agents.

As previously discussed, Telazol can be used as an induction agent, but an increased duration of action and poorer recovery scores should be considered when choosing this agent.

Ruminants should be kept sternal during induction until after intubation and after inflating the et-tube cuff (Figure 10.7). In goats and sheep, a long laryngoscope handle with the neck extended and head held up can help ease intubation. Due to a lack of opening of the mouth, sometimes a long stylet can be useful in aiding in intubation. Cows may require manual palpation of the arytenoids for intubation but can be achieved blindly with the head extended.

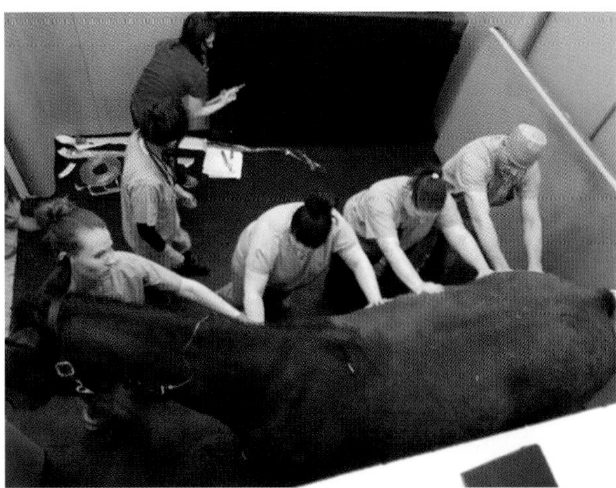

Figure 10.6 Induction of a horse requires multiple people with safety kept in mind.

Camelids can present more of a challenge in that they are more difficult to keep in sternal recumbency with the head elevated, the mouth opening is also narrow, and in camels, digital palpation is necessary to intubate. Alpacas and llamas have a small oral cavity and need to be intubated similar to goats and sheep, with the head elevated and a long laryngoscope available (Figure 10.8).

For all ruminants, an orogastric tube should be placed into the esophagus to allow for drainage of rumen contents. Rumination continues under anesthesia; this tube will aid in prevention of aspiration pneumonia. Suctioning prior to recovery is recommended.

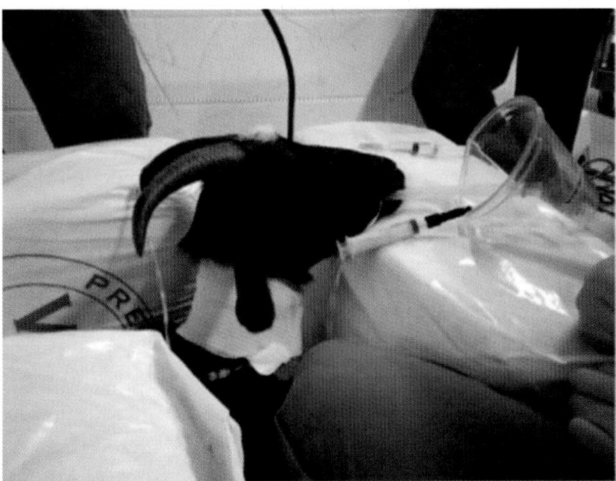

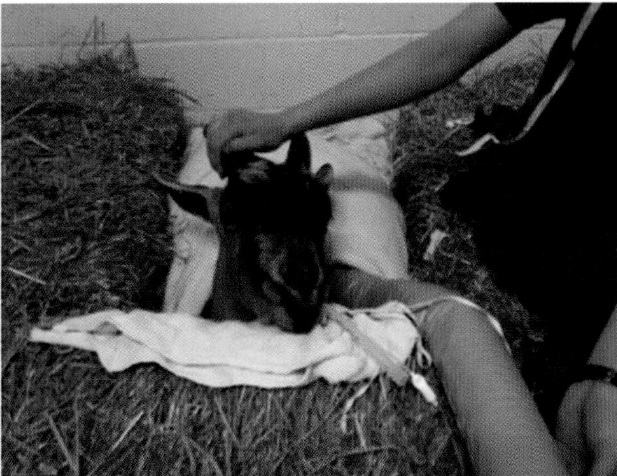

Figure 10.7 Ruminants should be kept in sternal through the induction and recovery phase. *Source:* Courtesy of Meagan Smith, RVT, VTS (Anesthesia).

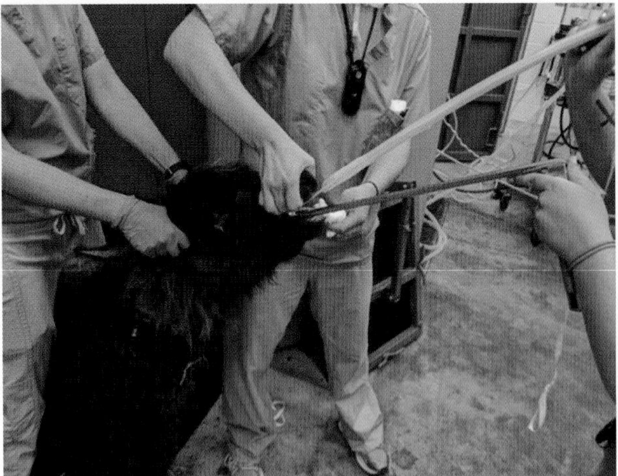

Figure 10.8 Camelids need to be in sternal with the head lifted while being intubated.

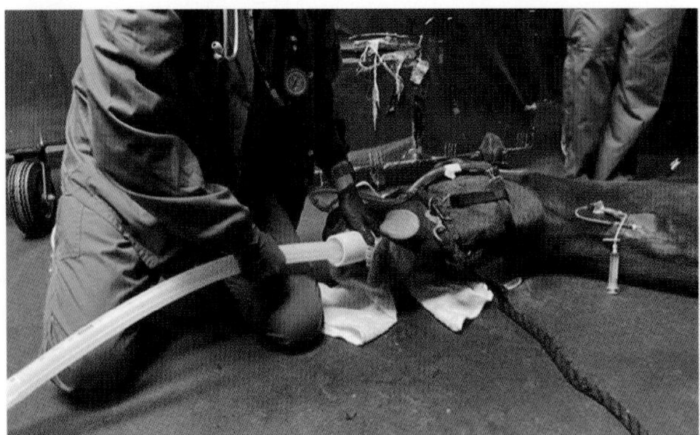

Figure 10.9 A horse being intubated.

Horses are intubated blindly in lateral with the head extended; after placing a speculum, a large silicon tube can be guided gently with a twist past the arytenoids (Figure 10.9). Be mindful of the back teeth to avoid tears in the cuff. After placing, inflate cuff and push on the chest to confirm air movement until capnography can be added, which will help ensure placement.

Foals can be intubated via nasal tracheal if too small to intubate traditionally. Lidocaine can be sprayed into the nostril to facilitate intubation and decrease irritation. Proper lubrication of the tube is required to decrease mucosal irritation. The tube should be directed ventrally to avoid hitting the ethmoid turbinate and causing hemorrhage.

Pigs can prove difficult to intubate as they have small tracheas and a pharyngeal diverticulum. Due to the diverticulum visual confirmation of intubation can be deceptive, and capnography should be used to confirm placement. The trachea of swine is delicate and prone to bleeding, which can lead to aspiration, blood clots preventing gas exchange, and obstruction of the airway (Figure 10.10).

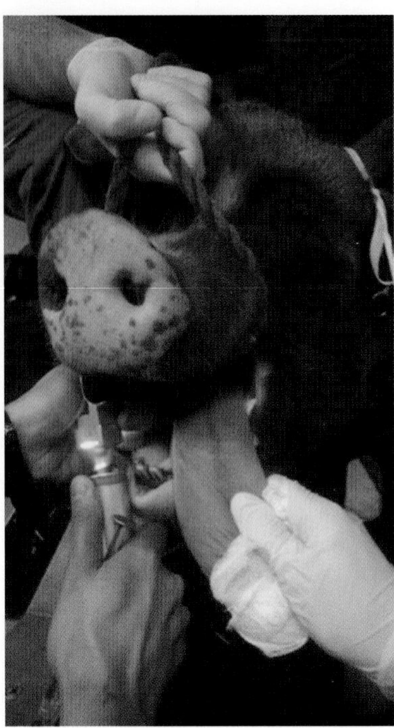

Figure 10.10 Pig intubation can be difficult due to their small trachea and a pharyngeal diverticulum.

When inhalant anesthesia is not an option for horses and cows or for a short procedure, triple drip with guaifenesin, ketamine, and xylazine can be used for up to 2 hr for total intravenous anesthesia (TIVA). Combined with local blocks, it provides adequate anesthesia and analgesia allowing tasks to be performed safely. Monitoring of the patients to ensure breathing and depth is necessary. The rate of the drip many need to be adjusted periodically to maintain proper depth, with the average being 1–2 ml/kg/hr. Patients recovering from TIVA with this combination should be kept down as long as possible with additional boluses of α_2 agonist and manual restraint when possible. Guaifenesin relaxes muscles and causes weakness that contributes to poor recoveries and injuries.

With all anesthetic events, patient monitoring is essential for the safety of the animal and staff. Anesthetic depth should be monitored every 15 min by checking ocular position, palpebral, and rectal tone if able. While recording an anesthesia record or observing, trends should be monitored for changes that could indicate a change in depth or foreseeable problem (Figure 10.11).

Whenever possible, all vitals should be monitored including heart rate, respiratory rate, capillary refill time, blood pressure, capnography, and carbon dioxide levels. Arterial blood pressure monitoring is considered the gold standard. A properly placed and secure arterial catheter can allow for easy sampling of arterial blood gases. An arterial blood gas should be checked hourly to ensure proper ventilation in larger species and electrolyte status (Figure 10.12).

Hypotension should be treated quickly to avoid decreased muscle perfusion as this will lead to a difficult recovery and increased lactic acid. Fluid boluses and a positive inotrope or vasopressor can be added for difficult cases. Dopamine or phenylephrine diluted and given to effect works rapidly but should be adjusted slowly to prevent arrhythmias and profound vasoconstriction. Constant rate infusions such as ketamine or dexmedetomidine can be added to decrease MAC of inhalant, therefore, further decreasing vasodilation.

Recovery for all species varies based on anesthetic time, metabolism, and temperature. All species should be safely kept down until nystagmus is no longer present and spontaneous breathing is occurring regularly. Any large species attempting to move or exhibiting nystagmus should be sedated to encourage a slow recovery to prevent injury.

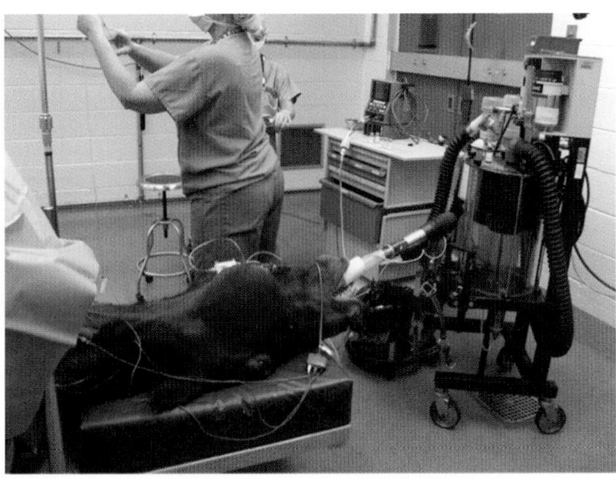

Figure 10.11 Anesthetized horse in dorsal recumbency.

Padded recovery stalls for horses, cows, and camelids are necessary to prevent injury as they may stumble or roll during recovery. Halters, bumpers, and ropes can be useful aids in assisting these larger species recoveries while keeping a safe distance and avoid being injured (Figure 10.13).

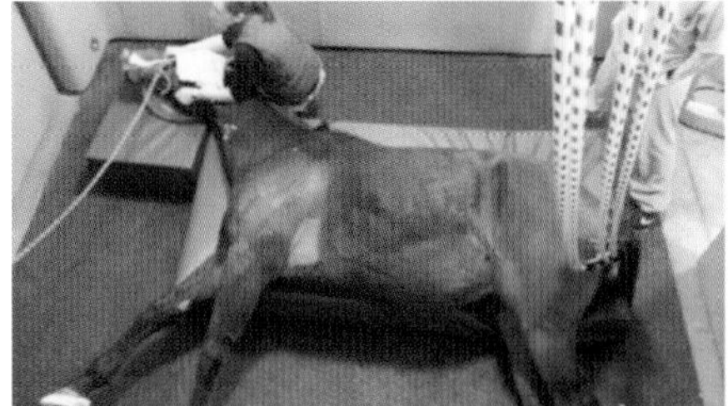

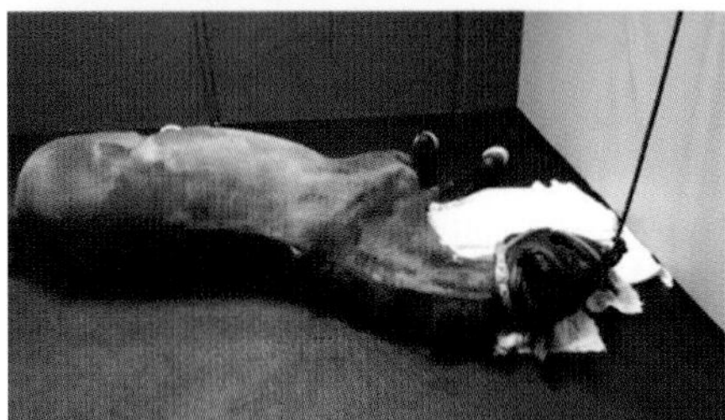

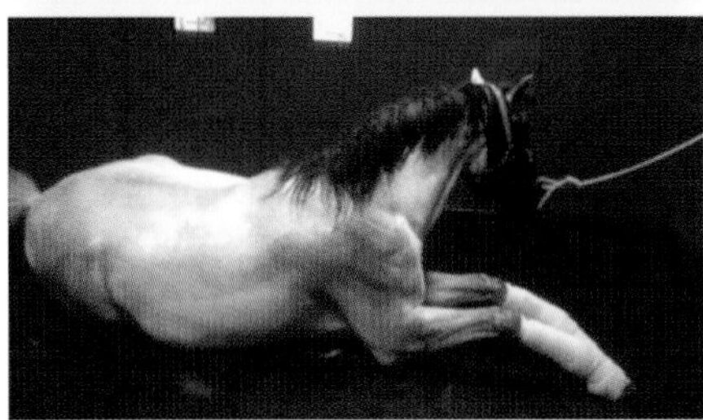

Figure 10.13 (Top) Horse still intubated, note the down leg is moved forward to prevent radial nerve damage. (Middle) Horse laying lateral after being extubated. (Bottom) You want the horse to stay sternal as long as possible during recovery. *Source:* Courtesy of Meagan Smith, RVT, VTS (Anesthesia).

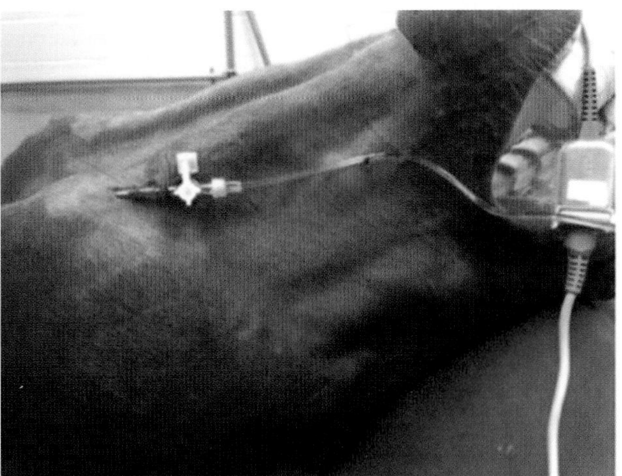

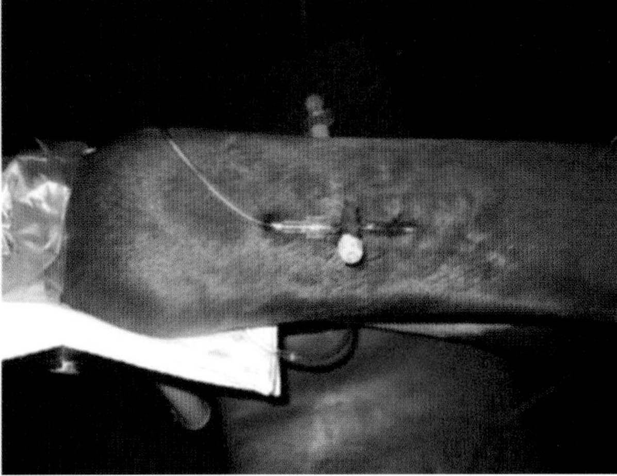

Figure 10.12 Arterial catheter placed in a horse; (left) facial artery; (right) metatarsal artery. *Source:* Courtesy of Meagan Smith, RVT, VTS (Anesthesia).

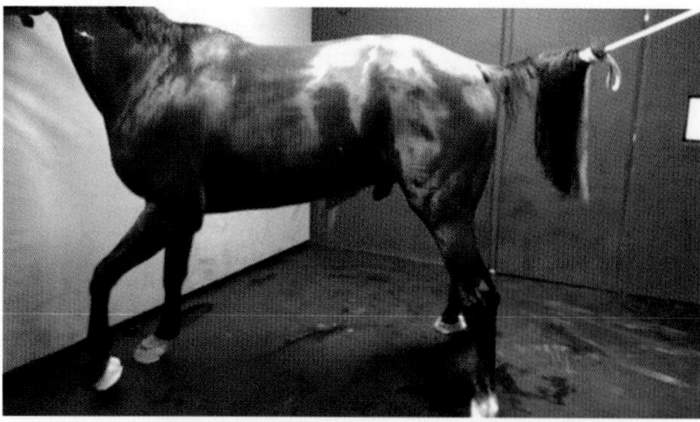

Figure 10.14 A horse standing in the recovery stall show signs of radial nerve paralysis in the left front leg. Prominent sign of radial nerve paralysis is the dropped elbow on the left front leg. *Source:* Courtesy of Meagan Smith, RVT, VTS (Anesthesia).

Positioning is equally important during recovery as in surgery. The front down leg should be pulled forward then released to prevent radial nerve damage, which could be catastrophic for the patient (Figure 10.14).

TECHNICIAN TIP 10.8: The surrounding area must be kept quite during recovery to help decrease stimulation.

Fluids are recommended in all anesthetic events to replace losses and compensate for any deficits. Decreased cardiac output due to medication administration or co-existing disease may require fluid boluses to compensate for vasodilation or losses. Electrolytes abnormalities and co-morbidities should be considered when choosing fluids for administration. The most common fluids to administer are isotonic (e.g. Plasma-Lyte, Lactated Ringer's Solution, Normosol-R).

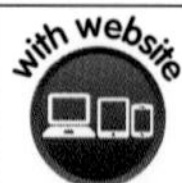

Check out additional surgeries

Equine Surgery

Colic Surgery

Relevant Anatomy

Colic is defined as abdominal pain, and it is perhaps the most common medical emergency we see in horses (Figure 10.16). The most common causes of colic in horses are impaction, large colon volvulus, right/left dorsal displacement, strangulating lipoma, and small intestinal intussusception. Although some colic episodes can be managed medically, others will require surgery to correct. Colic lesions are located within the gastrointestinal tract (Figure 10.18). This includes the stomach, mesentery, small intestine (duodenum, jejunum, ileum), cecum, and colon. It is important to note that some horses will display clinical signs of colic while having pain that originates outside of the abdominal cavity (i.e. pleural pneumonia, laminitis, etc.).

Indications

An exploratory celiotomy, or colic surgery, is indicated if the horses' pain is severe, persistent, and/or refractory to non-steroidal anti-inflammatory drugs (flunixin meglumine), α_2 agonists (xylazine, detomidine, romifidine), and opiates (butorphanol). Lack of response to medical management is also an indicator that surgery is the best course of action. However, if the colic lesion is known, and cannot be corrected medically, it is best to get the horse into surgery as soon as possible. These lesions include large colon volvulus, strangulating lipomas, and small intestinal intussusceptions.

Anesthesia and Surgical Preparation

Colic surgery is performed with the horse under general anesthesia. Before surgery, the horse's mouth should be rinsed to prevent aspiration of feed material during intubation, and the hair coat should be brushed to remove bedding and other debris.

An intravenous catheter is placed making it easier to administer perioperative and anesthetic medications. Preoperative medications should be given within 60 min of the surgery. Prophylactic antimicrobials will reduce the risk of incisional infections, septic peritonitis, and adhesions while anti-inflammatories will reduce surgical pain and treat endotoxemia.

Once anesthesia has been induced, an endotracheal tube is placed. The horse is then moved onto the surgery table and positioned in dorsal recumbency (Figure 10.17). Care must be taken to pad the horse appropriately and avoid pressure myopathies. The horse is maintained on inhalant anesthesia (isoflurane or sevoflurane) and positive pressure ventilation is used throughout the remainder of the surgery.

A urinary catheter is placed, and rectal sleeves are put over the patient's feet and tail to prevent contamination to the operating room. The abdomen is clipped from the xiphoid to the inguinal area and out to the edge of the ribcage. A rough preparation of the surgical field is done with betadine or chlorhexidine scrub for at least 5 min. The patient is then taken into the surgery area. Once positioned in the operating room, aseptic preparation of the surgical field is done with betadine or chlorhexidine scrub and alcohol.

Instrumentation

There are many instruments needed for an exploratory celiotomy. Some of the instruments used will depend on what lesion is being corrected and surgeon preference. A large

Drug	Route	Horse	Cattle	Camelids	Sheep	Goat	Pig
Romifidine	IV	0.04–0.1 mg/kg	0.003–0.02 mg/kg	0.04–0.12 mg/kg	0.003–0.04 mg/kg	0.003–0.04 mg/kg	
	IM	0.08–0.12 mg/kg	0.02–0.04 mg/kg		0.04–0.08 mg/kg	0.04–0.08 mg/kg	0.05–0.15 mg/kg
Xylazine	IV	0.5–1.0 mg/kg	0.01–0.1mg/kg	0.01–0.06 mg/kg	0.05–0.2 mg/kg	0.02–0.15 mg/kg	0.025–0.05 mg/kg
	IM	1–2 mg/kg	0.02–0.5 mg/kg	0.2–0.4 mg/kg	0.1–0.25 mg/kg	0.05–0.25 mg/kg	1–3 mg/kg
Detomidine	IV	0.01–0.02 mg/kg	0.003–0.01 mg/kg	0.02–0.04 mg/kg	0.01–0.02 mg/kg	0.05–0.02 mg/kg	0.02–0.04 mg/kg
	IM	0.02–0.04 mg/kg	0.005–0.02 mg/kg	0.02–0.04 mg/kg	0.02–0.03 mg/kg	0.02–0.03 mg/kg	0.04–0.08 mg/kg
Dexmedetomidine	IV	0.003–0.005 mg/kg	0.001–0.005 mg/kg	0.01–0.02 mg/kg	0.005–0.01 mg/kg	0.005–0.01 mg/kg	0.005–0.01 mg/kg
	IM		0.005–0.02 mg/kg	0.01–0.03 mg/kg	0.01–0.03 mg/kg	0.01–0.03 mg/kg	0.04–0.08
Acepromazine	IV	0.02–0.05 mg/kg	0.03–0.05 mg/kg	0.01–0.03 mg/kg	0.02–0.05 mg/kg	0.02–0.05 mg/kg	0.03–1 mg/kg
	IM	0.02–0.05 mg/kg	0.05–1 mg/kg		0.05–0.1 mg/kg	0.05–0.1 mg/kg	0.05–0.5 mg/kg
Midazolam	IV	0.02–0.06 mg/kg	0.05–0.2 mg/kg	0.1–0.5 mg/kg	0.2–0.6 mg/kg	0.2–0.6 mg/kg	0.1–0.5 mg/kg
	IM			0.5 mg/kg	0.4–1 mg/kg	0.4–1 mg/kg	0.2–0.4 mg/kg
Diazepam	IV	0.02–0.06 mg/kg	0.2–0.5 mg/kg	0.1–0.5 mg/kg	0.25–0.5 mg/kg	0.25–0.5 mg/kg	0.1–0.3 mg/kg
	IM						0.5–1 mg/kg
Ketamine	IV	2–3 mg/kg	0.05–0.5 mg/kg	1.1 mg/kg	1–2 mg/kg	1–2 mg/kg	0.2–6 mg/kg
	IM	1–2 mg/kg	0.1–0.5 mg/kg	2-5 mg/kg	10–15 mg/kg	1–1.5 mg/kg	1–12 mg/kg
Telazol	IV	0.7–1.0 mg/kg	1–2 mg/kg	1–2 mg/kg	2–4 mg/kg	1–5 mg/kg	1–2 mg/kg
	IM	0.5–1 mg/kg		2–4 mg/kg	6–12 mg/kg		1–8 mg/kg
Butorphanol	IV	0.01–0.04 mg/kg	0.05–0.1 mg/kg	0.05–0.1 mg/kg	0.05–0.5 mg/kg	0.05–0.5 mg-kg	0.1–0.2 mg/kg
	IM	0.01–0.02 mg/kg	0.2 mg/kg	0.05–0.2 mg/kg	0.2–0.4 mg/kg	0.2–0.4 mg/kg	0.1–0.5 mg/kg
Morphine	IV	0.1–0.2 mg/kg	0.05–0.1 mg/kg	0.05–0.1 mg/kg	0.01–0.05 mg/kg	0.05–2 mg/kg	
	IM	0.1–0.2 mg/kg	0.05–mg/kg	0.05–0.1 mg/kg			
Fentanyl	IV	0.004–0.01 mg/kg			0.002–0.01 mg/kg	0.002–0.01 mg/kg	
Propofol	IV	2–6 mg/kg	2–6 mg/kg	2–6 mg/kg	2–6 mg/kg	2–6 mg/kg	2–6 mg/kg
Phenylbutazone	IV, PO	1.1–4.4 mg/kg			5–6 mg/kg PO	5–6 mg/kg PO	5–6 mg/kg PO
Flunixin	IV,IM,PO	1.1 mg/kg	1.1–2.2 mg/kg	2.2 mg/kg	1.1 mg/kg IV	1.1 mg/kg IV	1–4 mg/kg IM, SC
Meloxicam		0.6 mg/kg IV	0.5–1 mg/kg PO	0.5 mg/kg IV	0.5 mg/kg	0.5 mg/kg	0.4 mg/kg PO, IM, SC
Carprofen		0.7 mg/kg IV	1.4 mg/kg IV		10.7 mg/kg IV	0.7 mg/kg IV	2 mg/kg PO, SC

Figure 10.15 Drug chart for multiple species.

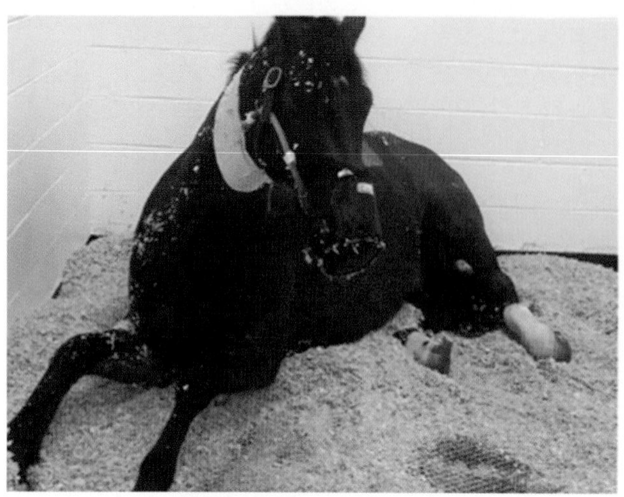

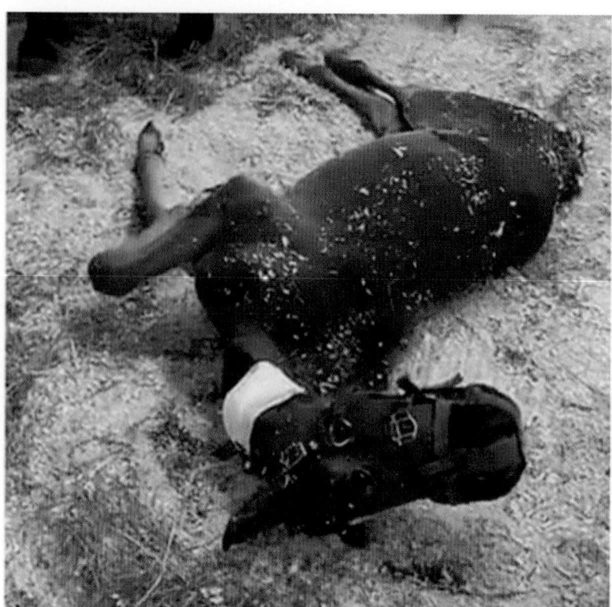

Figure 10.16 (Left) adult horse colicking; (right) foal colicking.

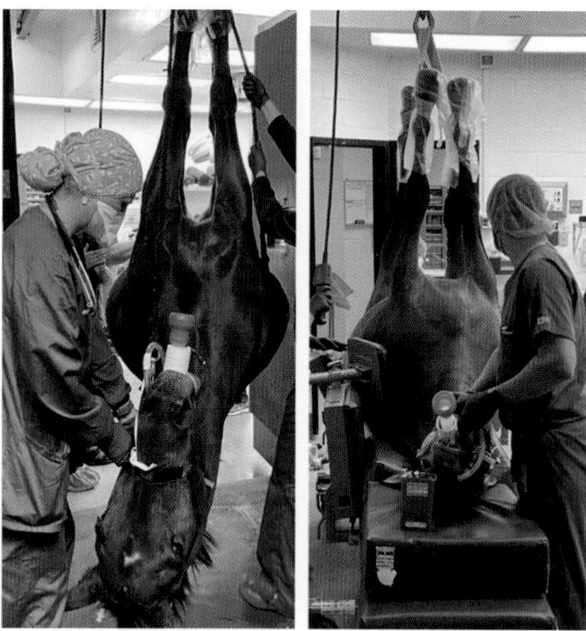

Figure 10.17 Horse being lifted from the induction stall and moved into surgery.

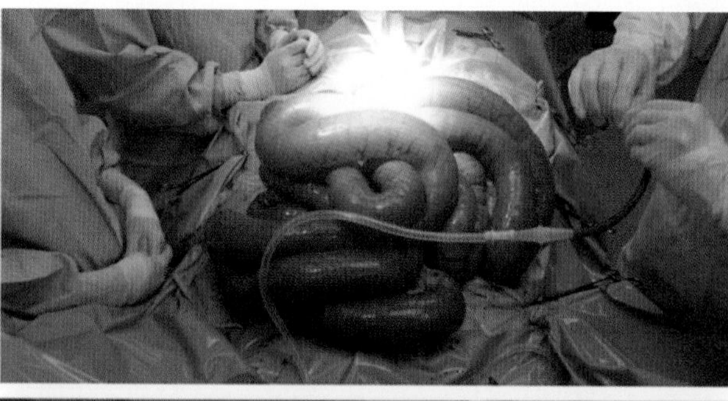

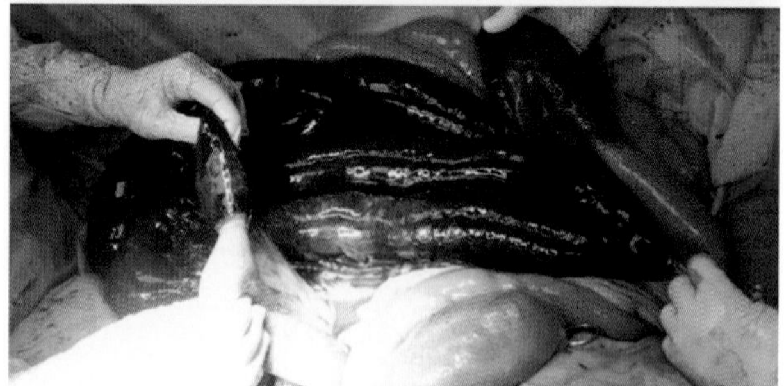

Figure 10.18 (Top) healthy small intestine; (bottom) dead small intestine with a clear demarcation line.

instrument pack containing scissors (Metzenbaum, mayo, suture), needle drivers, forceps (sponge, Allis, Kelly, mosquito, Brown-Adson, rat tooth), blade handles (#3 and #4) and Backhaus towel clamps will be needed for all colic surgeries. In addition, a suction set up with Poole suction tip, needle adapter for the suction line, lap sponges, sterile saline, bowl and syringe, hand towels, and suture are necessary. The surgeon(s) will wear sterile non-permeable gowns, sterile gloves, and sterile blue sleeves. Some surgeons like to use a visceral retainer, or FISH, when closing. This is used to retain the omentum and viscera when closing the peritoneal cavity. The FISH is made out of a wide, flexible rubber that can be easily folded to remove through a small space once the body wall has been almost completely sutured closed.

The following is a list of additional instruments and equipment needed for some lesions:

- Resection and anastomosis:
  - Ligasure unit and ligasure handles (20 cm 10 mm)
  - Sterile mayo stand cover or garbage bag
- Impaction/enterotomy:
  - Enterotomy table
  - Y-hose
  - Sterile mayo stand covers or garbage bags
  - Extra bottles of sterile saline

> **TECHNICIAN TIP 10.9:** Any instrument that is used on the enterotomy site will be considered dirty and cannot be used again throughout the remainder of the surgery.

> **TECHNICIAN TIP 10.10:** The surgeon(s) will also need new gowns and gloves once the enterotomy is complete (Figure 10.19).

Post-operative Management

Close post-operative monitoring is critical in patients with gastrointestinal disease. Although the primary condition was corrected, secondary problems frequently result from disease processes on other body systems or portions of the gastrointestinal tract near the original lesion. The frequency of monitoring will depend on the lesion identified in surgery, the health status of the horse, and the veterinarian's preference.

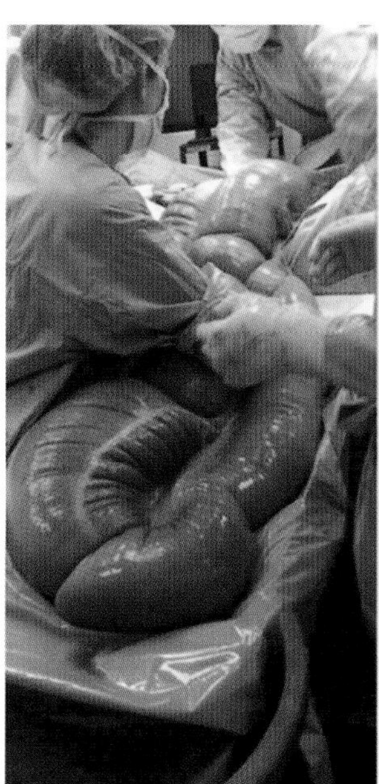

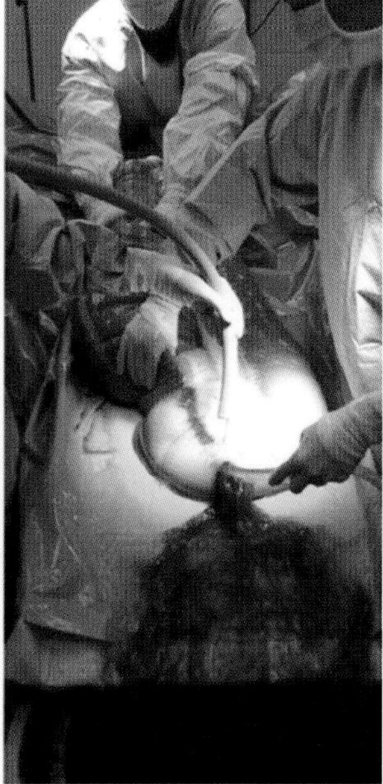

Figure 10.19 (Left) Full colon being placed on the enterotomy table. (Right) Colon enterotomy being performed.

Repeat physical exams will be done to fully assess the patient including mucous membrane color, heart and respiratory rate, urine and fecal production, digital extremity assessment, and rectal temperature. Gastrointestinal function is evaluated by parameters such as appetite, auscultating GI sounds, fecal production, and fecal consistency. It should be noted that if an enterotomy was performed, there may be less fecal output for a few days. Attention should be paid to pain indicators such as tachycardia, tachypnea, lack of GI motility, and behavioral signs such as abnormal posture, quiet demeanor, or traditional colic signs.

> **TECHNICIAN TIP 10.11:** A homemade strainer is a great way to filter feed stuff being evacuated from the caecum during an enterotomy.

It is important to frequently monitor the incision for signs of infection such as increased discharge or dehiscence. Excessive edema is also noteworthy. Any of these observations should be reported to the veterinarian immediately.

Dehydration and electrolyte imbalances are a common result of gastrointestinal disorders. Although the horse is stabilized and the primary lesion is corrected, replacement of fluid losses and electrolytes is critical. The daily fluid maintenance requirements for adult horses is 50–60 ml/kg and for foals is 70–80 ml/kg. Fluid supplementation must account for maintenance and any ongoing losses. Fluids available for replacement therapy include Lactated Ringers Solution, Normosol-R, and Plasma-Lyte.

Post-operative pain that is not addressed can cause suffering and distress, and result in poor GI motility, delayed wound healing, and weight loss. Flunixin meglumine provides post-operative analgesia and anti-inflammatory benefits. It is commonly administered for three to five days post-operatively. Intravenous lidocaine CRIs can be used for its analgesic, anti-inflammatory, and prokinetic affects as well (Figure 10.20).

> **TECHNICIAN TIP 10.12:** When using multiple IV fluid pumps, labeling them will keep them organized and reduce risk of errors.

Perioperative administration of broad-spectrum antimicrobials will assist in prevention of incisional infections, and together with anti-inflammatories may also help to prevent adhesion formation. Potassium penicillin and gentamicin are the most commonly used perioperative antimicrobials in horses undergoing GI surgery. The medications used and frequency/duration of administration will vary between surgeons and hospitals.

Complications and Prognosis

Recurrent abdominal pain is the greatest complication in the post-operative period. The risk is highest in the first 60 days after surgery, and surgical colic's are said to be at five times greater risk for recurrent colic than the general horse population. There can be many causes for post-operative colic, and it may resolve with conservative medical management. Common sources of pain include reoccurrence of the original lesion, adhesions, post-operative ileus, ongoing intestinal ischemia, incisional infections, or occurrence of a completely new lesion (Figure 10.21).

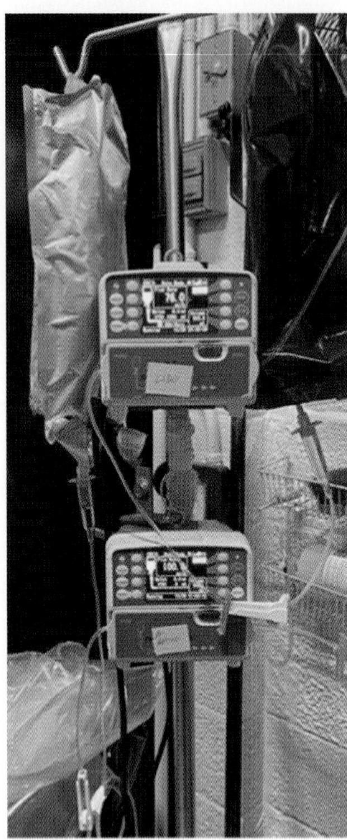

Figure 10.20 Amino acids and lidocaine CRI being delivered to a post-operative colic.

The prognosis for colic surgery patients is dependent on what the original colic lesion was, and the duration of their colic prior to surgical correction. As with most disease processes, early intervention is best. Age and physical condition can also affect outcome, although many older patients do very well. Because intense post-operative treatment is necessary, successful treatment is costly. A limiting factor in determining outcome can be a client's economic limitations.

Laparoscopy (Cryptorchids/Ovariectomies)

Relevant Anatomy

Laparoscopy is a surgical technique in which an abdominal surgery can be performed through a few small incisions (approximately 1 cm in length). Laparoscopies are commonly performed on horses to remove one or both ovaries (ovariectomy). An ovariectomy is indicated if an ovary is enlarged due to tumor, hematoma, or cyst, or for behavior modification when hormone therapy is unsuccessful. Granulosa cell tumors are the most common equine ovarian tumor. Affected mares may show anestrus, intermittent or continuous estrus (nymphomania), or stallion-like behavior. Generally, the affected ovary is enlarged, some-

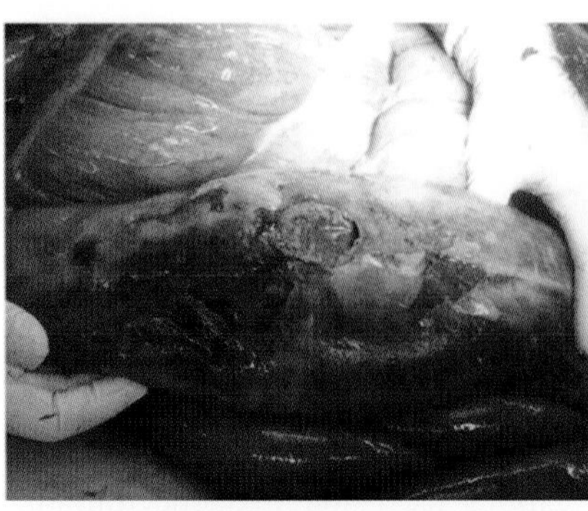

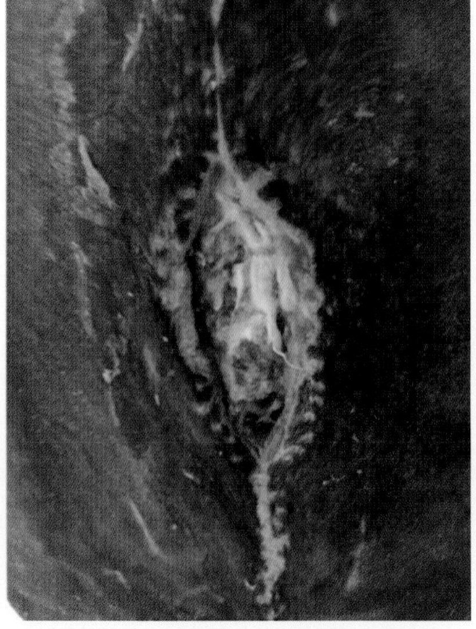

Figure 10.21 (Left) Perforation of the intestine (Right) Post-operative incisional infection with dehiscence.

times quite massively, and the contralateral ovary is usually small and inactive.

Removal of undescended testicles (cryptorchidectomy) can also be performed via laparoscopy. These testicles still produce testosterone, and therefore, the horse will display stallion-like behavior until the testicle is removed; however, cryptorchid testis are incapable of producing sperm. Unilateral cryptorchids are usually fertile but have reduced production of sperm, and horses affected with bilateral cryptorchidism are sterile.

Indications

Laparoscopies provide many benefits when compared with a traditional celiotomy. The incisions are much smaller, allowing for easier post-operative incisional care and faster recovery. In many cases, visualization is better with this approach as well. In addition, many laparoscopies can be done under standing sedation, eliminating the risks of general anesthesia.

Anesthesia and Surgical Preparation

Many laparoscopies can be done with standing sedation and local nerve blocks, while others require general anesthesia. Still others can be partially completed with the horse standing and then finished under general anesthesia.

Before surgery, feed should be withheld for 12–36 hr depending on surgeon preference. This will decrease the volume of ingesta in the intestines making visualization of the ovaries or testicle possible. It is important to note that disruption of the horses' diet or feeding schedule can increase the possibility of developing GI abnormalities such as colic or diarrhea.

An intravenous catheter is placed making it easier to administer perioperative medications and sedation or anesthesia throughout the procedure. The hair coat is brushed to remove bedding and other contaminants.

Perioperative anti-inflammatories and antimicrobials are indicated. It is recommended that the first dose be given within 60 min prior to surgery. Prophylactic antimicrobials will reduce the risk of incisional infections and septic peritonitis while anti-inflammatories will reduce surgical pain and inflammation.

Standing laparoscopy under sedation: The horse is positioned in the stocks and the flank is clipped from the 17th rib to just caudle to the distal border of the tuber coxae and from the dorsal midline down to the level of the stifle. This will give good margins around the incision(s) which will be in the paralumbar fossa (Figure 10.22). After clipping, a rough preparation of the surgical site is done with betadine or chlorhexidine scrub for at least 5 min. Once the rough prep is complete, the surgeon will do a local block of the incision sites. Many surgeons use mepivacaine, or a combination of

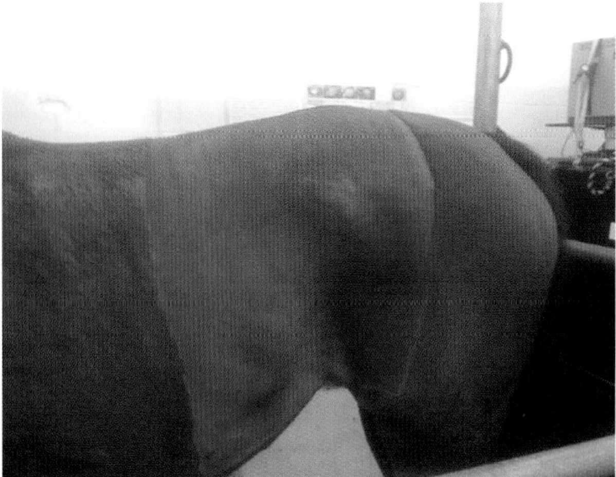

Figure 10.22 Horse that is clipped for a standing laparoscopy.

mepivacaine and lidocaine for this local block. Aseptic preparation with betadine or chlorhexidine scrub and alcohol follows the local block (Figure 10.23).

Throughout the surgery, the patient is maintained on a sedation CRI. Detomidine hydrochloride is the most commonly used drug for sedation and analgesia. It is commonly used in conjunction with butorphanol and xylazine. When used in combination with visceral and local anesthesia, this is very effective.

- Dorsal recumbency under general anesthesia: Once anesthesia has been induced; an endotracheal tube is placed. The horse is then moved onto the surgery table and positioned in dorsal recumbency. Care must be taken to pad the horse appropriately and avoid pressure myopathies. The horse is maintained on inhalant anesthesia (isoflurane or sevoflurane), and positive pressure ventilation is used throughout the remainder of the surgery.

A urinary catheter is placed, and rectal sleeves are put over the patient's feet and tail to prevent contamination to the operating room. The abdomen is clipped from the umbilicus to the inguinal area and out to the stifles. A rough preparation of the surgical site is done with betadine or chlorhexidine scrub for at least 5 min. The patient is then taken into the surgery area. Once positioned in the operating room, aseptic preparation of the surgical field is done with betadine or chlorhexidine scrub and alcohol.

When performing a laparoscopy in dorsal recumbency, the horse may need to be placed in Trendelenburg position. By tilting the head down and the hindquarters up, the surgeon is able to better visualize the caudal abdomen. There are two complications related to this. The viscera will slide forward due to gravity effects which puts pressure on the diaphragm and will cause breathing problems if the horse

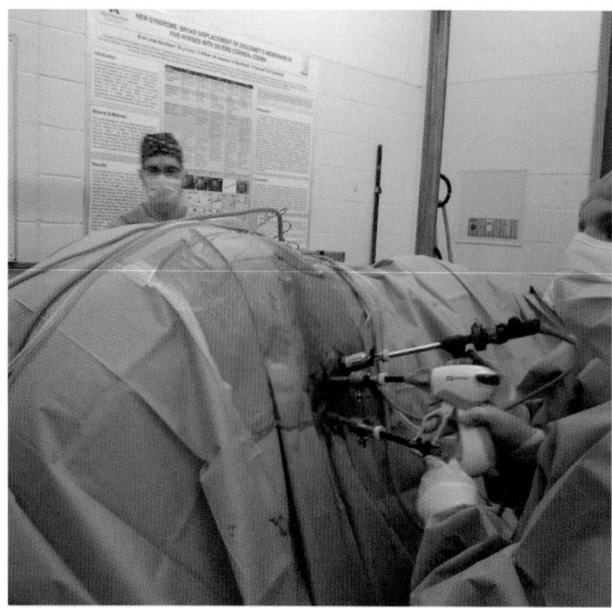

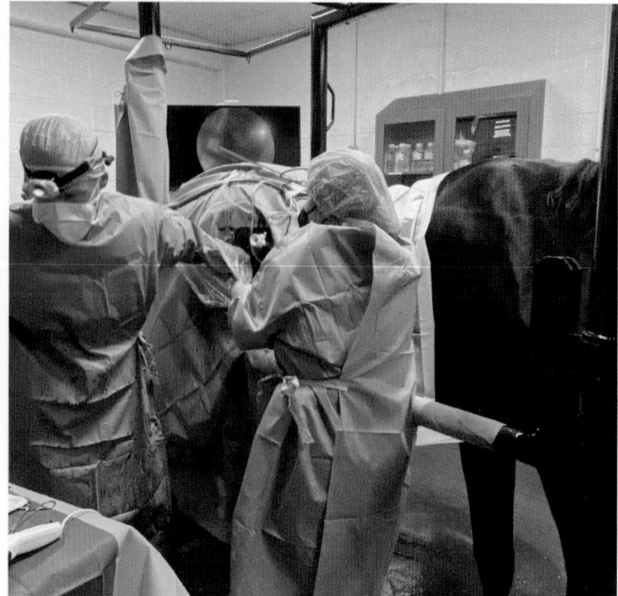

Figure 10.23 Two different views of a standing laparoscopy. Source: Courtesy of Kobi Derks, RVT.

is not ventilated. The horse also has the potential to slide off the table if not secured properly.

Instrumentation

Laparoscopies require a lot of instrumentation. A large instrument pack containing scissors (Metzenbaum, mayo, suture), needle drivers, forceps (sponge, Allis, Kelly, mosquito, Brown-Adson, rat tooth), blade handles (#3 and #4), and Backhaus towel clamps will be necessary for all laparoscopic surgeries (Figure 10.24). In addition, gauze, lap sponges, sterile saline, bowl and syringe, hand towels, and suture are needed. The surgeons will wear sterile gowns and sterile gloves.

In addition, the following laparoscopic equipment is needed:

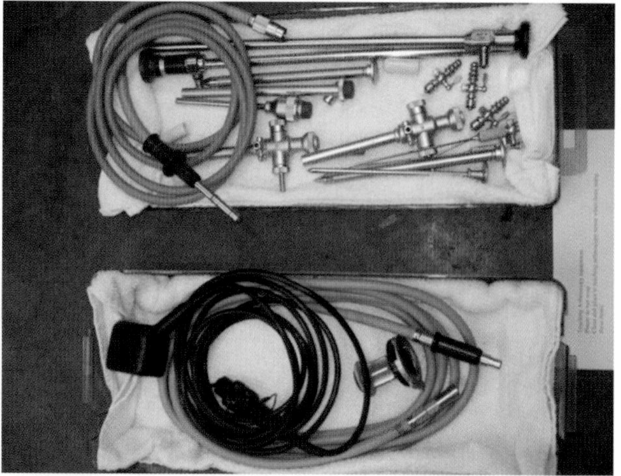

Figure 10.24 Laparoscopy pack.

- Laparoscopy tower – Holds the camera box, light source, insufflator and carbon dioxide tank, and viewing screen.
- Laparoscope – A rigid fiber optic scope inserted through the abdominal wall to view abdominal organs. Available with a 0° or 30° viewing lens.
- Camera – Attaches to the laparoscope and transmits the image to a screen on the laparoscopy tower for all who are involved to view.
- Light cord – Attaches to the laparoscope and the light source on the laparoscopy tower. Provides light in the abdomen. In a minimally invasive surgery, the room lights do not help with visualization.
- Insufflation – Attaches to the cannula and the insufflator unit on the laparoscopy tower. Carbon dioxide is passed through the tubing to insufflate the abdomen, creating pneumoperitoneum and giving the surgeon space to maneuver and work.
- Trocars – Trocars are made of two pieces, a cannula and an obturator. They allow instrumentation into the peritoneal space without loss of pneumoperitoneum.
- Laparoscopy instruments – Similar to instruments designed for open surgery, but they are longer, have smaller jaws and do not have inline handles to facilitate working through a cannula.
- Ligation and hemostasis – Ligation and hemostasis within the abdominal cavity is a critical part of a minimally invasive surgery. Techniques for accomplishing this include ligature, staplers, tie-raps, laser dissection, and monopolar and bipolar electrosurgical devices.

> **TECHNICIAN TIP 10.13:** It is important to realize that cannulated instruments and complex articulated instruments such as those used in laparoscopy surgeries have the ability to house infectious agents unless taken apart and very thoroughly cleaned.

> **TECHNICIAN TIP 10.14:** Reusable laparoscopy instrumentation is designed so that it can be taken apart to clean. Strict cleaning and sterilization processes should be followed.

Post-operative Management

Refeeding the horse post-laparoscopy is slower than most other surgeries due to the 24–36 hr pre-operative fasting. What is fed (mash vs. grass hay) and how soon after surgery will vary based on surgeon preference.

Close post-operative monitoring is critical for laparoscopy patients. These horses are prone to colic (most often in the 24–36 hr following surgery). This happens more frequently in ovariectomy than cryptorchidectomy patients due to ovarian pedicle pain and a larger vessel being severed. The frequency of monitoring will depend on the veterinarian's preference. Repeat physical exams will be done to fully assess the patient including heart and respiratory rate, urine and fecal production, and rectal temperature. Gastrointestinal function is evaluated by parameters such as appetite, auscultating GI sounds, fecal production, and fecal consistency. Attention should be paid to pain indicators such as tachycardia, tachypnea, lack of GI motility, and behavioral signs such as abnormal posture, quiet demeanor, or traditional colic signs.

It is important to monitor the incision for signs of infection such as increased discharge or dehiscence. Excessive edema is also noteworthy. Any of these observations should be reported to the veterinarian immediately. Some surgeons spray the suture line with Aluspray to help protect it from infection.

Perioperative administration of broad-spectrum antimicrobials and anti-inflammatory drugs will assist in prevention of incisional infections and reduce pain and inflammation. These patients are often sent home with trimethoprim sulfa and oral phenylbutazone or flunixin meglumine. The medications used and frequency/duration of administration will vary between surgeons and hospitals.

Complications and Prognosis

One of the most serious complications associated with laparoscopic procedures is bowel puncture. Decreasing the volume of gas and ingesta within the intestines by holding the horse off feed prior to surgery reduces the likelihood of this happening. Other complications include incisional infection, continued bleeding from the ovarian pedicle or castration stump, laceration of an artery while making portal incisions, and dropping the ovary or testicle after amputation but before removal from the abdomen.

In general, laparoscopic surgery is associated with better preservation of immune function and less inflammatory response than open surgery. With strict adherence to aseptic technique and a board-certified surgeon, the prognosis for these horses is great.

Tie-Back Surgery

Relevant Anatomy

Recurrent laryngeal neuropathy (RLN) affects the recurrent laryngeal nerves. Horses may develop bilateral or unilateral paralysis of the cricoarytenoideus dorsalis (CAD) muscle leading to dysfunction of the associated arytenoid cartilage but left-sided laryngeal paralysis is most common. The muscle paralysis results from a gradual loss of large myelinated axons in the laryngeal nerve. Most of these cases have a naturally occurring and unknown cause. However, the recurrent laryngeal nerve can also be damaged by perivascular jugular vein injection, strangles abscesses of the head and neck, impingement by neoplasms in the neck or chest, organophosphate toxicity, hepatic encephalopathy, and some diseases of the CNS. The goal of a tie-back surgery, or prosthetic laryngoplasty, is to attain some degree of permanent abduction of the affected arytenoid cartilage. Ideally, the result will be that the arytenoid cartilage is abducted enough to allow sufficient airflow during exercise, but not to allow saliva, food, or water into the trachea when swallowing.

Indications

Horses with RLN are unable to fully abduct the affected arytenoid cartilage and, therefore, are unable to sustain high-intensity exercise. Because of this, they develop hypoxia, hypercarbia, and metabolic acidosis more quickly than unaffected horses with similar workload. They may also make an abnormal noise, or "roar," on inspiration while exercising. If high-speed exercise is not expected, the horse may be able to tolerate and work despite the partial upper airway obstruction. Surgery may be indicated to allow the horse to perform to the owner's performance requirements.

> **TECHNICIAN TIP 10.15:** These horses are known as "roarers."

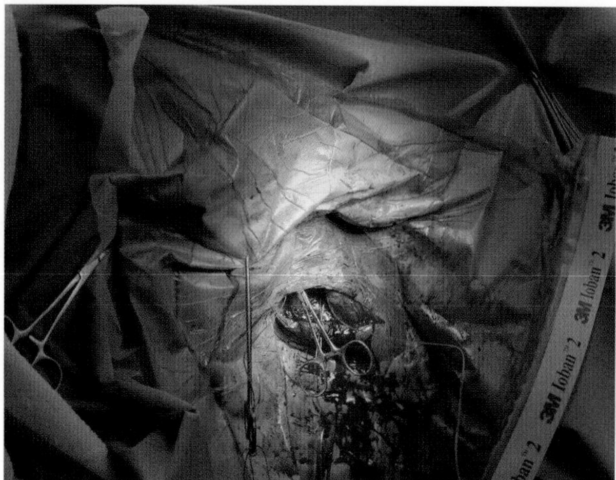

Figure 10.25 Standing tie-back surgery. *Source:* Courtesy of Molly Cripe Birt, RVT, VTS (EVN).

Anesthesia and Surgical Preparation

Prosthetic laryngoplasty, or tie-back surgery, is performed with the horse under general anesthesia. This surgery can also be performed standing (Figure 10.25). Before surgery, feed should be withheld for 6–8 hr and the horse's mouth should be rinsed to prevent aspiration of food material during intubation. The hair coat should be brushed to remove bedding and other debris.

An intravenous catheter is placed making it easier to administer perioperative medications. The catheter must be placed lower than normal due to the location of the surgical site. Pre-operative medications should be given within 60 min of the surgery. Prophylactic antimicrobials will reduce the risk of incisional infections while anti-inflammatories will reduce surgical pain and inflammation.

Once anesthesia has been induced, an endotracheal tube is placed. The horse is then moved onto the surgery table and positioned in lateral recumbency with the affected side up. The head and neck should be slightly extended. Care must be taken to pad the horse appropriately and avoid pressure myopathies. The horse is maintained on inhalant anesthesia (isoflurane or sevoflurane), and positive pressure ventilation is used throughout the remainder of the surgery.

A urinary catheter is placed, and rectal sleeves are put over the patient's feet and tail to prevent contamination to the operating room. The throat area is clipped from the mandible halfway down the neck and from the downside laterally past the jugular groove. A rough preparation of the surgical site is done with betadine or chlorhexidine scrub for at least 5 min. The patient is then taken into the surgery area. Once positioned in the operating room, aseptic preparation of the surgical field is performed with betadine or chlorhexidine scrub and alcohol.

Instrumentation

A large instrument pack containing scissors (Metzenbaum, mayo, suture), needle drivers, forceps (sponge, Allis, Kelly, mosquito, Brown-Adson, rat tooth), blade handles (#3), and Backhaus towel clamps will be needed. In addition, retractors (Weitlaner, army/navy, malleable, etc.), a suction set up with Yankauer tip, gauze, lap sponges, sterile saline, bowl and syringe, special tie-back instruments, hand towels, and suture are necessary. A 1M flexible endoscope should also be available in the operating room. This is passed transnasally and allows the surgeon(s) intraoperative viewing of the larynx. The surgeon(s) will wear sterile gowns and sterile gloves.

Post-op Management

Exactly when feeding begins post-surgery and the type of feed (mash vs. grass hay) will depend on surgeon preference. It is recommended that the feed be placed at the ground level to reduce laryngeal and upper tracheal contamination. This should be continued long term if possible. It should be noted that the horse may develop a chronic cough associated with eating. These horses should be closely monitored for dysphagia and coughing in the immediate post-operative period.

It is important to monitor the incision for signs of infection such as increased discharge or dehiscence. Excessive edema is also noteworthy and should be mentioned to the surgeon. Due to the anatomy involved in this surgery, careful attention must be paid to the horse's respiratory efforts. In some cases, a temporary tracheotomy must be performed to allow the horse to breathe comfortably until the inflammation goes down.

Perioperative administration of broad-spectrum antimicrobials and anti-inflammatory drugs will assist in prevention of incisional infections, and reduce pain and inflammation. In addition, most of these horses will be kept on antibiotics for an additional three to five days post-surgery since the large suture used to perform the tie-back is a foreign body. Topical administration of a pharyngeal medication (throat spray) is also recommended and usually administered BID for seven days. To administer throat spray, a #10 French catheter is advanced along the floor of the nasal passage into the nasal pharynx, and 20 ml of the solution is sprayed slowly through this catheter. In addition, the use of corticosteroids (20 mg Dexamethasone IV, SID for two to three days) is also often used. The medications used and frequency/duration of administration will vary between surgeons and hospitals.

Complications and Prognosis

In the first two weeks following surgery, the horse may experience wound infection, wound dehiscence, dysphagia, and coughing (usually) associated with eating. Loss of abduction (mild to severe) of the arytenoid cartilage is also possible. Severe or failed abduction may necessitate a revision laryngoplasty.

Possible chronic complications include persistent coughing; chronic airway contamination with feed, saliva, and water; chronic tracheitis and bronchitis; lung abscess formation; pneumonia; perilaryngeal abscess formation; suture pullout; progressive loss of abduction; and persistent nasal discharge of feed, water, and saliva.

The success rate of the laryngoplasty surgery varies and has been reported between 50 and 100%. This is due to different criteria used to measure success and the varied use of the horses. Although approximately 80% of racehorses have improved performance after surgery, the outcome is generally considered more successful in horses that are not intended to race after surgery.

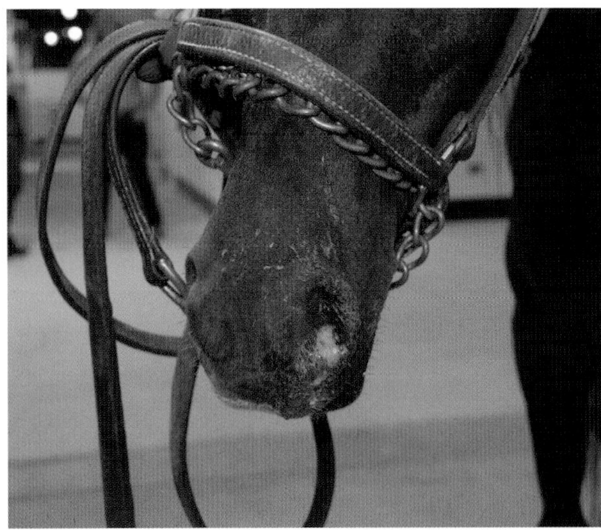

Figure 10.26 Purulent nasal discharge. *Source:* Courtesy of Kobi Derks, RVT.

Sinus Surgery

Relevant Anatomy

The horse has seven pairs of sinuses: the frontal, dorsal conchal, middle conchal (or ethmoidal), ventral conchal, caudal and rostral maxillary sinuses, and the sphenopalatine sinuses. The rostral and caudal maxillary sinuses communicate with the nasal cavity directly, while the other sinuses communicate indirectly through the maxillary sinuses. The paranasal sinuses are susceptible to infections that extend from the nasal cavity or from the upper cheek teeth. The maxillary sinus is more predisposed to infection than other sinuses due to its direct communication with the nasal cavity.

Indications

Clinical signs of paranasal sinus disease are unilateral nasal discharge, facial swelling, and decreased nasal airflow (Figure 10.26). Occasionally, external draining tracts, malodorous breath, ocular discharge, and stertor may occur.

Radiographic or CT imaging are the most useful diagnostic procedures to find the location and severity of paranasal sinus disease, although a tentative diagnosis is often made from the clinical signs, history, and physical exam. Abnormal radiographic findings pointing to paranasal sinus disease include increased opacity, free fluid accumulation, dental abnormalities, and related bone pathology.

Sinusitis is the most common disease of the paranasal sinuses and can be classified as primary or secondary, and acute or chronic. Primary sinusitis usually results from previous upper respiratory disease, whereas secondary sinusitis is often caused by dental disease, facial fractures, granulomatous lesions, or neoplasms. Secondary sinusitis is usually more difficult to treat and requires surgery to correct the primary problem.

Anesthesia and Surgical Preparation

The vast majority of sinus surgeries can be done with standing sedation and local nerve blocks, while others will require general anesthesia. If the surgery is being performed under general anesthesia, feed should be withheld for 6–8 hr prior to surgery depending on surgeon preference.

Before surgery, an intravenous catheter is placed making it easier to administer perioperative medications, and sedation or anesthesia throughout the procedure. The hair coat is brushed to remove bedding and other contaminants.

Pre-operative medications should be given within 60 min of the surgery. Prophylactic antimicrobials will reduce the risk of incisional infections while anti-inflammatories will reduce surgical pain and inflammation.

Trephination and bone flap are the two most common approaches to sinus surgery.

The surgery prep is the same for both:

- Standing under sedation: The horse is positioned in the stocks and the face is clipped with wide margins around the surgical site. This will vary based on which sinus is being accessed. After clipping, a rough preparation of the surgical site is done with dilute betadine solution (1 : 50) and sterile saline for at least 5 min. After the rough preparation is complete, the surgeon can do a local block of the incision site. Many surgeons use mepivacaine, or a combination of mepivacaine and lidocaine for this local block. After the local block is administered, aseptic preparation of the surgical field is done with dilute betadine solution (1 : 50) and sterile saline.

Throughout the surgery, the patient is maintained on a sedation CRI. Detomidine hydrochloride is the most commonly used drug for sedation and analgesia. It is commonly used in conjunction with butorphanol and xylazine.

- Lateral recumbency under general anesthesia: Once anesthesia has been induced; an endotracheal tube is placed. The horse is then moved onto the surgery table and positioned in lateral recumbency with the affected side up. Care must be taken to pad the horse appropriately and avoid pressure myopathies. The horse is maintained on inhalant anesthesia (isoflurane or sevoflurane), and positive pressure ventilation is used throughout the remainder of the surgery.

A urinary catheter is placed, and rectal sleeves are placed over the patient's feet and tail to prevent contamination to the operating room. The face is clipped with wide margins around the surgical site. This will vary based on which sinus is being accessed. A rough prep of the surgical site is done with betadine or chlorhexidine scrub for at least 5 min. The patient is then taken into the surgery area. Once positioned in the operating room, aseptic preparation of the surgical field is done with betadine or chlorhexidine scrub and alcohol.

Instrumentation

A large instrument pack containing scissors (Metzenbaum, mayo, suture), needle drivers, forceps (sponge, Allis, Kelly, mosquito, Brown-Adson, rat tooth), blade handles (#3), and Backhaus towel clamps will be needed. In addition, a suction set up with Poole and Yankauer suction tips, gauze, lap sponges, sterile saline, bowl and syringe, hand towels, and bandage material are necessary. Having bottles of saline on ice, Gelfoam, and/or phenylephrine on hand is recommended in case of hemorrhage. The surgeon(s) will wear sterile gowns and sterile gloves. The following is a list of additional instruments and equipment required for each approach.

- Trephination: (Figure 10.27)
  - Galt trephines (variety of sizes).
  - Foley catheters – May be used for indwelling lavage system.
  - Endoscope – May be inserted through the trephination site for better visualization of the sinus.
- Bone flap: Figure 10.28
  - Bone saw – Can be used to create the bone flap.
  - Carbon dioxide tank – Used to power the bone saw.
  - Osteotomes and mallet – Can be used in place of a bone saw.
  - Foley catheters – May be used for indwelling lavage system.

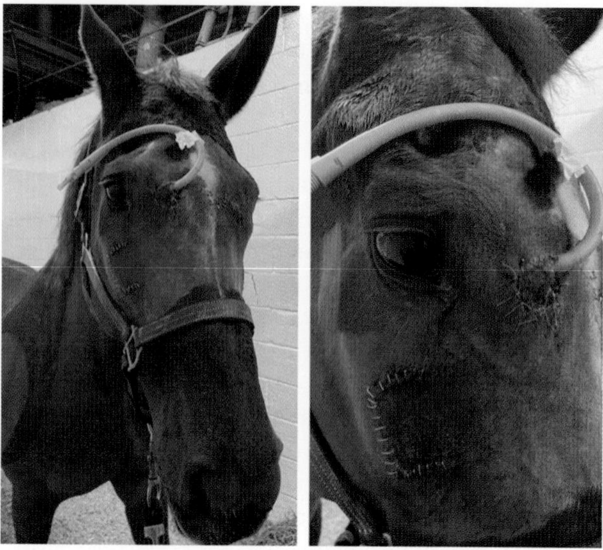

Figure 10.27 Horse with a bone flap and a trephine with foley catheter placed.

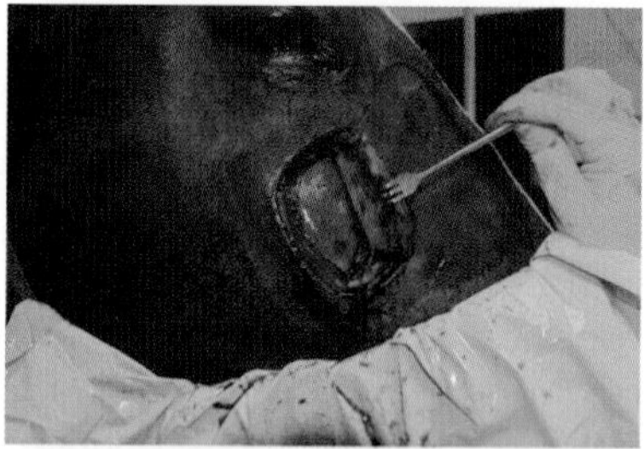

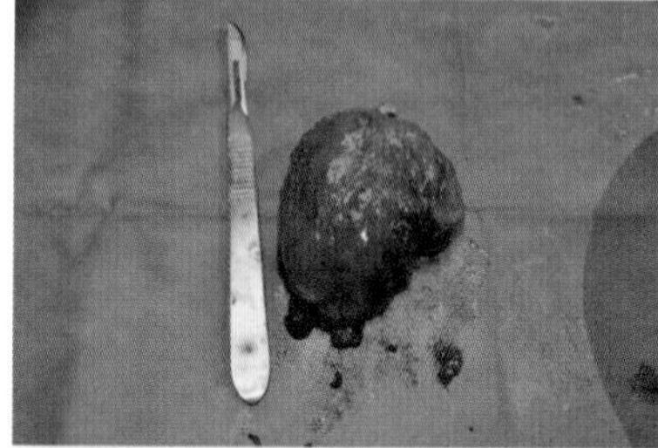

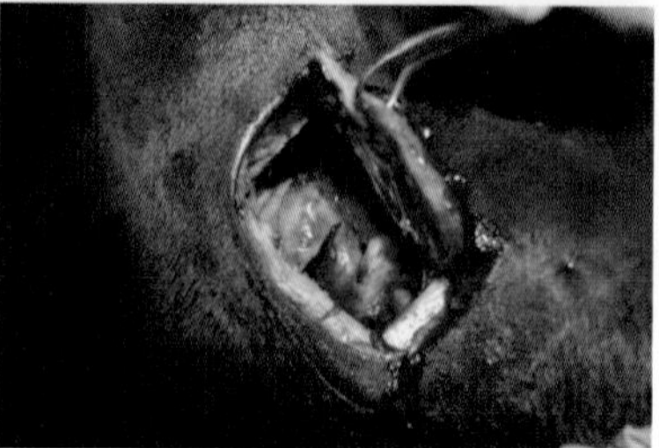

Figure 10.28 Ethmoid hematoma removal via bone flap. *Source:* Courtesy of Kobi Derks, RVT.

Post-Operative Management

If the surgery is performed standing, feeding of the regular diet can generally resume as soon as the sedation wears off. If the surgery is performed under general anesthesia, refeeding will vary based on surgeon preference.

It is important to monitor the incision for signs of infection such as increased discharge or dehiscence. Although some nasal drainage/bleeding is considered normal for the first week post-surgery, excessive bleeding is of concern and should be reported to the surgeon immediately.

Perioperative administration of broad-spectrum antimicrobials will assist in prevention of incisional infections and may be continued post-operatively as well. NSAIDS will reduce pain and inflammation and are usually continued for at least five days post-surgery. The medications used and frequency/duration of administration will vary between surgeons and hospitals.

A foley catheter is often sutured into the sinus during these surgeries to facilitate flushing. This is usually done one to two times per day until the sinus flushes consistently "clean." Some hospitals use saline, while others use saline with some betadine solution added. The foley catheter must be monitored to ensure the horse does not scratch it out when left unattended. Covering the foley with either bandage material and/or stockinette is recommended (Figure 10.29).

> **TECHNICIAN TIP 10.16:** It is important to note any strikethrough on the bandage to relay that to the veterinarian.

Complications and Prognosis

The biggest complication associated with equine sinus surgery is hemorrhage. When the surgery is performed standing, there is typically less blood loss because the horse's head is above its heart. Incisional infections are also possible but usually resolve with antibiotic treatment.

Horses with sinusitis typically have a good prognosis for return to function/athletic performance after appropriate treatment; however, prognosis correlates directly to the cause of the original sinus disease. For example, sinus cysts can be removed with an excellent prognosis, while neoplasia is generally malignant and carries a poorer prognosis.

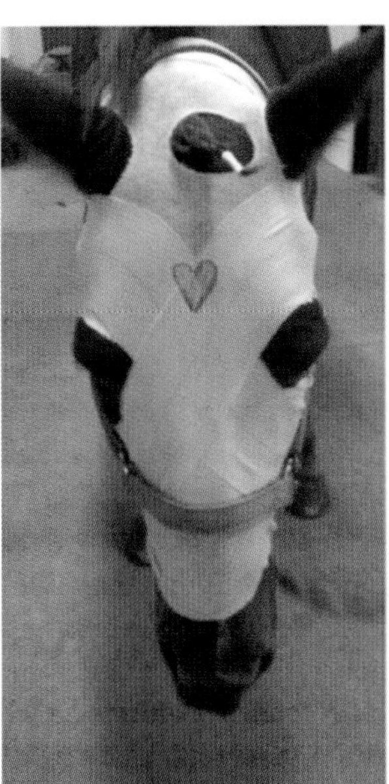
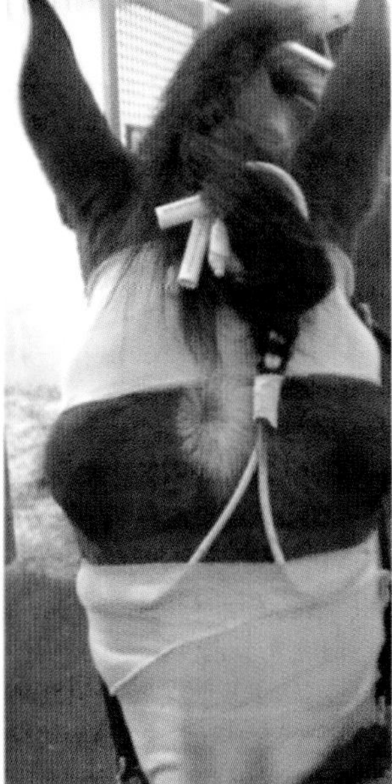

Figure 10.29 Incision and insertion site of foley catheters are covered with bandage material.

Tooth Removal

Relevant Anatomy

Foals normally have 24 deciduous teeth and adult horses have 36–42 permanent teeth. Every horse should have a thorough dental examination at least once a year in order to ensure the teeth are erupting normally and identify dental problems. Horses with recognized dental problems may need dental examinations two to three times per year in order to maintain good dental occlusion and mastication.

Indications

There are many possible indications for tooth removal. They include identification of draining tracts, periapical infections of the cheek teeth, retained deciduous teeth, supernumerary teeth, tooth fractures, equine odontoclastic tooth resorption and hypercementosis (EOTRH), diastemata, and less commonly, dental tumors. Some of these horses may have unilateral nasal discharge, a draining tract leading to the affected tooth, and/or a malodorous smell emanating from their mouth.

Anesthesia and Surgical Preparation

Oral extraction is the technique of choice for exodontia of most equine teeth as it can usually be done standing, and greatly reduces complications when compared with repulsion or buccotomy (Figure 10.30). However, if the surgery is being performed under general anesthesia, feed should be withheld for 6–8 hr prior to surgery depending on surgeon preference.

Before surgery, an intravenous catheter is placed making it easier to administer perioperative medications and sedation or anesthesia throughout the procedure. The hair coat is brushed to remove bedding and other contaminants.

Perioperative anti-inflammatories and antimicrobials are indicated. It is recommended that the first dose be given within 60 min prior to surgery. Prophylactic antimicrobials will reduce the risk of incisional infections while anti-inflammatories will reduce surgical pain and inflammation.

Oral extraction under standing sedation: The horse is positioned in the stocks. After clipping, a rough preparation

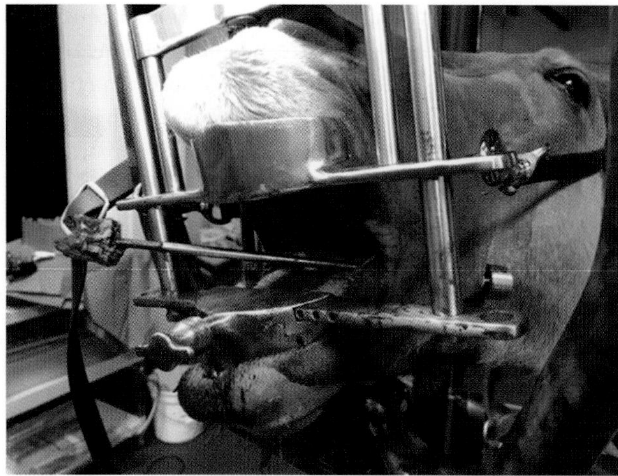
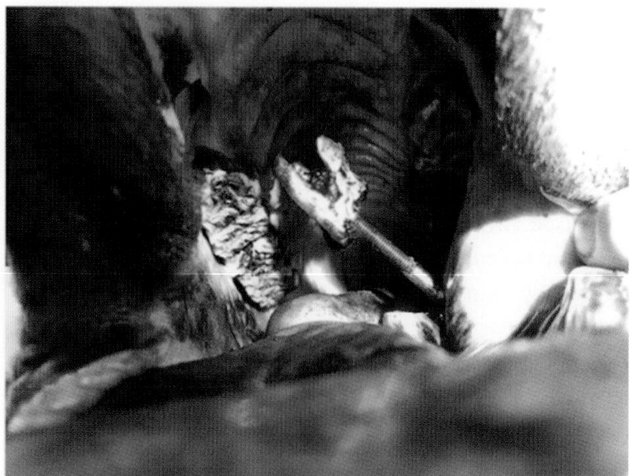

Figure 10.30 Removal of tooth via buccotomy. *Source:* Courtesy of Kobi Derks, RVT.

of the surgical site is done with dilute betadine solution (1 : 50) and sterile saline for at least 5 min. Scrubs, Chlorhexidine, and alcohol are toxic to the corneal epithelium, and therefore, their use should be avoided. After the rough preparation is complete, the surgeon can do a local block to prevent the horse from feeling the tooth removal. Many surgeons use mepivacaine, or a combination of mepivacaine and lidocaine for this local block.

Throughout the dental surgery, the patient is maintained on a sedation CRI. Detomidine hydrochloride is the most commonly used drug for sedation and analgesia. It is commonly used in conjunction with butorphanol and xylazine.

- Tooth repulsion under general anesthesia: Once anesthesia has been induced; an endotracheal tube is placed. The horse is then moved onto the surgery table and positioned in lateral recumbency with the affected side up. Care must be taken to pad the horse appropriately and avoid pressure myopathies. The horse is maintained on inhalant anesthesia (isoflurane or sevoflurane) and positive pressure ventilation is used throughout the remainder of the surgery.

The face is clipped with wide margins around the surgical site. This will vary based on which tooth is being repulsed. After clipping, a rough preparation of the surgical site is done with dilute betadine solution (1 : 50) and sterile saline for at least 5 min. Scrubs, Chlorhexidine, and alcohol are toxic to the corneal epithelium, and therefore, their use should be avoided. After the rough preparation is complete, the surgeon can do a local block to provide analgesia for the immediate post-surgical period. Many surgeons use mepivacaine, or a combination of mepivacaine and lidocaine for this local block. Aseptic preparation of the surgical field is then performed with dilute betadine solution (1 : 50) and sterile saline.

Instrumentation

- Oral extraction
  - Small instrument pack containing scissors (Metzenbaum, mayo, suture), needle drivers, forceps (mosquito, Brown-Adson, rat tooth), blade handles (#3), and Backhaus towel clamps will be needed. In addition, gauze, sterile saline, bowl and syringe, and hand towels are necessary. The surgeon will wear sterile gloves.
  - Head stand – Used to support the horse's head.
  - Dental speculum – Holds the horse's mouth open.
  - Bucket w/ mouth rinse and dosing syringe – Rinse feed material out of the mouth.
  - Head lamp – The surgeon will need extra light to visualize inside of the mouth while they are working.
  - Dental probes and mirrors – Helps to explore the mouth prior to and during extraction.
  - Dental elevators – Used to loosen the tooth prior to extraction.
  - Dental extraction forceps – Used to pull the tooth once it is loose.
  - Dental impression material – Can be used to fill the space left when the tooth is pulled until the tissue granulates in.
  - Radiograph equipment – Radiographs are taken to ensure there are no tooth fragments left behind.
- Repulsion
  - Large instrument pack containing scissors (Metzenbaum, mayo, suture), needle drivers, forceps (Allis, Kelly, mosquito, Brown-Adson, rat tooth), blade handles (#3), and Backhaus towel clamps will be needed. In addition, a suction set up with Yankauer suction tip, gauze, lap sponges, sterile saline, bowl and syringe, hand towels large body drape, and suture are necessary. The surgeon(s) will wear sterile gowns and sterile gloves.

- Bone saw – Used to make a bone flap over the tooth that needs to be repulsed.
- CO_2 tank – Powers the bone saw.
- Osteotomes – Can be used along with a mallet to make the bone flap if a bone saw is not available.
- Mallet – Used in combination with osteotomes or dental punches.
- Dental Punches – Used in combination with a mallet to repulse the tooth into the oral cavity.
- Curettes – Used to scrape tooth roots and eliminate remaining tooth material.
- Rongeurs – Used to clean up bone edges and remaining tooth material.
- Dental Impression Material – Can be used to fill the space left when the tooth is pulled until the tissue granulates in.
- Bandage material – Cover the sutured incision during the healing process.
- Radiograph equipment – Radiographs are taken to ensure there are no tooth fragments left behind.

> **TECHNICIAN TIP 10.17:** Chlorhexidine and alcohol are toxic to the corneal epithelium, and therefore, their use should be avoided when doing surgery around the eyes.

Post-operative Management

If the surgery is performed standing, feeding of the regular diet can generally resume as soon as the sedation wears off. If the surgery is performed under general anesthesia, exactly when feeding begins and the type of feed (mash vs. grass hay) will depend on surgeon preference.

If the tooth was repulsed, there will be an incision on the face where the flap was created. It is important to monitor the incision for signs of infection such as increased discharge or dehiscence. The diastema that was created by pulling the tooth is usually packed with dental impression material to prevent feed from being packed into that space as it granulates in. This packing should be checked (usually by the veterinarian) frequently to ensure it is still in place. While monitoring the patient, be sure to visually inspect the stall for this orange or pink dental impression material as it sometimes comes out while the horse is eating and can be found in the shavings.

Perioperative administration of broad-spectrum antimicrobials will assist in prevention of incisional infections and may be continued post-operatively as well. NSAIDS will reduce pain and inflammation and are usually continued for at least five days post-surgery. The medications used and frequency/duration of administration will vary between surgeons and hospitals.

A foley catheter can be sutured into the sinus during these surgeries to facilitate flushing. This is particularly important when pulling maxillary check teeth that had a severe tooth root infection. Flushing is usually done one to two times per day until the sinus flushes consistently "clean." Some hospitals use saline, while others use saline with some betadine solution added. The foley catheter must be monitored to ensure the horse does not scratch it out when left unattended. Covering the foley with bandage material and/or stockinette is recommended.

Complications and Prognosis

Complications most commonly occur after repulsion of apically infected cheek teeth in younger horses. Mechanical damage can occur to the supporting maxillary or mandibular bones due to the high and prolonged force required for repulsion. These complications include non-healing alveoli due to remaining dental fragments; supporting bone sequestra; osteomyelitis; damage to adjacent teeth; chronic sinusitis; oronasal, orofacial, and oromaxillary fistulae; and chronically draining facial tracts. In these cases, radiographic assessment will assist the veterinarian in selection of an appropriate treatment.

Horses typically have a good prognosis for return to function/athletic performance after tooth removal. Depending on which teeth were removed, there may need to be adjustments to their feeding plan.

Arthroscopy

Relevant Anatomy

Arthroscopy is a surgical technique in which surgery can be performed on a joint through a few small incisions (approximately 1 cm in length). Arthroscopies provide many benefits when compared with a traditional arthrotomy. The incisions are much smaller, causing less damage to the joint capsule and surrounding tissues. This leads to a faster recovery for the horse. In many cases, visualization is better with this approach as well.

Indications

Arthroscopy is both a diagnostic and therapeutic tool and is considered the gold standard for diagnosing equine joint problems. This surgery is most commonly performed on the fetlock, carpus, tarsus, and stifle to treat lesions such as osteochondritis dissecans, osteoarthritis, osteochondral fragments, and subchondral cysts (Figure 10.31).

Anesthesia and Surgical Preparation

Arthroscopies are performed with the horse under general anesthesia. Feed should be withheld for 6–8 hr depending on surgeon preference and before surgery, the horse's mouth should be rinsed to prevent aspiration of food material during intubation. The hair coat should be brushed to remove bedding and other debris.

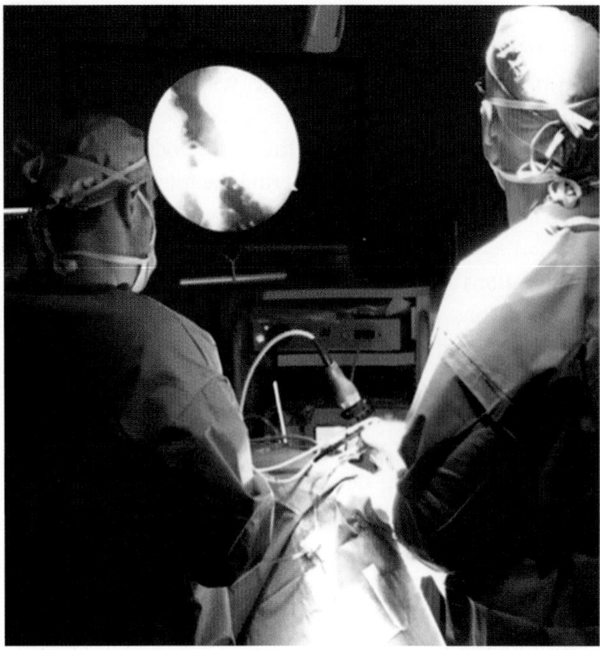

Figure 10.31 Arthroscopy surgery. *Source:* Courtesy of Catherine McDonald, LVT.

An intravenous catheter is placed making it easier to administer perioperative and anesthetic medications throughout the procedure. Pre-operative medications should be given within 60 min of the surgery. Prophylactic antimicrobials will reduce the risk of incisional infections, and anti-inflammatories will reduce surgical pain and inflammation.

Once anesthesia has been induced, an endotracheal tube is placed. The horse is then moved onto the surgery table and positioned in dorsal or lateral recumbency depending on the surgical lesion. Care must be taken to pad the horse appropriately and avoid pressure myopathies. The horse is maintained on inhalant anesthesia (isoflurane or sevoflurane), and positive pressure ventilation is used throughout the remainder of the surgery.

A urinary catheter is placed, and rectal sleeves are put over the patient's feet and tail to prevent contamination to the operating room. The joint(s) is clipped with wide margins around the incision site, and a rough preparation of the surgical site is done with betadine or chlorhexidine scrub for at least 5 min. The patient is then taken into the surgery area. Once positioned in the operating room, aseptic preparation of the surgical field is performed with betadine or chlorhexidine scrub and alcohol.

Instrumentation

Arthroscopies require a lot of instrumentation. A large instrument pack containing scissors (Metzenbaum, mayo, suture), needle drivers, forceps (sponge, Allis, Kelly, mosquito, Brown-Adson, rat tooth), blade handles (#3), and Backhaus towel clamps will be needed for all arthroscopic surgeries (Figure 10.32). In addition, sterile gauze, lap sponges, sterile saline, bowl and syringe, and hand towels are necessary. The surgeons will wear sterile gowns and sterile gloves.

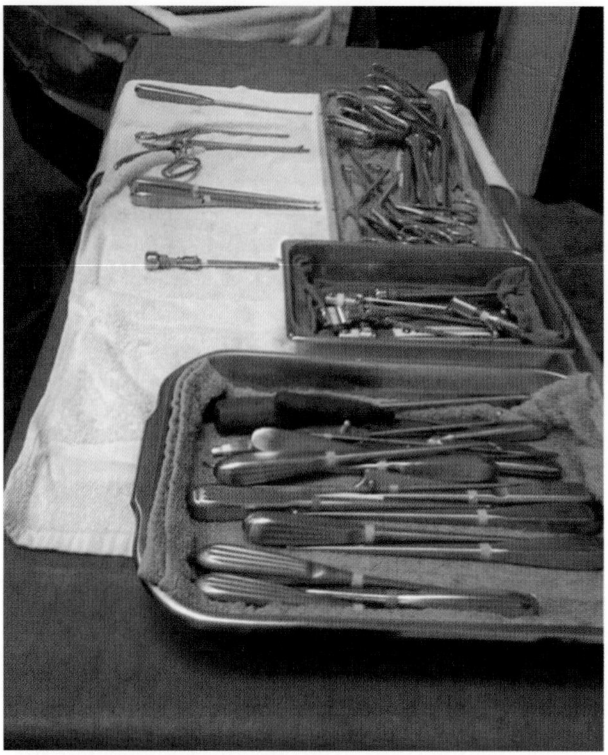

Figure 10.32 Arthroscopy pack.

The following arthroscopic equipment is also needed:

- Arthroscopy tower – Holds the camera box, light source, fluid pump, and viewing screen.
- Arthroscope – A rigid fiber optic scope inserted into the joint capsule to view the internal joint anatomy.
- Camera – Attaches to the arthroscope and transmits the image to a screen on the arthroscopy tower for all who are involved to view.
- Light cord – Attaches to the cannula and the arthroscopy tower. Provides light in the joint space. In a minimally invasive surgery, the room lights do not help with visualization.
- Fluid pump – Sterile fluids are used to distend the joint capsule, creating space for the surgeon to maneuver instruments and giving them better visualization of the joint. The fluid pump controls the rate at which fluids are pumped into the joint space.
- Trocars – Trocars are made of two pieces, a cannula and an obturator. They allow instrumentation into the joint space.

- Arthroscopy instruments – Similar to instruments designed for open surgery, but they have smaller jaws and do not have inline handles to facilitate working through a cannula.

TECHNICIAN TIP 10.18: It is important to realize that cannulated and complex articulated instruments such as those used in arthroscopy surgeries have the ability to house infectious agents unless taken apart and very thoroughly cleaned.

Post-operative Management

Feeding is usually resumed once the sedation and anesthesia is completely out of the horse's system. Exactly when feeding begins post-surgery and the type of feed (mash vs. grass hay) will depend on surgeon preference.

It is important to monitor the incision for signs of infection such as increased discharge or dehiscence. The patient will have a bandage over the incision. Monitoring for bandage complications such as slipping and strike through will be critical. Increased inflammation or lameness in the first few days after surgery may indicate a septic joint, and any observations of this nature should be reported to the veterinarian immediately.

Perioperative administration of broad-spectrum antimicrobials and anti-inflammatory drugs will assist in prevention of infections, reduce pain and inflammation. In addition, antibiotics may be continued post-operatively if the joint is thought to be septic. The medications used and frequency/duration of administration will vary between surgeons and hospitals.

TECHNICIAN TIP 10.19: It is important to keep the portal incisions clean and dry.

Complications and Prognosis

Post-operative arthroscopy complications include incisional infection, joint sepsis, lameness, and bandage complications.

Prognosis is dependent on the surgical lesion, and whether or not there is secondary arthritis or other joint damage as a sequela to that lesion. It is beyond the scope of this text to talk further about prognosis, as there are so many variables that can affect outcome.

Arthrodesis

Relevant Anatomy

Arthrodesis is the assisted fusion of a joint via removal of cartilage and stabilization of the joint with implants, which promotes fusion. In high motion joints, the goal is to alleviate pain associated with movement of the joint and extend the horses life as a non-athletic animal (brood mare or pet). Arthrodesis of low motion joints gives a better prognosis for athletic soundness.

Indications

Horses with severe degenerative joint disease, joints that have suffered loss of supporting soft tissue structures, or that have complex fractures involving joints may be candidates for an arthrodesis surgery. It is also a salvage procedure for some horses with joint pain that cannot be successfully managed in other ways (Figure 10.33).

Anesthesia and Surgical Preparation

Arthrodesis surgeries are performed with the horse under general anesthesia. Before surgery, the horse's mouth should be rinsed to prevent aspiration of feed material during intubation and the hair coat should be brushed to remove bedding and other debris.

An intravenous catheter is placed making it easier to administer perioperative and anesthetic medications throughout the procedure. Pre-operative medications should be given within 60 min of the surgery. Prophylactic antimicrobials will reduce the risk of incisional and joint infections, while anti-inflammatories will reduce surgical pain and inflammation.

Once anesthesia has been induced, an endotracheal tube is placed. The horse is then moved onto the surgery table and positioned in lateral recumbency with the affected limb up. Care must be taken to pad the horse appropriately and avoid pressure myopathies. The horse is maintained on inhalant anesthesia (isoflurane or sevoflurane) and positive pressure ventilation is used throughout the remainder of the surgery.

A urinary catheter is placed, and rectal sleeves are put over the patient's feet and tail to prevent contamination to the operating room. The leg is clipped with wide margins around the incision site and a rough preparation is done with betadine or chlorhexidine scrub for at least 5 min. The patient is then taken into the surgery area. Once positioned in the operating room, aseptic preparation of the surgical field is performed with betadine or chlorhexidine scrub and alcohol.

Instrumentation

Arthrodesis surgeries require a lot of instrumentation. A large instrument pack containing scissors (Metzenbaum, mayo, suture), needle drivers, forceps (sponge, Allis, Kelly, mosquito, brown-Adson, rat tooth), blade handle (#3), and Backhaus towel clamps will be needed for all laparoscopic surgeries. In addition, gauze, lap sponges, sterile gauze, sterile saline, bowl and syringe, and hand towels are necessary. The surgeons will wear sterile gowns and sterile gloves.

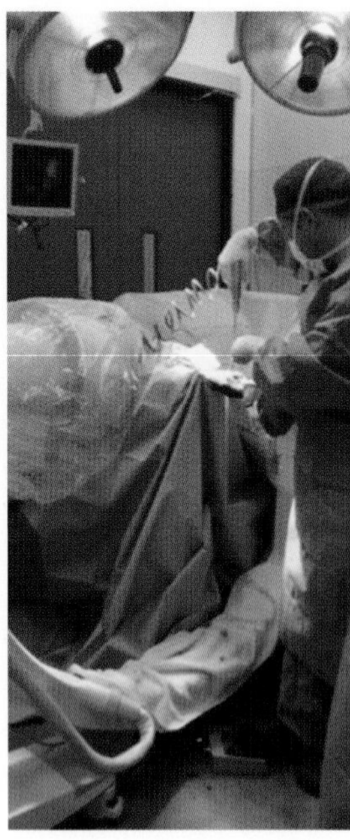
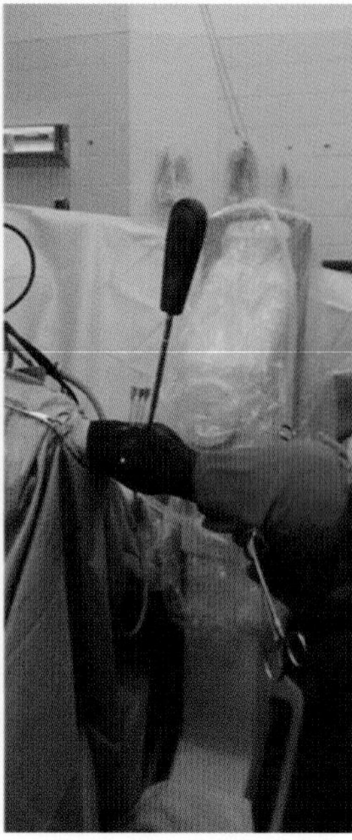
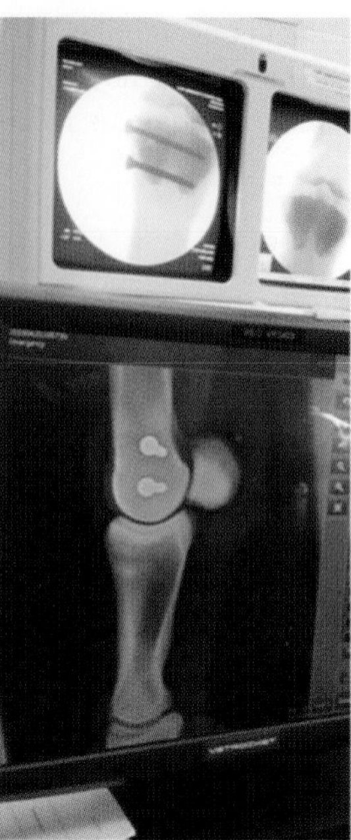

Figure 10.33 Fetlock arthrodesis surgery with guided screw placement.

In addition, the following orthopedic equipment is needed:

- AO Drill – Sterile drill that runs is run off of CO_2.
- Drill bits – Varying sizes.
- CO_2 Tank – Powers the drill if a wall hook up is not available in the operating room.
- Plate pack – Pack of plates in varying widths and lengths.
- Plate Bender – The plate must be bent to contour to the surface of the bone.
- 4.5 and 5.5 screws – The screws used will depend on patient size so having a variety of sizes and lengths is recommended.
- 4.5 and 5.5 Instruments – The size-specific instrument packs will include extra drill bits, taps, screw drivers, drill guides, and measuring tools.
- Bone clamps – Used to hold the plate in place on the bone before screws are inserted.
- Curettes – Used to scrape the cartilage off of the joint surface.
- Cast materials – A cast is applied to protect the surgical site during recovery and help to prevent hardware failure as well as support the soft tissue healing in the two weeks following surgery.

Post-operative Management

Feeding is usually resumed once the sedation and anesthesia is completely out of the horse's system. Exactly when feeding begins post-surgery and the type of feed (mash vs. grass hay) will depend on surgeon preference.

A cast is applied for the immediate post-operative period to protect the fixation during recovery and, most importantly, to support healing of the soft tissues. The cast is removed at about two weeks. The limb is then protected with a three-layer Robert Jones bandage. It is critical to monitor the cast for complications such as strike through, cracking/breaking, swelling proximal to the cast and cast sores. The subsequent bandage should be monitored for things such as strike through and slipping.

Perioperative administration of broad-spectrum antimicrobials and anti-inflammatory drugs will assist in prevention of incisional infections, and reduce pain and inflammation. In addition, these horses will be kept on antibiotics for an additional period post-surgery since the implants (plate and screws) are foreign bodies. The medications used and the frequency/duration of administration will vary between surgeons and hospitals.

Complications and Prognosis

Post-operative arthrodesis complications include infection, implant failure, support limb laminitis, chronic lameness, and the development of angular limb deformities.

Arthrodesis of a high motion joint is a salvage procedure. The goal is for the horse to be comfortable and pasture sound. Fusion of a low motion joint has a better prognosis for the horse to return to athleticism.

Patent Urachus

Relevant Anatomy

The urachus is a passageway through which urine passes from the fetal bladder into the allantoic cavity. The urachus normally closes during parturition. Incomplete closure is known as a patent urachus and occurs more frequently in foals than in other domestic species. Patent urachus results in urine leaking, either in drops or a stream, from the umbilicus.

Indications

Medical treatment is often pursued first and can be successful. Naval dips with dilute chlorhexidine solution and systemic antibiotics often lead to the urachus spontaneously closing. If the urine leakage does not decrease after five to seven days of medical therapy, or if ultrasound examination shows umbilical structure abnormalities, surgical resection of the urachus and umbilical vessels is indicated.

Anesthesia and Surgical Preparation

Umbilical resections are performed with the foal under general anesthesia. Before surgery, the foal's mouth should be rinsed to prevent aspiration of feed material during intubation, and the hair coat should be brushed to remove bedding and other debris.

An intravenous catheter is placed making it easier to administer perioperative and anesthetic medications throughout the procedure. Pre-operative medications should be given within 60 min of the surgery. Prophylactic antimicrobials will reduce the risk of incisional infections, and anti-inflammatories will reduce surgical pain and inflammation.

Once anesthesia has been induced, an endotracheal tube is placed. The foal is then moved onto the surgery table and positioned in dorsal recumbency. Care must be taken to pad the foal appropriately and avoid pressure myopathies. The foal is maintained on inhalant anesthesia (isoflurane or sevoflurane), and positive pressure ventilation is used throughout the remainder of the surgery.

Rectal sleeves are placed over the patient's feet and tail to prevent contamination to the operating room. The abdomen/inguinal area is clipped, and a rough preparation of the surgical site is done with betadine or chlorhexidine scrub for at least 5 min. The patient is then taken into the surgery area. Once positioned in the operating room, aseptic preparation of the surgical field is performed with betadine or chlorhexidine scrub and alcohol.

Instrumentation

There are many instruments needed for an umbilical resection. A large instrument pack containing scissors (Metzenbaum, mayo, suture), needle drivers, forceps (Allis, Kelly, mosquito, Brown-Adson, rat tooth), blade handles (#3), and Backhaus towel clamps will be needed. A suction set up with Poole suction tip, lap sponges, sterile gauze, sterile Vetrap, Doyen forceps, Babcock forceps, sterile saline, bowl and syringe, hand towels, and suture will also be necessary. The surgeon(s) will wear sterile gowns, and sterile gloves.

Post-operative Management

It is important to get the foal back in with the mare as soon as possible following surgery. Nursing is resumed once the sedation and anesthesia is completely out of the foal's system.

The foal will have a belly bandage over the incision. Monitoring for bandage complications such as slipping and strike through will be critical. Monitoring the foal for increased joint inflammation or lameness after surgery is also important, as it may indicate joint sepsis. Observations of this nature should be reported to the veterinarian immediately.

Perioperative administration of broad-spectrum antimicrobials and anti-inflammatory drugs will assist in prevention of incisional infections, and reduce pain and inflammation. In addition, antibiotics may be continued post-operatively because these foals are prone to joint sepsis. The medications used and the frequency/duration of administration will vary between surgeons and hospitals.

Complications and Prognosis

Common post-operative complications include incisional infections, and adhesion formation. These foals are also at higher risk for concurrent septic arthritis or pneumonia.

Prognosis for these foals is great, providing there are no further complications.

Castration

Relevant Anatomy

Castration is the surgical sterilization of a male horse, turning a stallion into a gelding. Also known as orchidectomy, orchiectomy, emasculation, and gelding; castration is one of the most common equine surgical procedures. Although stallions can be castrated at any age, most are castrated at one to two years.

Indications

Castrations are usually performed to sterilize horses unsuitable for breeding, and to eliminate stallion behavior. By removing the primary source of androgens, castration usually renders the horse more docile, even tempered, and manageable. Impotent or infertile breeding stallions can also be salvaged for other uses by castration (Figure 10.34).

Anesthesia and Surgical Preparation

Castrations can be performed under standing sedation but are more difficult and dangerous for the surgeon. Stallions with well-developed testes who are easily palpated without sedation are the best candidates for standing castration.

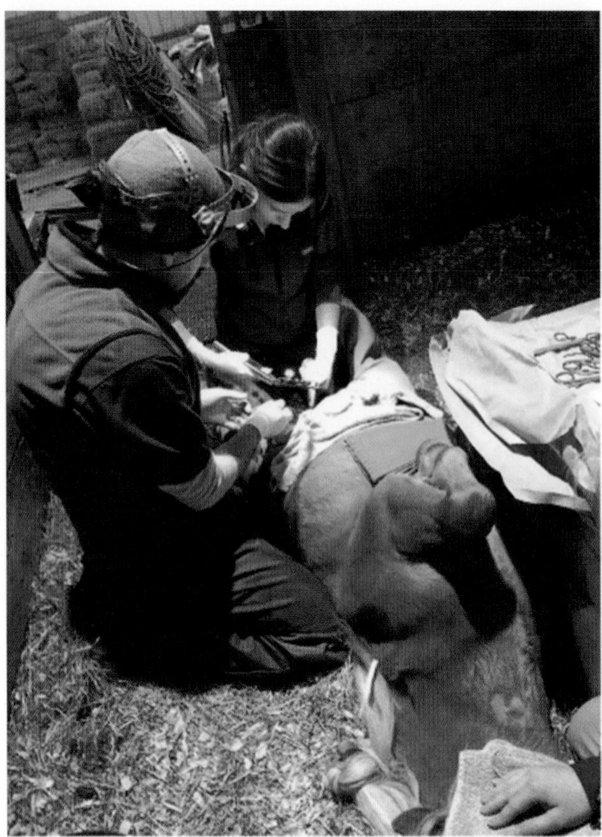

Figure 10.34 Equine castration. *Source:* Courtesy of Lauren Hughes, DVM.

Those who exhibit evasive or hostile behavior to palpation are best castrated under general anesthesia.

If the surgery is to be done under general anesthesia, an intravenous catheter is placed making it easier to administer perioperative medications and sedation or anesthesia throughout the procedure. The hair coat is brushed to remove bedding and other contaminants.

Perioperative anti-inflammatories and antimicrobials are indicated. It is recommended that the first dose be given within 60 min prior to surgery. Prophylactic antimicrobials will reduce the risk of incisional infections, while anti-inflammatories will reduce surgical pain and inflammation.

- Standing castration under sedation: The horse is positioned in the stocks with its head resting on a padded table or head stand. If necessary, the scrotum is clipped. After clipping, a rough preparation of the surgical site is done with betadine scrub and alcohol. Once the rough prep is complete, the surgeon will perform a local nerve block of the incision site and spermatic cord. Many surgeons use mepivacaine, or a combination of mepivacaine and lidocaine for these blocks. Another preparation with betadine scrub and alcohol follows the local block.

Throughout the surgery, the patient is sedated using detomidine hydrochloride. It is commonly used in conjunction with butorphanol and xylazine. When used in combination with regional anesthesia, this is very effective.

- Lateral recumbency under general anesthesia: Once anesthesia has been induced, the upper pelvic limb is lifted and secured with a rope before the scrotum is clipped. After clipping, a rough preparation of the surgical site is performed with betadine scrub and alcohol. Once the rough prep is complete, the surgeon will perform a local nerve block of the incision site and spermatic cord. Many surgeons use mepivacaine, or a combination of mepivacaine and lidocaine, for these blocks. Another preparation with betadine scrub and alcohol follows the local block.

TECHNICIAN TIP 10.20: Additional ketamine and xylazine can be administered to extend anesthesia time.

Instrumentation

An instrument pack containing scissors (Metzenbaum, mayo, suture), needle drivers, forceps (Kelly, mosquito, Brown-Adson, rat tooth), blade handles (#3), and Backhaus towel clamps will be needed. In addition, lap sponges, sterile gauze, emasculator, suture, and hand towels are necessary. The surgeon(s) will wear sterile gloves.

Post-operative Management

Feeding is usually resumed once the sedation or anesthesia is completely out of the horse's system. Exactly when feeding begins post-surgery and the type of feed (mash vs. grass hay) will depend on surgeon preference.

Monitoring for hemorrhage is very important. It should be noted that bleeding/dripping may occur and can be normal. A good rule of thumb is that if you can count the drips, it should be OK, and you can continue to monitor. If you cannot count the drips or it is a stream of blood, you should alert the veterinarian immediately.

Perioperative administration of broad-spectrum antimicrobials and anti-inflammatory drugs will assist in prevention of incisional infections, and reduce pain and inflammation. The medications used and the frequency/duration of administration will vary between surgeons and hospitals.

Complications and Prognosis

Post-operative complications include hemorrhage, edema, scrotal infection, septic funiculitis, septic peritonitis, hydrocele, and incomplete cryptorchid castration. Evisceration through the inguinal ring and open castration site is also a possibility but is uncommon and usually only happens in horses with unapparent inguinal hernias.

These hernias usually resolve by three to six months of age, so horses castrated before six months old are at higher risk for evisceration.

Prognosis for these geldings is great, providing there are no further complications.

Enucleation

Relevant Anatomy

Enucleation is the surgical removal of the eye and associated structures. The palpebral margins, nictitans, conjunctiva, and globe are completely removed in this surgery. This is the most commonly performed orbital surgery on the equine patient.

Indications

Enucleations are indicated for eyes that are painful, have severe corneal or intraocular infection, intraocular neoplasia, and globes with trauma that cannot be surgically repaired.

Anesthesia and Surgical Preparation

Most enucleations can be done with standing sedation and local nerve blocks, but if the patient is not a good candidate for standing surgery, it should be done under general anesthesia. If the surgery is to be done under general anesthesia, feed should be withheld for 6–8 hr depending on surgeon preference and the horse's mouth should be rinsed to prevent aspiration of food material during intubation.

An intravenous catheter is placed making it easier to administer perioperative medications and sedation or anesthesia throughout the procedure. The hair coat is brushed to remove bedding and other contaminants.

Perioperative anti-inflammatories and antimicrobials are indicated. It is recommended that the first dose be given within 60 min prior to surgery. Prophylactic antimicrobials will reduce the risk of incisional infections, while anti-inflammatories will reduce surgical pain and inflammation.

- Standing enucleation under sedation (Figure 10.35): The horse is positioned in the stocks with its head resting on a padded table or head stand. A topical anesthetic (Proparacaine or Tetracaine) should be applied to the corneal surface. A large part of the face is clipped allowing for good margins around the eye. After clipping, a rough preparation of the surgical site is done with dilute betadine solution (1 : 50) and sterile saline for at least 5 min. Scrubs, Chlorhexidine, and alcohol are toxic to the corneal epithelium, and therefore, their use should be avoided. Once the rough preparation is complete, the surgeon will perform auriculopalpebral, supraorbital, and retrobulbar blocks. Many surgeons use mepivacaine, or a combination of mepivacaine and lidocaine for these blocks. Aseptic preparation with dilute betadine solution and sterile saline follows the local blocks.

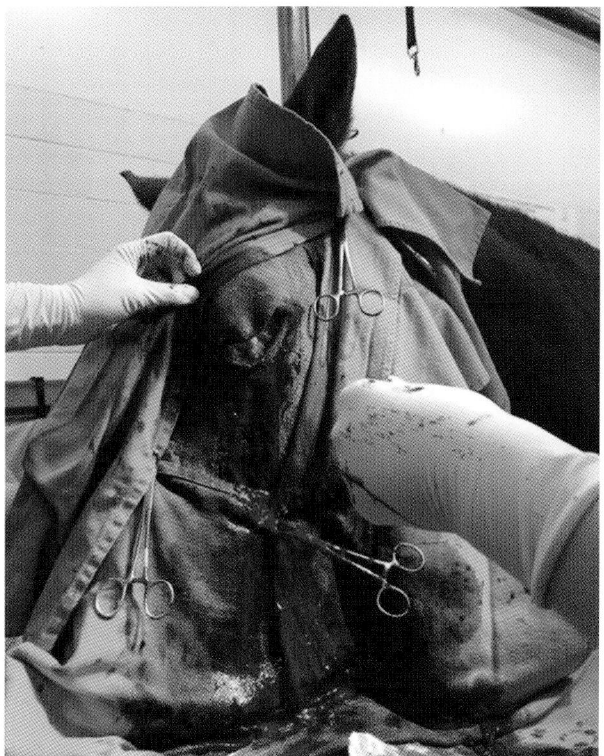

Figure 10.35 Standing enucleation.

Throughout the surgery, the patient is maintained on a sedation CRI. Detomidine hydrochloride is the most commonly used drug for sedation and analgesia. It is commonly used in conjunction with butorphanol and xylazine. When used in combination with regional anesthesia, this is very effective.

- Lateral recumbency under general anesthesia: Once anesthesia has been induced, an endotracheal tube is placed. The horse is then moved onto the surgery table and positioned in lateral recumbency with the affected side up. Care must be taken to pad the horse appropriately and avoid pressure myopathies. The horse is maintained on inhalant anesthesia (isoflurane or sevoflurane) and positive pressure ventilation is used throughout the remainder of the surgery.

A urinary catheter is placed, and rectal sleeves are put over the patient's feet and tail to prevent contamination to the operating room. The face is clipped with wide margins around the eye. A rough preparation of the surgical site is done with dilute betadine solution (1 : 50) and sterile saline for at least 5 min. The patient is then taken into the surgery area. Once positioned in the operating room, aseptic preparation of the surgical field is performed with dilute betadine solution (1 : 50) and sterile saline.

Instrumentation

An instrument pack containing scissors (curved Metzenbaum, curved mayo, suture), needle drivers, forceps (Allis, Kelly, mosquito, Brown-Adson, rat tooth), blade handles (#3), and Backhaus towel clamps will be needed. In addition, a suction set up with Yankauer tip, lap sponges, sterile gauze, sterile saline, bowl and syringe, and hand towels are necessary. The surgeon(s) will wear sterile gowns and sterile gloves.

Post-operative Management

If the surgery is performed standing, feeding of the regular diet can generally resume as soon as the sedation wears off. If the surgery is performed under general anesthesia, exactly when feeding begins and the type of feed (mash vs. grass hay) will depend on surgeon preference.

A pressure bandage will be placed immediately following the enucleation. This will assist with hemostasis and reduce post-operative swelling. The bandage should be closely monitored for slipping and strike through. Slight epistaxis may occur up to a week post-operatively and is to be expected due to drainage through the nasolacrimal duct.

Perioperative administration of broad-spectrum antimicrobials will assist in prevention of incisional infections and may be continued post-operatively as well for patients that already had an infection in the globe. NSAIDS will reduce pain and inflammation and are usually continued for at least five days post-surgery. The medications used and frequency/duration of administration will vary between surgeons and hospitals.

Complications and Prognosis

Enucleation complications include intra-operative and post-operative hemorrhage that could be severe, and formation of an orbital cyst (usually resulting from incomplete removal of lacrimal ducts and conjunctiva). Additionally, the globe may be ruptured intra-operatively. If the globe is infected, this may result in an orbital infection. If this is the case, the surgeon will obtain a culture, and lavage the orbit extensively. Systemic broad-spectrum antibiotics will be required based on results of the culture and sensitivity test.

Horses typically have a good prognosis for return to function/athletic performance after a unilateral enucleation.

Ruminant Surgery Considerations

Food and water restriction is critical in ruminants. Depending upon their position for surgery, the rumen places strain on the thoracic cavity, decreasing lung function and oxygenation capability. In addition, a large rumen allows for an increased chance of regurgitation during anesthesia, resulting in secondary aspiration. To help minimize these complications, roughage is typically removed for 48 hr prior to an elective surgery, and water is removed 12 hr before surgery. If emergency surgery is needed and the patient has severe abdominal distention, a Kingman Tube may be passed to allowed for the feedstuff and liquid rumen material to be removed, allowing for a deflated rumen with decreased thoracic compromise and risk of aspiration. In terms or neonatal ruminant species on a milk diet, there is no need for any food or water restrictions prior to anesthesia.

Due to the large size and skittish nature of some ruminant patients, patient positioning and surgical location are critical in the decision-making process. In a field setting, appropriate footing, light, and protection from any environmental conditions are necessary. For standing field surgeries, the patient needs to be restrained in such a way so as the clinician is not in any harm and can perform the surgery safely. Ideally, a chute system, or head catch with fence paneling would be ideal (Figure 10.36). A halter should be in place at all times with the head tied toward the flank that is being incised. This is in case the patient goes down during the surgical procedure; the incision and exposed abdominal cavity would be protected. For a recumbent field surgery, considerations for both the patient and surgeon are needed to be discussed. For a dorsal recumbency field surgery, the patient needs to be restrained adequately; allowing the patient to be supported by a strong structure, such as a wall or sturdy fence would be ideal. The patient would have their limbs restrained, such as they are being stretched out (Figure 10.37).

Padding under the down limb is critical to prevent any radial nerve damage. Cattle laying on their side need to be

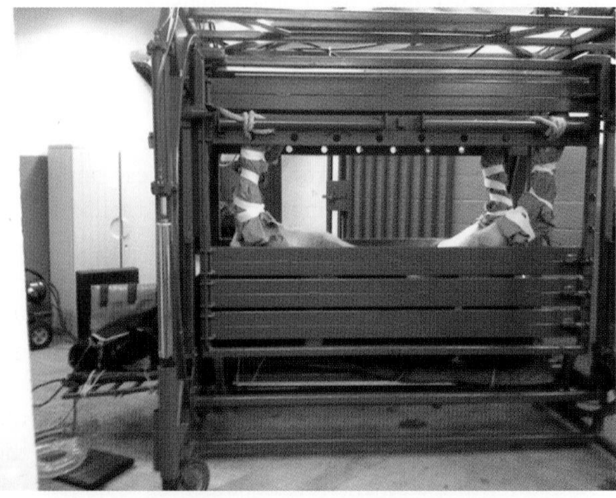

Figure 10.36 A bovine patient in dorsal recumbency. Notice the legs that are padded and tied to the squeeze chute.

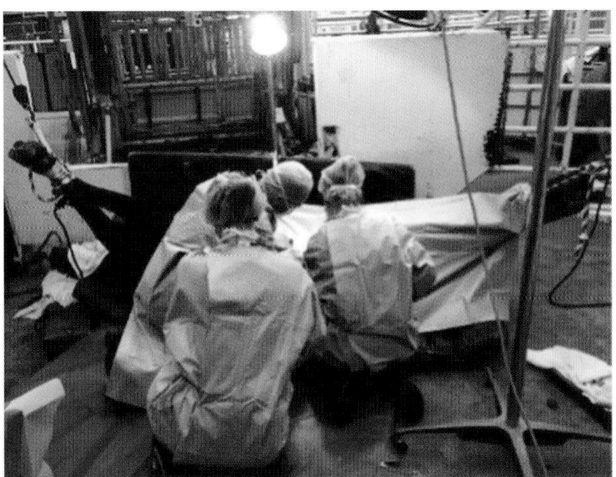

Figure 10.37 A bovine patient in dorso-lateral recumbency for a C-section. Note the restraints on the limbs and padding under the down forelimb. *Source:* Courtesy of Jennifer Halleran, DVM, DACVIM (LAIM).

watched for bloating; eructation is not possible in lateral or dorso-lateral recumbency. A halter should be in place at all times. Most hospital settings would have an appropriate chute for standing surgery or an area for recumbency surgery with padding.

In terms of pre-operative medications, antibiotics are indicated for patients that may have surgical contamination, are somehow compromised, or will be under anesthesia for a prolonged period of time. Consideration of the legal use of the antibiotics needs to be under observation to prevent any prolonged drug residue withdrawal intervals. Depending upon the surgery, patient position during surgery and the patient demeanor, different sedatives, anesthetics, or local analgesia can be utilized. Typically, local analgesia will usually be utilized during any surgical procedure. Lidocaine, bupivacaine, or Carbocaine can be used. Lidocaine is the least expensive and is readily available for food animal veterinarians. Lidocaine is available as a 2% solution, but a 1% solution can easily be made with sterile saline or sodium bicarbonate to decrease the stinging sensation with administration. It is important to note that there is a toxicity level associated with lidocaine, bupivacaine, or Carbocaine usage. In cattle, the toxic dose is 10 mg/kg and in small ruminants, the toxic dose is 5 mg/kg. Before use of any local anesthetic, the toxic dose should be determined and recorded to ensure the volume of lidocaine does not exceed that amount.

In addition to local anesthetics, injectable anesthesia or general anesthesia may be needed, depending upon the surgery, patient position, and patient demeanor. In terms of injectable anesthesia, the anesthetic drugs can be administered either subcutaneously, intramuscularly, or intravenously. Medications given intravenously will have the shortest duration of action, but also achieve sedation the quickest. Injectable anesthesia is advantageous in a field setting, for quick, non-complicated procedures and allow for minimal animal handling prior to the surgical procedure. However, with injectable anesthesia, the depth of anesthesia is difficult to control; patients may all react differently or not be affected by the anesthesia at all, may have more complications, or have a prolonged recovery time. In addition, many injectable anesthetics are not labeled for use in food animal medicine. These medications would be used in an extra label fashion which would require a Food Animal Residue Avoidance Databank (FARAD) submission for an extended meat and milk withdrawal interval. If a tail vein is used for injectable anesthesia administration, be aware of the possibility of intra-arterial or perivascular administration.

When performing injectable anesthesia, a multimodal drug approach is recommended. Ruminants handle some anesthetic drugs differently than other species. For example, ruminants are more sensitive to xylazine when compared to horses. Camelids, however, are more like horses in the use of alpha 2 agonists. Table 10.2 is a list of selected sedatives that are commonly utilized in food animal practice. Table 10.3 demonstrates different injectable anesthetic drug combinations.

Prior to surgery, the surgical site needs to be prepared. The tail of a bovine needs to be restrained prior to the start of any procedure to prevent contamination of the surgical field. This can be achieved by taping the tail to the leg or tying the tail with rolled brown gauze and applying a quick release knot around the neck. It is important to not restrain the tail by tying it to the chute to avoid breaking the tail. Brushing the animal clean of shavings and clipping the surgical site are the first steps. The hair should be removed as a large perimeter around the intended incision site. A rough scrub should be performed first with a cleaning solution, such as chlorohexidine or iodine. Please note, when performing surgery near the eyes, chlorohexidine should not be utilized. The rough scrub is completed with applying alcohol to the surgical site. At this time, any local blocks can be performed. After completion of the local blocks, a sterile scrub should be conducted. The individual scrubbing the site should wear a surgical cap, mask, and sterile gloves to apply the sterile scrub. The sterile scrub can be performed with either chlorohexidine or iodine and is again concluded with alcohol. At completion of the sterile scrub, draping can commence.

Most food animal surgeries will require the use of a bovine surgical pack. This would include the following instrumentation: towel clamps, a #3 and #4 scalpel blade handle, needle driver, suture scissors, sharp blunt scissors, mayo scissors, Metzenbaum scissors, Iris scissors,

Table 10.2 Commonly used medications for sedation in food animals.

Drug	Class	Route of administration	Dose	Sedation type	Notes (general)
Acepromazine	Phenothiazine-based tranquilizers	IM, IV, SQ, PO	Cattle: IV, 0.01–0.02 mg/kg	Mild	Onset typically 15–20 min after IV administration, about 30–45 min after IM administration
			Cattle: IM, 0.03–0.05 mg/kg	Mild	Lacks any analgesia, less sedative effect than xylazine
			SR: IM, IV, 0.05–0.1 mg/kg	Mild	
Butorphanol	Opioid	IM, IV, SQ, PO	Cattle: 0.02–0.05 mg/kg	Minimal	Used for analgesia
			SR: IV, 0.1–0.2 mg/kg		Best when used in combination with other sedation
			SR: IM, 0.2–0.4 mg/kg		May cause an excitatory response
Detomidine	Alpha 2 agonist	IM, IV, SQ, PO	Cattle: IV, 0.01–0.02 mg/kg	Moderate to profound, standing sedation	More potent than xylazine, increased chance of more profound cardiovascular and respiratory depression
			Cattle: IM, 0.02–0.05 mg/kg	Moderate, standing sedation	Complications: bradycardia, hyperglycemia, diuresis
			SR: IV, 0.05 mg/kg	Moderate	Reversal: atipamezole, yohimbine, tolazoline
Diazepam	Benzodiazepines	IV	Cattle: IV, 0.02–0.1 mg/kg	Mild to moderate	Minimal cardiovascular and respiratory effects; May produce ataxia or recumbency so typically not used in standing sedation
			SR: IV, 0.2 mg/kg	Mild to moderate	Muscle relaxant effects
					Used in combination with other sedatives
Ketamine	Dissociative anesthetic	IV	Cattle: IV, 2.2 mg/kg	Moderate to profound	Used for induction or procedures that require heavy sedation
			SR: IV, 2–4 mg/kg	Moderate to profound	Used in combination with other sedatives – a smaller dose will be utilized
					Recovery may include spastic movements
Midazolam	Benzodiazepines	IV	Cattle: IV, 0.02–0.1 mg/kg	Mild to moderate	Minimal cardiovascular and respiratory effects May produce ataxia or recumbency so typically not used in standing sedation
			SR: IV, 0.2 mg/kg	Mild to moderate	Muscle relaxant effects
					Used in combination with other sedatives

Morphine	Opioid	IM, IV, SQ	Cattle: IV, IM, SQ, 0.05–0.15 mg/kg	Minimal	Provides better analgesia than butorphanol
			SR: IV, IM, SQ, 0.05–0.15 mg/kg	Minimal	
			Epidural: 0.1 mg/kg		
Xylazine	Alpha 2 agonist	IM, IV, SQ, PO	Cattle: IM, 0.04–0.06 mg/kg	Mild to moderate, standing	Can be used alone or in combination with other medications. Ruminants are very sensitive, about 10 times more sensitive than horses
			Cattle: IV, 0.02–0.03 mg/kg	Mild to moderate, standing	May cause pulmonary edema in SR
			Cattle: IV, 0.05–0.1 mg/kg	Heavy, recumbency	Dose response depends on route of administration and demeanor of animal. More excitable animals will require a higher dose
			Llama: IV, IM, 0.4 mg/kg		Higher dose will result in recumbency
			Alpaca: IV, IM, 0.5–0.6 mg/kg		Complications: bradycardia, hyperglycemia, diuresis

Table 10.3 Commonly used sedation drug combinations in food animals.

Drugs	Dosage	Sedation type	Notes
Butorphanol/xylazine/ketamine	IV: 0.01 mg/kg/0.02 mg/kg/0.05–0.1 mg/kg	Standing in cattle	Called the ketamine stun. Depending upon route of administration, dose, and demeanor of animal, the sedation effect may vary. Intravenous administration will produce the quickest effect, but not last as long as when the injectable anesthetic is administered subcutaneously. This is called the 5-10-20 combination, as there is ultimately 5 mg of butorphanol, 10 mg of xylazine, and 20 mg of ketamine.
Butorphanol/xylazine/ketamine	SC, IM: 0.015–0.02 mg/kg/0.03–0.4 mg/kg/0.06–0.08 mg/kg	Standing in cattle	This is called the 10-20-40 combination, as there is ultimately 10 mg of butorphanol, 20 mg of xylazine, and 40 mg of ketamine. A 20-40-80 combination, 20 mg butorphanol, 40 mg xylazine and 80 mg of ketamine is recommended SC or IM for unruly patients.
Acepromazine/xylazine	IV: 0.02 mg/kg/0.02 mg/kg	Standing in cattle	Mild to moderate sedation.
Butorphanol/xylazine/ketamine	IV: 0.05–0.1 mg/kg/0.025–0.05 mg/kg/0.3–0.5 mg/kg	Recumbent sedation in cattle	Provides sedation and analgesia for about 15–20 min.
Butorphanol/xylazine/ketamine	SC, IzM: 0.025 mg/kg/0.05 mg/kg/0.1 mg/kg	Recumbent sedation in cattle	Onset in about 5 min with sedation and analgesia lasting for about 30–45 min.
Xylazine/ketamine	IV: 0.1 mg/kg/2 mg/kg	Recumbent sedation in cattle	Short duration of anesthesia, about 10–15 min.
Xylazine/ketamine	IM: 0.2 mg/kg/3–4 mg/kg	Recumbent sedation in cattle	Longer duration of anesthesia, about 15–30 min. A benzodiazepine can be added for muscle relaxation.
Xylazine/ketamine	IM, IV: 0.5 mg/kg, 5 mg/kg	Recumbent sedation in llamas	
Xylazine/ketamine	IM, IV: 0.6 mg/kg, 6 mg/kg	Recumbent sedation in alpacas	
Xylazine/ketamine	IM, IV: 0.3–0.5 mg/kg, 3–5 mg/kg	Standing sedation in alpacas	
Butorphanol/midazolam/ketamine	IV: 0.1 mg/kg/0.2 mg/kg/2–4 mg/kg	Recumbent sedation in goats	Commonly used for C-sections and blocked goat procedures.
Butorphanol/xylazine/ketamine	IM: 0.05 mg/kg/0.4 mg/kg/4 mg/kg	Llama sedation	

Adson-Brown thumb forceps, rat tooth forceps, DeBakey forceps, Allis forceps, and a variety of hemostats. Size 10 and 22 blades are normally used.

Post-operatively, depending upon the procedure performed, different analgesic drugs may need to be utilized. Currently, the only medication labeled for pain in food producing species is transdermal flunixin meglumine with the intended use to treat foot rot. There are currently no other medications approved to treat pain for food producing species in the United States. According to the Animal Medicinal Drug Use Clarification Act of 1994, in order to treat pain in a food producing species, another medication labeled for pain in either human or small animal medicine can be utilized in a food producing species. This enables for the use of flunixin meglumine intravenously, the most commonly used nonsteroidal anti-inflammatory in food animal medicine. Flunixin meglumine legally can only be administered intravenously; although labeled for intramuscular use in horses, the intramuscular administration can potentially lead to life-threatening clostridial myositis, as well as prolonged withdrawal intervals.

Doses for flunixin meglumine are typically given as either a 1.1 mg/kg IV dose every 12 hr, or 2.2 mg/kg IV dose every 24 hr. Intravenous administration may not be feasible for some animals; oral administration can be performed, but the dose needs to be doubled. The bioavailability and efficacy of flunixin is greatly decreased with oral administration. Meloxicam, another nonsteroidal anti-inflammatory can be administered orally. Gabapentin has also been noted to be efficacious in food producing species.

> **TECHNICIAN TIP 10.21:** Toxic lidocaine dose for cattle is 10 mg/kg.

Bovine Surgery

Cesarean Section

Relevant Anatomy

Aside from the body wall musculature, the relevant bit of anatomy is the uterus of the dam. The fetus will be palpated through the uterine wall.

Indications

Cesarean sections are performed in cattle to primarily assist with dystocia management. This includes fetal–maternal mismatching; emphysematous fetus and small pelvic diameter when fetotomy is not able to be performed; uterine or pelvic injury; or a severe vaginal prolapse. Deciding to perform a C-section has many variables, such as reproductive health of the dam, calf viability, economics, and restraint facilities available. These same variables will also help determine the position of the dam for the C-section to be performed. In cattle, C-sections can be performed standing or in lateral, dorsal, or latero-dorsal recumbency. The latter positions are typically used when the dam will not stay standing throughout the surgery or if a deceased calf is present in the uterus. The latter surgical position would allow for better and more complete exteriorization of the uterus from the abdominal cavity to minimize uterine fluid contamination from the dead fetus in the cow's abdomen.

Anesthesia and Surgical Preparation

As stated previously, there are four main surgical positions for performing a C-section in cattle: standing, lateral recumbency, dorsal recumbency, or dorso-lateral recumbency. Standing restraint requires a chute and head catch. This is typically done on cattle that will stay standing throughout the procedure and no known fetal compromise. Standing C-sections are performed on the left side – a right-sided approach would be difficult with the presence of the small intestines. A left-sided laparotomy encounters the uterus and the rumen, with the uterus being readily distinguished from the rumen due to the presence of the fetus. The left paralumbar fossa is clipped from the 13th rib to the pelvic bones, and from above, the transverse processes of the lumbar vertebrae down to the ventral abdomen. A surgical prep is performed as stated in the general introduction. With a standing surgery, a caudal epidural with lidocaine is performed to control tenesmus and pain associated with calf removal (Figure 10.38). If the patient is a bit nervous, xylazine can be added to the epidural.

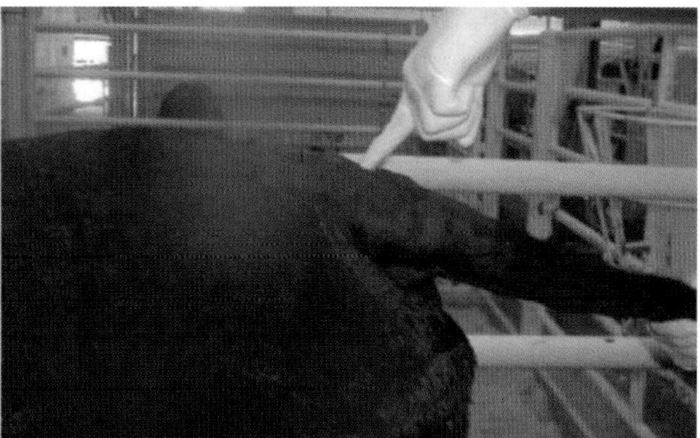

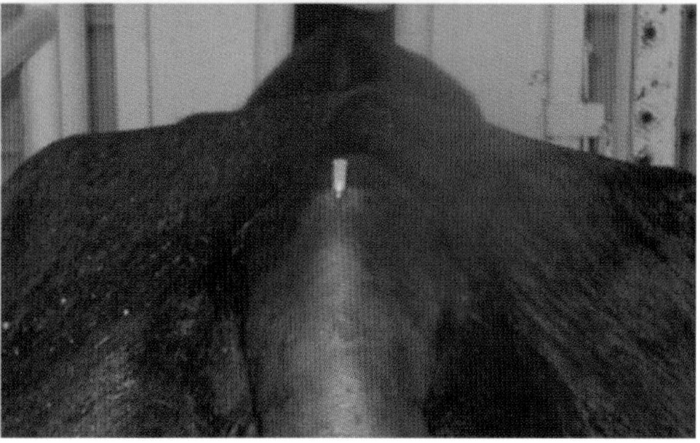

Figure 10.38 (Top) Location of a caudal epidural. Figure 3: Needle in the location for a caudal epidural. *Source:* Courtesy of Jennifer Halleran, DVM, DACVIM (LAIM).

Local analgesia, in terms of a distal paravertebral block, proximal paravertebral block, inverted L, or a line block with 2% lidocaine is used (Figure 10.39).

Lateral recumbency surgical positions can be achieved with minimal sedation, casting the bovine to the ground and proper foot restraint. Sedatives can cross the placenta barrier and cause a decreased conscious state in the fetus. The behavior of the dam will dictate how much sedation needs to be used. As stated in the general surgery introduction, a standing or recumbent combination of sedatives can be utilized to induce lateral recumbency. With lateral recumbency, it is again important to monitor abdominal distention, as this will cause a decrease in the thoracic ability to expand. The down forelimb should be placed as far cranial as possible with heavy padding underneath to prevent any radial nerve paralysis. Intravenous or intramuscular sedation will likely be used to allow for lateral recumbency. This will provide sedation and some analgesia,

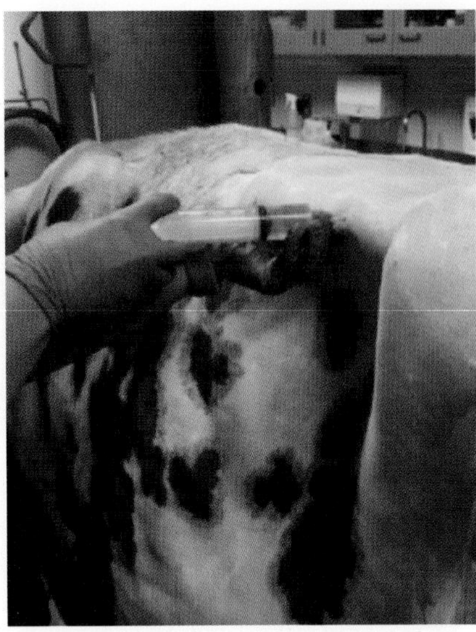
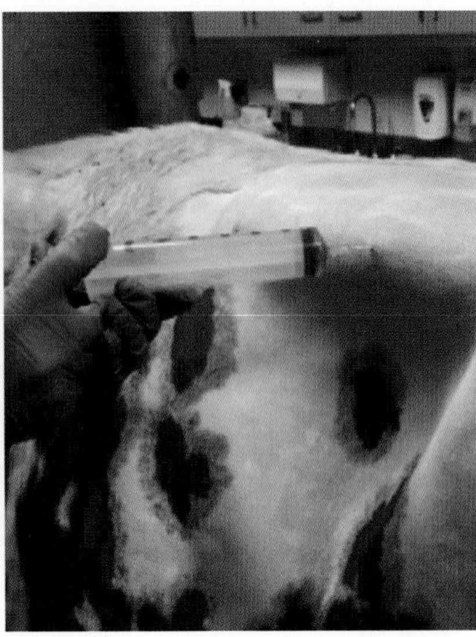

Figure 10.39 The needle and syringe administration of lidocaine for a distal paravertebral block. Source: Courtesy of Jennifer Halleran, DVM, DACVIM (LAIM).

but local anesthetics are warranted. Typically, a line block with 2% lidocaine would be performed in the area of the incision. With a patient in lateral recumbency, a flank, oblique, paramedian, or median incision can be made. Surgical preparation of the surgical site is the same as described above. The area to be clipped depends upon the surgical approach and incision site.

Dorsal recumbency will require the most hands-on deck to move and position the cow. This is a physically intensive surgical position to place the patient in. The same considerations as lateral recumbency are in place here in terms of monitoring for abdominal distension and radial nerve paralysis in the forelimb closest to the ground. Intravenous or intramuscular sedation would be required to induce recumbency. A dorsal recumbency surgical position would allow for a median abdominal incision; therefore, a line block of 2% lidocaine is the best method to provide local analgesia. The surgical preparation is the same as described above. Here, the surgical clip is from the xiphoid back to the mammary gland and as lateral on each side as can be obtained with the dam in the down position.

In general, bovine C-sections do not require general anesthesia. Sedation with local analgesia will facilitate the surgical procedure.

Instrumentation

As described above in the general surgery considerations, a bovine surgical pack is all that is required for this procedure. If a bovine surgery pack is not available, the surgeon will at least need a drape, towel clamps, scalpel handle, blade (both a 10 and 22 size blade), needle holders, suture scissors, and hemostats. Thumb forceps and Allis tissue forceps would be ideal to assist with tissue handling. In addition, surgeons would require the use of sterile sleeves; this would enable the surgeon to enter the abdominal cavity the entire length of the arm to retract and remove the uterus.

For some C-section surgical procedures, due to the position of the calf or the strength of the surgeon, the uterus may not be able to be brought outside the abdominal wall. In this case, the uterus will be opened within the abdominal cavity. Depending upon surgeon preference, sterile envelope openers may be used to make a clean, linear uterine incision. In terms of suture, this really depends upon surgeon preference. To close the uterus, a synthetic absorbable size two or three is used. The body wall is closed in a routine manner.

Post-operative Management

Post-operative management depends upon where the surgical incision was placed. For standing surgeries with a flank incision, routine surgical incision site monitoring is required. The most ventral aspect of the flank incision would be the most prone to infection due to gravity and ventral draining. Paramedian and median incisions would be the most troublesome post-operatively due to gravity, nursing behavior from the calf, and environmental contamination when the dam is in sternal recumbency. For patients with leg restraints, these should be removed, and the halter untied at the end. Depending upon the duration of surgery and sedation protocol used, cows should be standing within 15–20 min after finishing the surgical procedure.

The dam should receive pain analgesics such as flunixin meglumine or meloxicam. In addition, oxytocin should be administered to promote uterine contractions; this would allow for placental expulsion. In cattle, the placenta is typically passed within 24 hr of surgery. Depending upon the extent of vaginal manipulation and the contamination present during the surgery, systemic antibiotics should be continued post-operatively. Broad-spectrum antibiotics, such as ceftiofur products, are recommended. If the dam had a normal physical examination prior to surgery, fluid therapy is usually not warranted. If the dam was recumbent prior to surgery due to metabolic conditions, such as hypocalcemia, fluid therapy with calcium supplementation would be advised.

Caring for calf consumes most of the post-operative surgical time. After the calf has been removed from uterus, it important to ensure the calf has a patent airway, is breathing, and has adequate circulation. The calf should be placed in sternal recumbency, and the placental fluid should be removed from the calf's oral cavity. This can be done manually or with suction. A physical examination should be conducted to identify any cardiac or congenital abnormalities. The umbilicus should be dipped with a chlorhexidine/alcohol or iodine solution. Colostrum intake should occur within the first 2 hr of life, either by natural nursing, bottle feeding, or orogastric intubation.

Complications and Prognosis

For most routine bovine C-sections, the prognosis is very good with minimal complications. During surgery, abdominal contamination with uterine fluid resulting in peritonitis is the biggest complication. Surgery involving a deceased fetus increases the risk of abdominal contamination; this can be avoided by performing surgery in a lateral or dorsal recumbency position to allow for greatest exteriorization of the uterus to capture any uterine fluid leakage. Incision infections can occur. This would be most frequently encountered with incisions located in the ventral abdomen. Metritis and abdominal adhesions may also occur.

Displaced Abomasum

DA is a common medical condition in cattle. DAs occur as a result of management programs. The underlying etiology is complex, involving abomasal hypomotility, altered abomasal pH, potential electrolyte abnormalities, and increased space within the abdominal cavity due to the birth of the fetus one to four weeks prior. DAs frequently occur in recently freshened dairy cattle, having calved about one to four weeks prior. They can occur in calves, beef cows, and bulls, but not as frequently, and they are usually accompanied by concurrent metabolic conditions, such as retained placenta, metritis, ketosis, or mastitis.

There are three main syndromes that can occur with DAs: left displaced abomasum (LDA), right displaced abomasum (RDA), and a right abomasal volvulus (RAV). Right DAs can lead to RAV. The direction of the abomasum displacement may be dependent upon rumen fill; a full rumen would prevent the distended empty abomasum from swinging to the left side and result in a right DA. If the rumen is empty, the abomasum would swing to the left, causing an LDA. Left DAs are more common and not as problematic as RDA and RAVs. Cattle with LDAs present with decreased milk production and decreased feed intake. They may have abdominal distention. Most cattle have decreased fecal production, most notable with decreased feces present on a rectal sleeve during rectal examination. Diagnosis is made upon abdominal auscultation with positive percussion and succussion noted on the left side of the abdomen. Cattle with an LDA are not as systemically ill as cattle with an RDA or RAV; these patients may present more acutely with severe signs of depression, anorexia, and dehydration. A right-sided ping and splash would be appreciated. Right DAs and RAV are an emergency surgery. If left untreated, these conditions are fatal.

In addition to the DA, any concurrent medical conditions need to be diagnosed and treated. Electrolyte abnormalities may also be present, depending upon the duration of displacement and the position of the abomasum. A PCV/TS with a chemistry and urine dipstick would be considered a minimum database for this disease process. A PCV/TS would provide an objective view on hydration status. The chemistry would shed light on any electrolyte changes. With DAs, the most common electrolyte changes are a hypochloremic, hypokalemic metabolic alkalosis. Hypocalcemia may be present as a result of anorexia. Hypoglycemia may be present in patients with a concurrent ketosis. Ketosis can be diagnosed via urine collection and observation of ketones on a urine dipstick. Fluid therapy with electrolyte supplementation may be warranted during surgery and post-operatively.

There are many different surgical procedures that can be performed to fix LDAs, RDAs, and RAVs. The procedure performed depends on the location of the displacement, the health condition of the patient, the expertise of the surgeon, facilities present, and economics. Below, displaced abosmasums have been divided into the RDAs and LDAs. When needed, differences for RAVs will be discussed.

Right Displaced Abomasum

There are two main surgical approaches to correct RDAs and RAVs: a standing right flank omentopexy or pyloropexy, or a paramedian abomasopexy.

Relevant Anatomy

Ruminants have four compartments to their stomach, the reticulum, rumen, omasum, and abomasum. It is beyond the scope of this review to go over forestomach anatomy and function. The abomasum will be of focus here. The abomasum is the enzymatic stomach of ruminants. Although DAs occur infrequently in calves, neonatal gastrointestinal anatomy is important. Neonatal calves are essentially monogastric animals with the abomasum being the largest compartment. As calves age and increase concentrate feed intake, the size of the reticulum and rumen increase, so much so that around eight weeks of age, the abomasum and reticulorumen are about the same size. By two years of age, all compartments are at mature size, with the abomasum being the second largest, second to the rumen.

The abomasum is located on the right side of the abdomen ventrally. It has a greater and lesser curvature, with the distal aspect ending with the pyloric sphincter and entering into the duodenum.

Indications

Right DA and RAVs are not common as LDAs. Cattle present with decreased milk production, decreased appetite with decreased fecal output. The decreased fecal output is most noticeable during rectal examination by decreased manure present on the rectal sleeve. If present, the feces may appear to be loose or pasty. Cattle with RDAs are systemically sick. They have more pronounced depression, anorexia, and dehydration compared to cattle afflicted with LDAs. With RDAs, fluid is sequestered within the abomasum, resulting in severe dehydration and electrolyte imbalances. For an RDA, a ping ausculted upon percussion is heard on the right flank, spanning from the 10th rib to the 13th rib; the size of the ping depends upon degree of dilation of the abomasum. The location of the ping is important, as other fluid-gas interfaces within viscous structures on the right flank can result in a ping on percussion. These would include cecal dilation and torsion, gas in the duodenum or spiral colon, pneumoperitoneum, or pneumouterus.

In order to definitively diagnose and treat an RDA or RAV, surgery needs to be performed to prevent progression of the disease. There are two surgical approaches to correct an RDAs or RAV: a standing right flank omentopexy or pyloropexy and a right paramedian abomasopexy. Standing right flank omentopexy or pyloropexy is the most common surgical technique to correct an RDA or RAV. A right paramedian abomasopexy can be performed in adults; however, it is easier and preferred in calves.

Anesthesia and Surgical Preparation

For a standing right flank omentopexy and/or pyloropexy, the patient should be restrained in a chute or head catch apparatus. A halter should be applied and tied to the right side. For a standing technique, sedation is typically not required, unless the patient is fractious. Local analgesia with 2% Lidocaine and adequate restraint will allow for the surgical procedure to be performed. In order to provide analgesia, a distal paravertebral block, a proximal paravertebral block or inverted L block with lidocaine should be performed. The surgical site is the right paralumbar fossa; the right flank spanning from just cranial to the 13th rib and caudally to the hip bones should be clipped. Clipping should occur dorsally above the transverse lumbar spinal processes and span as far ventral as the restraint system allows. Surgical prep is performed as described above in the general surgical considerations section.

To facilitate a paramedian approach, injectable sedation is required to induce recumbency. The cow will be placed in dorsal recumbency with the limbs extended. Take care to monitor for increased abdominal distention/bloating or respiratory distress in this surgical position. The sedation will provide some analgesia, but a local block will be needed for the surgical incision. A line block with 2% lidocaine will be appropriate. The hair should be clipped along the entire ventral abdomen, spanning from the xiphoid caudally to the mammary gland and as lateral as can be achieved on each side. Surgical prep is performed as described above.

Instrumentation

A bovine surgical pack is needed. In addition, sterile rectal sleeves will be needed for abdominal exploration. For the standing right flank omentopexy and/or pyloropexy, a 2–3 in 14-gauge needle with suction tubing will be required to deflate and drain the abomasum. Suture typically used for both approaches is size three Chromic Cat Gut, but this is left to the surgeon's preference.

Post-operative Management

Prior to surgery, analgesia in the form of flunixin meglumine would likely be given, pending hydration status. Post-operatively, pain management should be continued with a nonsteroidal anti-inflammatory as long as the patient is well-hydrated. Again, depending upon presenting physical examination and clinical signs, pre-operative antibiotics were likely administered. The broad-spectrum antibiotics will likely be continued.

The surgical site for both approaches should be monitored. Because of the debilitating nature of RDAs and RAVs, return to normal feed consumption may take longer. Fluid therapy will likely be continued to correct any electrolyte imbalance. Any concurrent metabolic or disease conditions should be treated and monitored.

Complications and Prognosis

Return to function with an RDA or RAV is very dependent upon the degree of dilation and volvulus of the abomasum. The degree of dilation and volvulus correlates with tissue damage. If the cow was sick for a long period of time prior to presenting, the prognosis is guarded. If the DA was diagnosed early in the course of disease, complications should be minimal and prognosis is good.

Complications that can arise with correction of RDAs and RAVs include peritonitis, abomasal perforation, or altered abomasal function. The abomasum has the potential to displace again as well; this is more common in LDA corrections.

Left Displaced Abomasum

To correct an LDA, there are numerous techniques that can be performed. Deciding which technique to pursue will be dependent upon the cow's disease process, demeanor, experience of the veterinarian, and economics. They can be divided into two categories: minimally invasive and surgical technique. Minimally invasive techniques include: rolling, blind tack and toggle, and laparoscopic-assisted toggle pin placement. Surgical techniques include right flank omentopexy–pyloropexy, right paramedian abomasopexy, and left paralumbar fossa abomasopexy.

Relevant Anatomy

Please see the above section for normal abomasum relevant anatomy.

Indications

Left DAs are more commonly encountered in practice compared to RDAs and RAVs. As stated previously, LDAs are most commonly observed in dairy cattle, although they do occur in bulls, beef cattle, and calves. Left DAs normally occur within the first month of lactation and occur due to a combination of different events, such as recent parturition, feed changes, and any concurrent metabolic conditions that could have developed due to pregnancy or management principles. The abomasum in LDAs is primarily composed of gas as compared to the abomasum with an RDA or RAV pathophysiology.

Cattle with LDAs presented due to decreased milk production and decreased feed intake. Decreased fecal production is also observed, most notable on rectal examination. These animals are not as severely systemically ill as cattle with RDAs or RAVs. Diagnosis is based upon history of recent calving with the above-mentioned clinical signs. On physical examination, positive percussion and succussion is appreciated on the mid-left flank from rib 9 to 13. The size of the area of the ping is dependent upon the degree of dilation of the abomasum. There are other differentials for a positive percussion on the left flank. These include ruminal tympany, pneumoperitoneum, pneumouterus, and an empty rumen.

Anesthesia and Surgical Preparation

The method for correcting the LDA will dictate the position of the patient and, therefore, any need for injectable sedation and/or local analgesia to facilitate the procedure. The minimally invasive techniques rely on the underlying pathophysiology of LDAs, that the abomasum is gas filled and freely movable. This allows for the abomasum to be manipulated back into its normal anatomical location. The main disadvantage of these techniques is the inability of the surgeon to confirm the correct anatomical location. However, these techniques are economically more feasible for commercial operations and the time taken to correct the LDA is decreased compared to surgery.

Rolling is literally rolling the cow to allow for the gas-filled DA on the left to float back to the anatomically correct position on the right side of the abdomen. For this procedure, the cow should be clipped from the xiphoid to the umbilicus, from midline to just right lateral of the mammary vein. Ropes or other restraints will be needed to be placed on the down limbs. To induce recumbency and allow for rolling safely, intravenous injectable sedation is used. Animals are laid down in right lateral and then rolled clockwise. Once in right lateral, the clipped area can be surgically prepped.

The toggle and tacking procedure is a similar setup to rolling the cow. The clip area is the same. Sedation would be required to drop the cow and place in dorsal recumbency. Adequate limb restraints are needed to extend and restrain the limbs. Once in position, surgical prep can be conducted. With a toggle procedure, a local block with lidocaine is recommended.

When performing a laparoscopic-assisted toggle pin procedure, the patient is standing initially. After the first portion of the procedure, the patient will be placed in dorsal recumbency. A chute is needed for adequate restraint. The left paralumbar fossa and the 11th intercostal rib space are clipped and surgically prepped as described above. Local analgesia with 2% lidocaine should be used in the form of a line block at the placement of the laparoscope (paralumbar fossa) and trocar (11th intercostal space). After conclusion of the first part of procedure, the cow will then be sedated to induce recumbency and placed in dorsal recumbency. Leg restraints will be needed. At this time, the ventral abdomen is clipped and surgically prepared. Local analgesia will be required for placement of the laparoscope and instrument portal.

The surgical procedures are advantageous in that they allow for direct visualization of the abomasum, and the correction can be assessed. For the right and left paralumbar fossa approach, these animals are standing. A chute and halter are needed. The entire right or left paralumbar fossa should be clipped; this is from just cranial to the 13th rib, extending to the hip bones and spanning dorsally above

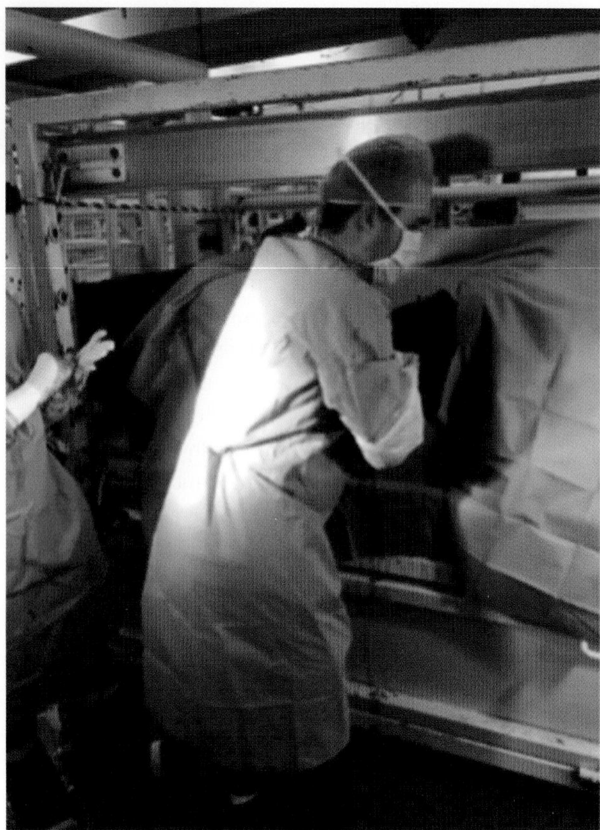

Figure 10.40 Left flank approach to the bovine abdomen. Source: Courtesy of Jennifer Halleran, DVM, DACVIM (LAIM).

the transverse lumbar spinal processes and as far ventral as the chute allows. The clipped area can be surgically prepared as described above. To facilitate surgery, a distal paravertebral block, a proximal paravertebral block, inverted L, or line block with 2% lidocaine can be administered. Due to the calm nature of dairy cattle, sedation not normally required. However, if the animal is fractious, sedation may be needed (Figure 10.40).

To perform a right paramedian abomasopexy, the cow needs to be in dorsal recumbency. This requires appropriate limb restraints. To allow for recumbency, injectable sedation is needed, unless the cow is quite docile and can be casted down. The ventral abdomen extending from the xiphoid to the mammary gland and laterally should be clipped. This area can be surgically prepped as described earlier. A line block or inverted L block with 2% Lidocaine is administered along ventral midline to facilitate the procedure.

Instrumentation

When rolling, aside from ropes for restraint, a large-gauged needle, a 14- or 16-gauge needle, 6–12 cm in length is needed to deflate the abomasum. If suction is available, that would assist in deflating the abomasum. When performing the toggle and tacking procedure, a toggle pin with cannula, trocar, and suture material is needed. A blind tacking can be performed with just suture material. Here, a large needle would be required with a long length of number 2 or 3 nonabsorbable suture. When performing a laparoscopic-assisted toggle pin procedure, a laparoscope is needed. A large trocar and toggle pin are required as well.

For the standing surgical procedures and right paramedian abomasopexy, a bovine surgical pack can be utilized. In addition, sterile rectal sleeves for abdominal exploration would be needed. A 2–3 in 14-gauge needle with suction tubing will be required to deflate the abomasum. Large sized suture, either two or three synthetic nonabsorbable suture would be needed to perform the omentopexy, pyloropexy, or abomasopexy.

Post-operative Management

Regardless of the procedure conducted, any concurrent medical conditions need to be diagnosed and treated. Analgesia in the form of flunixin meglumine would likely be given, pending hydration status, prior to the procedure. Post-operatively, pain management should be continued with a nonsteroidal anti-inflammatory as long as the patient is well-hydrated. Again, depending upon presenting physical examination and clinical signs, pre-operative antibiotics were likely administered. The broad-spectrum antibiotics will likely be continued.

At the conclusion of standing surgeries, it is a common practice to transfuanate or provide oral electrolyte solutions to the patient. This is typically done through orogastric tube placement. The rumen is then enlarged, occupying space on the left side of the abdomen, which may assist in preventing re-displacement if the pexy failed.

Complications and Prognosis

For patients that have been rolled, peritonitis from puncturing the abomasum and subsequent leakage into the abdominal cavity is possible. Puncture of the small intestines or rumen or other internal viscous structure is possible as well. Because the abomasum was not tacked, there is a chance for re-displacement. Blind tacking or toggle pin placement have similar complications compared to rolling cattle to fix LDAs. In addition, the placement of the toggle pin could result in a cellulitis, pexy a structure other than the abomasum or a partial to complete abomasal outflow obstruction. Again, there is a chance of re-displacement.

For patients undergoing a standing surgical procedure or the one in dorsal recumbency, complications are unlikely to arise. If so, incisional site infections, peritonitis, or re-displacement can occur. The incision site is well hidden in the right paramedian approach; however, a chance of incision site infection is more likely due to the location.

Teat Lacerations

Relevant Anatomy

The distal aspect of the teat has an opening. It is a straight, linear opening into the teat cistern. The teat cistern travels up to the gland cistern. There are many ducts that travel into the gland cistern that allow for milk production and milk collection.

Indications

Teat lacerations can occur for a variety of different reasons. Trauma is the main inciting cause. When the laceration or injury to the teat is noted, ice should be applied to reduce swelling. If the wound cannot be fixed quickly, a bandage should be applied to prevent further injury or contamination.

Anesthesia and Surgical Preparation

For most teat lacerations, standing procedures are performed. A chute and halter would be needed. Standing would decrease the risk of any further damage to the teat. If there is an extensive laceration, or extensive work needs to be conducted, lateral recumbency may be desired (Figure 10.41). Due to the calm nature of dairy cattle, sedation may not be necessary. If the animal is fractious or not used to being handled, sedation may be needed. If lateral recumbency is desired for the surgery, sedation may be required. There are some extensive nerve blocks that can be performed to provide anesthesia to the mammary gland; however, these blocks can affect motor function and result in ataxic movements. Therefore, individual teat anesthesia is typically performed. Ring blocks, inverted V blocks, or teat cistern infusions are commonly performed to an individual teat with 2% lidocaine. To facilitate safe application of any of the above-mentioned blocks, the cow may need to be tail jacked. The location of the blocked should be clipped (if there is hair present) and a rough scrub performed. For the teat cistern infusion, a rubber band or a tourniquet is needed to keep the lidocaine within the cistern. Prior infusion of lidocaine, the tip of the teat needs to be cleaned with iodine and alcohol. A sterile teat tube is required to infuse the lidocaine safely without damaging the teat cistern.

An intravenous regional limb infusion of lidocaine can be performed with administration of lidocaine in a venous plexus associated with the individual teat. A tourniquet is needed to clamp the base of the teat to allow for the venous plexus to engorge.

Cleanliness during teat surgery is critical. A potential complication is mastitis. Cleaning the teat, laceration, and orifice very well prior to a procedure will assist in decreasing the risk of mastitis.

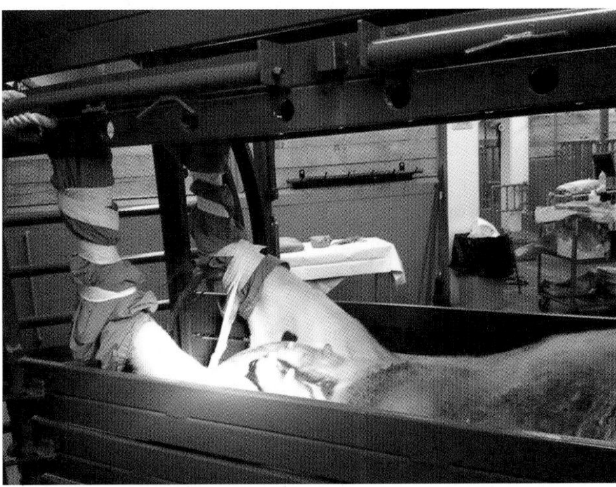

Figure 10.41 Teat surgery preparation on a lactating cow.

> **TECHNICIAN TIP 10.22:** It is optimal to perform the surgery after milking to avoid excess udder distention.

Instrumentation

For teat lacerations, a clean environment is needed. This cannot be stressed enough. Ample non-sterile and sterile gauze is needed. A scalpel handle with blade and a variety of scissors will be needed for debridement. Hemostats and gauze will be used to control hemorrhage. A tourniquet can be used at the base of the teat to assist with controlling hemostasis as well. A small size suture, determined by the laceration and the surgeon's preference should be used. The suture should be a synthetic absorbable suture material. Some clinicians may prefer a stapler for the skin compared to suture material.

Post-operative Management

A local block will provide analgesia during the repair and for a short time after. Nonsteroidal anti-inflammatories may be administered to decrease any swelling and assist in alleviating pain. These can be administered prior to or after the laceration repair. Antibiotics may be administered as well to prevent any bacterial infection or mastitis. It is important to take note of any drug residues and relay this information to the client. Machine milking is preferred to hand milking and milking should start again about two to three days after the laceration repair. Sutures can be removed in 10–14 days.

Complications and Prognosis

The prognosis for lacerations discovered and treated early is very good. The biggest complication associated with laceration repair is the development of mastitis. With appropriate antibiotic therapy and hygienic milking procedures, the risk of developing mastitis can be decreased.

Small Ruminant Surgeries

Urolithiasis

Urolithiasis is a complex disease process that affects male ruminants. It is beyond the scope of this section to delve into the pathophysiology of urolithiasis. But, briefly, ruminants develop urinary calculi due to diet. There are two main groups of stones: phosphatic stones and calcium carbonate stones. Phosphatic stones, known as struvite stones, are sandy in appearance. They develop due to high phosphate levels in the diet, such as high-concentrate feed consumption. Phosphatic stones develop in alkaline urine environments and can be readily dissolved by acidifying the urine. Calcium carbonate stones develop with high calcium diets, such as diets containing alfalfa or other legumes. These stones do not dissolve.

Stone development occurs in both males and females. Females have a shorter, wider urethra; they are able to pass urinary calculi easily. This is primarily a problem in males. Urinary calculi commonly obstruct the urethral process and the sigmoid flexure. To correct urolithiasis, there are numerous surgical options available. Deciding upon the surgical option depends on the job of the patient, how advanced the pathophysiology is, and economics. Tube cystotomies are considered the gold standard for correcting urolithiasis, but many new techniques have been developed. The focus of the section will be on tube cystotomies. Please see the recommended reading for other surgical methods to correct urolithiasis.

Relevant Anatomy

Male ruminants have similar urinary tracts. Kidneys are small, smooth, and bean shaped. They are connected to the urinary bladder via the ureters. The urethra has a sigmoid flexure present and urethral diverticulum located at the level of the ischium. A urethral process is located at the distal tip of the penis.

Indications

The primary indication for performing a tube cystostomy is to correct urolithiasis. The urinary calculi may be causing obstruction within the urinary bladder or the urethra. The bladder could possibly rupture due to prolonged obstruction with no urine voiding. Tube cystostomies do not affect the urethra in terms of the surgical procedure. This is important because this is one of the few surgical options for intact breeding males.

Tube cystostomies allow for healing and reduction of inflammation in the urogenital tract by means of voiding urine through a foley catheter that is placed surgically in the urinary bladder.

Anesthesia and Surgical Preparation

Tube cystostomies can be performed in a field setting. Hospital settings are preferred. General anesthesia is highly recommended. This procedure can be done under injectable sedation, but the patient may need to receive multiple doses of sedation throughout the surgical procedure. A lumbosacral epidural can be utilized to provide analgesia.

The patient will be placed in dorsal recumbency. The ventral abdomen should be clipped from the pubic and inguinal region up to the umbilicus and laterally. The necessary surgical prep as described in the general surgery considerations should be performed.

Blood work is performed prior to surgery. The patient's renal values, hydration status, and electrolytes need to be determined prior to general anesthesia. Patients with urolithiasis typically present with an azotemia (may be a combination of prerenal and post-renal azotemia), dehydration, and electrolyte abnormalities. The degree of electrolyte abnormalities depends upon the severity and duration of urolithiasis. Hyperkalemia is the most life-threatening electrolyte abnormality that may need to be corrected prior to surgery.

Instrumentation

A normal bovine or large animal surgical pack is needed. Suction would be useful for draining the urinary bladder. In addition, a sterile 6 ml syringe and needle would be used to collect a urine sample. A bladder spoon would be needed to remove the stones from the urinary bladder. A sterile foley catheter will be needed for placement within the urinary bladder. Usually, a 22 or 24 French catheter will be appropriate. Depending upon the surgeon, it is recommended to flush the urethra to resume patency. Red rubber catheters may be used for this.

Suture will be needed to place stay sutures in the urinary bladder (PDS). Suture will also be needed to correct any urinary bladder rupture and fix the tube in the urinary bladder. PDS can be used here as well. A nonabsorbable synthetic suture material should be used to fix the foley catheter to the skin. The abdomen will be closed in a routine fashion.

Post-operative Management

The goal of the surgery is providing relief to the urethra by means of voiding urine directly from the urinary bladder to the external environment via the foley catheter. The catheter needs to be monitored daily for urine drippage. The tube will remain in place for at least 7–10 days. This will provide ample time to reduce inflammation due to the obstruction or presence of stones within the penile urethra. Around 7–10 days, or if the patient is seen urinating from his penis, the foley catheter will be clamped. Initially, the catheter should be clamped for an hour period while the patient is being monitored for any signs of discomfort. These include straining, vocalization, restlessness, or pawing at the ground. If any of these signs are demonstrated, the tube should be unclamped. If not, the amount of time the tube is clamped can be increased gradually over a few days. The goal is to have the patient with the tube clamped for greater than 24 hr showing no signs of discomfort and urinating normally from the penis. Once this occurs, the tube can be removed by deflating the internal balloon and removing the suture keeping the balloon in place.

> **TECHNICIAN TIP 10.23:** It is very important to make sure there is urine dripping out of the tube when unclamped. If the patient is laying down for an extended amount of time, it is made to get up to make sure the tube is patent.

During this monitoring period, the urine can be collected, and the pH of the urine tested. Depending upon the type of calculi, an acidifying agent may be administered to assist in dissolving the urinary calculi. The most common acidifying agent administered is ammonium chloride. The abdominal incision and tube site should be monitored for any signs of inflammation (Figure 10.42).

Prior to surgery, the patient will have had blood work performed. Depending upon renal values and electrolytes, the patient may need to be continued on fluids with supplementation. Depending upon the hydration status, nonsteroidal anti-inflammatories may or may not be given. After completion of the surgery, NSAIDs may be given with the patient on fluids to assist in protecting the kidneys. Urinary bladder analgesics may be administered, such as phenazopyridine. To help with pain due to the surgical procedure, opioids are typically used. The author prefers to administer a dose of morphine post-operatively and place a fentanyl patch. The fentanyl patch will take about 12 hr to affect and last for 72 hr. These patients should have received a dose of antibiotics prior to surgery. Antibiotics will be continued the entire time the tube remains in place.

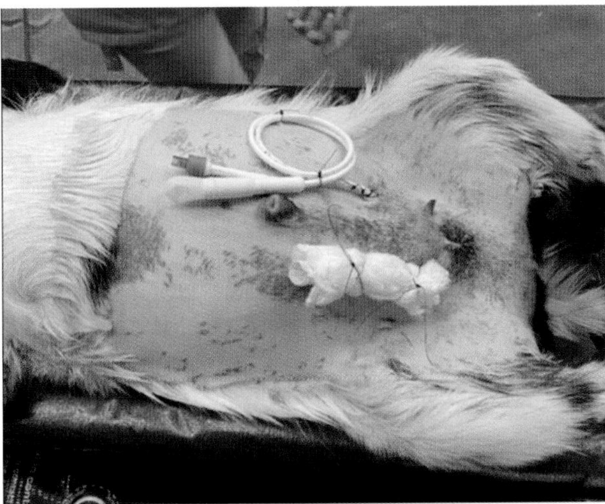

Figure 10.42 Post-operative tube cystotomy.

Complications and Prognosis

Complications associated with the disease process of urolithiasis include re-blockage with development of new urinary calculi, rupture of a region of the urinary tract due to blockage, stricture development, and abscess formation located in the region of the rupture. If the urinary bladder was ruptured prior to surgery, the patient is at risk for developing peritonitis. Complications associated with tube cystostomy include peritonitis, cystitis, or incision site infection.

The prognosis associated with tube cystostomies are quite variable. Some patients are able to have the tube removed within 10 days and have no problems. Other patients will re-obstruct and may need a second surgery. Others, they are patients that will live with a tube for the rest of their life. To aid in preventing the formation of new stones, the diet of the patient can be altered at home to exclude any alfalfa and/or concentrate. Increasing water consumption can also be useful in helping urinary calculi pass.

Cesarean Section

Relevant Anatomy

Small ruminants have a bicornuate uterus.

Indications

Cesarean sections are performed in small ruminants to assist with dystocia management. Dystocias in small ruminants most commonly occur due to fetal–maternal mismatching or all the fetuses are competing to exit the vaginal canal. Fetotomies may be difficult to perform on small ruminants, so if a dead fetus is present, C-sections are usually performed. Ring-womb, or failure of the cervix to have a complete dilation, is another indication for performing a C-section. Just as in cattle, deciding to perform a C-section has many variables, such as reproductive health of the dam, fetus viability, economics, and restraint facilities available. These same variables will also help determine the position of the dam for the C-section to be performed. Most facilities will be equipped to handle a small ruminant C-section. For small ruminants, C-sections are performed with the patient in sternal recumbency, right lateral recumbency, or dorsal recumbency. The latter surgical positions would allow for better and more complete exteriorization of the uterus from the abdominal cavity to minimize uterine fluid contamination from the dead fetus in the abdomen.

Anesthesia and Surgical Preparation

There are three main approaches: ventral paramedian, ventral midline, and a left flank approach. The first two would be performed with the small ruminant in dorsal recumbency. For a left flank approach, the patient can be in sternal or right lateral recumbency. All approaches may be facilitated through local analgesia, although sedation is usually needed. Please see the table in the general surgery considerations section for recommended drugs and dosages. In terms of local analgesia, a lumbosacral epidural or line block can be utilized with 2% lidocaine (Figure 10.43). Take note, the toxic dose of lidocaine is 5 mg/kg compared to 10 mg/kg in cattle. General anesthesia with endotracheal intubation can be performed for patients in dorsal recumbency. If that is not possible, flow-by oxygen is recommended due to the surgical position. Patients in dorsal recumbency may have compromised breathing due to the weight of the rumen and gravid uterus compressing the diaphragm.

For patients in dorsal recumbency, the limbs will need to be restrained to clear the surgical field. The patient should be clipped from the xiphoid down to the mammary gland and as lateral on each side as possible. A rough scrub should be performed prior to a line block, followed by a brief scrub, and then sterile scrub. For patients in sternal or right lateral recumbency, the left flank should be clipped and surgically prepped as described above, with the use of a line block and lumbosacral epidural for analgesia.

Instrumentation

A large animal surgery pack will be just fine for the surgical procedures performed. In addition, sterile rectal sleeves are needed for abdominal exploration and to retrieve the uterus for fetal extraction and delivery. If the fetuses are dead or known to be deceased prior to surgery, two packs of surgical instruments should be used to prevent any abdominal contamination. Suction and suction tubing will be needed, regardless of fetal viability or approach, for abdominal lavage. The uterus will be sutured using synthetic absorbable suture, size 0 or 1. The abdominal wall will be closed in a routine fashion.

Post-operative Management

Monitoring of the incision site is needed post-operatively. As with cattle, ventral abdominal incisions are more prone to infection or dehiscence due to environmental contamination and nursing behavior of the young.

The dam should receive pain analgesics such as flunixin meglumine or meloxicam. In addition, oxytocin should be administered to promote uterine contractions; this would allow for placental expulsion. Retained placentas are more problematic in small ruminants compared to cattle. Depending upon the extent of vaginal manipulation and the contamination present during the surgery, systemic antibiotics should be continued post-operatively. Broad-spectrum antibiotics, such as ceftiofur products, are recommended. If the dam had a normal physical examination prior to surgery, fluid therapy is usually not warranted. If the dam was recumbent prior to surgery due to metabolic conditions, such as pregnancy toxemia or hypocalcemia,

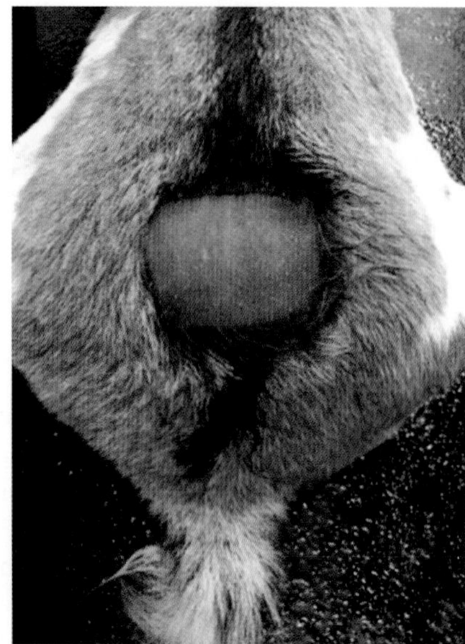
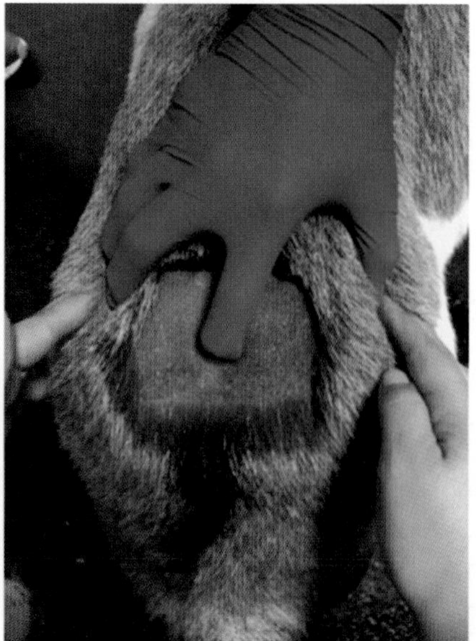

Figure 10.43 (Left) Clipped area for a lumbosacral epidural in a small ruminant. (Right) Location to perform a lumbosacral epidural in small ruminants.Source: Courtesy of Jennifer Halleran, DVM, DACVIM (LAIM).

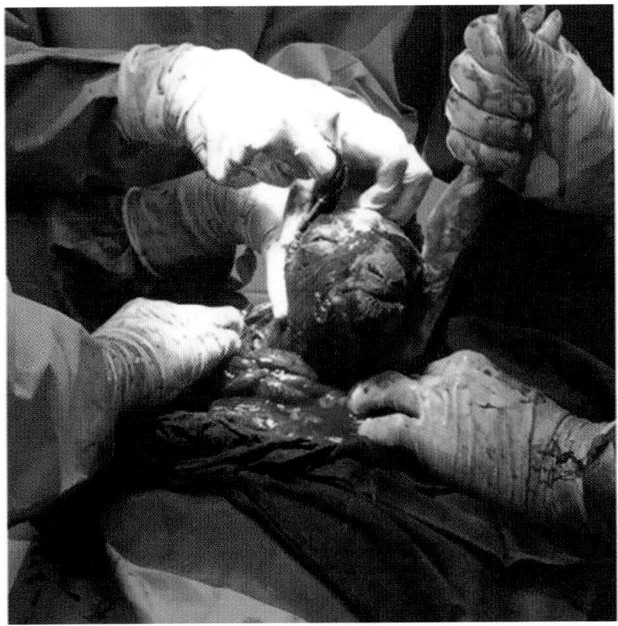

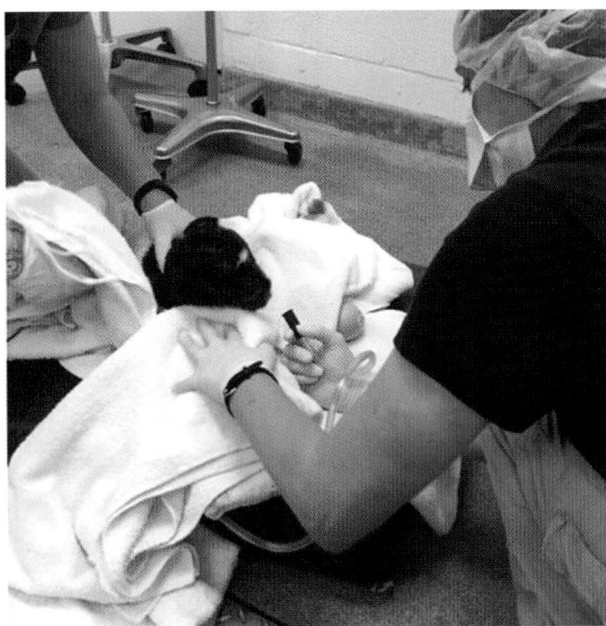

Figure 10.44 (Left) C-section in goat. (Right) Providing warmth and flow-by oxygen to a newborn goat delivered via C-section.

fluid therapy with calcium supplementation would be advised.

Caring for the goat kids or lambs will consume most of the post-operative surgical time. As with calves, ensuring a patent airway, breathing, and adequate circulation is imperative. The goat kids or lambs should be placed in sternal recumbency, and the placental fluid should be removed from the oral cavity. This can be done manually or with suction. A physical examination should be conducted to identify any cardiac or congenital abnormalities. The umbilicus should be dipped with a chlorhexidine/alcohol or iodine solution (Figure 10.44). Colostrum intake should occur within the first 2 hr of life, either by natural nursing, bottle feeding, or orogastric intubation.

TECHNICIAN TIP 10.24: It is important to set up for the goat kids or lambs while setting up for the actual surgery. This would include towels, suction bulb, and oxygen.

Complications and Prognosis

The prognosis is very good with minimal complications. During surgery, abdominal contamination with uterine fluid resulting in peritonitis is the biggest complication. Surgery involving a deceased fetus increases the risk of abdominal contamination; this can be avoided by performing surgery in a lateral or dorsal recumbency position to allow for greatest exteriorization of the uterus to capture any uterine fluid leakage. Incision infections can occur. This would be most frequently encountered with incisions located in the ventral abdomen. Metritis and abdominal adhesions may also occur.

Dehorning

Relevant Anatomy

The most important bit of relevant anatomy is the location of the nerves to be blocked. This is explained in detail below, but briefly, the cornual branch of the lacrimal nerve and the infratrochlear nerve needs to be blocked. Also different from cattle, the sinus is located directly below the horn base.

Indications

Disbudding or dehorning small ruminants is usually performed for safety concerns of other animals or handlers working with the animal. Trauma to the horn may also call for a dehorning to occur. The best age to disbud goat kids are from 7 to 14 days of age. Non-surgical techniques can then be used. For older goat kids, the base of the horn is very wide, and the entire base may not be removed, resulting in scur formation.

Anesthesia and Surgical Prep

For young goat kids, aged 7–14 days, the horns can be removed with hot iron dehorners. Depending upon the restraint available, sedation may be required. Tiny goat kit bud boxes are available. Local analgesia consists of a cornual nerve block and infratrochlear nerve block. Remember, the toxic dose of lidocaine is 5 mg/kg. In a small goat kid, this is not a large volume. If an increase in volume is needed, the solution can be made into a 1% lidocaine solution by diluting with equal parts of sterile water. Prior to application of the cornual nerve and infratrochlear nerve block, the horn base and skull region should be clipped of hair. The nerve block locations should be scrubbed with a dilute iodine solution. Chlorohexidine should not be used as this is caustic to the eye. After a rough scrub, the blocks can be administered, and another scrub can be performed.

For older goats or show goats, a cosmetic dehorn may be required. This would require heavier sedation, but the same local analgesics and prep. After a rough scrub, a sterile scrub will be conducted.

> **TECHNICIAN TIP 10.25:** Toxic lidocaine dose for small ruminants is 5 mg/kg.

Instrumentation

For simple disbudding, a hot iron is needed. For a cosmetic dehorn, a minor pack, consisting of scalpel handle, blade, hemostats, gauze, and thumb forceps are needed. In addition, OB wire and handles are needed for horn removal. A hot iron may be used for cautery after removal of the horn. Bone rongeurs may be needed to level the skull. The surgical site is closed with a large size (0) nonabsorbable suture material. For patients that do not undergo a cosmetic dehorn but have a large horn base and the horn is removed, the sinus cavity will be exposed. Bandage material will be needed to close and protect the sinus cavity.

Post-operative Management

Nonsteroidal anti-inflammatories should be administered prior to procedure and be continued after. Antibiotics can be given prior to the procedure. The sinus may or may not be entered; if it is, the sinus cavity should be bandaged, and antibiotics should be definitely administered. In addition, tetanus antitoxin is administered. Patients should be monitored for any head tilting, nasal discharge, sneezing, or signs of respiratory disease (Figure 10.45).

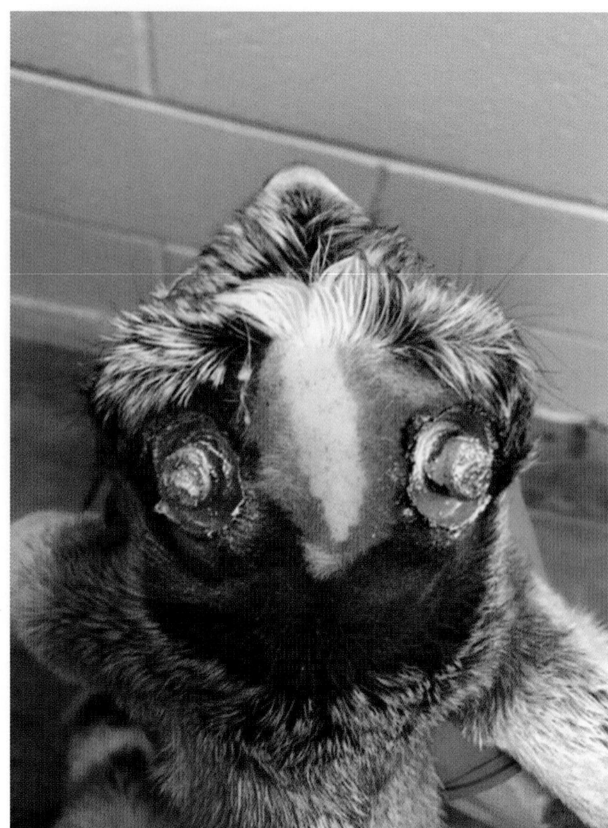

Figure 10.45 Post dehorning of a kid. Source: Courtesy of Lauren Hughes, DVM.

Complications and Prognosis

This is routine processing procedure of goat kids with a favorable outcome. The most common complication occurs when the sinus has been entered and the patient is at risk for developing sinusitis. If the whole horn base is not deadened by the hot iron or removed with surgery, a scur may develop.

Castration

Relevant Anatomy

The testicles are located within the scrotum. The scrotum is very pendulous.

Indications

In small ruminants, the time for castration is controversial. Castrating at younger age for production animals is recommended to alter behavior and prevent any unwanted pregnancies. However, castrating too early can influence urethral diameter and predispose the animal to urolithiasis. For pets, it is recommended to wait until six months of age for castration. This allows for testosterone to have its full effect in maturing the urethra. Waiting this long may pose complications, as the testicles and relevant anatomy are much larger, and hemorrhage may occur. Typically, the main indication for castration is to prevent any unwanted pregnancy, alter male behavior, and decrease the smell associated with bucks going into rut. There is very minimal effect on meat quality.

Anesthesia and Surgical Preparation

There are non-surgical and surgical forms of castration. Deciding upon the method is ultimately determined by economics. Surgical methods of castration may have more complications depending upon the size of the animal at the time of castration. Non-surgical methods tend to have a higher fail rate. Non-surgical castration methods for small ruminants include the use of either emasculatomes or elastrator bands. For non-surgical methods, providing local analgesia is usually not performed. It has shown to not be effective or show any difference in pain. Depending upon cost and the behavior of the patient, light sedation may be given. For the non-surgical techniques, there is no surgical prep work that needs to be performed.

For surgical castration, small ruminants should be sedated. They can be in lateral or dorsal recumbency. The testicles should be clipped, and a rough scrub applied. A testicular block with 2% lidocaine is performed. The block can be placed within the testicular tissue, the spermatic cord, or along the distal third of the scrotum where the incision will be made; be mindful of the toxic dose of lidocaine in small ruminants. After the local block has been performed, a sterile scrub can be applied.

Instrumentation

The instrumentation for non-surgical methods of castration depends upon the method to castrate the patient. If an emasculatome is used, this will be needed. Elastrator bands and apparatus to place the band will be needed. For surgical castration, a minor surgical pack is needed. This should include a scalpel handle, blade, gauze, hemostats, and suture. An emasculator can be used if desired. Suture is used to ligate the spermatic cord and associated vasculature. Chromic Cat Gut should be fine for this procedure.

Post-operative Management

Prior to castration, it is likely nonsteroidal anti-inflammatories will be administered. Anti-inflammatories can be continued after castration as well. Tetanus prophylaxis is recommended, especially with non-surgical methods of castration. Antibiotics are not warranted. The castration site should have fly spray applied to the area around it. The castration site should be monitored for any signs of inflammation or increased bleeding. Typically, the castration site is left open to allow for drainage. If the number of drops of blood cannot be counted, that is considered to be too much blood loss from the castration site.

Complications and Prognosis

For non-surgical methods of castration, the biggest complication is failure of proper castration. For surgical castration methods, hemorrhage is the most common complication. Typically, the prognosis is favorable for either castration method.

Camelid Surgeries

Tooth Removal

Relevant Anatomy

Llamas and alpacas have incisors, canines, premolars, and molars. The dental formula is as follows: I(1/3), C(1/1), PM(1-2/1-2), and M(3/3).

Indications

Retained incisors, removal of canine (fighting teeth), or tooth infection are the primary reasons for tooth removal. Removal of the canine teeth is a normal, routine procedure in camelids that are to be gelded. All camelids have canine teeth, but they are present in a mature state in intact males at a younger age. Camelids use the fighting teeth to well, fight other males, females, and possibly humans. Removal prevents injury to the neck, ears, scrotum, and other deep lacerations from occurring. Tooth root infection occurs when there is a loss of integrity of the gum line. A mandibular or maxillary fracture may also predispose the camelid to a tooth root infection. Clinical signs associated with a tooth root infection swelling over the area of the infected tooth root, hyporexia, or abnormal chewing pattern. A thorough oral exam along with skull radiographs would be warranted (Figure 10.46).

Anesthesia and Surgical Preparation

Sedation and general anesthesia may be needed depending upon the number and location of the teeth needing to be pulled. Depending upon the location and number of teeth, different nerve blocks may be implemented to assist in providing analgesia. Most extractions will occur through the oral cavity. However, if any part of the mandible or maxilla needs to be debrided, the area of the surgical site will need to be clipped and sterilely prepped.

Instrumentation

To remove canine teeth in a routine fashion, sedation will be needed. Obstetrical wire can be used to saw off the tooth flush to the gum line.

Camelid mouths do not open very wide. This makes removing teeth challenging. Small animal and equine dental equipment should be present, along with a general surgery pack. Different dental speculum may be needed to try out in order to see which one fits the camelid head comfortably. A Hauptner bovine speculum may work well. A chisel, mallet, curette, dental punch, periosteal elevator, and forceps should be on hand.

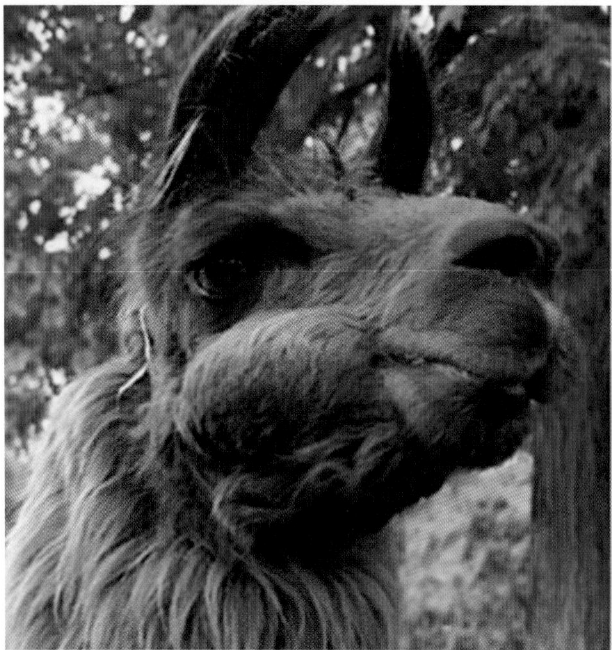
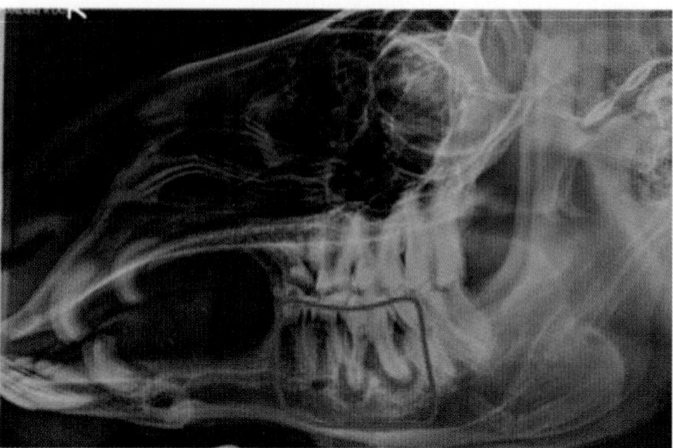

Figure 10.46 (Left) Swelling indicating a problem with a tooth. (Right) Radiograph confirming tooth root abscess on the mandible. Source: Courtesy of Shana Lemmenes, CVT, VTS (EVN).

Post-operative Management

Pain management may be difficult. Local blocks can be utilized, but they will not last for long periods of time. Nonsteroidal anti-inflammatories should be administered to control pain and inflammation. Depending upon the state of the tooth and if an infection is present, local antibiotic beads may be placed within the tooth socket. Culture and sensitivity should be performed in order to use appropriate antibiotics. Systemic antibiotics should be utilized, as well as daily mouth lavages. If the jaw was debrided, antibiotic beads may be placed in the surgical area. A bandage may be applied and changed daily.

Complications and Prognosis

For a simple canine tooth removal due to routine processing, there are minimal complications. If the pulp cavity is left and exposed, this could predispose the patient to a tooth infection. With infected teeth, managing the infection could potentially be difficult. If the infected root, tooth, or bone is not completely removed, a draining tract may develop.

Fractured Mandibles

Relevant Anatomy

Please see the preceding section for the dental formula to be aware of the teeth present on the mandible. The mandible itself is very similar to other species.

Indications

Mandibular fractures can be diagnosed in both males and females. They are usually the result of trauma, especially between fighting males. Fractures that are due to trauma are located just rostral to the cheek teeth. Mandibular fractures present with a malalignment of the mandible. The mandible and tongue may be hanging prolapse from the mouth. The patient will most likely demonstrate difficulty eating and pain upon jaw movement. Radiographs will confirm the diagnosis and assist with surgical preparation.

Anesthesia and Surgical Preparation

To correct and fix a mandibular fracture, general anesthesia is warranted. Depending upon the location of the fracture, different local blocks may be applied, such as a mental nerve block. This can be accomplished with 2% lidocaine. Depending upon the location of the fracture, the patient may be placed in lateral recumbency or dorsal recumbency. The area around the fracture on the face should have all the fiber clipped. The area should be surgically prepped as described in the general surgery considerations section. In addition, the mouth should be lavaged and rinsed with a chlorhexidine solution.

> **TECHNICIAN TIP 10.26:** IV catheter placement in camelids can be difficult due to the strong valves in the jugular vein.

Instrumentation

Instrumentation utilized to repair a fracture mandible will depend upon the preference of the surgeon and the severity of the fracture. Wire, bone pins, plates – they may all be utilized during this procedure. A large animal surgical pack and an orthopedic pack or quick access to orthopedic instruments should be considered prior to the start of surgery.

Post-operative Management

In the author's experience, pain is difficult to control with mandibular fracture repairs. Nonsteroidal anti-inflammatories need to be administered. Different local anesthetic blocks may be performed as well post-operatively, but they do not last for a long period of time. The use of opioids can be considered (morphine, fentanyl patch) as long as gastrointestinal stasis does not occur and fecal output is monitored.

The surgical site may or may not be bandaged. The oral cavity should be cleaned daily with gentle water pressure and chlorohexidine solution. Antibiotics should be given before surgery and for about 10–14 days after surgery.

For the first few days after surgery, the patient should be introduced to a mash or slurry of soft food to minimize any damage to the surgical site. If the patient does well, then they can gradually be re-introduced to their normal diet. As with other surgeries, the surgical site should be monitored for any signs of inflammation and draining.

Complications and Prognosis

Failure of the mandibular fracture correction can occur due to infection of the surgical site. Dehiscence or abscess formation can also occur. Healing of mandibular fractures may take some time, but the prognosis is generally favorable.

Castrations

Relevant Anatomy

The testicles sit within the scrotum. Camelid testicles are not as pendulous as small ruminants or cattle.

Indications

Castration of camelids is indicated for males that are not going to be breeding animals. When raised alone on the bottle, male crias will have socialization problems, believing humans are other male camelids. They may attack them as if they are other males in herd. Castration will decrease behavioral problems associated with fighting and, therefore, any injury they may arise. Castration of camelids can be performed as early as two weeks of age but is typically performed around two months of age.

Anesthesia and Surgical Preparation

The surgery is performed in right lateral recumbency. The left hind limb will need to be restrained forward to allow for access to the scrotum. Sedation will be required. Please the sedation recommendation in the general surgery section. In addition, a local testicular block with lidocaine will be performed. With the patient in lateral recumbency, the scrotum and surrounding area can be surgically prepped.

Instrumentation

There are many methods available to castrate camelids. Any method that is typically used in cattle, small ruminants or horses can be used in camelids. The method is dependent upon the surgeon's preference. The surgeon will at least need a scalpel handle, blade, gauze, hemostats, and suture (Figure 10.47).

Post-operative Management

Nonsteroidal anti-inflammatories should be administered prior to the surgery. NSAIDs can be continued for a few days after the procedure. Antibiotics should also be administered. The surgical site should have fly spray applied. The area is left open for drainage. If the number of drops of blood cannot be counted, that is considered to be too much blood loss from the castration site.

Complications and Prognosis

Hemorrhage is the most common complication. Typically, the prognosis is favorable for either castration method.

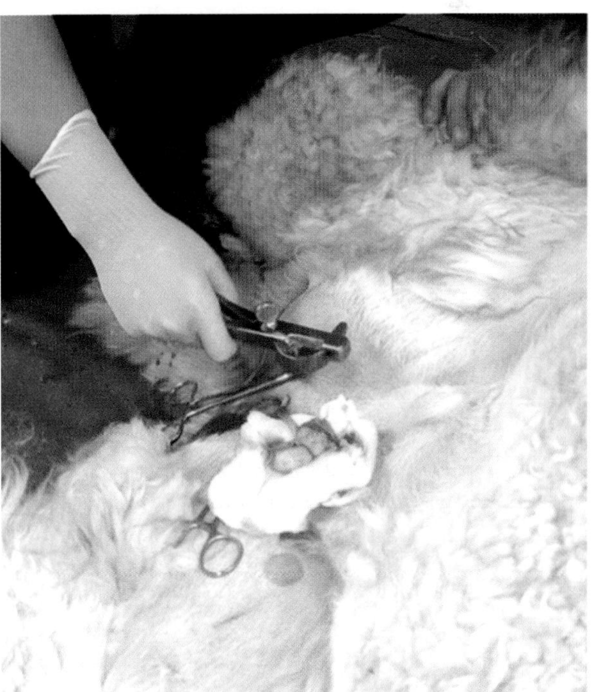

Figure 10.47 Camelid castration.

Cesarean Sections

Relevant Anatomy

The uterus of camelids is bicornuate and looks similar to mares.

Indications

Dystocias are not common in camelids. When a dystocia occurs, it is difficult to fix the dystocia vaginally due to the size of the cria and limited size of the dam. Crias are all legs, and with limited intrauterine space, retraction of the fetus is difficult. When dystocias arise, Cesarean sections are performed.

Anesthesia and Surgical Preparation

Cesarean sections can be performed with the patient in right lateral recumbency or dorsal recumbency. General anesthesia is required. If the surgery is performed in a field setting, injectable anesthesia can be used. A lumbosacral epidural can be performed to facilitate decreasing the amount of inhalant anesthesia. The left flank should be clipped for a left flank approach and the ventral abdomen should be clipped for a ventral midline approach. Surgical prep and scrub should be performed as described in the general surgery consideration section (Figure 10.48).

Instrumentation

A large animal or bovine surgical pack can be used. Sterile rectal sleeves will be required for abdominal exploration to remove the uterus and remove the fetus. If the fetus is dead or known to be deceased prior to surgery, two packs of surgical instruments should be used to prevent any abdominal contamination. Suction and suction tubing will be needed, regardless of fetal viability or approach, for abdominal lavage. The uterus will be sutured using synthetic absorbable suture, size 0 or 1. The abdominal wall will be closed in a routine fashion.

Post-operative Management

Monitoring of the incision site is needed post-operatively. As with cattle and small ruminants, ventral abdominal incisions are more prone to infection or dehiscence due to environmental contamination and nursing behavior of the young.

The dam should receive pain analgesics such as flunixin meglumine or meloxicam. In addition, oxytocin should be administered to promote uterine contractions; this would allow for placental expulsion. Depending upon the extent of vaginal manipulation and the contamination present during the surgery, systemic antibiotics should be continued post-operatively. Broad-spectrum antibiotics, such as

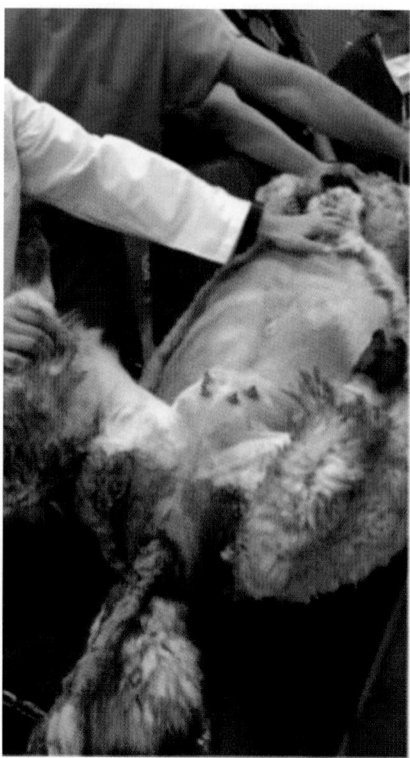
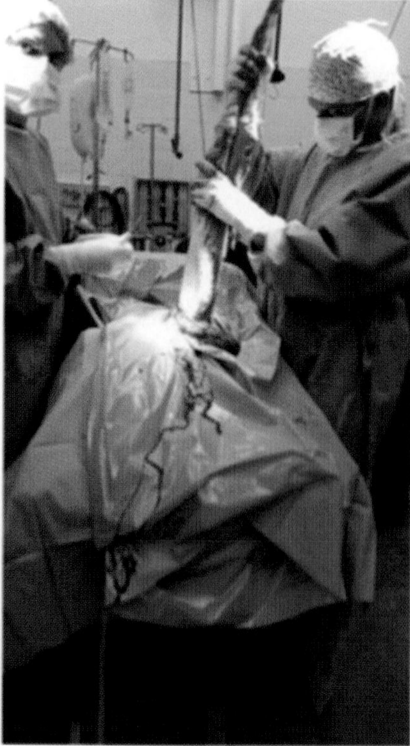

Figure 10.48 (Left) Leg of cria sticking out of vulva. (Right) Cria being pulled via C-section. Source: Courtesy of Shana Lemmenes, CVT, VTS (EVN).

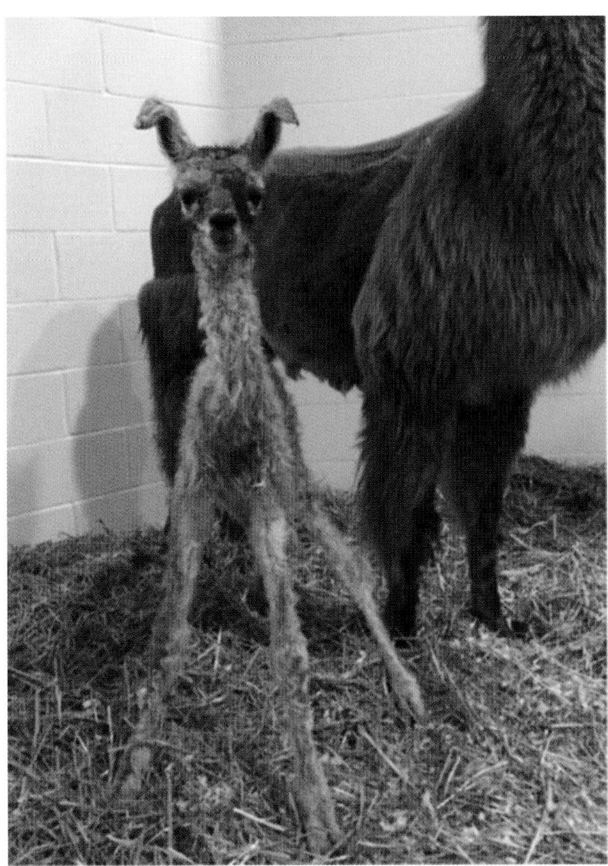

Figure 10.49 Caring for the cria will consume most of your post-operative time.

ceftiofur products, are recommended. If the dam had a normal physical examination prior to surgery, fluid therapy is usually not warranted.

Caring for the cria will consume most of the post-operative surgical time (Figure 10.49). As with calves and small ruminant neonates, ensuring a patent airway, breathing, and adequate circulation is imperative. The cria should be placed in sternal recumbency and the placental fluid should be removed from the oral cavity. This can be done manually or with suction. A physical examination should be conducted to identify any cardiac or congenital abnormalities. The umbilicus should be dipped with a chlorhexidine/alcohol or iodine solution. Colostrum intake should occur within the first 2 hr of life, either by natural nursing, bottle feeding, or orogastric intubation.

Complications and Prognosis

Camelids tend to develop adhesions with abdominal surgery, regardless of how clean the surgery was. During surgery, abdominal contamination with uterine fluid resulting in peritonitis is the biggest complication. Surgery involving a deceased fetus increases the risk of abdominal contamination; this can be avoided by performing surgery in a lateral or dorsal recumbency position to allow for greatest exteriorization of the uterus to capture any uterine fluid leakage. Incision infections can occur. This would be most frequently encountered with incisions located in the ventral abdomen. Metritis and abdominal adhesions may also occur.

Pig Surgeries

Spay

Relevant Anatomy

A spay, or ovariohysterectomy, is the surgical removal of the uterus and ovaries. This is rarely done in production swine but is frequently performed in pet pot belly pigs. It is recommended that pet pigs be spayed around six months old.

Indications

Pigs are spayed in order to prevent aggressive behavior, make management easier, sterilize animals intended for show, help prevent behavioral problems, and also to help prevent health problems such as pyometra and mastitis.

Anesthesia and Surgical Preparation

Pig spays are performed under general anesthesia. Before surgery, the pig should be held off-feed in order to help prevent regurgitation/aspiration and vomiting.

Pigs tend to be less stressed in their stall area, so administering IM sedation in the stall may be easiest. Once the pig is sedated, it will be easier to transport her to the surgery area and induce anesthesia. Once anesthesia has been induced, an endotracheal tube is placed, and the pig is maintained on inhalant anesthesia and positive pressure ventilation is used throughout the remainder of the surgery. An intravenous catheter is placed after anesthesia has been induced. This is due to the fact that pigs tend to be hard to restrain and will resist while awake.

Prophylactic antimicrobials will reduce the risk of infections and septic peritonitis while anti-inflammatories will reduce surgical pain and inflammation. It is important to remember that pigs, even pet pigs, are considered production animals, and therefore, many medications cannot be used. The FARAD website (www.farad.org) should be consulted for assistance selecting appropriate medications for these patients.

Once the pig is intubated and the catheter is placed, the pig can be positioned in dorsal recumbency. The abdomen/inguinal area is clipped, and a rough preparation of the surgical site is done with betadine or chlorhexidine scrub for at least 5 min. The patient is then taken into the surgery area. Once positioned in the operating room, aseptic preparation

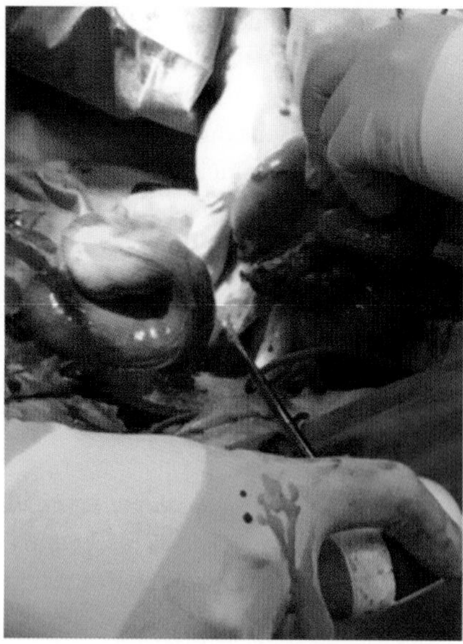
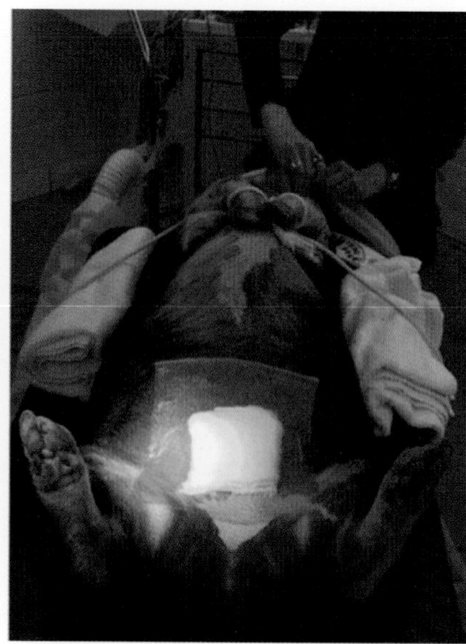

Figure 10.50 Pig spay. Source: Courtesy of Shana Lemmenes, CVT, VTS (EVN).

of the surgical field is performed with betadine or chlorhexidine scrub and alcohol (Figure 10.50).

Instrumentation

Pig spays require a lot of instrumentation. A large instrument pack containing scissors (Metzenbaum, mayo, suture), needle drivers, forceps (sponge, Allis, Kelly, mosquito, brown-Adson, rat tooth), blade handles (#3), and Backhaus towel clamps will be necessary. In addition, gauze, lap sponges, suction set up with Poole suction tip, sterile saline, bowl and syringe, hand towels, and suture are needed. The surgeons will wear sterile gowns and sterile gloves.

In addition, the following equipment is useful:

Ligasure – Handles come in various sizes and allow for both ligating and transecting vessels at the same time.

Post-operative Management

Feeding is usually resumed once the sedation and anesthesia is completely out of the pig's system. Exactly when feeding begins post-surgery and the type of feed (Mazuri, vegetable/fruit, etc.) will depend on surgeon preference. Pigs are prone to vomiting so care must be taken not to re-feed them too quickly.

Monitoring for incisional infection is very important. It should be noted that pigs are prone to herniation and if any signs of infection or herniation are noted, it should be reported to the veterinarian immediately.

Post-operative administration of broad-spectrum antimicrobials and anti-inflammatory drugs will assist in prevention of incisional infections, and reduce pain and inflammation. The medications used and the frequency/duration of administration will vary between surgeons and hospitals.

Complications and Prognosis

Post-operative complications include incisional infection, hemorrhage, septic peritonitis, and hernia.

Prognosis for these pigs is great, providing there are no further complications.

Neuter

Relevant Anatomy

Neuter, or castration, is the surgical sterilization of a male pig, or boar. It is recommended that piglets be neutered as early as possible. Most pet pot belly pigs are castrated before six months old. In comparison, male production piglets are usually neutered within the first 30 days of life.

Indications

Boars are neutered in order to prevent aggressive behavior, make management easier, sterilize animals intended for show, help prevent behavioral problems, and also to prevent health problems such as testicular cancer.

Anesthesia and Surgical Preparation

Pig neuters are performed under general anesthesia. Before surgery, the pig should be held off of feed in order to help prevent regurgitation of feed and vomiting.

Pigs tend to be less stressed in their stall area, so administering IM sedation in the stall may be easiest. Once the pig is sedated, it will be easier to transport him to the surgery area and induce with inhalant or injectable anesthesia.

If using inhalant, the pig is maintained on flow-by inhalant anesthesia throughout the remainder of the surgery.

Pre-operative medications should be given within 60 min of the surgery. Prophylactic antimicrobials will reduce the risk of infections while anti-inflammatories will reduce surgical pain and inflammation. It is important to remember that pigs, even pet pigs, are considered production animals, and therefore, many medications cannot be used. The FARAD website (www.farad.org) should be consulted for assistance with selecting appropriate medications for these patients.

The pig is positioned in dorsal or lateral recumbency. The inguinal area is clipped, and a rough preparation of the surgical site is done with betadine or chlorhexidine scrub for at least 5 min. The surgeon may perform a local nerve block of the incision site and spermatic cord. Many surgeons use mepivacaine, or a combination of mepivacaine and lidocaine for these blocks. Another preparation with betadine or chlorhexidine scrub and alcohol follows the local block.

Instrumentation

An instrument pack containing scissors (Metzenbaum, mayo, suture), needle drivers, forceps (Kelly, mosquito, Brown-Adson, rat tooth), blade handles (#3), and Backhaus towel clamps will be needed. In addition, lap sponges, sterile gauze, emasculator, suture, and hand towels are necessary. The surgeon(s) will wear sterile gloves.

Post-operative Management

Feeding is usually resumed once the sedation and anesthesia is completely out of the pig's system. Exactly when feeding begins post-surgery and the type of feed (Mazuri, vegetable/fruit, etc.) will depend on surgeon preference. Pigs are prone to vomiting so care must be taken not to refeed them too quickly.

Monitoring for incisional infection is very important. It should be noted that pigs are prone to herniation and if any signs of infection or herniation are noted, it should be reported to the veterinarian immediately.

Perioperative administration of broad-spectrum antimicrobials and anti-inflammatory drugs will assist in prevention of incisional infections, and reduce pain and inflammation. The medications used and the frequency/duration of administration will vary between surgeons and hospitals.

Complications and Prognosis

Post-operative complications include incisional infection, hemorrhage, abscess, scirrhus cord, inguinal hernia, and seroma or hematoma formation.

Prognosis for these pigs is great, providing there are no further complications.

Foreign Body

Relevant Anatomy

In cases of a foreign body, or gastrointestinal obstruction, a portion of the gastrointestinal tract is obstructed by a foreign object that the pig has consumed. Commonly affected portions of the gastrointestinal tract are the stomach, large and small intestine.

Indications

Surgery of the gastrointestinal tract is not commonly performed in production pigs, largely for economic reasons. Pot belly pigs are very busy and are prone to eating things they should not when left alone in the house or if they are upset due to changes in routine. They may exhibit clinical signs such as depression, vomiting, abdominal distension or decreased fecal production when obstructed.

Anesthesia and Surgical Preparation

Foreign body removal surgeries are performed under general anesthesia. Before surgery, the pig should be held off of feed in order to help prevent regurgitation of feed and vomiting.

Pigs tend to be less stressed in their stall area, so administering IM sedation in the stall may be easiest. Once the pig is sedated, it will be easier to transport it to the surgery area and induce anesthesia. Once anesthesia has been induced, an endotracheal tube is placed, and the pig is maintained on inhalant anesthesia and positive pressure ventilation is used throughout the remainder of the surgery. The intravenous catheter is placed after anesthesia has been induced. This is due to the fact that pigs tend to be hard to restrain and will resist while awake.

Prophylactic antimicrobials will reduce the risk of infections and septic peritonitis while anti-inflammatories will reduce surgical pain and inflammation. It is important to remember that pigs, even pet pigs, are considered production animals and therefore many medications cannot be used. The FARAD website (www.farad.org) should be consulted for assistance selecting appropriate medications for these patients.

Once the pig is intubated and the catheter is placed, the pig can be positioned in dorsal recumbency. The abdomen/inguinal area is clipped, and a rough preparation of the surgical site is done with betadine or chlorhexidine scrub for at least 5 min. The patient is then taken into the surgery area. Once positioned in the operating room, aseptic preparation of the surgical field is performed with betadine or chlorhexidine scrub and alcohol.

Instrumentation

Abdominal surgeries require a lot of instrumentation. A large instrument pack containing scissors (Metzenbaum, mayo, suture), needle drivers, forceps (sponge, Allis, Kelly, mosquito, brown-Adson, rat tooth), blade handles (#3) and Backhaus towel clamps will be necessary. In addition, gauze, lap sponges, suction set up with Poole suction tip, sterile saline, bowl and syringe, hand towels and suture are needed. The surgeons will wear sterile gowns and sterile gloves.

The following equipment is also useful:

Ligasure – Handles come in various sizes and allow for both ligating and transecting vessels at the same time.
Intestinal forceps – Carmaults, Babcocks.

Post-Operative Management

Feeding is usually resumed once the sedation and anesthesia is completely out of the pig's system. Exactly when feeding begins post-surgery and the type of feed (Mazuri, vegetable/fruit, etc.) will depend on surgeon preference. Pigs are prone to vomiting so care must be taken not to refeed them too quickly.

The pig's fecal output should be monitored to ensure that the obstruction has been successfully cleared and the gastrointestinal system is functioning properly post-operatively. It is also a good idea to keep towels, stuffed beds and blankets away these pigs, as they will sometimes chew on them and could re-obstruct if they ingest that material.

Monitoring for incisional infection is very important. It should be noted that pigs are prone to herniation and if any signs of infection or herniation are noted, it should be reported to the veterinarian immediately.

Perioperative administration of broad-spectrum antimicrobials and anti-inflammatory drugs will assist in prevention of incisional infections and reduce pain and inflammation. The medications used and the frequency/duration of administration will vary between surgeons and hospitals.

Complications and Prognosis

Post-operative complications include incisional infection, hemorrhage, intestinal ileus, septic peritonitis and hernia.

Prognosis for these pigs is great, providing there are no further complications and they are kept from ingesting foreign bodies in the future.

References

Ames, N.K. (2006). *Noordsy's Food Animal Surgery*. Wiley.

Auer, J. and Stick, J. (2019). *Equine Surgery*, 5e. Elsevier.

Edmondson, M.A. (2016). Local, regional, and spinal anesthesia in ruminants. *VCNA Food Animal* 32: 535–552.

Fowler, M. (2010). *Medicine and Surgery of Camelids*. John Wiley and Sons.

Fubini, S.L. and Ducharme, N.G. (2004). *Farm Animal Surgery*. Saunders.

Hendrickson, D.A. and Baird, A.N. (2013). *Turner and McIlwraith's Techniques in Large Animal Surgery*. John Wiley and Sons.

Seddighi, R. and Doherty, T.J. (2016). Field sedation and anesthesia of ruminants. *VCNA Food Animal* 32: 553–570.

Tighe, M. and Brown, M. (2020). *Mosby's Comprehensive Review for Veterinary Technicians*, 5e. Elsevier.

Clinical Case Resolution 10.1

Recording a thorough history is vital to resolution of patient problems. Items that must be recorded are:

- number of breedings this season;
- breeding method used;
- intervention or therapy used thus far;
- amount and frequency of exercise or training;
- number of live offspring produced;
- type and number of breedings used to produce live offspring;
- any instances of dystocia;
- other health problems;
- diet;
- housing;
- any history of travel; and
- immunizations.

Activities

Multiple Choice Questions

(Answers can be found in the back of the book.)

1. Pre-operative blood work will include all of the following except:
   - **A** CBC
   - **B** Sedimentation Rate
   - **C** PCV
   - **D** TS

2. Which drug is considered a dissociative anesthetic?
   - **A** Morphine
   - **B** Butorphanol
   - **C** Ketamine
   - **D** Flunixin

3. Alpha$_2$ agonist can be reversed by all the following except:
   - **A** Acepromazine
   - **B** Yohimbine
   - **C** Tolazoline
   - **D** Atipamezole

4. Duration of action of mepivacaine is:
   - **A** 1–2 hr
   - **B** 1–3 hr
   - **C** 4–6 hr
   - **D** 2–4 hr

5. Complications of a post-operative colic include all of the following except:
   - **A** post-operative ileus
   - **B** incisional infection
   - **C** adhesions
   - **D** foot abscess

6. What is the Trendelenburg position?
   - **A** tilting head down and hindquarters up
   - **B** tilting head up and hindquarters down
   - **C** right lateral recumbency
   - **D** sternal recumbency

7. Complications of a tie-back surgery include all of the following except:
   - **A** wound dehiscence
   - **B** coughing
   - **C** shaking of head
   - **D** lung abscess formation

8. Toxic lidocaine dose for cattle is:
   - **A** 2 mg/kg
   - **B** 5 mg/kg
   - **C** 8 mg/kg
   - **D** 10 mg/kg

9. Toxic lidocaine dose for small ruminants is:
   - **A** 2 mg/kg
   - **B** 5 mg/kg
   - **C** 8 mg/kg
   - **D** 10 mg/kg

10. Complications of a pig foreign body surgery include all of the following except:
    - **A** intestinal ileus
    - **B** septic peritonitis
    - **C** tooth root abscess
    - **D** hernia

Test Your Learning

1. Prior to the start of any anesthetic procedure, certain considerations must be thought out. What are some of these considerations?
2. It is very important to know which drugs can be reversed after given. List these drugs and their reversal.
3. You are asked to get instruments together for a standing ovariectomy. What extra equipment is needed beyond the large instrument pack?
4. When a cow is admitted to the hospital for an elective surgery, why is it important to know when they last had access to food and water?
5. A pig comes in for emergency foreign body surgery. What should you do before you administer any drugs to pigs?

Answers can be found in the back of the book.

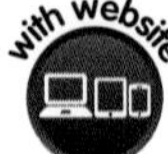

Extra review questions, case studies, and a breed ID image bank can be found online at http://www.wiley.com/go/lienvettech.

Chapter 11

Neonatology

Laura Lien, MS, CVT, VTS (LAIM), Kimberly Schreiber Young, BS, DVM, and Sue Loly, LVT, VTS (EVN)

Learning Objectives

- Describe the importance of addressing passive transfer of immunoglobulins.
- List body systems that must be assessed during the perinatal period.
- Compare ways to test and treat neonates for failure of passive transfer.
- List characteristics and clinical signs of prematurity in large animal neonates.
- Describe the types of systems that are used to deliver medications and treatments to neonates.
- Describe diagnostic procedures and treatments used for septicemic neonates.

Key Terms

Asphyxia
Auscultation
Bacteremia
Brooder
Dysmature
Electrocardiography
Epitheliochorial placenta
Failure of passive transfer
Glucometer
Holosystolic
Immunoglobulins
Neonate
Obligate nasal breather
Parenteral nutrition
Sepsis
Shock
TPR

Clinical Case Problem 11.1

A two-day-old Arabian foal presents to the hospital with inability to rise. What items should you prepare to receive this foal and why?

See Clinical Case Resolution 11.1 at the end of this chapter.

Introduction

The neonatal period is defined as the first three to five days of life. This is a crucial time period where producers and the veterinary team must be vigilant in recognizing and attending to patients whose needs can change in a very short period of time. When caring for the large animal neonate, the veterinary team must be concerned with addressing species-specific management, husbandry, and treatment needs. The veterinary technician caring for the sick neonate must establish baseline parameters on the respiratory, cardiac, and gastrointestinal system, so that any changes in status can be communicated to the clinician and immediately addressed.

Large Animal Medicine for Veterinary Technicians, Second Edition. Edited by Sue Loly and Heather Hopkinson.

Companion website: www.wiley.com/go/loly/veterinary

TECHNICIAN TIPS 11.1: The neonatal period is defined as the first three to five days of life.

Perinatal Period

The time immediately before and after birth is the perinatal period. During the birthing process, the fetus is still dependent on the dam for homeostasis – oxygen, nutrition, temperature, and circulatory support. The fetus can suffer significant damage if there is any disruption in delivery of oxygen. This is also true during the transition to neonatal status if there is any deprivation of oxygen supply to cells, tissues, organs, or the brain.

While in utero, the fetus lives in a highly regulated, safe environment. At birth, the neonate moves to a less stable thermoregulated environment, as it possesses decreased body insulation. The new environment's temperature, humidity, and wind or drafty conditions, which are much colder than the uterus, tax the neonate's ability to survive. The skin and coat must dry before it is of benefit to maintain body temperature. Further, piglets do not have sufficient brown fat stores to maintain normal blood glucose levels, and premature neonates can suffer from hypothermia due to decreased body fat stores and coat insulation.

TECHNICIAN TIPS 11.2: Premature foals have decreased body fat stores and insulating body coat.

Assessment

Evaluation at birth or at presentation requires assessment of cardiac function, respiratory function, thermoregulation, fluid balance, immune status, and blood glucose levels. Any values outside of normal parameters that are not quickly addressed can have disastrous results. Recognition and treatment early in the assessment process can have a significant influence on patient outcomes. Typically, "ABC" evaluation is followed; airway, breathing, and circulation, which are addressed below as cardiac and respiratory function. Gestational length, parturition stage length, history of dystocia, and neonatal behaviors can provide vital information about their overall health status (Figure 11.1).

TECHNICIAN TIPS 11.3: ABC = Airway, Breathing, and Circulation

Cardiac Function

Without sufficient circulatory support cells, tissues, and organs cannot properly sustain life. Auscultation of the heart and palpation of the pulse provide information as to heart rhythm, rate, and perfusion. Electrocardiography can provide valuable information on status and response to therapy. Chest compressions and administration of medications to stimulate and maintain cardiac output are vital not only to immediate patient status, but also for an overall positive treatment outcome.

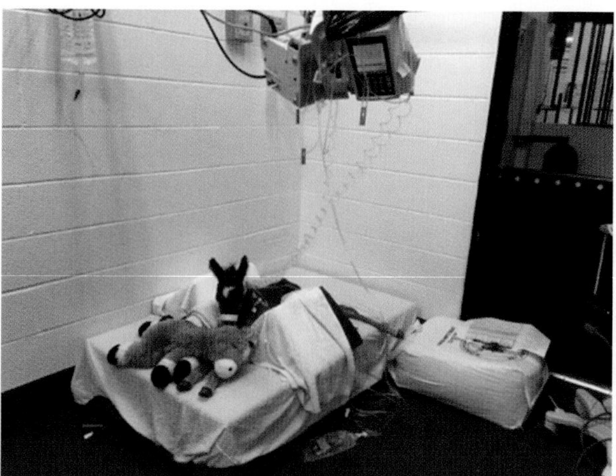

Figure 11.1 Initial assessment and treatment could have significant influence on patient outcomes.

The ductus arteriosus is present in the fetus to bypass the pulmonary circulation to oxygenate the blood supply. At varying times after birth, dependent on species, the ductus arteriosus will close. In foals, it can be heard for periods of up to five days after birth. Patent ductus arteriosus may be auscultated as a holosystolic, grade 2–5/6 murmur at approximately the third intercostal space. The murmur is caused by left to right shunting of blood from the aorta to the pulmonary artery.

Respiratory Function

Varying degrees of asphyxia can occur in utero, during or after parturition, due to multiple factors (Table 11.1). Chronic or acute placental insufficiency or separation, umbilical cord occlusion or torsion, or problems associated with the fetus' or dam's systemic health can all contribute to oxygen deprivation in utero. Assessing the dam during gestation can provide information that will alert the veterinary team that intervention may be necessary during and immediately after parturition to assist the neonate's transition to its new environment. Shortly after birth, the neonate can suffer from asphyxiation from complications in utero or from physical barriers to inspiration or expiration, such as lack of patent airway, lack of surfactant due to prematurity/dysmaturia, failure of spontaneous respiration, or the neonate's position in a stall. Lack of oxygen can result in hypoxemia, ischemia, or death. Equine and

Table 11.1 Parturition normals for large animal species.

Species	Normal gestation length	Minimum viable gestational age (days)	First-stage labor	Second-stage labor	Third-stage labor	Number of offspring	Average birth weight (lb)	Time to stand	Time to suckle
Equine	11 months	300	240 min	30 min	30–180 min	1	Breed Variations	0–1 h	0–2 hr
Bovine	Nine months	240	6 hr	1–2 hr	4–6 hr	1	Breed Variations	15–30 min	1–2 hr
Caprine	150 days	140	Up to 12 hr	1/2–2 hr	2–3 hr	1–3	Breed Variations	30 min–2 hr	30 min–2 hr
Ovine	150 days	138	1–4 hr	1/2–2 hr	2–3 hr	2–3	7–12	min	min
Porcine	114 days	108	Up to 24 hr	2–12 hr	4–6 hr	7–15	3–4	min	min
Camelid	11 months	>321	1–6 hr	30 min–1 h	4–6 hr	1	Llama 20–35; Alpaca 15	1–2 hr	6–8 hr

camelids are obligate nasal breathers; therefore, their nares must be unobstructed for normal breathing to occur. Clearing air passageways immediately after birth can be accomplished by using resuscitation pump action devices that aspirate mucus and amniotic fluid and then deliver room air or 100% oxygen to the neonate. Simple obstructions at the nares can also be manually removed or suctioned with bulb syringes if other resuscitation devices are not available. If mucus or fluids in the respiratory tract are not a concern, then 100% oxygen can also be delivered via mask, insufflation, or endotracheal tube (Figure 11.2).

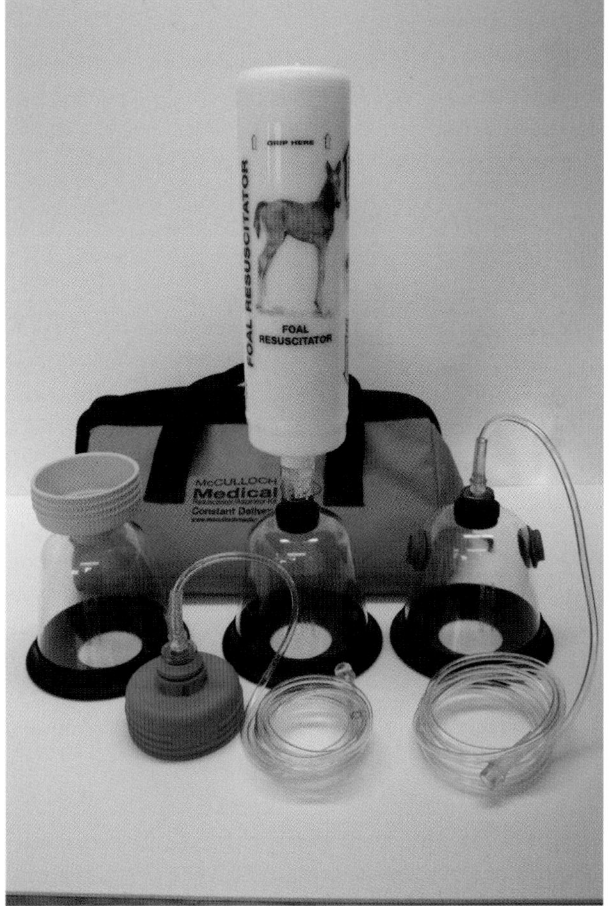

Figure 11.2 McCulloch foal aspirator/resuscitator. *Source:* Reproduced with permission of McCulloch Medical NZ Ltd.

Thermoregulation

To prevent or treat hypothermia, provide clean, dry bedding in a draft-free pen. Blankets or rugs can be used to conserve body heat. Supplemental heat sources, such as heat lamps or warm air blankets, may be used. The technician must be mindful that heat sources, such as heat lamps, are in good working order, are well secured, and not close to combustible items or within reach of the neonate or dam. The neonate should be checked regularly to monitor ongoing need for supplemental heat, as overheating can occur (Figure 11.3).

TECHNICIAN TIPS 11.4: When using heat sources to warm a patient, body temperature must be checked frequently to prevent hyperthermia.

Fluid Regulation

Dehydration of neonates can coincide with lack of suckle and inability to nurse, but also many other common conditions including hypoxic ischemic encephalopathy (HIE) and diarrhea. Hydration status can be assessed from a thorough history, observation of decreased skin turgor, sunken eyes, tacky mucous membranes, decreased urine production, increased urine-specific gravity, decreased pulse quality, elevated blood lactate, tachycardia, and abnormal PCV/TP values. Dehydration can have detrimental effects on kidney function as well as other body processes.

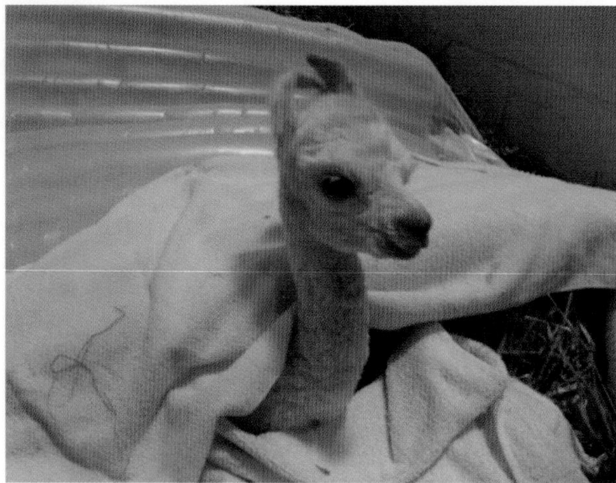

Figure 11.3 Premature cria with a Bair Hugger and towels to help with thermoregulation.

Intervention to address current hydration status and ongoing maintenance and fluid losses must be assessed and implemented along with ongoing observations and evaluation so that over hydration does not occur.

Glucose

Most compromised neonates will have lower than normal blood glucose levels, as they are often too sick and weak to nurse or appropriately regulate their metabolism (Table 11.2). With a lack of sufficient milk intake, they also suffer from dehydration. Low glucose levels starve cells, tissue, and organs of energy to function and grow. This is especially true of an already compromised and often septic neonate. In addition, neonates have increased need for glucose in cases of shock, infection, and asphyxia. The low end of normal glucose levels in the neonate varies by species. Portable glucometers and 50% dextrose with compatible diluent should be available at admission to evaluate and treat hypoglycemia. It is imperative that 50% dextrose should never be administered without appropriate diluent to prevent cellular lysis.

> **TECHNICIAN TIPS 11.5:** When working with neonates, any change in behavior or values outside of parameters must be communicated to the clinician.

Table 11.2 Minimum neonatal blood glucose levels.

Equine	<60 mg/dl
Porcine	<50 mg/dl
Bovine	<40 mg/dl

Neonatal Infections

Production losses from neonatal infections are significant to the owner/producer. Providing a clean, draft-free rearing environment and sufficient nutrients and hydration, as well as assuring sufficient oxygenation and cardiac perfusion, satisfy the immediate needs of the neonate. Ongoing concerns for the newborn include adequate acquired immune protection.

Immune Status

An epitheliochorial placenta nourishes the large animal fetus. This type of placenta, which has more layers of separation between maternal and fetal circulation than other species, does not allow the transfer of immunoglobulins to the fetus. The neonate must receive IgG, IgA, and IgM immunoglobulins through ingestion of colostrum because of this placental barrier. Ideally, this should occur within a few hours of life, as neonatal intestinal absorption rates decrease significantly over time. References state that the closure of the intestinal lining begins when the neonate consumes colostrum, but that the ability to absorb macromolecules such as IgG drastically diminishes or closes at 24 hr postpartum. Other factors that influence neonatal IgG levels are quantity and quality of the colostrum.

Whenever possible, colostrum should be tested. Traditionally, colostrum is tested by colostrometer, which is still a reliable, easy, and low-cost method to determine quality, but requires approximately one pint of colostrum. Samples should be at room temperature (72 °F), as samples at lower temperatures overestimate IgG concentrations and at higher temperatures underestimate concentrations. Good-quality colostrum should measure greater than 50 mg/ml or within the green colored zone marked on the meter.

Other testing methods include colorimetry, refractometer, ELISA, and glutaraldehyde, and are useful when sample volume is a concern with a colostrometer. The Brix refractometer was originally designed to measure sucrose in solution, but these same values have been associated to colostral IgG. If samples show a Brix value of 22%, this correlates to 50 mg/ml, a level of IgG that should under optimum circumstances provide sufficient protection to the neonate.

Dairies may experience shortages of colostrum due to several factors, many directly linked to the cow's health during the gestational period. Colostrum replacement and supplement products have recently been developed to combat these shortages. Early research has shown that quantity and quality of the IgG concentrations vary widely in these products. The use of fluid (natural, maternal) colostrum carries a biosecurity concern for dairy producers, as colostrum should only be used from multiparous cows testing negative for *Mycobacterium paratuberculosis*, bovine leukosis virus, bovine viral diarrhea virus, *Neospora caninum*, *Salmonella dublin*, and *Mycoplasma bovis*. Using replacement or supplemental products decreases this concern but further study is warranted to determine their place in combating failure of passive transfer.

Equine breeding facilities can experience the same frustrations for quality and quantity of colostrum. Breeders across the United States may access electronic database colostrum banks via the World Wide Web. Drawbacks to this type of system are that the colostrum may not provide immunity to local pathogens and the quality of the colostrum cannot be guaranteed.

Failure of Passive Transfer

Failure of passive transfer occurs when less than optimum levels of IgG are found in the circulation of neonates. Neonates should be tested for adequate levels of IgG (Table 11.3). Calves can be quickly and easily screened by testing total plasma protein. Levels >5.2 mg/dl are considered adequate. Foals can be tested using ELISA tests and all species via RID (radial immunodiffusion) testing.

The gold standard for treating FPT is the use of commercially available species-specific plasma. Commercially produced plasma is often harvested from donors that are vaccinated to produce a hyperimmune plasma product. Drawbacks to the use of plasma are product and administration expenses. Administering plasma is an invasive procedure compared to oral products, and it carries the risk of transfusion reaction and complications from intravenous injection or catheterization. Clinicians may administer plasma via nasogastric tube in equine neonates or via intraperitoneal route to camelid neonates to speed administration time and to reduce instances of antigen reaction, but much is dependent on the age of the neonate and whether, in the case of nasogastric administration, the gut has closed. There is some evidence that nasogastric administration does not confer similar immunity as the intravenous route. While the procedure is less invasive, there is still risk when considering inappropriate intubation, esophageal rupture, and aspiration.

Table 11.3 Assessing passive transfer of immunity.

	PFPT or FPT	Adequate levels	FPT plasma treatment
Equine	<400–800 mg/dl	>800 mg/dl	1–21
Bovine	TP <5.2 mg/dl	TP > or = 5.2 mg/dl	1–21
Caprine	<600 mg/dl	1600 mg/dl	10% of BW
Ovine	<1600 mg/dl	1600 mg/dl	10% of BW
Camelid	TP <5.0 g/dl	TP 6.0 g/dl	20–40 ml/kg

Plasma products must be handled with care both in frozen and thawed states. Frozen plasma should not be placed in frost-free freezers, as these types of freezers raise and lower temperatures to accomplish their frost-free status. Commercially available bags should remain in their cardboard box or cushioned wrap to avoid causing holes in bags if dropped or otherwise jostled in the freezer. Plasma should be stored at −4° to −40 °F (−20° to −40 °C) for up to one year.

Plasma is thawed with a warm water bath, using temperatures <100 °F (37 °C). Higher temperatures during the thawing process will denature proteins. If any cloudiness or clumping in the plasma is observed, the plasma should be discarded. Administration is accomplished using a blood administration set utilizing a mesh filter (150–260 μm) (Figure 11.4). The technician should obtain a baseline TPR of the patient and repeat every 10 min during the first hour. Any observations of tachypnea, tachycardia, agitation, or urticaria should be reported to the clinician and

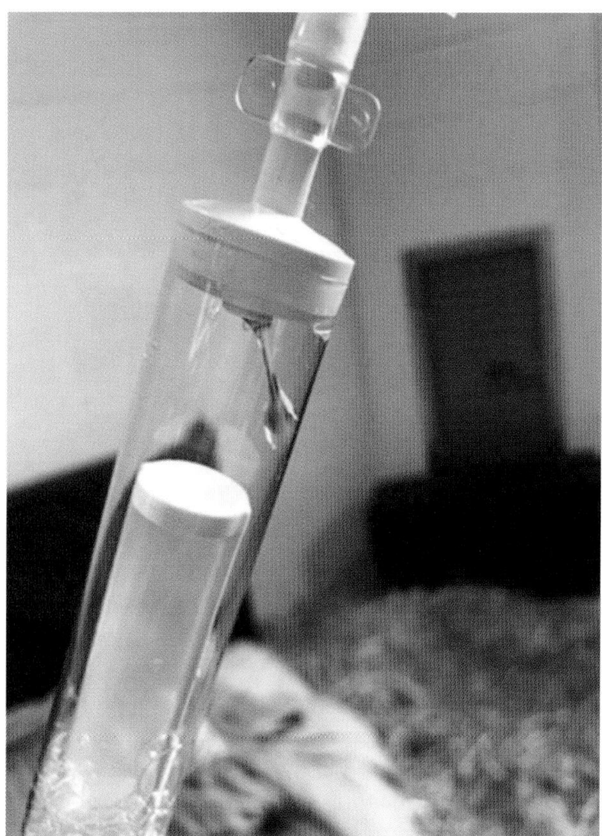

Figure 11.4 Plasma must be administered using a filter administration set.

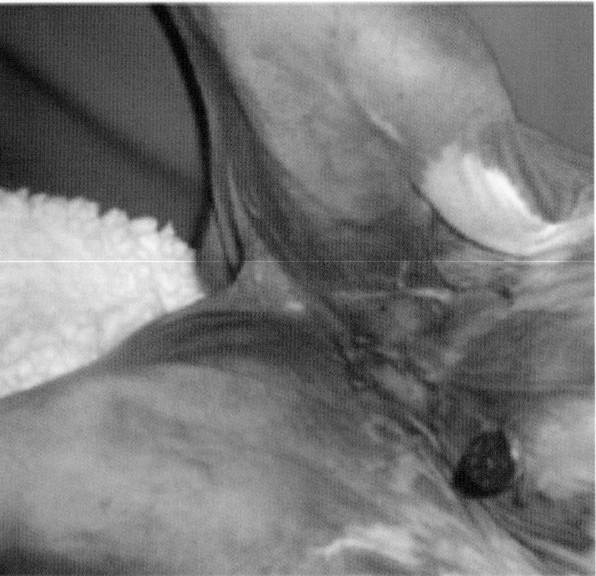
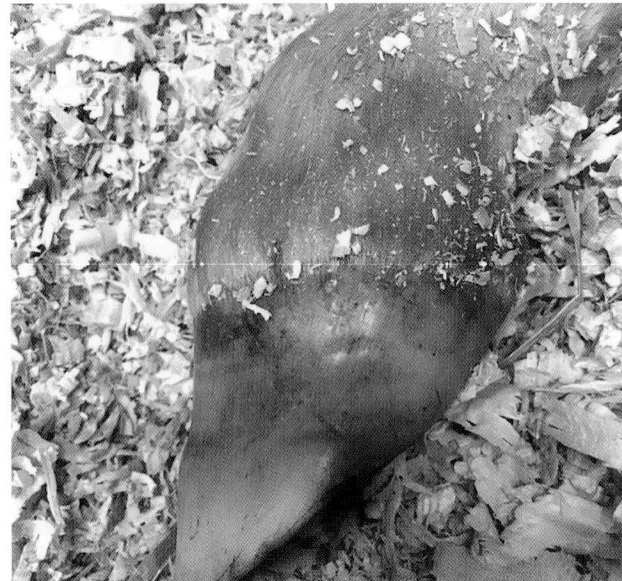

Figure 11.5 Petechial hemorrhage and septic hoof line on a premature foal.

administration stopped until further assessment has been performed. Administration rates begin at 20–40 ml over 30 min, and the rate is gradually increased during the first hour of administration. Neonates or adults receiving multiple units of plasma from different donors have an increased risk of reaction. When administering from multiple donors, the initial monitoring period must be repeated with each subsequent donor bag. If multiple liters are being administered, attempts to use those with similar lot numbers may decrease risk.

> **TECHNICIAN TIPS 11.6:** Plasma must be thawed in *warm*, not hot water and not in the microwave.

Sepsis

Bacteremia is the presence of bacteria in the blood, whereas septicemia or sepsis is a syndrome characterized by a severe systemic inflammatory response to such an insult, often resulting in multiple organ dysfunction syndrome (MODS). Bacteria have high metabolic needs and deplete available nutrients from the neonate causing hypoglycemia. As bacteria grow, reproduce, and die, they produce endotoxins and other substances causing degeneration of healthy tissue and organs. The inflammation associated with the body's response to these events (sepsis or SIRS) can have other deleterious effects on the body. Without timely, sufficient, and aggressive treatment with antimicrobials, anti-inflammatory medications, hydration support, and other supportive care, the neonate will likely suffer organ failure and death. Initial clinical signs of sepsis in neonates include malaise, inability to rise or suckle, fever, tachycardia, petechial hemorrhage, scleral injection, and hyperemia (Figure 11.5). Diagnosing sepsis in the neonate can be accomplished through the use of Sepsis Score Sheets (Figure 11.6). To determine the most appropriate antimicrobial therapy, blood cultures are collected at admission. Best results can be obtained if the samples are drawn before antimicrobial administration, though removal devices are available. Strict adherence to aseptic technique is crucial, as environmental and procedural contaminants can skew results. Blood is collected from a large vessel, usually the jugular vein. Bacteremia can be intermittent, so negative blood cultures do not mean a foal is not septic. In foals, some clinicians prefer to obtain two samples 30 min apart from different aseptic sites to enhance the chance of growth and to clarify pathogenic growth versus environmental contamination (Figure 11.7).

Premature Neonates

Although prematurity can affect any large animal species, the species of great concern for prematurity is the foal. Body systems have insufficient time to prepare for life outside of the uterus and predispose the neonate to problems of respiratory, metabolic, and immune systems as well as infectious disease. Prematurity is defined as a foal born prior to 320 days of gestation. Dysmature foals are those individuals that are immature and undersized with placental insufficiency including placentitis as a frequent cause.

Neonatal Sepsis Score

Foals's Name ______________________ Date ____________ Total Score ____________
Check one: ☐ admission ☐ day # ____________ subsequence to admission ☐ Date # ____________

Number of points to assign:

Information collected:		4	3	2	1	0	Score
I. CBC 1. Neutrophil count	Record <u>exact</u>		<2,000/mm^3	2,000–4,000 or >12,000	8,000–12,000	Normal	
2. Band neutrophil count			>200/mm^3	50–200		<50	
3. Doehle bodies, toxic, granulation, or vacuolization in neutrophilis		Marked	Moderate	Slight		None	
4. Fibrinogen				>600	500–600	<400	
II. Other Laboratory Data 1. Hypoglycemia				<50 mg/dl	50–80	>80	
2. IgG test		<200	200–400	401–800		>800	
3. Arterial oxygen			<40 Torr	40–50	51–70	>70	
4. Metabolic acidosis			Yes			No	
III. Clinical Examination 1. Petechiation or scleral injection not secondary to eye disease or trauma			Marked	Moderate	Mild	None	
2. Fever				>102°F	<100°F	Normal	
3. Hypotonia, coma, depression, convulsions				Marked	Mild	Normal	
4. Anterior uveitis, diarrhea, respiratory distress, swollen joints, open wounds			Yes			No	
IV. Historical Data 1. Placentitis, vulvar discharge prior to delivery, dystocia			Yes			No	
2. Prematurity			<300 days	300–310	310–330	>330	
						Total Points	________

A sepsis score of 12 or higher will accurately predict sepsis 93% of the time, while a score of 11 or less will predict non-sepsis correctly 88% of the time.

The sepsis score should be repeated daily in the following instances:

1 The score is in the questionable range on day 1 (11–14).
2 The foal's zinc sulfate test registers under 800 or the globulins are less than 1.5.
3 The foal's clinical condition has not improved at all by day 2 or is deteriorating.

Figure 11.6 Neonatal sepsis score sheet. *Source:* Courtesy University of Minnesota.

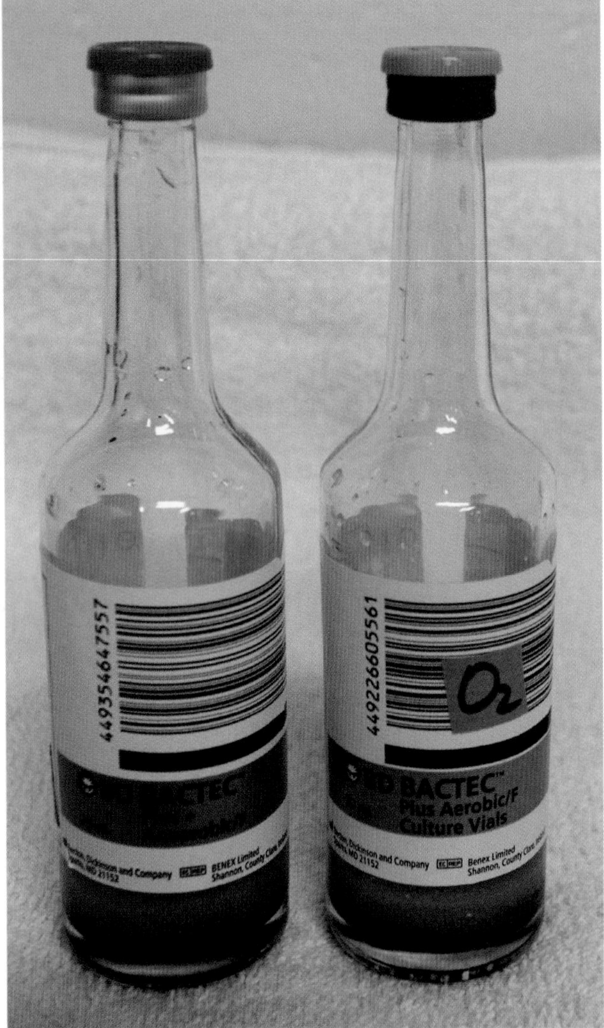

Figure 11.7 These blood culture tubes require 8–10 ml of blood for inoculation.

These foals have a normal gestational length. Most veterinary practitioners and breeding facilities keep strict records of breeding and due dates of mares. Keeping records of gestation length in multiparous mares assists the facility in planning for parturition and possible intervention. Complete breeding records, and careful preparation for foaling season can assist in the delivery of healthy foals.

Despite the best-laid plans, premature and dysmature foals can surprise even the most experienced foaling team. They will typically present with the following signs: low birth weight, generalized weakness, short, silky hair coat, pliable ears, bulging forehead, increased range of motion or hyperflexion of limb, increased chest wall compliance leading to atelectasis, and partial to complete lack of ossification of tarsal and carpal bones (Figures 11.8–11.10). Baseline radiographs of the thoracic cavity, lateral tarsal,

Box 11.1 Collecting Blood Cultures

- sterile gloves
- needles
- syringe
- povidone-iodine scrub
- isopropyl alcohol
- gauze sponges
- clippers with #40 blade

Clip and prep the area over the collection site as for inserting an intravenous catheter using povidone-iodine scrub and alcohol sponges.

Prep the tops of the blood collection bottles just as you would for prepping the collection site using povidone-iodine scrub and alcohol sponges. Place a fresh alcohol sponge over the prepared bottle tops.

Open sterile glove package and place a sterile syringe and at least three needles of appropriate size on the glove's sterile field. If needles are encased in plastic, have an assistant open the needles in an aseptic fashion for phlebotomist to retrieve in a sterile manner.

Perform venipuncture while maintaining aseptic technique. Remove venipuncture needle and discard. Place a new sterile needle on the syringe and place an amount of blood appropriate to the size of bottle into the anaerobic bottle first. Remove needle. Place a new sterile needle on the syringe and place an amount of blood appropriate to the size of bottle into the aerobic bottle. If intravenous catheterization is being performed simultaneously, the blood culture can be obtained through a sterile catheter site.

Properly label bottles and discard syringes and sharps in appropriate containers. If multiple samples are to be taken, include time and order of draw in your labeling (Box 11.1).

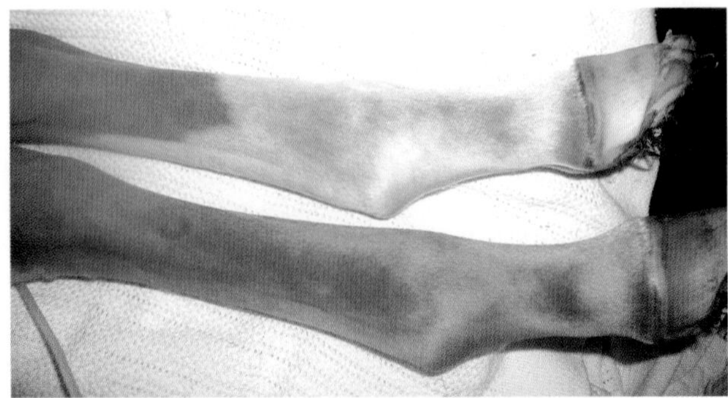

Figure 11.8 Thin hair coat on premature foal.

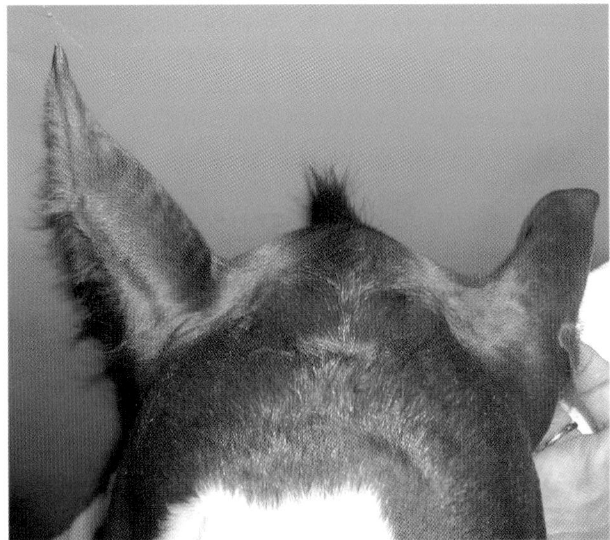

Figure 11.9 Premature foal showing pliable ears and bulging forehead.

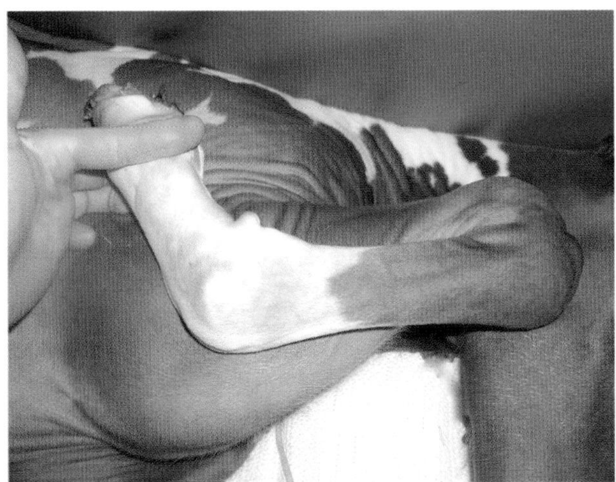

Figure 11.10 Hyperflexion of the forelimb typically seen in the premature foal.

and D/V carpal joints provide a wealth of information on status of the premature equine neonate. Radiographs should be performed prior to allowing the foal to stand if prematurity or dysmaturity is a clinical concern to prevent crushing of cuboidal bones.

Premature foals require excellent nursing skills to identify and address their compromised conditions.

The respiratory system of the premature neonate is often compromised, as the lungs do not have sufficient surfactant for the lungs to work normally. Atelectasis and hypoxemia usually result. Respiratory dysfunction requires adequate support through the use of nasal insufflation or positive pressure ventilation. With atelectasis risk at a very high level, foals must be kept in sternal recumbency to facilitate expansion of all lung fields and provide oxygen to all body systems. Positioning aids are invaluable in keeping neonates properly positioned.

Incomplete ossification of carpal and tarsal joints necessitates restricting exercise and/or applying bandages and splints to transfer weight around the affected joints (Figure 11.11). Lack of proper support can collapse the joint capsule leading to malformation of developing cuboidal bones and subsequent orthopedic problems. These

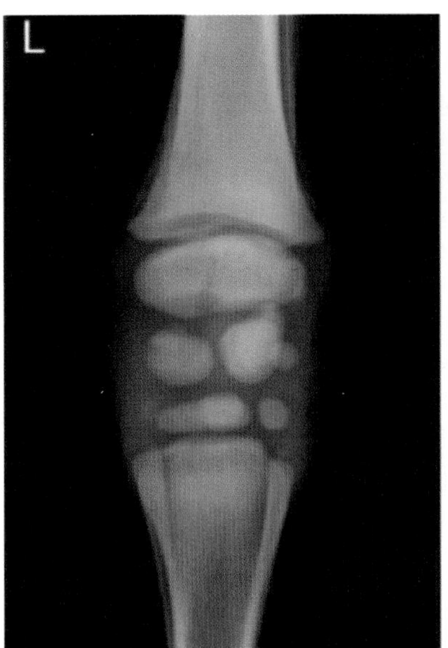

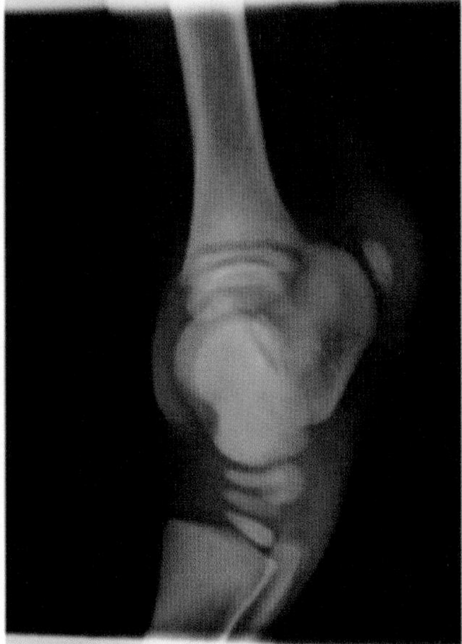

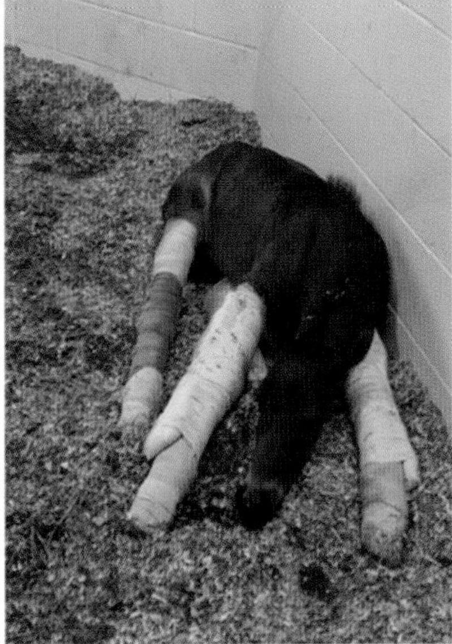

Figure 11.11 Left front (left) and left hind (middle); 20 days premature, bilateral incomplete ossification. *Source:* Reproduced with permission of Amy S. Lang, B.A., R.T.R. (Right) Foal in bandages and splints to help transfer the weight.

types of support wraps and splints must be kept clean and dry. Reapplication is expensive and usually occurs more than once per week.

TECHNICIAN TIPS 11.7: Down foals have a high risk of atelectasis; therefore, it is important to keep them sternal and/or flip them every other hour.

Due to lack of sufficient body fat and hair coat to insulate the premature neonate, patients will almost certainly require thermal support and glucose supplementation at presentation. A first choice would be to provide mare's milk or colostrum if available from the dam or a plausible surrogate via nasogastric tube. If not available or if glucose levels are dangerously low, 50% dextrose with diluent is given slowly intravenously. This type of supplement usually provides sufficient energy until the neonate is settled in its stall and placed on a feeding schedule or on a CRI of IV dextrose. Frequent monitoring is required.

Premature neonates will often lack sufficient suckle reflex and require an orogastric tube or nasogastric tube, indwelling or temporary. If the dam is with the neonate, the dam will often need to be milked, as most premature neonates have difficulty standing to nurse let alone possess sufficient suckle reflex to remove milk from the udder. This milk can be administered to the neonate via nasogastric tube or an orogastric feeding bag for calves (Figure 11.12). Excess milk can be stored in clean containers in the refrigerator or frozen and thawed for later use. Milk can be warmed in the microwave, but the temperature should be slightly below body temperature to avoid burns. Substitute milk replacers are readily available and are manufactured in species-specific formulations. Reconstitution must follow manufacturer's directions and dry powder stored in a clean, dry place.

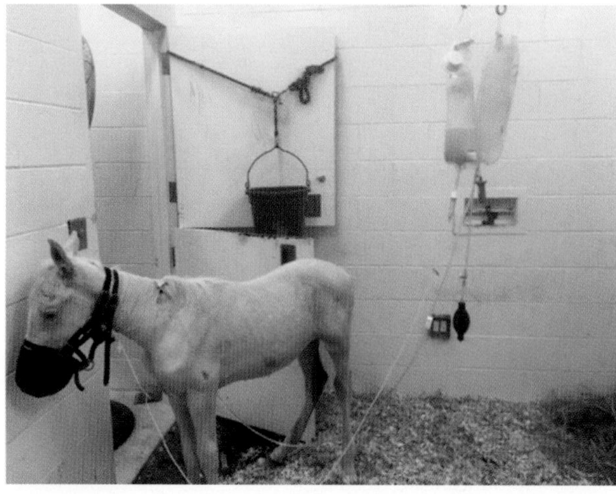

Figure 11.12 Foal being fed via gravity system through a nasal gastric tube.

Freezers can act as long-term storage for milk replacer if heat or humidity is a concern. Only enough milk replacer should be reconstituted for each feeding, as it may spoil in a short period of time, but follow the manufacturer's directions. Rapid changes in diet or milk replacer may result in nutritional diarrhea. Some premature foals have immature gastrointestinal tracts and need to be monitored closely during enteral supplementation for signs of colic.

Items used for mixing and storing of milk and milk replacers must be kept clean. Rinse all utensils with water before allowing to drain and dry. Frequent cleaning and disinfection of these items assures that microorganisms will not be a cause for concern for an already compromised neonate.

Nursing Care

The technician has many concerns when caring for neonates, whether normal or ill. Providing a safe, clean, warm, and dry environment can be challenging, depending on climate and season. Different types of bedding may be used alone or in combination, and their use is dependent on local availability, absorbency, dustiness, and cost. These can include wood shavings, hemp, shredded paper, or clean, dry straw. Recumbent neonates, especially premature neonates, require deep, soft bedding to reduce decubital ulcer formation. Additional actions to reduce ulcer formation are frequent checks to maintain sufficient bedding underneath them, maintaining them in sternal recumbency, and frequently changing them from laying on one rear limb to the other. Removal of wet bedding and replacing with additional dry bedding is crucial to keep the neonate dry and free of urine or fecal scalding. Additional items may be used with bedding to keep neonates dry, such as disposable pads, bed sheets, towels, or blankets. These are imperative to cover items that could otherwise increase the risk of ulcer formation like foam troughs or foal mats (Figure 11.13). Keeping the neonate's skin clean and dry, especially in case of diarrhea, can be accomplished by use of rinse-free shampoo and using a hair dryer to thoroughly dry the hair and skin.

If the neonate is not receiving CRI treatments, it may remain in the same stall as the dam dependent on husbandry techniques for that species or breed. If frequent treatments, providing a place to perform those treatments is essential to efficiently and safely administer medications or perform procedures. If there are multiple procedures being performed, there should be a separate area less accessible to the dam, but one where she can see and/or touch the neonate with her nose. This area provides a place where the technician can safely restrain and complete treatments. Without this area, additional physical and/or chemical restraint may be necessary for the dam so that treatments can be completed (Figure 11.14).

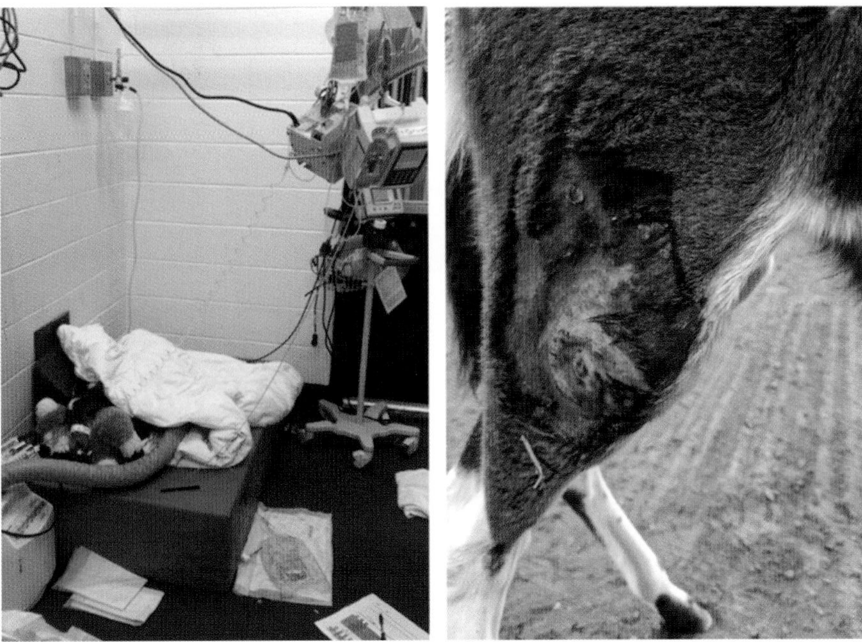

Figure 11.13 Down foals (left) must be kept on soft bedding and turned/flipped every other hour to avoid decubital ulcers (right).

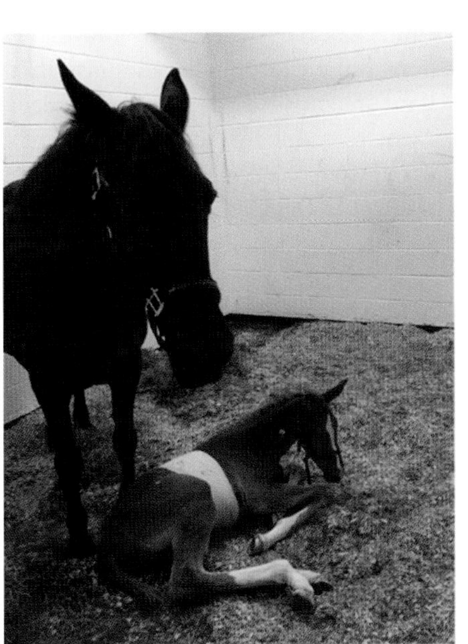

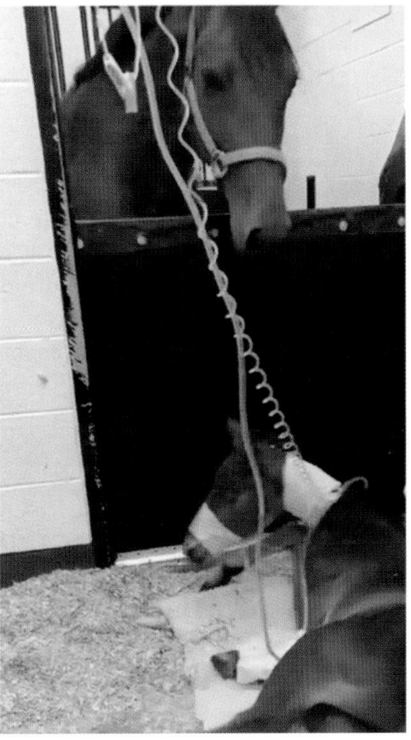

Figure 11.14 Foals can be in same stall as their dam (left) or in separate stall depending on how intensive they are and safety for all (right).

Catheter Placement and Care

Many medications used to treat ill neonates require the use of an intravenous catheter. Material choices for catheters are dependent on the expected duration of treatment. For short-term treatment, a catheter made of polypropylene may be used for two to three days but are used infrequently for long-term care of sick neonates. Other choices include Teflon®, polyurethane, and silicone. These materials are less thrombogenic but are more costly. If total or partial parenteral nutrition (TPN/PPN) treatment is expected,

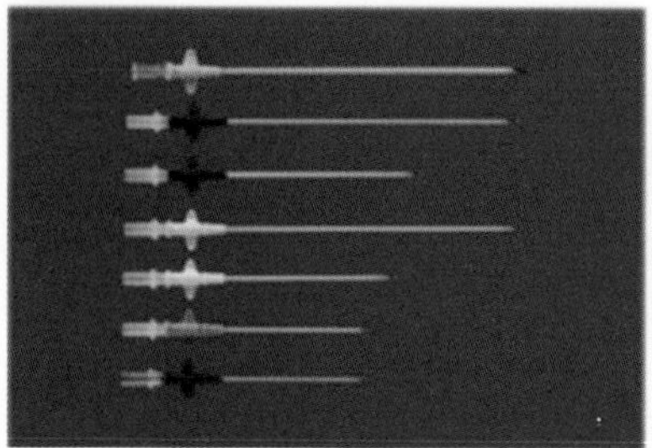

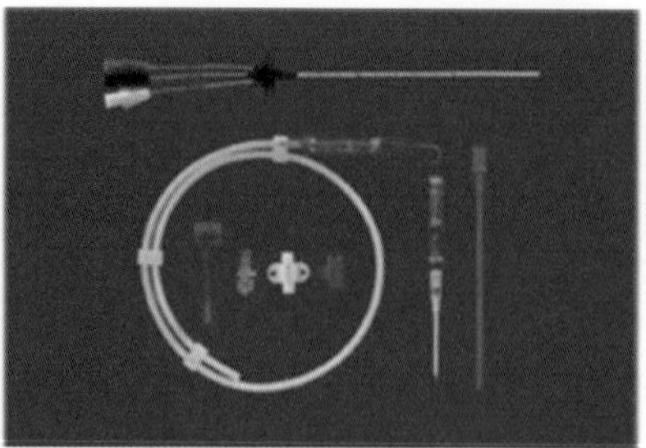

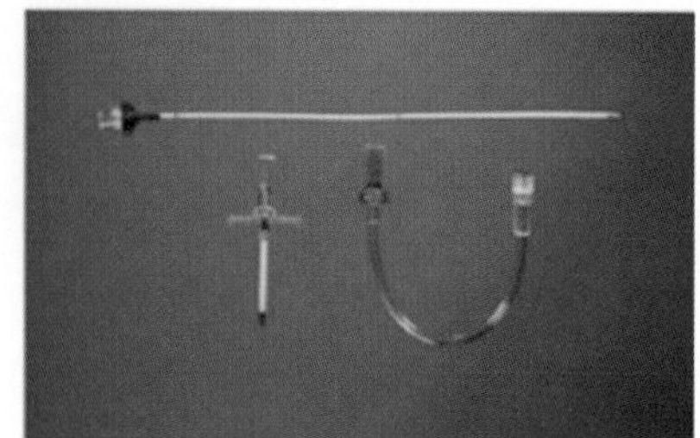

Figure 11.15 Extended use of polyurethane over-the-needle catheters (left). Long-term, over-the-wire, multi-lumen, polyurethane catheter (middle). Long-term, peel-away introducer catheter (right). *Source:* Courtesy of MILA International, Inc.

multi-lumen catheters are the best choice for administration (Figure 11.15). This removes the concern of disconnecting fluid lines to administer medications, as most parenteral nutrition fluids contain high levels of dextrose, a perfect medium for bacterial growth. Insertion methods for these catheters include over-the-needle, over-the-wire, and peel-away adaptors. Catheters may also have antimicrobial coatings with bactericidal properties to reduce complications from catheter-related infections.

Using sterile catheter placement methods and ongoing, frequent catheter care are crucial to reducing catheter reaction and site infection. Sterile catheter placement includes the use of surgical prep of the area, wearing sterile gloves, and strict adherence to aseptic technique (Figure 11.16). Catheter wraps are helpful to keep the catheter site clean, as neonates frequently lay in lateral position exposing the catheter and catheter site to contaminated bedding and fecal material, but should be changed regularly (Figure 11.17). Catheters should be flushed with heparinized saline QID to maintain patency. Catheters, sutures, and the catheter site must be inspected each time medications are given or whenever catheters are flushed. Intermittent infusion plugs should be changed daily.

Any sign of heat, swelling, loss of patency, or pain would require removal of the catheter, but must be communicated to the clinician who will decide whether the catheter will be replaced or perhaps treatment protocols changed to reflect permanent removal of an intravenous catheter. If replacement is chosen, the contralateral jugular vein is used if available. Catheters that have been removed for site reactions or thrombosis usually require hot pack application to speed healing.

Intravenous Fluids and Medications

Clinicians often prescribe intravenous fluids or medications using CRI or bolus administration. Intravenous fluid lines are changed per hospital protocol but typically every 48 hr, or more frequently dependent on the fluid being administered. TPN/PPN fluid lines are changed every time the bag is changed. Changing fluid lines includes three-way stopcocks and any extension sets between bag and

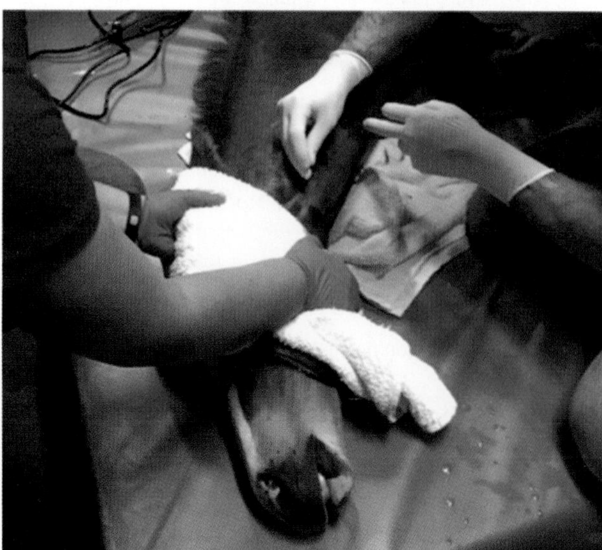

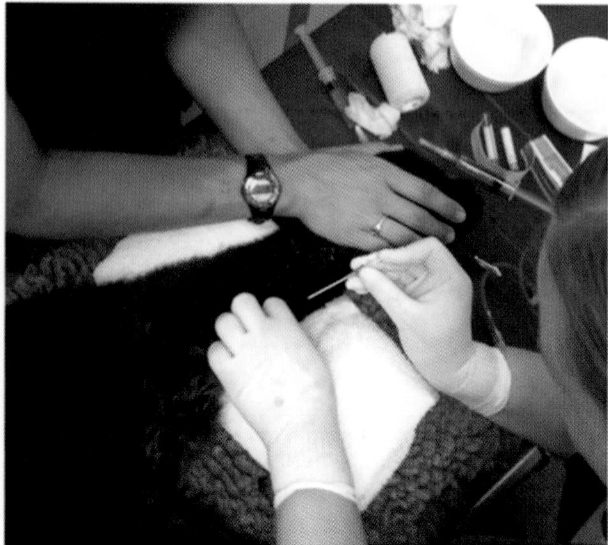

Figure 11.16 Sterile jugular catheter placement on foal (left) and cria (right).

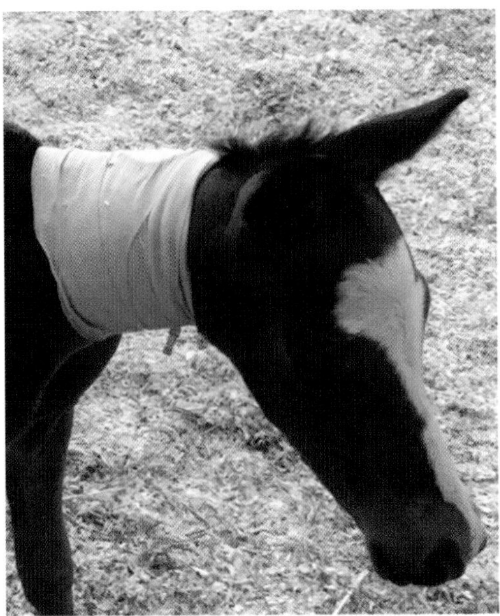
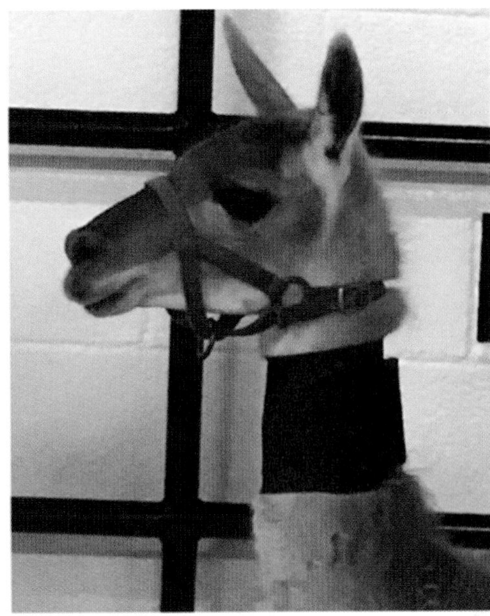

Figure 11.17 Catheter wraps must be changed every day and must not be wrapped too tight.

patient. If multiple fluids or CRI medications are administered, labeling the fluid lines and IV infusion pumps can reduce the risk of medication mistakes.

> **TECHNICIAN TIPS 11.8:** Intravenous fluid and oxygen insufflation lines must be changed every 48 hr; glucose lines every 24 hr; PPN and TPN lines are changed at every bag change.

Administration of intravenous medications to sick neonates usually requires the discontinuation and disconnection of IV fluid lines to access catheter ports. Precautions to decrease the likelihood of contamination would include the use of exam gloves and the wiping of catheter ports with alcohol. To reduce the possibility of complications of IV fluid and drug compatibility issues, sufficient catheter flush should be used before, between, and after administration of each medication. Each time a fluid line or syringe is applied or removed, the catheter must be clamped or closed to eliminate the introduction of air into the vein. If the patient is not on CRI IV fluids, then the catheter is flushed before, between, and after each medication and the catheter infusion plug replaced.

Feeding Tubes

When a neonate cannot suckle from the dam, other methods must be implemented. Unless closely monitored and replaced, rubber nipples become weak and holes become elongated or enlarged allowing for passage of large quantities of milk, which the neonate cannot properly swallow. In addition, staff holding the bottle may hyperextend the head and neck allowing milk to flow unrestricted to the back of the pharynx. Both situations increase the risk of aspiration pneumonia. Whenever possible, dependent on species, bucket or pan feeding should be employed. If the neonate is too weak to suckle or use a pan, then an indwelling nasogastric tube is indicated.

Tubes left in place for extended periods of time should be made of materials that reduce irritation, typically polyurethane. Most tubes have stylets to help with placement and radiopaque markings to help identify proper placement on radiographs; therefore, the timing of tube placement should be just prior to baseline radiographs of the thoracic cavity. Tubes may or may not have fenestrations or weights at the distal end. The tube must be measured for placement either in the distal esophagus or stomach, dependent on clinician orders. Water is flushed through the tube before placement to ease removal of the stylet after successful placement. The distal end of the tube should be lubricated to ease passage.

The neonate is restrained in sternal recumbency with head flexed and the tube passed up the nares ventromedially. If the neonate cannot swallow, then an endoscope may be indicated to provide additional visualization in placing the tube. Tubes can be taped or sutured to the nares using the Chinese Finger Trap Suture technique and the remaining length of the tubes taped to a halter fitted to the neonate made from 2 in flexible wrap bandage such as Velcro®. Mark the tube at the suture line to provide a visual verification each time the tube is used to confirm it has not moved in or out from the prescribed depth. Tubes can also be palpated via the jugular groove as a separate tubular structure in the neck. Other methods of confirmation of placement include checking for negative pressure while passing

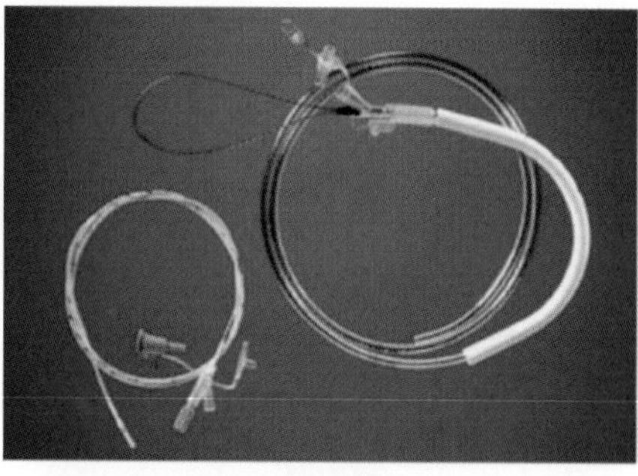

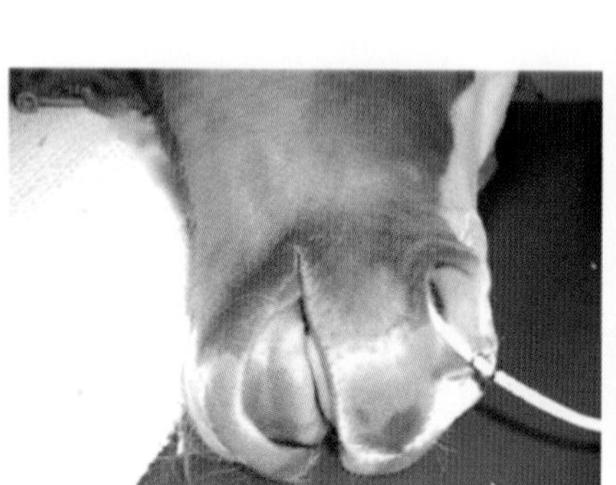

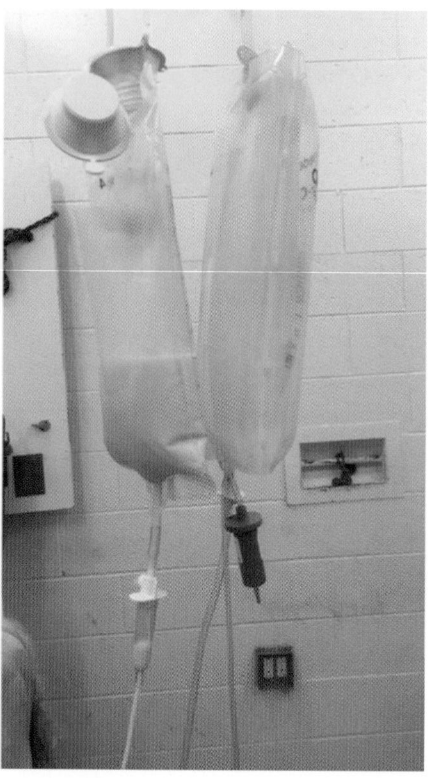

Figure 11.18 Nasogastric feeding tubes with stylet (top left). *Source:* Courtesy of MILA International, Inc. Indwelling nasogastric tube secured with a Chinese Finger Trap Suture (bottom left). Milk fed via gravity system (right).

through esophagus, obtaining gastric contents, and checking for presence of tracheal rattle (Figure 11.18).

CRI milk feedings have been used historically but current methods include the use of feedings every 1–2 hr. The tube should be checked for reflux before milk is administered. Any reflux must be reported to the clinician before feeding begins. Gravity feedings use extension sets and appropriately sized vessels, either syringe barrel or bags. Milk should be added to the vessels and air bled from the entire line before it is attached to the feeding tube. With tubes placed in the distal esophagus, the milk enters the tube and the level in the vessel will drop as the esophagus fills, then it temporarily stops until the esophageal sphincter opens, then the cycle repeats. When the milk empties from the vessel, water should be used as flush so that the indwelling tube contains water between feedings. Tubes must be kept capped between feedings. All items used to feed neonates or mix and store milk must be thoroughly rinsed and allowed to air-dry between feedings. Utensils and adaptics should be replaced with new disinfected items every 48 hr.

TECHNICIAN TIPS 11.9: Indwelling feeding tubes must be flushed with water after milk is administered.

The dam's milk is the best nutrient for the neonate but other replacement milk may have to be used. There are tools that are commercially sold to aid in milking the mare out and saving milk for the foal (Figure 11.19). Commercial powdered milk replacers are readily available for many large animal species. Goat's milk is a very palatable replacement milk and is easily stored frozen and thawed quickly for use. Occasionally, thawed milk may contain flakes, but these flakes can be removed with an electric blender. Powdered milk replacers should be stored in a clean, dry place so that moisture or heat does not render it useless. Dependent on clinician orders, the dam's milk, powdered replacers, or goat's milk may be supplemented with high-fat plain yogurt to provide additional calories and fat if appropriate.

TECHNICIAN TIPS 11.10: Always follow the manufacturer's directions for reconstitution and storage of powdered milk replacers.

Other Oral and Parenteral Treatments

Oral medications should be administered when the neonate is fully awake, able to swallow, and in sternal recumbency

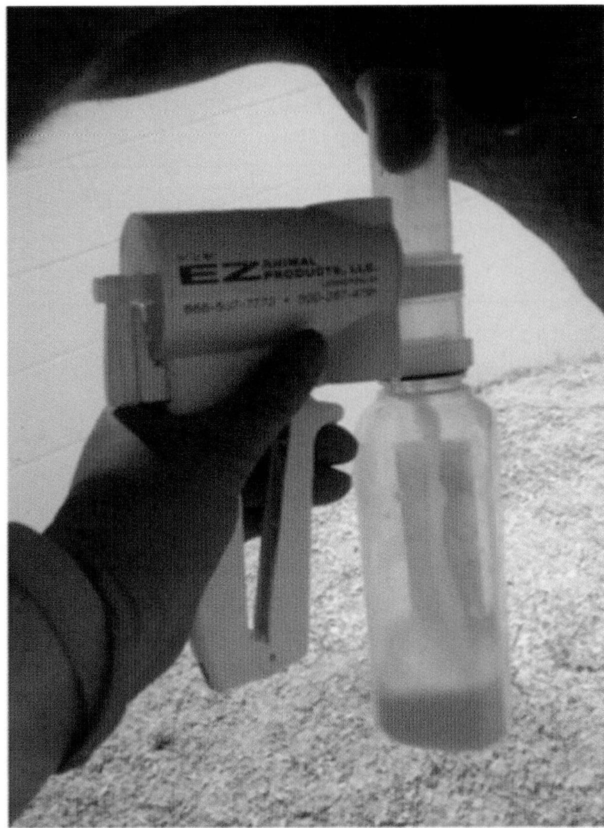

Figure 11.19 Udderly EZ is a commercially sold product to aid in milking out.

to avoid aspiration. If the foal is unable to swallow, the indwelling nasogastric tube may be utilized, but extreme caution must be used that the medication is ground to a powder that will easily move through the tube otherwise the tube may become clogged and require replacement. Medications delivered via SQ (subcutaneous) or IM (intramuscular) routes may be given to sick neonates. While areas for SQ injections are easily found on neonates, most IM injections are best given in the semimembranosus or semitendinosus muscles, as cervical muscles are less developed than on adult animals. Care should be taken when giving any parenteral injection that the site is properly prepared and aseptic technique used during the procedure.

Oxygen Treatments

Dependent on level of treatment, neonates requiring oxygen therapy require that the patient and the dam be separated to reduce problems of oxygen lines or equipment being disconnected or of patient entanglement. Oxygen can be supplied from an oxygen compressor, H or E tanks, or oxygen drops. Care must be taken with any portable tank to ensure it is out of the reach of the patient, is properly secured to a wall or cart to prevent accidental breakage and is stored upright.

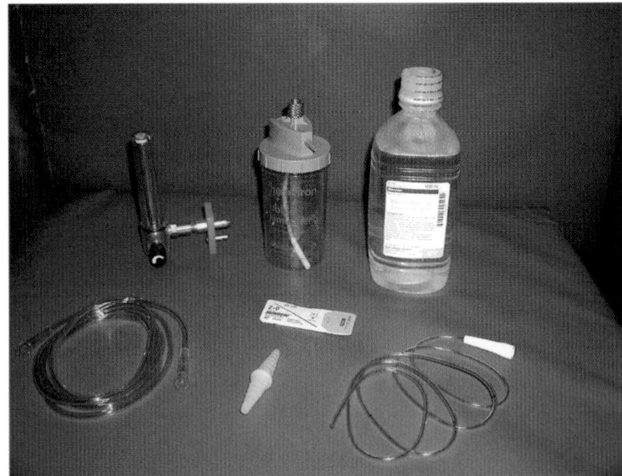

Figure 11.20 Items for oxygen insufflation.

Oxygen is delivered to the patient through the use of a ventilator or nasal insufflation. Ventilators require a high level of the technician's time, as patients are under constant monitoring and increased frequency of treatment and maintenance schedules. Nasal insufflation is used frequently and delivers humidified oxygen via a nasal catheter sized to the neonate. The necessary patient items are shown in Figure 11.20 and assembled as shown in Figure 11.21. Nasal catheters should be measured to reach the medial canthus and can be sutured using a Chinese Finger Trap Suture technique to the lateral aspect of the nares or taped to a halter fitted to the neonate made from 2 in flexible wrap bandage such as Velcro.

Maintenance of nasal insufflation systems includes BID cleaning of the nasal catheter. Great care must be taken when removing the catheter from the nares so as not to rip out sutures or dislodge tape holding the catheter in place, as patients often dislike any movement of the catheter in the nares. Dry or moistened gauze sponges can be used to remove dried mucus and dirt. All fenestrations should also be inspected to ensure that they are open. Humidifiers, Christmas tree adaptors, supply lines, and sterile water should be replaced every 48 hr.

TECHNICIAN TIPS 11.11: The distal end of nasal insufflation tubes should be cleaned BID.

Blood Sampling

Veins commonly used for blood sampling on neonates include the jugular, cephalic, and saphenous veins. Whenever possible, the jugular veins should be avoided as

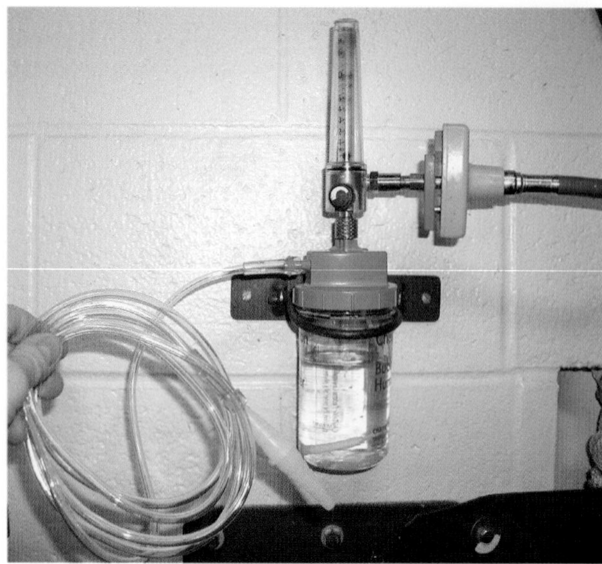

Figure 11.21 Items for oxygen insufflation, assembled.

these veins should be reserved for catheter placement. To avoid injury to any vein being used for catheters or frequent blood sampling, proper restraint is necessary. Choosing the proper size of needle is dependent on the amount of blood needed for testing; the smallest gauge should be used to avoid injury, but it should also be large enough to reduce blood sample problems including hemolysis.

Chicken Hatchling Management

Newly hatched chicks should be housed in a brooder pen, whether they are being reared by a hen or by humans. The bedding should be 2–4 in deep, highly absorbent, non-toxic, and reduce thermal conductivity. Things like wood shavings, pine sawdust, or paper by-products are the most common but additional options include chopped straw, ground corn cobs, sand, or leaves. Avoid cardboard, plastics, and free of contaminants. The bedding should be kept clean and dry in order to avoid caking.

Supplemental heat should be provided until the birds are fully feathered, approximately four to six weeks of age. Depending on climate and season, heat may need to be provided for longer. The ideal temperature for chicks during the first week should be around 90–95 °F and can generally be reduced by 5 °F weekly. A heat lamp, hanging approximately 18–24 in above the bedding is recommended. Use a 100-W bulb for small brooders and 250-W for larger brooders. A red bulb reduces the chance of the birds pecking each other. Use a lamp with a ceramic socket to avoid melting plastic from the heat. One must watch the birds' behavior and positioning around the heat source to get an indication of its effectiveness. If it is too warm, the chicks will be scattered away from the source and if it is too cool, the chicks will cluster together as close to the heat source as possible. Extreme conditions for chicks can quickly result in death (Figure 11.22).

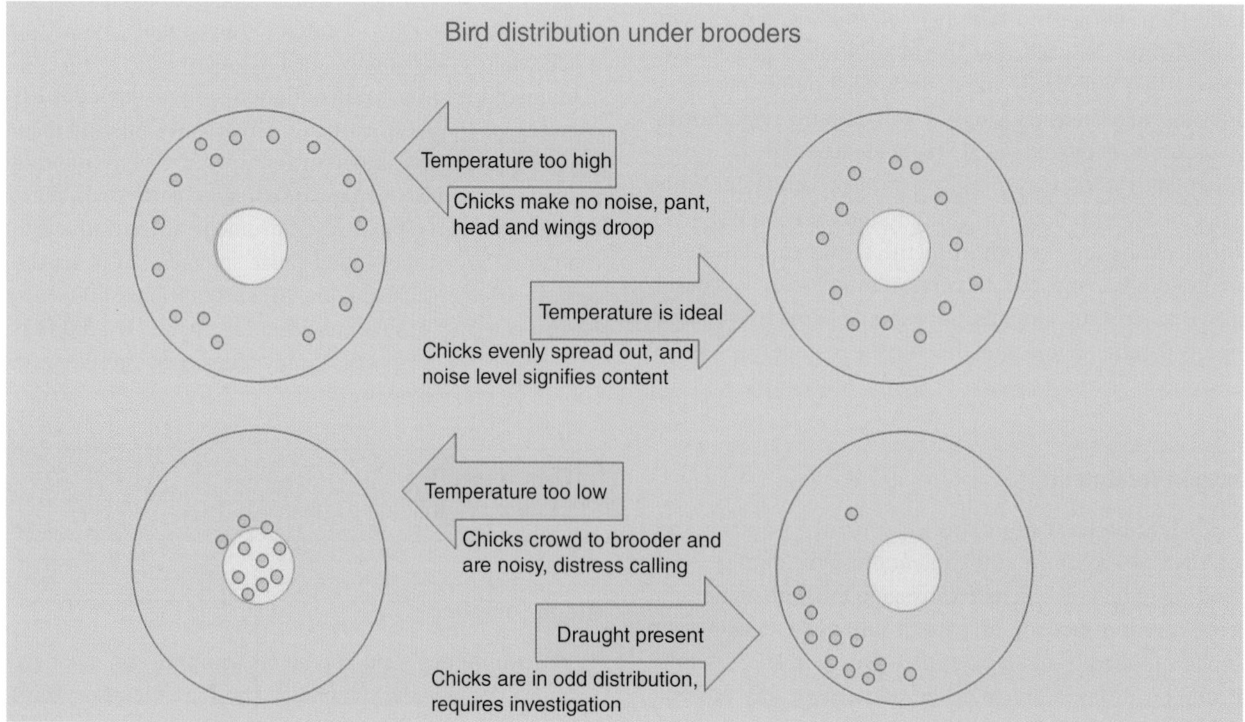

Figure 11.22 Bird distribution under heat lamps.

Age of Chick	Floor Space	Feeder Space	Waterer Space
0–4 weeks	½ sq ft/chick	0.12 ft/chick	0.04 gal./chick
4–8 weeks	1 sq ft/chick	0.20 ft/chick	0.10 gal./chick
8–12 weeks	2 sq ft/chick	0.30 ft/chick	> 0.10 gal./chick
>12 weeks	3–4 sq ft/chick	0.40 ft/chick	> 0.10 gal./chick

Figure 11.23 Space requirement of chicks.

Food and water should not be too far from the heat source, nor should it be too deep where the chicks could drown. When first introduced to the environment, one can dip the beak of each chick into the water so they learn where the source is. In terms of lighting, it should meet the biological requirements of the bird, which will vary according to life stage and type of production. Intensity duration and quality of the lighting all matter (Figure 11.23).

References

Chucri, T., Monteiro, J., Lima, A. et al. (2010). A review of immune transfer by the placenta. *Journal of Reproductive Immunology* 87 (1–2): 14–20.

Fowler, M. (2010). *Medicine and Surgery of Camelids*. Ames, Iowa: Wiley Blackwell.

Jones, C. (2011). *Tools for measuring IgG useful in managing colostrum*. Penn State University. Retrieved from http://www.das.psu.edu/researchextension/dairy/dairy-digest/articles/dd201104-01

Koterba, A., Drummond, W., and Kosch, P. (1990). *Equine Clinical Neonatology*. Baltimore, Maryland: Williams & Wilkins.

Polsen, K., Foley, A., Collins, M., and McGuirk, S. (2010). Comparison of passive transfer of immunity in neonatal dairy calves fed colostrum or bovine serum-based colostrum replacement and colostrum supplement products. *Journal of American Veterinary Medical Association* 237 (8): 949–954.

Pugh, D. and Baird, A. (2012). *Sheep and Goat Medicine*. Maryland Heights, Missouri: Elsevier Saunders.

Radostits, O., Gay, C., Hinchcliff, K., and Constable, P. (2007). *Veterinary Medicine: A Textbook of the Disease of Cattle, Horses, Sheep, Pigs and Goats*. Philadelphia, Pennsylvania: Saunders Elsevier.

Taylor, S. (2015). A review of equine sepsis. *Equine Veterinary Education* 27 (2): 99–109.

Tennent-Brown, B. (2011). Plasma therapy in foals and adult horses. *Compendium: Continuing Education for Veterinarians*, Vetstreet Inc. 33 (10): E1–E4.

Clinical Case Resolution 11.1

There are items that should be assembled and prepared when receiving a sick neonatal foal. Other items may be needed based on ambient temperature.

- Padded cart to transport foal
- Oxygen delivery system
- Crash cart and emergency drugs
- IV catheter placement items and material for neck wrap if desired
- Glucometer
- Items to perform PCV/TP
- Collection tubes for complete blood count, chemistry, and blood cultures
- 50% dextrose and diluent
- IV fluids and drip sets
- Plasma ready to thaw and adaptics
- Items to milk dam
- Items to administer milk or milk replacer to foal
- Hot air blankets
- Bedded stall

Activities

Multiple Choice Questions

(Answers can be found in the back of the book.)

1. Dairies can quickly assess transfer of IgG in calves by using which of the following tests?
A ELISA
B total protein
C RID
D FTP

2. Water bath temperature for thawing plasma should be below:
A 130 °F
B 120 °F
C 110 °F
D 100 °F

3. What type of administration sets should be used to deliver plasma to patients?
   A 10 ggt/ml set
   B 60 ggt/ml set
   C 150–260 μm filter set
   D extension set

4. Which of the following IgG tests is easily used with foals to determine adequate passive transfer of immunoglobulins?
   A ELISA
   B total protein
   C colorimeter
   D glutaraldehyde

5. Hypoglycemia in the large animal neonate is often the result of:
   A being too sick and weak to nurse
   B dehydration
   C excess ingestion of milk
   D the inability of dam to produce milk

6. Hyperflexion of the limbs is a clinical sign of what condition?
   A prematurity
   B umbilical occlusion
   C chronic hypoglycemia
   D hypoxemia

7. Milk from a mare can be refrigerated or frozen for future use. Which of the following is a true statement?
   A The milk is warmed only using a warm water bath.
   B The milk can be warmed in a microwave.
   C Milk should be warmed to a temperature above normal body temperature.
   D Milk should be fed cold.

8. The neonatal period is:
   A The first 30 days of life.
   B The first 15 days of life.
   C The first 10 days of life.
   D The first 3–5 days of life.

9. An initial assessment of a neonate at birth should include which items?
   A cardiac function, respiratory, and gastrointestinal system
   B cardiac function, thermoregulation, and respiratory system
   C thermoregulation, fluid balance, and integumentary system
   D thermoregulation, fluid balance, and endocrine system

10. Chronic or acute placental insufficiency or separation can cause which disease process?
    A endocrine insufficiency
    B asphyxia
    C valgus
    D failure of passive transfer

Test Your Learning

1. When an equine neonate is present for admission to the hospital, what body systems should be evaluated? How are they evaluated?
2. Describe parts of a neonate's history that would influence hydration and glucose status.
3. Why do large animal neonates require colostrum for acquired immunity?
4. Name two ways that colostrum can be tested.
5. Compare and contrast bacteremia and sepsis.

Answers can be found in the back of the book.

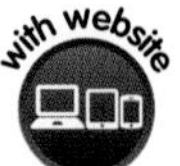

Extra review questions, case studies, and a breed ID image bank can be found online at www.wiley.com/go/loly/veterinary.

Chapter 12

Diseases

Fernando J. Marqués, DVM, DACVIM (LAIM), William Gilsenan, VMD, DACVIM (LAIM), Amy L. Johnson, DVM, DACVIM (LAIM & Neurology), Shirley Sandoval, BAS, LVT, VTS (LAIM), Sian Durward-Akhurst, BVMS, Lauren Hughes, DVM, Stephanie Rutten-Ramos, DVM, PhD, Sue Loly, LVT, VTS (EVN), Heather Hopkinson, RVT, VTS (EVN), CCRP, Derek Foster, DVM, PhD, DACVIM (LAIM), and Danielle Mzyk, DVM, PhD

Learning Objectives

- List causative agents of large animal diseases.
- Describe clinical signs of large animal diseases.
- Outline preventative methods for large animal diseases.
- Describe treatment available for large animal diseases.
- Understand zoonotic potential of specific diseases.

Key Terms

Agalactic
Ataxia
Autogenous
Base-narrow stance
Base-wide stance
Blepharospasm
Brachygnathia
Cervical radiography
Colibacillosis
Cytopathic
Desquamation
Endophyte
Encephalitides
Exenteration
Gangrene
Gastroscopy
Hematogenously
Hematopoietic
Hyphema
Hypotrichosis
Incipient
Meningitis
Mucopurulent
Multifocal
Myelography
Odontoprisis
Peracute
Persistently infected
Proprioceptive deficits
Pseudohyphae
Recrudescence
Strabismus
Torticollis
Transketolase
Typhlocolitis
Xanthochromia

Introduction

Preventing and treating disease processes occupies a significant portion of the veterinary team's day; therefore, understanding relevant details of a specific disease is important for any veterinary technician. Fomites at a dairy must be identified to control or prevent the spread of Johne's disease. Pregnant mares must be vaccinated at specific times so they will produce transferrable antibodies in their colostrum to their offspring. Classifications of disinfectants must be identified to process confinement facilities that may be experiencing disease outbreaks. Clients may need reassurance that specific diseases are self-limiting as they are noninfectious in nature. When the veterinary technician can recall this information, they are a valuable asset to their practices and clientele.

Large Animal Medicine for Veterinary Technicians, Second Edition. Edited by Sue Loly and Heather Hopkinson.

Companion website: www.wiley.com/go/loly/veterinary

Organization of this chapter is alphabetical by common name. Species affected are shown by symbols immediately before the disease name. Further study may be warranted; therefore, an extensive reference list is provided at chapter's end.

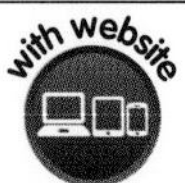

check out more images

Clinical Case Problem 12.1

A seven-year-old quarter horse gelding is being brought to the clinic with a history of aggressive and unpredictable behavior that started 24 hr ago. His vaccination history is not known. What precautions should be taken before evaluating the horse? What medications may the veterinarian need? What diagnostic tests may the veterinarian need to perform?

See Clinical Case Resolution 12.1 at the end of this chapter.

Actinobacillus Pleuropneumonia (APP)

Definition

Contagious bacterial pleuropneumonia caused by *Actinobacillus pleuropneumoniae.*

Cause

A. pleuropneumoniae, a gram-negative coccobacillus with serovars 1, 3, 5, and 7 responsible for most disease.

Systems Affected

Respiratory.

Transmission

Direct contact; nose-to-nose including vertical exposure.

Signs

Clinical signs are most often observed in growing pigs. In naïve populations, peracute presentation is dead pigs. Acute presentations include respiratory distress with "thumping" pattern in breathing and high fevers (>105 °F). Nasal and oral discharge may appear frothy and bloodstained. Chronically affected pigs display a "thump" in their respiration.

TECHNICIAN TIP 12.1: Growing pigs most often show clinical signs of *Actinobacillus pleuropneumonia.*

Onset

Bacteria colonize the upper respiratory tract. Disease emerges when bacteria enter the lower respiratory tract.

Prevalence/Geographical Distribution

Worldwide distribution.

Diagnosis

Postmortem lesions include extremely dense, hemorrhagic lung lobes with bloody froth in airways and from cut surfaces along with fibrinous pleuritis. Chronically affected pigs will have pleural adhesions. Culture of *Actinobacillus* pleuropneumonia (APP) requires a nurse colony such as *Staphylococcus aureus.* Serology can be used to identify serovar-specific antibodies.

Treatment

APP is generally susceptible to penicillin's and it is common to treat entire groups of exposed animals to limit the extent of an outbreak.

Recovery

Recovered animals may carry the organism in their nasal cavities, thereby serving as a reservoir for naïve animals.

Zoonotic Potential

No zoonotic potential.

Genetic Prevalence

No genetic prevalence known.

Prevention

APP-naïve animals should be used to establish new swine populations. For herds with endemic APP, killed vaccines with appropriate serovars can be used, strategic antibiotic application before stressful events (i.e. nursery-to-finisher transportation) and biosecurity practices such as all-in, all-out movement of groups.

Actinobacilosis – See Wooden Tongue

Actinomycosis – See Lumpy Jaw

Acute Hypocalcemia – See Milk Fever

Anaplasmosis

Definition

Intraerythrocytic infection with *Anaplasma marginale* (a rickettsial organism) causing progressive anemia.

Cause

A. marginale. Anaplasma marginale subspecies *centrale* (a.k.a. *Anaplasma centrale)* induces mild disease.

Systems Affected

Erythropoietic system; erythrocytes become infected with the organism, which can be detected by microscopic examination of a blood smear.

TECHNICIAN TIP 12.2: Erythrocytes become infected with *Anaplasma marginale*, which can be observed on a stained blood smear.

Transmission

Persistently infected animals are an important reservoir for transmission. The bacteria are transmitted by vectors, such as Ixodidae ticks, including *Dermacentor* and *Rhipicephalus*, and biting insects. Also, iatrogenic infection can occur by using contaminated needles, dehorning, castration, and ear-tagging instruments during herd-wide procedures.

Signs

The signs range from acute and severe disease to subclinical infection, depending on the virulence of the strain and animal susceptibility. Calves and young cattle are usually either resistant to infection or are mildly affected, whereas adult animals tend to have more severe disease. In adult cattle, the disease is characterized by an initial fever, anorexia, and lethargy. A sudden decrease in milk production and decreased ruminations are seen in dairy cattle. Mucous membranes are pale and icteric. If animals survive the acute stage, they show weight loss and icterus as main clinical signs. Recovered cattle become persistently infected for life, are typically asymptomatic, and act as reservoir of anaplasmosis.

Onset

Progressive anemia with clinical signs occurring when more than 1% of erythrocytes become infected.

Prevalence/Geographical Distribution

The disease is most prevalent in temperate regions and is the most prevalent tick-borne infection in cattle around the world. Geographical distribution is mainly determined by vector distribution and activity.

Diagnosis

In the acute stage, definitive diagnosis is made by the identification of *A. marginale* in red blood cells in addition to a substantial decrease in PCV. Persistently infected animals are diagnosed by serology (cELISA). The absence of hemoglobinuria helps to rule out other hemolytic diseases such as babesiosis, bacillary hemoglobinuria, and so forth.

Treatment

Oxytetracycline is the treatment of choice in the acute stage, although complete clearance of the bacteria from the infected animal is not achieved.

Recovery

The recovery rate is variable depending on the susceptibility of the animal and the pathogenicity of the strain. The immune system can clear the acute bacteremia but is not able to completely clear the infection because of the development of antigenic variants of the organism.

Zoonotic Potential

No zoonotic potential.

Genetic Prevalence

No genetic prevalence known.

Prevention

In the United States, a modified live vaccine is licensed for use only in California. Other live vaccines are used in other countries but are not licensed for use in the United States. Tick and biting fly control, such as insecticide-impregnated ear tags and sprays, are recommended.

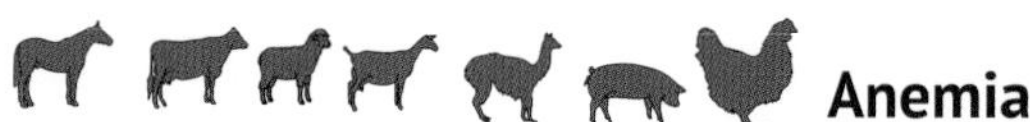

Anemia

Definition

Insufficient hemoglobin levels in the blood due to nutritional deficiency.

Cause

Most commonly caused by iron deficiency in neonatal pigs. In other species, it is most typically caused by parasite overload.

> **TECHNICIAN TIP 12.3:** Piglets are iron deficient at birth, and this is exacerbated by rapid growth.

Systems Affected

Hematopoietic.

Signs

Pallor and lethargy in suckling piglets. Lethargy and dullness in all species.

Onset

Progressive from birth. Piglets are iron deficient at birth and this deficiency becomes exacerbated by rapid growth on an exclusive diet of iron-poor sow's milk. Anemia can be found in all species at different times of onset.

Prevalence/Geographic Distribution

Worldwide, though more pronounced in piglets farrowed off-dirt.

Diagnosis

Clinical signs and low hemoglobin levels.

Treatment

Prophylactic administration of up to 200 mg iron in the first week of life. Anemia not responding to iron dextran should be checked for deficiencies of vitamin E. Other species may receive blood transfusions.

Recovery

Piglets respond well to parenteral iron administration.

Zoonotic Potential

No zoonotic potential.

Genetic Prevalence

No genetic prevalence known.

Prevention

As noted above, piglets should be given early access to iron, either orally or via injection.

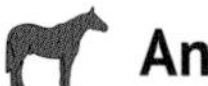

Anterior Uveitis

Definition

Uveitis is inflammation of the iris and ciliary body (anterior uveitis) and/or choroid (posterior uveitis). Uveitis is often an acute and extremely painful disorder. Equine recurrent uveitis (ERU) is characterized by recurrent episodes of uveitis. Horses affected by ERU often do not demonstrate the classical signs of pain associated with anterior uveitis and, therefore, often present further into the disease process with potentially irreversible changes. Anterior uveitis is one of the most common ophthalmic problems encountered in the horse.

Cause

Anterior uveitis has numerous initiating causes including trauma (blunt or penetrating) or underlying systemic disease (including leptospirosis [primarily, *Leptospira interrogans* serovar Pomona-often associated with ERU], *Streptococcus equi* infection, onchocerciasis, and influenza virus). ERU is an immune-mediated disease, the precise factors leading to the development of signs is unknown; there appears to be a genetic component, with Appaloosas being overrepresented. It is often a chronic process, and the protracted disease process is thought to be secondary to deposition of antibody–antigen complexes in the anterior chamber.

Systems Affected

Ocular. May be unilateral or bilateral.

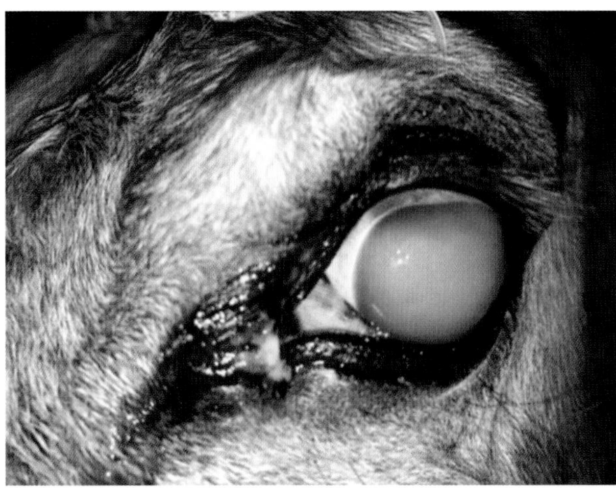

Figure 12.1 Corneal edema. *Source:* Photo courtesy of Lauren Hughes, DVM.

Signs

Clinical signs for patients with acute onset are miosis, photophobia, blepharospasm, chemosis, aqueous flare, and reduced intraocular pressure. For chronic onset, signs include corneal edema, which leads to scarring, synechiae formation (adhesions between the iris and lens or cornea), atrophy of the corpora nigra, cataract formation, lens luxation. Chronic onset may lead to glaucoma, retinal detachment, blindness, and phthisis bulbi (Figure 12.1).

Onset

May be acute or chronic.

Prevalence/Geographical Distribution

Any age. Worldwide distribution.

Diagnosis

To reach a diagnosis, a physical examination is performed (to identify any systemic illness present), ophthalmic examination, serological analysis to detect conversion to Leptospira species, and tonometry. In acute cases, a tonometry result where intraocular pressure readings are low is diagnostic.

Treatment

- Systemic flunixin meglumine (anti-inflammatory) – ensure the horse is adequately hydrated; side effects include gastric ulceration, right dorsal colitis, and nephrotoxicity.
- Systemic aspirin (some evidence that chronic use decreases frequency and severity of episodes) – side effects are similar to flunixin, but also include prolonged clotting times.
- Topical atropine (promote mydriasis and decrease synechiae formation) – side effects include ileus (rare).
- Topical steroids (e.g. prednisolone; decrease inflammation) – check with fluorescein that no corneal ulceration is present; side effects include the development of melting ulcers if damage to the cornea occurs.
- Topical Cyclosporine A (moderates the immune response).
- Long-term management – surgical placement of an intravitreal, suprachoroidal, or subconjunctival cyclosporine A implant (can be done standing or under general anesthetic).
- Fly masks to reduce UV radiation entry into the eye.

Watch for corneal ulceration with prolonged topical steroid usage. When combining nonsteroidal anti-inflammatory drugs, there is an increased risk of right dorsal colitis. Monitor closely for signs of recurrent uveitis, treatment should be maintained for as long as signs of uveitis are present, and then gradually reduced, and the horse should be monitored closely for recurrence of signs.

> **TECHNICIAN TIP 12.4:** When using topical steroids for a prolonged period of time, corneal ulcerations may result.

Zoonotic Potential

No zoonotic potential.

Genetic Prevalence

None known for anterior uveitis, though ERU is extremely common in Appaloosas.

Prevention

Prevent eye trauma, manage systemic disease, and watch closely for signs of uveitis and treat aggressively and early on in the disease process.

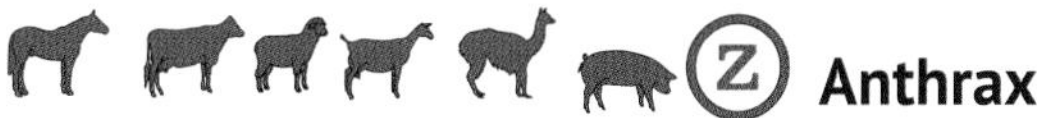

Anthrax

Definition

A soil-borne bacterial zoonotic disease-causing acute septicemia and high mortality rates.

Cause

Bacillus anthracis, a large, rectangular-shaped, gram-positive rod in the vegetative form. Under unfavorable conditions, the bacteria forms spores that are very resistant, can survive and persist infectious in the environment for decades.

TECHNICIAN TIP 12.5: *B. anthracis* can form spores that can survive in the environment for decades.

Transmission

Ingestion of spores from the soil when grazing contaminated pastures is the most common mode of transmission. Once in the gastrointestinal tract, the spores are able to cross mucosal membranes and are transported by macrophages to regional lymph nodes. Spores become vegetative in the host and are able to escape phagocytic mechanisms. There is a fast multiplication of the organism causing severe septicemia, multiorgan dysfunction, toxic shock, and death.

Signs

Due to the peracute onset and rapid progression of the disease, clinical signs are usually not seen. Cattle are commonly found dead. When clinical signs are seen, they are usually unspecific with fever and lethargy. In some animals, bloody diarrhea and swelling of specific parts of the body can be noted.

In animals that die from the disease, bloody exudates from body orifices and incomplete rigor mortis are commonly seen. Blood typically does not clot fully, and rapid decomposition of the carcasses is common.

Onset

Peracute onset, with rapid progression and death.

Prevalence/Geographical Distribution

The disease has been endemic in many countries and continents. The disease is still common in some Mediterranean countries, and in some focal areas of the United States and Canada, some countries of Central and South America, central Asia, several African countries, and western China. Sporadic cases and outbreaks continue to occur elsewhere.

Diagnosis

Suspect animals dying from anthrax should not be opened in the field, or moved from the area where they were found, to prevent bacterial sporulation and dissemination of the disease. As a precaution, farmers and other people should not handle carcasses suspected of being infected with anthrax. It is recommended that in any suspect anthrax case, diagnosis should be done by laboratory personnel in charge of the diagnostic testing, after contacting the appropriate local or state veterinary regulatory officials. Examination of direct blood smears and bacterial isolation and identification are the most common diagnostic tests, in addition to rapid molecular-based techniques used mainly in bioterrorism surveillance programs.

Anthrax is a reportable disease both in the United States and Canada; therefore, veterinarians and producers must notify local and federal health departments, federal animal health officials and the CDC's National Center for Infectious Disease in the United States, and the Canadian Food Inspection Agency (CFIA) in Canada, of all suspected or confirmed cases.

Treatment

Most animals are found dead with no chance of therapeutic intervention. Because of the peracute characteristic of the disease, affected animals must be treated very early in the course of the disease. Administration of penicillin or tetracycline is the treatment of choice, although animals usually succumb despite therapy.

Recovery

High mortality rates.

Zoonotic Potential

Anthrax is a zoonotic disease. In humans, the disease can present in three forms depending on the route of exposure: cutaneous (the most common form), gastrointestinal, and inhalational.

Genetic Prevalence

No genetic prevalence known.

Prevention

Bacterial spores survive in the soil and persist in an infectious state for decades. Handling carcasses is a key factor in preventing spread of the disease and further outbreaks. Carcasses should not be opened or moved. They must be buried deeply and covered with quicklime or burned, which is the latest method of choice.

Protective clothing and physical barriers, including gloves, gowns, and facemasks, should be used by personnel obtaining samples or handling carcasses. Vaccination is used to protect animals in endemic areas.

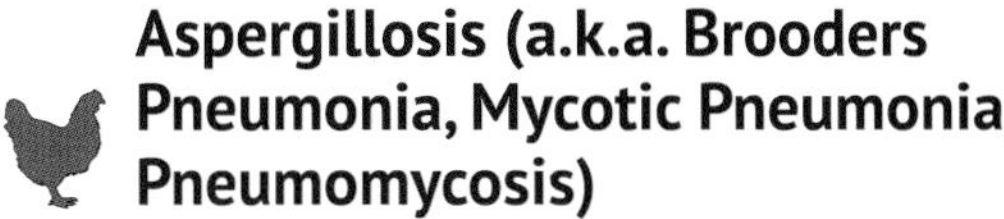

Aspergillosis (a.k.a. Brooders Pneumonia, Mycotic Pneumonia, Pneumomycosis)

Definition

An infection generally of the lung and air sacs and often occurs after other respiratory diseases like fowl cholera.

Cause

Contracted from normal spores of Aspergillus fumigatus in the environment.

Systems Affected

Respiratory tract.

Transmission

This infection does not pass from bird to bird like the bacterial and viral diseases discussed, but rather is contracted from normal spores of Aspergillus fumigatus in the environment that get out of control under poor sanitation situations.

Signs

Dyspnea, labored breathing, fever, inappetence, emaciation, and torticollis.

Diagnosis

Through observation of clinical signs and identification of numerous white to yellow granulomas in the respiratory tissue. May also be confirmed through histology or cultures.

Treatment

None.

Recovery

Depends on the progression of the disease. Removal from a contaminated environment and improving ventilation may help.

Zoonotic Potential

No zoonotic potential.

Genetic Prevalence

No genetic prevalence known.

Prevention

Avoiding wet litter, providing clean feed, having adequate ventilation, and disinfecting feed and water containers should be implemented to prevent and control diseases. Taking the time to make sure chickens have clean dry bedding, clean food and water, and good ventilation can save on costs for avoiding and treating disease. Many of these issues can also be avoided in free-range setups but most urban backyard chicken owners do not have that opportunity as owner education is key.

Atrophic Rhinitis

Definition

Contagious upper respiratory infection in swine causing contortion and/or disfigurement of the snout.

> **TECHNICIAN TIP 12.6:** Atrophic rhinitis can cause permanent disfigurement of the pig's snout.

Cause

Bordetella bronchiseptica causes a regressive form of rhinitis; *Pasteurella multocida* (type A and D) causes a progressive form.

Systems Affected

Upper respiratory, with potential involvement of upper digestive.

Transmission

Nose-to-nose; inhaled.

Signs

Initial infections present as persistent sneezing with tear stains below the eyes. In the case of progressive *P. multocida*, the snout twists to the side and shortens, affecting apposition of upper and lower jaws. Effects on growth are considered minimal.

Diagnosis

Antemortem diagnosis can be made on the basis of clinical signs. Postmortem diagnosis is done by evaluating the nasal septum and turbinates on cross-section at the second premolar tooth (as during slaughter check). The causative agent can be identified through bacterial culture. Cytomegalovirus is a virus that causes rhinitis but is not associated with turbinate atrophy.

Treatment

Strategic vaccination may be used to reduce clinical signs. Pre-farrow vaccinations generate strong maternal immunity (through colostral transfer) that may interfere with piglet vaccination. Antibiotic application according to sensitivity is an uncommonly employed control measure.

Recovery

Although antibiotics may effectively eliminate infection from the nasal cavity, structural and anatomical changes are permanent.

Zoonotic Potential

P. multocida can infect mammals and birds.

Genetic Prevalence

No genetic prevalence known.

Prevention

Establish new swine populations from AR-free stock and do not introduce animals from herds with a history of AR. *Note:* Both *B. bronchiseptica* and *P. multocida* are potential causes of pneumonia independent of AR, although *P. multocida* most commonly presents as a secondary pathogen.

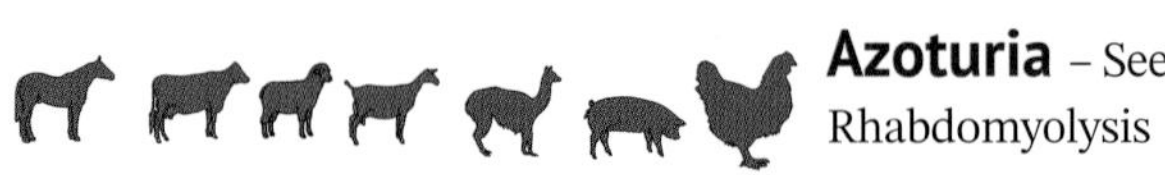

Azoturia – See Rhabdomyolysis

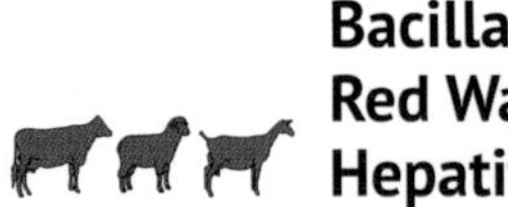

Bacillary Hemoglobinuria (a.k.a. Red Water Disease, Clostridial Hepatitis)

Definition

The name Red Water Disease or Bacillary Hemoglobinuria comes from the classic red color of the urine in affected animals. This is due to the presence of hemoglobin from lysed (ruptured) red blood cells. This infection can easily be confused with several other diseases, including blackleg, anthrax, or leptospirosis.

Cause

The gram-positive anaerobic bacteria *Clostridium haemolyticum* becomes absorbed by the gastrointestinal tract to the liver, where it proliferates and secretes toxins and causes hemolysis.

Systems Affected

The liver is primarily affected after absorption from the gastrointestinal tract.

Transmission

The *C. haemolyticum* bacteria in the soil become ingested while grazing on poorly draining pastures. The bacteria then fester in areas of the liver that have been previously damaged liver flukes or other disorders.

Signs

- Jaundice
- Hemoglobinuria
- Necrotic areas in the liver
- Abdominal pain
- Dark feces and/or urine
- Labored breathing

Onset

Incubation period of this disease is 7–10 days.

Prevalence/Geographical Distribution

Red Water is found primarily in the western part of the United States and occasionally in the southern states. It is also associated with poorly draining pastures that also contain liver fluke populations.

Diagnosis

Diagnosis is based on clinical signs or postmortem examination.

Treatment

Antibiotic therapy that may include penicillin or tetracycline. Antitoxic serum may be given simultaneously as well.

Preventative

Provide adequate drainage for grazing pastures or avoid usage when pastures are wet. Remove any carcass from the area that may have been affected. Necropsy any fatalities to ensure proper diagnosis. A vaccine is also available, and high-risk areas should vaccinate up to every three to six months.

Recovery

Affected animals will rarely improve without medical intervention, including antibiotic therapy.

Zoonotic Potential

No zoonotic potential.

Genetic Prevalence

No genetic prevalence known.

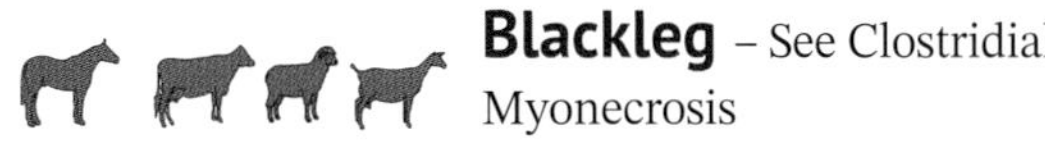

Blackleg – See Clostridial Myonecrosis

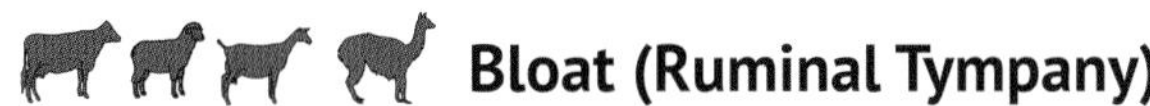

Bloat (Ruminal Tympany)

Definition

A dysfunction of eructation or outflow leading to free gas or froth accumulation in the rumen.

Causes

Neurological, such as vagal nerve damage, and ileus; metabolic, such as hypocalcemia; esophageal damage or choke; infectious disease, such as tetanus; and dietary factors, such as over ingestion of green forages leading to froth formation, which negatively influences eructation.

Signs

Distention of the left paralumbar fossa as the rumen becomes distended with free gas or froth. When the ruminal distention is severe, both the upper and lower left abdominal quadrants become distended. In severe cases, dyspnea can be observed due to diaphragm compression by the distended viscus.

With free gas bloat, a distinct ping can be ausculted on the left paralumbar fossa, and when passing an orogastric tube, bloat is readily relieved. It is important to detect other clinical signs related to the underlying disease process (hypocalcemia, esophageal injury, etc.) leading to gas accumulation in the rumen (bloat).

With frothy bloat, a ping in the left paralumbar fossa is not as evident as it is with free gas bloat, and the bloat is not relieved when passing an orogastric tube.

Onset

Acute or chronic.

Prevalence/Geographical Distribution

Worldwide distribution.

Diagnosis

Clinical signs and the use of an orogastric tube are essential for establishing the diagnosis.

Treatment

The main goals are to relieve the ruminal gas distention and to treat the underlying disease process. Passing an orogastric tube relieves free gas bloat, and frothy bloat can be treated with drench administration containing surfactant products, such as poloxalene or vegetable oil, to break down the froth in the rumen.

Other specific treatments should be initiated based on the underlying condition leading to free gas bloat. Parenteral calcium solutions are used to treat hypocalcemia; esophageal choke should be relieved by gentle manipulation or under anesthesia in severe cases, and so forth.

Recovery

Good to poor depending on the severity of the case and underlying primary disease. Severe cases can occur within a few hours and become life threatening.

Zoonotic Potential

No zoonotic potential.

Genetic Prevalence

No genetic prevalence known.

Prevention

Avoiding succulent alfalfa, sweet clover, red clover, and diets rich in chloroplast membrane fragments and soluble proteins can prevent frothy bloat.

Other preventative measurements are based on the specific underlying diseases leading to ruminal free gas bloat.

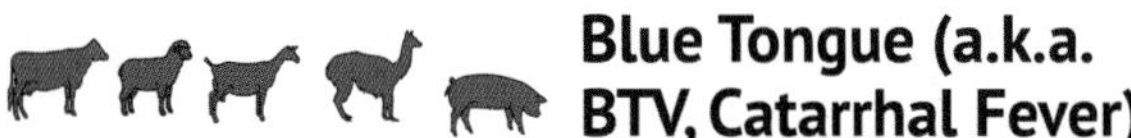

Blue Tongue (a.k.a. BTV, Catarrhal Fever)

Definition

BTV is a vector transmitted viral disease that affects ruminants, camelids, and pigs.

Cause

Orbivirus.

Systems Affected

Systemic vascular disease (vasculitis) that also affects the skeletal muscles, and respiratory and cardiac systems.

Transmission

The virus is spread through the bite of an infected insect vector of the genus *Culicoides.*

Signs

Goats rarely show clinical signs; camelids may show respiratory distress and abortion. Susceptible sheep present with fever; nasal discharge; pulmonary edema; pneumonia; vasculitis, which leads to necrosis of the cardiac and skeletal muscles; lips, oral, and nasal mucosa that become congested then necrotic. They may demonstrate coronary band necrosis resulting in lameness and possible sloughing of the hooves.

Onset

Incubation period is 7–10 days.

Prevalence/Geographical Distribution

Disease is more prevalent in animals previously exposed (sensitized). Although many ruminant species are infected, sheep appear to demonstrate clinical disease most commonly, with meat breeds the most susceptible. BTV is found in the Americas, Europe, Africa, the Middle East, Australia, and parts of Asia.

> **TECHNICIAN TIP 12.7:** Although many ruminant species are infected with BTV, meat breeds of sheep demonstrate clinical disease most often.

Diagnosis

Clinical signs and viral isolation.

Treatment

Supportive therapy, antibiotics for secondary bacterial infections.

Recovery

Sheep will maintain a resistance to the specific serotype of the virus for which they are infected for a few months.

Zoonotic Potential

No zoonotic potential.

Prevention

Vaccines are available in some areas but are only effective against the specific serotypes.

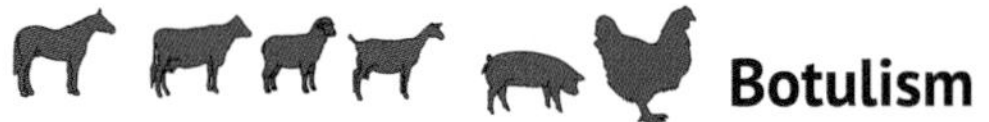

Botulism

Definition

Botulism is a disease that is caused by the action of neurotoxins produced by the bacterium *Clostridium botulinum.* Like other Clostridia, it is an obligate anaerobic bacterium. Consequently, its typical state in the environment is its sporulated (dormant) form. The neurotoxin can be released when under specific suitable conditions, spores germinate.

> **TECHNICIAN TIP 12.8:** Botulism is caused by *C. botulinum* neurotoxins.

There are three major mechanisms by which large animals can be exposed to the neurotoxin and consequently develop clinical signs of botulism.

1) The toxicoinfectious route of infection most commonly occurs in foals. Foals are often affected between one and three months of age, but signs can be observed in foals as young as seven days of age. Infection occurs via this route when foals ingest spores that multiply within the gastrointestinal tract and elaborate neurotoxin.
2) Infection can occur via ingestion of the preformed neurotoxin in spoiled feed materials. This is the most common route of exposure for adult horses and ruminants.
3) Contamination of wounds with *C. botulinum* spores can, under appropriate conditions, allow bacterial

proliferation and elaboration of neurotoxin in the tissues. The effect of the neurotoxin is to prevent release of acetylcholine into nerve synapses at the neuromuscular junction of skeletal muscle fibers. Acetylcholine is necessary for muscle contraction to occur. Therefore, the toxin results in what is termed flaccid paralysis and characterized by signs of weakness.

Systems Affected

The neuromuscular junction of skeletal muscle is affected. As a result, all skeletal muscles are involved, which includes the diaphragm and intercostal muscles.

Onset/Signs

Onset is typically rapid. Clinical signs do not vary based on route of infection or type of botulinum spore (e.g. type A, B, C) involved in intoxication. Exposure to greater amounts of toxin may result in faster onset and progression of clinical signs. Common initial signs include weakness, muscle fasciculations, and dysphagia. Eyelid, tongue, and anal tone may be decreased (Figure 12.2). Because affected animals often lie down and are dysphagic, clinical signs can be confused with colic.

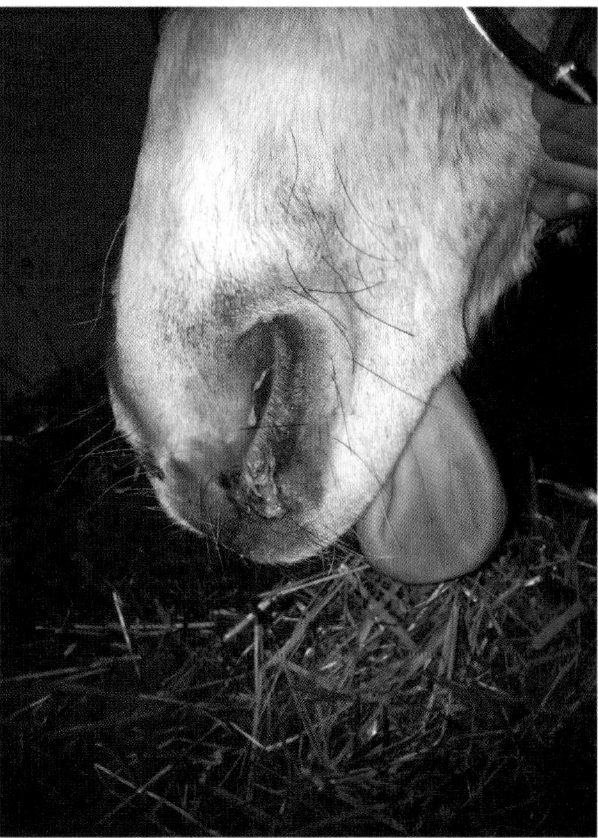

Figure 12.2 Decreased tongue tone may be one of the earliest clinical signs in large animals affected with botulism. *Source:* Reproduced with permission of Dr. Michelle Abraham.

Prevalence/Geographical Distribution

Worldwide, but clinical cases are most frequently observed in the mid-Atlantic region of the United States and Kentucky. The most prevalent type of botulism varies geographically. Type B botulinum spores are most frequently isolated from the mid-Atlantic region of the United States and Kentucky. Type A botulinum spores are identified more commonly in the Western United States, where occasional cases occur. Type C botulinum spores are associated with carrion and are seen sporadically across the United States.

Diagnosis

Diagnosis is presumptively made based on consistent clinical signs, particularly in an endemic area, when history of vaccination is absent. Upper airway endoscopy and cerebrospinal fluid (CSF) collection may be performed to rule out other causes of dysphagia and neurologic deficits. Clinical laboratory work, including CBC, biochemical analysis, and CSF analysis typically yields normal findings.

The "grain test" is a helpful ancillary test to heighten or decrease suspicion of clinical botulism. A horse should be offered 8 oz of sweet feed in a flat feeding pan. A normal horse is expected to eat this entire portion within 2 min; the majority of horses should finish it within 1 min. In cases of botulism, affected horses do not finish this portion and the grain often becomes mixed with saliva because the horse cannot swallow. This leaves a ring of grain in the feed pan and on the horse's muzzle. This test does not confirm a diagnosis of botulism, but the aforementioned findings would support this diagnosis. The tongue (stress) test can also be performed. While holding the horse's mouth closed with one arm, the other hand gently pulls the horse's tongue out of the side of the mouth. Normal horses quickly retract their tongues with one or two tugs, while affected horses retract their tongues slowly if at all.

Identification of the botulinum toxin or spores in feed, gastrointestinal contents, feces, or plasma can be attempted for more definitive diagnosis but is often unrewarding.

Treatment

Treatment with botulinum antitoxin is strongly encouraged to neutralize any circulating toxin. The importance of early antitoxin administration cannot be overstated and should be considered a high priority. Botulinum antitoxin is available in the form of hyperimmune plasma. Antitoxin is available in either monovalent or multivalent forms. Monovalent forms are only effective against a single type of botulinum toxin (usually, type B or C); there is no cross-protection between types. Multivalent antitoxins are effective against a wider spectrum of botulism cases. Without antitoxin therapy, most cases will invariably worsen; death typically ensues secondary to respiratory arrest following paralysis of the respiratory muscles. If possible, botulinum antitoxin should be administered prior to shipping an affected animal to a hospital for supportive care.

The patient's neurologic status will continue to worsen for 24–48 hr even after administration of antitoxin due to irreversible binding of botulinum toxin to existing nerve terminals. Once botulinum antitoxin has been administered, the cornerstone of therapy is supportive care.

Prognosis

Clinical signs are expected to continue to worsen for 36–48 hr following antitoxin administration. If a horse is recumbent prior to administration of antitoxin, prognosis is poor (<15%). Without antitoxin, most affected horses die secondary to respiratory paralysis. Early identification and therapeutic intervention is crucial and significantly improves prognosis (~70% survival if antitoxin administered before recumbency occurs). Prognosis for affected foals, even those requiring mechanical ventilation, is good if antitoxin is administered, as long as supportive care is financially possible. Costs associated with treatment are often very high and financial constraints may become the limiting factor in achieving a successful outcome. Outcome does seem to be related to the amount of toxin that is present.

Zoonotic Potential

Botulism can affect humans, but the toxin cannot be transmitted from animals to humans.

Prevention

Vaccination is an extremely effective method of prevention and strongly recommended in endemic areas. Owner education regarding proper feeding management is important, as use of haylage and silage to feed horses is not recommended.

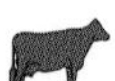 Bovine Coronavirus (BCV)

Definition

A viral infection causing calf diarrhea, winter dysentery, and contributing in the pathogenesis of bovine respiratory disease complex.

Cause

Bovine coronavirus, a single-stranded ribonucleic acid (RNA) virus.

Transmission

Oral and respiratory routes. The virus is shed in the feces of diarrheic calves for about a week, and nasal shedding occurs in animals with respiratory disease for up to two weeks.

Signs

Diarrhea in calves five days to one month of age. The virus causes a mucohemorrhagic enterocolitis, affecting both the small and large intestine. Dehydration, metabolic acidosis, electrolytes derangements, and recumbency occur in severe cases.

Respiratory signs in calves are mild and include sneezing and coughing. In adult cattle, the virus contributes with other viral and bacterial pathogens to cause bovine respiratory disease. Affected animals show lethargy, anorexia, and serous to mucopurulent nasal discharge.

Onset

Acute.

Prevalence/Geographical Distribution

Coronavirus is commonly isolated from affected animals during outbreaks, but it is also commonly found in normal dairy and beef cattle. Worldwide distribution.

Diagnosis

Clinical signs in addition to antigen-capture ELISA, RT-PCR (reverse transcriptase-polymerase chain reaction) assays, and viral isolation.

Treatment

Supportive care for diarrhea in calves and treatment for bronchopneumonia in cases of bovine respiratory disease complex.

Recovery

Good to poor depending on the severity of the disease.

Zoonotic Potential

No zoonotic potential.

Genetic Prevalence

No genetic prevalence known.

Prevention

Good husbandry and hygiene is the best prevention. Isolation of affected animals is important in preventing the spread of the virus.

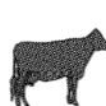

Bovine Herpes Virus 1 Infection (Infectious Bovine Rhinotracheitis [IBR])

Definition

A viral infection of the upper respiratory tract characterized by high fevers, nasal discharge, and white plaque formation in the nasal and tracheal mucosa (respiratory form, also known as infectious bovine rhinotracheitis [IBR]). Other forms of the disease include infectious pustular vulvovaginitis (IPV), infectious balanoposthitis, conjunctivitis, abortions, and neonatal encephalitis. The virus also contributes with other viruses and bacteria to the pathogenesis of bovine respiratory disease complex.

Cause

Bovine herpes virus type 1 (BHV1).

Transmission

The routes of infection are direct contact or aerosol. The virus is capable of establishing latent infection in neural tissue, and stress or steroid administration to infected animals can reactivate the latent virus.

Signs

The respiratory form is characterized by fever, tracheitis, and rhinitis. Pustules are found in the nasal mucosa and later on diphtheria white plaques form. Only the upper respiratory tract is affected unless there is a secondary bacterial infection in the lungs. The virus causes epithelial cell damage of the respiratory tract and immunosuppression, which predisposes for secondary bacterial pneumonia. Conjunctivitis with corneal opacity and serous ocular discharge may be the only manifestation of the disease (conjunctival form).

Onset

Chronic and latent infection with recrudescence.

Prevalence/Geographical Distribution

Based on serologic studies, the virus is widely distributed.

Diagnosis

Clinical signs in addition to paired serology, indirect immunofluorescence antibody testing (IFA) and viral isolation.

Treatment

Supportive treatment and prophylactic antibiotic administration to prevent secondary bacterial bronchopneumonia.

Recovery

Good unless secondary bacterial bronchopneumonia develops. The disease has high morbidity and low mortality rates.

Zoonotic Potential

No zoonotic potential.

Genetic Prevalence

Genetic factors seem to play a role in host susceptibility.

Prevention

Avoid management practices that induce stress. Parenteral and intranasal vaccines are available to protect cattle from the disease.

> **TECHNICIAN TIP 12.9:** Intranasal vaccines are available for BHV1.

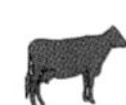

Bovine Leukemia Virus (BLV); Adult Lymphosarcoma

Definition

A lifetime viral infection causing the vast majority of lymphosarcoma cases in cattle. Nonetheless, only a small percentage of bovine leukemia virus (BLV) infected cows develop lymphosarcoma.

Cause

BLV.

Transmission

Horizontal and vertical transmissions occur. Close contact between infected and susceptible animals promotes horizontal transmission of the virus. Iatrogenic infection can occur by using contaminated needles, dehorning, castration, and ear-tagging instruments during herd-wide procedures. The role of insects in horizontal transmission is controversial. Calves may become infected in their first days of life by the ingestion of colostrum or milk from infected cows. Vertical transmission of the virus during pregnancy is possible, thus calves can also be infected in utero.

TECHNICIAN TIP 12.10: Iatrogenic infection of BLV can be transmitted via fomites used during herd-wide procedures.

Signs

Less than 5% of BLV-infected cows develop lymphosarcoma or show clinical signs. Most cattle with lymphosarcoma show unspecific clinical signs such as anorexia, weight loss, and decreased milk production in dairy cows. Generalized lymphadenopathy is commonly seen. Depending on the location of the tumor, many forms of the disease are recognized. Common anatomical areas for lymphosarcoma development are abomasum, heart (right atrium), uterus, spinal cord (epidural location), and retrobulbar. Clinical signs are related to specific organ or anatomical site involvement. With abomasal involvement, signs of vagal indigestion, melena, or weight loss may occur. Cardiac arrhythmias, murmurs, and signs of congestive heart failure may be seen in cases of cardiac lymphosarcoma. Neurologic signs are common in cases of spinal cord involvement. Retrobulbar lymphosarcoma leads to exophthalmos development.

Onset

Chronic. It is a lifetime viral infection.

Prevalence/Geographical Distribution

Prevalence increases in herds during confinement or when infected cattle are introduced to a susceptible BLV-negative herd. Herd size also appears to be related to prevalence, the larger the herd the higher the prevalence.

Diagnosis

Clinical signs in addition to serologic testing identifying antibodies against the viral envelope glycoprotein "gp51" are used for diagnosis. Traditionally, agar gel immunodiffusion (AGID) has been used for serologic diagnosis. Commercial ELISA test kits are available to be used with serum or milk samples. PCR (polymerase chain reaction) is also used to detect BLV nucleic acid.

Treatment

No effective treatment is available.

Recovery

When clinical signs of lymphosarcoma are evident, affected animals usually die in a few weeks to a few months.

Zoonotic Potential

No zoonotic potential.

Genetic Prevalence

A possible genetic predisposition exists. Certain families of infected cattle appear predisposed to lymphoma development.

Prevention

Currently, there are no vaccines to effectively protect against the disease. Reduction of iatrogenic blood transmission is recommended along with segregation of infected animals.

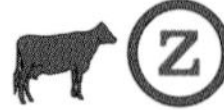

Bovine Papular Stomatitis (BPS)

Definition

A viral proliferative stomatitis that affects young cattle, usually between 1 and 12 months of age. The virus has also been associated with the "rat tail" syndrome in feedlot cattle.

Cause

Parapoxvirus.

Transmission

Direct contact.

Signs

The infection is usually asymptomatic. Affected animals present lesions characterized by raised papules on the nose, muzzle, lips, oral mucosa, hard palate, and esophagus.

When the lesions regress, they leave a brown or yellow area for some time. "Rat tail" syndrome of feedlot cattle is characterized by alopecia of the end of the tail, along with decreased weight gain, diarrhea, and salivation.

Onset

Acute. Typical lesions develop in a few hours and regress in about one to three weeks. Chronic disease may occur.

Prevalence/Geographical Distribution

Worldwide distribution.

Diagnosis

By clinical signs.

Treatment

No effective treatment is available.

Recovery

Raised papules regress in a matter of weeks but secondary lesions can occur in chronic cases.

Zoonotic Potential

The virus can cause painful proliferative lesions in humans limited to the site of infection, usually the hands.

Genetic Prevalence

No genetic prevalence known.

Prevention

Avoid direct contact between infected and noninfected animals. Local strains of the virus can be used for developing a vaccine.

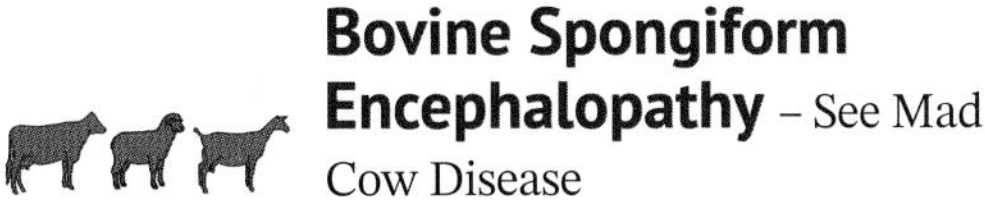

Bovine Spongiform Encephalopathy – See Mad Cow Disease

Bovine Viral Diarrhea (BVD)

Definition

A viral disease causing a variety of clinical syndromes depending on a number of host factors and viral differences. It is a cause of economic losses because of decreased milk production, reproductive failure, secondary infectious diseases, and so forth.

Cause

BVD virus (BVDV), of the family *Flaviviridae*, genus *Pestivirus*, biotype cytopathic (CP) and noncytopathic (NCP), genotype type 1 and type 2.

Transmission

Direct contact with body fluids from persistently infected (PI) cattle is the most effective mode of transmission. Indirect transmission also occurs by means of insects, contaminated needles, and so forth, and vertical transmission (transplacental infection) and horizontal transmission (frozen semen) can also occur.

> **TECHNICIAN TIP 12.11:** BVD transmission is most effective via direct contact with body fluids from PI cattle.

PI animals are the main source of the virus in a herd; they shed large numbers of virus for a long period of time in contrast to acutely infected animals that shed fewer viruses for a limited period of time.

Signs

Numerous clinical signs and syndromes can occur depending on multiple factors, that is, age of the animal, reproductive and vaccination status, concurrent stressful conditions, and presence of PI animals in the herd. Also, viral factors play a role on clinical disease manifestation (i.e. strain and biotype of the virus).

Persistent Infection (PI)

It is caused by fetal infections with noncytopathic-BVDV before 125 days of gestation. PI animals are usually asymptomatic, but some PI calves may show weakness, poor growth rate, and some may die shortly after birth. PI animals superinfected with cytopathic-BVDV strains can develop "mucosal disease."

Acute BVD Infection

It occurs in non-PI animals usually between 2 and 24 months of age. Clinical signs include fever, lethargy,

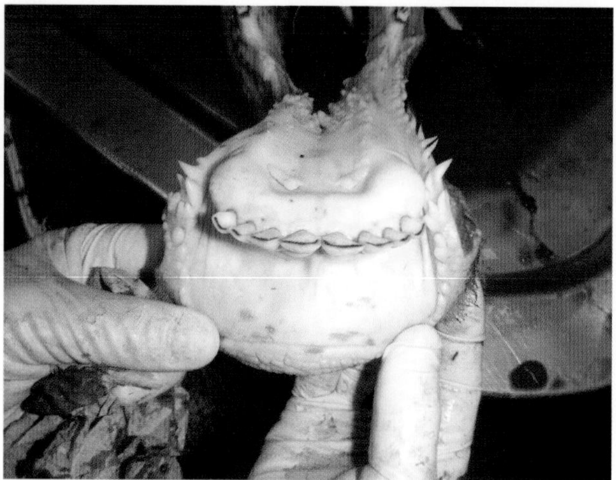

Figure 12.3 Oral ulcers typically seen with acute onset of BVD. This 1½-year-old Charolais heifer clinically presented with diarrhea and weight loss.

anorexia, diarrhea, oral erosions and ulcers, and decreased milk production in dairy cows (Figure 12.3). Acute BVD infection causes immunosuppression, which is a predisposing factor for secondary infectious diseases, particularly that of the respiratory tract (i.e. bacterial and viral pneumonias) and the gastrointestinal tract (i.e. salmonellosis, *Escherichia coli, coronavirus*, and *rotavirus* infections).

Hemorrhagic Syndrome

This syndrome is associated with noncytopathic-BVDV type 2 infections. It is characterized by virus-mediated thrombocytopenia leading to bloody diarrhea, epistaxis, hyphema, hemorrhages from mucosal surfaces, bleeding from injection sites, and so forth.

Reproductive Implications

The virus can cause infertility, early embryonic deaths, and abortions during any time of gestation. Fresh or frozen semen from infected bulls can serve as a source of infection.

Congenital Disease

Infection of the fetus in the second term of gestation can cause congenital abnormalities such as hydrocephalus, cerebellar hypoplasia, microphthalmos, cataracts, retinal atrophy, hypotrichosis, brachygnathia, skeletal anomalies, and pulmonary hypoplasia.

Mucosal Disease

This occurs when PI cattle are infected with a CP-BVDV strain. Antigenic characteristics of the NCP-BVDV (causing the PI state) and the CP-BVD strain determine different clinical forms of mucosal disease – the closer the antigenic homology between the two strains, the more severe the disease. Mucosal disease is characterized by biphasic fever, tachycardia, tachypnea, profuse diarrhea, and erosive lesions in mucosal surfaces, such as the oral cavity and vulva, in addition to interdigital spaces and teats. Affected cattle usually develop secondary bacterial infections and die within a few days.

Onset

Acute or chronic.

Prevalence/Geographical Distribution

The seroprevalence ranges between 20 and 90% in many countries around the world.

Diagnosis

Serology, viral isolation, PCR, fluorescent antibody testing, immunohistochemistry, and antigen-capture ELISA are used for the diagnosis of specific clinical forms of the disease.

Treatment

No specific treatment is available.

Recovery

Variable depending on the form or clinical manifestation of the disease.

Zoonotic Potential

No zoonotic potential.

Genetic Prevalence

No genetic prevalence known.

Prevention

Vaccination is used to restrict the disease after infection by limiting viral replication within the host. Identifying PI animals is an important tool to reduce the source and rate of infection within a herd.

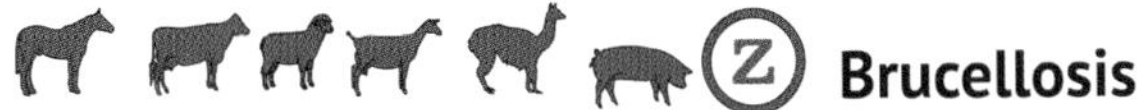 Brucellosis

Definition

A zoonotic bacterial infection causing abortions after the fifth month of gestation in cattle. The disease is less common in sheep and goats, and other mammals such as bison, elk, deer, swine, horses, and other ruminants.

> **TECHNICIAN TIP 12.12:** PPE should be used whenever handling products of conception, as brucellosis is a zoonotic disease.

Cause

Brucella abortus. Brucellosis in sheep is caused by *Brucella melitensis* and *B. ovis*.

Transmission

By ingestion.

Signs

The typical clinical sign is abortion after the fifth month of gestation. Other clinical signs include orchitis, epididymitis, mastitis, and lameness. Affected animals become carriers for life.

Onset

Chronic.

Prevalence/Geographical Distribution

The disease has almost been eradicated in the United States and Canada, although some natural wildlife reservoirs are still present.

Diagnosis

Bacterial culture, PCR, and serology are used for diagnosis. Surveillance of *B. abortus* in dairy cattle is conducted by the milk ring test assessing the presence of agglutinating antibodies in the milk.

Treatment

Treatments are not effective; oxytetracycline and streptomycin have been used to reduce shedding and to treat the infection. Affected cattle are rarely treated and may be sent to slaughter to eradicate the disease.

Recovery

Cattle who abort their first pregnancy are capable of carrying subsequent pregnancies to term but remain chronic carriers.

Zoonotic Potential

Humans can become infected and develop "undulant fever" by ingesting unpasteurized milk products or by handling contaminated body fluids or tissues.

Genetic Prevalence

No genetic prevalence known.

Prevention

Vaccination to young heifers before pregnancy and surveillance methods.

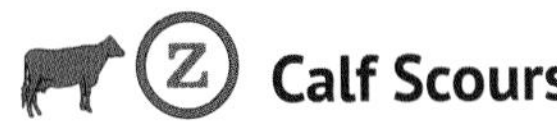 Calf Scours

Definition

Infectious or parasitic diarrhea in calves within the first 30 days of life.

Cause

A wide spectrum of bacterial, viral, and parasitic organisms can induce diarrhea in neonatal calves, although the most common agents are enterotoxigenic *E. coli* (ETEC), *Salmonella*, rotavirus, coronavirus, and cryptosporidium.

Transmission

Fecal-oral route. Partial or total failure of passive transfer (FPT) of antibodies, due to decreased colostrum intake or decreased colostrum quality, is a main predisposing cause of diarrhea in young calves. Environmental factors also play a role in predisposing young animals to infection.

> **TECHNICIAN TIP 12.13:** Partial or total FPT is a main cause of diarrhea in young calves.

Signs

Profuse watery diarrhea, lethargy, reduced suckle reflex, dehydration, tachycardia, progressive weakness, and recumbency are common clinical signs, depending on the severity of the disease and the etiologic agent.

Onset

Acute or peracute.

Prevalence/Geographical Distribution

Worldwide distribution and high prevalence in beef and dairy cattle.

Diagnosis

Clinical signs and specific tests are used to achieve a specific etiologic diagnosis, including bacterial and viral isolation, antigen specific immunoassays, microscopic examination of fecal preparations, electron microscopy, and so forth.

Treatment

Supportive and medical treatment includes intravenous fluids, anti-inflammatories, antimicrobials, and enteral or parenteral nutrition. Correction of dehydration, acid–base (i.e. metabolic acidosis), and electrolyte imbalances is warranted.

Recovery

Good with appropriate treatment in non-septic calves.

Zoonotic Potential

Cryptosporidium can affect humans via the fecal-oral route, inducing diarrhea.

Genetic Prevalence

No genetic prevalence known.

Prevention

Adequate colostrum quality and intake, in addition to hygiene of the pens or area where calves are housed, are important tools to prevent diarrhea in neonatal calves.

ETEC vaccination to cows in late gestation is used to increase specific antibodies (anti-K99 antibodies) in colostrum, and thus to reduce the disease in calves. There are also *Salmonella*-modified live attenuated vaccines to be used in calves. Oral rotavirus and coronavirus vaccines for calves and intramuscular vaccine formulations for cows are available for preventing diarrhea in calves.

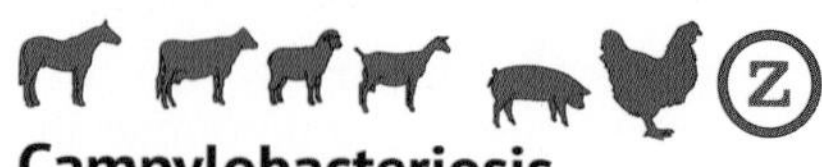

Campylobacteriosis

Definition

A zoonotic disease-causing enterocolitis in many species.

Cause

Campylobacter jejuni (formerly, *Vibrio jejuni*), a gram-negative motile rod.

Transmission

Fecal-oral route. *C. jejuni* is a normal inhabitant of the gastrointestinal tract of animals and humans.

Signs

Varies from unapparent infection to severe diarrhea, fever, and dehydration in both calves and cattle. Clinical signs are unspecific and not different from any other cause of diarrhea. The backyard chickens may not show any signs of infection, but it can still be spread to humans.

Onset

Acute.

Prevalence/Geographical Distribution

One of the most common causes of diarrhea in people worldwide.

Diagnosis

Clinical signs in addition to isolation of the organism in feces without involvement/isolation of other pathogens.

Treatment

Supportive treatment includes fluid therapy, anti-inflammatories and correction of acid–base and electrolyte imbalances.

Recovery

Prolonged recovery period of one to two weeks in severe cases. Asymptomatic carriers are possible.

Zoonotic Potential

The organism is a main cause of enterocolitis in humans. Consumption of unpasteurized milk and improperly cooked meat are common sources of infection.

Genetic Prevalence

No genetic prevalence known.

Prevention

Hygiene is the best prevention.

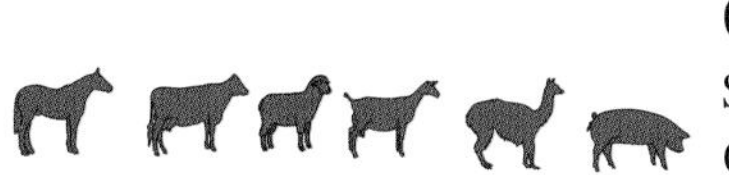

Cancer Eye – Squamous Cell Carcinoma

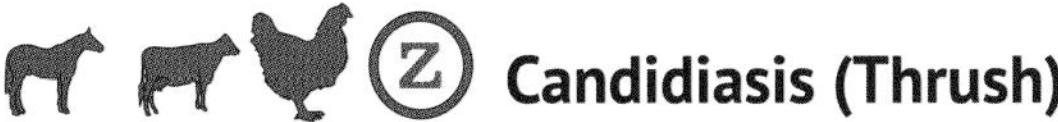

Candidiasis (Thrush)

Systems Affected

Alimentary and genital tract (common flora of mucous membranes).

Transmission

Overgrowth of normal flora.

1) Host is compromised/immunocompromised with chronic disease; antibiotics have adjusted the flora causing *Candida* overgrowth.
2) Ingested via contaminated feed.
3) Inoculated at birth or when very young.

Signs

Gastrointestinal – anorexia, diarrhea, may include death. Dermal – thick, crusty skin lesions in the areas of the body with thin or no fur/fiber. Axillary, inguinal, peritoneal, and muzzle are the most common areas affected. Also commonly referred to as thrush in poultry, most of the time occurs from prolonged antibiotic use or in poultry raised under adverse conditions. It is from the yeast *Candida albicans* and most often affects the mouth, crop, gizzard, and vent of birds. Like aspergillosis, it is not contagious between birds but birds living in the same environment are likely to all have it as a consequence of the environment.

Onset

Acute onset after chronic primary problem.

Prevalence/Geographical Distribution

Worldwide distribution.

Diagnosis

Difficult to diagnose as it is considered normal flora; therefore, a positive culture would not be indicative of disease. Positive skin cytology demonstrates budding yeast and pseudohyphae.

Treatment

Treatment should include topical and/or oral antifungal medications.

Recovery

The health of the animal and owner compliance both play important roles in the ability for a patient to recover from Candidiasis. Successful treatment can take a long time.

Zoonotic Potential

Rare but possible.

Genetic Prevalence

No genetic prevalence known.

Prevention

Monitor the use of long-term antibiotics. Ensure they are efficacious for the disease process being treated and are not causing overgrowth of *Candida*.

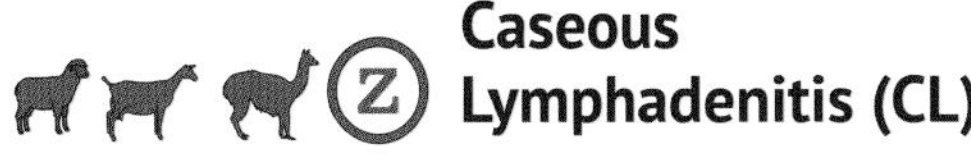

Caseous Lymphadenitis (CL)

Definition

A contagious disease of sheep, goats, and camelids that affects the lymph nodes, both internal and external, which has zoonotic potential (although rare).

> **TECHNICIAN TIP 12.14:** Caseous lymphadenitis has a rare zoonotic potential.

Cause

Corynebacterium pseudotuberculosis.

Systems Affected

Lymph nodes are primarily affected, but it can infect any organ through the lymph or blood systems.

Transmission

From direct contact:

- Intact skin and open wounds, abrasions, or sores with the bacteria from ruptured lesions.
- Respiratory secretions if abscesses are in the lungs.
- Through fomites such as shearing equipment, infectious material left on walls, feeders, and so forth, in the environment.
- May be transmitted to humans via contact (shearing) or contaminated raw milk.

Signs

Encapsulated abscesses of the superficial lymph nodes, presenting as a firm mass or series of masses filled with thick pus (Figure 12.4). Internal abscesses cause symptoms consistent with the affected system.

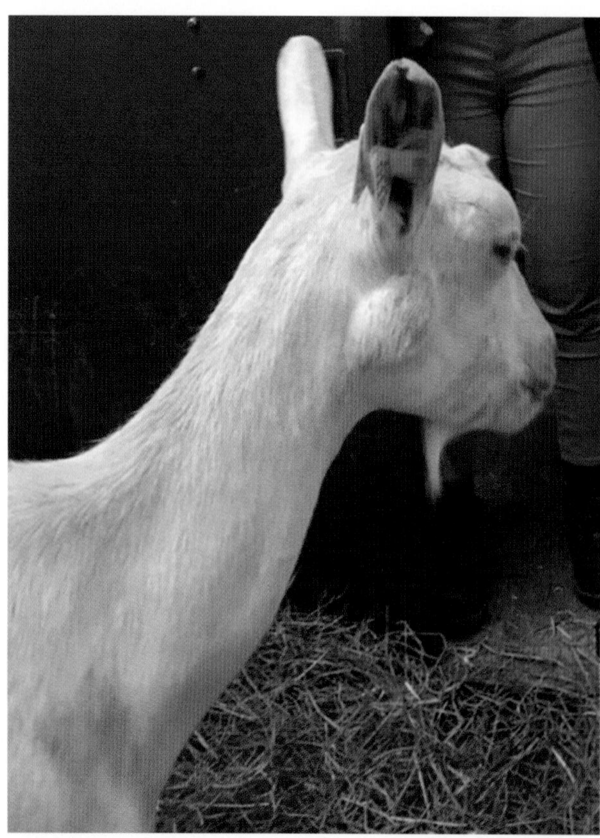

Figure 12.4 Caseous lymphadenitis goat presenting with firm mass on the right side. *Source:* Photo courtesy of Erin Elder, DVM.

- Respiratory
- Coughing
- Pneumonia
- Gastrointestinal
- Wasting
- Renal
- Pyelonephritis
- Hepatic
- Anorexia
- Diarrhea
- Abdominal distension
- Ventral edema

Onset

Acute or chronic.

Prevalence/Geographical Distribution

The prevalence of CL in individual animals increases as the animals age. It is found in North and South America, Australia, New Zealand, South Africa, Britain, Northern, and Southern Europe.

Diagnosis

- Bacterial culture of abscess material.
- Serological testing to detect *C. pseudotuberculosis* specific antibodies.

Treatment

These lesions are rarely treated. The organism is susceptible to penicillin, however, because the abscesses are encapsulated, there is little penetration. Some lesions may be surgically removed or drained.

Prevention

- Test and cull.
- Cleaning and disinfection of all instruments used in processing sheep/goats.
- Cleaning and disinfection of environment when abscesses are opened.

Recovery

None. Test and cull.

Zoonotic Potential

Rare, most common with those who work closely with the animals, such as sheep shearers.

Genetic Prevalence

No genetic prevalence known.

Prevention

Vaccination can decrease the number of sheep affected. The vaccine is more efficacious in sheep than in goats.

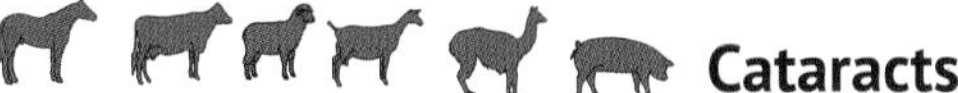 Cataracts

Definition

A condition in which the lens of the eye becomes progressively opaque.

Cause

Cataracts can be congenital, inherited, or acquired and are defined as opacified areas of the lens. Cataracts are the most common congenital abnormalities in foals and often accompany other anomalies including persistent pupillary membranes, microphthalmia, or lens coloboma. Acquired cataracts are most common secondary to inflammation within the eye (esp., ERU in horses) and trauma. Their development has been associated with bovine viral diarrhea virus (BVD) and hypovitaminosis A in cattle and may be related to development of the eye in utero.

Systems Affected

Ocular – lens.

Signs

Cataracts can be congenital, juvenile, or geriatric depending on when they present. The rate of progression and severity vary largely based on cause. They can range from focal incipient cataracts that cause small lesions within the lens to widespread diffuse opacification of the lens. This opacification may be visible at all times or only during ophthalmic examination. Additional signs of decreased vision (bumping into objects, shying/spooking) may be present associated with the affected eye (Figure 12.5).

Prevalence/Geographical Distribution

Cataracts are reported to be the most common congenital ocular abnormality in foals. Worldwide distribution.

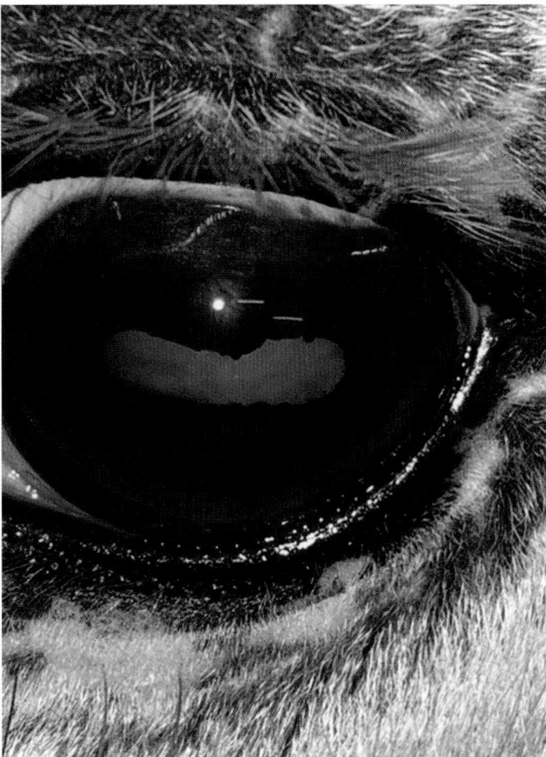

Figure 12.5 Equine cataract. *Source:* Photo courtesy of Lauren Hughes, DVM.

Diagnosis

Diagnosis can be made during ophthalmic examination, and the location, size, and distribution of the cataract will help determine the extent of vision deficits. Dilation of the pupil during examination is recommended to fully evaluate the lens. Close examination of the remaining ocular structures is recommended to aid in determining the cause and concurrent ocular conditions.

Differentials

Differentials will include additional congenital or acquired ocular abnormalities that change the appearance of structures within the eye. Nuclear sclerosis, the normal aging progress of the lens, can be misdiagnosed as a cataract.

Treatment

No medical treatment exists to resolve or delay progression of cataracts. Prompt identification and appropriate treatment of ERU will aid in controlling inflammation within the eye and potentially may decrease cataract development. Surgical treatment using phacoemulsification with aspiration allows for removal of the opacified lens and replacement with a commercial product. A variety of post-operative complications can develop, and success rates are highest in congenital cases.

Zoonotic Potential

No zoonotic potential.

Genetic Prevalence

Inherited cataracts have been documented in Thoroughbreds, Quarter Horses, Morgans, and Rocky Mountain horses. Congenital cataracts have been identified in Holstein, Romagnola, and Ayrshire cattle breeds.

Prevention

Regular ophthalmic examinations will aid in prompt identification of ocular conditions that may be associated with cataract development.

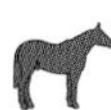

Cervical Vertebral Stenotic Myelopathy (CVSM, a.k.a. Wobbler's Syndrome)

Definition

Cervical vertebral stenotic myelopathy (CVSM) is a cause of spinal ataxia in horses.

Cause

The cause of CVSM is multifactorial. Clinical signs result from stenosis of the cervical vertebral canal leading to compression of the spinal cord. This probably develops due to the rate of cartilage formation exceeding bone ossification in the vertebrae (osteochondrosis). It is most often seen in rapidly growing horses receiving a high plane of nutrition. Micronutrient imbalance (excessive carbohydrates, excessive zinc, and deficient copper) further predisposes osteochondrosis. Spinal cord compression may be static (constant impingement) or dynamic (impingement only in certain neck positions).

TECHNICIAN TIP 12.15: Multiple factors cause CVSM.

Onset/Signs

CVSM is characterized by spinal ataxia in all four limbs. Ataxia in the hindlimbs is generally more pronounced than that in the forelimbs. Affected horses often assume a base-wide stance when at rest and may be reluctant to back up when asked. Toe-dragging and stumbling of the feet may result in scuffing and chipping of the hooves at the toe.

Diagnosis

A provisional diagnosis of CVSM is made following gait analysis and cervical radiographs. Intravertebral and intervertebral sagittal ratios have been established to help screen for CVSM. Myelography under general anesthesia remains the best antemortem diagnostic test and is a more reliable method to identify compressed segments compared to plain cervical radiography (Figures 12.6 and 12.7). Definitive diagnosis can only be made postmortem.

Treatment

Neurologic deficits are unlikely to resolve without surgical management or dietary changes. Surgical procedures used to treat CVSM include cervical vertebral interbody fusion

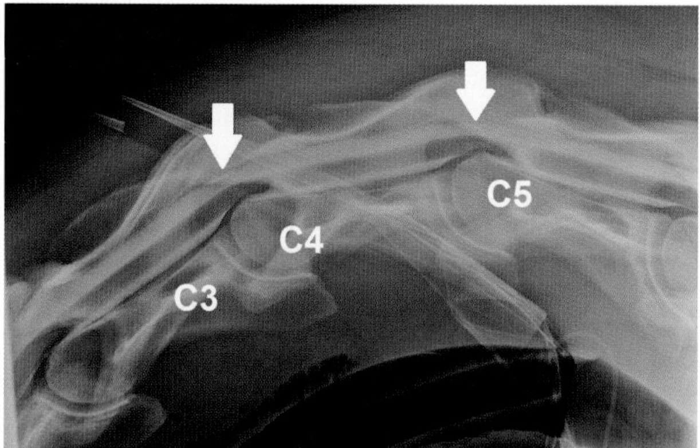

Figure 12.6 Myelogram of a horse not affected with CVSM. This image was captured with the horse's neck maximally flexed. The radio-opaque dorsal myelographic column is not obliterated at the articulation of any of the cervical vertebrae in this image. Normal dorsal myelographic column is denoted by arrows.

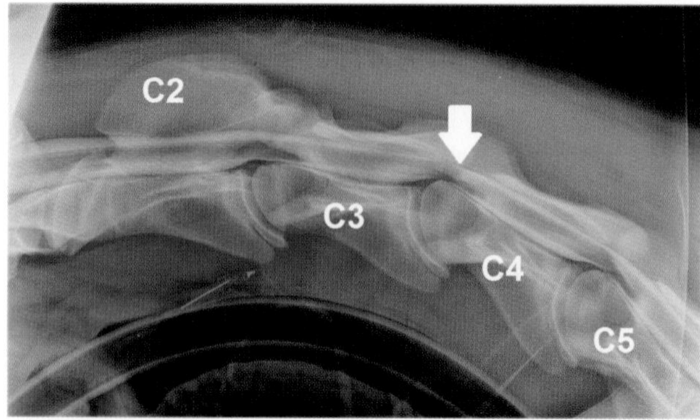

Figure 12.7 Myelogram of a horse affected with CVSM. This image was captured with the horse's neck maximally flexed. Note the obliteration of the radio-opaque dorsal myelographic column at the articulation of the fourth and fifth cervical vertebrae (denoted by arrow).

and dorsal laminectomy. It is contraindicated to perform these procedures without first performing myelography to confirm the compression location(s). Interbody fusion is considered a safer technique and involves fixing the abnormal vertebrae in extension to stop repetitive trauma to the spinal cord. Dorsal laminectomy involves removing portions of the dorsal lamina, ligamentum flavum, and joint capsule at the compressed site. Although dorsal laminectomy provides rapid decompression of the traumatized spinal cord, it is frequently associated with severe and potentially fatal complications and is rarely performed.

Horses that undergo either surgical procedure require extensive rehabilitation time, up to 6–12 months. Horses are only expected to improve one or two neurologic grades based on a scale of five.

Horses less than one year of age may be treated conservatively with a "paced diet" program restricting protein and carbohydrates while providing a balanced amount of vitamins and minerals, including vitamin A, vitamin E, and selenium. Because surgical management may not be financially feasible and not without complications, euthanasia may be elected for affected horses due to concerns for safety, quality of life, and inability to use the horse as intended.

Prognosis

Without intervention, neurologic deficits generally will not resolve. Prognosis is poor for return to athletic function but affected horses may be kept on pasture without being ridden if their clinical signs do not continue to worsen.

Zoonotic Potential

No zoonotic potential.

Prevalence/Geographical Distribution

Two forms of CVSM exist. One form affects younger horses, generally between six months and three years of age. Thoroughbreds are overrepresented. Males are more commonly affected than females. Young horses being fed a diet that is rich in carbohydrates and/or is deficient in copper are at greater risk of developing CVSM. The other form affects older horses and is often related to malarticulation of the synovial articulations with degenerative joint disease (e.g. arthritis).

Prevention

Although not proven, a heritable basis of CVSM is strongly suspected. Consequently, if a breeding animal or stallion-mare pairing consistently produces offspring affected with CVSM, removal from breeding stock should be considered.

Young horses should be monitored for signs of spinal ataxia. Cervical vertebral radiography could be considered as a screening technique for young horses suspected to be "at risk" for CVSM. Ensure that mineral balances (specifically, copper and zinc) are appropriate for a growing foal's diet.

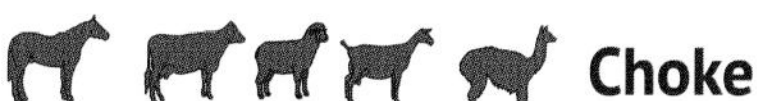

Choke

Definition

Choke is an obstruction of the esophagus.

Cause

There are numerous causes of choke; the most common presentation is impaction of feed material, such as unsoaked beet pulp, leafy alfalfa or grass hay, and so forth. Previous esophageal injury and poor dentition predispose animals to developing choke. Foreign bodies, intra or extraluminal masses, and congenital abnormalities can all lead to food impaction and the signs associated with choke. The obstruction tends to occur at areas where the esophagus is narrow, that is, the cervical esophagus, thoracic inlet, and heart base.

Systems Affected

Gastrointestinal.

Signs

Clinical signs show patients as anxious and extremely distressed, food material appearing from both nostrils, ptyalism, violently extending the neck (appear to retch), and coughing. In severe cases, swelling and emphysema is associated with esophageal rupture.

Prevalence/Geographical Distribution

Common in all ages, particularly old horses with bad teeth. Worldwide distribution.

Diagnosis

Diagnostics include palpation, if the obstruction is in the cranial esophagus, inability to pass a nasogastric tube into the stomach, and endoscopy (Figure 12.8). Further diagnostics may include ultrasound and radiographs.

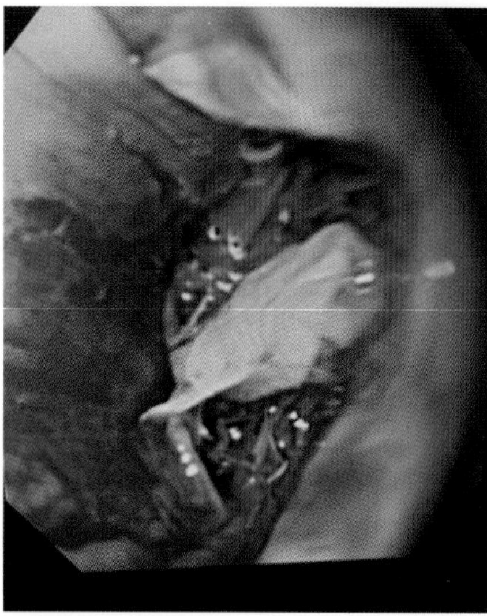
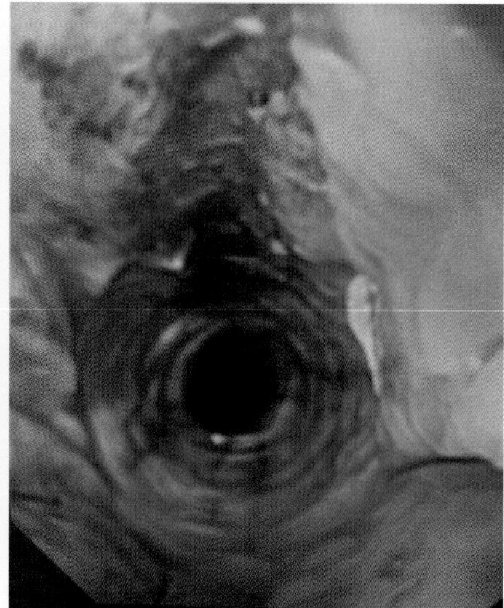

Figure 12.8 **Left:** Obstructed esophagus with grass wad. **Right:** Choke resolved, and endoscopy shows the lining of the esophagus is inflamed and irritated.

Radiographs may require contrast media to visualize distended esophagus and location of choke.

Laboratory work may initially be unremarkable. With chronic choke, electrolytes and acid–base changes may be associated with decreased feed intake and ptyalism (increased hematocrit, hyponatremia, hypochloremia, and metabolic alkalosis).

Treatment

Patients must be held off-feed and water in an unbedded stall. Sedation, anti-inflammatories, and smooth muscle relaxants can be instituted. More invasive intervention could include heavy sedation so that the horse hangs their head with simultaneous lavage of small volumes of water via nasogastric tube. Side effects of this treatment may include aspiration pneumonia. An esophagostomy can help to remove impacted food material. Horses with severe choke may need intravenous fluid therapy to correct dehydration, and electrolyte and acid–base imbalances.

> **TECHNICIAN TIP 12.16:** Patients diagnosed with choke must be held off-feed and water in an unbedded stall.

Withhold food for at least 12–24 hr following clearance of the choke. Endoscopy can be used to assess damage to the esophagus following clearance. Prophylactic antimicrobials may be indicated to minimize severity of aspiration pneumonia. Two important concerns for severe choke are: excessive force with the nasogastric tube can lead to esophageal perforation; and aspiration pneumonia. Follow up after a choking episode includes a dental examination and a dietary evaluation to ensure the horse is being fed an appropriate diet. Choke can recur, particularly following severe cases. Some horses that repeatedly suffer from choke require soft liquid diets and no hay.

Zoonotic Potential

No zoonotic potential.

Genetic Prevalence

No genetic prevalence known.

Prevention

Regular dental care, do not feed dry beet pulp to horses, and avoid feeding horses immediately following exercise. Horses that gulp their feed should be fed small amounts frequently.

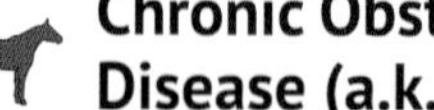

Chronic Obstructive Pulmonary Disease (a.k.a. Heaves, COPD, RAO)

Definition

COPD is a common inflammatory condition of the equine respiratory system, typically characterized by repeated episodes of increased respiratory rate and effort leading to chronic changes in the lungs and the development of a heave line (due to hypertrophy of the external abdominal oblique muscle).

TECHNICIAN TIP 12.17: Recurrent airway obstruction (RAO) is also known as heaves and COPD.

Cause

The exact cause of COPD is yet to be established; however, it appears to be a hypersensitive reaction to organic dusts and molds found in hay and straw (particularly those of poor quality). Inhalation of these spores and dust particles causes an accumulation of neutrophils and mucous in the airways as well as significant bronchospasm. Often the signs are initiated due to inhalation of high concentrations of dust and mold, but as the disease progresses and the hypersensitivity worsens, even very low levels of allergen can cause severe signs.

Systems Affected

Respiratory tract.

Signs

Clinical signs include mucopurulent nasal discharge, chronic cough, hypertrophy of the external abdominal oblique and rectus abdominis muscles, tachypnea at rest, respiratory distress, exercise intolerance, weight loss, and nostril flaring.

Diagnosis

Diagnosis includes bronchoalveolar lavage, endoscopy, and thoracic radiographs. Arterial blood gases may show hypoxemia in severe cases (PaO2 < 85 mmHg).

Treatment

Treatment includes management changes: provide maximum duration of outdoor turnout, provide low dust bedding (e.g. shavings), change from round bale hay to small bales ± steam/soak the hay, avoid mucking out and grooming while the horse is in the stable, increase ventilation of the stable if possible. With acute exacerbation, intravenous atropine may be warranted (relieve bronchospasm), and if that is insufficient then intravenous dexamethasone should relieve signs followed by oral prednisolone for seven days. Long-term therapy may include inhalant fluticasone and albuterol/salmeterol. Ideally parenteral therapy should only be maintained while management changes are made, and inhaled therapy instigated. Horses with COPD can often be managed well with management changes alone; however, the owners should have access to inhaled therapies to use prophylactically during high-risk periods. Some horses require constant drug therapy to prevent acute exacerbations, particularly horses that have been affected for a long time before treatment was started.

Prevalence/Geographical Distribution

Adult horses and ponies. Worldwide distribution.

Zoonotic Potential

No zoonotic potential.

Genetic Prevalence

None known. It does appear to be a genetic link and can occur in families, but the exact mutation is not known.

Prevention

Prevention includes providing low dust/mold environments, providing routine vaccination against common respiratory pathogens, monitoring closely for respiratory signs, and treating early on in the disease process.

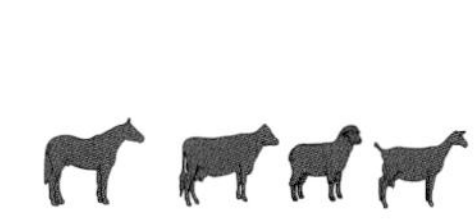

Clostridial Myonecrosis (a.k.a. Clostridrial Myositis, Blackleg, Malignant Edema, Gas Gangrene)

Definition

A bacterial infection that produces tissue gas in gangrene.

Cause

Clostridial myonecrosis can occur due to a variety of infectious organisms including *Clostridium chauvoei, Clostridium septicum, Clostridium sordelli, Clostridium novyi, Clostridium perfringens* and *Clostridium carnis.* Infection can occur via an intramuscular injection, inoculation through a wound, or via the alimentary tract.

Systems Affected

Infection can be localized to muscle or systemic and involve multiple body systems.

Signs

This disease can affect animals of varying breeds, ages, and genders. Depending on the route of infection, signs can be variable and include local signs (i.e.: muscle swelling, pain on palpation, heat) or systemic signs (i.e.: fever, tachycardia, tremors, ataxia, recumbency). Disease progression can be extremely fast (12–24 hr) and animals may be found dead. Mortality can approach 100% in affected animals.

Prevalence/Geographical Distribution

Prevalence depends on immunization protocols and exposure to the inciting organisms in ruminants. Infection in horses is relatively rare and most commonly associated with a wound or intramuscular injection. Worldwide distribution.

Diagnosis

Presumptive diagnosis can be made when muscles are enlarged, hard, painful or have crepitus present at a previous intramuscular injection site or wound. Ultrasound can be supportive with identification of gas and inflammation within the muscle. Alternatively, infection can be diagnosed at postmortem exam and animals often have blood staining and gas bubbles present within muscles and fascial planes. Hemorrhage may be present in many organs. Dark discoloration of the muscle can occur, and rancid odors are often present.

Lab Work

Elevated muscle enzymes including creatinine kinase (CK) and aspartate aminotransferase (AST) may be present depending on the timeline of infection.

Differentials

Differentials would include other disease processes that cause toxemia and/or rapid death.

Treatment

In many cases, infection is fatal, and treatment may not be attempted. Treatment can be successful in individual cases, and involves a combination of aggressive antimicrobial therapy, surgical debridement, supportive care (IV fluids, antipyretics, analgesics, anti-inflammatories), and administration of antitoxins if available. Infections with *C. perfringens* in horses tend to have the best prognosis for survival.

Associated Conditions

Large areas of muscle and tissue necrosis often occur along with skin sloughing. Systemic infection can lead to a variety of organ dysfunction, toxemia, coagulopathies and rapid death.

Zoonotic Potential

No zoonotic potential.

Genetic Prevalence

No genetic prevalence known.

Prevention

Ruminants are routinely vaccinated for protection against a variety of clostridial organisms. In horses, proper injection technique as well as avoiding intramuscular injections of irritating substances is the mainstay of prevention.

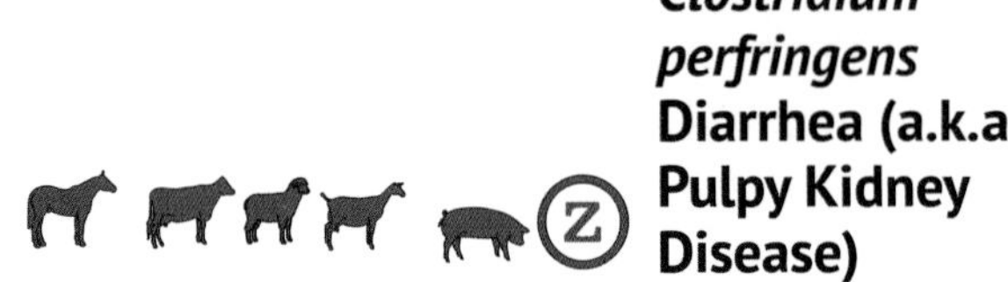

Clostridium perfringens Diarrhea (a.k.a. Pulpy Kidney Disease)

Definition

A contagious gastrointestinal disease caused by an infection with the bacterium *C. perfringens.*

Cause

C. perfringens type B and C, a gram-positive rod.

Transmission

Oral, as with fecal-oral or contaminated skin surface.

Signs

In piglets one to three days of age, *C. perfringens* causes a bloody diarrhea; piglets three to five days of age experience a watery diarrhea. Piglets three to five days or older and chronically infected piglets experience chronic, discolored diarrhea with noticeable wasting. On necropsy, small intestines are dark red, content is bloody liquid. In older infections, pockets of gas may be observed in the jejunal wall, and a necrotic membrane may be present on the mucosal surface.

Onset

Diarrhea appears within 12–14 hr of infection.

> **TECHNICIAN TIP 12.18:** Swine infected with *C. perfringens* may show clinical signs within 12 hr of infection.

Prevalence/Geographical Distribution

Worldwide distribution.

Diagnosis

Intestinal lesions at necropsy with gram-positive rods on the mucosal surface or culture of organism are diagnostic.

Treatment

After the onset of diarrhea, no treatments are considered effective. Prophylactic antibiotic or antitoxin can be effective if administered within 2 hr of birth.

Recovery

Recovered animals may continue to shed *C. perfringens*.

Zoonotic Potential

Puncture or open wounds may be contaminated by *C. perfringens*.

Genetic Prevalence

No genetic prevalence known.

Prevention

Sows may be vaccinated prior to farrowing with attention paid to cleanliness of the sow and farrowing environment.

> **TECHNICIAN TIP 12.19:** Another neonatal clostridial diarrhea, caused by *Clostridium difficile*, is associated with over-administration of antibiotics early in life.

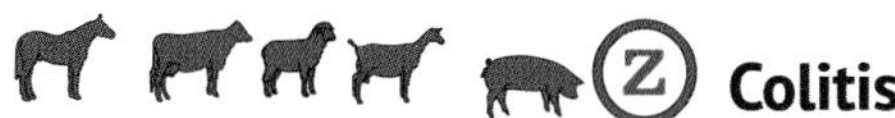

Colitis

Definition

Colitis is diarrhea secondary to inflammation and mucosal injury of the large colon (and cecum in typhlocolitis).

Cause

The diarrhea is caused by increased water loss through the large colon; this may be due to malabsorption or hyper secretion, or a combination of the two. Intestinal secretion is controlled by at least four mechanisms: hormonal secretion, the enteric nervous system, bacterial enterotoxins, and the immune system.

Systems Affected

Large intestine.

Signs

Clinical signs include inappetence/anorexia; colic signs; fever; lethargy; profuse watery, sometimes hemorrhagic, diarrhea (may not show signs until 24–48 hr after initial symptoms); endotoxemic signs. Further signs that may develop are laminitis and severe hypovolemia.

Diagnosis

Diagnostics include clinical signs, blood work, abdominal ultrasound, Potomac horse fever using whole blood PCR or serology, fecal culture for *Salmonella* species, demonstration of *Clostridium* toxin in feces.

> **TECHNICIAN TIP 12.20:** Causes of colitis can include Potomac horse fever, Salmonellosis, and Clostridia.

Lab Work

- CBC: neutropenia, lymphopenia, leucopenia, toxic changes to the neutrophils ± left shift. Often see elevated fibrinogen and hematocrit, thrombocytopenia.
- Chemistry: azotemia, elevated hepatocellular enzymes and serum lactate (hypoperfusion), hypoproteinemia, hypokalemia, hyponatremia, hypochloremia, hypocalcemia, metabolic acidosis.

Treatment

Treatment may include fluid therapy, anti-inflammatories, antimicrobials, antiendotoxic therapy, nutrition, and absorbent powders.

Recovery

Once recovered, any dietary changes should be made gradually, and caution should be used when using antimicrobials. Horses with salmonellosis may be at risk of shedding *Salmonella* again; however, this is rarely clinically significant. Owners should be warned that the horse may shed *Salmonella* at stressful times.

Prevalence/Geographical Distribution

Any age. Worldwide distribution.

Zoonotic Potential

May be zoonotic if animal is shedding *Salmonella*.

Genetic Prevalence

No genetic prevalence known.

Prevention

Careful management changes, good fiber diet, and careful monitoring.

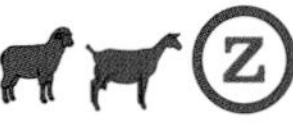

Contagious Ecthyma (a.k.a. Orf, SoreMouth)

Definition

Highly contagious zoonotic disease that affects lambs and kids, self-limiting; may also infect susceptible adults.

> **TECHNICIAN TIP 12.21:** Orf is a highly contagious zoonotic disease.

Cause

Parapoxvirus.

Systems Affected

Integument, mucocutaneous junctions, areas of low fur/wool. Secondary effects: alimentary and respiratory tract, ophthalmic.

Transmission

From contact, rapidly spread through herd or flock by processing of young animals: ear-taggers, emasculators, or hands of workers. Also, may be spread via nursing if the dam has an infected udder.

Signs

Pustules, ulcerations, scabs, and inflammation of infected areas. Most commonly affects the mucocutaneous junction at the commissure of the mouth and spreads to the nose; may spread to the coronary bands, ears, vulva, scrotum, or anus. Severe infections can infect the alimentary or respiratory.

Onset

Acute or chronic.

Prevalence/Geographical Distribution

May occur at any time, but more prevalent in dry areas. Distribution is unknown but thought to be wherever sheep and goat populations exist. Disease also affects some wildlife.

Diagnosis

Via clinical signs, identification of lesions.

Treatment

Supportive care for clinical symptoms.

Recovery

Morbidity rates near 100% while mortality rates are less than 15%. Mortality rates increase in animals with secondary infections. Animals that recover are immune to reinfection for two to three years.

Zoonotic Potential

High, although self-limiting. Most commonly affect the hands via direct contact.

Genetic Prevalence

No genetic prevalence known.

Prevention

Vaccine.

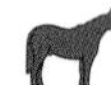

Contagious Equine Metritis (CEM)

Definition

CEM is an acute, highly communicable venereal disease of horses.

Cause

CEM is caused by the gram-negative, microaerophilic coccobacillus *Taylorella equigenitalis*. There is only one serotype of this organism, but it has been found that there are two different strains. One of the strains is sensitive to streptomycin while the other has been found to be resistant. Susceptible mares have the potential to contract both strains of CEM. There is another closely related organism, *Taylorella asinigenitalis*, which has been identified in donkeys, yet has shown no cause of significant disease in horses.

System Affected

Reproductive System.

Transmission

The most likely method of transmission is during sexual intercourse between undetected mares and stallions. CEM may also be transmitted through fomites during artificial insemination and collection of the stallion. The transmission rate is extremely high in which every mare that comes in contact with an infected stallion will contract the disease. Some reasons for transmission during collection from stallion to stallion can be due to not using a disposable AV (artificial vagina) liner, sharing of penis washing equipment, and not using a protective disposable barrier on the rear of the breeding dummy. Mares can be bred with infected semen during the artificial insemination process.

Signs

Chronically infected mares and infected stallions rarely show any clinical signs of disease. The incubation period is between 2 and 14 days, but typically the mare will show signs between day 10 and 14. CEM is a serious disease because it is highly contagious, and it can have a devastating effect on reproductive efficacy resulting in substantial economic loss. One of the first clinical signs in the mare is the inability to become pregnant, typically after more than one breeding. There are three different degrees of infection in the mare. The acutely infected mare will present with an inflamed uterus, which causes an obvious thick purulent discharge from the vulva. These mares will often return to estrus earlier than anticipated. The chronically infected mare will have a less inflamed uterus, which in turn will have less of a purulent discharge. These mares typically are more difficult to treat, and it is more difficult to eliminate the infection in them. The carrier mare shows no clinical signs but harbors the organism in her reproductive tract. It is difficult to get rid of the infection in these mares and they may remain carriers for months. Stallions display no clinical signs and may carry the organism on their external genitalia for years.

> **TECHNICIAN TIP 12.22:** Chronically infected mares and stallions rarely show clinical signs of CEM.

Prevalence/Geographical Distribution

The first cases of CEM were observed in the spring of 1977 in England and Ireland in Thoroughbreds. Mares were found unable to conceive, having shorter diestrus periods, and having a purulent discharge from the vulva. There are many countries affected by CEM, even though strict import/export policies have been put in place. No equine death has been associated with CEM.

Diagnosis

Diagnosis depends strictly on laboratory isolation of *T. equigenitalis*. There are two other common genital infections that will cause similar clinical signs and must be ruled out. These common infections are caused by *Klebsiella* and *Pseudomonas spp*. bacteria. Swabs from the mare should be taken from the cervix during estrus from the clitoral sinuses and clitoral fossa. Swabs from the stallion should be taken from the sheath, urethral sinus, and fossa glandis. *T. equigenitalis* grows optimally on chocolate agar. The colonies are usually shiny, waxy, and grayish white. Stallions should be tested at least three times to be declared CEM free. Because stallions also carry a low number of organisms, they should also be bred to test mares, which in turn can be tested for CEM.

Treatment

Treatment in the mare and the stallion consists of cleaning of the external genitalia with a 2% chlorhexidine solution and then application of topical antibiotics. This should be done once daily for five consecutive days. Although you can treat the external genitalia of the mare, she cannot be successfully treated until the bacteria are cleared from the uterus, which may take upward of two weeks. Systemic antibiotics may also be used.

Zoonotic Potential

No zoonotic potential.

Genetic Prevalence

No genetic prevalence known.

Prevention

There are strict importation regulations in most countries to help prevent outbreaks. Prevention includes quarantine of all mares, fillies, and stallions that are of foreign origin until tested and cleared. Testing for the stallion includes testing the first three mares that he has bred. The current prevalence of CEM is low and there is no evidence that it infects humans.

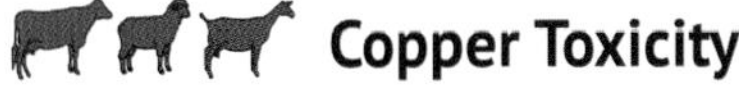

Copper Toxicity

Definition

Ingestion of excess copper that exceeds an animal's essential requirement affecting small ruminants, swine, poultry, livestock, and horses.

Cause

Two forms: Chronic and Acute Ingestion of copper

Chronic form – Excessive amounts of copper are ingested over a prolonged period of time but below toxicity threshold. Copper is stored in the liver and when released suddenly, can cause intravascular hemolysis. The hemolytic crisis may be precipitated by many factors, including transportation, handling, weather conditions, pregnancy, lactation, strenuous exercise, or poor plane of nutrition, including diets low in molybdenum and sulfur. Primary chronic toxicity is seen most commonly in sheep when excessive amounts of copper are ingested over a prolonged period.

Acute form – Occurs when an animal ingests high levels of copper, for example when sheep/camelids ingest cattle rations, which contain higher levels of copper or drink contaminated water sourced from copper plumbing.

Systems Affected

Gastrointestinal, hepatic, respiratory, cardiovascular.

Signs

- Increased respiration
- Depression
- Hemoglobinuria
- Sudden death
- Necropsy findings include icterus and "gun-metal blue" kidneys

Onset

Acute or chronic.

Prevalence/Geographical Distribution

Copper toxicity occurs more often in sheep than in goats. Worldwide distribution.

Diagnosis

Blood and liver copper concentrations may be increased during the hemolytic crisis. Since copper is mainly stored in the liver, serum copper levels can be unreliable. If serum copper levels are elevated (>2.0 ppm), this is diagnostic for copper toxicity.

Treatment

Treatment is often not successful and affected animals generally have a poor prognosis. Several drugs have been used to treat copper toxicity, including penicillamine and ammonium tetrathiomolybdate. Supportive care may be needed due to acute hemolysis.

Zoonotic Potential

No zoonotic potential.

Genetic Prevalence

No genetic prevalence known.

Prevention

Restriction of copper intake is the most effective preventative measure. Molybdenum supplementation and sodium thiosulfate has been shown to decrease copper accumulation/increase copper excretion.

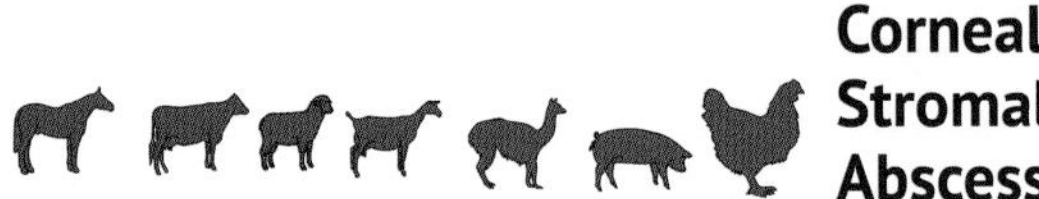

Corneal Stromal Abscess

Definition

An accumulation of white blood cells as a result of the cornea being infected.

Cause

Most corneal stromal abscesses appear to occur when epithelial cells migrate over a defect in the cornea trapping infectious agents. Neutrophils migrate into the cornea stimulating inflammation. Topical medical administration may not penetrate the cornea effectively, and trapped organisms can then proliferate and continue to incite inflammation and secondary uveitis can result.

Systems Affected

Ocular – cornea.

Signs

This disease can affect animals of varying breeds, ages, and genders. Typically present with mild signs initially that progress to more fulminant uveitis. Signs of ocular discomfort including blepharospasm, excessive tearing, redness, and corneal edema may be present. The abscess is identified as a focal white to yellow opacity within the cornea and can have well-demarcated or wispy margins.

Prevalence/Geographical Distribution

Increased prevalence reported in recent years. Unclear whether this is a true increase or due to increased recognition and diagnosis of the condition. Worldwide distribution.

Diagnosis

Diagnosis is based on appearance on ophthalmic examination. Fluorescein stain is often negative. Evidence of infiltrate within the cornea and secondary uveitis may be present.

Differentials

Differentials would include other diseases that cause corneal opacification (keratitis, foreign body, granulation tissue), lipid or mineral deposition, and neoplastic conditions.

Treatment

Early and aggressive medical treatment using a combination of antimicrobials, mydriatics, and anti-inflammatory drugs may be successful in superficial cases. These medications are often needed for a prolonged time period and are given multiple times daily. The insertion of a subpalpebral lavage system (SPL) can be beneficial and aid in treatment. Antifungals have been injected into and around the lesions within the cornea with variable successes.

Deep or fungal abscesses often require additional surgical intervention, which can include a variety of grafts and multiple lamellar keratoplasty procedures.

Associated Conditions

Secondary uveitis can lead to a variety of other changes within the structures of the eye.

Recovery

Recovery rate depends on aggression of lesion and aggression of treatment.

Zoonotic Potential

No zoonotic potential.

Genetic Prevalence

No genetic prevalence known.

Prevention

Prompt and appropriate treatment for corneal ulceration can decrease the likelihood for development of stromal abscesses.

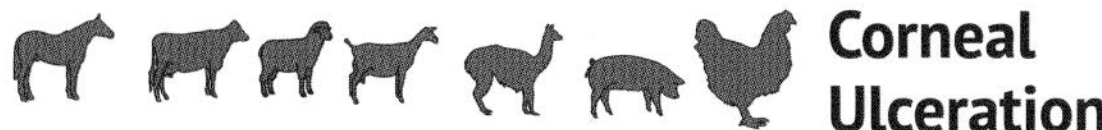

Corneal Ulceration

Definition

Ulceration of the cornea most commonly occurs due to a lack of protective mechanisms, mechanical/chemical trauma, or infectious agents. The cornea is protected by tear film, and deficiencies in tear film leave the cornea exposed and susceptible to trauma. Underlying infectious agents can also weaken the cornea leading to ulceration. Ulceration in horses is most common secondary to trauma, whereas infectious bovine keratoconjunctivitis (IBK, pink eye) is the most common cause in cattle. Additional causes can include secondary to entropion, eyelid defects, facial nerve paralysis, or ocular neoplasia.

> **TECHNICIAN TIP 12.23:** A corneal ulcer is any disruption of the normal corneal epithelium.

Systems Affected

Ocular – cornea.

Signs

This disease can affect animals of varying breeds, ages, and genders. Ocular signs will be present and depend on the chronicity and severity. Blepharospasm, excessive tearing, redness, and photophobia are often present. Focal corneal edema surrounding the ulcer may progress to widespread edema, and infection of the corneal ulcer can progress to suppurative discharge, corneal vascularization, keratomalacia (corneal melting), and corneal rupture (Figure 12.9).

Onset

Primarily acute.

Prevalence/Geographical Distribution

Prevalence depends on immunization protocols and exposure to the inciting organisms in ruminants. Ocular ulcerations are relatively common in horses and occur at a high prevalence in all populations. Worldwide distribution.

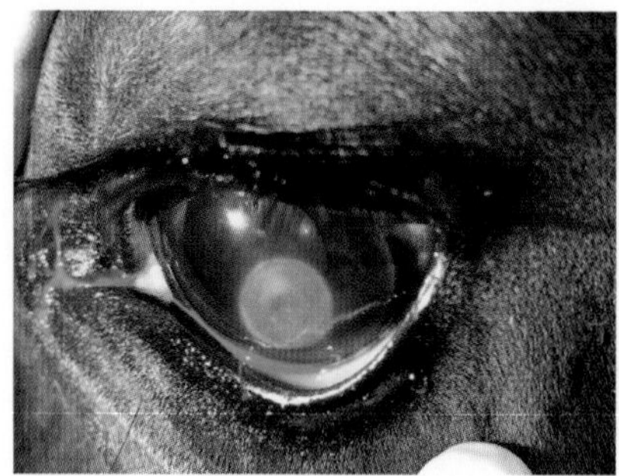
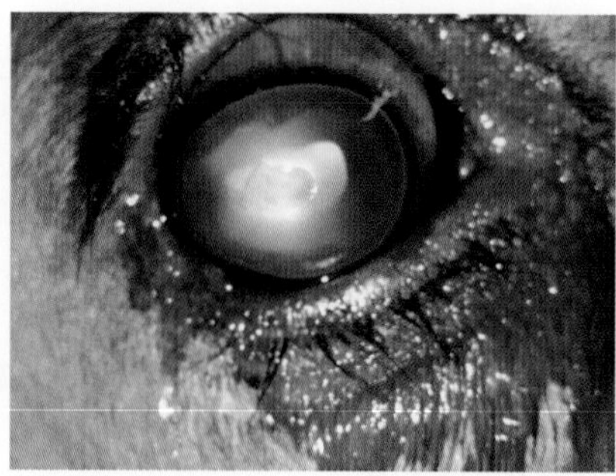
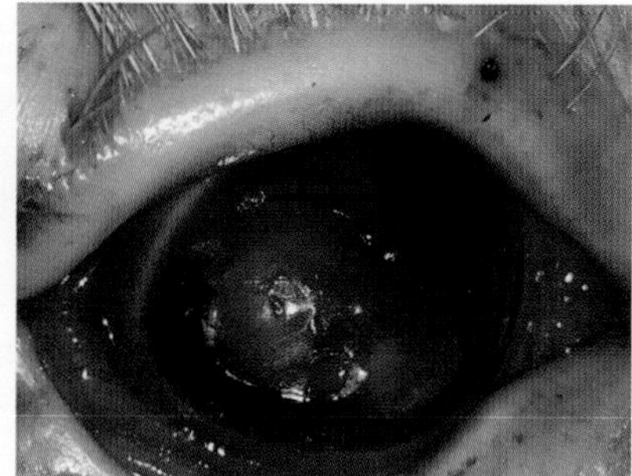

Figure 12.9 **Left:** Equine corneal ulcer. **Middle:** Bovine corneal ulcer with neovascularization. **Right:** Swine corneal ulcer. *Source:* Photo courtesy of Kimberly Young, DVM and Lauren Hughes, DVM.

Diagnosis

Fluorescein stain uptake, as the corneal stroma takes up fluorescein and stains green. Deep ulcers to Descemet's membrane or the endothelium do not take up stain. Fungal/bacterial cultures should be collected and checked for secondary anterior uveitis.

Differentials

Differentials include other disease processes that affect the cornea including keratitis (immune-mediated, bacterial, fungal, eosinophilic, etc.), mineral or lipid infiltrate, and corneal neoplasia.

Treatment

Treatment is dependent on cause and severity of the ulcer. Topical or systemic antimicrobials and antifungals are used in combination with NSAIDs, mydriatic agents, and anti-collagenase products. Treatment of underlying conditions (entropion, facial nerve paralysis) are necessary, or the condition will recur. Protection of the globe through homemade or commercially available masks/eye cups is recommended to prevent further trauma and infection. In some cases, surgical grafting becomes necessary to protect and bring blood supply to the affected cornea.

Associated Conditions

Ulcer development can occur secondary to conditions that affect normal eyelid function (facial nerve paralysis, eyelid defects, entropion).

Zoonotic Potential

No zoonotic potential.

Genetic Prevalence

No genetic prevalence known.

Prevention

Avoid sharp objects in the stall. Manage any reasons that the animal may be pruritic. Carefully monitor for any signs of ocular pain. The sooner these ulcers are recognized and treated the better the prognosis. Ruminants can be vaccinated for *Moraxella bovis*, the causative agent of infectious bovine keratoconjunctivitis.

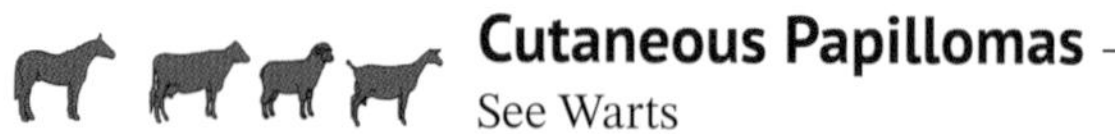

Cutaneous Papillomas –

See Warts

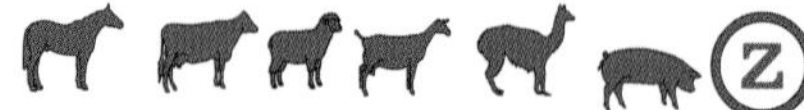

Dermatophilosis (a.k.a. Rain Scald, Rain Rot, Cutaneous Streptothricosis, Lumpy Wool)

Definition

A bacterial skin infection.

Cause

Normal healthy skin is resistant to infection. When skin becomes compromised, most commonly through excessive moisture or abrasions, this bacterial infection can occur. The causative organism, *Dermatophilus congolensis*, enters the compromised skin causing lesions.

Systems Affected

Integumentary.

Transmission

Can be spread to other animals via direct contact, vectors (flies, ticks), or fomites (brushes, tack, shears).

Signs

Disease can affect animals of varying breeds, ages, and genders. Infection generally leads to crusting and clumping of hair with moist lesions present at skin surface. Lesions are most commonly located on the dorsum of the back or the distal extremities due to more exposure to excessive moisture and trauma (Figure 12.10).

Prevalence/Geographical Distribution

Relatively common condition with the prevalence varying depending on environment and management of animals. Worldwide distribution, more common in climates that have higher rainfall.

Diagnosis

Most commonly diagnosed via Gram stain on an impression smear when the gram-positive cocci are identified in a classic "railroad track" appearance. The organism can also be diagnosed via histopathology or bacterial culture.

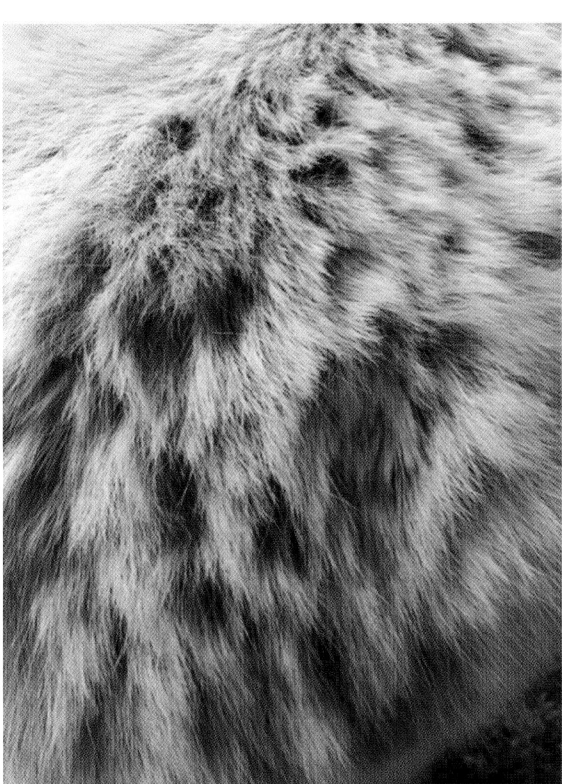

Figure 12.10 Rain rot on a horse. *Source:* Photo courtesy of Erin Elder, DVM.

Differentials

- Dermatitis caused by other organisms (bacterial, fungal)
- Atopy
- Ectoparasites

Treatment

Treatment is variable depending on the severity of infection and is often a combination of eliminating exposure to continued moisture, removal of the crusts, bathing (most commonly with iodine or lime sulfur), and topical or systemic antimicrobials. Recovery generally occurs in two to three weeks, although chronic infections can occur.

Associated Conditions

Secondary bacterial or fungal infections of the affected skin can occur.

Zoonotic Potential

Zoonotic potential and can lead to lesions of the skin in humans.

Genetic Prevalence

No genetic prevalence known.

Prevention

Prevention includes keeping skin healthy and intact as well as avoiding excessive moisture by ensuring animals have access to shelter and avoiding muddy conditions. Limit the sharing of potential fomites (i.e.: brushes, tack, blankets/sheets, shears) between animals and ensure ectoparasite control programs are in place.

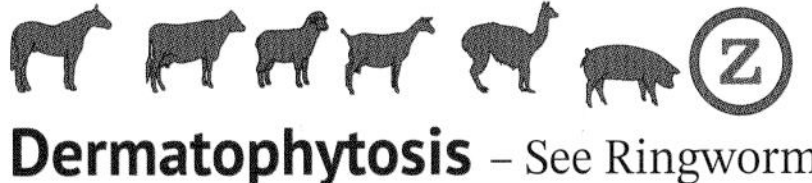

Dermatophytosis – See Ringworm

Digital Dermatitis (Hairy Heel Wart, Papillomatous Digital Dermatitis, Mortellaro's Disease)

Definition

An infectious and contagious infection of the digital skin of dairy cattle characterized by lameness and lesions typically occurring in the plantar aspect of the hind limbs, proximal to the heel bulbs.

TECHNICIAN TIP 12.24: Hairy heel warts are an infectious and contagious disease found on the plantar aspect of the hind limbs, proximal to the heel bulbs.

Cause

A multifactorial disease. Anaerobic organisms and spirochetes from the genus *Treponema* along with environmental and host factors play a role in the development of the disease. Rough, dirty, and wet floorings are predisposing factors.

Transmission

The exact mode of transmission is not clear. Affected cows and fomites serve as source of infection to susceptible animals and naïve herds.

Signs

Skin lesions usually develop on the plantar aspect of the pastern region. Lesions in the early stages are circular with raised and well-demarcated borders. The periphery of the lesions is characterized by the presence of matted long hairs. The surfaces of the lesions are typically filiform in appearance or have a granular aspect. In a more advanced stage, lesions grow as raised papillomatous masses. Lameness is more often seen in second or third lactation cows in an endemically infected herd.

Onset

Acute to chronic.

Prevalence/Geographical Distribution

The disease is more prevalent in the United States and Europe.

Diagnosis

Clinical signs.

Treatment

Topical antibiotics and footbaths are used to treat and control the disease.

Recovery

Relapses after successful treatment are common as the disease is difficult to eradicate once it is established in a herd.

Zoonotic Potential

No zoonotic potential.

Genetic Prevalence

No genetic prevalence known.

Prevention

Improving environmental predisposing factors and hygiene. Claw-trimming tools and other fomites should be properly cleaned and disinfected between animals and between herds to control the spread of the disease.

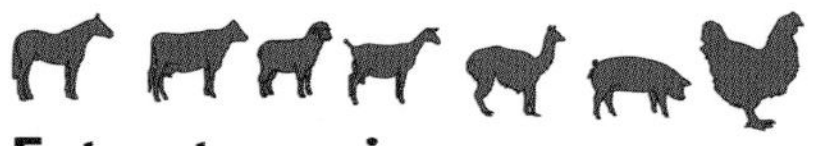

Enterotoxemia

Definition

Blood poisoning caused by an enterotoxin.

Cause

Enterotoxemia is a broad term that encompasses a wide variety of syndromes caused by *C. perfringens* type A, B, C, D, and E. *C. perfringens* is an anaerobic, Gram-positive, spore-forming rod that can be commonly found in the intestinal tract and environment of ruminants and horses.

Systems Affected

Primarily gastrointestinal, though neurologic signs can be seen in sheep and goats with *C. perfringens* type D (overeating disease, pulpy kidney disease).

Onset

Incubation appears to be short as enteric disease can appear in the first few days of life. Progression can be extremely rapid, and many animals will be found dead without any premonitory clinical signs.

Transmission

As the organism can commonly be found in the intestine and environment of healthy animals, it is believed to a normal inhabitant of the intestine of ruminants and horses. Disease occurs when there is a rapid growth of *C. perfringens* with toxin production. This is believed to be associated with changes in the intestinal microbiota and/or undigested, rapidly fermentable carbohydrates entering the small intestine.

Signs

Many animals may be found dead due to the rapid progression of clinical signs. Diarrhea in animals ranging from a few days to a few weeks of age is commonly seen and is often accompanied by significant abdominal distension and abdominal pain.

Prevalence/Geographical Distribution

Enterotoxemia is seen worldwide in all ruminants and horses. Disease is most commonly seen in young animals.

Diagnosis

Diagnosis is most commonly made based on clinical signs or at necropsy. Fecal culture of the organism with specific testing for toxin production is confirmatory.

Treatment

Specific antitoxin is available for *C. perfringens* type D in sheep and goats, but often animals die prior to administration. Systemic and oral penicillin should be administered along with supportive fluid therapy.

Recovery

Prognosis is poor for severely affected animals, while those with mild intestinal disease can recover with appropriate therapy.

Zoonotic Potential

No zoonotic potential.

Genetic Prevalence

No genetic prevalence known.

Prevention

Specific vaccinations are available, economic and appear to be effective in ruminants. As rapidly fermentable carbohydrates appear to be a risk factor, reducing grain in the diet may reduce risk of disease. Specific antitoxin is available for sheep and goats and can be used in cases of herd outbreaks.

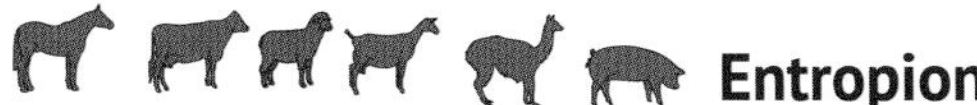

Entropion

Definition

A condition affecting the eyelids.

Cause

Entropion can occur as a congenital or acquired condition. Most commonly involves the lower eyelid but can involve both and be unilateral or bilateral. The inward rolling of the eyelid causes eyelashes to rub on the cornea and often leads to secondary conditions including conjunctivitis, keratitis, or corneal ulceration.

Systems Affected

Ocular – eyelids.

Signs

Entropion can be identified on examination with no accompanying clinical signs or recognized when signs of ocular pain are present. Excessive tearing, blepharospasm, and redness may accompany keratitis or corneal ulceration secondary to mechanical trauma from entropion.

Prevalence/Geographical Distribution

Relatively common condition in foals (4–10%). Worldwide distribution.

Diagnosis

Diagnosis is made on clinical examination, and a full ophthalmic examination should be performed including fluorescein stain to rule out secondary conditions.

Differentials

Additional congenital ocular abnormalities can look similar including coloboma, dermoid, or ciliary abnormalities. Acquired entropion needs to be differentiated from microphthalmia, eyelid trauma, or other causes of keratitis/ulceration.

Treatment

Treatment method depends on the severity and chronicity of entropion. Temporary repair can be performed with subcutaneous injection of penicillin G, silicone, or hyaluronic acid. Temporary eversion of the eyelids and tacking with sutures or staples is commonly performed and only necessary for days to weeks. Rarely a permanent surgical correction (Holz-Celsus procedure) is needed in congenital cases.

Additionally, treatment including frequent ocular lubrication and/or topical antibiotic treatment for secondary ulceration is warranted.

Associated Conditions

Can be associated with other congenital ocular abnormalities.

Zoonotic Potential

No zoonotic potential.

Genetic Prevalence

Unknown genetic predisposition. Inheritance suspected in Thoroughbreds and Quarter Horses.

Prevention

Prompt and regular examination of the eyelids in foals is recommended to identify and initiate treatment.

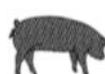

Eperythrozoonosis

Definition

A vector-borne bacterial disease that causes hemolytic anemia in swine.

Cause

Mycoplasma suis (formerly known as *Eperythrozoon suis*), an obligate intracellular bacterium.

Systems Affected

Hematopoietic.

Transmission

Vectors including arthropods, such as lice and mosquitos, contaminated needles, or surgical equipment, and vertical in utero.

Signs

Infected pigs become febrile and ataxic or paralyzed and exhibit severe wasting. Pigs become icteric with pale mucous membranes. Reproductive failure may be observed in adult animals, and surviving suckling piglets are weak. Spleens are enlarged.

Onset

Clinical signs appear with moderate anemia or stressful events and mild anemia.

Prevalence/Geographical Distribution

Worldwide distribution.

Diagnosis

Clinical signs, gross lesions, and demonstration of the organism in blood smear to diagnose.

Treatment

Tetracyclines are the treatment of choice since the organism is intracellular.

Recovery

Recovery depends upon severity of infection before treatment and effectiveness of treatment. Incomplete recovery results in asymptomatic carriers.

Zoonotic Potential

No zoonotic potential.

Genetic Prevalence

No genetic prevalence known.

Prevention

Most efforts focus on elimination of arthropod vectors, especially lice.

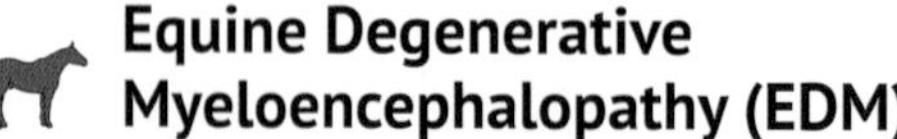

Equine Degenerative Myeloencephalopathy (EDM)

Definition

Equine degenerative myeloencephalopathy (EDM) is a noninfectious non-compressive cervical spinal cord and brainstem disease that results from neuronal degeneration.

Cause

The exact cause of EDM is not fully understood. Pathogenesis is probably multifactorial and may be related to low plasma concentration of vitamin E, and it is likely partially genetic in nature.

> **TECHNICIAN TIP 12.25:** The exact cause of EDM is not fully understood.

Onset/Signs

Characteristic clinical signs are spinal ataxia affecting all four limbs, including weakness, knuckling and dragging of the toes, circumduction of the limb when turning, and pivoting of the foot when turning instead of lifting it off the ground.

Prevalence/Geographical Distribution

Cases have been reported throughout North America since the disease was initially recognized in the 1970s. Prevalence of the disease is suspected to have decreased considerably since 1990.

Diagnosis

Diagnosis requires postmortem histology. Suspicion of this disease is increased by ruling out other neurologic diseases that result in similar clinical signs (CVSM, EHM, equine protozoal myeloencephalitis [EPM]). Cervical radiography should be performed to rule out CVSM; cervical radiographs are normal in cases of EDM as well as white blood cells and total protein levels in CSF. Plasma vitamin E concentration may be within the normal range. A low plasma vitamin E concentration is supportive of a diagnosis of EDM with consistent clinical signs.

Treatment

Supplementation with oral vitamin E is the current therapy of choice, but therapy cannot be expected to reverse spinal ataxia.

Prognosis

Neurologic damage caused by EDM is generally considered irreversible. Progression of spinal ataxia may cease by two to three years of age and supplementation with oral vitamin E may halt progression or even yield mild improvement in ataxia. However, the prognosis should be considered guarded to poor. Euthanasia may become warranted if ataxia worsens to an unsafe level.

Prevalence/Geographical Distribution

EDM primarily affects horses less than one year of age. This disease is known to affect many breeds.

Zoonotic Potential

No zoonotic potential.

Genetic Prevalence

A genetic component is suspected but the characteristics of any pattern of inheritance have not been identified.

Prevention

Allowing foals access to green pasture has been documented as a protective measure. Exposure to insecticides and wood preservatives has been demonstrated as a risk factor. Vitamin E supplementation should be considered when access to green pasture is unavailable.

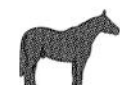 Equine Gastric Ulcer Syndrome

Definition

Inflammation, and in more severe cases erosion and ulceration, of the stomach wall. Lesions in adult horses are most commonly found on the non-glandular (squamous) portion of the stomach adjacent to the margo plicatus and are usually initially found along the lesser curvature of the stomach. Lesions can also be found in the distal esophagus, in the glandular portion of the stomach, around the pylorus, and in the proximal duodenum.

> **TECHNICIAN TIP 12.26:** Equine gastric ulcer syndrome is an inflammation and/or erosion and ulceration of the stomach wall.

Cause

It occurs when the equilibrium between acid production and the protective mechanisms of the stomach are disrupted. This can be due to decreased protective mechanisms: mucous and bicarbonate layer, prostaglandin E_2, epidermal growth factor, and gastroduodenal motility; or increased gastric acid production: mainly hydrochloric acid but also bile acids and pepsin. Gastric ulceration can reliably be induced in horses starved for periods over 24 hr.

Risk factors:

- High-concentrate diet (even with normal amounts of fiber supplementation)
- Long periods of time between feeds
- Exercise
- Stress (stall confinement, transport, horses that crib bite)
- Nonsteroidal anti-inflammatory drugs

Systems Affected

Gastrointestinal. Stomach, including distal esophagus and proximal duodenum.

Signs

Clinical signs can be vague and nonspecific to anorexia, chronic/intermittent colic (often postprandial), and bruxism. Foals may have diarrhea.

Diagnosis

Gastroscopy requires a 3-m endoscope (Figure 12.11). Response to treatment (omeprazole).

Treatment

There are multiple treatments recommended for gastric ulcers.

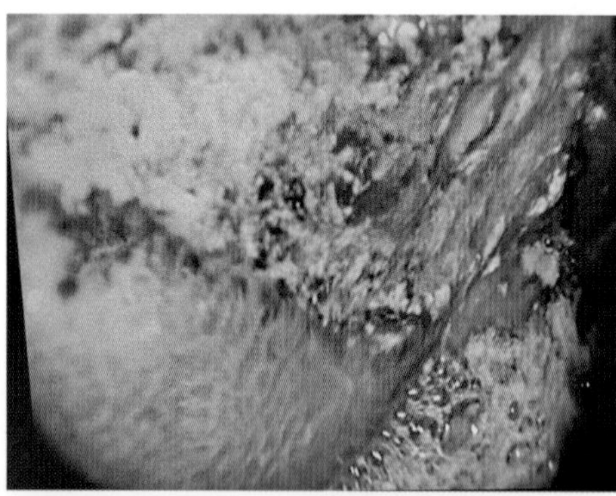

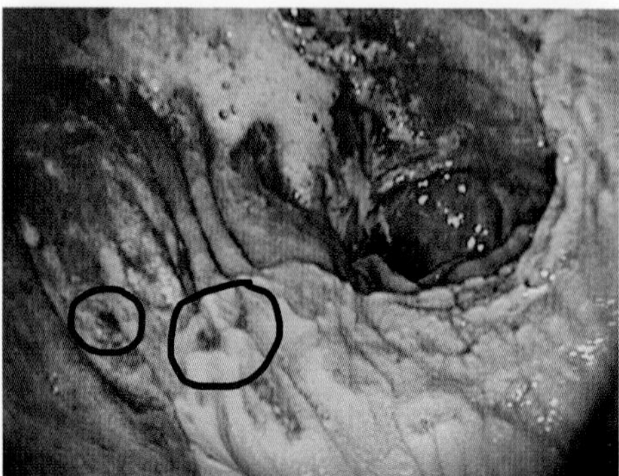

Figure 12.11 Gastric ulcers visualized during a gastroscopy using a 3-m endoscope.

Box 12.1

Scoring system from the Equine Gastric Ulcer Council:

- Grade 0: Intact epithelium, no appearance of hyperemia or hyperkeratosis
- Grade 1: Intact mucosa with areas of hyperemia or hyperkeratosis (squamous)
- Grade 2: Small single or multifocal lesions
- Grade 3: Large single or multifocal lesions or extensive superficial lesions
- Grade 4: Extensive lesions with areas of deep ulceration

- Omeprazole given for at least 28 days (repeat gastroscopy before terminating treatment is recommended).
- Sucralfate given for a short-term treatment in severe cases.

Other drugs include H_2 agonists (ranitidine or cimetidine) and pantoprazole. Foals with suspected delayed gastric emptying can be given prokinetics such as bethanechol and erythromycin.

Zoonotic Potential

No zoonotic potential.

Genetics Prevalence

No genetic prevalence known.

Prevalence/Geographical Distribution

Equine gastric ulcer syndrome is extremely common and is estimated to be present in over 70% of racing Thoroughbreds. Most common in performance animals but can affect any horse. Neonatal foals are at increased risk if hospitalized, and ulcers are a common sequel to a primary disease elsewhere. Worldwide.

Prevention

Adequate dietary fiber, low grain diets for horses with severe gastric ulceration, periods of pasture turn out, prophylactic use of omeprazole during periods of stress.

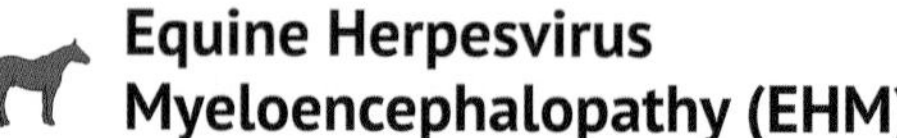

Equine Herpesvirus Myeloencephalopathy (EHM)

Cause

EHM is an uncommon consequence of infection with equine herpesvirus type 1 (EHV-1). The pathogenesis involves viral infection of endothelial cells within the central nervous system with subsequent vasculitis, microthrombosis, local hemorrhage, and spinal cord ischemia. Note that there is no evidence that clinical signs result from direct viral infection of neurons. EHV-4 strains affect primarily the respiratory system and rarely affect the neurologic system or result in abortion.

Systems Affected

EHV-1 is more commonly associated with respiratory disease, abortion, and neonatal disease. Consequently, clinical signs associated with these problems may be observed in the patient or, more commonly, in other horses on the premises. Ocular disease including uveitis, hypopyon, and mydriasis may also be observed.

Onset/Signs

Onset of clinical signs is typically acute. Fever is usually present just before clinical signs and may persist once clinical signs are apparent. Signs include ataxia, decreased tail and anal tone, and urinary incontinence. "Dog-sitting" might be observed as with other disease processes affecting the spinal cord. Clinical signs usually do not progress after the first one to two days (Figure 12.12).

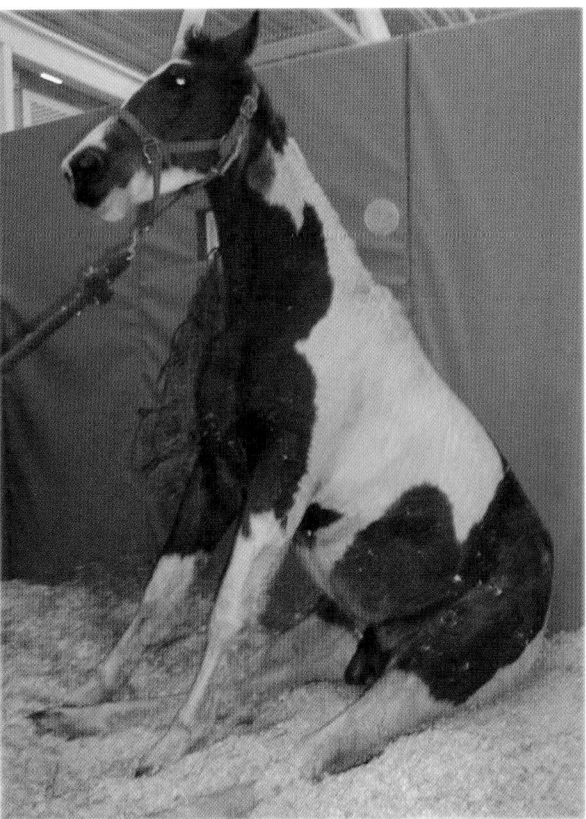

Figure 12.12 Horses affected with EHM and other spinal cord diseases may occasionally "dog-sit." *Source:* Reproduced with permission of Dr. Katherine Wilson.

Prevalence/Geographical Distribution

EHV-1 is ubiquitous. It is believed that most horses are exposed to EHV-1 at a young age and develop a latent infection. Compared to the prevalence of EHV-1 infection, EHM is uncommon. EHM might result from recrudescence of latent EHV-1 infection or a new EHV-1 infection and can occur as an isolated case or as an outbreak of neurologic disease.

> **TECHNICIAN TIP 12.27:** EHV-1 is ubiquitous in the environment.

Diagnosis

Initial clinical signs include an acute onset of fever, hindlimb ataxia, decreased tail and anal tone, and urine dribbling. A tentative diagnosis should be made if multiple horses on the premises are affected, particularly if there is a recent history of travel, fever, abortion, or respiratory disease within the herd. If clinical signs are observed in one or more horses, nasal swabs or blood samples (buffy coat) should be tested via PCR to identify EHV-1 DNA. Positive results with compatible clinical signs are strongly suggestive of EHM.

CSF analysis can help support a diagnosis of EHM. Typical findings include xanthochromia with increased total protein concentration (100–500 mg/dl) and normal cellularity. These changes are reflective of vasculitis and protein leakage into CSF. None of these changes are specific to EHM and these findings (or their absence) neither confirm nor rule out EHM or other causes of neurologic disease.

Serum antibody titers (either serum neutralization or complement fixation tests) can be used to support a diagnosis of EHM. In EHM, antibody titers against EHV-1 are expected to increase by a magnitude of fourfold or greater. Acute and convalescent samples should be sampled 7–21 days apart. Limitation of this testing method is that antibody titers rise rapidly and may have peaked by the time the acute sample is obtained; as a result, a fourfold or greater increase may not be measured. Antibody titers have an increased lag time for results compared to PCR.

Treatment

Supportive care is the cornerstone of treatment. Routine evacuation of the bladder and rectum may be necessary. Sling management may be necessary in recumbent or severely ataxic horses (Figure 12.13). Corticosteroids may

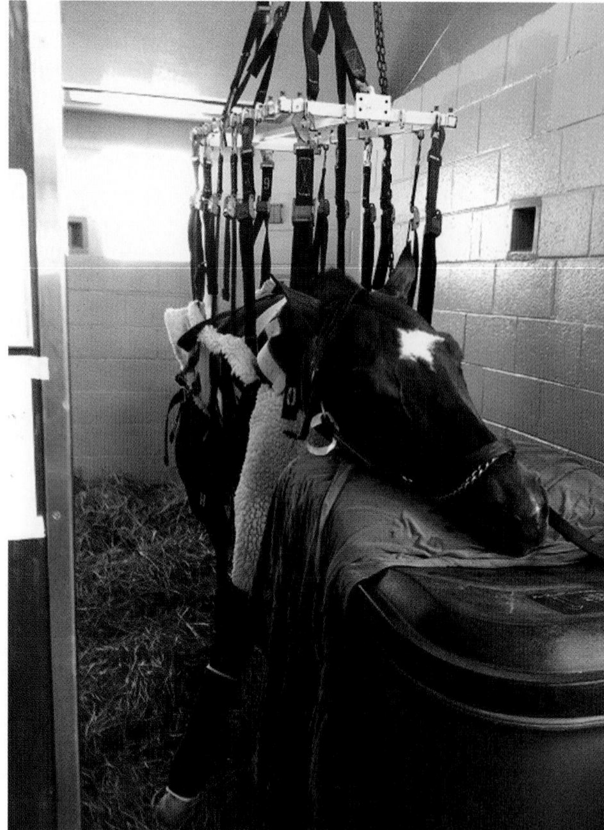

Figure 12.13 Slings can be used to help regain muscle strength in horses recovering from EHM. *Source:* Reproduced with permission of Dr. Michelle Abraham.

be beneficial for severe cases. Antiviral medications (acyclovir or valacyclovir) can be considered, although valacyclovir may be cost-prohibitive. Antibiotic therapy is indicated in patients requiring urinary catheterization or showing evidence of secondary bacterial respiratory disease.

Prognosis

Prognosis is more favorable for those horses that do not become recumbent. Neurologic deficits typically improve over a period of weeks to months. Complete resolution of neurologic deficits may be achieved, but it is possible that ataxia and urinary incontinence may persist. Prognosis is guarded for horses that become recumbent, in part due to complications including myonecrosis, decubital ulcers, and gastrointestinal dysfunction.

Zoonotic Potential

No zoonotic potential.

Genetic Prevalence

No genetic prevalence known.

Prevalence/Geographical Distribution

Horses of any signalment may be affected. Worldwide distribution.

Prevention

The propensity of EHM to occur as an outbreak places this reportable disease among those of utmost concern for horse owners, caretakers, and veterinarians. Highly suspect and confirmed cases must be immediately reported to the state veterinarian, who will assist in management of the facility to attempt to limit spread of the virus. Strict biosecurity and quarantine procedures must be enacted whenever a case or outbreak of EHM is suspected. The virus can spread readily via direct contact, fomites, and aerosol. Aborted fetuses and placenta carry a high viral load and become an important source for spread of the virus. These biological tissues should be disposed of swiftly, either by burning or submission to a diagnostic laboratory. Stalls and equipment must be cleaned thoroughly and disinfected with an iodophor or phenolic compound. Used stalls should be kept empty for several weeks. Affected animals should be isolated immediately in a well-ventilated area far from other members of the herd. Horses in contact with the affected horse should also be quarantined for a minimum of 21 days. Human and horse traffic should be kept to an absolute minimum.

All personnel working with EHM suspects and confirmed cases must understand the gravity of an outbreak and must be educated on the high potential for EHV-1 to spread. Outbreaks can spread even in a hospital setting using extremely strict biosecurity protocols and physical isolation of affected horses – highlighting how readily this disease can spread; therefore, lapses in biosecurity protocols have fatal implications for horses that become infected either in the field or hospital setting.

None of the currently available vaccines against equine herpesvirus claim to prevent EHM. Because many horses are latently infected with EHV-1, stress can cause recrudescence of the viral infection and shedding of the virus. To limit dissemination of the virus, isolating newly arrived horses for at least 21 days before introduction to the remainder of the herd may be effective.

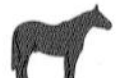 Equine Infectious Anemia (EIA)

Cause

Equine infectious anemia (EIA) is a retroviral, blood-borne infection in which natural transmission of blood with blood-feeding insects is the predominant cause of infection.

Transmission

The horse and deer flies of the *Tabanidae* family are responsible for transmitting the infection and appear to be the most efficient vectors because of their painful bites. Due to their painful bites, their meals are often interrupted, and they continue to seek a host to finish the meal. This may be on the same host or one that is nearby. These flies can hold up to 10 ml of blood in their mouths, which can be transferred to the next host, although they are not able to transfer the virus if the next feeding is delayed by 4 hr. The virus does not appear to shed in urine or saliva but can be found in semen and milk. Venereal transmission is very rare. Using blood-contaminated instruments on different horses, such as needles and surgical instruments, may transmit EIA.

> **TECHNICIAN TIP 12.28:** Horse and deer flies of the *Tabanidae* family are responsible for transmitting EIA.

Signs

There are different degrees of infection. The acute phase may happen initially or during any subsequent attacks. These horses typically die within two to three weeks after onset. An elevated body temperature of 104–108 °F characterizes the acute phase. Other characteristics of this phase include rapid loss in physical condition, inappetence, petechial hemorrhages of the mucous membranes, and severe lethargy. The chronic carriers have clinical signs that are severe and appear frequently. These horses often have thrombocytopenia, pale mucous membranes, hemolytic anemia, and weight loss with dependent edema. Most of the horses are inapparent carriers, which may revert to acute or chronic carriers at any time, especially during times of stress. Once a horse contracts EIA, they are considered infective for life. Enlarged lymph nodes and petechiae on internal organs are noted upon necropsy.

Onset

The incubation period is 1 week to 45 days, where some patients may not show clinical signs until stressed.

Prevalence/Geographical Distribution

EIA can affect every member of the Equidae family, including zebras. EIA was first identified in France in 1843 and first diagnosed in the United States in 1888. This disease has been found worldwide and appears to be absent in only a few countries, including Japan and Iceland.

Diagnosis

Until the 1970s, there was no effective test to diagnose EIA. The agar gel immunodiffusion (AGID) or Coggins test is able to test for antibodies and, therefore, can identify virus carriers. There is also an ELISA test available, but it has a high occurrence of false positive results; therefore, the results are confirmed with the AGID test. There are other tests that are available, but the Coggins test has been recognized internationally as the "gold standard." EIA is considered a reportable disease and must be reported to state and federal animal health authorities.

Treatment

None.

Recovery

If a horse is positive for EIA, several things may be done, but the most common choice is humane euthanasia. They may be shipped in a sealed trailer to a research facility. If neither one of these options is chosen, the horse must be permanently identified with a lip tattoo or brand and be quarantined with a 200-yard separation from other horses. There is no vaccine or specific treatment for identified EIA horses.

Many countries have programs in place to control the movement of identifiable diseases including EIA. Horses must have a negative Coggins test to be allowed entry into most countries. Testing is required for horses for interstate travel, entering competitions or auctions, and change of ownership. Testing should also be included with yearly vaccines. Prevention includes the testing and isolation or destruction of positive cases of EIA.

Zoonotic Potential

No zoonotic potential.

Genetic Prevalence

No genetic prevalence known.

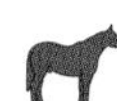

Equine Leukoencephalomalacia –

See Moldy Corn Disease

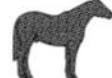

Equine Motor Neuron Disease (EMND)

Cause

The pathogenesis of equine motor neuron disease (EMND) is not completely understood but seems to be related to free radical damage sustained by neurons secondary to a vitamin E deficiency.

Systems Affected

Nervous and musculoskeletal systems.

Onset/Signs

Clinical signs include generalized weakness, a base-narrow stance ("elephant on a ball" stance), muscle tremors, sweating, raised tail, frequent weight shifting, excessive recumbency, muscle atrophy, and weight loss. Although horses may be weak, they are not ataxic. Signs are usually worse when standing versus moving.

Prevalence/Geographical Distribution

EMND is a sporadic disease that can occur worldwide. Cases are most common in areas with limited green pasture and poor-quality hay.

> **TECHNICIAN TIP 12.29:** Cases of EMND are most common in areas with limited green pasture and poor-quality hay.

Diagnosis

Diagnosis is often based on clinical signs and a history of risk factors, particularly a lack of access to grass or good-quality hay. Serum biochemistry analysis may indicate mild to moderate increases in creatine kinase and aspartate aminotransferase. Plasma vitamin E concentration is typically low. Biopsy of the tailhead muscle (sacrocaudalis dorsalis medialis) or spinal accessory nerve can be performed to confirm the diagnosis antemortem. Ophthalmic examination may reveal brown pigmentation in the fundus indicative of lipofuscin deposits.

Treatment

Although not proven to be efficacious, oral supplementation of vitamin E is the recommended course of action. Corticosteroids may be beneficial.

Prognosis

While oral vitamin E supplementation may yield some improvement and stabilization of clinical signs, full recovery is uncommon due to death of affected neurons. Muscle mass is often not regained and as such prognosis for return to athletic function is guarded to poor. A minority of horses will continue to deteriorate and necessitate euthanasia. Moreover, relapse of clinical signs is possible.

Zoonotic Potential

No zoonotic potential.

Genetic Prevalence

No genetic prevalence known.

Prevention

Horses without access to green forage (grass or good-quality hay) for extended periods (greater than one year) are at risk of developing the disease. Routine testing of plasma vitamin E concentration and oral supplementation of vitamin E in at-risk horses is an effective means of prevention.

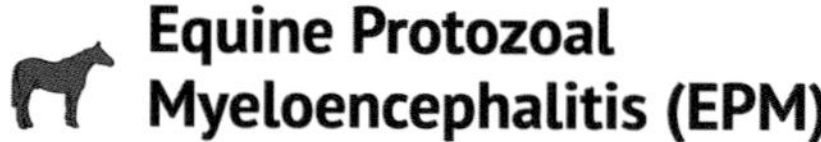

Equine Protozoal Myeloencephalitis (EPM)

Cause

EPM is a multifocal neurologic disease affecting the central nervous system. The disease is most often caused by the infection of neurons with *Sarcocystis neurona*, a protozoal parasite. *Neospora hughesi*, another protozoal species, has also been identified as a less common cause of EPM.

> **TECHNICIAN TIP 12.30:** EPM is most often caused by *Sarcocystis neurona*, a protozoal parasite.

Transmission

Ingesting *S. neurona* sporocysts in feed or water contaminated from opossum (definitive host) feces infects horses.

Signs

EPM can cause multifocal neurologic deficits. Due to the multifocal nature of the disease, EPM can present with a variety of clinical signs; clinical signs can vary significantly across cases. Potential clinical signs include spinal ataxia (usually, asymmetric), weakness, dysphagia, changes in mentation, urinary incontinence, and seizures. Atrophy may develop in muscle groups innervated by affected neurons.

Onset

Onset of clinical signs can range from acute to insidious.

Prevalence/Geographical Distribution

True prevalence is difficult to estimate due to the complicated nature of diagnosis of the disease. Moreover, EPM can only be definitively diagnosed postmortem, hampering diagnosis in cases that seem to respond to therapy. However, EPM is believed to be a common cause of equine neurologic disease in North America. Cases have also been reported in South America. There are several risk factors associated with this disease, many of which are related to the likelihood of exposure to opossums. Additionally, stressors (changes to environment, shipping, illness) might play a role in the development of clinical signs.

Diagnosis

Current understanding of this disease indicates that many horses are exposed to either *S. neurona* or *N. hughesi* or both, although only a minority (possibly <1%) develops neurologic disease as a result. Currently available antemortem diagnostic tests can only assess exposure to the disease, making accurate diagnosis of EPM quite challenging. Consequently, horses should only be tested for EPM if they have clinical signs consistent with EPM as determined by a neurologic examination. An effort should be made to rule out other diseases that can cause similar neurologic deficits in a specific case. Multifocal and asymmetric neurologic disease is suggestive of EPM.

Several antemortem testing methods are currently available and can be performed on serum and CSF. One method compares the antibody titers of serum versus those of CSF. Testing serum alone is less helpful, as so many horses are exposed and so few develop neurologic disease due to the protozoa. Recommended tests include the SAG-2, 4/3 ELISA, IFAT, and Western blot test. The SAG-1 ELISA is not typically recommended due to low sensitivity of the test in certain areas of the country. Definitive diagnosis can only be made via postmortem examination.

Treatment

There are several antiprotozoal medications available for treatment of EPM. The first FDA-approved medication was ponazuril and is administered orally once daily. Treatment should be administered for at least 28 days when a diagnosis of EPM is made. Improvement may not be seen until the completion of a 28-day course. Treatment should not be discontinued before this time simply due to a failure of the patient to improve. If a horse responds to therapy, treatment with ponazuril beyond 28 days may be warranted. In lieu of treatment with ponazuril, other available approved antiprotozoal medications include diclazuril combined with sulfadiazinepyrimethamine.

Additional considerations include NSAIDs and/or corticosteroids. Dimethyl sulfoxide (DMSO) may be used to increase absorption of ponazuril. Vitamin E supplementation may be helpful based on its antioxidant properties. Supportive care is necessary, and specifics of management will vary widely based on the patient's specific neurologic deficits. Potential considerations would include recumbency, urine/feces retention, and dysphagia. If the patient has changes in mentation or is having seizures, safety measures must be taken.

Prognosis

It is estimated that 60% of horses will improve by 1 or more neurologic grades following a course of therapy, and approximately 20% of horses will experience complete resolution of neurologic disease. Relapse of clinical signs has been observed following discontinuation of treatment.

Zoonotic Potential

No zoonotic potential.

Genetic Prevalence

No genetic prevalence known.

Preventative

Prevention of EPM is difficult. Storing feed in rodentproof containers should limit access of opossum to feed and, in turn, minimize exposure. There is no effective vaccine available at this time.

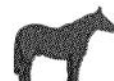

Equine Recurrent Uveitis

Definition

Recurrent inflammation of the uvea.

Cause

ERU is defined as episodes of intraocular inflammation that persist and recur over time. The specific cause is unknown, but the disease appears immune-mediated with evidence of a delayed hypersensitivity reaction present within the eye. Development has been associated with leptospirosis as well as additional viral or bacterial infections.

Systems Affected

Ocular – uveal tract (iris, ciliary body).

Signs

This disease can affect animals of varying breeds, genders, and ages and often initially presents between the age of 5–10. Condition can consist of acute episodes with period of quiescence in between or consistent low-grade inflammation over time. Acute episodes include pain, blepharospasm, redness, and excessive tearing. The cornea and structures within the eye may appear cloudy due to the influx of inflammatory cells, and corneal edema may develop. In chronic, the corpora nigra will atrophy, iris will become hyperpigmented, and synechia can be present. Chorioretinitis may be present on fundic examination. This disease is progressive and leads to diminished vision and ultimately blindness in affected horses. The number, severity, and length of episodes vary.

Prevalence/Geographical Distribution

Relatively common condition especially in certain breeds and the leading cause of blindness in horses. Worldwide distribution.

Diagnosis

Diagnosis is based on chronic, recurrent history of episodic inflammation within the eye and consistent ocular lesions on ophthalmic examination. Intraocular pressure may be low during episodes of inflammation and additional ocular abnormalities including synechia, and cataracts may develop. Serum titers and aqueous humor testing for *Leptospira* serovars is recommended. Additional testing for other bacterial or viral antigens may be warranted depending on clinical case.

Differentials

Primary uveitis, herpesvirus or immune-mediated keratitis, glaucoma, and stromal abscessation may appear similar.

Treatment

Prompt and effective treatment is important to diminish inflammation within the uveal tract. Treatment consists of reduction of inflammation using systemic NSAIDs or corticosteroids, ocular NSAIDs or corticosteroids, and mydriatic agents to assist in pupil dilation. Antibiotics may be needed to treat bacterial conditions including leptospirosis. Intravitreal injection with gentamicin has been performed to control inflammation or intravitreal injection with tissue plasminogen activator (tPA) to accelerate fibrinolysis.

Surgical implantation of cyclosporine sustained-release devices is used to decrease the number and severity of episodes but does not control active inflammation or cure the disease. Vitrectomy has also been performed with varying results.

Associated Conditions

Development of synechia and cataracts are common secondary to ERU.

Recovery

Recovery rate depends on aggression of lesion and aggression of treatment.

Zoonotic Potential

No zoonotic potential.

Genetic Prevalence

Recent study showed 8× increased prevalence in Appaloosas compared to all other breeds. Also present at higher rates in some Warmblood and draft breeds.

Prevention

Vaccination for leptospirosis has been used with varying results.

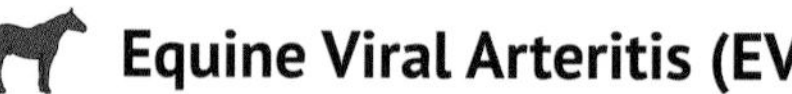

Equine Viral Arteritis (EVA)

Cause

This is a contagious viral respiratory pathogen.

Systems Affected

Respiratory and reproductive tract of mares and stallions.

Onset

Clinical symptoms generally begin three to seven days post infection.

Transmission

The principal route of transmission is through the respiratory system. Venereal and congenital routes or indirect means, such as via fomites common on breeding farms, can also facilitate transmission. The virus can be spread through artificial insemination and the use of fresh-cooled or frozen semen. Limited evidence suggests that the virus can also be transmitted via embryo transfer, where the donor mare is bred with infective semen from a carrier stallion. The natural host of EVA is restricted to equids, but there is limited data to suggest that llamas and alpacas also have been associated.

Signs

Clinical signs include fever, depression, anorexia, leukopenia, dependent edema (especially of the lower hind extremities, scrotum, and prepuce in the stallion), infertility, conjunctivitis, and nasal discharge (Figure 12.14). It can also clinically cause abortion in pregnant mares and, although uncommon, death in young foals. Many carriers of the disease can remain subclinical.

Diagnosis

Laboratory confirmation is required for diagnosis.

Treatment

There are no specific antiviral treatments for this disease. All affected patients should recover naturally. Instead, treatment is targeted at improving the clinical symptoms that arise (antipyretic, anti-inflammatory, and diuretic drugs).

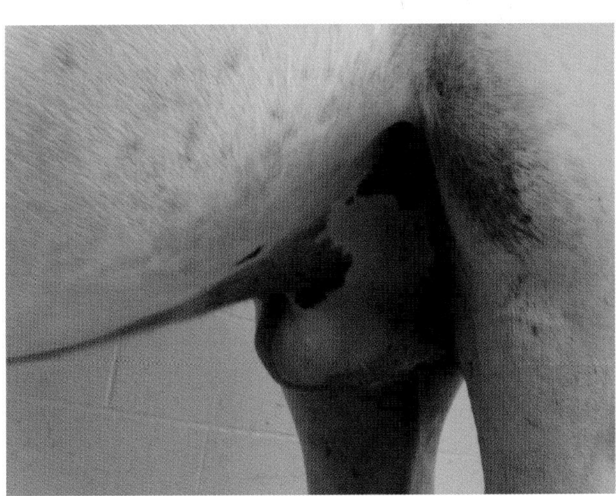

Figure 12.14 Swollen sheath in a 10-year-old gelding.

Recovery

Complete recovery should occur naturally.

Zoonotic Potential

No zoonotic potential.

Genetic Prevalence

No genetic prevalence known.

Prevalence/Geographic Distribution

EVA can affect any horse breed, with higher seropositivity rates occurring in Standardbreds and Warmbloods. Worldwide distribution.

Prevention

In the case of any positive test confirmation or even suspicion of EVA, all breeding activities should be ceased, and restriction of horse movement should be put in place. Sound farm management practices are essential to gain control and eliminate the disease, including minimizing or eliminating direct or indirect contact of unprotected horses with infected animals. Vaccinations are also available to protect stallions against infection and subsequent development of the carrier state; to immunize seronegative mares before being bred with EVA-infective semen; and to curtail outbreaks in non-breeding populations. Vaccination in the face of an EVA outbreak has been successful in controlling further spread of the virus within 7–10 days. This is a USDA reportable disease.

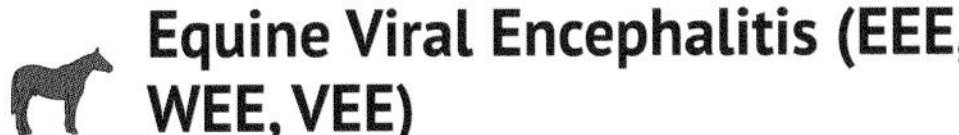

Equine Viral Encephalitis (EEE, WEE, VEE)

Cause

Eastern equine encephalitis (EEE), Western equine encephalitis (WEE), and Venezuelan equine encephalitis (VEE) comprise a group of diseases in the *Alphavirus* genus. VEE is considered a foreign animal disease in the United States.

Transmission

The life cycle of the viral encephalitides involves a reservoir host and vectors. Birds are the primary reservoir host for these diseases. The virus is transmitted by and replicated in an arthropod vector (mosquitos). Infection occurs when a vector carrying the virus inoculates the horse through a bite. A low-grade viremia results that is sufficient to cause disease but is insufficient to infect other vectors, so horses generally are not responsible for spread of these diseases. The exception to this rule is VEE; horses infected with VEE develop viremia to a magnitude great enough to infect other vectors.

Signs

Acute clinical signs of EEE and WEE include fever, anorexia, dullness, and stiffness. The acute stage may not be noticed because of subtle clinical signs and may last as long as five days. Disease progression may halt after this stage in cases of WEE. Progression to neurologic disease is more common in cases of EEE. Signs include somnolence, dullness, hyperesthesia, and aggression. Clinical signs observed later in the course of disease include head pressing, blindness, circling, muscle fasciculations, and seizures, ultimately progressing to recumbency, coma, and death (Figure 12.15).

Prevalence/Geographical Distribution

Disease typically occurs in the summer months in temperate regions due to the requirement of a vector for disease transmission. Disease may occur year-round in tropical areas. Disease is restricted to the Western Hemisphere. Both EEE and WEE outbreaks have occurred in the United States. EEE predominates in the Eastern United States and along the coast of the Gulf of Mexico. WEE predominates west of the Mississippi River. Outbreaks of VEE have occurred throughout central and southern Mexico. One of these outbreaks spread to Texas in 1971. EEE, WEE, and VEE are reportable diseases. VEE is a foreign animal disease and has federal reporting requirements.

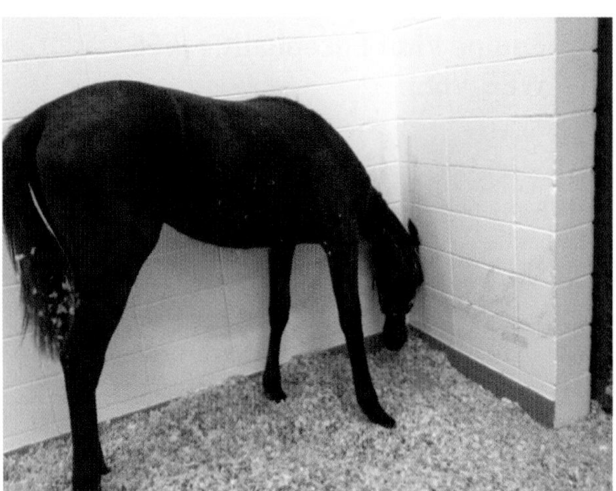

Figure 12.15 A horse head pressing against the wall. *Source:* Photo courtesy of Amy Stieler Stewart, DVM, PhD, DACVIM (LAIM).

Diagnosis

Antemortem diagnosis can be difficult to achieve. Tentative diagnosis can be made based on compatible clinical signs, lack of appropriate vaccination, and positive surveillance for the virus in the patient's area. Cerebrospinal fluid analysis may indicate increased cellularity (predominantly, mononuclear cells) and protein concentration, as is seen in other viral encephalitides. EEE is unique in that white blood cells in CSF are typically predominantly neutrophilic.

Measurement of antibody concentrations in serum can be performed; IgM antibody titers should be measured to assess for recent infection (titer >1:400). IgM antibody titers can also be measured in CSF. Paired IgG titers (acute and convalescent) can be performed to support a diagnosis if the horse survives beyond the acute stage of disease. It is not typically possible to isolate the virus from blood once clinical signs arise. In applicable cases, identification of virus in brain tissue should be attempted postmortem.

Treatment

No known effective specific therapy currently exists but supportive therapy is warranted. Anti-inflammatory therapy and intravenous fluid therapy can be considered. Anticonvulsant therapy (pentobarbital, phenobarbital, diazepam, or phenytoin) may become necessary in patients that develop seizures.

Prognosis

Survival is rare once a horse is infected with EEE and most horses die three to five days following onset of clinical signs. Estimated mortality for WEE (20–50%) and VEE (40–80%) is lower. In horses that do recover, gradual resolution of neurologic signs is noted over the course of weeks to months.

> **TECHNICIAN TIP 12.31:** Horses infected with EEE rarely survive and die three to five days following onset of clinical signs.

Zoonotic Potential

Humans are susceptible to EEE and WEE, but cases result from direct exposure to mosquitos, as horses are dead-end hosts and do not amplify the virus. Horses do amplify VEE once infected and are, therefore, important with respect to spread to other horses and people, although the mosquito vector is still essential for transmission.

Genetic Prevalence

No genetic prevalence known.

Prevention

Vaccination is highly effective and a bivalent vaccine against EEE and WEE is commercially available. Following two immunizations one month apart, annual or biannual boosters are recommended depending on the length of the vector season. Mosquito control in the environment and spraying horses with permethrin-based products are helpful complements with vaccination.

Recovery

May occur spontaneously, or over short periods of time with treatment.

Erysipelas

Definition

Highly contagious, systemic bacterial disease in swine caused by *Erysipelothrix rhusiopathiae.*

Cause

E. rhusiopathie, a gram-positive rod.

Systems Affected

Hematopoietic, integumentary, and skeletal.

Signs

Because of standard vaccination programs, erysipelas most commonly presents in growing/finishing pigs. Infected animals develop septicemia, which may generate diamond-shaped skin lesions (from bacteria occluding local blood supply), arthritis, and/or vegetative valvular endocarditis. In acutely infected animals, fevers exceed 104 °F. Pregnant sows may abort from high fevers. Nursing sows may become agalactic.

> **TECHNICIAN TIP 12.32:** Animals infected with erysipelas are septicemic, developing diamond-shaped skin lesions.

Onset

In peracute cases, pigs doing well present dead. Acute cases present with fever and sometimes skin lesions. Arthritis is most common in chronic cases.

Prevalence/Geographical Distribution

Worldwide distribution.

Diagnosis

In acute case, the organism can be cultured or identified in blood smears. Diamond-shaped skin lesions and response to penicillin within 24 hr may also be considered diagnostic.

Treatment

E. rhusiopathiae is highly responsive to penicillins and potentiated penicillins.

Recovery

Recovery rate is generally good with prompt treatment, provided initial fevers do not exceed compatibility with life.

Zoonotic Potential

Rare but has the potential to be zoonotic.

Genetic Prevalence

No genetic prevalence known.

Prevention

Both killed injectable and modified live oral vaccines are available. Because of the effectiveness of vaccine, sow herd immunization is standard practice in the United States. Growing/finishing pig vaccination may be employed seasonally or year-round, depending on regional disease patterns.

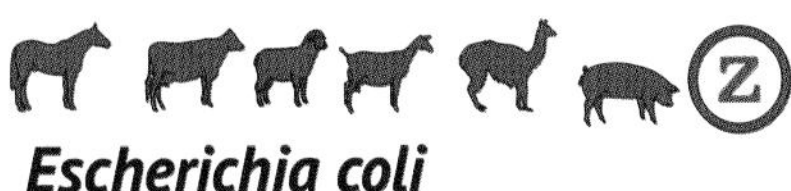

Escherichia coli

Definition

Contagious infection with certain enterotoxin-producing strains of *E. coli.*

Cause

E. coli with pillus antigens K88, K99, or F18 cause colibacillosis; *E. coli* with virulence factors O138, O139, or O141 among others.

Systems Affected

Gastrointestinal in colibacillosis; gastrointestinal, nervous, and vascular in edema disease.

Transmission

Fecal-oral.

Signs

Edema disease is generally observed in the fastest-growing animals one to two weeks post weaning. Pigs may present with death, neurological signs, swelling in the face, and unwillingness to eat. Colibacillosis is generally observed in the farrowing crate or shortly after weaning, and characterized by profuse, watery diarrhea that creates a localized, distinctly humid environment. It is very hard to tell if a chicken is affected by *E. coli* because it shows up in the normal flora of the intestine of the chicken.

Onset

Edema disease is rapid in onset and associated with high feed consumption by newly weaned pigs; colibacillosis is generally observed in the first week of young piglets in a new environment (i.e. farrowing crate or nursery).

Prevalence/Geographical Distribution

Worldwide distribution.

Diagnosis

Disease is confirmed through pure-growth *E. coli* from intestinal culture and associated clinical signs and necropsy lesions (i.e. edema in stomach, mesentery, and colon). Isolates may be serotyped at diagnostic laboratories.

Treatment

For edema disease, treatment is limited, and efforts should focus on prevention. For colibacillosis, treatment with sensitive antibiotics is appropriate and action to prevent spread to adjacent litters imperative.

> **TECHNICIAN TIP 12.33:** Prevention is the best treatment.

Recovery

Outbreaks of edema disease may impact as much as one-third of the population, with mortality approaching half among those affected. Recovery from colibacillosis is dependent on the extent of fluid and electrolyte loss in affected piglets. Pigs recovering from colibacillosis may experience short-term stunting on account of intestinal damage.

Zoonotic Potential

E. coli can infect humans and other animals if ingested.

Genetic Prevalence

Some genetic lines have been identified as having genes that confer *E. coli* resistance.

> **TECHNICIAN TIP 12.34:** Some porcine genetic lines have been identified as having genes that confer resistance to *E. coli*.

Prevention

Hygiene is the best prevention. Crates and pens should be thoroughly cleaned and disinfected between litters and groups, with special attention to mats and other reservoirs of fecal material. Affected litters should be in de facto isolation with sick piglets treated only after newborn, younger, and healthy litters treatment is complete. Equipment should be cleaned and disinfected, and workers must change clothes, wash boots, wash hands, and so forth, before working with potentially naïve animals. Vaccines to boost maternal immunity are available.

Exertional Rhabdomyolysis (ER; a.k.a. Monday Morning Disease, Azoturia, Equine Rhabdomyolysis Syndrome, Tying-up, Chronic ER)

Definition

A syndrome that results in muscle cramps after exercise or physical exertion.

Cause

Several types of ER have been identified. Sporadic ER can be related to muscle trauma, overexertion, and sudden increase in exercise activity, toxicity, exhaustion, or dietary and electrolyte imbalances. One form of the chronic disease known as resting energy requirement (RER) is commonly identified in Thoroughbreds and Standardbreds and is caused by abnormal regulation of muscle contraction and relaxation.

Systems Affected

Musculoskeletal system.

Signs

- Profuse sweating
- Trembling
- Stilted and stiff gait
- Reluctance to move

Onset

Onset of clinical signs is usually directly related to some sort of exercise event, although in sporadic cases, clinical signs may only be identified a very few times in the horse's life.

Prevalence/Geographical Distribution

More research is needed to identify all related prevalence to ER. The chronic version, RER, has been found to be more prevalent in Thoroughbreds and Standardbreds, and in females more than males, and it is also more common in nervous horses than calm horses.

Diagnosis

In part, the diagnosis of ER can be made by ruling out many other similar diseases or disorders, including but not limited to PSSM, HYPP, hypothyroidism, acute viral influenza, tetanus, botulism, lactic acidosis. Diagnostics include:

- Thorough history and physical examination paying close attention to muscle mass and symmetry as well as muscle tone.
- Exercise test.
- Blood chemistry: elevated blood serum CK and AST, hyponatremia, hypochloremia, hypocalcemia, hyperkalemia, and hyperphosphatemia.
- A caffeine or halothane muscle contracture test.

Treatment

Eventually, the treatment for ER will depend on the underlying factors. Treatment for clinical episodes of ER should address the active symptoms, including rehydration with balanced electrolytes and in some cases administration of nonsteroidal anti-inflammatories (NSAIDs)

Long-term treatment plans for ER patients should include regular conditioning/exercise, access to fresh water supplemented with electrolytes, decrease carbohydrate intake, and in some cases, supplementation of vitamin E and selenium. Chromium is also suggested to calm horses and improve their response to exercise testing of the use of dantrolene is also being performed and thought to be useful.

Recovery

Horses that have exhibited a severe episode of rhabdomyolysis may develop muscle fibrosis resulting in difficulty returning to the activity level they previously performed at. Milder cases of ER can recover back to normal function over time and with proper maintenance and conditioning.

Zoonotic Potential

No zoonotic potential.

Genetic Prevalence

Breeding trials have confirmed a genetic prevalence, though the specific genome has yet to be identified in Thoroughbreds. A heritable basis for RER in Standardbreds was supported by equine lymphocyte antigen profiles in affected horses. Research on these diseases is ongoing and complex due to the variety of causes.

Preventative

The development of ER is unavoidable; however, the prevention of tying-up type occurrences can be mitigated.

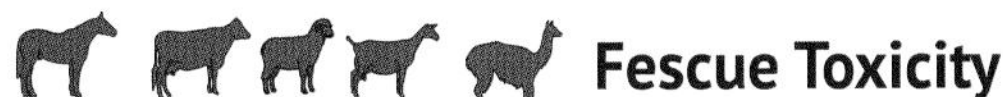 Fescue Toxicity

Definition

Contaminated tall fescue pastures that seasonally become infested with an endophyte, whereby ingestion may cause mycotoxicosis resulting in peripheral vasoconstriction.

Causes

Neotyphodium coenophialum.

Systems Affected

Vascular.

Transmission

Ingestion of fungus contaminated tall fescue grass.

> **TECHNICIAN TIP 12.35:** Fescue toxicity is caused by ingestion of tall fescue grass contaminated with fungus.

Signs

Sheep may present with lameness and a hunched appearance. Chronic severe cases can demonstrate possible gangrene of the distal limbs and tail. Diarrhea may also be present. Camelids may show weight loss, rough fiber coat, agalactia, and hyperthermia. Goats and horses present with weak parturition, failure to dilate, thick placentas, thick umbilical cords, and agalactia.

Onset

Acute to chronic.

Prevalence/Geographical Distribution

A major portion of the tall fescue in the United States is contaminated with the endophyte.

Diagnosis

Test pasture or blood.

Treatment

Remove animals from infected feed.

Recovery

Common.

Zoonotic Potential

No zoonotic potential.

Genetic Prevalence

No genetic prevalence known.

Prevention

Limit access to contaminated pastures.

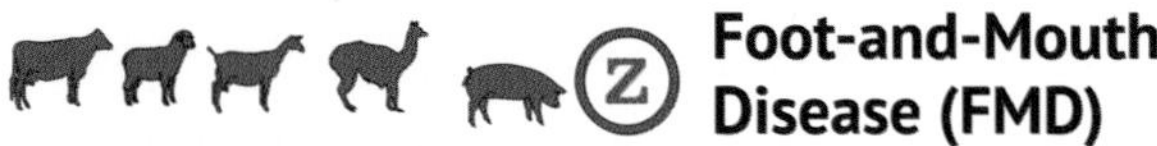

Foot-and-Mouth Disease (FMD)

Definition

A highly contagious vesicular disease affecting cloven-hoofed animals. The disease is characterized by high morbidity and low mortality rates. Cattle and swine are most susceptible, whereas sheep and goats tend to develop mild signs.

Cause

FMD virus, a picornavirus of the genus *Aphthovirus*. There are at least 7 immunologically different types of virus, with more than 60 subtypes.

Transmission

By direct contact, aerosol, and fomites. People can spread the disease by carrying the virus in their clothes, shoes, hands, and body. The disease is highly contagious and spreads rapidly. Recovered animals continue to shed the virus for approximately two weeks or longer. Semen of infected animals can contain the virus. The virus can survive in raw and pasteurized milk, and fresh and frozen meat.

Signs

Vesicular lesions, erosions, and ulcers in the oral cavity, muzzle, teats, coronary band, and interdigital space are the typical signs. Affected animals can appear lame as well. Lameness and foot lesions are the main manifestation of the disease in small ruminants. Blisters in affected areas rupture in 48 hr, leaving erosive lesions with sloughing of the oral mucosa. Animals are febrile, lethargic, and reluctant to eat with excessive salivation.

Young animals, although rare, can die due to viral induced cardiac damage.

Onset

Acute.

Prevalence/Geographical Distribution

The disease is endemic in many areas of Europe and South America, Asia, and Africa. United States, Canada, Great

Britain, Japan, New Zealand, and Australia are considered FMD-free.

Diagnosis

Clinical signs and laboratory confirmation using ELISA, complement fixation, virus neutralization, agar gel precipitation, or fluorescent antibodies. Local and federal authorities must be contacted when the disease is suspected in the United States and Canada.

> **TECHNICIAN TIP 12.36:** Local and federal authorities must be contacted when FMD is suspected in the United States or Canada.

Treatment

There is no specific treatment. Antibiotics are sometimes used to prevent or treat secondary bacterial mastitis.

Recovery

The recovery rate is high, but rarely some young animals can die due to viral-mediated cardiac disease. Affected animals usually stop eating and milking, abort, or lose weight leading to main economic losses.

Zoonotic Potential

Rarely, the disease can be transmitted to humans.

Genetic Prevalence

No genetic prevalence known.

Prevention

Vaccination programs using type-specific vaccines in endemic areas. Early identification of diseased animals, quarantine, and nursing care are important prevention tools.

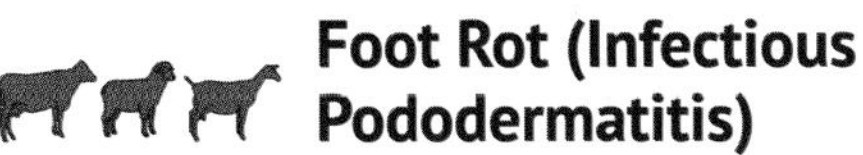

Foot Rot (Infectious Pododermatitis)

Definition

An anaerobic infection of the soft tissues of the interdigital space causing lameness.

Cause

Fusobacterium necrophorum, along with other organisms such as *Prevotella melaninogenicus*. *Dichelobacter nodosus* is also involved in the development of contagious foot rot in small ruminants.

Transmission

Wet and humid conditions predispose to the disease. Factors that lead to skin damage of the digit (i.e. walking on hard surfaces or exposure to dirty and wet flooring) are predisposing factors for bacterial penetration through the skin and subsequent infection.

Signs

Lameness with initial swelling and heat of the interdigital soft tissues is seen. The disease usually affects only one limb. The inflammation progresses toward the coronary band and ultimately the fetlock. Fissures and necrosis with a foul odor are noted in the interdigital area without significant discharge from the lesion. Deeper tissues, such as bone, tendons, and joints, can also be affected in severe and advanced cases.

Onset

Acute to chronic.

Prevalence/Geographical Distribution

A common cause of lameness in beef cattle and confined dairy cows. The disease has a worldwide distribution.

Diagnosis

Clinical signs and infrequently bacterial cultures are pursued.

Treatment

Several parenteral antibiotics (sodium penicillin, ceftiofur, oxytetracycline, etc.) are effective.

Recovery

Favorable when there is early recognition and early treatment of the disease process.

Zoonotic Potential

No zoonotic potential.

Genetic Prevalence

Bos indicus breeds are more susceptible to the disease, whereas *Bos taurus* breeds are more resistant.

Prevention

Housing management. Footbaths are used by some producers.

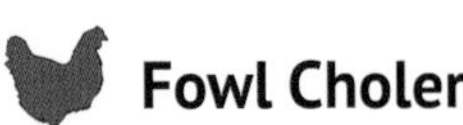

Fowl Cholera

Cause

Caused by *P. multocida* bacteria.

Systems Affected

Vast internal and external systems can be affected. Acute mortality and suppurative necrosis.

Transmission

Ingestion of contaminated food or water or from biting insects.

Signs

Depression, anorexia, mucoid discharge from the mouth, ruffled feathers, increased respiratory rate, lameness, swollen wattles, pneumonia, sudden death but can also be asymptomatic. Also, can be identified via postmortem lesions.

Onset

Five to eight days incubation period.

Prevalence/Geographical Distribution

Worldwide.

Diagnosis

Via bacterial culture testing, PCR, or serology or even clinical signs.

Treatment

Can be sensitive to some antibiotic therapies based on culture and sensitivity provided disease is not too far advanced.

Recovery

There is a high morbidity and mortality rate.

Zoonotic Potential

No zoonotic potential.

Genetic Prevalence

No genetic prevalence known.

Prevention

Attenuated live and adjuvanted vaccines available or eradication through depopulation and deep cleaning between flocks.

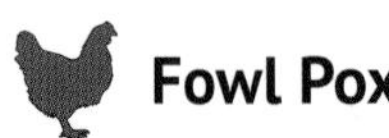

Fowl Pox

Cause

Caused by the fowl pox virus which is a part of the DNA virus family Poxviridae.

Transmission

This disease spreads easily among flocks via natural infection, the most common form being cutaneous pox.

Signs

Cutaneous pox typically forms inflamed lesions on areas of exposed skin on the head, legs, feet, or toes of the bird, but can be seen in feathered areas as well.

Onset

Incubation period is 4–10 days. Lesions or nodules appear 5–8 days after infection.

Prevalence/Geographical Distribution

Worldwide distribution.

Diagnosis

Identification of lesions. Additional symptoms may include buildup of plaque in the mucosa of the upper respiratory and digestive systems.

Treatment

None.

Recovery

In most cases, the bird will survive, and the lesions will heal in three to four weeks.

Zoonotic Potential

No zoonotic potential.

Genetic Prevalence

No genetic prevalence known.

Prevention

Utilizing proper stock density aids in preventing the spread of the virus, as there is less chance for injury which increases a bird's susceptibility to the disease. The most effective steps in preventing fowl pox include vaccination at 0–6 weeks of age, proper management, and intentional sanitation measures.

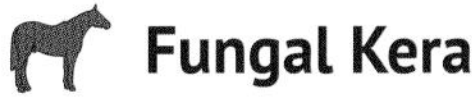

Fungal Keratitis

Definition

Infection of the cornea caused by a fungus.

Cause

Fungal organisms are commensal to the equine cornea, and fungal keratitis can present with a variety of conditions. Fungal organisms can lead to tear film disorders, nonulcerative corneal abrasions, ulcerations, fungal plaques, or stromal abscesses. *Fusarium* and *Aspergillus* spp. can be aggressive fungi and lead to widespread corneal disease. Additionally, fungi can become implicated in existing bacterial ulcerative keratitis.

Systems Affected

Ocular – cornea.

Transmission

None.

Signs

Fungal keratitis can affect animals of varying breeds, ages, and genders. Fungal lesions can present as small multifocal abrasions throughout the cornea, thick raised fungal plaques, ulcerative lesions, or focal opacifications within the cornea. At times, fungal organisms will have a raised appearance off the surface of the cornea, appear wispy, and can range in color. Ocular clinical signs can vary from mild discomfort to severe blepharospasm, excessive tearing, redness, and ranging corneal opacification and lesions.

Prevalence/Geographical Distribution

Relatively common with increased prevalence in warm/wet climates with higher fungal organism burdens. Worldwide.

Diagnosis

Presumptive diagnosis based off clinical history and ophthalmic examination. Confirmative diagnosis based on cytology and/or culture. Fungal culture can take multiple weeks so empirical antifungal therapy is normally started prior to culture results.

Differentials

Differentials would include other disease processes that affect the cornea including keratitis (immune-mediated, bacterial, herpesvirus, eosinophilic, etc.), trauma, mineral or lipid infiltrate, and corneal neoplasia.

Treatment

Antifungal therapy is initiated with topical and/or systemic antifungals. Additional medications including systemic NSAIDs are added to decrease corneal and intraocular inflammation. Surgical therapy may be necessary to remove the fungal organisms and resulting inflammation via keratectomy and grafts can be used to stabilize the compromised cornea.

Recovery

Recovery rate depends on aggression of lesion and aggression of treatment.

Zoonotic Potential

No zoonotic potential.

Genetic Prevalence

No genetic prevalence known.

Prevention

Prompt and aggressive medical treatment of ulcerative bacterial keratitis may prevent fungal invasion.

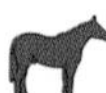

Gastric Ulceration – See Equine Gastric Ulceration Syndrome

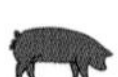

Glässer Disease (*Haemophilus parasuis*)

Definition

Contagious systemic bacterial infection caused by the bacterium *Haemophilus parasuis*; historically referred to as "Glässer's disease."

Cause

H. parasuis.

Systems Affected

Nervous, skeletal.

Transmission

Aerosol.

TECHNICIAN TIP 12.37: Glässer's disease is transmitted via aerosolization.

Signs

Peracute infections present as deaths of apparently healthy animals. Acutely infected animals exhibit high fever (>104 °F) with exquisitely painful joints, difficulty breathing, or neurologic signs. Chronically infected pigs may display arthritis and/or lesions consistent with polyserositis.

Onset

Clinical signs generally follow a stressful event, with incubation less than a week and as quickly as 24 hr.

Prevalence/Geographical Distribution

Worldwide, though naïve populations may be developed through double caesarian-derived populations.

Diagnosis

Necropsy lesions include polyserositis, including pleuritis, pericarditis, and peritonitis. Fibrin is present in joint fluid. The organism may be cultured successfully from joint fluid or CSF of acutely infected pigs. Serology is also available.

Treatment

H. parasuis is generally responsive to penicillin's and potentiated penicillin's.

Recovery

Recovery rate is good among timely treated animals, though lameness may persist, and carriers will develop, since not all animals clear the infection.

Zoonotic Potential

No zoonotic potential.

Genetic Prevalence

No genetic prevalence known.

Prevention

Autogenous vaccines may be the method of choice to prevent and control severe cases of *H. parasuis*. Strategic use of feed-grade antibiotics can also control *H. parasuis* flares precipitated by predictable stressor events (i.e. weaning).

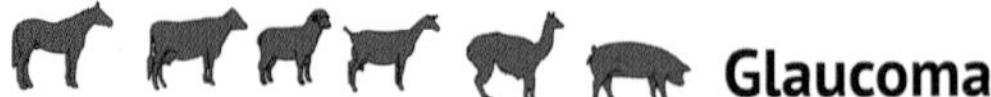

Glaucoma

Definition

A condition of increased pressure within the eye.

Cause

Can occur as a congenital, primary or secondary condition. Obstruction of the outflow of aqueous humor within the eye leads to an increase in intraocular pressure. This increased pressure causes loss of retinal ganglion cells and degeneration of the optic nerve which ultimately leads to loss of vision. Secondary development of this condition occurs after physical obstruction of the aqueous outflow tract most commonly due to inflammation, trauma, fibrosis, synechia, lens luxation, or prolapse of the vitrea or iris. In horses, glaucoma is most commonly a secondary condition and due to ERU. Glaucoma is rare in cattle and most commonly secondary to neoplasia or trauma.

Systems Affected

Ocular.

Transmission

None.

Signs

This disease can affect animals of varying breeds, ages, and genders. In acute phases, focal or diffuse corneal edema is present along with ocular pain, episcleral injection, mydriasis, and decreased menace. As the condition progresses, enlargement of the globe (buphthalmos) and diffuse corneal edema is often present (Figure 12.16). The pupil may be fixed in dilation, and the lens may luxate. The retina and optic nerves show degeneration, and retinal detachment may occur.

Prevalence/Geographical Distribution

Congenital and primary glaucoma is relatively rare. Majority of large animal cases are secondary to inflammation, infection, or trauma. Worldwide distribution.

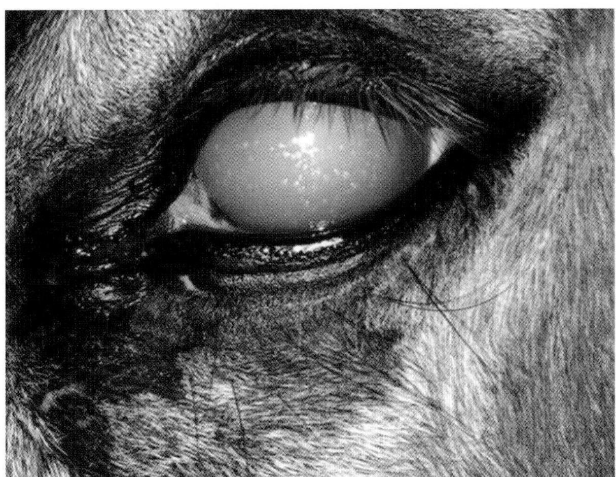

Figure 12.16 Equine glaucoma. *Source:* Photo courtesy of Lauren Hughes, DVM.

Diagnosis

Ophthalmic examination may reveal changes within the eye consistent with glaucoma as well as potential causes for its development. Elevated intraocular pressures would be expected using tonometry.

Differentials

Differentials include other conditions that create corneal opacity/scarring including fungal, immune-mediated, or infectious keratitis. Intraocular or retrobulbar tumors may also affect intraocular pressure.

Treatment

Treatment can include both medical and surgical management. Medical therapy aims to reduce intraocular pressure by decreasing production of aqueous humor or increasing outflow. Drugs typically used include topical beta-adrenergic blockers (timolol maleate), topical/systemic carbonic anhydrase inhibitors (dorzolamide, brinzolamide, acetazolamide), and topical prostaglandin analogs (latanoprost). Surgical treatment is used when medical therapy cannot achieve controlled IOP and includes laser cyclophotoablation, placement of a gonioimplant device, or chemical ciliary body ablation. Enucleation may be performed in cases where medical and/or surgical management fail or vision has already been lost.

Associated Conditions

Glaucoma is often secondary and associated with ERU or trauma in horses and trauma or neoplasia in cattle.

Zoonotic Potential

No zoonotic potential.

Genetic Prevalence

Congenital glaucoma has been reported in Thoroughbred, Arabian, and Standardbred foals.

Prevention

Controlling primary ocular conditions and regularly monitoring intraocular pressures during ophthalmic examinations may prevent conditions from progressing to development of glaucoma.

Grass Tetany

Definition

Metabolic disease due to low magnesium concentration, affecting lactating cattle, ewes, and does causing tetanic spasms and convulsions.

> **TECHNICIAN TIP 12.38:** Grass tetany is a metabolic disease due to low magnesium concentration.

Cause

Hypomagnesemia. Lactating animals grazing on lush pastures with high levels of potassium and nitrogen, and low levels of magnesium and sodium during spring or fall are at risk. Ewes are generally affected on their second to fourth week of lactation. They usually are hypomagnesemic and hypocalcemic.

Transmission

It is not a transmissible disease.

Signs

Affected animals show lethargy and muscular twitching, progressing to staggering, tetany, convulsions, and eventually death.

Onset

Acute.

Prevalence/Geographical Distribution

A common disease with a worldwide distribution.

Diagnosis

Clinical signs and confirmation with measurement of magnesium concentrations in CSF or vitreous humor. Serum magnesium concentration is not a reliable diagnostic method because intracellular magnesium can be released due to muscular damage during convulsions or tetany.

Treatment

Affected animals should be treated immediately with intravenous magnesium administration. Some animals may require to be treated a second time because relapses are common.

Recovery

After treatment, the recovery is rapid, in about 1 h. Relapses are common 12 hr after the first treatment.

Zoonotic Potential

No zoonotic potential.

Genetic Prevalence

No genetic prevalence known.

Prevention

Oral magnesium supplementation to a herd or flock from which an individual animal was diagnosed with the disease.

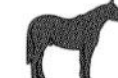

Guttural Pouch Empyema

Definition

Guttural pouch empyema occurs as a result of *Streptococcus equi* subspecies *equi* infection.

Cause

Swelling and subsequent bursting of the retropharyngeal lymph nodes into the guttural pouches. It may occur secondary to other upper respiratory tract infections, for example, *Streptococcus equi* subspecies *zooepidemicus*. Involving the guttural pouch, the disease may clear as the animal's infection improves or may persist for weeks or months due to the poor drainage. If the pus becomes inspissated it leads to chondroid formation.

> **TECHNICIAN TIP 12.39:** Guttural pouch empyema is caused by swelling of and subsequent bursting of retropharyngeal lymph nodes into the guttural pouches.

Systems Affected

Guttural pouches.

Signs

Clinical signs include persistent purulent nasal discharge, swelling in the retropharyngeal area, dysphagia, dyspnea, and inspiratory stridor at rest.

Diagnosis

Endoscopy of the guttural pouches or radiography of the head.

Treatment

Lavage the guttural pouches until clear. Repeated flushes may be needed, and placement of an indwelling Foley catheter may be warranted. Endoscope may be required to remove chondroids, or a surgical removal of the chondroids using a Viborg's triangle approach may be needed.

Prevalence/Geographical Distribution

Young horses less than five years old. Worldwide.

Zoonotic Potential

No zoonotic potential.

Genetic Prevalence

No genetic prevalence known.

Prevention

Hot pack the retropharyngeal area. If during endoscopy enlarged retropharyngeal lymph nodes are visualized, recheck frequently to treat earlier and try to minimize chondroid formation.

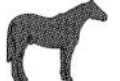 Guttural Pouch Mycosis

Definition

Fungal plaques develop most commonly on the roof of the medial compartment of the guttural pouch associated with the internal carotid artery. Can occur on the lateral wall of the lateral pouch associated with the external carotid or external maxillary artery. The most common fungus is Aspergillus species.

Cause

The exact cause is unknown; it is more common in middle-aged to older horses. It is thought that fungi proliferate in the guttural pouch leading to erosion of the underlying mucosa, vascular compromise, and hemorrhage. Secondarily, injury to the adjacent nerves and dysfunction may occur. It is usually unilateral.

TECHNICIAN TIP 12.40: Guttural pouch mycosis is more common in middle-aged to older horses.

Systems Affected

Guttural pouches.

Signs

Clinical signs most commonly seen are spontaneous epistaxis, less frequent is nasal discharge. Patients are typically dysphagic with recurring laryngeal neuropathy, Horner's syndrome, abnormal head extension, swelling in the parotid region, facial nerve paralysis, and mycotic encephalitis.

Onset

Acute.

Prevalence/Geographical Distribution

Usually adult horses. Worldwide.

Diagnosis

Endoscopy of the guttural pouches with visualization of yellow/green proliferative mass – most commonly over the blood vessels inside the pouches (Figure 12.17).

Treatment

Medical management, topical lavage with antifungals, surgical management by implanting a coil or intravascular balloon proximal and distal to the fungal lesion hoping to

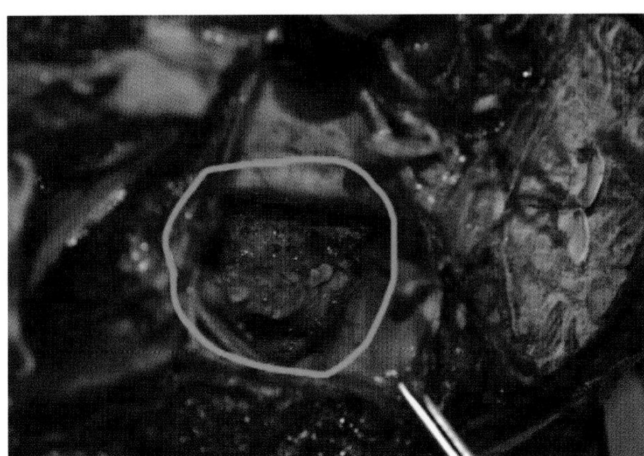

Figure 12.17 Circle denotes area of erosion within the guttural pouch.

obliterate the arterial flow. Treat secondary complications particularly any aspiration pneumonia.

Recovery

Monitor for signs of recurrence of infection, prognosis is worse with signs of dysphagia or recurrent laryngeal neuropathy.

Zoonotic Potential

No zoonotic potential.

Genetic Prevalence

No genetic prevalence known.

Prevention

Minimize prolonged uses of antimicrobials.

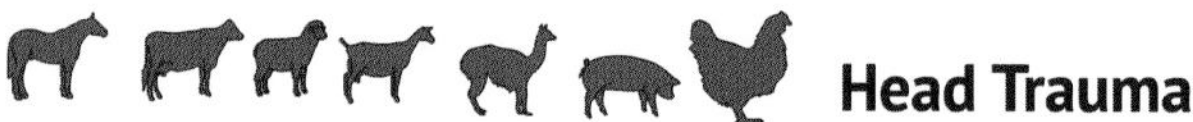

Head Trauma

Definition

Head trauma refers to mechanical or external force to the head, resulting in injury.

Cause

Causes of head trauma vary widely dependent on the disease process or traumatic incident.

> **TECHNICIAN TIP 12.41:** Causes of head trauma vary widely dependent on the disease process or traumatic incident.

Onset/Signs

Clinical signs and onset can vary dramatically based on the region of the head that becomes traumatized and the force with which it is traumatized (Figure 12.18). Many clinical signs result from either increased intracranial pressure (ICP) or due to damage of central nervous system (CNS) tissue. A complete neurologic examination must be performed as completely as the patient's status allows. Because the forebrain (cerebrum) is typically involved, often a change in mentation is noted. Seizures and a decreased response to noxious stimuli might be observed. Behavioral changes include pacing, head pressing, blindness, and circling. Signs of vestibular disease may be present. More severely affected animals may be obtunded to comatose. Patients may have dangerous derangements of heart rate, heart rhythm, blood pressure, and respiratory pattern due to brain injury. Patients should be assessed for evidence of hemorrhage from the ears, mouth, or nostrils. In some instances, CSF can be seen leaking from the ear or wounds.

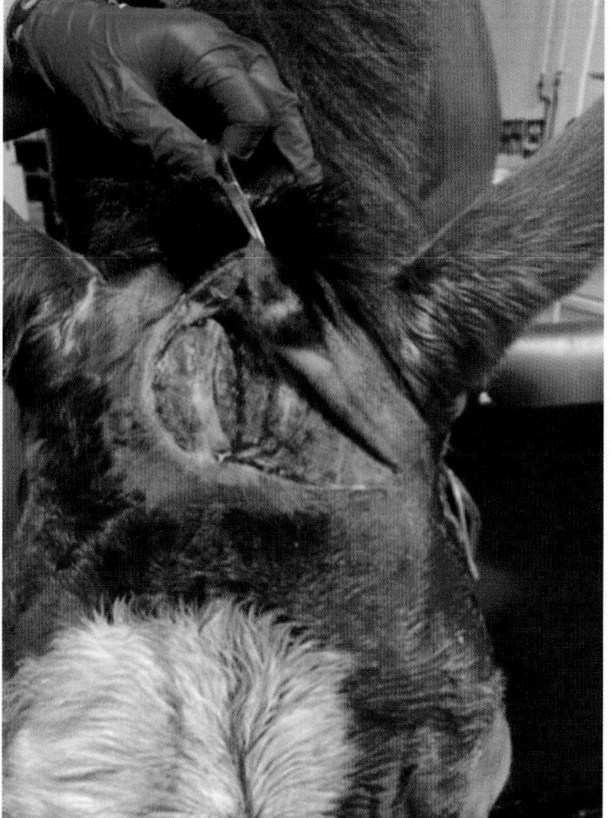

Figure 12.18 Open skin flap on the top of a horse's head.

Diagnosis

Diagnosis is usually based on clinical signs and history. Changes on hematology and biochemistry panels may include an elevated blood glucose and white blood cell count secondary to stress. Muscle enzyme activities may be increased secondary to trauma. Cerebrospinal fluid can be collected to assess for evidence of hemorrhage in the CNS.

Skull radiography is recommended if a skull fracture is suspected. Skull fractures can be difficult to detect by radiography, and normal skull radiographs do not preclude presence of a skull fracture. While computed tomography (CT) and magnetic resonance imaging (MRI) offer more information and superior imaging, the cost and need for general anesthesia is a consideration.

Cerebrospinal fluid collection can be performed in the acute phases of disease to exclude other causes of CNS disease, but risks and benefits must be considered as CSF collection may increase the risk of damage to neural structures while not aiding in disease management.

Treatment

Initial therapy is aimed at stabilizing the patient as necessary. This includes ensuring that the patient's cardiovascular and respiratory systems are functioning properly. Aggressive intravenous fluid therapy may be the best means of maintaining blood pressure and ensuring adequate blood flow to the CNS. A patent airway may need to be established and oxygen supplementation required. Additional therapies that may be indicated are corticosteroids, hypertonic saline, mannitol, or DMSO. If seizures are noted, anticonvulsants might include diazepam and phenobarbital. Patients should be monitored for changes in mentation; sedation may be required if aggressive and potentially dangerous behavior is observed. Surgical reduction of depression fractures of the frontal and parietal bones of the skull can be considered. Prophylactic antimicrobial therapy should be instituted due to risk of secondary bacterial meningitis. Time and adequate supportive care are essential treatment components.

Prognosis

Prognosis is heavily dependent on the severity and duration of clinical signs and the initial response to treatment. Prognosis is grave for stuporous or comatose patients and is guarded for those patients that have some change in mentation.

Prevalence/Geographical Distribution

Younger horses are probably more susceptible due to their more excitable demeanor. Likewise, variation in temperament among breeds may influence breed susceptibility. Regardless, all species and all ages are susceptible to head trauma.

Zoonotic Potential

No zoonotic potential.

Genetic Prevalence

No genetic prevalence known.

Prevention

Safe handling techniques is the most important facet of prevention.

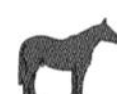

Heaves – See Chronic Obstructive Pulmonary Disease

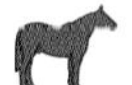 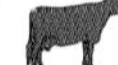

Hepatic Encephalopathy

Definition

Hepatic encephalopathy (HE) is a term used to describe a manifestation of severe liver disease and, sometimes, liver failure. HE is not considered a disease in its own right but, rather, a sign of underlying disease.

Cause

The exact mechanism by which HE occurs is not known. The pathogenesis of HE is probably a result of lack of detoxification of substances by the liver. Failure of the liver to convert ammonia to urea is believed to be important to the development of HE. The resulting alteration of the biochemical environment in the CNS leads to dysfunction of neuro-transmitter activity.

Systems Affected

Signs of neurologic disease are representative of underlying hepatic disease.

Onset/Signs

Clinical signs of HE ranges from subtle to dramatic. Yawning has been considered a common initial sign in horses. Behavioral changes and changes in demeanor are frequently noted. Affected animals might become dull or excitable. Head pressing is occasionally observed. In more severe stages of the disease, affected animals can become unpredictable, aggressive, and dangerous to handle. Seizure activity may be present. In advanced stages of the disease, the affected animal is stuporous to comatose. Concurrent signs of liver disease, such as icterus, might be noted on physical examination.

Prevalence/Geographical Distribution

There is no geographic predilection as the causes of HE and hepatic failure are extensive. However, certain plant toxins (example: pyrrolizidine alkaloids) can cause hepatic failure; availability of these plants poses a risk factor.

Diagnosis

Suspicion of HE should arise in an animal with changes in mentation. To support a diagnosis of HE, assessment of serum liver enzyme and hepatic functional indicators (gamma glutamyltransferase [GGT], aspartate aminotransferase [AST], sorbitol dehydrogenase [SDH], conjugated and unconjugated bilirubin, and bile acids) should yield abnormal findings.

> **TECHNICIAN TIP 12.42:** Blood samples for certain hepatic enzyme activity levels and ammonia concentration require special handling and submission requirements.

Additionally, measurement of blood ammonia concentration should be performed; blood ammonia concentration must be measured shortly after collection and requires specialized laboratory equipment, so this diagnostic tool may not be readily available. Changes in mentation with normal serum liver enzyme activities and normal blood ammonia concentration (<55 μmol/l) does not support a diagnosis of HE.

Treatment

Sedation should be considered for aggressive or convulsing horses. Diazepam may worsen signs of HE and is, therefore, a poor choice for sedation in these animals. Xylazine and detomidine are more appropriate options; phenobarbital can be used if necessary. Cerebral edema may accompany HE and can be treated with a slow infusion of mannitol (0.5–1 g/kg intravenously over 15–30 min) or hypertonic saline.

> **TECHNICIAN TIP 12.43:** Diazepam should be avoided in horses suspected of having hepatic encephalopathy.

Prognosis

Prognosis is heavily dependent on the underlying cause of disease. Severity of HE is associated with the severity of hepatic insufficiency, but this is not necessarily associated with the reversibility of disease.

Zoonotic Potential

No zoonotic potential.

Genetic Prevalence

No genetic prevalence known.

 Hog Cholera (Classical Swine Fever)

Definition

Highly contagious viral-borne disease of swine.

Cause

Hog cholera virus, a pestivirus of the family *Flaviviridae*, with considerable variation in severity by strain.

Systems Affected

Gastrointestinal, reproductive, nervous, vascular.

Transmission

Oral through consumption of contaminated tissue and body fluids.

Signs

In acute infections, pigs become febrile, anorexic, and inactive with constipation followed by diarrhea. If vasculitis occurs, extremities can appear purple and the nervous system can be affected, leading to ataxia or convulsions. Deaths occur 1.5–3 weeks post infection. In chronic cases, pigs appear to recover following fever but then relapse. Sow herds may experience reproductive failure.

Onset

Incubation ranges from two to six days, followed by appearance of clinical signs and progressive decline of affected animals.

Prevalence/Geographical Distribution

Latin America, some Caribbean Islands, and parts of Asia.

Diagnosis

In addition to virus isolation and/or PCR from blood and serologic testing, characteristic necropsy lesions include widespread petechial and ecchymotic hemorrhages in lymph nodes, kidneys, spleen, bladder, and larynx, and splenic infarction.

Treatment

In countries without endemic hog cholera, hog cholera is a reportable disease to the government and OIE (World

Organization for Animal Health). Control measures are designated by governmental authorities.

TECHNICIAN TIP 12.44. Hog cholera is a reportable disease in those countries without endemic hog cholera.

Recovery

Recovered animals may carry the virus.

Zoonotic Potential

No zoonotic potential.

Genetic Prevalence

No genetic prevalence known.

Prevention

Do not feed uncooked swill. Garbage feeding is a potential source of spread, since the virus is not deactivated by curing (i.e. salt and smoke treatment to make bacon or ham).

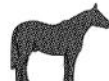 Hyperkalemic Periodic Paralysis (HYPP)

Definition

Hyperkalemic periodic paralysis (HYPP) is a genetic disorder that occurs primarily in Quarter Horses but may be apparent in other breeds such as Appaloosas and Paint Horses. This genetic defect has been traced back to the American quarter horse sire, Impressive. Impressive had many desirable traits, such as musculature, which led him to be a leading sire during his time.

TECHNICIAN TIP 12.45: The HYPP genetic defect has been traced back to the American quarter horse sire, Impressive.

Cause

HYPP is an autosomal dominant trait; it is not sex linked and can be inherited from either parent. Homozygous affected horses typically show more severe clinical signs than heterozygous horses.

System Affected

The primary system affected by HYPP is the musculoskeletal system.

Transmission

This disease is not infectious but an inherited disorder. Even though the name suggests high potassium blood levels found during HYPP episodes, the disease is due to a mutation in the sodium channels on the muscle cells surface. The muscle becomes overly excited and contracts when the sodium channels become "leaky." When there are small changes in blood potassium, it causes the sodium channels to open and start to leak sodium, which in turn causes the cells to leak potassium and cause an excess of potassium in the blood stream. At first, this leads to a hyperexcitable muscle, which trembles and contracts to the point where there is more and more potassium in the bloodstream and the muscles are unable to contract.

Signs

The most common clinical sign that will be seen during an episode is muscle fasciculations. This trembling typically occurs in the neck, shoulders, and flank areas. Generalized weakness, especially in the hind end, could be noted, as well as a prolapsed third eyelid. Episodes may be accompanied by an abnormal whinny or increased breathing noises due to paralysis of the upper airway muscles. Complete collapse and acute death may occur in the most severe cases due to cardiac arrest or respiratory failure. The patient's heart rate and respiratory rate are normal during an episode or might be slightly increased. Episodes may last anywhere from 20 min to 4 hr, with the most common ones lasting from 30 min to 1 h.

Onset

Onset of this disease typically occurs at two to three years of age.

Prevalence/Geographical Distribution

Published estimates suggest that approximate 4% of the quarter horse breed is affected but currently all affected animals trace their heritage to Impressive.

Diagnosis

A definitive diagnosis of HYPP is a genetic test. DNA can be extracted from equine hair or whole blood samples. In the past, veterinarians administered a potassium challenge test. During these tests, the horse was given potassium orally to see if they had any reactions. This test produced a lot of false negatives and was rather dangerous. The potassium that was given orally could induce a severe HYPP episode. If your veterinarian is present during an episode and is able to collect blood, it will show increased potassium levels. The genetic tests can be reported as three different results: homozygous normal (N/N), heterozygous (N/H), and homozygous affected (H/H). The clinical signs of HYPP can be apparent in both the heterozygous and the homozygous affected.

Treatment

If a patient has already been diagnosed with HYPP, mild episodes can typically be treated at home with success. A mild episode could be characterized as nonrecumbency with muscle fasciculation and no abnormal respiratory signs. Treatment for a mild episode includes light exercise and feeding a readily absorbable source of carbohydrates (light corn syrup). Insulin is released when sugar is introduced into the body, which in turn drives the potassium back into the cells. When feeding a carbohydrate, it is recommended to avoid molasses because of its high potassium content. For a moderate to severe HYPP episode, a veterinarian should be called for emergency treatment. Treatment by a veterinarian typically first includes the administration of fluids with 5% dextrose intravenously. This drives the potassium back into the cells. These fluids may or may not contain insulin, bicarbonate, or calcium as well. Bicarbonate has an additive effect when combined with dextrose and calcium as it may help counter the effects of the potassium on the body. The veterinarian may also administer acetazolamide, which is a diuretic that promotes the loss of potassium in the urine and may also stimulate insulin secretion.

Zoonotic Potential

No zoonotic potential.

Recovery and Prevention

Horses affected with HYPP can be managed in a way to help to decrease the frequency and the severity of episodes via diet. Avoid all the feeds that are high in potassium, such as molasses-infused feed and alfalfa hay. These horses do much better on grains such as corn and oats with beet pulp added. Timothy and Bermuda grass hay are alternatives for the alfalfa hay. Feeding smaller and more frequent meals has shown a benefit, as well as regular exercise and access to a large paddock turnout. Acetazolamide also may be recommended as a daily medication. To completely eradicate HYPP, every horse must be tested. Heterozygous or homozygous horses should be eliminated from any breeding program.

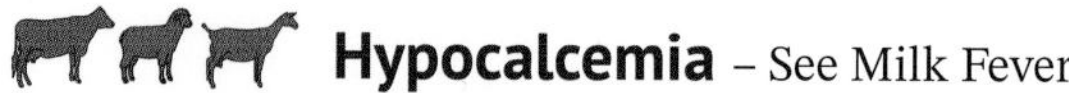

Hypocalcemia – See Milk Fever

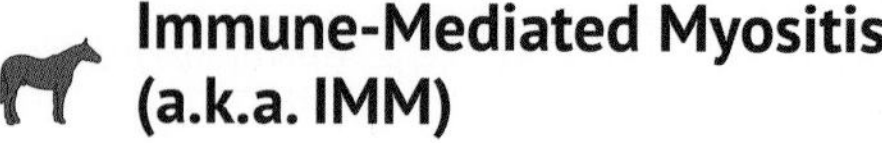

Immune-Mediated Myositis (a.k.a. IMM)

Definition

An immune-mediated disease that causes rapid muscle wasting.

Cause

Immune-mediated myositis occurs when inflammatory cells, predominantly lymphocytes, infiltrate the muscle fibers and surround blood vessels. The type 2× fibers in skeletal muscles are targeted leading to profound atrophy.

Systems Affected

Musculoskeletal.

Signs

IMM is most common in Quarter Horses and related breeds with up to 40% having a "triggering" event. These triggers can include recent exposure to a respiratory pathogen, most commonly strangles (*Streptococcus equi* var. *equi*) or recent vaccination. Affected horses often present with sudden onset and significant muscle atrophy, most commonly along the topline and hindquarters. Horses may also exhibit soreness/stiffness, lethargy, and weakness.

Prevalence/Geographical Distribution

Highest prevalence in Quarter Horse and related breeds. Worldwide distribution.

Diagnosis

Diagnosis is obtained via muscle biopsy of the gluteal or epaxial muscles. Lab work can be supportive of concurrent infection or muscle damage but may also be normal. Genetic testing is available for identified MYH1 mutation.

Lab Work

Elevated muscle enzymes including CK and AST may be present. If concurrent infection is present, inflammatory changes may also be present including leukopenia/leukocytosis, hyperfibrinogenemia, and hyperglobulinemia.

Differentials

- Vitamin E-deficient myopathy or equine motor neuron disease (EMND)
- Equine Cushing's disease (pituitary pars intermedia dysfunction, PPID)
- Neurogenic muscle atrophy

Treatment

The mainstay of treatment for IMM is corticosteroid therapy. Supportive therapy may be necessary in horses with lethargy, weakness, or prolonged recumbency. Treatment of concurrent respiratory infections with antimicrobials may be warranted depending on the etiologic agent and severity.

Associated Conditions

Severe muscle atrophy can lead to weakness, prolonged recumbency, and the development of secondary pressure sores.

Zoonotic Potential

No zoonotic potential.

Genetic Prevalence

A mutation in the MYH1 gene has been identified in Quarter Horse and related breeds with genetic testing available.

Prevention

Genetic testing of Quarter Horse and related breeds can demonstrate the susceptibility for development of IMM, allowing closer monitoring of at-risk individuals.

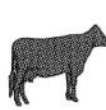

Infectious Bovine Keratoconjunctivitis (IBK, "Pink eye")

Definition

A bacterial infection of the eye causing conjunctivitis ("pink cyc") and corneal damage.

Cause

Pathogenic strains of *M. bovis*, a gram-negative bacterium.

Transmission

Factors affecting the integrity of the cornea such as trauma from plant awns, in addition to the presence of face flies (i.e. *Musca autumnalis*) and increased sun exposure are predisposing factors.

Signs

Affected animals show conjunctivitis, corneal edema and ulceration, photophobia, blepharospasm, eyelid swelling, and lacrimation. The disease is most common in calves and heifers and tends to affect only one eye.

> **TECHNICIAN TIP 12.46:** Pink eye is most common in calves and heifers and tends to affect only one eye.

Onset

Acute.

Prevalence/Geographical Distribution

The most common ocular disease of cattle worldwide.

Diagnosis

Clinical signs. Bacterial culture can be used to achieve a definitive diagnosis.

Treatment

Although not very practical in a farm setting, individual animals can be treated with local and frequent administration of antibiotics, atropine, and anti-inflammatories.

Recovery

In mild cases, recovery with or without scarring of the cornea can occur. More severe cases can progress to corneal rupture and iris prolapse.

Zoonotic Potential

None.

Genetic Prevalence

A higher incidence has been reported in the Hereford breed and a lower incidence in Brahmans.

Prevention

Fly control (e.g. insecticide-impregnated ear tags), routine clipping of mature pastures, and vaccination with bacterins and other novel vaccines are used to reduce the incidence of the disease.

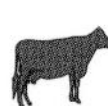

Infectious Bovine Rhinotracheitis – See Bovine Herpesvirus

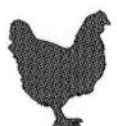

Infectious Bronchitis Virus (IBV)

Definition

A viral disease that impacts the upper respiratory tract of poultry.

Cause

Infectious bronchitis virus (IBV).

System Affected

Respiratory tract.

Transmission

This is a highly contagious disease that is spread easily via direct contact with infected birds or direct inhalation of the virus from respiratory secretions of feces. May also be found in peafowl and pheasants.

Signs

IBV infections cause upper respiratory problems in younger chickens, as well as weight and hunger loss. When layer chickens are infected, the eggshell quality is significantly reduced, and egg production may be decreased up to 70%.

Onset

Incubation period is typically 24–48 hr.

Prevalence/Geographical Distribution

When IBV is present in a flock, the entire flock will become infected and up to 82% can die as a result.

Diagnosis

ELISA and hemagglutination inhibition (HI) testing for serum antibodies, as well as virus detection by RT-PCR and virus isolation in embryonated eggs.

Treatment

Antimicrobials may reduce mortality from bacterial complications.

Recovery

The mortality rate depends on the age and immunity of each bird, as well as the specific strain of the virus. Morbidity for flocks affected is typically 100%.

Zoonotic Potential

No zoonotic potential.

Genetic Prevalence

No genetic prevalence known.

Prevention

Two different types of vaccines are used, a live version and an inactivated virus version. These vaccines are used widely across the poultry industry and are considered to be the most effective step in the prevention. Strict sanitation procedures are also essential in prevention.

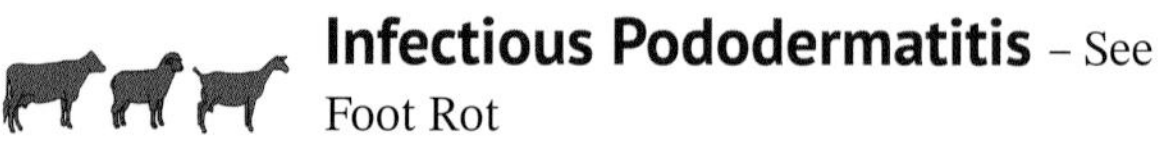

Infectious Pododermatitis – See Foot Rot

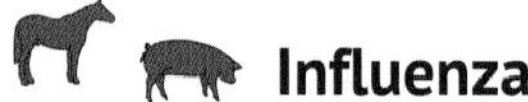

Influenza

Definition

Influenza is a viral disease.

Cause

The influenza virus is categorized into three types. Type A can affect many species, though in regard to the context of this book, includes horses and swine. Type B and C only affect humans.

Systems Affected

Respiratory tract.

Transmission

Influenza is highly contagious and is spread as aerosolized droplets dispersed via coughing from the infected individual. Horses can also become subclinically infected and shed virus.

Signs

Clinical signs of this disease and their severity can vary between individuals. They are also relative to the particular strain of the virus and the immune strength of the individual patient. The most common symptoms include fever, depression, coughing, and purulent nasal discharge. In severe cases, pneumonia can develop as a secondary complication.

Onset

Typically, affected horses will generally develop symptoms within 3–5 days of exposure, but can incubate as long as 14 days.

Prevalence/Geographical Distribution

This disease is widely and quickly spread among groups of horses, particularly in young groups.

Diagnosis

Nasopharyngeal swabs are obtained for virus isolation and antigen detection. Thoracic ultrasound or radiographs will not be helpful in specific virus isolation but can be very useful diagnostic tools for determining the severity of the symptoms and for developing a course of treatment.

Treatment

Primary treatment of this disease includes basic supportive care according to the specific symptoms they are exhibiting. Antipyretics can be administered for fevers and intravenous fluids may be necessary for maintaining hydration status.

Recovery

It can take three weeks or more to redevelop epithelium and cilia in the respiratory track. Severe cases, including those that develop pneumonia, can take up to six months or longer to gain full respiratory function or recovery. It is important to counsel clients about returning a horse back to work too soon to avoid replace or secondary complications.

Zoonotic Potential

No zoonotic potential.

Genetic Prevalence

No genetic prevalence known.

Prevention

Vaccines are available; however, they are short-lived. There are two inactivated and a modified live vaccine available for horses, unless the animals live in a closed or isolated facility. Avoiding frequent contact with large numbers of other horses can also reduce the chances of exposure. Individuals can continue to be infectious even days after clinical symptoms have resolved.

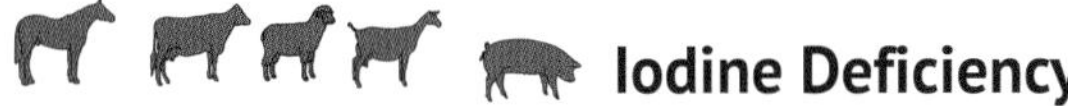

Iodine Deficiency

Definition

Decrease in bioavailability of iodine.

Cause

Insufficient iodine levels in the diet or ingestion of substances that interfere with the absorption of iodine.

Systems Affected

Thyroid, reproductive, mammary, and integument.

Transmission

Dietary.

Signs

Enlarged thyroid (goiter), dry skin, alopecia, weakness, fetal loss (abortion storms), neonatal loss, infertility, pregnancy toxemia, and retained placenta. Some babies are born with fine hair or are hairless (Figure 12.19).

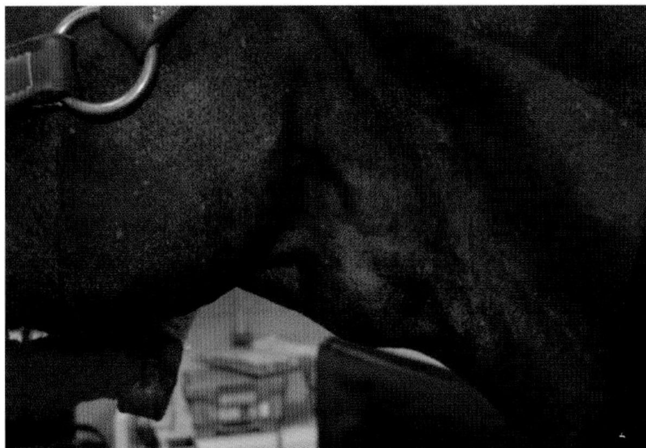

Figure 12.19 Enlarged thyroid in a horse.

Onset

Varies.

Prevalence/Geographical Distribution

Prevalence depends on the geographical location of the animals and/or feed sources; however, it is more common in the Northern tier states of the United States.

TECHNICIAN TIP 12.47: Iodine deficiency is more common in the Northern tier states of the United States.

Diagnosis

Serum or plasma thyroxine status.

Treatment

Iodine added to the diet, usually in the form of mineral salt (loose or block). Lactating dams have a higher iodine requirement than non-lactating animals. Topical application of iodine (Lugol's solution) is also a known treatment method.

Recovery

Requires attaining and continuing appropriate iodine levels in the animals.

Zoonotic Potential

No zoonotic potential.

Genetic Prevalence

Incidence is higher in certain Merino sheep, and Nubian, Angora, and Dutch goats.

Prevention

Iodine in the diet.

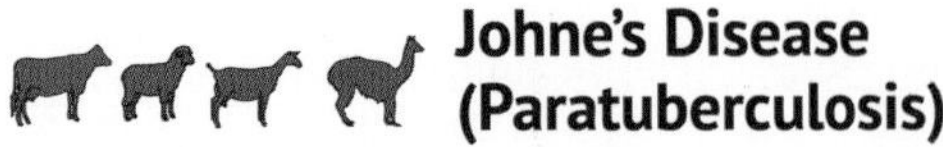

Johne's Disease (Paratuberculosis)

Definition

An insidious chronic disease affecting ruminants and other animals, causing weight loss and diarrhea.

Cause

Mycobacterium avium subspecies *paratuberculosis*. Different strains are recognized, such as the cattle strain, sheep strain, bison strain, and others.

Transmission

Fecal-oral route is the most important mode of transmission. Animals typically become infected during the perinatal period when suckling from teats stained with manure containing the bacteria. The organism is ingested, infects the small intestinal mucosa, and then spreads to regional lymph nodes. Subsequently the infection becomes systemic. The infection can also be transmitted in utero and can be passed through colostrum and milk.

Signs

Most infected animals are asymptomatic. Clinically affected animals initially show gradual weight loss, despite normal appetite, and decreased milk production. As the disease progresses, the fecal consistency becomes looser, progressing to intermittent profuse watery diarrhea. At this stage, animals appear cachectic, with intermandibular ("bottle jaw") and ventral edema due to hypoalbuminemia.

There is a classification in four stages based on the progression of the disease process. *Stage I* represents "silent" infection, *stage II* represents inapparent carrier state in adult animals, *stage III* represents animals with clinical disease, and *stage IV* represents animals with advanced clinical signs. For every mature cow showing advanced signs of the disease, it is estimated that around 15–25 others from the herd are infected. This is what is called "the iceberg effect," where animals with clinical signs are at the tip of the iceberg (what you can actually see).

The most common clinical signs in sheep and goats are weight loss and diarrhea and occur in approximately 20% of the clinical cases. Submandibular edema is also common. Clinical signs are apparent after two years of age and tend to exacerbate after parturition or another stressful situation.

Onset

Chronic and insidious onset with a long incubation period (longer than two years).

Prevalence/Geographical Distribution

A common disease with a worldwide distribution in many species.

Diagnosis

Fecal culture is the gold standard. The downside of this diagnostic technique is the long incubation period of 12–16 weeks. ELISA test is commonly used for diagnosis. Other tests include agar gel immunodiffusion (AGID) and PCR.

Treatment

No effective treatment is available.

Recovery

There is no recovery; animals with advanced clinical disease die due to cachexia and dehydration. Usually, affected animals are sent to slaughter before they develop advanced clinical signs.

Zoonotic Potential

There is an association between *M. avium* subspecies *paratuberculosis* and Crohn's disease in humans, but the possibility of a causative relationship is still unclear.

> **TECHNICIAN TIP 12.48:** There is an association between Johne's disease and Crohn's disease in humans, but a causative relationship is still unclear.

Genetic Prevalence

No genetic prevalence known.

Prevention

Biosecurity measurements aimed at reducing the exposure of young animals to the organism are important to control the spread of the disease. Monensin added to the ration is used as a preventative because it helps in diminishing the progression of the disease process.

A killed vaccine is available in some states of the United States and should be used through an accredited veterinarian with the approval of a state veterinarian. The vaccine does not eliminate infection but reduces the fecal shedding and delays the onset of clinical signs. Cattle vaccine can be used extra labeled in sheep and goats with the approval of a state veterinarian. There is no licensed vaccine available in Canada.

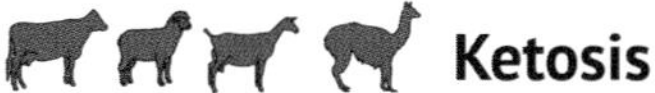 Ketosis

Definition

A metabolic disease characterized by increased levels of ketone bodies in serum and body fluids. Ketone bodies are normally a metabolic substrate for energy source in ruminants, but when its absorption and production exceed their use, clinical signs arise. Subclinical ketosis is also possible and leads to decreased milk production and associated peripartum diseases.

Cause

Elevated concentrations of ketone bodies can occur as a consequence of a negative energy balance during early lactation, that is, three to six weeks postpartum (*Type I ketosis* or primary ketosis), or secondary to over conditioning and fatty liver, usually seen immediately after parturition and before peak milk production (*Type II ketosis*).

> **TECHNICIAN TIP 12.49:** Ketone bodies can be elevated as a consequence of a negative energy balance during early lactation.

Transmission

It is a metabolic disease and, therefore, it is not transmissible.

Signs

Subclinical ketosis leads to decreased milk yield and increased incidence of peripartum conditions. Clinical ketosis is characterized by gradual inappetence and decrease in milk production. Lethargy and decreased rumen contractions are also common. A characteristic odor can be perceived in the milk or breath of affected animals. Displaced abomasum, metritis, traumatic reticuloperitonitis, and mastitis are common underlying conditions triggering secondary ketosis. There is also a nervous form of ketosis characterized by peculiar neurologic signs, including circling, head pressing, apparent blindness, hyperesthesia, bellowing, and so forth.

Onset

Acute.

Prevalence/Geographical Distribution

A prevalent disease in the dairy industry with a worldwide distribution.

Diagnosis

Measurement of ketone bodies in urine, plasma, or milk.

Treatment

Secondary ketosis is resolved when the underlying condition is corrected. Primary clinical ketosis can be treated with intravenous administration of dextrose, oral propylene glycol, corticosteroids, and insulin.

Recovery

Spontaneous resolution of clinical signs can occur when a balance between milk yield and feed intake is reached.

Zoonotic Potential

No zoonotic potential.

Genetic Prevalence

There is a genetic correlation between milk yield and ketosis.

Prevention

Dietary management in dry cows during the last three to four weeks prepartum. Excessive energy and reduced fiber intake should be avoided during the early dry period and immediately post calving.

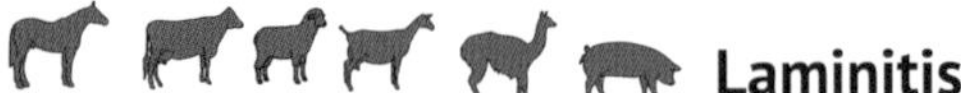 Laminitis

Definition

Inflammation and degeneration of the sensitive laminae of the hoof.

Cause

Variable, including systemic illnesses, or high-concentrate or lush feeds.

Systems Affected

Integument, specifically the epidermal and dermal laminae.

Signs

Lameness, increased temperature of the hooves, claws can become deformed over time.

> **TECHNICIAN TIP 12.50:** Clinical signs of laminitis include lameness and increased temperature of the hooves and claws.

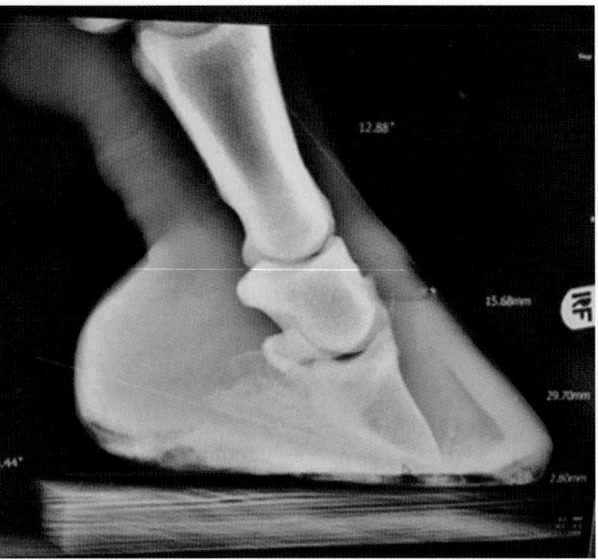

Figure 12.20 Coffin bone close to penetrating the sole of the foot.

Onset

Acute or chronic.

Prevalence/Geographical Distribution

Worldwide.

Diagnosis

Physical examination and radiographs (Figure 12.20).

Treatment

Therapy for the primary cause(s), anti-inflammatory drugs.

Recovery

Depends on the initial insult, and the initiation and success of treatment.

Zoonotic Potential

No zoonotic potential.

Genetic Prevalence

No genetic prevalence known.

Prevention

Ensure feed is properly contained to prevent accidental engorgement, acidosis. Keep susceptible animals off lush feed.

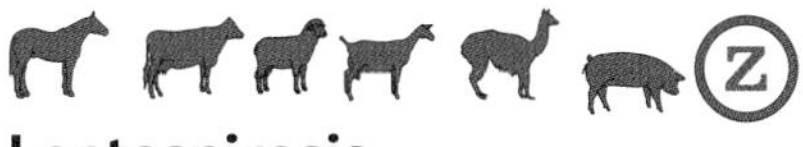

Leptospirosis

Definition

A chronic infection with hematogenous spread into multiple organs and renal colonization, causing hemolytic anemia, mastitis, and reproductive problems, including abortions. Multiple wild animals, rodents, and small ruminants can also be affected.

Cause

Pathogenic *Leptospira* species. There are host-specific and non-host-specific serotypes. There are 13 named species and 4 genomospecies of pathogenic *Leptospira* that have been characterized. Cattle are the maintenance host reservoir for *L. interrogans* serovar *hardjo* and *L. borgpetersenii* serovar *hardjo*.

Transmission

Direct contact or indirect contact with contaminated urine or aborted fetus.

Signs

Most infections are asymptomatic or subclinical. Clinical signs include abortion during the last trimester of gestation, reproductive failure, fever, lethargy, decreased milk production, mastitis, hemolytic anemia, and hemoglobinuria. Clinical signs in small ruminants are similar to those of cattle. In swine, problems of leptospirosis are observed in breeding herds and present as late-term abortions, between 85 and 100 days' gestation. Affected piglets surviving pregnancy may be stillborn or weak, dying soon after.

Onset

Acute or chronic.

Prevalence/Geographical Distribution

A high prevalence in dairy cattle with a worldwide distribution.

Diagnosis

Microscopic agglutination test (MAT) is used for serological testing. Urinary shedding or presence of *Leptospira* in semen can be assessed by phase-contrast microscopy, dark-field microscopy, fluorescent antibody, PCR, and so forth.

Treatment

Clinical cases can be treated with supportive treatment and antibiotics such as oxytetracycline, amoxicillin, and so forth.

Recovery

Treatment is generally unsuccessful. Chronic cases with renal colonization carry a good prognosis for life, but are a threat for other animals in the herd, because of bacterial shedding.

Zoonotic Potential

Humans are considered incidental hosts.

> **TECHNICIAN TIP 12.51:** Leptospirosis is a zoonotic disease.

Genetic Prevalence

No genetic prevalence known.

Prevention

Vaccination commencing at an early age with annual boosters is recommended against species-specific serovars. Other measurements, such as reducing the exposure of cattle and their feed and water to wild animals and rodents, are also important for prevention. Swine facility designs that reduce animal contact with urine are also helpful.

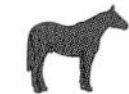

Equine Leukoencephalomalacia – See Moldy Corn Disease

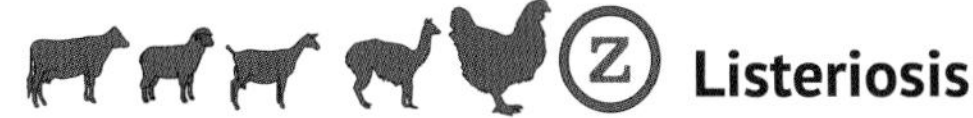

Listeriosis

Definition

A bacterial disease affecting the CNS of cattle and small ruminants.

Cause

Listeria monocytogenes, a gram-positive bacterium, ubiquitous in the environment.

Transmission

The bacterium is shed by asymptomatic carriers and clinically affected animals, and proliferates in spoiled silage, decaying forage, or rotting hay with a pH above 5.4. After penetrating through lesions or abrasions in the oral or nasal mucosa, the organism gains access to the CNS through the cranial nerve rootlets or hematogenously.

Signs

The disease can induce different clinical forms, such as septicemia, abortion, neonatal death, ophthalmitis, and neurologic disease (meningoencephalitis). It usually affects individual animals and only one clinical form is apparent. Neurologic signs include lethargy, conscious proprioceptive deficits, head pressing, propulsive walking, or compulsive circling, along with multiple cranial nerve dysfunctions. Depending on the cranial nerve affected, neurologic signs can include dropped jaw, drooped ear, strabismus, nystagmus, decreased lip tone, and so forth.

TECHNICIAN TIP 12.52: Clinical signs of listeriosis include head pressing and compulsive circling.

Sheep and goats tend to develop more acute disease than cattle with a higher case-fatality rate. Goats can demonstrate torticollis. Lambs may develop spinal cord dysfunction without brainstem involvement (Figure 12.21).

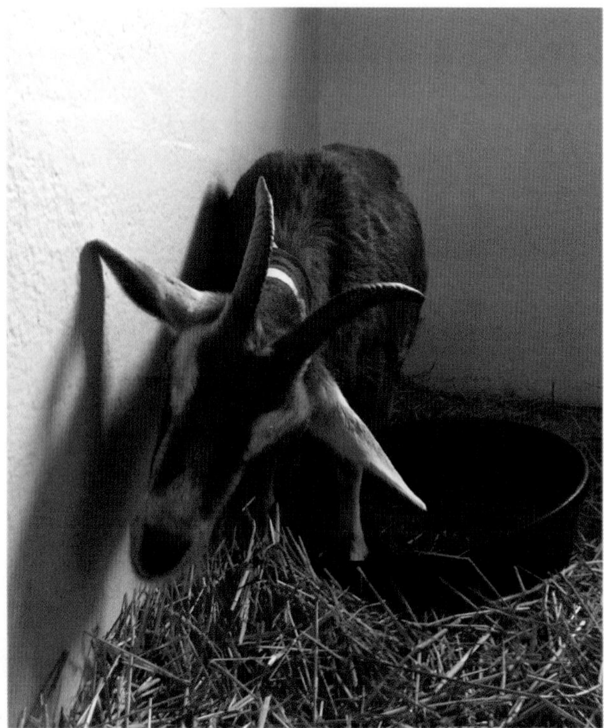

Figure 12.21 A head tilt is a common clinical sign associated with listeriosis in small ruminants. *Source:* Reproduced with permission of Dr. Gemma Tyner.

Onset

Acute.

Prevalence/Geographical Distribution

A disease with a low prevalence and a worldwide distribution. In temperate areas, the disease has a higher prevalence.

Diagnosis

Clinical signs. CSF analysis typically reveals increased protein concentration and total nucleated cell count, with more than 50% of the nucleated cells being mononuclear cells.

Treatment

Nursing and supportive care in addition to medical treatment, including antibiotic therapy (i.e. oxytetracycline or penicillin), early in the disease process.

Recovery

Mortality rate is high in untreated animals. Convulsing or comatose animals have a grave prognosis, and treatment is generally unsuccessful.

Zoonotic Potential

The disease can affect humans causing meningoencephalitis. Consumption of contaminated milk is a main concern for public health.

Genetic Prevalence

No genetic prevalence known.

Prevention

Avoid feeding improperly fermented silage or rotting hay with a pH higher than 5.4.

Lumpy Jaw (Actinomycosis)

Definition

A bacterial infection of the bone of the mandible of cattle causing firm, non-painful, and immovable masses. Occasionally, sheep and goats can also be affected.

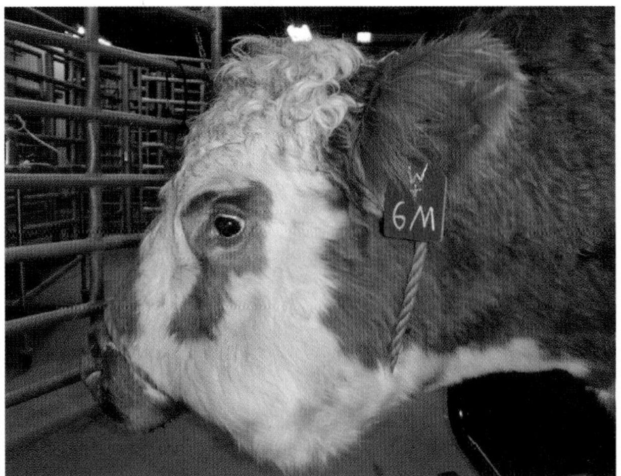

Figure 12.22 Actinomycosis or lumpy jaw in a beef steer.

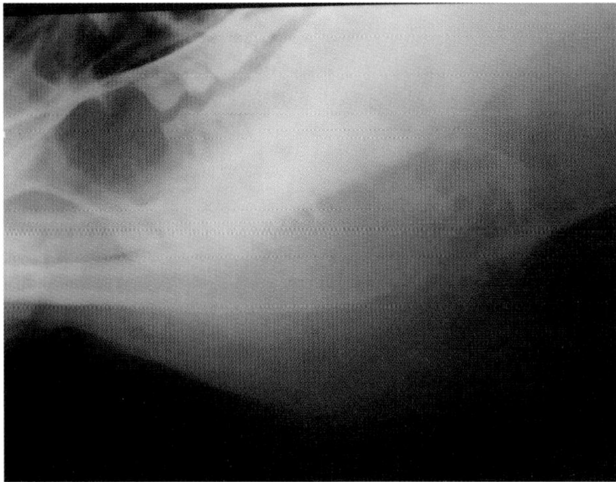

Figure 12.23 Radiograph of same patient showing inflammation and abscessation in the mandible.

Cause

Actinomyces bovis, a gram-positive bacterium, and normal inhabitant of the ruminant oral cavity.

> **TECHNICIAN TIP 12.53:** Lumpy jaw is caused by *A. bovis*, a normal inhabitant of the ruminant oral cavity.

Transmission

The bacterium penetrates the oral mucosa through erosions or lesions (punctures, openings, and abrasions) invading the mandible (or less frequently the maxilla).

Signs

Typically, the disease is manifested as firm, non-painful, immovable masses in the horizontal ramus of the mandible (Figures 12.22 and 12.23). Rarely, the bacteria can cause lesions in other parts of the body, including soft tissues, with clinical signs related to the area involved.

Onset

Chronic.

Prevalence/Geographical Distribution

A sporadic disease with worldwide distribution.

Diagnosis

Clinical signs. Bacterial culture and Gram stain are sometimes performed to confirm the diagnosis. The bacterium appears as a gram-positive, branching, and filamentous organism. "Sulfur granules" are commonly seen.

Treatment

Medical treatment aimed at arresting the disease process includes intravenous sodium iodide and antibiotic therapy (i.e. penicillin). Curettage of the area is performed in cases where fistulous tracts are present.

Recovery

Regression of the mass cannot be accomplished with medical treatment. Prognosis for life is good.

Zoonotic Potential

No zoonotic potential.

Genetic Prevalence

No genetic prevalence known.

Prevention

Avoid feeding rough hay containing plant awns or other materials capable of inducing oral mucosal damage.

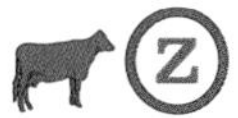

Mad Cow Disease (a.k.a. Bovine Spongiform Encephalopathy)

Definition

A progressive neurologic disease of cattle.

Cause

Protein known as a prion gets ingested by cattle that eat meat and bone meal made of cattle.

Systems Affected

Neurologic.

Transmission

Ingested.

Signs

Weight loss, trouble walking, unable to move, abnormal behavior, unable to stand.

Onset

Long onset of four to five years after exposure.

Prevalence/Geographical Distribution

Worldwide distribution.

Diagnosis

Suspect on clinical signs and confirmed on necropsy.

Treatment

None.

Recovery

None, death within weeks to months.

Zoonotic Potential

Yes, in humans known as Creutzfeldt–Jakob disease.

Genetic Prevalence

No genetic prevalence known.

Prevention

Not allowing older animals to enter the food supply.

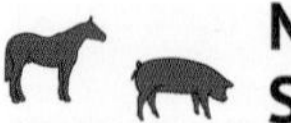

Malignant Hyperthermia (Porcine Stress Syndrome)

Definition

Disease of the skeletal muscle resulting in excessive muscle contracture.

Cause

Autosomal recessive genetic mutation affecting the Ca^{2+} channels.

Systems Affected

Musculoskeletal and cardiovascular.

Transmission

Inherited.

Signs

Upon a stressor event, muscles become rigid or twitch excessively and sinus tachycardia develops. Core body temperature rises rapidly (up to 113 °F); dyspnea ensues followed by death from cardiac arrest.

Onset

Episodes are triggered by stressful situations (e.g. loading or unloading animals), inhalant anesthetics, or depolarizing muscle relaxants.

Prevalence/Geographical Distribution

Worldwide distribution.

Diagnosis

Diagnosis consists of clinical syndrome combined with pale, soft, wet muscle on necropsy (or PSE [pale, soft exudative] muscle on slaughter); DNA tests can be used to identify gene carriers.

> **TECHNICIAN TIP 12.54:** DNA tests can be used to identify gene carriers of malignant hyperthermia.

Treatment

Treatment in the field consists of immediate removal of stress from the affected animal (i.e. allow it to rest). In surgical situations where the trigger is inhalant anesthesia, immediately remove gas anesthetic agent and administer dantrolene sodium IV; provide respiratory support, fluid therapy, and bicarbonate to correct acidosis; and apply cooling practices.

Recovery

Success of recovery is dependent on the extent to which an episode progresses.

Zoonotic Potential

No zoonotic potential.

Genetic Prevalence

The trait is most common in Pietrain, but also observed in Landrace, Duroc, and other breeds. Most common in Quarter Horses when compared with other breeds.

Prevention

Employ breeding programs to reduce gene prevalence and prevent production of homozygous carrier animals. Use injectable and local anesthesia.

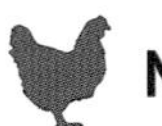

Marek's Disease

Definition

Disease of the immune system where the nerves are infiltrated by lymphocytes. This results in suppressed immune system and neurological disorders in the infected chickens.

Cause

Caused by an alphaherpesvirus known as Marek's disease virus (MDV).

Systems Affected

Immune system.

Transmission

Highly contagious oncogenic and neuropathic disease of chickens. It is also contagious between poultry, turkeys, and wild birds. The virus is most spread by contaminated litter or from feather dust and dander as well as bird to bird via airborne transmission.

Signs

Neurological deficits including transient leg paralysis is a hallmark sign of Marek's disease. Mortality as well as atherosclerosis can also be noted.

Onset

Incubation period is approximately 14 days with clinical signs appearing around 3–6 weeks.

Prevalence/Geographical Distribution

Worldwide distribution.

Diagnosis

Primarily identified by clinical signs and gross pathology. Quantitative PCR and serology also available.

Treatment

None.

Recovery

None.

Zoonotic Potential

No zoonotic potential.

Genetic Prevalence

No genetic prevalence known.

Prevention

Isolating the chicks for the first few months helps ensure sanitary conditions when the birds are most vulnerable to the disease and prevents possible spread from outside sources – thus also building the genetic resistance of the birds. Vaccination has proven to be the most effective lifelong approach to prevention. The vaccine, found to be over 90% effective, is recommended at 18 days' incubation or when the chick is less than 24 hr old.

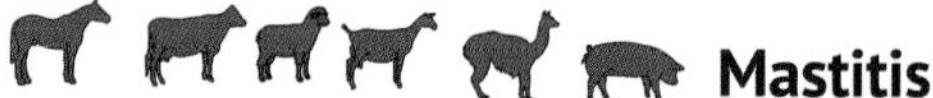

Mastitis

Definition

Clinical or subclinical infection of the mammary gland.

TECHNICIAN TIP 12.55: Mastitis infections can be clinical or subclinical.

Cause

Both contagious organisms and environmental pathogens can cause infection of the mammary gland. Contagious organisms infect the mammary gland and spread to other animals through milking machines and milkers, in contrast to environmental pathogens that do not normally gain access to the mammary gland except when the milking machine, teats, or udder are contaminated.

In cattle, contagious organisms include *Streptococcus agalactiae*, *Streptococcus dysgalactiae*, *Mycoplasma*, and so forth. Environmental pathogens include *E. coli*, *Pseudomonas spp.*, *Proteus spp.*, *Serratia spp.*, *Klebsiella pneumoniae*, and so forth.

The most common cause of clinical mastitis in sheep and goats is *S. aureus* and the most common cause of subclinical mastitis is coagulase-negative staphylococci in addition to *St. aureus*, *Streptoccocus spp.*, *Enterococcus spp.*, and *Mycoplasma spp.*

Retroviruses responsible for ovine progressive pneumonia (OPP) in sheep and caprine arthritis encephalitis (CAE) in goats can cause interstitial mastitis.

Transmission

The main reservoir of *contagious* organisms is the mammary gland of affected animals, and transmission occurs by milking machines, personnel, and milking procedures. Contamination of teats, udder, and milking machines is the principal mode of transmission for *environmental* pathogens. Also, new infections with environmental pathogens can be established during the dry period.

Signs

Subclinical and clinical mastitis occur, but subclinical mastitis represents the majority of cases in cattle, sheep, and goats.

Mild clinical cases are characterized by alterations of the milk from the affected quarter/half (change in color, viscosity, and/or consistency). In moderate cases, the mammary gland seems inflamed along with alteration of milk appearance. Animals with severe clinical mastitis not only show milk and mammary gland alterations, but also systemic signs of disease such as lethargy, anorexia, weakness, and so forth.

Although most cases of mastitis are subclinical in small ruminants, clinical mastitis can cause severe systemic illness or can lead to a chronic state with abscess formation in the mammary gland. *S. aureus* tend to cause more severe clinical signs or gangrenous mastitis ("blue bag") in sheep and goats compared to cattle. *Mycoplasma mycoides sp. mycoides* is an important cause of clinical mastitis in goats causing severe illness, reduced milk production, abnormal milk quality, and swollen udder. Subclinical mastitis can also occur.

An abnormal gait in lactating ewes and can also be a sign of mastitis. The abnormal gait is explained by the abduction of the hind limbs in an attempt to keep its limbs away from a painful mammary gland.

Retroviral mastitis in sheep and goats is characterized by a firm, but not swollen, udder. Milk from affected animals appears normal at gross inspection.

Onset

Acute or chronic.

Prevalence/Geographical Distribution

A prevalent disease in dairy cattle and small ruminants causing substantial economic losses. The disease has a worldwide distribution.

Diagnosis

Screening tests to detect subclinical mastitis are California Mastitis Test (CMT), somatic cell count (SCC), and electrical conductivity of milk (Figure 12.24). Diagnosis of clinical cases is done by clinical signs and bacterial cultures.

Treatment

Antibiotic therapy and supportive treatment in severe cases. Frequent milk-out is recommended to remove secretions from the affected mammary gland.

Recovery

Good to poor depending on the organism involved, and the severity of the disease process.

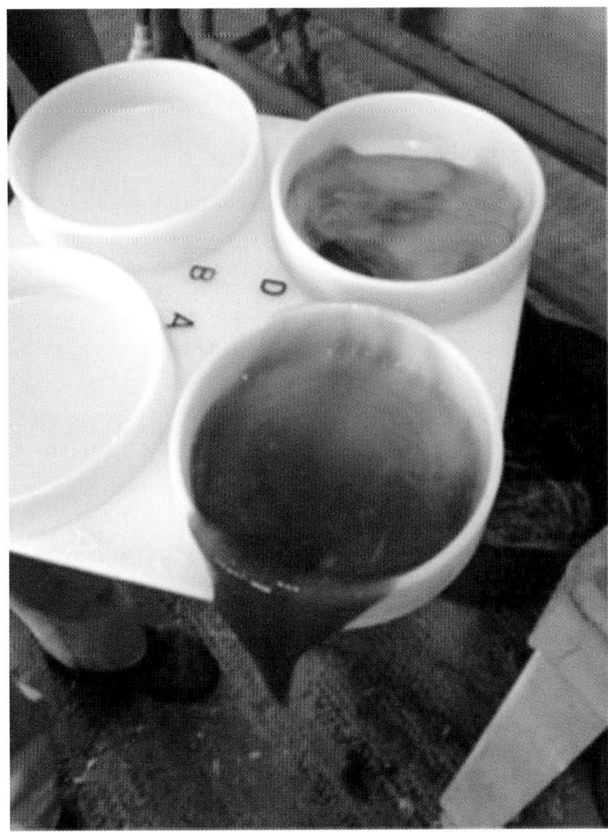

Figure 12.24 Positive (purple) results on a California Mastitis Test. *Source:* Photo courtesy of Amy Stieler Stewart, DVM, PhD, DACVIM (LAIM).

Zoonotic Potential

Many pathogens present in raw milk can be transmitted to people. Pasteurization is used to reduce the risk of milk-related foodborne illness in humans.

Genetic Prevalence

Some general resistance factors are thought to have a genetic component. Genetic selection for mastitis resistance is possible in sheep flocks.

Prevention

Predipping, germicidal teat disinfection after milking, and antibiotic therapy of dry cows, in addition to other control measures (use of individual cloth to prepare teats for milking, use of gloves by milkers, milking fresh heifers before adult cows, frequently removing manure from lots, avoid overstocking, etc.) are important to prevent the disease.

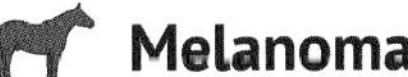

Melanoma

Definition

A melanoma is a neoplasm arising from the dermal melanocytes or melanoblasts. They can be benign or malignant.

> **TECHNICIAN TIP 12.56:** A melanoma is a benign or malignant neoplasm arising from the dermal melanocytes or melanoblasts.

Cause

The underlying cause is not yet known. As with any cancer, the affected cells are induced to replicate, and do not follow the normal cell cycle. Three growth patterns are recognized:

1) Slow growth without metastasis
2) Slow growth with sudden metastasis
3) Rapid growth and malignancy from the onset

Gray horses are heavily overrepresented, and they are most commonly seen in horses over the age of 15 years. The exact genetic mutation that increases the likelihood of developing melanomas has not been identified.

Systems Affected

Integumentary; it occurs most commonly under the tail and around the genitals, around the lips and eyes, and in the region of the parotid gland.

Signs

Single or multiple black (usually) nodules most commonly found on the perineum or ventral surface of the tail.

Diagnosis

Diagnosis is usually based on the clinical signs and signalment, though punch or excisional biopsy would be definitive. Iris melanomas can be diagnosed with ocular ultrasound. Melanomas are solid soft tissue structures, whereas iris cysts are usually fluid filled (Figure 12.25).

Treatment

The recommendations for treatment of melanomas are highly controversial. In the past, people have recommended

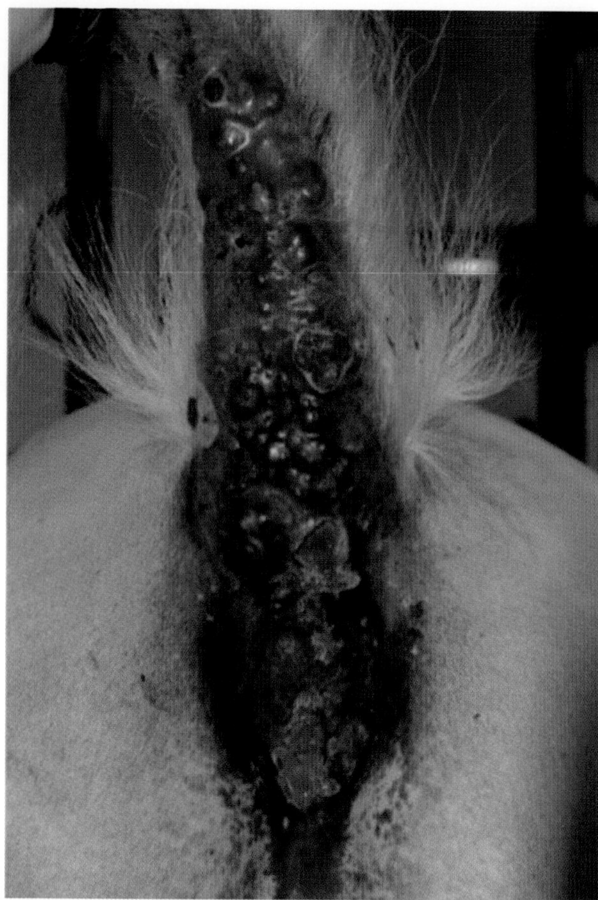

Figure 12.25 Multiple melanomas on the ventral surface of the tail.

not to treat them unless they are causing a problem. Now, some schools of thought believe that early surgical excision may limit the potential for metastasis.

- Cimetidine has been reported to cause partial and sometimes complete regression, it can then be continued as maintenance therapy.
- Surgical excision if the mass is causing a problem – problems with healing and recurrence.
- Cryotherapy can be effective.
- Iris melanomas are usually monitored; surgery can be attempted by a skilled ophthalmologist.

Recovery

None. Horses with one melanoma are more likely to develop multiple melanomas, although they do not always cause problems. Monitoring and assessing rapidity of growth will help to determine a prognosis.

Prevalence/Geographical Distribution

Melanomas are common in older gray horses. Worldwide.

Zoonotic Potential

No zoonotic potential.

Genetic Prevalence

Most common in Arabian and Percheron horses.

Prevention

None.

Milk Fever (Hypocalcemia)

Definition

An acute decrease in serum calcium levels typically seen in cattle 24 hr before and 72 hr after parturition ("milk fever"), and in ewes during the last two weeks of gestation (especially, ewes carrying twins). Beef cows also show clinical signs of hypocalcemia during late gestation. High-producing dairy goats commonly show clinical signs of hypocalcemia after parturition, similarly to dairy cattle.

> **TECHNICIAN TIP 12.57:** Due to increased calcium demands during fetal maturation, colostrum production, and incipient lactation in late gestation, decreases in serum calcium are seen. Development of milk fever results.

Cause

A decrease in serum calcium concentration due to increased demands from fetal maturation, colostrum production, and incipient lactation in late gestation.

Transmission

Milk fever is not a transmissible disease, but a metabolic disease.

Signs

Affected cows initially appear excitable and restless, progressing to show inability to regulate their body temperature, generalized weakness, diminished rumen contractions, and bloat. As the disease process advances, cattle become recumbent and are unable to rise. Affected animals if left untreated eventually die within 12 hr of the onset of signs. Clinical signs in small ruminants are similar to those in cattle except that they occur in late gestation.

Onset

Acute.

Prevalence/Geographical Distribution

A prevalent metabolic disease with a worldwide distribution.

Diagnosis

Clinical signs and measurement of serum calcium concentration can be used to confirm the clinical diagnosis.

Treatment

Parenteral administration of calcium borogluconate. Oral calcium-containing products can be used when affected animals still have a normal swallow response in order to prevent aspiration into the airways.

Recovery

Good with appropriate treatment in a timely manner.

Zoonotic Potential

No zoonotic potential.

Genetic Prevalence

Some general resistance factors are thought to have a genetic component.

Prevention

Nutritional management of dairy cows in the dry period is important to prevent the disease.

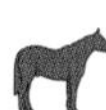

Moldy Corn Disease (a.k.a. Equine Leukoencephalomalacia)

Cause

Leukoencephalomalacia is caused by ingestion of fumonisins (fumonisins B1 and B2), which are neurotoxins produced by a mold known as *Fusarium moniliforme*. The mold has a predilection for corn. The onset of clinical signs is dependent on the amount of toxin ingested. This period may last several months but can be as short as five days. Repeated exposure to the toxin appears to be strongly associated with the development of clinical signs, as compared to a single large dose.

Systems Affected

In addition to neurologic disease, evidence of hepatic insufficiency is common, including icterus and petechiation of mucous membranes. Clinical laboratory work often indicates increased liver enzyme levels.

Clinical Signs

Clinical signs develop due to liquefactive necrosis of the white matter of the cerebrum caused by neurotoxins. Onset of clinical signs is typically peracute to acute. Clinical signs include somnolence, ataxia, head pressing, mania, blindness, and seizures. Affected horses are unpredictable and may be dangerous, so appropriate protective action should be taken.

Prevalence/Geographical Distribution

Leukoencephalomalacia occurs worldwide. Cases occur most commonly during winter and early spring.

Diagnosis

Diagnosis is based on consistent clinical signs and a history of exposure to moldy corn.

Treatment

Treatment is supportive in nature for both neurologic and hepatic disease. Attempts at decontamination are unlikely to improve outcomes due to the delay in onset of clinical signs after exposure.

Prognosis

Prognosis for affected horses is grave. The majority of affected horses die within 24 hr of developing neurologic signs. Those that survive are likely to have permanent neurologic damage.

Zoonotic Potential

No zoonotic potential.

Genetic Prevalence

No genetic prevalence known.

Prevalence/Geographical Distribution

Any horse of any gender, sex, or age is susceptible. Older horses may be more sensitive to the neurotoxin.

Prevention

Access to corn and corn products is the greatest risk factor for ingestion of fumonisins. Production of fumonisins is greater when weather conditions are dry during the corn-growing season, and moist and cool during pollination and kernel formation. Contamination with fumonisins is less common during storage.

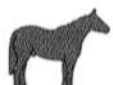 Navicular Disease

Definition

A chronic degenerative condition of the navicular bone.

Cause

A wide variety of conditions can lead to pain in the heel or foot of the horse, and many of these are commonly known as *navicular syndrome*. This term can be used to reference changes to the navicular bone or bursa as well as lesions affecting adjacent coffin and pastern bones, associated tendons, ligaments, joints, or the collateral cartilages.

Systems Affected

Musculoskeletal.

Signs

This disease is most common in Quarter Horses, warmbloods, and Thoroughbreds. Horses often present middle-aged (8–15 years old) but can be much younger or older at the time of diagnosis. At the time of presentation, horses display acute or chronic forelimb lameness and may have a shortened stride or "choppy" gait.

Prevalence/Geographical Distribution

Prevalence varies depending on breed, age, and use of horse. Worldwide distribution.

Diagnosis

Clinical signs and measurement of serum calcium concentration can be used to confirm the clinical diagnosis.

Differentials

- Hoof abscess
- Laminitis
- Trauma
- Other injuries/conditions of the forelimb leading to lameness

Treatment

A large variety of treatment options exist for navicular disease and depend on the structures involved and the lesions identified. Treatment is most successful when definitive diagnosis of the lesions is obtained so treatment can be directed. Medical treatment can include any combination of rest and rehabilitation, therapeutic trimming and shoeing, intra-articular medications (coffin joint, navicular bursa, or digital flexor tendon sheath), systemic drug therapy (NSAIDS, isoxsuprine, hyaluronan, polysulfated glycosaminoglycans, bisphosphonates), and extracorporeal shockwave treatment. Surgical treatment may be needed in select cases and includes a palmar digital neurectomy, navicular bursoscopy, or collateral sesamoidean desmotomy. Success of treatment depends on severity of the disease at the time of diagnosis, lesions/structures involved, and the desired performance level of the affected horse.

Associated Conditions

Depending on the severity of the pain in the heel or foot of the horse, contralateral lameness and/or laminitis can occur. Also, lesions in and potential rupture of the deep digital flexor tendon can accompany disease of the navicular bone.

Zoonotic Potential

No zoonotic potential.

Genetic Prevalence

This syndrome may be potentially heritable with certain breeds more commonly diagnosed. However, the extent of the genetic association is not known at this time.

Prevention

Poor hoof conformation may be a risk factor for development of this condition as well as excessive stress placed on the structures of the hoof through exercise.

Ovine Progressive Pneumonia (OPP), Maedi-Visna

Definition

Chronic fatal viral respiratory disease of small ruminants.

Cause

Retrovirus.

Systems Affected

Respiratory.

Transmission

Lateral and vertical.

Signs

Respiratory disease as adults, with exercise intolerance, ill thrift, loss of condition, and mastitis.

Onset

Infection as lambs/kids most common, however, clinical signs present around two years of age or later.

> **TECHNICIAN TIP 12.58:** Lambs and kids are infected at a young age though clinical signs are delayed into adulthood.

Prevalence/Geographical Distribution

Prevalence varies between areas, farms, and flocks. The virus is found in most sheep producing countries. It has been eradicated from Finland and Iceland. It is not found in Australia or New Zealand.

Diagnosis

Clinical signs, serology (PCR), and necropsy.

Treatment

None.

Recovery

Fatal.

Zoonotic Potential

No zoonotic potential.

Genetic Prevalence

No genetic prevalence known.

Prevention

Test and cull seropositive ewes.

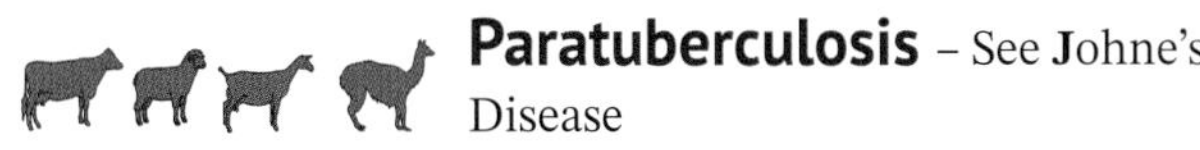

Paratuberculosis – See Johne's Disease

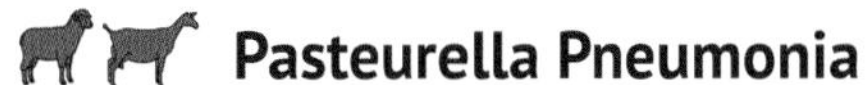

Pasteurella Pneumonia

Definition

Opportunistic pneumonia of sheep and goats with prior respiratory insult or those housed/managed under stressful conditions.

Cause

Mixed pathogens, *P. multocida*, and *Mannheimia haemolytica*.

Systems Affected

Primarily respiratory tract, but can also cause systemic disease, localizing in the joints and mammary gland, among other sites.

Transmission

P. multocida and *M. haemolytica* are normal flora of the upper respiratory tract in most small ruminants. Initial insult of viral or bacterial respiratory disease may interfere with the ability of the upper respiratory tract to clear inhaled pathogens. However, these pathogens may also be spread by direct contact with the agents via nose-to-nose exposure or by lambs nursing from infected mammary glands.

Signs

Animals present as febrile, anorexic, pyrexic, with coughing, nasal discharge, tachypnea, and sudden death. Individuals may separate from the herd or flock.

Onset

Clinical signs begin 10–14 days after initial insult.

Prevalence/Geographical Distribution

Stressful events surrounding neonates, commingling, and/or shipping of animals. Worldwide distribution.

Diagnosis

History, clinical signs, physical exam, culture of tracheal swabs/wash, or culture of lesions at necropsy.

Treatment

Treatment protocols should be established from a culture and sensitivity of the agent. Select antibiotics and supportive therapy with judicious use of anti-inflammatory drugs to prevent gastric ulcers.

Prevention

Minimize stressful events such as commingling and shipping. House with adequate ventilation and animal density to decrease weather or temperature-related stressors.

Recovery

Dependent on chronicity of the disease process, area(s) affected, and the efficacy of the treatment for eradication of the disease. Animals with extensive tissue damage (lungs, joints, mammary gland) may not come back to full potential as production animals.

Zoonotic Potential

No zoonotic potential.

Genetic Prevalence

No genetic prevalence known.

Prevention

No vaccines available.

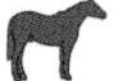 Pemphigus Foliaceus

Definition

An autoimmune disorder that the horse makes antibodies that attack their own skin.

Cause

Unknown.

Systems Affected

Integument.

Signs

Hair loss, crusting of skin, blisters (Figure 12.26).

Onset

Varied.

Geographical Distribution

Worldwide distribution.

Diagnosis

Diagnosis is only confirmed with a biopsy.

Treatment

Treatment is with drugs that suppress the immune system including steroids. Steroids do have serious side effects to include laminitis.

Prevention

None.

Recovery

Prognosis is guarded. Treatment tends to be lifelong. Some will be euthanized due to uncontrollable pain and laminitis.

Zoonotic Potential

No zoonotic potential.

Genetic Prevalence

No genetic prevalence known.

Prevention

No vaccines available.

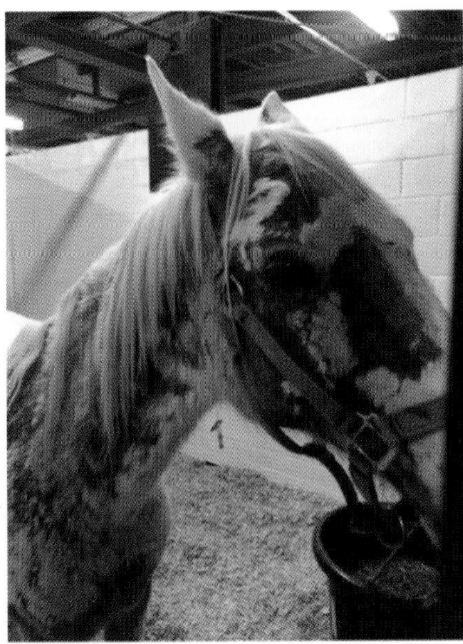
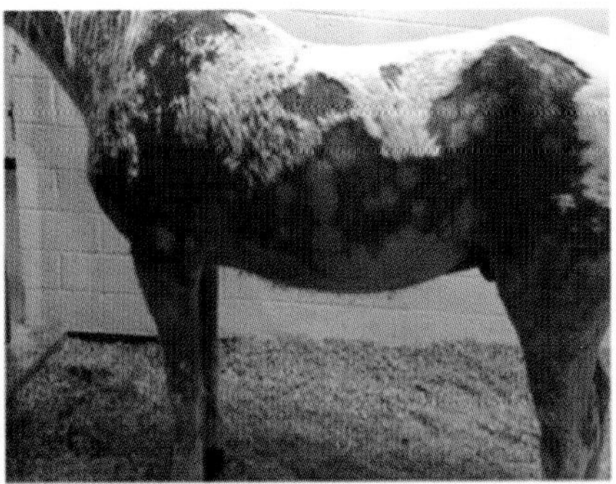

Figure 12.26 Horse with pemphigus that has affected the entire body. Source: Photo courtesy of Erin Elder, DVM.

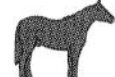 Phenylbutazone Toxicity

Definition

Adverse effects of phenylbutazone usage include gastrointestinal disease (gastric ulceration or right dorsal colitis) and renal disease. Side effects are usually secondary to prolonged high dose therapy; however, they can occur with any duration of therapy at any dose. Horses that are hypovolemic, or with hepatic or renal dysfunction, are most likely to show signs.

> **TECHNICIAN TIP 12.59:** Horses that are hypovolemic or with hepatic or renal dysfunction are more likely to show signs of phenylbutazone toxicity.

Cause

Nonsteroidal anti-inflammatory drugs are cyclooxygenase (COX) inhibitors. The complete function of the separate COX enzymes is not fully understood. However, COX 1 is mainly thought to have a homeostatic role and COX 2 is thought to be more inducible during inflammatory processes. There appears to be a large degree of overlap between the COX enzymes, and for this reason, no NSAID is completely safe. Phenylbutazone is a nonselective COX inhibitor; some of the COX 2 selective NSAIDs are reported to be less toxic. The main detrimental effect of inhibition of COX is inhibition of certain prostaglandins (most importantly PGE_2 and PGI_2) that have regulatory effects in the body. In the gastrointestinal tract, inhibition of COX enzymes leads to: decrease in gastric acid pH; decrease in protective, and repair mechanisms. Prostaglandins are important in regulation of blood flow in the kidney, mainly promoting vasodilatation when there is decreased perfusion. Therefore, NSAID renal toxicity mainly occurs in hypovolemic patients, or those already suffering from renal disease.

Systems Affected

Gastrointestinal tract (especially, stomach and right dorsal colon) and kidneys.

Signs

Gastric ulceration: bruxism, mild colic signs, reluctance to eat grain; right dorsal colitis: anorexia, lethargy, diarrhea, fever, signs of endotoxemia, colic; ventral edema, may see weight loss; renal toxicity: often see RDC (right dorsal colitis) first followed by anuria/oliguria.

Diagnosis

Often presumptive with clinical signs and history of phenylbutazone use. Gastroscopy shows ulcers usually on the glandular mucosa. Ultrasound of the right dorsal colon shows thickening (>0.5 cm). Renal damage: isosthenuric urine, decreased/absent urine production, renal casts, or hematuria; if chronic may see changes on ultrasound (increased echogenicity of the renal crest and debris in the renal pelvis).

Treatment

Discontinue nonsteroidal anti-inflammatory usage. Treatment of RDC, renal disease, and supportive care.

Prevalence/Geographical Distribution

Any age. Worldwide.

Zoonotic Potential

Dependent on infectious agents passed in feces.

Genetic Prevalence

No genetic prevalence known.

Prevention

Use appropriate doses of nonsteroidals and try to limit the duration of use, always using the lowest possible dose. Use extra caution in hypovolemic patients.

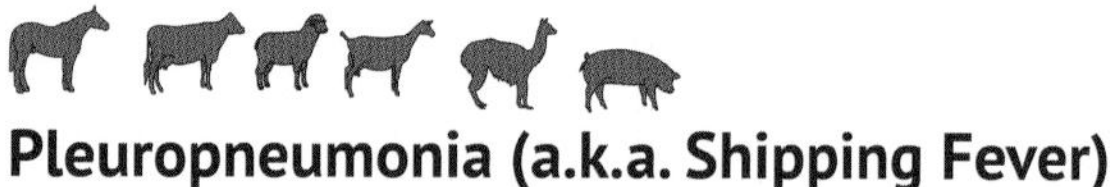

Pleuropneumonia (a.k.a. Shipping Fever)

Definition

Inflammation of the lungs and the pleura.

Cause

Bacterial infections of the lower respiratory tract most commonly occur due to the aspiration of normal bacterial flora from the upper respiratory tract. These infections are termed pleuropneumonia when they affect the lung parenchyma and extend to the pleura. Infections occur when bacterial loads are high and/or pulmonary defenses are compromised by stress, viral infections, malnutrition, dust or gas exposure, or an immune deficiency.

Systems Affected

Respiratory.

Signs

Pleuropneumonia can affect horses of any age, breed, or gender. Infections are more common in young horses with multiple risk factors identified including recent travel, prolonged period of confinement with head elevated (trailering), high-intensity exercise, or recent general anesthesia. Initially, clinical signs may be vague and include lethargy, decreased appetite, and a fever. Signs will progress to nasal discharge, cough, tachypnea, increased respiratory effort, pleurodynia, and occasionally respiratory distress (Figure 12.27).

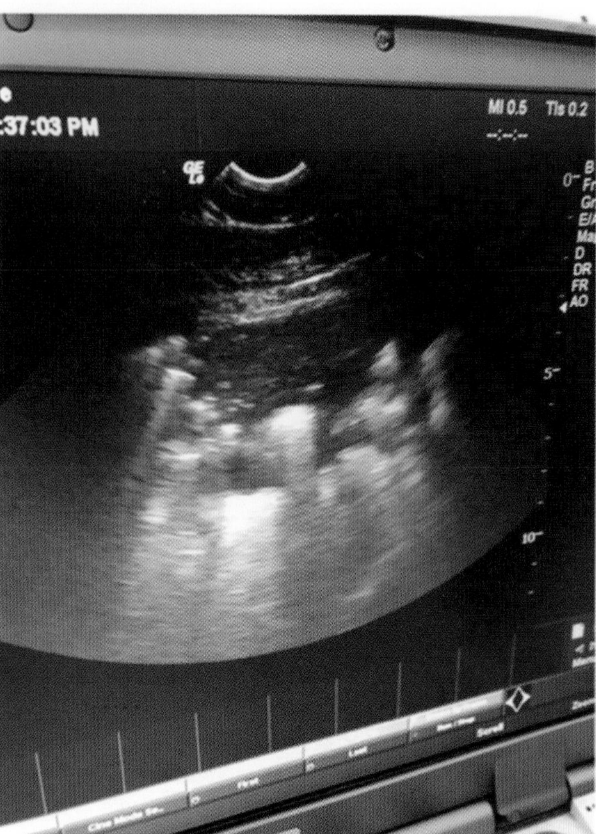

Figure 12.27 Ultrasound of the pleura shows severe pulmonary consolidation. *Source:* Photo courtesy of Kimberly Schreiber Young, DVM.

Prevalence/Geographical Distribution

Higher prevalence in Thoroughbreds than Standardbreds and in younger horses. Worldwide distribution.

Diagnosis

A presumptive diagnosis is often made based on history of recent travel/anesthesia and development of clinical signs. Diagnostics including physical exam, rebreathing exam, bloodwork, thoracic ultrasound, radiographs, and airway sampling can be confirmative. Bacterial culture of both the airway (transtracheal wash) and pleural effusion is recommended to determine the causative organism and antimicrobial susceptibility.

Lab Work

Lab work may be consistent with infection including leukopenia/leukocytosis, neutropenia/neutrophilia, presence of band neutrophils, hyperfibrinogenemia, hyperglobulinemia, and hypoalbuminemia.

Differentials

- Equine multinodular pulmonary fibrosis (EMPF)
- Inflammatory airway disease (IAD)
- Pulmonary aspergillosis
- Parasitic pneumonia
- Smoke inhalation
- Pneumothorax
- Pulmonary edema
- Idiopathic interstitial pneumonia
- Neoplasia

Treatment

Treatment of pleuropneumonia depends on the severity and disease progression at the time of diagnosis. A combination of systemic antimicrobials, aerosolized antimicrobials, pleural drainage ± pleural lavage, fibrinolytic agents, and supportive therapy (IV fluids, NSAIDs, anti-endotoxics, distal limb cryotherapy, analgesics, oxygen therapy) is often needed. Aggressive treatment is warranted at the time of diagnosis based on the potential for the disease to progress and risk for secondary complications to develop. In severe cases, surgery including thoracoscopy or thoracotomy with rib resection, may be needed to facilitate removal of fibrin and lung abscesses (Figure 12.28).

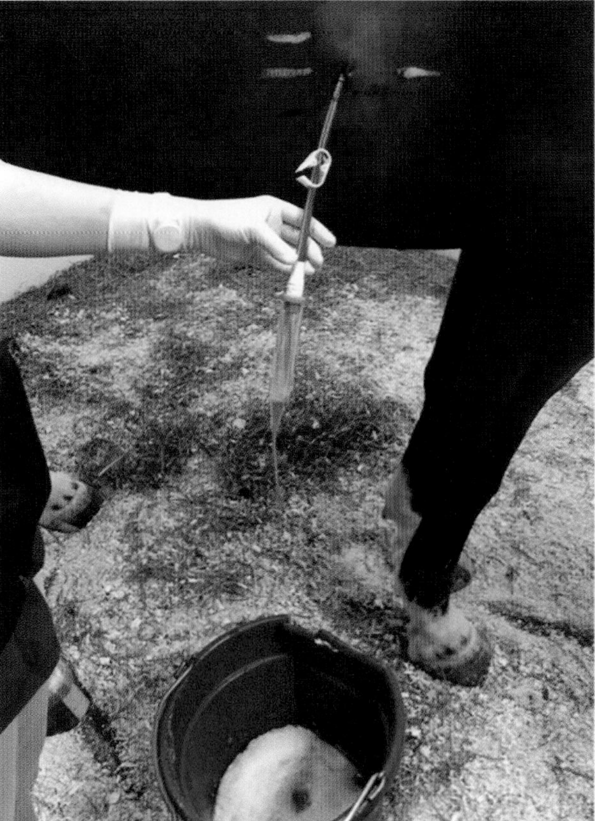

Figure 12.28 Pleural lavage with indwelling drain into the chest. *Source:* Photo courtesy of Lauren Hughes, DVM.

Associated Conditions

Secondary complications are common including jugular vein thrombophlebitis, diarrhea, pericarditis, coagulopathies, pneumothorax, bronchopleural fistulas, and laminitis.

Zoonotic Potential

No zoonotic potential.

Genetic Prevalence

No genetic prevalence known.

Prevention

Prevention is aimed at minimizing known risk factors. Avoiding prolonged travel and ensuring horses are able to lower the head regularly during travel are important to aid in normal clearance of bacterial organisms from the airway. Close monitoring (including rectal temperatures) of horses that recently underwent travel or general anesthesia is recommended to help identify pleuropneumonia in the earlier stages and initiate treatment.

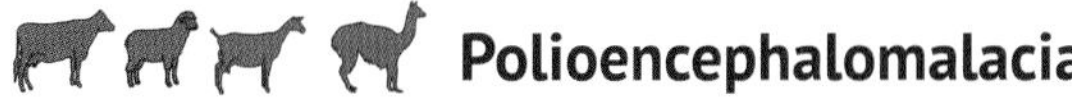

Polioencephalomalacia

Definition

A metabolic disease characterized by degeneration and necrosis of the gray matter of the cerebral cortex, leading to neurologic signs. The disease affects cattle and small ruminants.

Cause

Thiamine deficiency is believed to be the leading cause, although other causes such as sulfur toxicity, lead poisoning, osmolality derangements, and so forth can also induce the disease.

> **TECHNICIAN TIP 12.60:** Thiamine deficiency is believed to be the leading cause of polioencephalomalacia.

Particular diets, especially those with high-grain and low fiber composition and plants containing thiaminase activity, are associated with the development of the characteristic lesions in the brain.

Transmission

It is not a transmissible disease.

Signs

Initially affected animals are seen separated from the herd or flock, walking with the head erect and slightly hypermetric. Central blindness, head pressing, muscle tremors, and odontoprisis are common clinical signs. As the disease progresses opisthotonos, dorsomedial strabismus, nystagmus, recumbency, seizures, and coma occur.

Onset

Subacute and acute.

Prevalence/Geographical Distribution

A prevalent disease with a worldwide distribution.

Diagnosis

Clinical signs. Laboratory confirmation can be achieved by measuring erythrocyte transketolase activity, or fecal and ruminal thiaminase concentrations. Histologic evaluation of necropsy brain specimens is helpful for establishing a definitive diagnosis.

Treatment

Parenteral thiamine administration.

Recovery

Aggressively treated animals may recover from mild disease when treated in the initial stages. More advanced cases carry a grave prognosis. Untreated animals usually die in one to four days.

Zoonotic Potential

No zoonotic potential.

Genetic Prevalence

No genetic prevalence known.

Prevention

Nutritional factors should be evaluated in affected animals and/or herds. The addition of thiamine in the diet is used with variable success.

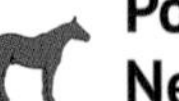

Polyneuritis Equi (Cauda Equina Neuritis)

Cause

Polyneuritis equi is an inflammatory disease of unknown origin affecting horses. An autoimmune etiology is suspected but has not been proven.

> **TECHNICIAN TIP 12.61:** Polyneuritis equi is an inflammatory disease of unknown origin, which may have an autoimmune component.

Systems Affected

Inflammatory changes can occur in various nerve roots but those of the cauda equina and cranial nerves are affected most frequently.

Onset/Signs

Onset of clinical signs is gradual. Initial clinical signs may include rubbing and chewing of the region around the tail head. Decreased to absent sensation of the tail and perineum ultimately develops. As a result of nerve dysfunction, weakness of the tail, rectum, anal sphincter, and bladder develops. Urine dribbling, urine scalding of the hindlimbs, and retention of feces in the rectum are often observed. The disease is also characterized by hindlimb weakness and ataxia.

If cranial nerves are affected, signs of facial paralysis may be present. Typically, cranial nerves V and VII are the most commonly affected, but others are occasionally involved (Figure 12.29).

Prevalence/Geographical Distribution

Polyneuritis equi is a sporadic disease with no known geographic patterns.

Diagnosis

Diagnosis is based on consistent clinical signs. Cerebrospinal fluid analysis may indicate an increase in

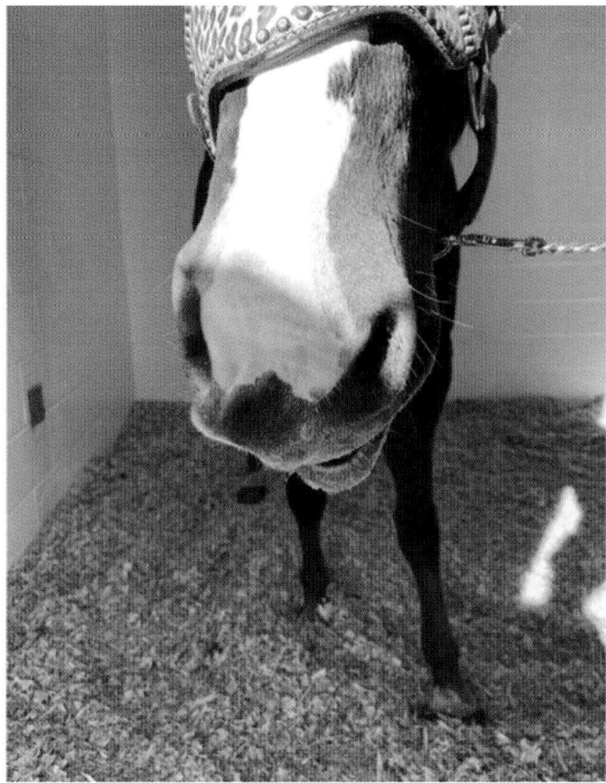

Figure 12.29 Horse with left-sided facial paralysis. *Source:* Photo courtesy of Kimberly Schreiber Young, DVM.

both cellularity and total protein concentration. A mononuclear or neutrophilic pleocytosis may be noted.

Treatment

Treatment is supportive in nature. Nursing care, such as evacuation of the bladder and rectum, may be necessary. Corticosteroid therapy may be attempted but is typically not effective. Azathioprine, an immunosuppressive drug, has anecdotally led to some improvement.

Prognosis

Prognosis is considered poor, as patients generally do not respond to therapy and, as a result, continue to deteriorate to the point where euthanasia is required.

Zoonotic Potential

No zoonotic potential.

Prevalence/Geographical Distribution

The disease typically affects adult horses; no breed or gender has been identified.

Prevention

Because it is a sporadic disease of unknown etiology, no recommendations regarding prevention are available.

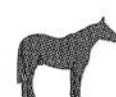 Polysaccharide Storage Myopathy (a.k.a. PSSM, EPSM, EPSSM)

Definition

This is a genetic carbohydrate metabolism disorder that causes episodes of rhabdomyolysis. Commonly confused with musculoskeletal-type diseases including vitamin E or selenium deficiency, HYPP, or ER.

Cause

Currently two separate forms of PSSM have been identified: type 1 and type 2. Some horses have been found to have one or the other, or both types. PSSM type 1 is the most common type of those diagnosed with the disease, effecting about 90% of PSSM cases. It occurs as a result of a genetic mutation in a glycogen synthesis enzyme gene. It manifests enhanced insulin sensitivity and increased synthesis of muscle glycogen.

Systems Affected

Skeletal muscle, carbohydrate metabolism.

Symptoms

Clinical symptoms can vary widely between cases and vary according to the severity, exercise regime, and diet. Common symptoms include muscle pain, stiffness, weakness, laziness, shifting lameness, flank tremors, profuse sweating, firm hard muscles, and reluctance to move. Symptoms may appear shortly after light exercise or as infrequent as a few times per year in mild cases. Dark colored urine may be noted after an episode.

Transmission

Genetic inheritance.

Onset

While a horse acquires the disease through genetics and is born with the trait, typical onset is acute and tends to develop after initial training has started or after a layup period of rest.

Prevalence/Geographical Distribution

Both types of the disease have been found in 20 different breeds of horses with the highest prevalence in Quarter Horses, American Paints, and Appaloosas, but also having been found in draft breeds and warm bloods.

Diagnosis

- Exercise tolerance test with serum CK evaluated at baseline and after 15 min of trotting.
- Genetic testing of whole blood sample (PSSM type 1).
- Evaluation and testing of muscle biopsies (see Chapter 7, Diagnostic Procedures) for PSSM type 2.
- Fractional electrolyte excretion testing for Na, K, Cl, Ca, Mg, PO4.
- It is also recommended to concurrently test serum vitamin E and selenium.

Treatment

During or after individual episodes of rhabdomyolysis, there should be cessation of exercise and rest for at least 24 hr. Provide fresh water and electrolytes. Consult a veterinarian regarding the possibility of administration of anti-inflammatories. Discontinue any grain supplements until return to normal function. After 24 hr, provide small paddock turnout and gradually reintroduce exercise.

Severe episodes may require supportive care, including intravenous fluid therapy and intravenous anti-inflammatories.

Recovery

Elimination of the disease is not possible, as it is a hereditary myopathy.

Zoonotic Potential

No zoonotic potential.

Genetic Prevalence

PSSM type 1 has been confirmed as a dominant genetic trait transmissible to offspring. PSSM type 2 is still being researched, although initial research indicated similar genetic links.

Preventative

Development of this disease is unavoidable in horses that carry the genes; however, severe episodes can be minimized with regular daily exercise and a diet low in starch and high in fat. Frequency of episode occurrences appears to be decreased in horses housed outdoors where they can move about freely throughout the day.

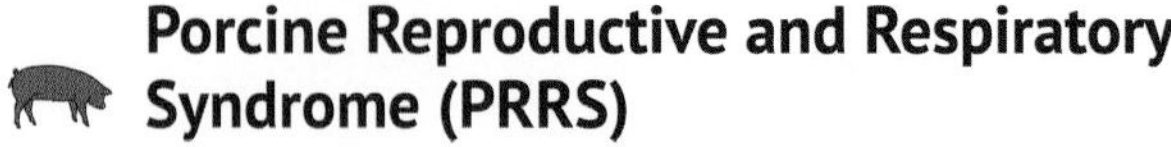

Porcine Reproductive and Respiratory Syndrome (PRRS)

Definition

Contagious viral disease of swine that causes interstitial pneumonia in all ages and affects the reproductive systems of mature swine.

Cause

Porcine reproductive and respiratory syndrome virus (PRRSv), an enveloped virus of the family *Arteriviridae*.

Systems Affected

Respiratory, reproductive, and occasionally vascular.

Transmission

Aerosol, fomite (i.e. dirty trailer), and vector (e.g. needle, biting insects).

> **TECHNICIAN TIP 12.62:** Aerosol, fomites, and vectors are the primary transmission modes for PRRSv.

Signs

Suckling piglets may exhibit respiratory distress, but in otherwise healthy herds, most commonly present with nonresponsive diarrhea and high mortality. Nursery and finishing pigs experience transient fevers, pneumonia, and increased susceptibility to secondary infections. Depending on strain severity and coinfections, mortality from acute and chronic infections in growing and finishing pigs may increase 2–10%. With some strains, vasculitis in the ear pinnae results in a bluish appearance, although this is more common with European strains (where the disease is also referred to as "blue-eared pig disease"). Sexually mature boars may shed PRRSv in semen from days to months postinfection. The sow herd may experience rolling anorexia as well as abortions (possibly due to fever), preterm farrowings (day 108–111), stillbirths, mummies, or weak-born piglets – some of which may be viremic.

Onset

In naïve sow populations, outbreaks are identifiable within 7–14 days of the index animals displaying clinical signs.

Prevalence/Geographical Distribution

Worldwide, except Australia and New Zealand.

Diagnosis

PRRSv can be detected through PCR or virus isolation on serum, semen, tissue homogenate, or oral fluids, or immunofluorescence on histopathology. Serology is used to detect antibodies to the virus.

Treatment

Treatment is limited to supportive care including antipyretics (such as liquid aspirin) and prevention of secondary infections.

Recovery

The majority of nursery and finisher pigs recover within two to three weeks assuming uncomplicated infection, although a small number of animals may continue to shed virus for months post infection. Sow herd outbreaks typically last three to four months (enough time for every sow to farrow once), with ongoing low-level infection persisting thereafter unless a herd cleanup strategy is employed. Cleanup strategies include herd closure, whole-herd vaccination, and depopulation/repopulation.

Zoonotic Potential

Experimental infection of mallards.

Genetic Prevalence

No genetic prevalence known.

Prevention

Only PRRSv-naïve genetic material (gilts, boars, and semen) should be brought into sow herds or used to establish new herds. Potential breeding stock should be isolated a minimum of 21 days and verified PRRSv-naïve prior to entry. Farm biosecurity practices should be designed to prevent exposure of animals to PRRSv-containing material (such as manure, arthropods, and airborne particles) and to eliminate all unnecessary traffic.

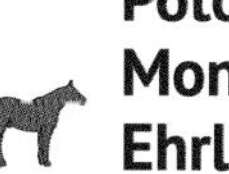

Potomac Horse Fever (a.k.a. Equine Monocytic Ehrlichiosis, Equine Ehrlichial Colitis, Ditch Fever, PHF)

Cause

Neorickettsia risticii (formerly, *Ehrlichia risticii*).

Systems Affected

Gastrointestinal tract (small and large colon).

Transmission

Known to be associated with pastures bordering creeks or rivers that carry freshwater snails and isolates from trematodes released from the snails.

Symptoms

Clinical signs are variable but may include:

- Lethargy or depression
- Fever
- Mild to severe diarrhea
- Laminitis
- Mild colic or abdominal discomfort
- Decreased abdominal sounds
- Late-term abortion (though uncommon)

Onset

This disease is generally seasonal, occurring between late spring and early fall in temperate areas. Most cases occur during the onset of hot weather in July, August, and September. The incubation period ranges from 10 to 18 days.

Prevalence/Geographical Distribution

This disease originated by the Potomac River but has since expanded to other areas of the United States and Canada.

Diagnosis

Primarily based on season, geographical location, and clinical signs.

- There is a high prevalence of false positive serological testing.
- A definitive diagnosis of PHF should be based on isolation or detection of *N. risticii* from the blood or feces of infected horses.

- Newly developed real-time PCR assay allows the detection of *N. risticii* DNA within 2 hr using both a blood and fecal sample.

Treatment

Oxytetracycline is the antibiotic recommended for this type of infection for a minimum of five days. Additional supportive therapies including intravenous fluids and anti-inflammatories may also be warranted. Due to the related clinical symptoms of the disease, secondary concerns such as laminitis should be considered.

Recovery

Early recognition and treatment will result in a quick recovery. Delay in treatment can complicate symptoms and prolonged recovery.

Zoonotic Potential

No zoonotic potential.

Genetic Prevalence

No genetic prevalence known.

Preventative

Commercial killed adjuvanted vaccine products are available as stand-alone vaccines or in combination with rabies vaccination. Initial inoculation should be followed up with a booster. Thereafter, annual vaccination is recommended every 6–12 months, depending on risk of exposure in the environment.

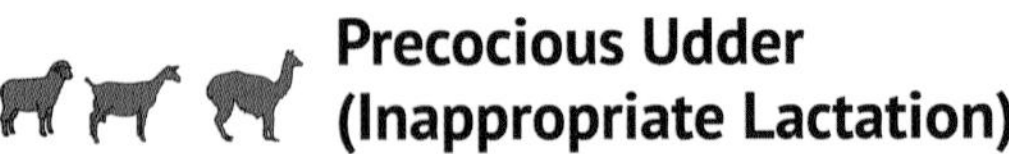

Precocious Udder (Inappropriate Lactation)

Definition

Inappropriate development and spontaneous lactation of nulliparous or unbred female small ruminants, predominantly goats.

Cause

Not all causes are known, however, the following have been implicated in cases of inappropriate lactation of small ruminants: hormonal influences from onset of puberty in high-producing dairy breeds, endocrine tumors (or removal of endocrine tumors), pseudopregnancy, or consumption of estrogenic feed stuff.

Systems Affected

Mammary and reproductive.

Transmission

A decrease in progesterone with an increase in prolactin is necessary for lactogenesis.

Signs

Udder enlargement, spontaneous lactation in spite of lack of parturition.

Onset

Acute.

Prevalence/Geographical Distribution

Prevalence in the pet goat population and in high-producing dairy goats. Distribution is worldwide.

Diagnosis

Physical exam. Diagnostic ultrasound and hormone assays may demonstrate the presence of an endocrine mass.

Treatment

Removal of hormone producing mass. Decrease consumption of feeds and grain that promote milk production. Use of antiprolactin drugs (dopamine agonists) has limited efficacy. Do not milk, rather treat for mastitis prevention and allow to dry off. Mastectomy may be necessary; however, these animals should not be bred postmastectomy, as there is a documented predilection toward prolonged parturition and dystocia. Also, there is an increased rate of FPT for the newborn kids if colostrum supplementation is not available.

Prevention

Do not feed moldy grain or legumes, as they are estrogenic.

Recovery

Dependent on success of the treatment.

Zoonotic Potential

No zoonotic potential.

Genetic Prevalence

Yes, in high-producing dairy goat lines.

Prevention

None.

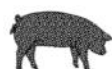 Pseudorabies (PRV, Aujeszky's Disease)

Definition

Highly contagious herpes virus infection of swine.

Cause

Pseudorabies virus of the family *Herpesviridae*.

Systems Affected

Nervous, lymphatic, respiratory.

Transmission

Nose-to-nose or fecal-oral.

Signs

Mortality approaches 100% in young piglets, with suckling piglets displaying neurological signs, including shaking and paddling in lateral recumbency. Nursery pigs are more likely to exhibit sneezing and labored breathing along with moderate fever; mortality can reach 50%. Finisher pig and sow mortality is minimal.

Onset

Incubation period is short, with viral shedding observed in all body fluids within two to five days of infection.

Prevalence/Geographical Distribution

Worldwide, with exceptions of Canada, Australia, and Africa, and domestic swine in the United States.

Diagnosis

Characteristic lesions on histopathology along with virus isolation, PCR, immunofluorescence, and serology able to distinguish vaccine from field infection are diagnostic.

Treatment

In the United States, pseudorabies is a federally regulated disease, with treatment and control directed by federal authorities. In countries with endemic PRV, vaccine can be used to reduce shedding and improve survival.

> **TECHNICIAN TIP 12.63:** In the United States, pseudorabies is a federally regulated disease.

Recovery

Although clinical recovery occurs, latent PRV infections remain in nervous tissue.

Zoonotic Potential

Cattle, sheep, goats, dogs, cats, raccoons, skunks, opossums, and other rodents are dead-end hosts (become infected and exhibit neurologic signs but cannot shed virus).

Genetic Prevalence

None.

Prevention

Introduce only PRV-negative animals into herds; prevent contact with feral swine, and use vaccine where PRV is endemic.

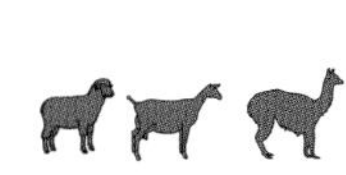 Pulpy Kidney Disease (Type D Enterotoxemia, Overeating Disease)

Definition

A clostridial disease that causes enterotoxemia primarily in small ruminants.

Cause

C. perfringens type D.

Systems Affected

Gastrointestinal, neurological, and systemic.

Transmission

C. perfringens type D is considered a normal flora of the GI tract in ruminants. Problems occur when animals consume large quantities of feed resulting in an overgrowth of the organism and subsequent endotoxin production.

> **TECHNICIAN TIP 12.64:** Pulpy kidney disease occurs when animals consume large quantities of feed resulting in an overgrowth of *C. perfringens* type D and subsequent endotoxin production.

Signs

Sudden death, acute neurological signs, ± diarrhea.

Onset

Acute in young; peracute to chronic in goats.

Prevalence/Geographical Distribution

Most common among large single, fit lambs, or feeder lambs when switched to grower rations.

Diagnosis

Identification of toxin in GI fluid during necropsy.

Treatment

No treatment.

Prevention

Vaccination of dams prior to parturition.

Recovery

None.

Zoonotic Potential

No zoonotic potential.

Genetic Prevalence

No genetic prevalence known.

Prevention

Vaccination of dams prior to parturition and/or vaccination of lambs/kids prior to being placed on high plain of nutrition (feedlot, grower scenario).

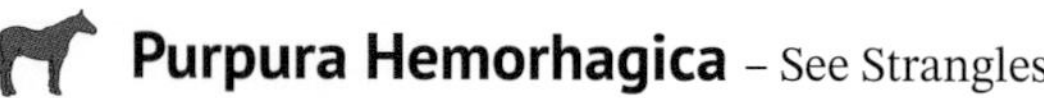

Purpura Hemorhagica – See Strangles

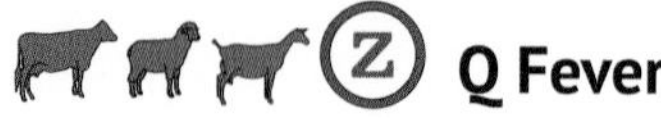

Q Fever

Definition

A zoonotic disease capable of causing abortions in cattle, sheep, and goats.

Cause

Coxiella burnetii, an obligate intracellular rickettsia.

> **TECHNICIAN TIP 12.65:** Q Fever is caused by *C. burnetii*.

Transmission

Aerosolization. Cattle, sheep, and goats are the primary reservoirs of the organism. A high concentration of the organism is found in fetuses and fetal membranes, and fluids, placenta, milk, feces, and urine of symptomatic and asymptomatic animals. Ticks can contribute in spreading the infection. The organism is very resistant in the environment and contaminated material, beddings, wool, and so forth, provide a source of aerosol infection to humans.

Signs

The infection is usually asymptomatic in cattle, sheep, and goats. Clinical disease is characterized by placentitis and abortions.

Late-term abortions or weak newborn lambs can be seen in affected flocks during a two- to four-week period. Up to 50% of the flock may abort during an outbreak. The placenta of aborted does and ewes present a characteristic thickening with white to soft gray plaques and brown exudates.

Onset

Acute to chronic.

Prevalence/Geographical Distribution

A prevalent disease with worldwide distribution.

Diagnosis

Complement fixation tests.

Treatment

Tetracyclines are used to treat the disease in small ruminants and humans.

Recovery

Infected animals are usually asymptomatic. A carrier state can occur after an abortion. Goats are more likely to abort in subsequent pregnancies compared to sheep.

Zoonotic Potential

Personnel in contact with cattle and small ruminants (veterinarians, technicians, and farm workers) are at risk. Consumption of raw milk is an additional risk for human infection. Affected people usually recover after treatment, although granulomatous hepatitis, pneumonia, myocarditis, and neurologic damage can occur.

Genetic Prevalence

No genetic prevalence known.

Prevention

Proper disposal of aborted fetuses and placentas of affected animals. Awareness in veterinarians of potential exposure during obstetric procedures and in people of the risk associated with consuming unpasteurized milk or milk products.

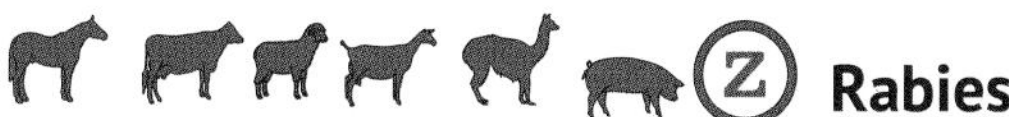

Rabies

Cause

Rabies is a viral disease of the family *Rhabdoviridae* affecting the CNS. Feral reservoir hosts primarily propagate the disease with occasional transmission to domestic animals. Typical reservoir hosts in the United States include raccoons, skunks, bats, and foxes.

Transmission

Rabies is spread by exposure to infected saliva, usually through a bite wound or saliva penetration of an open wound on the body. Transmission via mucous membranes is possible but rare. Wild animals accounted for 92% of reported cases of rabies in 2010. The Centers for Disease Control and Prevention report that, in 2010, 36.5% of all reported cases were raccoons, with most of the remainder consisting of skunks, bats, and foxes. Other wild animals, including rodents, only account for 1.8%. Once an animal has been inoculated, the virus travels via the nervous system to the brain. Once the disease reaches the brain, death is imminent within days.

Signs

Signs vary greatly between patients, especially those exhibiting early signs. Clinical signs may include lameness, fever, anorexia, blindness, dysphagia, hypersensitivity, muscle twitching, paralysis, ataxia, incontinence, self-mutilation, or death. The equine patient may exhibit colic signs while the ruminant may exhibit bloat. There are three different forms that may be exhibited: furious, paralytic, and dumb forms.
Furious form:
Patients showing these signs are often dangerous, exhibiting very aggressive behaviors such as charging the stall door without provocation.
Dumb form:
Also referred to as *paralytic form* and often presents as lethargy with excessive salivation.
Paralytic form:
Patients exhibit lameness, ataxia, and weakness that progress to paralysis and recumbency within days.

Onset

Rabies may initially be difficult to diagnose as it mimics other large animal diseases. The more the disease progresses, the more severe the symptoms; this allows other diseases on the differential diagnosis list to be ruled out.

Prevalence/Geographical Distribution

In 2006, there were 547 cases of rabies reported in domestic animals. Horses and mules accounted for 53 of these cases. In recent years, the number of equid cases has decreased; there were 37 cases in 2010. Cases of rabies occur worldwide, except in Hawaii, Australia, New Zealand, the British Isles, and Japan, among others.

> **TECHNICIAN TIP 12.66:** In the United States, 547 cases of rabies were reported in domestic animals in 2006.

Diagnosis

Incubation period is variable but usually is three to eight weeks from the time of patient exposure. Patients exhibiting symptoms for longer than 10 days can generally have rabies ruled out. Clients should be questioned on vaccination status, how the patient is housed, and potential for exposure to species that carry the rabies virus. No antemortem test can be performed to confirm a rabies diagnosis. History is an important part of diagnosis. Postmortem examination of the brain using immunofluorescence is necessary to confirm diagnosis.

Treatment

There is neither adequate treatment nor a cure for rabies.

Prognosis

Rabies is a universally fatal disease and affected patients die within days.

Zoonotic Potential

- Rabies is zoonotic and has the potential to affect any mammal.
- Persons in contact with a suspect rabies patient must take precautions to limit exposure. Appropriate precautions include the use of gloves and facemasks.
- Animals showing acute neurologic signs should be considered rabies suspects, particularly in the absence of appropriate vaccination history.

Predispositions

There are no known gender, age, or breed predilections. All mammals are susceptible.

Prevention

There are commercial inactivated vaccines that are available for use in horses and livestock in the United States. Horses should receive vaccinations annually after an initial series.

When handling an animal that is suspected of having rabies, personal protective equipment (PPE) of gloves and protective eye wear must be worn by all personnel. A written record should be established for all personnel who come in contact with the patient. Equipment exposed to the patient with potential rabies can be processed using a standard decontamination process and common disinfectants, which will inactivate the virus.

Vaccination against rabies is generally recommended and sometimes required by institutions for individuals working with animals. It is recommended to recheck antibody titers approximately every two years to evaluate an individual's titer levels. Only personnel that have protective titer levels should be allowed to work with rabies suspect patients.

Any individual who has been potentially exposed (through bites or contact with saliva on cuts or mucous membranes) to a confirmed case of rabies should seek attention from a medical doctor as soon as possible. This applies to vaccinated persons as well.

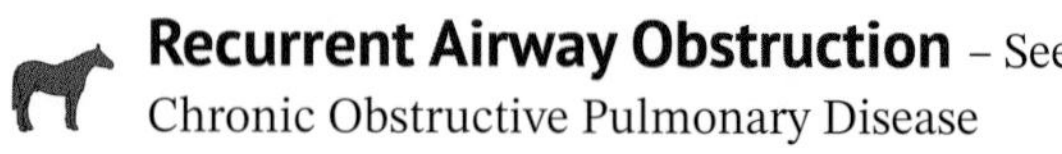

Recurrent Airway Obstruction – See Chronic Obstructive Pulmonary Disease

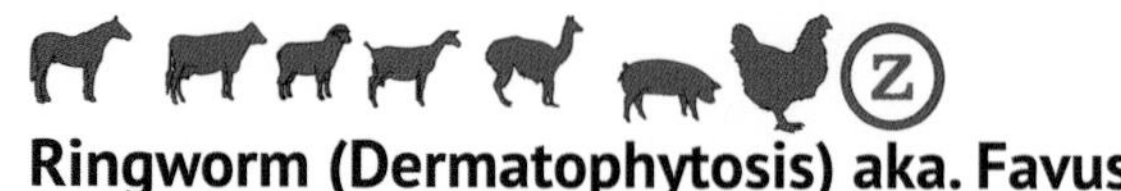

Ringworm (Dermatophytosis) aka. Favus

Definition

A non-pruritic, contagious, fungal infection of the stratus corneum of the skin, causing damage to the hair shaft and alopecia.

Cause

Trichophyton verrucosum (the most common organism), and *Trichophyton mentagrophytes.*

Transmission

By direct contact or indirect contact through fomites, such as feed bunks, fences, and so forth. Host and environmental factors play a role in the development of the disease. Young animals are more predisposed to develop clinical signs, and warm and humid weather play a role in the incidence of the disease. The condition is more prevalent in winter months.

Lanolin prevents fungal invasion of the skin of sheep, which explains the low prevalence of the disease in this species. Show lambs that are sheared short are predisposed to the disease.

Signs

Circular alopecic areas starting on the face and around the eyes, spreading to the head, neck, and shoulder. The lesions appear dry and crusty with desquamation and alopecia (Figure 12.30).

In sheep, lesions in wooled regions are characterized by hyperemic areas in the skin that are covered by matted wool. Lesions in hairy areas are similar to those of cattle (i.e. circular, alopecic, and crusty patches). When it affects poultry, it can also be referred to as "favus." Owners need to

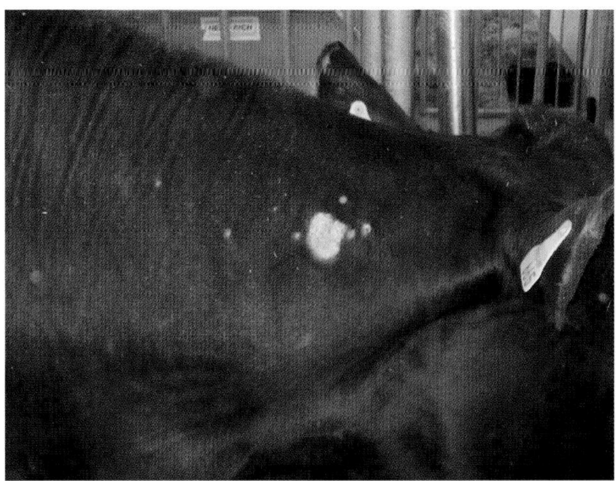

Figure 12.30 A typical dermatophytosis lesion on the right cervical area of a cow. Most ringworm lesions are from the genus *Trichophyton*. *Source:* Reproduced with permission of Dr. Kamal Gabadage.

be diligent about their hand washing and handling practices to avoid also contracting it from their birds. Other birds within the flock are also at risk of contracting it. Ringworm on chickens is most commonly seen on the comb, head and neck areas as scaly or crusty patches. The disease is usually self-limiting.

Onset

Acute.

Prevalence/Geographical Distribution

A very common disease of cattle, less common in goats, and rare in sheep, with a worldwide distribution.

Diagnosis

Clinical signs, fungal culture, and direct microscopy of hair.

Treatment

Local treatment with antifungals such as enilconazole (available in Canada and Europe) is effective. Other topical treatment options include lime sulfur 2–5% and 0.5% sodium hypochlorite.

Recovery

Spontaneous regression can occur in approximately one to four months.

Zoonotic Potential

This disease can affect humans with heightened risks for immune-suppressed individuals.

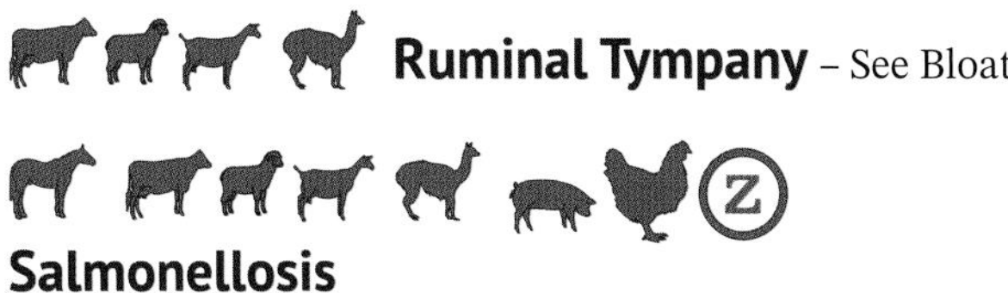

TECHNICIAN TIP 12.67: Ringworm can affect immune-suppressed individuals.

Genetic Prevalence

No genetic prevalence known.

Prevention

Isolation of affected animals is recommended to limit the spread of the disease. A cattle vaccine against *T. verrucosum* is available is Europe.

Ruminal Tympany – See Bloat

Salmonellosis

Definition

Contagious bacterial disease caused by *Salmonella* spp.

Cause

Salmonella cholerasuis is associated with septicemia and enteritis; *Salmonella typhimurium* is predominantly associated with enteritis.

Systems Affected

Gastrointestinal, vascular.

Transmission

Fecal-oral.

Signs

With *S. cholerasuis* infection, pigs experience profound fever (up to 108 °F), with or without diarrhea, cyanosis of extremities including the ears, inappetence, and reluctance to move. With *S. typhimurium* infection, profound enterocolitis and diarrhea develop. On necropsy, button ulcers may be found in the cecum, and enteric lymph nodes will be markedly enlarged.

Onset

Clinical signs appear within 24–48 hr of exposure.

Prevalence/Geographical Distribution

Worldwide distribution.

Diagnosis

Isolation of *Salmonella spp.* from fecal culture, mesenteric lymph nodes, or tissue homogenate, or demonstration of characteristic lesions on histopathology is diagnostic.

Treatment

Antibiotics may be administered according to culture sensitivity.

Recovery

Recovery is dependent on age of the animal, level of exposure and ongoing exposure, and effectiveness of treatment. In severe outbreaks, mortality and culls can exceed 20%.

Zoonotic Potential

Salmonella can infect humans, cattle, horses, rodents, birds, and other species. The most common occurrence of this is the handling of baby chicks. Humans can get sick from *Salmonella* by touching live poultry or their environment the chickens live in. Ways to protect yourself from these most common bacterial diseases are washing your hands every time you come in contact with live poultry and their environment.

> **TECHNICIAN TIP 12.68:** Prevention strategies for Salmonellosis include vaccination, vermin control, disinfection, and other management practices.

Genetic Prevalence

No genetic prevalence known.

Prevention

Vaccines are available for use where facilities do not permit removal of exposure sources. Do not allow birds and rodents access to feed. Thoroughly clean and disinfect housing between groups to prevent exposure to fecal-contaminated surfaces. Procure *Salmonella*-free breeding stock. Do not feed uncooked garbage to swine.

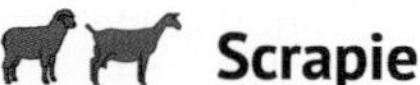 Scrapie

Definition

Transmissible spongiform encephalopathy of goats and sheep.

Cause

Prion protein.

Systems Affected

Central nervous system.

Transmission

From the placenta to the lamb/kid, however, not in utero as C-section lambs to scrapie dams do not contract the disease. Scrapie can be spread via blood transfusion or sheep-to-sheep contact. In goats, scrapie occurs spontaneously. In infected sheep, scrapie prions have also been found in milk and urine.

Signs

The clinical signs for scrapie are variable between animals. Although infected at a young age, the clinical signs do not develop until animals are two to five years old. Damage to the nervous system causes behavioral changes that include tremors, rubbing or scratching, abnormal gait, and ataxia, which progresses with the disease process and may become more pronounced when the animal is stressed. In the final stages, animals may become recumbent and have convulsive type activity before death occurs.

Onset

Chronic, slow progressive disease. It takes years until the animals exhibit the first clinical signs.

Prevalence/Geographical Distribution

The predominant breed of sheep affected is Suffolk; however, other purebred and crossbred sheep are susceptible. Scrapie is found worldwide with the exception of New Zealand and Australia.

Diagnosis

History and clinical signs play a role in the diagnosis. Definitive diagnosis: presence of scrapie prion.

- Live animals – biopsy of lymph tissue from the inside of the third eyelid.
- Dead animals – histological examination of the brain.

Treatment

There is no treatment for scrapie.

Recovery

None.

Zoonotic Potential

No zoonotic potential.

Genetic Prevalence

Certain alleles (amino acid sequences) at codon 171 (a specific point on the DNA) have been recognized as being linked to a sheep's susceptibility or resistance to scrapie. These alleles are known as "Q" and "R." Animals acquire one allele from each parent. With respect to scrapie, the most susceptible coding is "QQ," while the most resistant is "RR."

Prevention

No vaccine is available. Genetic strengthening of a flock or herd may be accomplished by using an "RR" ram. This will create a flock where all offspring are coded at least "QR," if not "RR." Replacement animals should be taken from this pairing. Ideally, ewes would also be tested and only "RR" animals are maintained. This is not a guarantee, but does increase the chances of resistance if the flock is challenged with the scrapie prion.

> **TECHNICIAN TIP 12.69:** Genetic strengthening of a flock or herd against scrapie may be accomplished by using an "RR" ram.

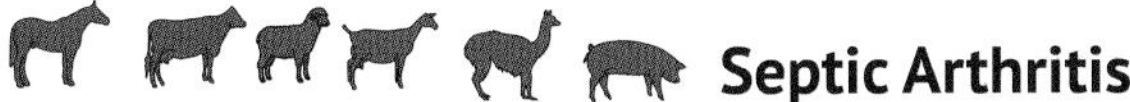

Septic Arthritis

Definition

Bacterial infection of the joint(s), most commonly in neonates, but can also occur in adults with penetrating joint trauma or sepsis.

> **TECHNICIAN TIP 12.70:** Septic arthritis affects neonates and adults, and its causation has many possible factors.

Cause

Multiple bacterial agents, ticks, trauma, septicemia.

Systems Affected

Skeletal, specifically joints.

Transmission

Bacterial infection, trauma, ticks.

Signs

Lameness, hot, swollen joints (usually, the carpus, tarsus, and stifle).

Onset

Acute and chronic.

Prevalence/Geographical Distribution

Primarily a neonatal problem across large animal species but can affect adults. Higher incidence among animals with FPT or omphalitis; also, can occur with penetrating trauma or septicemia.

Diagnosis

Culture and cytology of joint fluid.

Treatment

Culture and sensitivity results would dictate the appropriate antibiotic. Joint lavage may also be efficacious.

Recovery

Guarded, depends on the severity and response to treatment and early intervention.

Zoonotic Potential

No zoonotic potential.

Genetic Prevalence

No genetic prevalence known.

Prevention

Ensure passive transfer and maintain a clean environment for birthing.

Sheep and Goat Pox

Definition

A highly contagious group of viral diseases that affects multiple tissues.

> **TECHNICIAN TIP 12.71:** Sheep and goat pox is highly contagious and is reportable in the United States.

Cause

Capripoxvirus.

Systems Affected

Integument and mucous membranes of the respiratory, genital, and alimentary tracts.

Transmission

Variety of possible transmissions: the virus can remain in the environment for up to six months in shaded, protected spaces, and may remain virulent in the wool for up to three months. Infectious scabs may fall off and reinfest the environment.

- Animal-to-animal contact via the respiratory tract or through abrasions or other mucous membranes
- Fomite – contaminated articles
- Mechanical – stable flies

Signs

There is an incubation period of 4–21 days. Initial signs include a high fever, lethargy, anorexia, swollen lymph nodes, and nasal and ocular discharge. Skin lesions appear beginning as papules and progress into hard nodules that subsequently develop necrotic centers and finally scab over. The lesions are more common in the non-wool/hair areas, such as the axilla, ears, nose, lips, around the eyes, under the tail, teats, and udder. Young animals may die before reaching the skin lesion phase of the disease.

Internal lesions may occur resulting in clinical signs consistent with the system affected. Lesions in the respiratory tract will result in coughing, nasal discharge, and difficulty breathing; while lesions in the digestive tract may result in diarrhea, anorexia, and dehydration. Affected animals are predisposed to secondary bacterial infections such as pneumonia. Mild forms of the illness may affect adults in endemic areas.

Onset

Acute.

Prevalence/Geographical Distribution

North and Central Africa, Middle East, India, China, parts of the former Soviet Union, and sporadically in Europe. In the United States, this disease is considered an agent that could be used for agroterrorism and is reportable.

Diagnosis

Clinical signs and history; endemic in some areas. Disease is more severe in newly introduced animals than indigenous herds.

- Live animals – biopsy skin lesions for viral isolation; PCR – blood.
- Necropsy – collect and test lesions located on the skin, lymph nodes, respiratory tract, alimentary tract, and reproductive tract.

Treatment

There is no treatment. Animals may require supportive care for the viral disease and preventative care to avoid secondary infections.

Recovery

Depending on the naivety of the animal, there is a 30–50% mortality rate.

Zoonotic Potential

No zoonotic potential.

Genetic Prevalence

No genetic prevalence known.

Prevention

Vaccine available.

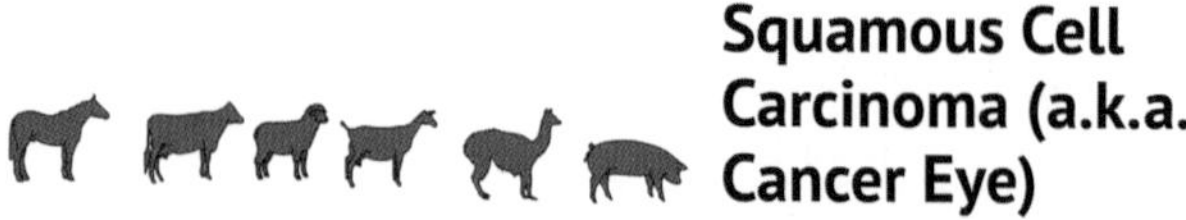

Squamous Cell Carcinoma (a.k.a. Cancer Eye)

Definition

A common ocular tumor affecting cattle in the United States and Canada, leading to carcass rejection, in addition to treatment and production losses.

Cause

Most common neoplasm of the head in horses and cattle. The tumor arises from epithelial surfaces of the conjunctiva or cornea. Pathophysiology is unknown with genetic, environment, and potential viral agents risk factors.

> **TECHNICIAN TIP 12.72:** Decreased pigmentation around the eyes and increased exposure to UV light are factors for ocular SCC formation.

Systems Affected

Can be local or disseminate/metastasize to other structures of the head and organs.

Signs

This disease can affect animals of varying breeds, ages, and genders. Tumors often start as small raised or ulcerated lesions around the eyelids, third eyelid, conjunctiva, or cornea. They appear discolored and may be white or reddened in appearance. Depending on malignancy, these tumors progress at variable rates and can invade into other ocular structures, other structure of the head or metastasize to other organs (rare). Clinical signs may be restricted to the tumors themselves, or more general including blepharospasm, redness, tearing, and tissue destruction. Swelling may be present as well as local tissue inflammation/ulceration (Figure 12.31).

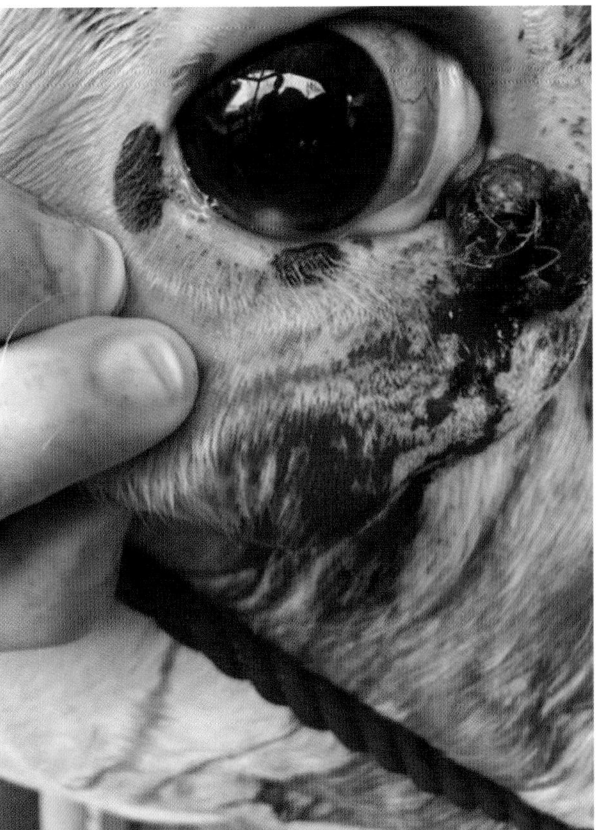

Figure 12.31 Bovine squamous cell carcinoma. *Source:* Photo courtesy of Lauren Hughes, DVM.

Onset

Acute to chronic.

Prevalence/Geographical Distribution

Prevalence is dependent on UV exposure, pigmentation, and genetics. Animals with a lack of pigment surrounding the eyes are at an increased risk including Hereford cattle, Paints, and Appaloosas. Worldwide distribution.

Diagnosis

Diagnosis is made off clinical signs, appearance, and histopathology of lesions. Imaging (x-rays, CT) can aid in determining the extent of lesions and lymph node aspirates can be performed if metastasize is suspected.

Differentials

Differentials would include trauma, infectious bovine keratoconjunctivitis, or additional neoplasms.

Treatment

Depending on the extent of the lesions, surgical removal may be curative. Multiple local therapies including cryotherapy, intralesional injections, photodynamic therapy, chemotherapeutic agents, or radiation have been used. Enucleation or exenteration may be warranted.

Associated Conditions

Squamous cell carcinomas are often aggressive, and locally invasive tumors that can affect other structures of the head and/or metastasize to other organs, although metastasis is rare.

Zoonotic Potential

No zoonotic potential.

Genetic Prevalence

Genetic association in Belgian horses and Haflingers has been documented.

Prevention

Protection from UV light is important and achieved through UV blocking face masks. Eyelids can also be tattooed but the efficacy of this is contemplated.

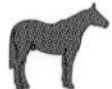 Strangles (Purpura Hemorrhagica)

Definition

Strangles is a highly contagious bacterial infection primarily affecting the upper respiratory tract.

Cause

Streptococcus equi subspecies *equi*.

Systems Affected

Primarily upper respiratory tract, occasionally may spread around the body by the hematogenous or lymphatic routes (bastard strangles).

Transmission

Highly contagious. Either by direct contact with nasal, ocular, or lymph node secretions from infected horses or by exposure to contaminated objects, including brushes, clothing, feed buckets, and equipment (including veterinary tools).

Bacteria are either inhaled or ingested and gain entry via the pharyngeal tonsil to the associated lymphoid tissue. Rapidly translocated to lymphatic system and draining lymph nodes. The complement system interacts with bacterial peptidoglycan and large numbers of neutrophils are attracted to the affected area leading to lymphadenitis and abscess formation. Virulence factors in the antiphagocytic capsule of the organism stimulate release of cytokines leading to inflammation. The incubation period is 2–10 days.

Signs

Horses are often pyrexic (103 °F or higher); show signs of lethargy; have serous nasal discharge that develops to mucopurulent. Mucopurulent ocular discharge may also occur. There is marked lymphadenopathy of the submandibular and retropharyngeal lymph nodes, initially they are firm, but become soft and apparently fluid filled before bursting. Retropharyngeal lymph nodes may rupture into guttural pouches: dysphagia, empyema, and chondroid formation. The lymphadenopathy can cause dysphagia, stridor, and potentially respiratory distress. May see a soft cough.

TECHNICIAN TIP 12.73: Strangles patients may have lymphadenopathy, which can cause dysphagia, stridor, and potentially respiratory distress.

Onset

Acute.

Prevalence/Geographical Distribution

Common in young horses (<five years) and on farms with a high number of horses arriving or leaving frequently. Usually occurs in young animals (one to five years of age), although it can affect any age or sex. Worldwide distribution.

Diagnosis

Diagnosis includes aspiration from an affected lymph node, nasopharyngeal swab, or lavage of the guttural pouch – culture and/or PCR. Serology includes SeM (*Streptococcus equi* M protein gene) specific antibody that is only useful to diagnose previous history of strangles infection, or with concerns about the development of purpura hemorrhagica or a bastard strangles abscess (Figure 12.32).

Lab work includes CBC (a marked neutrophilic leukocytosis, hyperfibrinogenemia, hyperglobulinemia, and occasionally anemia). Chemistry profiles are usually unremarkable.

Treatment

Treatment includes stopping all movement of horses on and off premises, identifying symptomatic and

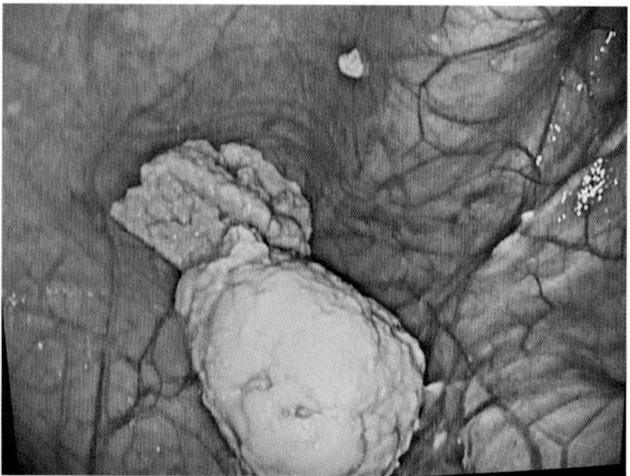

Figure 12.32 Mucopurulent substance seen in the guttural pouches on endoscopy.

asymptomatic carriers, isolating and treating infected horses, and monitoring the "in-contact" group (horses with no clinical signs but were close to the infected individuals – monitoring temperatures twice daily). Once signs have resolved via three negative nasopharyngeal swabs or a single negative guttural pouch wash, clean contaminated equipment and stalls with 1:200 dilution of phenol, povidone-iodine, chlorhexidine, and glutaraldehyde.

For horses showing clinical signs, treatment may include nonsteroidal anti-inflammatory drugs and hot pack for enlarged lymph nodes. Once lymph node abscesses are ready to burst, lance them to facilitate drainage.

For horses that are systemically ill, dysphagic, or in respiratory distress, treatment may include tracheotomy, procaine penicillin, or potassium penicillin, and treatment for secondary infections. Dysphagic may require intravenous fluid therapy ± nutritional support.

Horses with strangles complications (e.g. purpura hemorrhagica, bastard strangles) may need prolonged courses of systemic penicillin.

Recovery

Average course is usually 21–28 days; in the majority of horses, signs resolve and shedding ceases by four to six weeks. Contact horses may be assumed to be negative based on three nasopharyngeal swabs (taken seven days apart) or bilateral guttural pouch lavage (samples submitted for PCR and culture) – they then may be taken out of isolation. Complication rate is approximately 20%, mostly related to hematogenous or lymphatic spread. Complications include internal abscessation, purpura hemorrhagica-aseptic necrotizing vasculitis; if re-exposed to *S. equi* infection by vaccination or natural exposure, guttural pouch empyema, chondroid formation, and septicemia.

Zoonotic Potential

No zoonotic potential.

Genetic Prevalence

No genetic prevalence known.

Prevention

Vaccination – protein rich acid and enzyme extract product – administered parenterally or attenuated live *S. equi* via the intranasal route. Short-lived immunity: vaccinate high-risk horses every three months and normal horses every four months. Do not administer intranasal vaccination with other parenteral injections – can lead to abscessation.

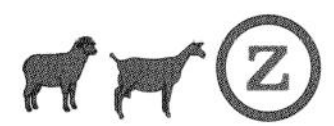

Streptococcal Infections

Definition

Bacterial infection by a member of the genus *Streptococcus*, a gram-positive coccus.

Causes

Streptococcus suis (most common) causes polyserositis and meningitis; *Streptococcus equisimilus* causes polyserositis and endocarditis; Group E *Streptococcus* can cause lymphadenitis and abscessed lymph nodes.

Systems Affected

Musculoskeletal, nervous, lymphatic.

Transmission

Colonization during passage through the birth canal, inhaled, contact with wound.

Signs

Str. suis type 1 and 2 presents most often as nursery pigs with meningitis with or without swollen joints. Pigs with meningitis are unable to stand and most often lie on their sides, neck arched and paddling. In more chronic infections, pigs become unthrifty and, upon necropsy, are found to have fibrin in their abdomen and/or pericardial sac. Occasionally, vegetative valvular endocarditis develops. Clinical signs are similar with *Str. equisimilus* but tend to be confined to the joints and heart. Group E Streps are potential causes of lymph node abscesses, particularly in the jowl region when pigs are exposed to abrasive feeders.

Onset

Streptococcal infections are rarely peracute. Untreated, meningitis infections persist four to seven days before pigs die. Chronic infections lead to unthriftiness and wasting.

Prevalence/Geographical Distribution

Worldwide distribution.

Diagnosis

Clinical signs with identification or isolation of gram-positive cocci from lesion sites.

Treatment

Streptococcal infections should be treated according to culture sensitivity, though they are generally responsive to penicillins and potentiated penicillins.

Recovery

For systemic infections, recovery rate varies according to duration and severity of infection. Acutely infected pigs generally respond well to treatment; chronically infected animals have poor prognosis. Strep infections walled in abscesses result in trim loss.

Zoonotic Potential

Humans and domesticated animals.

Genetic Prevalence

No genetic prevalence known.

Prevention

Minimize stresses that predispose (already colonized) animals to infections (i.e. poor ventilation, temperature extremes, etc.). Keep pens, feeders, and alleyways free of sharp edges that predispose pigs to skin cuts. Clipping of needle teeth may also be a source of bacteria introduction. Autogenous vaccines may be used in extreme cases.

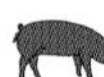

Swine Fever – See Hog Cholera

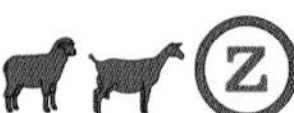

Swine Influenza

Definition

Contagious, highly infectious, and potentially zoonotic viral disease affecting the respiratory tract of swine.

Cause

Type A influenza virus of the family *Orthomyxoviridae*.

Systems Affected

Respiratory.

Transmission

Aerosol; nose-to-nose.

Signs

Pigs infected with influenza develop fever, sometimes in excess of 104 °F, temporary loss of appetite, and interstitial pneumonia that results in a “honking” type cough. Animals may also appear reluctant to move. On necropsy, affected lungs will be purple in color and heavy with fluid. Non-affected lung can be emphysematous. Trachea and bronchi contain excessive amounts of mucous, and local lymph nodes are swollen.

> **TECHNICIAN TIP 12.74:** Pigs infected with swine influenza develop fever, sometimes in excess of 104 °F.

Onset

Typical outbreaks occur quickly, with the entire herd displaying clinical signs within one to three days of infection. In the absence of secondary infections, pigs recover within a week, with a slight increase in mortality (1–4%) and abortions among bred animals spiking high fevers.

Prevalence/Geographical Distribution

Worldwide distribution.

Diagnosis

Clinical signs with histopathologic lesions and identification of viral antigen through virus isolation or PCR are diagnostic, although virus is usually only identifiable in acutely infected animals. Serology can be used to detect exposure.

Treatment

Treatment consists of minimizing additional stressors and prevention of secondary infections.

Recovery

Recovery is good in uncomplicated cases with minimal increases in mortality. A few animals may remain persistently affected and be a reservoir.

Zoonotic Potential

Birds and humans.

Genetic Prevalence

No genetic prevalence known.

Prevention

Killed vaccines are available. Prevent contact between pigs and birds, especially migrating waterfowl. Humans experiencing influenza should not work around naïve animals.

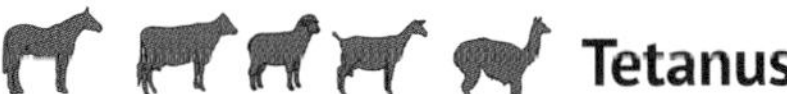 Tetanus

Definition

An infectious disease causing generalized muscular stiffness and death in multiple animal species, including cattle, horses, sheep, goats, and also humans.

Cause

Clostridium tetani, an anaerobic, spore-forming bacterium. The bacteria are commonly present in the intestinal contents of livestock and are ubiquitous in the soil. Horses are especially sensitive to the bacterium.

TECHNICIAN TIP 12.75: *Clostridium tetani* is an anaerobic, spore-forming bacterium.

Transmission

The organism can gain access through the uterus of cattle. Skin lesions or wounds caused by elastrator bands, tail docking, dehorning, puncture wounds to feet, and so forth are also ports of entry for the bacterium. Once the bacteria enter the host's tissue where anaerobic conditions exist, it transforms to a vegetative form and produces toxins (i.e. tetanospasmin, tetanolysin, and nonspasmogenic toxin) responsible for the tissue damage and neurologic clinical signs.

Signs

Affected animals initially show a stiff gait and extended head position, and by 24 hr a generalized spasticity becomes evident. The limbs are held in an extended and rigid position with the characteristic "saw horse" stance. The tail is seen elevated, and bloat is commonly noted. All the facial muscles are contracted causing the jaw to be shut very tightly (*trismus mandibularis*) and the lips to be held in a retracted position (*sardonic grin*). The ears are usually held caudally. Spastic muscular contractions can be triggered by mild tactile, auditory, or visual stimulation. Affected animals are unable to swallow, thus accumulation of frothy saliva is seen in the mouth, and aspiration pneumonia is a common complication. The respiratory muscles are also affected causing progressing hypoxemia with subsequent death (Figure 12.33).

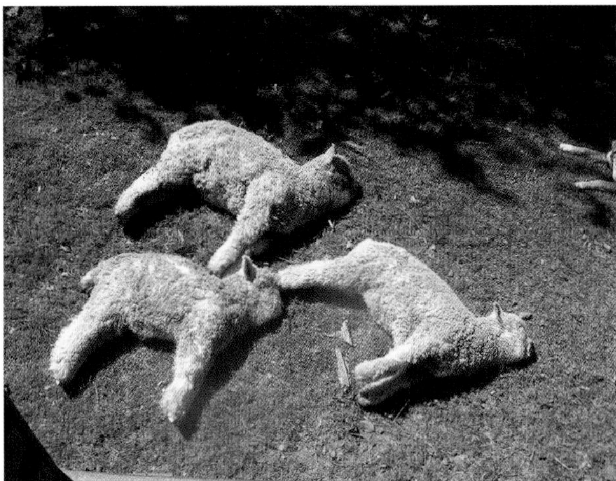

Figure 12.33 Typical tetanic posture in lambs affected by *Clostridium tetani*. *Source:* Reproduced with permission of Dr. Eduardo Battistessa.

Onset

Acute.

Prevalence/Geographical Distribution

A prevalent disease with a worldwide distribution.

Diagnosis

Clinical signs.

Treatment

Parenteral administration of tetanus antitoxin to neutralize the unbound toxin, tetanus toxoid to induce an active immune response, penicillin to eliminate the infection, and acetylpromazine or other sedatives to provide muscle relaxation and to reduce muscle spasms. Providing excellent footing and maintaining hydration and nutritional requirements are also very important components of the treatment protocol.

Recovery

The disease carries a poor prognosis. The faster the progression, the poorer the prognosis. Some animals may recover with aggressive and early treatment, but clinical signs may persist for a several weeks because of the irreversible binding of toxin to neurons. About half of the affected cattle die from the disease.

Zoonotic Potential

None, though tetanus affects animals and humans.

Genetic Prevalence

No genetic prevalence known.

Prevention

Vaccination is commonly performed in small ruminants and horses. Cattle are not regularly vaccinated because they seem more resistant to the disease compared to sheep, goats, and horses.

 Ulcerative Dermatosis

Definition

Highly contagious ulcerative disease of sheep, self-limiting.

Cause

Virus, related to, but distinct from, the *parapoxvirus*, which causes contagious ecthyma.

Systems Affected

Two scenarios:

- Integument of the face and limbs
- Reproductive – glans penis and vulva

Transmission

From direct contact, spread through flock by processing of animals when cuts or abrasions occur during shearing, or during breeding when animals may receive abrasions.

Signs

Ulcerative lesions with scabs not associated with mucocutaneous junctions, but on the lips, nose, eyelids, interdigital space, and above the coronary band. Also, the genital lesions affect the glans penis or the vulva.

Onset

Acute.

Prevalence/Geographical Distribution

In the United States, ulcerative dermatosis is most common in the western states.

Diagnosis

Via clinical signs and identification of lesions.

Treatment

Topical treatment for the lesions. Preventative measures to avoid secondary bacterial infections.

Recovery

Morbidity rate of 15–20%. Mortality rates are low in treated animals in otherwise good health.

Zoonotic Potential

No zoonotic potential.

Genetic Prevalence

No genetic prevalence known.

Prevention

None.

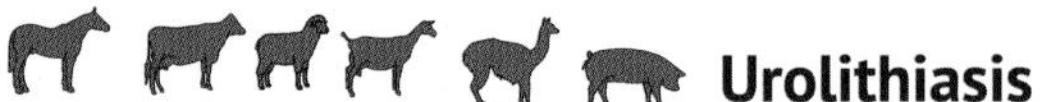 Urolithiasis

Definition

Urinary tract diseases caused by the development of urinary calculi.

Cause

Nutritional, environmental, and husbandry.

Systems Affected

Urinary tract.

Transmission

Crystal formation within the kidneys and urinary bladder caused by ingestion of high-concentrate feed, water, or various environmental factors (pasture). Alternate factors may include low water consumption, urinary pH, and other systemic disease factors that may affect mineral concentrations in urine production.

Signs

Urinary track obstruction. Most females pass the calculi without incident. However, males may be off-feed, colicky,

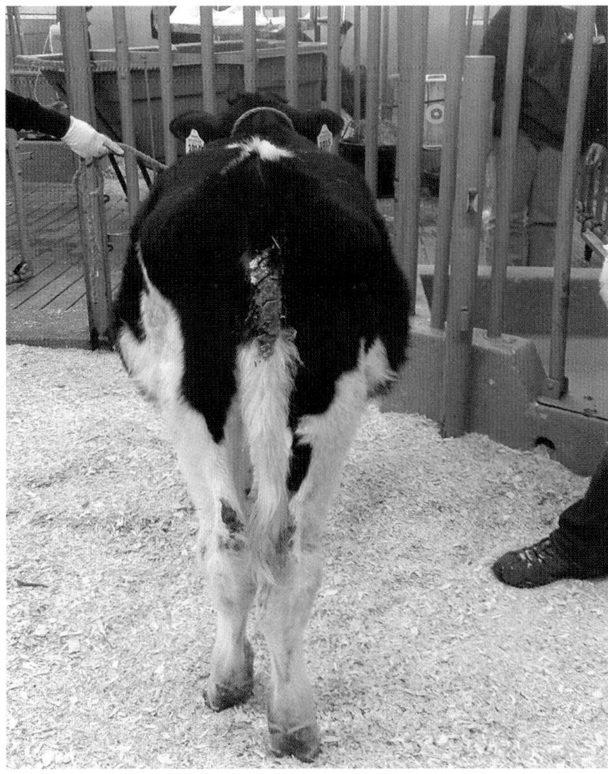

Figure 12.34 Abdominal distention in a six-month-old Holstein steer.

posturing to urinate without success, or have a small intermittent stream; they may be kicking at their belly, vocalizing, demonstrate bruxism, have prepucial swelling, or abdominal distention (Figure 12.34).

Onset

Subacute, acute.

Prevalence/Geographical Distribution

Urolithiasis is most commonly found in young, castrated male feeder animals or pets, but is also common in intact male small ruminants and South American Camelids due to anatomical narrowing of the urinary tract at the sigmoid flexure and urethral process. Distribution is worldwide.

> **TECHNICIAN TIP 12.76:** Urolithiasis is most commonly found in young, castrated male feeder animals or pets.

Diagnosis

Physical examination; clinical signs; presence of calculi; absence of urine; ultrasound demonstrating an enlarged bladder or ruptured bladder and uroabdomen; pulsation of the pelvic urethra upon rectal examination. Serum chemistries will demonstrate an increase in urea nitrogen and creatinine levels.

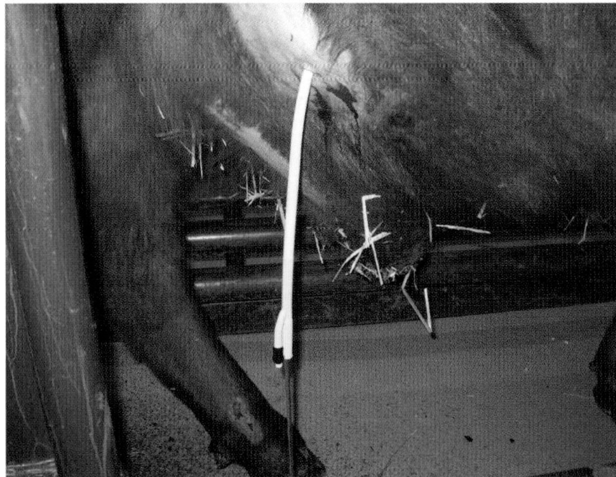

Figure 12.35 A steer affected by urolithiasis and uroperitoneum. Urine is being drained from the abdomen with a Foley catheter after abdominal drainage surgery was performed.

Treatment

Analgesics, muscle relaxants, and/or sedation, being careful to use products that will not promote urine production. Relieve the obstruction by amputating the urethral process, perineal urethrostomy, or tube cystotomy to remove offending calculi. Once the blockage is clear, fluid therapy to correct electrolyte imbalances, anti-inflammatory drugs to decrease swelling/inflammation, and antibiotics to prevent infection of traumatized tissues may be warranted (Figures 12.35 and 12.36).

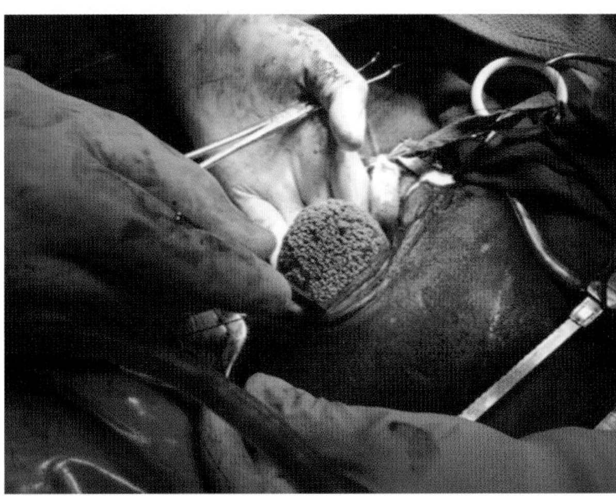

Figure 12.36 Bladder stone being surgically removed. *Source:* Photo courtesy of Lauren Hughes, DVM.

Prevention

Feed a balanced diet with a calcium phosphors ration of 1.2:1 to 2:1; provide salt supplementation to increase water intake.

Recovery

Surgical treatment of urolithiasis is considered a salvage procedure; the incidence of reoccurrence is high.

Zoonotic Potentia

No zoonotic potential.

Genetic Prevalence

No genetic prevalence known.

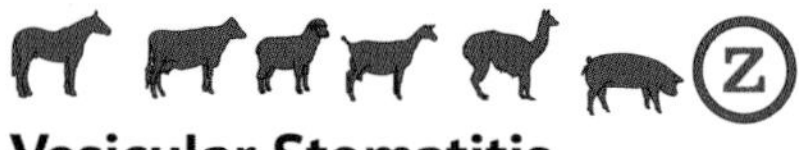

Vesicular Stomatitis

Definition

A viral vesicular disease affecting cattle, horses, sheep, goats, and swine. The disease is characterized by high morbidity and low mortality rates, and clinical signs are undistinguishable to those of FMD. In contrast to FMD, vesicular stomatitis can also affect horses.

Small ruminants are less susceptible to vesicular stomatitis compared to cattle.

Cause

Vesicular stomatitis virus (VSV), genus *Vesiculovirus*, family *Rhabdoviridae*, with two serotypes Indiana and New Jersey, is the causative agent.

Transmission

The virus is spread by aerosol and penetrates the oral mucosa and skin through abrasions or small injuries. Arthropod vectors are also thought to play a role in the transmission of the disease as well as a transovarian route.

Signs

Increased salivation, fever, severe lameness, and teat lesions are characteristic. Affected animals show vesicles in the oral cavity, coronary band, and teats. Vesicular lesions rupture leaving deep erosions with sloughed mucosa. Sheep and goats tend to develop mild lesions. Outbreaks in the United States usually occur in summer and fall.

Onset

Acute onset and may correspond to the rapidity of vesicle development.

Prevalence/Geographical Distribution

The disease is endemic in the southwest part of the United States, Central and South America.

Diagnosis

Clinical signs. In the United States and Canada, vesicular stomatitis is a reportable disease because of similarities to foreign animal diseases such as FMD, vesicular exanthema, and swine vesicular disease. Complement fixation and fluorescent antibody staining are used for diagnosis.

> **TECHNICIAN TIP 12.77:** Vesicular stomatitis is a reportable disease in the United States and Canada.

Treatment

There is no specific treatment. Prevention of secondary infections in rupture vesicle sites is important.

Recovery

Good. Most animals recover in less than two weeks, but viral recrudescence is possible. Economic losses occur because of the risk of mastitis in dairy cattle as a consequence of incomplete milk-out due to painful teats.

Zoonotic Potential

Humans may become infected and develop clinical disease (i.e. headache, fever, and muscular aches).

Genetic Prevalence

No genetic prevalence known.

Prevention

Restrict animal movement in and out of outbreak areas. Clean and disinfect vehicles, trailers, and other potential fomites. Vaccines are also available.

Warts (Cutaneous Papillomas)

Definition

A viral disease of the skin affecting cattle, and less frequently goats and sheep.

Cause

Species-specific papilloma viruses (papovaviruses). More than 10 bovine strains are recognized and named BPV-1 through BPV-10, and 1 strain is recognized in goats and sheep.

> **TECHNICIAN TIP 12.78:** More than 10 bovine strains of bovine papilloma virus are recognized and named BPV-1 through BPV-10.

Transmission

The virus can be transmitted directly (direct contact between animals), or indirectly by fomites (e.g. tattooing, tagging, and dehorning instruments).

Signs

Single or multiple small, white, or tan, protruding masses in the skin. The disease usually affects young animals. Warts also occur on the teats of adult cattle and goats, and predisposes to mastitis.

Onset

Acute.

Prevalence/Geographical Distribution

A prevalent disease with a worldwide distribution.

Diagnosis

Clinical signs.

Treatment

There is no effective treatment.

Recovery

In general, warts spontaneously regress in 4–12 months with no clinical significance.

Zoonotic Potential

No zoonotic potential.

Genetic Prevalence

No genetic prevalence known.

Prevention

Disinfect tattooing, dehorning, and tagging instruments between animals, and isolate affected animals. Autogenous vaccines have variable efficacy.

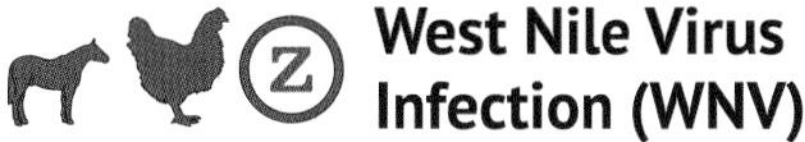

West Nile Virus Infection (WNV)

Definition

West Nile virus (WNV) is a viral disease that causes inflammation of the CNS (encephalomyelitis).

Cause

WNV is caused by a flavivirus. The disease was foreign to the United States prior to 1999.

Transmission

Transmission involves a life cycle that includes a reservoir host and a vector species. A reservoir host is an animal that can amplify the virus. Many species of birds are capable of functioning as reservoir hosts, including crows, American robins, and house sparrows. The vector species can feed off the reservoir's blood, thus becoming a carrier of the virus. *Culex* spp. mosquitos are the vector species responsible for spreading WNV. Once the vector species is infected, it is able to infect other susceptible animals via subsequent blood feeding. Both horses and humans can be affected by WNV but are considered "dead-end" hosts. This means that the virus does not replicate in their body to an extent that it will infect vectors.

Onset/Signs

Viremia occurs three to five days after initial inoculation. Initial signs that occur during viremia are nonspecific and may include dullness, inappetence, and fever. It has been estimated that approximately 10% of infected horses will develop neurologic signs due to translocation of the virus into the CNS. Neurologic signs occur 7–10 days after inoculation. Signs consistent with WNV encephalomyelitis include ataxia, weakness, and muscle fasciculations. Changes in behavior and mentation (hyperexcitability or somnolence) are occasionally noted. Neurologic deficits can be asymmetric. Ataxia and weakness might progress to recumbency.

> **TECHNICIAN TIP 12.79:** Approximately 10% of WNV-infected horses will develop neurologic signs due to translocation of the virus into the CNS.

Prevalence/Geographical Distribution

Because transmission of the virus requires a vector, a reservoir incidence of the disease is seasonal (late summer until early autumn) in temperate regions. Transmission may be year-round in tropical and subtropical climates. WNV has been reported in all 48 contiguous states of the United States.

Diagnosis

A diagnosis of WNV is considered in endemic areas at the time of year the disease is expected to occur. Signs supporting a diagnosis of WNV include a history of recent fever combined with an onset of neurologic disease. Fine muscle fasciculations, or tremors, are a common component of WNV encephalomyelitis. Consideration of other risk factors (vaccination status and exposure to mosquitos) is also important if WNV encephalomyelitis is suspected.

CBC and serum chemistry are generally unremarkable, although a low lymphocyte count may be present. Increased total protein and white blood cell count are common on CSF analysis. Testing of serum ± CSF via WNV IgM capture ELISA is recommended to determine if recent exposure has occurred; preexisting titers from vaccines should not interfere with interpretation of this test.

Treatment

Therapy is primarily supportive in nature. West Nile virus-specific hyperimmune plasma is available in the United States as a treatment for the disease, but its efficacy has not been proven. Corticosteroids, such as dexamethasone, are often recommended to decrease inflammation in the CNS, but their use remains controversial. Mannitol or DMSO may be used when cerebral edema is suspected. Management of a recumbent horse may become necessary.

Prognosis

Severity of disease is quite variable. It is estimated that disease progresses to recumbency in 30–40% of affected horses. The majority of these horses are euthanized or die. Horses that remain standing are expected to improve within three to seven days of onset of clinical signs. Approximately 90% of these horses are expected to make a good recovery, although residual ataxia or weakness may persist.

Zoonotic Potential

WNV is a disease that can infect humans, but there is little risk of transmission directly from horses to humans. There is a possibility of transmission from inappropriate handling of infected tissues on postmortem examination. PPE should be worn when handling potentially infected tissues.

Prevalence/Geographical Distribution

Identified risk factors include vaccination status, turnout at dusk and dawn, season, residence in an endemic area, and the status of mosquito control programs. Horses are considered the primary livestock species susceptible to WNV, but the disease has been reported in camelids and sheep.

Prevention

Vaccination is recommended once to twice annually depending on geographic location. Management of the environment is another important means of prevention. Methods include elimination of standing water (change water tanks at least once weekly) and limiting turnout of horses at dusk and dawn. Likewise, treatment of the environment with insecticides is a means of reducing breeding of mosquitos that will, in turn, limit spread of the virus.

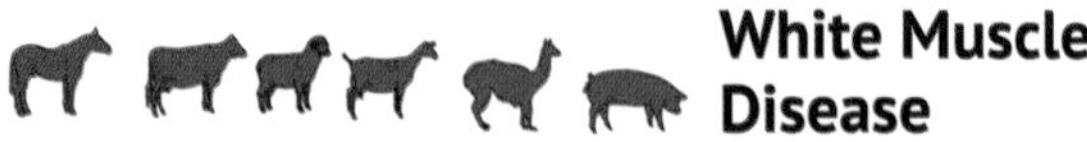

White Muscle Disease

Definition

Regional nutritional disease of large animals.

Cause

Deficient levels of vitamin E and selenium in the diet.

> **TECHNICIAN TIP 12.80:** White muscle disease is caused by deficient levels of vitamin E and selenium in the diet.

Systems Affected

Skeletal and cardiac muscles.

Signs

Stiff gait, lameness, hunched appearance, reluctance to move. Sudden death due to cardiac muscle disease.

Onset

Acute or chronic.

Prevalence/Geographical Distribution

High prevalence in selenium deficient areas in animals not on supplementation. Regional soil selenium levels vary from deficient to toxic worldwide.

Diagnosis

Serum selenium, liver biopsy, gross skeletal and cardiac muscle lesions upon necropsy.

Treatment

Vitamin E and selenium supplementation, overdosing can be fatal.

Prevention

Monitor selenium levels in feed and supplement accordingly.

Recovery

Recovery is dependent upon severity of disease when treatment is initiated.

Zoonotic Potential

No zoonotic potential.

Genetic Prevalence

No genetic prevalence known.

Prevention

Selenium supplementation to dams prior to parturition or to neonates.

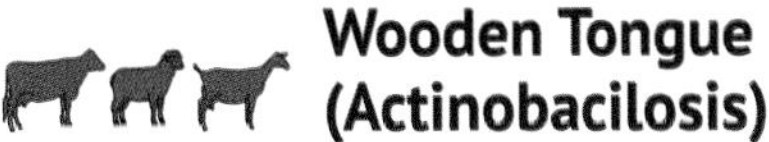

Wooden Tongue (Actinobacilosis)

Definition

An infectious disease affecting the tongue and causing granulomatous abscessation with a hard and diffuse nodular swelling ("wooden tongue"). It is more common in cattle, less common in sheep, and rare in goats.

Cause

Actinobacillus lignieresii, a gram-negative rod, and normal inhabitant of the mouth and rumen of cattle and small ruminants.

Transmission

The organism enters the soft tissues through lesions or abrasions of the tongue.

> **TECHNICIAN TIP 12.81:** Wooden tongue is caused by a bacterium normally found in the mouth but causes disease when it enters the tissues through lesions or abrasions of the tongue.

Stemmy coarse feed with plant awns or thistles predispose the development of lesions in the tongue and, therefore, predispose the occurrence of disease.

Signs

Salivation and inability to prehend feed are the initial signs seen on distant exam. On close inspection, the tongue appears firm and painful to the touch with nodular lesions. Atypical locations for the lesions (granulomatous abscesses) can occur (i.e. lymph nodes of the head, lips, nose, etc.). Atypical locations are associated with previous injury or lesions at the site. Sheep usually develop lesions in the lips and face.

Onset

Acute to chronic.

Prevalence/Geographical Distribution

A sporadic disease with a worldwide distribution.

Diagnosis

Clinical signs. Biopsy and culture of the organism can be performed to confirm the diagnosis.

Treatment

Parenteral sodium iodide administration. Antibiotic therapy is warranted in severe cases or in cases with atypical lesion location.

Recovery

Rapid recovery after treatment with sodium iodide. Within two days after starting treatment, the swelling on the tongue decreases and affected animals return to eat.

Zoonotic Potential

No zoonotic potential.

Genetic Prevalence

No genetic prevalence known.

Prevention

Avoid feeding abrasive feedstuffs.

References

Acres, S., Saunders, J., and Radostits, O. (1977). Acute undifferentiated neonatal diarrhea of beef calves: the prevalence of enterotoxigenic *E. coli*, reo-like (rota) virus and other enteropathogens in cow-calf herds. *Can. Vet. J.* 18: 133.

Alban, L. (1995). Foul-in-the-foot (interdigital necrobacillosis) in Danish dairy cows: frequency and possible risk factors. *Prev. Vet. Med.* 24: 73.

American Association of Equine Practitioners. (2012). *Potomac Horse Fever (Equine Monocytic Ehrlichiosis, Equine Ehrlichial Colitis)*. Retrieved from http://www.aaep.org/potomac_fever.htm

American Association of Equine Practitioners. (2012). *Rabies*. Retrieved from www.aaep.org

Amstutz, H., Anderson, D., Armour, J. et al. (eds.) (1998). *The Merck Veterinary Manual*, 8e. Whitehouse Station, NJ: Merck & Co., Inc.

Anderson, D. and Badzioch, M. (1991). Association between solar radiation and ocular squamous cell carcinoma in cattle. *Am. J. Vet. Res.* 52: 784.

Anderson, T., Cheville, N., and Meador, V. (1986). Pathogenesis of placentitis in the goat inoculated with *Brucella abortus* II, ultrastructural studies. *Vet. Pathol.* 23: 219.

Anderson, M., Barr, B., and Conrad, P. (1994). Protozoal causes of reproductive failure in domestic ruminants. *Vet. Clin. North Am. Food Anim. Pract.* 10 (3): 439.

Bailey, C., Hanks, D., and Hanks, M. (1990). Circumocular pigmentation and incidence of ocular squamous cell tumors in *Bos taurus* and *Bos indicus x Bos taurus* cattle. *J. Am. Vet. Med. Assoc.* 196: 1605.

Bassert, J. and McCurnin, D. (2010). *McCurnin's Clinical Textbook for Veterinary Technicians*, 7e. St. Louis, MO: Saunders-Elsevier.

Bergonier, D., de Cremoux, R., Rupp, R. et al. (2003). Mastitis of dairy small ruminants. *Vet. Res.* 34: 689.

Berri, M., Rousset, E., Champion, J. et al. (2007). Goats may experience reproductive failures and shed *Coxiella burnetti* at two successive parturitions after a Q fever infection. *Res. Vet. Sci.* 83: 47.

Bharti, A., Nally, J., Ricaldi, J. et al. (2003). Leptospirosis: a zoonotic disease of global importance. *Lancet Infect. Dis.* 3: 757.

Blanton, J., Palmer, D., Dyer, J., and Rupprect, C. (2010). Rabies surveillance in the United States during 2010. *J. Am. Vet. Med. Assoc.* 239 (6): 773–783.

Bulgin, M., Ward, A., Barrett, D. et al. (1989). Detection of rotavirus and coronavirus shedding in two beef cow herds in Idaho. *Can. Vet. J.* 30: 235.

Buttenschon, J. (1989). The occurrence of lesions in the tongue of adult cattle and their implications for the development of actinobacillosis. *J. Vet. Med. Assoc.* 36: 393.

Canadian Food Inspection Agency (CFIA). (2012). *Anthrax*. Retrieved September 18, 2012, from http://www.inspection.gc.ca/animals/terres-trial-animals/diseases/reportable/anthrax eng/1330045348336/1330045807153

Castillo-Olivares, J. and Wood, J. (2004). West Nile virus infection of horses. *Vet. Res.* 35: 467–483.

Centers for Disease Control and Prevention (CDC). (2011). *Q Fever*. Retrieved September 21, 2012, from http://www.cdc.gov/qfever/symptoms/index.html

Centers for Disease Control and Prevention (CDC). (2011). *Rabies*. Retrieved from http://www.cdc.gov ncidod/dvrd/rabies/

Centers for Disease Control and Prevention (CDC). (n.d.). *Anthrax*. Retrieved September 18, 2012, from http://www.bt.cdc.gov/agent/anthrax

Centers for Disease Control and Prevention (CDC); National Center for Emerging and Zoonotic Infectious Diseases. (2010). *Campylobacter*. Retrieved on October 1, 2012, from http://www.cdc.gov/nczved divisions/dfbmd/diseases/campylobacter/

Cieslak, T. and Eitzen, E. (1999). Clinical and epidemiologic principles of anthrax. *Emerg. Infect. Dis.* 5: 552.

Clark, B., Stewart, D., and Emery, D. (1985). The role of *Fusobacterium necrophorum* and *Bacteroides* melaninogenicus in the aetiology of interdigital necrobacillosis in cattle. *Aus. Vet. J.* 62: 47.

Coetzee, J., Apley, M., Kocan, K. et al. (2005). Comparison of three oxytetracycline regimes for the treatment of persistent *Anaplasma marginale* infections in beef cattle. *Vet. Parasitol.* 127: 6.

Collins, D., Gabric, D., and de Lisle, G. (1990). Identification of two groups of *Mycobacterium paratuberculosis* strains by restriction endonuclease analysis and DNA hybridization. *J. Clin. Microbiol.* 28: 1591.

Constable, P.D. (ed.) (2004). *Ruminant Neurologic Diseases in Veterinary Clinics of North America: Food Animal.* Philadelphia, PA: Saunders.

Contreras, A., Luengo, C., Sanchez, A. et al. (2003). The role of intramammary pathogens in dairy goats. *Livest. Prod. Sci.* 79: 273.

Corley, L. and Stephen, J. (eds.) (2008). *The Equine Hospital Manual.* West Sussex, UK: Blackwell Publishing.

Crossley, B., Zagmutt-Vergara, F., Fyock, T. et al. (2005). Fecal shedding of *Mycobacterium avium* subsp. *paratuberculosis* by dairy cows. *Vet. Microbiol.* 107: 257.

Dill, S., Correa, M., Erb, H. et al. (1990). Factors associated with the development of equine degenerative myeloencephalopathy. *Am. J. Vet. Res.* 51 (8): 1300–1305.

Dirikolu, L., Karpiesiuk, W., Lehner, A. et al. (2009). Synthesis and detection of toltrazuril sulfone and its pharmacokinetics in horses following administration in dimethylsulfoxide. *J. Vet. Pharmacol. Ther.* 32 (4): 368–378.

Divers, T. and Peek, S. (2007). *Rebhun's Diseases of Dairy Cattle.* St. Louis, MO: Elsevier Health Services.

Doyle, M. (1987). Survival of *Listeria monocytogenes* in milk during high-temperature, short-time pasteurization. *Appl. Environ. Microbiol.* 53: 1433.

Duffield, T. (2000). Subclinical ketosis in lactating dairy cattle. *Vet. Clin. North Am. Food Anim. Pract.* 16 (2): 231.

Edwin, E. and Jackman, R. (1970). Thiaminase I in the development of cerebrocortical necrosis in sheep and cattle. *Nature* 228: 772.

Erskine, R. (1992). Mastitis control practices in dairy herds with high prevalence of subclinical mastitis. *Compend. Contin. Educ. Pract. Vet.* 14: 969.

Freestone, J. and Carlson, G. (1991). Muscle disorders in the horse: a retrospective study. *Equine Vet. J.* 23: 86–90.

Furr, M. and Reed, S. (2008). *Equine Neurology.* Ames, IA: Blackwell.

Gerloff, B. (2000). Dry cow management for the prevention of ketosis and fatty liver in dairy cows. *Vet. Clin. North Am. Food Anim. Pract.* 16 (2): 283.

Goehring, L., van Winden, S.C., van Maanan, C., and Sloet van Oldruitenborgh-Oosterbaan, M. (2006). Equine herpesvirus type 1-associated myeloencephalopathy in The Netherlands: a four-year retrospective study (1999–2003). *J. Vet. Intern. Med.* 20: 601–607.

Goehring, L., Landolt, G., and Morley, P. (2010). Detection and management of an outbreak of equine herpesvirus type 1 infection and associated neurological disease in a veterinary teaching hospital. *J. Vet. Intern. Med.* 24 (5): 1176–1183.

Goff, J. (2000). Pathophysiology of calcium and phosphorus disorders. *Vet. Clin. North Am. Food Anim. Pract.* 16 (2): 319.

Goodger, W. and Skirrow, S. (1986). Epidemiologic and economic analysis of an unusually long epizootic of trichomoniasis in a large California dairy herd. *J. Am. Vet. Med. Assoc.* 189: 772.

Gronstol, H. (1979). Listeriosis in sheep: isolation of *Listeria monocytogenes* from grass silage. *Acta Vet. Scand.* 20: 492.

Hansen, D., Thurmond, M., and Thorburn, M. (1985). Factors associated with the spread of clinical vesicular stomatitis in California dairy cattle. *Am. J. Vet. Res.* 46: 789.

Haskell, S. (ed.) (2009). *Blackwell's Five-Minute Veterinary Consult: Ruminant.* Ames, IA: Wiley-Blackwell.

Heeney, J. and Valli, V. (1985). Bovine ocular squamous cell carcinoma: an epidemiological perspective. *Can. J. Comp. Med.* 49: 21.

Herdt, T. (2000). Ruminant adaptation to negative energy balance. Influences on etiology of ketosis and fatty liver. *Vet. Clin. North Am. Food Anim. Pract.* 16 (2): 215.

Heringstad, B., Chang, Y., Gianola, D., and Klementsdal, G. (2005). Genetic analysis of clinical mastitis, Milk fever, ketosis, and retained placenta in three lactations of Norwegian red cows. *J. Dairy Sci.* 88 (9): 3273–3281.

Hoet, A., Nielsen, P., Hasoksuz, M. et al. (2003). Detection of bovine torovirus and other enteric pathogens in feces from diarrhea cases in cattle. *J. Vet. Diagn. Investig.* 15: 205.

Houe, H. (1995). Epidemiology of BVDV. *Vet. Clin. North Am. Food Anim. Pract.* 11: 521.

Johnson, A., Lamm, C., and Divers, T. (2006). Acquired cervical scoliosis attributed to *Parelaphostrongylus tenuis* infection in an alpaca. *J. Am. Vet. Med. Assoc.* 229 (4): 562–565.

Johnson, A., Burton, A., and Sweeney, R. (2010). Utility of 2 immunological tests for antemortem diagnosis of equine protozoal myeloencephalitis (*Sarcocystis neurona* infection) in naturally occurring cases. *J. Vet. Intern. Med.* 24 (5): 1184–1189.

Jolley, W. and Bardsley, K. (2006). Ruminant coccidiosis. *Vet. Clin. North Am. Food Anim. Pract.* 22: 613.

Jones, C. (2003). Herpes simplex virus type 1 and bovine herpesvirus 1 latency. *Clin. Microbiol. Rev.* 16: 79.

Knottenbelt, D. (2006). *Saunders Equine Formulary.* St. Louis, MO: Elsevier.

Larkin, M. (2010). JAVMA news: high prevalence of EEE in Michigan. *J. Am. Vet. Med. Assoc.* 237 (9): 1001.

Laven, R. and Logue, D. (2006). Treatment strategies for digital dermatitis for the UK. *Vet. J.* 171: 79.

Lavoie, J. and Hinchcliff, K. (2008). *Blackwell's Five-Minute Veterinary Consult: Equine*, 2e. Ames, IA: Wiley-Blackwell.

Lentz, L., Valberg, S., Balog, E. et al. (1999). Abnormal regulation of muscle contraction in horses with recurrent exertional rhabdomyolysis. *Am. J. Vet. Res.* 60: 992–999.

Loew, F. and Dunlop, R. (1972). Induction of thiamine inadequacy and polioencephalomalacia in adult sheep with Amprolium. *Am. J. Vet. Res.* 33: 2195.

Loneragan, G., Thomson, D., Montgomery, D. et al. (2005). Prevalence, outcome, and health consequences associated with persistent infection with bovine viral diarrhea virus in feedlot cattle. *J. Am. Vet. Med. Assoc.* 226: 595.

Machackova, M., Svastova, P., Lamka, J. et al. (2004). Paratuberculosis in farmed and free-living wild ruminants in the Czech Republic in the years 1999–2001. *Vet. Microbiol.* 101: 225.

Maclachlan, N., Drew, C., Darpel, K., and Worwa, G. (2009). The pathology and pathogenesis of bluetongue. *J. Comp. Pathol.* 141 (1): 1–16.

Mars, M., de Jong, M., van Maanen, C. et al. (2000). Airborne transmission of bovine herpesvirus 1 infections in calves under field conditions. *Vet. Microbiol.* 76 (1).

Martens, H. and Schweigel, M. (2000). Pathophysiology of grass tetany and other hypomagnesemias. Implications for clinical management. *Vet. Clin. North Am. Food Anim. Pract.* 16 (2): 339–367.

McAllister, M., Gould, D., Raisbeck, M. et al. (1997). Evaluation of ruminal sulfide concentrations and seasonal outbreaks of polioencephalomalacia in beef cattle in a feedlot. *J. Am. Vet. Med. Assoc.* 15 (211): 1275.

McKenzie, E., Valberg, S., Godden, S. et al. (2003). Effect of dietary starch, fat, and bicarbonate content on exercise responses and serum creatine kinase activity in equine recurrent exertional rhabdomyolysis. *J. Vet. Intern. Med.* 17: 693–701.

Menzies, F., McBride, S., McDowell, S. et al. (2000). Clinical and laboratory findings in cases of toxic mastitis in cows in Northern Ireland. *Vet. Rec.* 147: 123.

Merck Veterinary Manual. (2012). *Potomac Horse Fever*. Retrieved from http://www.merckvetmanual. com/mvm/index.jsp?cfile=htm/bc/22204.htm

Nataraj, C., Eidmann, S., Hariharan, M. et al. (1997). Bovine herpesvirus 1 downregulates the expression of bovine MHC class I molecules. *Viral Immunol.* 10: 21.

Nicoletti, P., Milward, F., Hoffmann, E., and Altvater, L. (1985). Efficacy of long-acting oxytetracycline alone or combined with streptomycin in the treatment of bovine brucellosis. *J. Am. Vet. Med. Assoc.* 187: 493.

Oetzel, G. (2000). Management of dry cows for the prevention of milk fever and other mineral disorders. *Vet. Clin. North Am. Food Anim. Pract.* 16 (2): 369.

Ogawa, T., Tomita, Y., Okada, M. et al. (2004). Broad-spectrum detection of papillomaviruses in bovine teat papillomas and healthy teat skin. *J. Gen. Virol.* 85: 2191.

Pavlik, I., Bejcková, L., Pavlas, M. et al. (1995). Characterization by restriction endonuclease analysis and DNA hybridization using IS900 of bovine, ovine, caprine and human dependent strains of mycobacterium paratuberculosis isolated in various localities. *Vet. Microbiol.* 45: 311.

Pennsylvania's West Nile Virus Control Program. (2012). *What Horse Owners Should Know about West Nile Virus*. Retrieved from http://www.west-nile.state.pa.us/animals/horses.htm

Pugh, D. and Baird, A. (2001). *Sheep and Goat Medicine*. St. Louis, MO: Elsevier Health Services.

Pugh, G. and Hughes, D. (1968). Bovine infectious keratoconjunctivitis: carrier state of *Moraxella bovis* and development of preventive measures against the disease. *J. Am. Vet. Med. Assoc.* 167: 310.

Pugh, G. and Hughes, D. (1972). Bovine infectious keratoconjunctivitis: *Moraxella bovis* as the sole etiologic agent in a winter epizootic. *J. Am. Vet. Med. Assoc.* 161: 481.

Read, D. and Walker, R. (1998). Papillomatous digital dermatitis (Footwarts) in California dairy cattle: clinical and gross pathologic findings. *J. Vet. Diagn. Investig.* 10: 67.

Rebhun, W., Fubini, S., Miller, T. et al. (1988). Vagus indigestion in cattle: clinical features, causes, treatments, and long-term follow-up of 112 cases. *Compend. Contin. Educ. Pract. Vet.* 10: 387.

Reed, S., Bayly, W., and Sellon, D. (2010). *Equine Internal Medicine*, 3e. St. Louis, MO: SaundersElsevier.

Reeder, D. and Zimmel, D. (2009). *AAEVT's Equine Manual for Veterinary Technicians*. Ames, IA: Wiley-Blackwell.

Reynolds, D., Morgan, J., Chanter, N. et al. (1986). Microbiology of calf diarrhoea in Southern Britain. *Vet. Rec.* 119: 34.

Saglam, Y., Temur, A., and Aslan, A. (2003). Detection of Leptospiral antigens in kidney and liver of cattle. *Dtsch. Tierarztl. Wochenschr.* 110: 75.

Simard, C., Richardson, S., Dixon, P. et al. (2000). Enzyme-linked immunosorbent assay for the diagnosis of bovine leukosis: comparison with the agar gel immunodiffusion test approved by the Canadian food inspection agency. *Can. J. Vet. Res.* 64: 101.

Smith, B. (2008). *Large Animal Internal Medicine*, 4e. St. Louis, MO: Elsevier Health Services.

Thurmond, M., Ardans, A., Picanso, J. et al. (1987). Vesicular stomatitis virus (New Jersey strain) infection in two California dairy herds: an epidemiologic study. *J. Am. Vet. Med. Assoc.* 191: 965.

Torioni de Echaide, S., Knowles, D., McGuire, T. et al. (1998). Detection of cattle naturally infected with *Anaplasma marginale* in a region of endemicity by nested PCR and a competitive enzyme-linked immunosorbent assay using recombinant major surface protein 5. *J. Clin. Microbiol.* 36: 777.

Tranas, J., Heinzen, R., Weiss, L., and McAllister, M. (1999). Serological evidence of human infection with the protozoan *Neospora caninum. Clin. Diagn. Lab. Immunol.* 6 (5): 765–767.

Tumbull, P. (2002). Anthrax history, disease and ecology. *Curr. Top. Microbiol. Immunol.* 271: 1.

Valberg, S. and Mickelson, J. (1997). Polysaccharide storage myopathy: one important cause of exertional rhabdomyolysis in horses. *J. World Equine Health Net.* 3: 32–37.

Valberg, S., McCue, M., & Mickelson, J. (2008). Proceedings from AAEP Focus Meeting, Austin, TX; First Year of Life *Review of Genetic Muscle Disorders in Foals of Quarter Horse-related Breeds.*

Van Biervliet, J., deLahunta, A., Ennulat, D. et al. (2004). Acquired cervical scoliosis in six horses associated with dorsal grey column chronic myelitis. *Equine Vet. J.* 36 (1): 86–92.

Van der Maaten, M. and Miller, J. (1978). Susceptibility of cattle to bovine leukemia virus infection by various routes of exposure. *Comp. Res. Leukemia Rel. Dis. Proc.* 8: 29.

Wakelin, D., Rose, M., Hesketh, K. et al. (1993). Immunity to coccidiosis: genetic influences on lymphocyte and cytokine responses to infection with *Eimeria vermiformis* in inbred mice. *Parasite Immunol.* 15 (1): 11.

Westbury, H., Doughty, W., Forman, A. et al. (1988). A comparison of enzyme-linked immunosorbent assay, complement fixation and virus isolation for foot-and-mouth disease diagnosis. *Vet. Microbiol.* 17: 21.

Whitlock, R. (1984). Preclinical and clinical manifestations of paratuberculosis (including pathology). *Vet. Clin. North Am. Food Anim. Pract.* 12: 345.

Wilkins, P. and Palmer, J. (2003). Botulism in foals less than 6 months of age: 30 cases (1989–2002). *J. Vet. Intern. Med.* 17 (5): 702–707.

Wilson, D. (2012). *Clinical Veterinary Advisor: The Horse*. St. Louis, MO: Elsevier-Saunders.

Winkler, M., Doster, A., and Jones, C. (2000). Persistence and reactivation of bovine herpesvirus 1 in the tonsils of latently infected calves. *J. Virol.* 74: 5337.

World Health Organization (WHO). (2008). *Anthrax in Humans and Animals*. Retrieved September 18, 2012, from http://www.who.int/csr/resources/publi-cations/anthrax_web.pdf

Yilma, T. (1980). Morphogenesis of vesiculation in foot-and-mouth disease. *Am. J. Vet. Res.* 41: 1537.

Clinical Case Resolution 12.1

Because the horse's vaccination history is not known, it must be considered a rabies suspect. Rabies can be transmitted through contact of the infected animal's saliva with cuts, bite wounds, or mucous membranes. Proper personal protective equipment (PPEs), therefore, includes face shields (to protect the eyes and mouth) and gloves. Because it is impossible to definitively diagnose rabies antemortem, it is very important to maintain a list of all individuals that have handled or contacted the rabies suspect so that appropriate postexposure prophylaxis can be pursued if rabies is diagnosed postmortem.

Items that should be available include blood collection tubes and an intravenous catheter setup. Sedation (xylazine, detomidine, butorphanol) may be necessary as the horse might be extremely dangerous to handle and as such sedation should be readily available. Anticonvulsants, such as phenobarbital or diazepam, may be requested if the veterinarian diagnoses seizures. If possible, the horse should be housed in a secure padded stall to avoid injury to itself or staff. Other items or medications that may be potentially used include mannitol, dextrose, dexamethasone, oxygen supplementation equipment, and intravenous fluids (crystalloids). The veterinarian may wish to perform a cerebrospinal fluid collection, so spinal needles (18-gauge, 3.5–8 in needles), materials for sterile site preparation, and sterile gloves should be available.

Primary concerns are hydration, oxygenation, and most importantly, safety of staff and patient. Clinical laboratory work will likely include CBC and biochemistry panel. Assessment of electrolyte levels and liver function are particularly important.

Activities

Multiple Choice Questions

(Answers can be found in the back of the book.)

1. Which of these sedatives would be a poor choice for use in a horse with hepatic encephalopathy?
   - **A** diazepam
   - **B** xylazine
   - **C** detomidine
   - **D** butorphanol
2. Which of the following diseases is zoonotic?
   - **A** leukoencephalomalacia
   - **B** white muscle disease
   - **C** polioencephalomalacia
   - **D** rabies
3. Which of these diseases is most strongly associated with poor-quality nutrition?
   - **A** equine degenerative myeloencephalopathy (EDM)
   - **B** Eastern equine encephalitis (EEE)
   - **C** rabies
   - **D** equine herpesvirus myeloencephalopathy (EHM)
4. Which of these statements is true regarding the zoonotic potential of West Nile virus?
   - **A** WNV can be readily transmitted from infected horses to humans via bites.
   - **B** Transmission of WNV from infected horses to humans is unlikely but PPE should be worn when handling infected tissues.
   - **C** It is impossible to transmit WNV from infected horses to humans.
   - **D** The risk of transmission of WNV from infected horses to humans is high because the horse acts as a reservoir host, aiding transmission of the virus to vector species.
5. Which of these neurologic diseases is NOT generally prevented by vaccination?
   - **A** tetanus
   - **B** rabies
   - **C** Eastern equine encephalitis
   - **D** equine herpesvirus myeloencephalopathy
6. Which of these neurologic diseases can be spread from affected horses to healthy horses by contaminated personnel in a hospital setting?
   - **A** equine herpesvirus myeloencephalopathy
   - **B** rabies
   - **C** botulism
   - **D** equine protozoal myeloencephalitis
7. Which of the following is true regarding collection of cerebrospinal fluid from a horse?
   - **A** CSF can be collected from the atlantooccipital space safely from the standing horse.
   - **B** Sedation should be avoided during CSF collection because drugs such as xylazine and detomidine can interfere with the flow of CSF.
   - **C** CSF can be collected from the lumbosacral space safely from the standing horse.
   - **D** Collection of CSF should never be performed in stocks because this method of restraint may make horses nervous.
8. Which of the following is true regarding cervical vertebral stenotic myelopathy (CVSM)?
   - **A** Cervical radiography of the standing horse is the best method of diagnosis.
   - **B** The genetic basis of CVSM has been definitively identified.
   - **C** Complete resolution of neurologic deficits is expected in most cases following surgical management of CVSM.
   - **D** CVSM is most likely caused by a combination of genetic and environmental factors.
9. Which of the following is true regarding equine protozoal myeloencephalitis (EPM)?
   - **A** In cases of EPM, improvement is unlikely if not observed within seven days of institution of therapy with ponazuril.
   - **B** Most horses that are exposed to the causative agent of EPM, *S. neurona*, develop signs of clinical EPM.
   - **C** Clinical signs of EPM are highly variable and can include ataxia, seizures, and dysphagia.
   - **D** Horses likely become infected with EPM due to exposure to its primary host, the white-tailed deer.
10. If managing a number of cases in a hospital, which of these equine patients should be handled and treated BEFORE the other cases in the hospital are handled and treated?
    - **A** 13-year-old Warmblood gelding with diarrhea and laminitis
    - **B** Nine-year-old Thoroughbred broodmare with ataxia and suspected EHM
    - **C** Three-year-old Standardbred filly that is recumbent and thought to have botulism
    - **D** Two-year-old Thoroughbred colt with swollen retropharyngeal lymph nodes and suspected strangles

Test your Learning

1. What are some measures that should be taken by personnel to minimize exposure to a potentially rabid horse?
2. What are important management and monitoring considerations when working with a recumbent large animal?
3. How can rabies be ruled out as a potential cause of disease?
4. What are some measures that should be taken for animals with mentation changes?
5. Which neurologic diseases of large animals are zoonotic?
6. Which neurologic diseases of large animals are contagious?

Answers can be found in the back of the book.

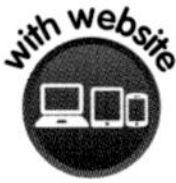

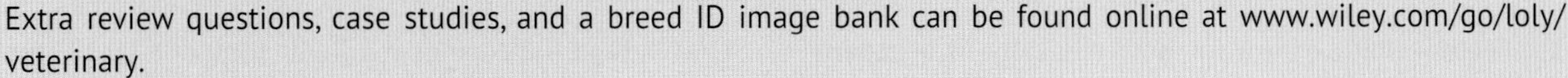

Extra review questions, case studies, and a breed ID image bank can be found online at www.wiley.com/go/loly/veterinary.

Multiple Choice Questions Answer Bank

Chapter 1 Hospital Biosecurity

1) Factors that account for how clinically ill a patient may become include:
C) virulence of the pathogen

2) What host factor will not affect disease prevention?
B) mode of transmission

3) Good antibiotic stewardship refers to which of the following:
B) Give the right antibiotics, at the right dose, at the right time, and for the right duration.

4) Which of the following is not considered a portal of exit for pathogens:
D) central nervous system

5) Patients in the hospital should be separated according to which factor?
A) their risk level of spreading or acquiring infectious diseases

6) Which of the following precautions should be used for hospitalizing a patient with EHV-1?
D) strict isolation precautions

7) What is the number one way to prevent transmission of disease?
C) hand hygiene

8) In order for steam sterilization to be effective the following conditions must be met:
B) type of steam, pressure, temperature, and time

9) In order to kill all pathogens, spores, and heat resistant organisms, the steam inside of the autoclave must contain a relative humidity of:
D) 97–99%

10) Which of the following is not true of methicillin-resistant *Staphylococcus aureus* (MRSA)?
D) species specific

Chapter 2 Restraint

1) While at the edge of the flight zone of a small ruminant, moving from the front to the rear of the animal will make the animal:
B) move forward

2) While at the edge of the flight zone of a small rumi nant, moving from the rear to the front of the animal will make it:
A) move backward

3) Which of the following will not prevent a sheep from moving forward?
D) a well-lit opening where it can see herd mates

4) A llama or alpaca:
B) should have a well fitted halter with the nose band high on the nose resting on bone

5) Acceptable methods of catching a goat include all of the following except:
D) using a shepherd's crook on a hind leg

6) Restraining an adult sheep is easily done by all but:
C) hanging on to handfuls of wool

7) Where is the best place to stand while restraining an alpaca?
B) at the shoulder near the body

8) Why do you need to point the nose of the sheep upward while restraining?
C) because it is much more powerful when its head is down

9) When setting up a sheep, you should
C) use its weight to shift it off balance and slide it down your legs to the floor

10) Signs of increased agitation and displeasure include all except
D) tail curved all the way forward over the back

Large Animal Medicine for Veterinary Technicians, Second Edition. Edited by Sue Loly and Heather Hopkinson.

Companion website: www.wiley.com/go/loly/veterinary

11) What is not true regarding use of nose tongs in cattle?
B) may be used in place of anesthesia for significantly painful procedures

12) What is true regarding use of a halter and chain for restraint on horses?
A) pressure should always be removed as a reward when they do what they are asked

Chapter 3 History

1) Which of the following is part of the signalment?
B) age, breed, sex

2) Biosecurity refers to:
B) measures taken to prevent transmission of disease to other animals

3) When taking a thorough history for an equine emergency exam, one must include the following:
C) if the horse is insured

4) Bloat refers to:
A) gas distension of the rumen, stomach, or cecum

5) Animals in a herd environment:
C) share common resources that can increase disease transmission

6) Caprine refers to which species?
B) goats

7) Ovine refers to which species?
C) sheep

8) Camelid refers to which species?
D) alpacas

9) Which of the following species is not a ruminant?
A) horse

10) Which species are more likely to be kept individually and have an extensive travel history?
C) equine

11) History questions that are common among all species include all of the following except?
D) herd health status

Chapter 4 Physical Exams

1) Where do you properly take a camelid's pulse?
A) ventral coccygeal artery

2) What is the normal rectal temperature of feeder pigs in degrees Celsius?
A) 38.9–40.0

3) Which cardiovascular defects can be ausculted on the right side of a patient?
B) ventricular septal defects (VSD)

4) In sheep, the presence of ketone bodies in the urine is indicative of what malady?
A) pregnancy toxemia

5) What is the pathophysiology behind polioencephalomalacia in the adult ruminant?
A) thiamin deficiency

6) What are the chambers in the camelid designated as?
A) C1-3

7) What pathologic conditions are associated with a severe jugular pulse found during a physical exam?
B) right-sided heart failure

8) Which of the following heart valves can be auscultated on the right side of the patient?
C) tricuspid

9) When ausculting heart sounds on a normal patient, which ones are frequently heard?
A) S1 and S2

10) A clinical sign that may indicate septicemia is:
B) brick red mucous membranes

Chapter 5 Nutrition

1) What is one way to determine protein quality?
A) measuring the biologic value

2) What is the most common source of carbohydrates found in pet and livestock foods?
A) cereal grains

3) How can good-quality roughage be determined?
D) all of the above

4) What is considered to be the foundation of an equine feeding program?
C) roughages

5) If a decision is made to enterally supplement a 450 kg horse with a slurry via a nasogastric feeding tube, what is the maximum amount the horse should be fed?
B) 1.5 to 2 gallons

6) What is considered normal rumen pH of cattle?
C) 6.5

7) How many stomach compartments does the camelid have?
C) 3

8) What is important to know when providing water to camelids in cold climates?
   C) Camelids will not break through the ice to get to a water source.

9) How many pounds of feed does it take to produce approximately 1 lb of pork?
   B) 2 to 2.5 lb

Chapter 6 Clinical Procedures

1) Which of the following would be the most appropri ate catheter choice for an adult horse that will be on fluids for several days following colic surgery?
   D) 14-gauge, 13-cm (5.25-in), polyurethane, over-the-needle

2) Which of the following is not a sign of a possible transfusion reaction?
   C) increased urination

3) Which of these patients should not have PO medication administered?
   C) an adult mare with 4 L of gastric reflux every 4 hr

4) Which of the following statements about plasma is true?
   A) Frozen plasma can safely be stored at −4 °C for 1 year.

5) Which of these routes of administration would be least appropriate for antibiotic treatment of a patient with an infected metacarpophalangeal joint (fetlock)?
   D) topical/transdermal

6) Which of the following anatomic structures is not encountered during proper passage of a nasogastric tube?
   B) ethmoid turbinates

7) Which location is most appropriate for intramuscular administration of drugs in a beef cow?
   A) neck muscles

8) What is the approximate fluid deficit for a 550-lb pony estimated to be 8% dehydrated?
   B) 20 l

9) Which of the following is not an important safety precaution to take when performing routine dentistry in horses?
   A) resting the horse's head on an assistant's shoulder to reduce movement

10) Which of the following fluids will increase osmotic pressure in the vasculature?
   C) 7.2% saline

Chapter 7 Diagnostic Procedures

1) Aseptic preparation should be used for each of the following procedures except:
   D) skin biopsy

2) Which specialized tool could be used for a muscle biopsy?
   D) Bergström

3) Which cycle is the most preferred during the sampling for a uterine biopsy?
   A) diestrus

4) Mineral deficiencies, acute hepatitis, or icterus may warrant which of the following tests:
   A) liver biopsy

5) Normal activated clotting time for a cow is:
   C) 145 S

6) Which cardiac abnormality is commonly found in athletic horses?
   A) atrial fibrillation

7) Besides checking total protein levels and cell counts, peritoneal fluid may also be tested for:
   D) glucose, lactate, and pH

8) Which cerebral spinal fluid tap location will be more likely to yield a large sample?
   A) atlantooccipital space

9) How many times should RBCs be washed for a Coomb's test?
   B) twice

10) Which of the following crossmatches should be per formed for a pregnant mare or previously transfused patient?
   B) minor crossmatch

Chapter 8 Medical Imaging

1) Which of the following is not a principle of radiation safety?
   B) power

2) A racehorse presents with a hot, swollen, and thick superficial digital flexor tendon (bowed tendon). Which is the best imaging modality to use to examine this?
   C) ultrasonography

3) How does increasing the gain change an ultrasound image?
   C) makes it brighter

4) Which of the following is not considered a standard radiographic view of the tarsus?
A) flexed lateral

5) Which of the following is not an indication to perform a nuclear scintigraphy bone scan?
D) to accurately evaluate the extent of a fracture line for surgical planning

6) When making radiographs of the foot, you see a thin radiolucent line extending across the navicular bone on the D60P view. What do you do next?
C) This could be a gas artifact from packing, but it would be significant if it were a real fracture line. It is important to know the difference. Repack the sole and repeat the view.

7) To perform a suspensory ligament ultrasound, what would be the ideal ultrasound transducer to use?
B) a mid-to-high frequency linear array probe

8) Which of the following is the minimum amount of information that should be included with a patient's musculoskeletal ultrasound exam?
A) the patient's and owner's names and the specific structure being imaged

9) Why is radiography the mainstay of equine imaging?
D) It is widely available, affordable, and gives good bone detail.

10) Which of the following does not degrade the quality of an equine bone scan?
B) too high a dose of 99mTc

Chapter 9 Reproduction

1) The hormone that causes the release of FSH and LH is:
A) GnRH

2) The hormone that causes the destruction of the CL is:
D) luteinizing hormone

3) Specially adapted tubule that gathers the ova release from the ovary is:
B) oviduct

4) A BSE concentrates on:
D) adequate quantity and quality of semen

5) The instrument used to manually count sperm in a quantity of ejaculate is:
B) hemocytometer

6) Which of the following species is a seasonal breeder that responds to decreasing day-length?
B) ovine

7) The part of the estrous cycle where follicular development and increasing estrogen leads to demonstration of sexual characteristics is called:
B) proestrus

8) The species that possesses a musculocavernous penis is:
D) equine

9) The stage of labor where the cervix relaxes and the fetus is positioned for delivery is:
A) stage 1

10) The stage of labor where the placenta is passed is:
C) stage 3

Chapter 10 Anesthesia and Surgery

1) Pre-operative blood work will include all of the following except:
B) Sedimentation Rate

2) Which drug is considered a dissociative anesthetic?
C) Ketamine

3) Alpha$_2$-agonist can be reversed by all the following except:
A) Acepromazine

4) Duration of action of Mepivacaine is:
B) 1–3 hr

5) Complications of a post-operative colic include all of the following except:
D) foot abscess

6) What is the Trendelenburg position?
A) tilting head down and hindquarters up

7) Complications of a tie-back surgery include all of the following except:
C) shaking of head

8) Toxic lidocaine dose for cattle is:
D) 10 mg/kg

9) Toxic lidocaine dose for small ruminants is:
B) 5 mg/kg

10) Complications of a pig foreign body surgery include all of the following except:
C) tooth root abscess

Chapter 11 Neonatology

1) Dairies can quickly assess transfer of IgG in calves by using which of the following tests?
B) total protein

2) Water bath temperature for thawing plasma should be below:
D) 100 °F

3) What type of administration sets should be used to deliver plasma to patients?
C) 150–260 μm filter set

4) Which of the following IgG tests is easily used with foals to determine adequate passive transfer of immunoglobulins?
A) ELISA

5) Hypoglycemia in the large animal neonate is often the result of:
A) being too sick and weak to nurse

6) Hyperflexion of the limbs is a clinical sign of what condition?
A) prematurity

7) Milk from a mare can be refrigerated or frozen for future use. Which of the following is a true statement?
B) The milk can be warmed in a microwave)

8) The neonatal period is:
D) The first 3–5 days of life)

9) An initial assessment of a neonate at birth should include which items?
B) cardiac function, thermoregulation, and respiratory system

10) Chronic or acute placental insufficiency or separation can cause which disease process?
B) asphyxia

Chapter 12 Diseases

1) Which of these sedatives would be a poor choice for use in a horse with hepatic encephalopathy?
A) diazepam

2) Which of the following diseases is zoonotic?
D) rabies

3) Which of these diseases is most strongly associated with poor-quality nutrition?
A) equine degenerative myeloencephalopathy (EDM)

4) Which of these statements is true regarding the zoonotic potential of West Nile virus?
B) Transmission of WNV from infected horses to humans is unlikely but personal protective equipment should be worn when handling infected tissues.

5) Which of these neurologic diseases is NOT generally prevented by vaccination?
D) equine herpes myeloencephalopathy

6) Which of these neurologic diseases can be spread from affected horses to healthy horses by contaminated personnel in a hospital setting?
A) equine herpes myeloencephalopathy

7) Which of the following is true regarding collection of cerebrospinal fluid from a horse?
C) CSF can be collected from the lumbosacral space safely from the standing horse.

8) Which of the following is true regarding cervical vertebral stenotic myelopathy (CVSM)?
D) CVSM is most likely caused by a combination of genetic and environmental factors.

9) Which of the following is true regarding equine protozoal myeloencephalitis (EPM)?
C) Clinical signs of EPM are highly variable and can include ataxia, seizures, and dysphagia.

10) If managing a number of cases in a hospital, which of these equine patients should be handled and treated BEFORE the other cases in the hospital are handled and treated?
C) Three-year-old Standardbred filly that is recumbent and thought to have botulism

"Test Your Learning" Answer Bank

Chapter 1 Hospital Biosecurity

1) **Describe three things that factor into a pathogen's success.**
The environment, the pathogen itself, and the host it needs. In some cases, an intermediate host can also play a role in a pathogen's success. Mode of transmission can also play a part in the completion of a pathogen's life cycle.

2) **Describe what a dead-end host is and its effect.**
A dead-end host is one that accidentally ends up on or in the wrong host species in transmission. Typically, the pathogen is not strongly species specific and may be able to cause some level of disease to its host, but it will not be able to complete its replication process.

3) **Describe the three common routes of disease transmission.**
Contact transmission includes animal-to-animal contact, which may be in the form of grooming, biting, or just touching, or where the pathogen is transported to a new host through a fomite or object, which may include medical equipment, grooming supplies, or even via staff.
Aerosol transmission is for pathogens that are transmitted through tiny droplets of moisture through the air from one animal to another.
Vector-borne transmission is a pathogen that travels through an intermediate host like a mosquito, fly, or tick.

4) **Describe the difference between disinfection and sterilization.**
Disinfection is a process that eliminates many or all pathogenic microorganisms on inanimate objects.
Sterilization is a process that destroys or eliminates all forms of microbial life via physical or chemical methods.

5) **List the key components of an infectious disease program.**
Determining which diseases are to be controlled and understanding the ecology of these diseases.
   - Grouping animals based on their infection status.
   - Maintaining hygiene of the facility, personnel, and patients.
   - Monitoring the occurrence of infectious disease.
   - Instituting an immunization program for patients and staff.
   - Optimizing the overall health of the animals by minimizing stressors, nutritional status, specific immunity through vaccination, and minimizing treatments that may make the animal more susceptible to disease.

Chapter 2 Restraint

1) **When working with animals in a race/chute system, what are the best ways to get and keep the animals moving forward?**
Have the alleyway free of shadows and dark corners or dead ends. A curve works better than a right-angle turn. Animals prefer to move into light rather than darkness. Keep race free of distractions especially at animal level – remove junk on floor, flapping or swinging coats, or tarps.
   - Keeping the race full so the animals can always see somebody to follow.
   - If you must "help," work at the rear of the animal – lift the tail and push but remember you will now be in front of the point of balance for the animal behind the one you are trying to get to go forward, making the animal behind back up.

Large Animal Medicine for Veterinary Technicians, Second Edition. Edited by Sue Loly and Heather Hopkinson.

Companion website: www.wiley.com/go/loly/veterinary

- Walking along the raceway from front to back makes the animals move forward as you pass by each of their points of balance.
- Stand far enough away that you are outside of their flight zone.

2) **What does it mean to use minimal restraint?**
Using only as much restraint as needed to accomplish the desired task.
- Not keeping the animal restrained for longer than necessary.
- Calm and quiet environment and handlers.
- Reevaluating plan if things are not going well. May need to change tactics or use a different approach.
- Chemical restraint or sedation is indicated if the animal cannot safely be restrained for whatever reason – physical limitations, environment, painful procedure.

3) **Why must an alpaca or llama halter be well fitted?**
If the halter is not appropriately sized and fitted, the noseband can slide down from its correct position just below the eyes. When the noseband slides down off the bony portion of the nose, it compresses the cartilage and soft tissue, occluding the nasal passageways. This makes it hard for the animal to breathe and causes the animal to fidget and struggle more and eventually panic.

4) **List the different handling points where your hands and legs should go when holding sheep and goats.**
To control the head, one hand on jaw (nose tilted upward), fingers wrapped around muzzle or between mandibles.
Second hand:

- Around muzzle
- Behind ears
- On rump
- Grasping tail base
- Skinfold in opposite flank
- Beard (goats only, not preferred)

Goats only: horn base
Never ears or horn scurs.
Legs/Knees:

- In flank
- Behind elbow
- Straddling, pressed into shoulders

5) **Describe two ways crias could be restrained.**
Lateral recumbency, arm over neck holding fore legs with other arm over hips holding rear legs.
- Straddling a kushed cria and holding head in hands.
- Pushed against a wall by several people, elevated off ground by handler's knees underneath belly.
- One arm around chest and other hand holding tail or on rump.

6) **Describe two restraint methods that can be used to inspect a cow's foot.**
Front leg hopple
- Hindleg restraint
- Tilt table
- Casting

Chapter 3 History

1) **Why is it important to note food and water sources in the history?**
Animals may have limited access to water, have a contaminated access, or, due to unforeseen circumstances, may not have access at all. Feed can also be a source of contamination. Abrupt feed changes may cause digestive upsets such as colic or bloat as well.

2) **Why is it important to understand management practices when taking a history?**
Being knowledgeable in the management practices will allow you to understand how animals are handled, vaccinated, and dewormed. It will also guide you when asking questions pertaining to housing of the animals.

3) **Why is biosecurity so important in our large animal species?**
Large animals are many times kept in herd situations that allow for contact with many animals at once allowing for increased prevalence in disease transmission.

4) **Large animal medicine leans more toward herd health, how is this different than small animal medicine?**
Herd health looks at the group of animals as a whole rather than an individual. If there is disease in the herd, common resources must be looked at. Sick animals may be necropsied to obtain diagnostic information that can help the herd.

5) **Why is the intended use of the animal important to note in the history.**
If the animal is not intended for food, there are certain medications that can be utilized; if the animal is intended for slaughter, withdrawal times for drugs must be taken into account.

Chapter 4 Physical Exam

1) **When a pyrexic five-month-old gilt with diarrhea and dehydration is presented for admission to your hospital, what body systems should be evaluated first? How should you approach the rest of the herd?**
All body systems must be assessed but the cardiovascular system would be a first concern, as this patient is a young animal who may suffer from hypovolemic shock and collapse. All other herd mates must be evaluated as they may be in the early stages of the disease. Earlier intervention will reduce financial losses.

2) **Describe how you would complete a technician's lameness assessment on a three-week-old cria with valgus deformity.**
A technician would determine the affected limbs. The patient should be restrained and the affected limbs examined ventral to dorsal. All observations would be reported to the doctor who would make his/her own assessment and diagnosis.

3) **Why do small ruminants require a more sedate environment to complete your physical examination?**
Small ruminants are easily agitated if they are not properly restrained or placed in an area where they can escape. Excessive agitation leads to elevated physical parameters, which may mislead the diagnosis.

4) **List the areas on a horse where a technician would assess Body Condition Score.**
Nuchal crest, withers, caudal to point of elbow, over the ribs, croup, and lumbar spine.

5) **Outline the use of a rebreathing examination to assess the respiratory system.**
A plastic bag is placed over the animal's nose for 3–5 min to mimic the animal under stress or exercise. This results in deep breaths. The person ausculting the lungs should listen to all lung fields and the trachea during this time. Any abnormalities should be noted. When the bag is removed, the animal will take several large breaths to return to a normal state and these breaths may reveal additional information.

Chapter 5 Nutrition

1) **Define the term kilocalorie.**
A unit to measure energy, 1000 cal.

2) **What determines the amount of protein an animal needs?**
Species, the animal's age, and the quality of the protein.

3) **What are the three main categories of horse feeds?**
Roughages
- Concentrates
- Complete feeds

4) **What is considered to be the foundation of an equine feeding program?**
Roughage

5) **Name two things that may develop if excess concentrates are fed.**
Laminitis
   1) Rhabdomyolysis
   2) Developmental orthopedic disease
   3) Obesity

6) **List the factors that will influence the growth rate of growing horses.**
Protein level
   1) Protein quality
   2) Vitamin level
   3) Mineral level

7) **List two ways the critically ill can receive nutrition.**
Enterally or parenterally

8) **How many hours can the healthy adult horse withstand food deprivation (simple starvation) with little systemic effects?**
24–72 hr.

9) **List two indications for feeding a patient parenterally?**
The gastrointestinal tract is obstructed.
   1) The gastrointestinal tract is dysfunctional.
   2) The gastrointestinal tract is damaged.
   3) The gastrointestinal tract is painful.

10) **What types of questions should healthcare team members ask when documenting the patient's nutritional history?**
Has there been movement of animals from one field to another?
   1) Has there been a change from pasture to cereal grazing?
   2) Has there been a change from unimproved to improved pasture?
   3) Have there been periods of bad weather or transportation?
   4) Has there been a change to new/unfamiliar feeds?

5) Have there been changes occurring rapidly versus gradually – especially in pregnant and lactating ruminants, as metabolic diseases are more likely to occur in these animals (i.e. hypocalcemia, hypoglycemia, hypomagnesemia)?
6) What is the availability of drinking water?

11) What is the most important nutrient for all animals, especially sheep and goats?
Water

12) Why should trace mineral blocks be avoided in sheep?
To avoid copper toxicity

13) What is important regarding the practice of grinding feeds to increase feed efficiency in swine?
If the grain is ground too finely, digestive problems in the pig may result.

Chapter 6 Clinical Procedures

1) List four ways in which proper placement of a nasogastric tube in the stomach can be confirmed.
1) Visualize passage of the tube on the left side of the neck.
2) Blow air through the tube and hear gurgling when ausculting the stomach.
3) Odor of gastric contents (sweet to fetid).
4) Obtain gastric contents through the tube by establishing a siphon effect.

2) Calculate the approximate amount of fluids to be given in the first 12–24 hr for an adult Quarter Horse mare weighing 950 lb, estimated to be 7% dehydrated on presentation, and producing 4 l of gastric reflux every 4 hr.
Fluid deficit: $\sim 430\,\text{kg} \times 0.07$(estimated 7% dehydration) $\approx 30\,\text{l}$
Maintenance needs: $\sim 430\,\text{kg} \times 60\,\text{ml/kg/day} \approx 25\,800\,\text{ml} = 25.8\,\text{l}$
Ongoing losses: $1\,\text{l/hr} \times 24\,\text{h} = 24\,\text{l}$
TOTAL: $30\,\text{l} + 25.8\,\text{l} + 24\,\text{l} = 79.8\,\text{l}$
Thus, approximately 80 l of intravenous fluids should be administered over the first 12–24 hr. Response to therapy should be periodically reassessed and the plan changed as needed.

3) A yearling Thoroughbred weighing 454 kg is presented with a severe laceration to the axillary region that occurred the night before. Packed cell volume (PCV) is 14%. How much whole blood would be needed to raise the PCV to 22% in this individual? Would a single donor weighing 550 kg with a PCV of 40% be sufficient to provide this volume?

$$Volume\ to\ be\ infused(L) = \frac{(22\%\ \ 14\%)}{40\%} \times (454\,\text{kg} \times 0.08) \approx 7\,\text{L}$$

Yes, this volume can easily be collected from a single donor (up to 10 l can be collected from *a horse of this weight*).

4) What are the major risk factors for the development of thrombophlebitis?
Presence of endotoxemia, hypoproteinemia, sepsis, and other systemic illness; turbulent blood flow at the catheter tip; excessive vessel trauma during placement; infection secondary to contamination during placement (failure to follow aseptic technique), leaving a catheter in for too long; use of a catheter made of a thrombogenic material. Many of these factors are under the direct control of members of the veterinary care team.

5) Compare and contrast crystalloid and colloid fluids, and explain why a combination of the two might be useful in a fluid plan.
Crystalloids contain salts or other water-soluble molecules that can freely pass through the vascular walls into the interstitium, while colloids contain molecules that are too big to pass through the vascular walls and thus exert osmotic pressure in the vascular space. Thus, colloids will expand vascular volume by more than their own volume by drawing fluid in from the interstitium and/or intracellular fluid compartment. In contrast, crystalloids will rapidly equilibrate between the vasculature and the rest of the extracellular fluid space, so approximately 3× the volume must be given to achieve the desired expansion. Of the crystalloids, hypertonic saline can also draw fluid into the vasculature, but its effects are shorter-lived than those of colloids. Colloids alone are cost-prohibitive for volume expansion in large animals. For patients that are severely hypovolemic (especially, if they are hypoproteinemic) it can be useful to give an initial bolus of 1–2 l of colloids (±hypertonic saline) to immediately boost vascular volume and then follow up with large volumes of crystalloids to replace the remainder of the fluid deficit.

6) Describe physical exam findings that might be suggestive of pathology related to the teeth.
Soft or hard swelling of the maxilla or mandible (may or may not be painful to palpation); restricted or painful movement of the jaw; malodorous/purulent nasal

discharge; halitosis; palpation and/or visualization of sharp points or malocclusions; abrasions/lacerations of the tongue or buccal mucosa; pocketed food between the caudal cheek teeth; evidence of dropped, partially masticated food.

Chapter 7 Diagnostic Procedures

1) **Describe three diagnostic procedures that may be performed on a patient with an airway disease.**
   Brochoalveolar lavage (BAL) sample cells from the distal lung fields
   a) Transtracheal wash (TTW) sample cells from the upper airway
   b) Endoscopic evaluation of the upper airway

2) **Describe the different sites that can be used for abdominocentesis in a small ruminant patient.**
   Caudal to the xiphoid and 2–5 cm to the right and/or left of midline or cranial to the mammary gland or scrotum, also 2–5 cm to the right and/or left of midline.

3) **Describe the process for culturing a milk sample.**
   Wash teats with individual paper towels, cleaning the teats farthest away from you first then scrubbing the closer teats. Dry teats with individual paper towels. Wipe each teat end with an alcohol-soaked cotton ball or swab.
   When taking the milk samples, start sampling the closest teats first followed by the teats farthest away last. When taking milk from each teat, discard the first two squirts then put the next two to four streams into a culture vial. Only a small amount of milk is needed. Securely cap the vial closed. Be sure to record proper patient intradermal (ID) on the lid of the vial, along with the teat location, farm name, and date.

4) **Name two key functions of bone marrow and list two locations that may be commonly used for the collection of bone marrow.**
   Bone marrow is responsible for the production of erythrocytes, leukocytes, and platelets.
   Bone marrow can be sampled from either the xiphoid (8–10 cm caudally and 2 cm lateral of the sternal midline) or the ilium (approximately 8 cm cranial to the caudal most aspect of the ilium).

5) **Describe each of the following and what they represent in an electrocardiogram (ECG) tracing: P wave, PR interval, QRS complex, T wave, ST segment, baseline.**
   P wave represents atrial depolarization. This is followed by a period of conduction delay, which corresponds to the PR interval. The ventricles are depolarized, resulting in the QRS complex. Repolarization of the ventricles is represented by the T wave. The time between the QRS complex and T wave is known as the ST segment, which represents the time the ventricles are resistant to other electrical stimulus. The area between the T wave and the next P wave is known as the baseline.

Chapter 8 Medical Imaging

1) **Explain the importance of properly preparing a horse for an ultrasound exam.**
   Hair traps gas and dirt and degrades the image quality. Clipping the hair and washing the skin provides better contact of the probe with the skin. Eliminating the dirt and oil will also improve the ability of the sound waves to penetrate the skin. Allowing gel to soak in will hydrate the skin and also improve sound wave penetration. These steps will allow for better image quality.

2) **Why is nuclear scintigraphy useful in cases of multi-limb lameness?**
   Nuclear scintigraphy allows for evaluation of the entire skeleton. Areas of increased bone turnover (sites of inflammation or disease) will have increased radiopharmaceutical uptake. Nuclear scintigraphy provides a global view; however, while it is very sensitive, it is not specific for disease, and the areas of increased uptake must be further evaluated for clinical significance.

3) **Give three examples of how to put the principle of time, distance, and shielding to use.**
   Use lead gloves and aprons, rotate who holds the plate, increase body distance from the plate, minimize repeat or unnecessary radiographs, ensure that the X-ray tube is properly maintained, use the lowest exposure technique necessary for a good-quality image.

4) **Why is it important to have a full radiographic study of an affected joint?**
   All views highlight different areas of the joint. Excluding views leads to the risk of missing, underestimating, or misdiagnosing a lesion.

5) **Describe some of the limitations of ultrasonography.**
   It is very user dependent. Not all machines are the same, and image quality will vary significantly with user experience and machine quality. Poor patient preparation will also affect image quality. While very good for soft tissue, it does not have the contrast resolution of magnetic resonance imaging (MRI) and provides only limited information regarding boney pathology.

Chapter 9 Reproduction

1) **A male porcine patient must have a semen evaluation. What procedures must be accomplished during a breeding soundness examination (BSE)? What species-specific concerns should a veterinary technician be aware of?**
A BSE on a boar does not differ from any other species, except for the semen collection procedure. A thorough history must be recorded, which includes general health and husbandry questions, as well as libido and adequate quantity and quality of semen. Boars can be collected via manual technique putting pressure on the distal glans penis.

2) **When collecting a stallion for semen evaluation, is there any collection method that cannot be used on this species?**
Electroejaculation should not be used with a stallion.

3) **You are asked to perform a semen evaluation. List the areas of concern when performing the laboratory portion of the evaluation?**
All items that interact with the sperm must be warmed to avoid abrupt changes in temperature. Physical characteristics should be recorded. After taking a portion for analysis, the remainder should be extended to maintain viability of the remainder.

4) **A cow visits the hospital for a BSE. What items would need to be assembled to assist the veterinarian to perform the evaluation?**
Restraint of the cow is important to keep all parties safe. Equipment that should be set up could include tail tie, items for cleansing the vulva, vaginoscope, endometrial biopsy instrument, culture and cytology tubes, ultrasound machine, and blood collection materials.

5) **You are attending to a dystocia at a cattle ranch. The cow is in the pasture with a dead fetus. The veterinarian needs to perform a fetotomy. What concerns are there for this procedure?**
The cow needs to be restrained for this procedure. Stocks in a well-lit area with all disinfection and surgical instruments need to be assembled to increase the chances for a successful outcome.

Chapter 10 Anesthesia and Surgery

1) **Prior to the start of any anesthetic procedure, certain considerations must be thought out. What are some of these considerations?**
First, all patients need to have a thorough history collected and a physical examination conducted. For the physical examination, at least, a temperature, heart rate, respiratory rate and rumen contraction needs to be evaluated. Respiratory pattern, abdominal distention, and a rectal examination are also warranted. Under certain emergency situations, this limited physical examination would be all that can be performed; however, if the situation is not emergent, a complete and thorough physical examination should be conducted to ensure the patient is deemed healthy and fit and for surgery and anesthesia. For patients undergoing general anesthesia, relevant clinical diagnostics are warranted. These would include a PCV and total solids (TS), a complete blood chemistry (CBC), and a biochemistry profile.

2) **It is very important to know which drugs can be reversed after given. List these drugs and their reversal.**
Romifidine – Yohimbine
Xylazine – Yohimbine/Tolazoline
Detomidine – Atipamezole
Dexmedetomidine – Atipamezole
Diazepam – Flumazenil
Midazolam – Flumazenil
Morphine – Naloxone
Butorphanol – Naloxone

3) **You are asked to get instruments together for a standing ovariectomy. What extra equipment is needed beyond the large instrument pack?**
Laparoscopy tower
Laparoscope
Camera
Light cord
Insufflation
Trocars
Laparoscopic instruments
Ligation and hemostasis

4) **When a cow is admitted to the hospital for an elective surgery, why is it important to know when they last had access to food and water?**
Depending upon their position for surgery, the rumen places strain on the thoracic cavity, decreasing lung function and oxygenation capability. In addition, a large rumen allows for an increased chance of regurgitation during anesthesia, resulting in secondary aspiration. To help minimize these complications, roughage is typically removed for 48 hr prior to an elective surgery and water is removed 12 hr before surgery.

5) **A pig comes in for emergency foreign body surgery. What should you do before you administer any drugs to pigs?**
Consult the FARAD website (www.farad.org) for assistance in selecting appropriate medications because pigs, even pet pigs, are considered production animals.

Chapter 11 Neonatology

1) **When an equine neonate is present for admission to the hospital, what body systems should be evaluated? How are they evaluated?**
Cardiac function, respiratory, thermoregulation, fluid balance, immune status, and blood glucose levels are systems that should be evaluated on every neonate at admission.
Cardiac function can initially be evaluated via auscultation and capillary refill time (CRT). Dependent on results, further diagnostic procedures may be warranted. Respiratory function can also be evaluated via auscultation and mucus membrane color. Thermoregulation status is easily evaluated via rectal temperature. Fluid balance can initially be evaluated through skin turgor test and further from PCV (packed cell volume) value. Immune status requires additional steps as blood must be drawn and tested. Stall-side tests are available. Glucose values also require venous blood. Stall-side glucometers are available for rapid results.

2) **Describe parts of a neonate's history that would influence hydration and glucose status.**
The ability of the neonate to suckle, whether from the dam or a bottle will directly influence hydration and glucose status. Inability to stand and nurse would be a red flag that the neonate has not yet nursed and consumed both fluids and nutrients, including sugars.

3) **Why do large animal neonates require colostrum for acquired immunity?**
Large animal species do not pass immunoglobulins through the placenta. All immunoglobulins are found in colostrum and must be transferred to the gastrointestinal system of the neonate to be effective in bolstering the immune status of the neonate.

4) **Name two ways that colostrum can be tested.**
Colostrum can be tested with a Brix refractometer, with a colostrometer, or with several types of stall-side tests.

5) **Compare and contrast bacteremia and septicemia.**
Bacteremia is a disease condition where bacteria are present in the bloodstream. Septicemia differs in that the bloodstream contains bacteria and the by-products of bacterial reproduction. These substances cause considerable damage to cells and tissues.

Chapter 12 Diseases

1) **What are some measures that should be taken by personnel to minimize exposure to a potentially rabid horse?**
Wear gloves.
   - Wear facemasks (protect the eyes and other mucous membranes).
   - Limit handlers to those who have already been vaccinated for the disease and have adequate titers.
   - Keep a record of every individual who has been in contact with the animal.
   - Note specifically if an individual was "exposed" to the animal (via an animal bite or contact of bodily fluid with cuts or mucous membranes).

2) **What are important management and monitoring considerations when working with a recumbent large animal?**
Pressure necrosis of muscles is a major concern in a large (>500 lb) animal. This complication adds significant morbidity to disease so great attention should be paid by veterinary technicians to preventing it. Means of prevention include providing deep bedding continuously and alternating recumbency (left/right lateral) at least every 4–6 hr as possible.
   - Decubital ulceration occurs for the same reasons as pressure necrosis of muscles does. As such, prevention of decubital ulcers is the same for that of pressure necrosis. Treatment of decubital ulceration includes protecting wounds and applying topical therapy, such as silver sulfadiazine cream.
   - Some animals will neither defecate nor urinate when recumbent; this may be related to the primary disease or may simply be secondary to recumbency. The animal's fecal and urine output should be monitored closely; if either is absent, a veterinarian should be notified, as evacuation of the bladder and/or rectum may be required.
   - Recumbent large animals might be at an increased risk for developing nosocomial disease due to prolonged time lying down and thus increased exposure to hospital-borne pathogens.
   - Recumbent animals may require slinging therapy at the discretion of the attending veterinarian. Slinging can be quite dangerous with untrained personnel, so it should only be undertaken under the direction of a veterinarian.

3) **How can rabies be ruled out as a potential cause of disease?**
   - Because there is no definitive antemortem diagnostic test, rabies cannot be ruled out in any case of acute neurologic disease.
   - Animals with neurologic disease due to rabies, however, do not improve and these animals also die within several days of the onset of clinical signs. Therefore, any animal whose status is improving, or has been clinical for greater than 10 days can be considered a very unlikely rabies case.

4) What are some measures that should be taken for animals with mentation changes?

Large animals with changes in mentation are inherently dangerous to manage. Their behavior is unpredictable and may be aggressive. If at all possible, the animal should be restricted to an enclosed and secure area, such as a stall. Ideally, the stall's walls should be padded to preempt self-inflicted injury. Foam "helmets" are available for horses and should be utilized to minimize self-inflicted injury.

- Only experienced personnel should assist with management of the patient and should never handle the patient alone.
- Sedation may be necessary but of course should only be given by a veterinarian's orders.

5) Which neurologic diseases of large animals are zoonotic?

- Rabies

6) Which neurologic diseases of large animals are contagious?

- Equine herpesvirus myeloencephalopathy

Glossary

Active surveillance Collecting swabs and cultures looking for specific organisms of interest that could threaten the hospital population.

Aerosol transmission Animal-to-animal transmission of pathogens through the air, such as coughing or sneezing.

Agalactic Unable to produce milk.

Alloantibodies An antibody that occurs naturally against foreign tissues from another individual of the same species.

Amino acid Class of organic compounds containing one amino group and one carboxyl group, building blocks of proteins.

Analgesia The inability to feel pain.

Antibiotic stewardship A program that encourages judicious use of antibiotics.

Antiseptics Antimicrobial substances applied to the skin or mucous membranes to reduce the number of microbial florae.

Aortic stenosis (AS) Narrowing of the aorta.

Arrhythmia Without rhythm.

Artifact A structure or an appearance that is not normally present on the radiograph and is produced by artificial means.

Artificial insemination (AI) Injection of semen into the vagina or uterus by means other than coitus.

Aseptic technique Refers to a procedure that is performed under sterile conditions.

Asphyxia Lack of oxygen.

Assessment The act of evaluation.

Asymptomatic carrier A patient that serves as a host for an infectious agent but who does not show any apparent signs of the illness.

Ataxia Lack of voluntary coordination of muscular movement.

Atrial fibrillation Rapid irregular contractions of the atria.

Auscultation Listening to body sounds, usually through use of a stethoscope.

Autogenous Arising from within.

Average daily gain Weight gain of animals over a period of time divided by the total number of days during the period.

Bacteremia The presence of bacteria in the bloodstream.

Bacterial endocarditis Inflammation of the inner layer of the heart caused by bacterial infection.

Ballottement A diagnostic technique to determine the amount of solid objects surrounded by fluid.

Base-narrow stance Abnormal placement of feet close together.

Base-wide stance Abnormal placement of feet further lateral from midline.

Basilar Located at or near the base.

Biological value Expressed as a value, the nutritional effectiveness of a protein.

Biosecurity The precautions taken to protect against harmful biological agents.

Blepharospasm An involuntary, forced closure of the eye.

Body condition score (BCS) A subjective evaluation communicated through a numeric value given to an individual animal to determine distribution of muscle mass and fat. May be used for assessing a patient's nutritional status.

Borborygmi Rumbling or gurgling sounds of the gastrointestinal tract.

Bowline A knot that does not slip or tighten and is commonly used to create loops.

Brachygnathia It is where the mandible is shorter than the maxilla. Also called an overbite or parrot mouth.

Breeding soundness exam (BSE) Fertility evaluation of the male or female.

Bright alert responsive (BAR) Subjective assessment of a patient's awareness or attentiveness.

Large Animal Medicine for Veterinary Technicians, Second Edition. Edited by Sue Loly and Heather Hopkinson.

Companion website: www.wiley.com/go/loly/veterinary

Bright-field microscopy Procedure where illumination is transmitted from below and observed from above the sample.

Brooder A heated house for chicks or piglets.

Bruxism Grinding or clenching of teeth.

Buphthalmos General term for an enlarged eye.

Capillary refill time (CRT) Subjective assessment of perfusion status done typically by blanching the gum against the tooth root and timing the return of normal gum color.

Carina The area of the trachea where it branches into two bronchi.

Caseous Resembling cheese-like or cottage cheese-like consistency made up of leukocytes, pathogens, and cellular debris.

Casting A method used on cattle to force them to lie down on the ground.

Catch pen Small enclosure used to hold the gathered flock, herd group, or subset, which enables individual animals to be caught while bunched in a tight group rather than chased around in a larger pen. To work best, the pen should be kept full.

Central nervous system (CNS) Controls most functions of the body and mind. Consists of two parts: the spinal cord and the brain.

Cervical radiography Radiographic images of the cervical vertebrae.

Chemical restraint Provides a range of reactions from slowing an animal down, through head-hanging sedation, to full injectable anesthesia.

Chute (See Race) The area at the end of a race or a separate piece of equipment that is used to restrain an individual animal. It is a narrow passage or enclosure and generally has sides that are removable for access to the animal, as well as head restraint (cross ties, head gate, etc.).

Clove hitch Used as the basis for many other types of knots; can slip when used by itself.

Cognition Act or process of knowing.

Colic A clinical sign indicating pain and usually related to pain occurring in the abdomen. There is an extensive list of medical causes that can result in symptoms of colic including gastrointestinal impactions, ulcerations, and colitis.

Colloids Solution containing large insoluble molecules that can rarely cross the capillary membrane barrier.

Colostrum First milk produced by the dam that transfers immunoglobulins to the neonate.

Complete feeds A type of food preparation that provides all necessary nutrients.

Computed tomography (CT) A series of X-ray views taken from different angles and processed by a computer to create cross-sectional images of bones and soft tissue structures inside the body.

Concentrates Feeds containing high density of nutrients, low in crude fiber.

Cornea The transparent part of the eye that covers the front portion of the eye.

Corpus luteum Structure remaining after release of mature egg; involved in the production of progesterone and estradiol.

Costochondral Pertaining to the area between the ribs and costal cartilage.

Coupage A technique helpful at mobilizing respiratory secretions by using a cupped hand and gently but rapidly taping the patient's chest wall repeatedly.

Cow kick Reaching forward and backward using back legs.

Cryoprotectant An agent that allows cells to survive the freezing and thawing process.

Cryptorchidism The absence of testis from the scrotum.

Crystalloids Aqueous solutions of mineral salts or other water-soluble molecules that can cross the capillary membrane barrier.

Cush See Kush.

Cytopathic Related to disease or degeneration or pathologic changes to cells.

Cystoscopy Endoscopic procedure to view the urinary bladder and urethra.

Daily energy requirement Amount of energy required per day.

Daily sperm output Semen collection once daily for 7–10 days; an average of the total sperm number of the last three collections is then used to estimate DSO.

DAMNIT system A clinical investigation plan acronym: D = degenerative/developmental; A = allergic/autoimmune; M = metabolic/mechanical; N = nutritional/neoplastic; I = inflammatory/autoimmune/iatrogenic/ischemic/idiopathic; T = toxic/traumatic.

Days in milk The interval between parturition and the drying-up period, also known as lactation.

Dehydration A condition that occurs when the loss of body fluids, mostly water, exceeds the amount that is taken in.

Demand valve A mechanism that delivers oxygen flow when an animal inhales.

Dental float The process of filing sharp edges, ramps, or waves from a horse's mouth to achieve a flat grinding surface between the upper and lower teeth.

Depolarization Atrial or ventricular contraction.

Descemet's membrane The basement membrane that lies between the stroma and the endothelial layer of the cornea.

Desquamation Shedding of outermost layer or membrane.

Developer A solution used in the darkroom for developing radiographs.

Diastema A space separating teeth of different functions.

Diestrus Luteal phase that follows estrus and ovulation.

Differential interference contrast microscope Optical microscope using an illumination technique to increase contrast from a sample.

Digestible energy A food's gross energy minus the energy that is nonabsorbable and lost in the feces.

Direct contact transmission Animal-to-animal transmission such as biting, touching, and grooming.

Disinfection Process that eliminates many or all pathogenic microorganisms on inanimate objects.

Distance Increasing the distance between personnel and the radiation source to help decrease exposure to radiation.

Doppler A method of echocardiography used for evaluating blood flow within the heart.

Dry matter The remainder of a specific feed after all water is removed.

Ear-ing Method of restraint for camelids applied by grasping the base of the ear and firmly squeezing up. Not appropriate for goats or sheep.

Electrocardiography The process to record electrical activity of the heart.

Embryo transfer Moving a developing embryo from or to the uterus of a surrogate dam.

Endometrial cytology A procedure where cells from the endometrium are harvested for examination.

Endophyte A plant that lives inside another plant, especially a fungus.

Enteral nutrition Food that is fed via the alimentary tract.

Enterocentesis Surgical puncture during an abdominocentesis, which enters the gastrointestinal tract.

Epidemiologic data Facts or statistics that describe the distribution or outcome of a specific disease.

Epitheliochorial placenta Female organ of large animal species that provides for transfers of nutrients, oxygen, and waste products, but disallows transfer of IgG from maternal to fetal circulation.

Estradiol A hormone that causes proliferation and thickening of tissue and blood vessels of the endometrium.

Estrogen Female hormone capable of inducing estrus and secondary female sex characteristics and preparing the uterus for accepting the fertilized ovum.

Estrous Period of time composed of proestrus, estrus, metestrus, and diestrus.

Estrus Period of sexual receptivity of the female; heat.

Eutocia Normal parturition or birthing

Evaluation The act of appraising.

Exodontia A branch of dentistry that deals with the extraction of teeth.

Exenteration Surgical removal of an organ or structure.

Extracellular fluid Usually denotes all body fluid outside of cells.

Failure of passive transfer Inadequate absorption of immunoglobulins from colostrum to neonatal circulation.

Feedback mechanism Can be positive or negative; involved in regulating hormones.

Fetotomy Dissection of a dead fetus in utero.

Flight zone The area around the animal that is its safety zone and personal space where it feels comfortable and unthreatened.

Flocking instinct The set of instinctive behaviors best exhibited by sheep, and to a lesser degree by goats and camelids, that lead the animals to bunch together when threatened, follow one another readily, and need to be in visual contact with other herd mates.

Fodder Food stuff for livestock, given to them instead of them foraging it. Particularly, dried hay or grasses.

Follicle-stimulating hormone (FSH) Hormone causing growth and maturation of ovarian follicles.

Freshening The process of a dairy animal giving birth and milk let down into the teats.

Front leg hopple (hobble) Used for inspecting the front feet for injury or to help keep the back legs from kicking.

Gantry A frame housing the X-ray tube, collimators, and detectors in a CT or radiation therapy machine.

Gametes Mature sexual reproductive cell.

Gangrene Localized death and decomposition of body tissue, resulting from a bacterial infection.

Gastric reflux Duodenal contents can readily reflux or flow back into the stomach of equine patients.

Gastrointestinal (GI) Pertaining to the stomach and the intestines.

Gastroscopy Endoscopic procedure to view the gastrointestinal tract from pharynx to duodenum.

Gauss A small unit of magnetic flux density.

Glucometer Instrument that measures circulating glucose.

Gonadotropin-releasing hormone (GnRH) Hormone that causes release of FSH and LH.

Gonads A sex gland in which gametes are produced; testes or ovaries.

Half hitch Valuable component of many other hitches, bends, and knots.

Halter A head collar made of rope, nylon, or leather straps that fits behind the ears and around the muzzle of an animal and is used to lead or secure the animal.

Haploid A single set of chromosomes.

Hazard identification Identifying what infectious and zoonotic diseases are most likely to affect the hospital.

Hematogenously Produced by the blood.

Hematopoietic The formation of blood or of blood cells in the living body.

Hemocytometer An instrument for manually counting cells.

Herd health Planned animal health and production management program that uses a combination of regularly scheduled veterinary and herd management activities designed to optimize animal health and productivity.

Holosystolic Abnormal heart sound occurring throughout the entire ventricular contraction phase.

Holter monitor A device used to record ECG readings over a period of time.

Hormone Chemical messengers.

Hounsfield scale The attenuation value of the X-ray beam in a given voxel, minus the attenuation of water, divided by the attenuation of water multiplied by 1000.

Hydrophilic Having a tendency to mix and dissolve in water.

Hydrophobic Having a tendency to repel or fail to mix with water.

Hypercapnia A buildup of carbon dioxide in the bloodstream.

Hyperimmune plasma Plasma that contains high levels of antibodies.

Hypertonic Has a greater concentration or osmolality than intracellular fluid. Administration causes fluid to draw out of cells into the extracellular system, decreasing the intracellular fluid volume.

Hyphema Accumulation of blood in the anterior chamber of the eye.

Hypopion Pus or pus-like fluid in the anterior chamber of the eye.

Hypotrichosis Less than normal amount of hair on the body.

Hypoxemia An abnormally low concentration of oxygen in the bloodstream.

Hysteroscopy Endoscopic procedure to view the uterus.

Immunoglobulins Antibodies produced from plasma cells.

Incipient Initial stage.

Incubation period The time period between exposure to an infectious agent and the appearance of the first clinical signs.

Indirect contact transmission Occurs by contact with a contaminated piece of equipment, surface, or objects.

Inhibin A hormone responsible for suppressing FSH levels and limiting the number of ovulatory follicles to an appropriate level.

Insoluble Incapable of being dissolved.

Interpretation Explanation of meaning.

Intracellular fluid Denotes all fluid inside of cells.

Isotonic Fluid that matches the osmotic makeup of normal intracellular fluid.

Kilocalorie (kcal) A unit to measure energy, 1000 cal.

Kilovoltage (kVp) The peak potential applied to the X-ray tube, which accelerates electrons from the cathode to the anode in radiology or CT.

Kush Sternal recumbency in camelids with all four legs tucked tightly underneath. Default position of submission or indignation.

Lactation Secretions of fluid or milk originating in the mammary gland.

Lameness Refers to a disabled movement of gait that may be in response to pain, strain, or serious injury. Affects the cadence of an animal's gait and the rhythm of ambulation.

Laryngoscope An instrument for examining the larynx or for inserting a tube.

Left displaced abomasum (LDA) Disease process where the abomasum moves from its usual place in the lower right side of the abdomen to the upper left side of the abdomen. More common than an RDA.

Luteinizing hormone (LH) Hormone that causes ovulation of mature follicles and formation of the CL.

Magnetic resonance imaging (MRI) A noninvasive procedure that produces very detailed pictures of body soft tissue, bone, and organs without using ionizing radiation.

Meningitis Inflammation of the meninges.

Mentation Mental activity.

Metabolizable energy (ME) The amount of energy in a feed minus the energy excreted via feces or urine.

Milliampere-seconds (mAs) A measure of radiation produced over a set amount of time.

Minimal alveolar concentration (MAC) The concentration of inhaled anesthetic within the alveoli at which 50% of people do not move in response to a surgical stimulus.

Mitral valve insufficiency (MVI) A disease process where the mitral valve does not function at its normal capacity.

Morphology Study of form or structure.

Mucopurulent A discharge containing both mucus and pus.

Multidrug-resistant organism (MDRO) An organism whose susceptibility panels have three or more antibiotic classes that are completely resistant.
Multifocal More than one focus or location.
Myelography A type of radiographic image that uses contrast medium to visualize structures in the spinal cord.
Nasal obligate breather Normal anatomy within a species that prevents oral breathing.
Neonate Newborn.
Neuroleptanalgesia Administration of a tranquilizing drug and an analgesic especially for relief of surgical pain.
Nonprotein nitrogen (NPN) Dietary energy from sources other than protein.
Normovolemic Normal blood volume.
Nose tongs A restraint tool used on bovids, which pinches the nasal septum to help them remain still.
Nosocomial Acquired or occurring in a hospital.
Nuclear scintigraphy The use of radiolabeled isotopes to detect areas of increased bone turnover. Nuclear scintigraphy is a physiologic imaging modality.
Nutrients Providing nourishment.
Odontoprisis Grinding of teeth or bruxism.
Off-feed An animal's food intake is less than normal or completely absent.
Open Not pregnant.
Open-ended question A question that is not easily answered with a simple and nonspecific answer such as yes or no. Answers to open-ended questions require the responder to elaborate with descriptive terminology.
Oviducts Fallopian tubes.
Oxytocin Hormone that signals the uterus to contract as well as milk letdown.
Parenteral The introduction of nutrition, a medication, or other substance into the body via a route other than the mouth, may include injection or implantation.
Parenteral nutrition Providing nourishment delivered via intravenous route.
Paroxysmal A severe attack or sudden increase in a disease process.
Parturition The act of giving birth.
Passive surveillance Gathering, organizing, and analyzing data that is already present to ensure that nosocomial events are not occurring.
Patent ductus arteriosus (PDA) Congenital heart defect where the neonate's ductus arteriosus does not close shortly after birth.
Pathophysiology Functional changes associated with a disease or syndrome.
Peracute Excessively acute onset.
Percussion Tapping a body surface to produce an auscultable tone used for diagnostic purposes.
Persistently infected Disease state where the individual is not cleared of the virus, which remains in specific cells for life.
Personal protective equipment (PPE) Safety equipment or clothing used by staff to protect themselves and/or the animal from spreading disease.
Phase-contrast microscopy The procedure where a microscope's optics make objects appear brighter or darker, which increases color contrast with the surrounding mounting medium.
Point of balance Usually located at the animal's shoulder. Determines what direction the animal will move as one enters the animal's flight zone. If entering in front of this point, the animal will move backward. If behind, the animal will move forward.
Problem list A part of a medical record listing the patient's conditions that require diagnostic or therapeutic intervention.
Proestrus Period of estrous cycle before sexual receptivity.
Proprioceptive deficits Lack of knowledge of the position or weight as they relate to the body.
Prostaglandin F2 alpha (PGF2 alpha) Hormone that destroys the CL.
Pseudohyphae Newly dividing cells through budding. Related to fungi.
Pulmonic stenosis (PS) Obstruction of blood flow from the right ventricle to the pulmonic artery.
Pupillary light response (PLR) Reduction of pupil size in response to direct light.
Quick release knot A knot that can be quickly untied in case of an emergency by pulling the loose end of the rope.
Quiet alert responsive (QAR) Subjective assessment of a patient's awareness or attentiveness.
Race A single-file lane or alleyway for moving livestock. Consists of parallel walls spaced just wide enough to allow the animal to pass through without being able to turn around. This allows the animals to line up single file and move forward.
Radiation safety The practice of minimizing the exposure of personnel and patients to ionizing radiation.
Radiography The use of X-rays or gamma rays to produce an image. This modality is best suited for the evaluation of bone.
Recrudescence Recurrence of symptoms.
Repolarization Period where atria or ventricles relax.
Respiratory Acidosis Low pH. A condition that occurs then the lungs cannot remove all of the carbon dioxide the body produces.

Respiratory Depression A breathing disorder characterized by slow and ineffective breathing.

Reticulopericarditis Disease process often involving traumatic perforation of the reticulum, diaphragm, and pericardial sac.

Retroflex To bend backward.

Rhythm strip A printed form of an ECG reading.

Right displaced abomasal torsion (RTA) Additional sequelae of an RDA where the abomasum rotates on its axis.

Right displaced abomasum (RDA) Disease process where the abomasum moves from its usual place in the lower right side of the abdomen to the upper right side of the abdomen. Less common than an LDA.

Rickets A condition resulting in soft, weak bones.

Risk communication Ensuring that all personnel understand, support, and adopt the protocols and procedures developed to improve hospital infection control.

Risk management Process of identifying, selecting, and implementing measures that can be applied to reduce the level of risk.

Risk perception Real or perceived risk for infectious or zoonotic disease.

Roughages Coarse or rough feed for livestock.

Ruminant A mammal that digests plant-based feeds through various stages in a compartmentalized complex stomach.

Rut A periodic and often annually recurring state of certain male animals during which behavior associated with the urge to breed is displayed.

Scur A small rounded portion of horn tissue attached to the skin of the horn pit of a polled animal.

Sepsis The body's overwhelming and life-threatening response to infection that can lead to tissue damage, organ failure, and death.

Septicemia Blood condition where pathogenic microorganisms and the toxins they produce are present.

Sertoli cells Cell within the seminiferous tubules that act as nurse cells to sperm.

Setting up Method of restraint used in sheep, in which they are sitting on their rump, slightly off center and leaning back into the holder's legs with their back. They often relax, and the head and legs may be left free, allowing the handler to perform other tasks on the sheep (blood sample collection, foot trim).

Sheet bend Used to tie together two lines of equal size.

Shepherd's crook A hind leg catch tool used on sheep.

Shielding Use of lead aprons, thyroid shields, and lead gloves, which help minimize exposure.

Shock Inadequate tissue perfusion.

Sigmoid flexure Anatomical area of the non-erect penis that is bent into an S shape.

Skin twitch Neck twitches are an effective manner to distract the horse from an event for a short time. Grabbing a handful of skin at the junction of the neck and shoulder of a horse and pulling firmly applies the neck twitch.

Soluble Dissolvable.

Somnolent Sleepy or drowsy.

Spectrophotometry Instrument for producing a spectrum and measuring photometric intensity of wavelengths present.

Spermatogenesis Process in the seminiferous tubules where male sex cells are formed.

Square knot A common knot used to join two lines together.

Stanchion (See Chute) For ruminants, the two upright poles in a chute that press against the shoulder to prevent forward movement.

Sterilization Process that eliminates all forms of microbial life.

Strabismus Abnormal eye position.

Subjective objective assessment plan (SOAP) A documentation method for patient medical records.

Superovulation To produce more than the normal number of ova through the use of pharmaceuticals.

Tail tie A knot used to safely secure an animal's tail out of the way.

Telemetry To transmit automatically and at a distance between a ground and mobile unit.

Tenesmus Straining to urinate or defecate.

Temperature pulse respiration (TPR) Basic objective data on a patient's physiologic status.

Tesla A unit of measurement to define the magnetic flux density.

TPR Temperature, pulse, respiration.

Thalamocortical Relating to the thalamus and cerebral cortex.

Thrombophlebitis Inflammation and formation of a clot within a vein.

Time The amount of time an individual is exposed to radiation.

Torticollis A condition in which the head becomes persistently turned to one side, often associated with muscle spasms.

Total intravenous anesthesia (TIVA) The use of intravenous agents for induction and maintenance of anesthesia.

Transducer A device used to perform ultrasonography.

Transketolase An enzyme that assists with glycolysis.

Transrectal ultrasonography Procedure where a picture is produced using sound waves through the use of a probe placed in the rectum.

Tricuspid valve insufficiency (TVI) A disease process where the tricuspid valve does not function at its normal capacity.

Twitch A device that can be applied to the horse's nose to provide restraint.

Typhlocolitis Inflammation of both the cecum and the colon.

Ultrasonography The use of sound waves to produce images. This is a dynamic modality that is excellent for evaluation of soft tissue structures.

Utrecht guidelines Methodology used to treat dystocia.

Vaginoscopy Procedure to view the vagina.

Vasoconstriction The narrowing of blood vessels, which increases blood pressure.

Vas deferens Tubule where spermatozoa move from the epididymis to the urethra during ejaculation.

Vasodilation The widening of blood vessels, which decreases blood pressure.

Vector-borne transmission Occurs by indirect transmission of an infectious agent, as by a vector biting or touching, for example, by an insect bite.

Ventricular septal defect (VSD) Physical communication between the left and right ventricles.

Verrucous surfaces Areas whose appearance is wart-like.

Within normal limits (WNL) Values obtained during patient assessment fall within established normal parameters.

Xanthochromia Yellowish appearance of cerebrospinal fluid.

Zoonotic diseases Diseases communicable from animals to humans.

Index

Large Animal Medicine for Veterinary Technicians, Second Edition. Edited by Sue Loly and Heather Hopkinson.

Companion website: www.wiley.com/go/loly/veterinary

C

q

r

w

x

y

z